Color Atlas & Synopsis of

PEDIATRIC DERMATOLOGY

Color Atlas & Synopsis of

PEDIATRIC DERMATOLOGY

Fifth Edition

Sandipan Dhar
MBBS MD DNB FRCP(Edinburgh)
Professor and Head
Department of Pediatric Dermatology
Institute of Child Health
Kolkata, West Bengal, India

Maitreyee Panda
MBBS MD
Professor
Department of DVL
Institute of Medical Sciences (IMS) and SUM Hospital
Bhubaneswar, Odisha, India

JAYPEE

JAYPEE BROTHERS MEDICAL PUBLISHERS
The Health Sciences Publisher
New Delhi | London

Jaypee Brothers Medical Publishers (P) Ltd

Headquarters
EMCA House
23/23-B, Ansari Road, Daryaganj
New Delhi 110 002, India
Landline: +91-11-23272143, +91-11-23272703
+91-11-23282021, +91-11-23245672
E-mail: jaypee@jaypeebrothers.com

Corporate Office
Jaypee Brothers Medical Publishers (P) Ltd.
4838/24, Ansari Road, Daryaganj
New Delhi 110 002, India
Phone: +91-11-43574357
Fax: +91-11-43574314
E-mail: jaypee@jaypeebrothers.com

Overseas Office
JP Medical Ltd.
83, Victoria Street, London
SW1H 0HW (UK)
Phone: +44-20 3170 8910
Fax: +44(0)20 3008 6180
E-mail: info@jpmedpub.com

Website: www.jaypeebrothers.com
Website: www.jaypeedigital.com

Inquiries for bulk sales may be solicited at: jaypee@jaypeebrothers.com

***Color Atlas & Synopsis of Pediatric Dermatology* / Sandipan Dhar, Maitreyee Panda**

First Edition: 2003
Fifth Edition: 2025
Revised and Reprint: 2025

ISBN: 978-93-5696-801-1

Printed at: Samrat Offset Pvt. Ltd.

Dedication

To all those innocent children who bear the stigma of untouchability of skin diseases, silently tolerating the humiliation and ostracism of the civilized society…in whom the blemish disappears with time but the scar lingers on the mind…

Preface to the Fifth Edition

The fourth edition of the book has evoked spontaneous and overwhelming response, much more than the first three editions. I have received innumerable e-mails containing valuable feedback about the book from various pediatricians and dermatologists across the country. In fact, the book ran out of print and a huge void was felt. These have inspired me to update the book and come up with the fifth edition. I feel privileged to have Dr Maitreyee Panda, an erudite colleague, a successful teacher, a great pediatric dermatologist and researcher, as my co-author for the book. In the current edition, we have introduced two new chapters pediatric dermatology–oncology interface, cutaneous manifestations in pediatric COVID. The topic of "patient/parents' education and counseling" has been elaborated further. Sixty-new entities and 600 new illustrations have been added to it. The "Suggested Readings" and the "Index" have been updated. We have added a new feature "What's New" to update our readers about the recent development on the subject. Altogether, a new set of quotable quotes cater to nearly (574) pages of the book. We are sure that now the book will be even more useful to the pediatricians, dermatologists, and all those involved in pediatric skin care. We believe that there is still scope for further improvement of this book. We will appreciate feedback (e-mail: doctorsandipan@gmail.com/pandamaitreyee@gmail.com) from the readers.

Sandipan Dhar
Maitreyee Panda

Preface to the First Edition

Dermatology in relation to children has far-reaching new connotations. There have been extensive research and rapid developments in the field of pediatric dermatology in the last two decades. It is now recognized as a separate subspecialty in most countries. Nearly 50% of all skin problems pertain to pediatric age group.

Diseases like atopic dermatitis, vitiligo and other pigmentary disorders are to be seen in a different light in relation to children as they are not intellectually mature to deal with the psychological aspect of the diseases. The concept of pediatric dermatology is a unifying one where the subjects of pediatrics and dermatology shake their hands for a better understanding of the skin diseases in infants, children and adolescents. There are a number of textbooks and color atlases on pediatric dermatology published from UK and USA which obviously do not address the difference in presentation of pediatric dermatoses in types IV and V skins. Therefore, there has been a growing need for such a color atlas in Indian context among the pediatricians in particular (as I have been insisted by my pediatrician friends and colleagues). That is why I have taken up this endeavor.

The chapters compiled in this book make an attempt to give a visual impression and important clues to diagnose a dermatosis. Most of the common (and some rare) skin diseases have been incorporated.

This book is basically meant for the pediatricians, beginners in dermatology and all those involved in the care of children. I am sure that the book will serve its purpose. The 'quotable quotes' have been incorporated to provide relief in-between the serious readings. Despite my best possible efforts, there may be some unwanted errors and some shortcomings in this book, which I promise to rectify in its future edition.

You may give your valuable feedback about this book to me (e-mail: babyd@vsnl.net).

Sandipan Dhar

Acknowledgments

I am deeply indebted to a host of individuals who have made innumerable contributions toward the completion of this book, some identified below and others, with apologies, perhaps unwittingly overlooked.

First, I wish to extend my sincere gratitude and thanks to Subhra, my best friend and wife. But for her active support and help, this book would have remained in the realm of unreality. She has contributed 50%, if not more, of the total work toward completion of this title.

It is my proud privilege to keep on record my deep respect and gratitude to Late Dr AK Dutta, former Professor and Head, Pediatric Dermatology Unit, Institute of Child Health, Kolkata, for inspiring me to take up this challenging task.

I like to convey my warm regards and sincere gratitude to Dr Apurba Ghosh, Professor of Pediatrics and Director, Institute of Child Health (ICH), Kolkata, for giving me all liberty to preach and practice pediatric dermatology. Many of the illustrations in this book are contributed by him. I hereby express my heartfelt gratitude to Dr GK Mehrotra, Late Dr U Sarkar, Dr (Mrs) Maya Mukhopadhyay, Dr Ritabrata Kundu, Professors of Pediatrics, ICH, Kolkata, for always being kind and supportive to me.

I have been fortunate to get a number of good friends and well-wishers who have been very supportive in all my endeavors including this. Dr Rajeev Sharma, Dr Arun Inamadar, Dr Arunaloke Bhattacharya, Dr Swapan Roy, Dr Raghubir Banerjee, and Dr Rajib Malakar are to name a few. A special note of thanks to Dr Mandira Roy and Mr Debraj Roy for compiling and arranging the "quotable quotes". Special thanks to Dr Samujjala Deb, Dr Abhijit Saha, and Dr Rashmi Agarwal.

We sincerely thank Dr Jayakar Thomas, Dr Sudip Das, Dr Rahul Mahajan, Dr Ram Gulati, Dr Bornali Dutta, Dr Debjit Kar, Dr Swetalina Pradhan, and Dr Sahana M Srinivas for their contribution.

A special thanks to Mr Tapas Kayal, my shadow in all my academic endeavors over the last 25 years!

I am very grateful to the whole team of M/s Jaypee Brothers Medical Publishers (P) Ltd, New Delhi, India, with whom my association is for nearly 25 years, especially Shri Jitendar P Vij (Group Chairman), Mr Ankit Vij (Managing Director), Mr MS Mani (Group President), Ms Chetna Malhotra (Senior Director—Professional Publishing, Marketing and Business Development), Mr Sabyasachi Hazra (Associate Director, Publishing and Digital Sales), and Ms Himani Pandey (Senior Development Editor) for all their tremendous support to work in this project and make it a great success.

I (MP) am eternally grateful to my mentor Dr Sandipan Dhar for trusting me and giving me this exceedingly important opportunity to co-author this book. His presence in my life has made all the differences.

I (MP) am blessed to have a solid support system and backbone of my existence which is my Family. I thank my parents Hrushikesh Panda and Chandrika Panda, my sister Vasudha, my husband Dr Mrutunjay Dash, and my son Tridivesh Dash for everything.

Finally, we thank all the ardent readers (both pediatricians and dermatologists) for more than two and half decades to have trust in us.

Sandipan Dhar
Maitreyee Panda

Special Acknowledgments

I (MP) am forever thankful to my dependable team consisting of my talented and committed juniors, namely Dr Nibedita Patro, Dr Akash Agarwal, Dr Asritha CVV, and Dr Aditya Prakash for their unwavering support and assistance.

Maitreyee Panda

Contents

CHAPTER

1

Basics of Skin and Neonatal Dermatoses

STRUCTURE OF SKIN

Skin is the largest organ of the body. It is a very complex structure composed of three layers viz., epidermis, dermis, and subcutaneous tissue. It is also composed of various appendages. The outermost layer or the epidermis is further composed of four layers, stratum corneum, stratum granulosum, stratum spinosum, and stratum basale. There are melanocytes situated at the basal cell layer and Langerhans cells throughout the epidermis.

The dermis is predominantly composed of collagen and elastic fibers. There are cell types including fibroblasts, macrophages and mast cells in the dermis. Various structures situated in the dermis are composite structure of hair follicle with sebaceous gland known as pilosebaceous apparatus, and eccrine or sweat glands. Beneath the dermis, there is a layer of fat known as subcutaneous tissue. In the dermis, there are dermal capillaries and venules which comprise dermal vasculature. There are also lymphatics and nerve endings situated in the dermis.

FUNCTIONS OF SKIN

The outermost layer or stratum corneum performs the barrier function and maintains the hydration of skin. It also prevents the penetration of irritants, toxins, and organisms through the epidermis into the dermal capillaries from the environment. The rest of the epidermis acts as protective layer. Melanocytes of the epidermis confer color of the skin by transferring melanin to the basal keratinocytes. It also protects the skin from deleterious effect of ultraviolet light. Langerhans cells present antigen to the immunological unit of the skin. Hence, it is considered as the first line of immunologic defense.

The collagen and elastic fibers act as a tough, leathery, mechanical barrier against cuts, bites, abrasions, and bruises. Its collagenous matrix provides structural support for various cutaneous appendages. Hair grows from follicles placed in the deep dermis and imparts beauty to the individual. It also protects the scalp from the sunlight and various environmental allergens. Sebaceous glands produce oily secretions, lubricate the skin and contribute to the protective function of epidermal barrier. Eccrine glands produce sweat which secrete on the skin surface through eccrine ducts. Thus, it acts as an important organ responsible for thermoregulation. Cutaneous capillaries, venules, and lymphatics act as perfusion unit of skin. The skin also contains specialized receptors for heat, pain, touch, and pressure. Sensory inputs from these structures help to protect the skin surface against environmental trauma and noxious agents. The subcutaneous fat acts as a protective cushion for the skin and stores energy and provides insulation to the body. To summarize, various functions of the skin are as follows:

- *Protection:* It protects the body from physical, chemical, and biological injuries.
- *Perception:* It perceives various sensations such as pain, touch, temperature, and vibration.
- *Temperature regulation:* Eccrine sweat glands and dermal vasculature play important role in thermoregulation.
- *Barrier function:* Skin acts as a permeability barrier that regulates the diffusion of substances particularly water and electrolytes, etc.
- *Secretory function:* Synthesis of vitamin D3 is an important secretory function with the help of sunlight.
- *Storage function:* The dermis and subcutaneous fat act as a storage center for energy and other compounds.
- *Excretory function:* Some of the harmful substances are excreted through the skin.
- *Immunological function:* Recognition of antigens and elicitation of immunological response is done by skin.
- *Cosmetic function:* Color and texture of skin along with the hair and nail play an important role in esthetic appeal of an individual.

"Real knowledge is to know the extent of one's ignorance." —**Confucius**

SKIN TYPES AND SKIN COLOR

Skin color is of two types: Constitutive skin color and facultative skin color.

Constitutive skin color is the basic skin color of an individual and is genetically determined. Facultative skin color is the skin color that results from ultraviolet ray (UVR) exposure. It is basically tanning of the skin. Depending on the response of the skin to UVR, various skin phototypes (SPTs) have been described and different races with different SPTs possess different types of skin color. **Table 1** highlights color of skin and response to UVR in different SPTs.

Three types of melanin in humans have been demonstrated—eumelanin (brown-black melanin), pheomelanin (yellow-red melanin), and neuromelanin (black). While in most of the melanocytes there is a minimal admixture of pheomelanin and eumelanin, in red hairs exclusively pheomelanin is present. Neuromelanin is present in nerve cells. Neuromelanin is formed by an enzymatic pathway different from that of eumelanin or pheomelanin synthesis. Hence, in oculocutaneous albinism (OCA) there is presence of pigment in substantia nigra.

BASIC MORPHOLOGY OF SKIN LESIONS

Various morphologies of the lesions have been divided into three types—primary lesions, secondary lesions, and special lesions.

Primary Lesions

Different types of primary lesions are:

- *Macule*: It is only the change of color of skin, texture remaining unaltered. A macule can be hyperpigmented, hypopigmented or erythematous.
- *Papule:* It is a circumscribed solid lesion measuring <1 cm in diameter. A papule can be erythematous, skin-colored or of any other color. The surface may be flat, verrucous, or umbilicated.
- *Plaque:* It is a solid elevation >1 cm in diameter. There may be associated follicular plugging, telangiectasia, atrophy, etc.
- *Nodule:* It is a deep-seated solid three dimensional lesion which may be hard, firm, soft, fleshy, tender or nontender, fixed or mobile. The surface of the nodule can be smooth, keratotic, ulcerated or fungating.
- *Pustule:* It is a circumscribed elevated lesion containing pus. Sometimes it may be sterile.
- *Vesicle and bullae:* A vesicle is a circumscribed raised lesion containing fluid and <1 cm in diameter. Bulla is a circumscribed raised lesion containing fluid, >1 cm diameter. Vesicle or bullae may be tense or flaccid and on rupture leave behind raw area.
- *Wheal:* It is a transient or evanescent elevated plaque-like lesion with erythema, edema, and central pallor.
- *Cyst:* It is a sac that contains liquid or semisolid material.
- *Abscess:* It is a collection of pus either in the dermis or subcutaneous plane or both.

Table 1: Color of skin and response to ultraviolet ray in different skin phototypes (SPTs).

SPT	*Reaction to moderate sun exposure*	*Skin color*
I	Burn and no tan	Pale white
II	Burn and minimal tan	Pale white
III	Burn but good tan	White
IV	Severe tan but no burn	Light brown
V	Moderate tan but no burn	Brown
VI	Minimal tan but no burn	Dark brown

Secondary Lesions

These are lesions which are basically modified primary lesions induced by scratching, rubbing or secondary bacterial infections. Various secondary lesions are:

- Scales are formed as a result of increased or abnormal keratinization. They may be fine powder-like or large silvery white or even fish like.
- Crust is a collection of dried exudates, dead tissues, and microorganisms. Crust may be brown/brownish-yellow, may be adherent or friable.
- Excoriation or scratch marks are predominantly seen in pruritic disorders.
- Erosion is a superficial ulceration covered with serous exudates and heals without scarring.
- Ulcer is the result of breach in the continuity of skin with loss of epidermis and a part of dermis. Ulcer always heals with scarring.
- Lichenification is thickening, increased criss-cross markings, and mild hyperpigmentation. It is the end result of chronic eczema.
- Atrophy is thinning of skin which appears shiny wrinkled with prominent blood vessels underneath.

"In the practice of tolerance, one's enemy is the best teacher." **—The Dalai Lama**

Special Lesions

Some of the lesions are pathognomonic of certain diseases as follows:

- *Burrows* are tunnel-like serpiginous lesions seen in the superficial part of the skin.
- *Comedones* are the result of plugging of the pilosebaceous duct by internal secretion. Comedones may be open (black) or closed (white).
- *Milia* are small superficial cysts 1–2 mm in diameter, commonly seen on the face.
- *Telangiectasia* means distinctly visible dilated superficial blood vessels.

Configuration of the Skin Lesions

Characteristic configuration of lesions may suggest a diagnosis. Some classical examples are:

- *Linear:* Lesions are present in a line. Examples are epidermal nevi, lichen striatus, warts, psoriasis, incontinentia pigmenti, etc.
- *Dermatomal:* Lesions are present in a dermatome. Examples are herpes zoster, vitiligo, nevus depigmentosus, and PWS.
- *Serpiginous:* Lesions follow a serpiginous track. Examples are cutaneous larva migrans, and elastosis perforans serpiginosa.
- *Annular:* Lesions present with central clearing with peripheral border. Examples are tinea, granuloma annulare, erythema annulare centrifugum, and erythema marginatum.
- *Herpetiform:* Grouped lesions or clustered lesions. Examples are herpes simplex infection, herpes zoster, and dermatitis herpetiformis.
- *Reticulated:* Means net-like. Examples are cutis marmorata, livedo reticularis, and erythema ab igne.
- *Filiform:* Means thread-like. Examples are filiform warts, dermatosis papulosa nigra, and skin tags/acrochordons.
- *Geographic*: Examples are geographic tongue, psoriasis, and erythema annulare centrifugum.

NEONATAL DERMATOSES AND CARE OF NEWBORN SKIN

Most of the newborn disorders are transient in nature requiring only symptomatic treatment. They can be divided into physiological, acquired, congenital infections and developmental disorders **(Table 2)**.

Table 2: Classification of neonatal dermatoses.

Physiological changes	• Vernix caseosa • Peripheral cyanosis • Erythema neonatorum • Harlequin color change • Cutis marmorata • Bronze baby syndrome • Physiological exfoliation of newborn **(Figs. 1E and F)** • Suckling blister • Neonatal occipital alopecia • Hair shedding in infancy (Telogen effluvium) • Milia • Sebaceous hyperplasia • Neonatal acne • Miniature puberty • Hyperpigmentation disorders (linea alba, Mongolian spot, scrotal hyperpigmentation, linear/reticulate hyperpigmentation) • Oral findings (Epstein's pearl, Suckling pads)
Developmental defects	• Aplasia cutis congenita • Polythelia • Median raphe cyst • Sternal cleft with umbilical raphe • Amniotic band syndrome • Congenital cysts (Dermoid cyst, branchial cleft cyst, Thyroglossal cyst bronchogenic cyst, urachal cyst) • Cephalocele • Nasal glioma • Congenital fistulas of lower lip • Skin dimpling defect • Preauricular pits • Accessory tragi
Acquired conditions	• Miliaria • Subcutaneous fat necrosis • Sclerema neonatorum • Neonatal erythroderma • Transient neonatal pustular melanosis • Acropustulosis of infancy • Granuloma gluteale infantum • Cutis marmorata telangiectatica congenita • Congenital erosive and vesicular dermatosis • Dermatitis (seborrheic dermatitis, diaper dermatitis, intertrigo, irritant/allergic contact dermatitis, acrodermatitis enteropathica, psoriasis)
Congenital infections	• Congenital rubella • Congenital varicella syndrome • Neonatal herpes • Congenital syphilis • Congenital toxoplasmosis • Congenital parvovirus B19 infection • Congenital Epstein–Barr virus infection • Congenital cytomegalovirus infection

Mongolian Spot (Figs. 1A to F)

It is the most common type of congenital dermal melanocytosis noted in 90% of Asians. It presents as macular blue-gray pigmentation at birth most commonly on the lumbosacral area in normal infants of darker-skinned races. They are rounded or oval in shape, in variable sizes and usually single or multiple. Less common sites include buttocks, flanks, and shoulders. The pigmentation develops in fetal life, increases in depth for a period after birth and then diminishes. It usually disappears in the first decade of life.

Natural History

It is considered as one of the physiological skin changes of the newborn. When Mongolian spots are associated with bilateral Nevus of Ota, they take much longer time to disappear spontaneously. Persistent and giant *Mongolian* spots are seen in Niemann-Pick disease, type 1 gangliosidosis, Hurler, and Hunter disease.

Management

Explanation of the condition and its natural history to the parents helps to reassure them.

Neonatal Acne (Figs. 2 and 3)

The sebaceous glands of neonates produce a considerable amount of sebum in first few weeks of life influenced by maternal androgen. There is increased production of dehydroepiandrosterone (DHEA) by fetal adrenal glands. Neonatal acne mostly affects male infants and is seen at birth or within first week of life. Clinically presents as erythematous papules, pustules, and occasionally with comedones distributed on face, more over the cheeks and forehead. Pustular eruption in neonatal

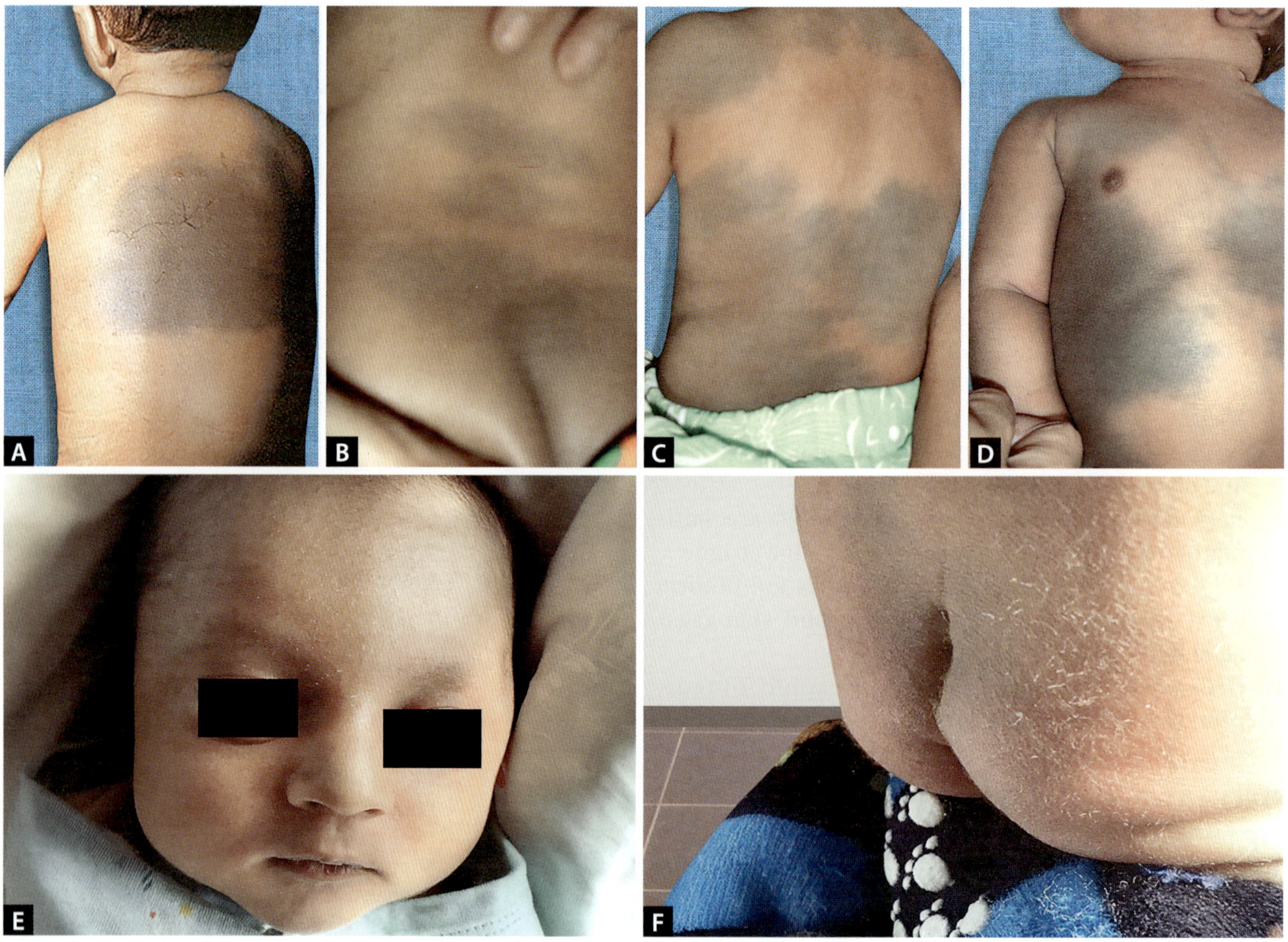

Figs. 1A to F: (A) Bluish-black hyperpigmented patch of Mongolian spot over back; (B) Mongolian spots over back in a newborn; (C) Mongolian spots over back; (D) Extensive Mongolian spots; (E) Physiological exfoliation in newborn marked on forehead; (F) Same child with physiological exfoliation on back.

"You don't need to see the whole staircase, just take the first step." —**Martin Luther King Jr**

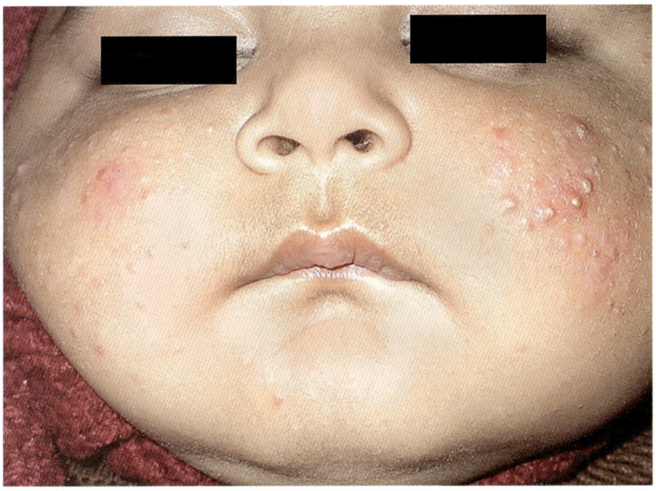

Fig. 2: Neonatal acne (inflammatory papules and pustules).

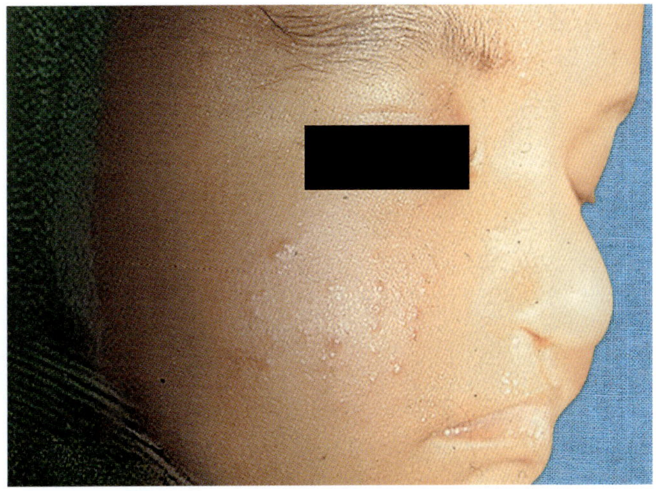

Fig. 3: Close-up view of neonatal acne.

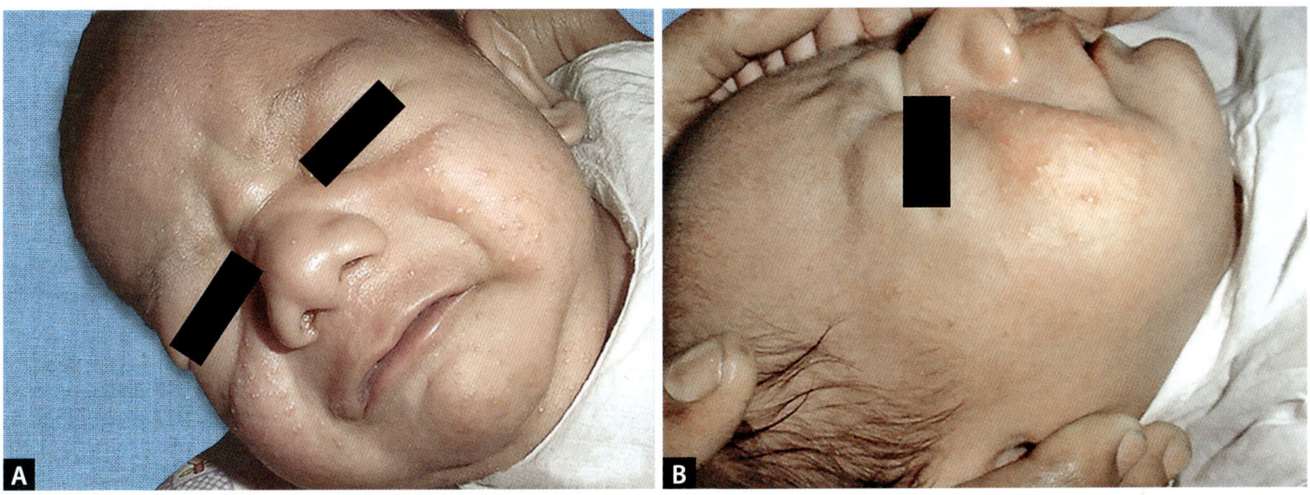

Figs. 4A and B: Neonatal milia.

acne has been termed as neonatal cephalic pustulosis secondary to colonization of *Malassezia* species. Child should be evaluated for underlying virilizing tumors or adrenal cortical hyperplasia if there are other signs of hyperandrogenism.

Management

The lesions are self-limiting and tend to subside by 2–3 weeks and require no treatment. It can persist for 1 year. Benzoyl peroxide 2.5% or 1% salicylic acid has been tried.

Neonatal Milia (Figs. 4 to 6)

Milia are one of the most common transient findings in the cutaneous survey in neonates seen in 40–50% of healthy newborns. These consist of 2–3 mm white or yellow papules on the nose, chin, cheeks, and forehead. Milia are epidermal cysts derived from the pilosebaceous follicle of vellus hair and contain concentric layers of keratin. Widespread and persistent milia can be associated with epidermolysis bullosa, type 1 oro-facial-digital syndrome, and pachyonychia congenita.

Natural History

They are normally spontaneously extruded in a few weeks.

Toxic Erythema of the Newborn (Erythema Toxicum Neonatorum) (Figs. 7A to D)

The cause of toxic erythema of the newborn is unknown and is seen in 48–72% of full-term newborn. In majority, the

"The invariable mark of wisdom is to see the miracles in the common." —**Ralph Waldo Emerson**

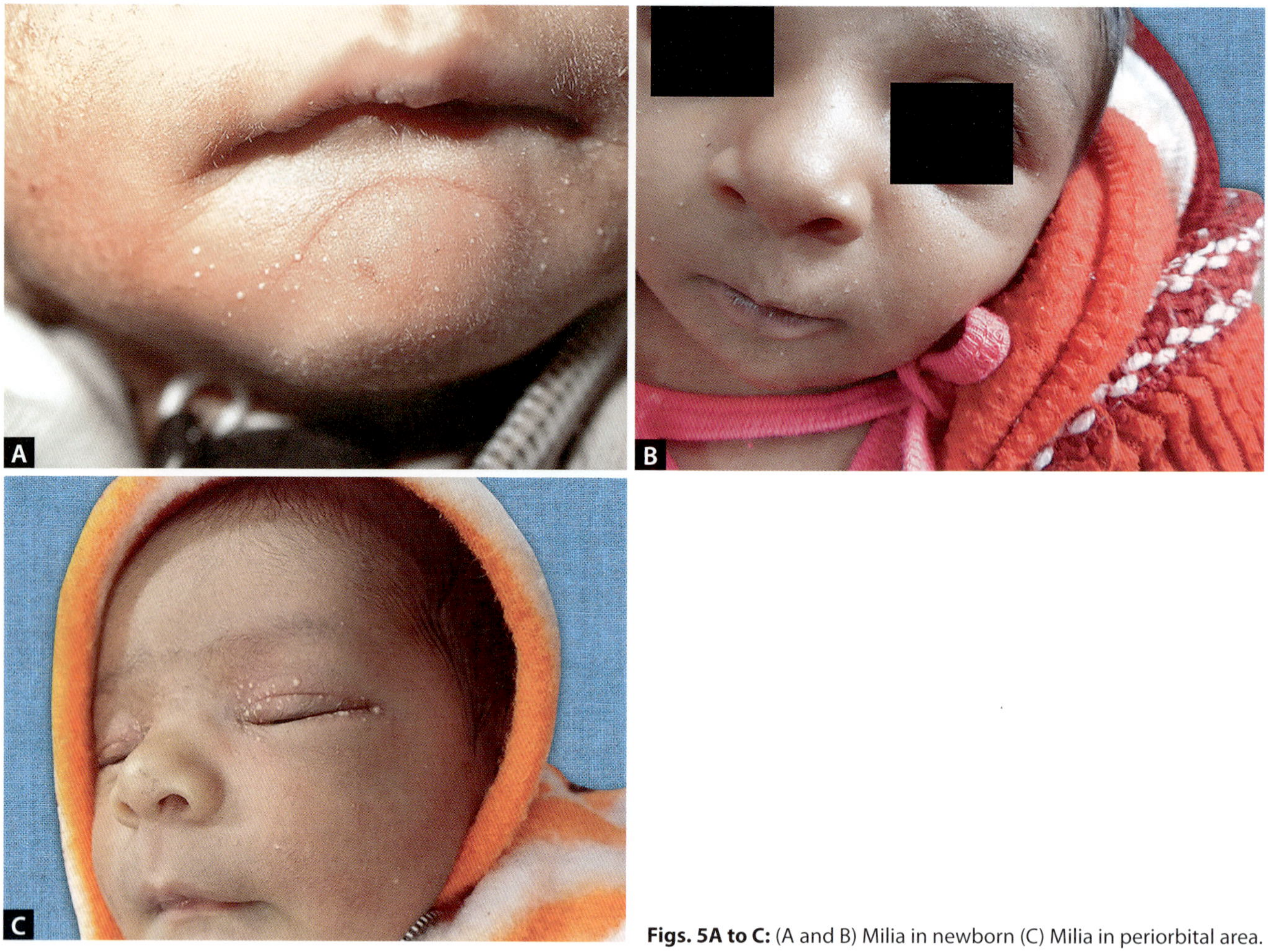

Figs. 5A to C: (A and B) Milia in newborn (C) Milia in periorbital area.

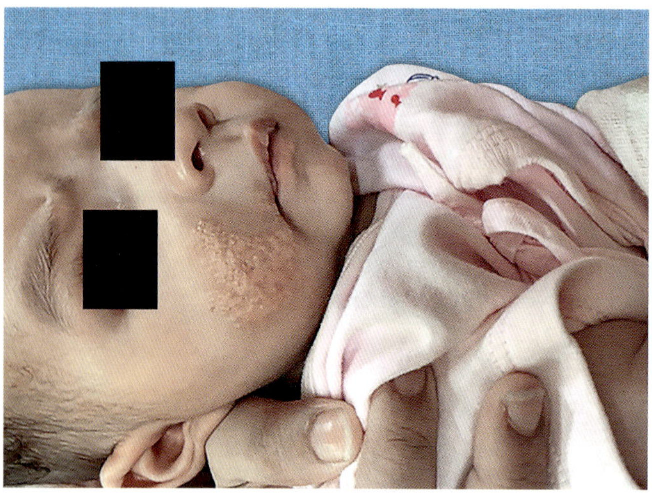

Fig. 6: Neonatal milia en plaque.

onset is during the first 48 hours after birth or up to 3 weeks. The eruption can appear as a blotchy macular erythema initially and later develop multiple erythematous papules, their number varying from one to several hundred, most profuse on the anterior trunk, rapidly spreading to involve the face, chest, and extremities. They are often described as "flea bitten appearance" or papules surrounded by a sea of erythema. In severe cases, urticarial papules develop which in 10% cases are surmounted by pustules measuring 2–4 mm in diameter.

Differential Diagnosis

These lesions have to be distinguished from milia, miliaria, transient neonatal pustular melanosis, infantile acropustulosis, incontinentia pigmenti, herpes simplex virus infection, varicella, and impetigo.

Diagnosis

Toxic erythema can be diagnosed by microscopic examination of a smear of pustular contents stained with Giemsa and in doubtful cases, cultures to rule out infective

"The true sign of intelligence is not knowledge but imagination." —**Albert Einstein**

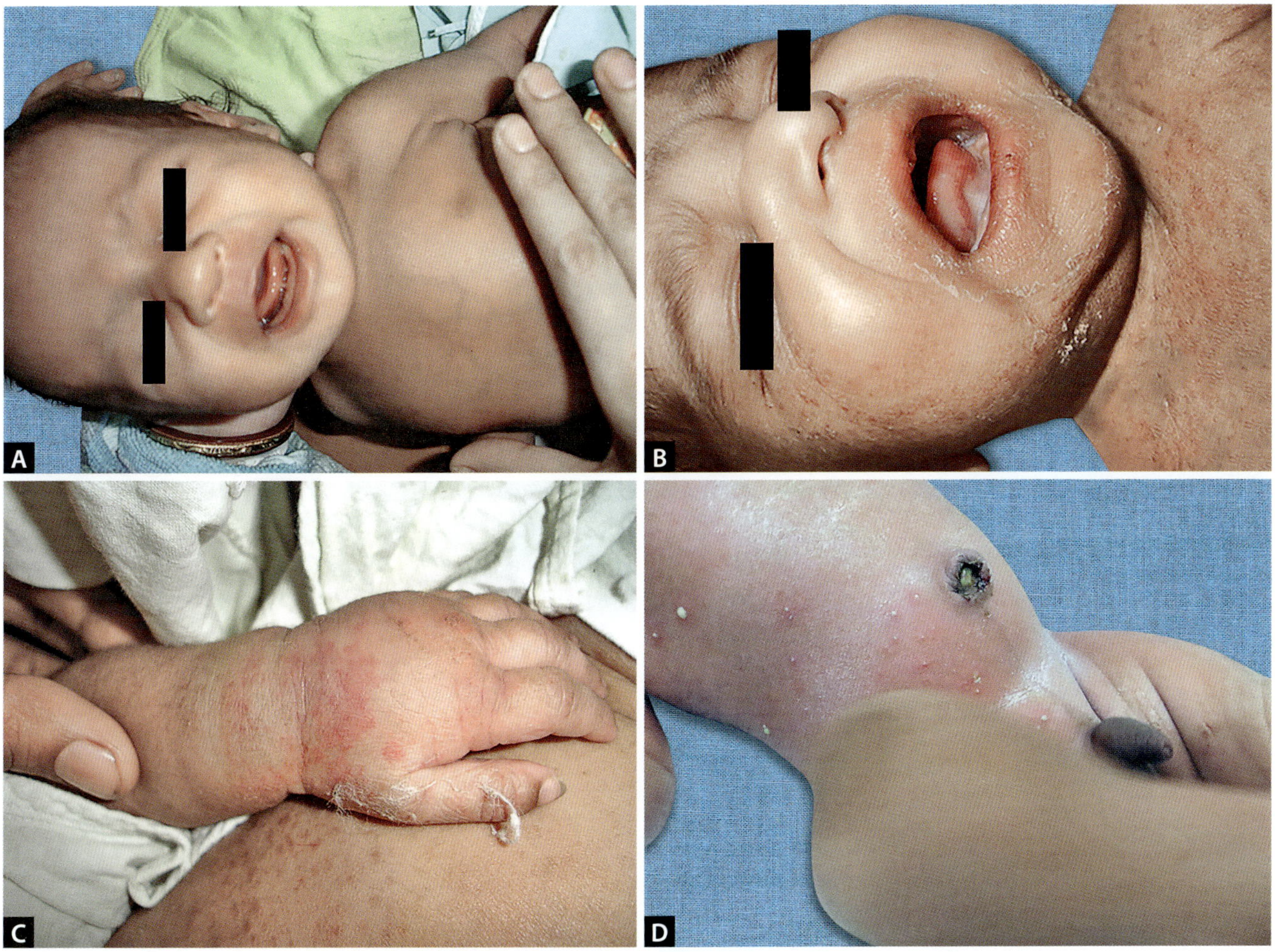

Figs. 7A to D: (A) Toxic erythema of newborn; (B) Close-up view of lesions; (C) Blotchy macular erythema and satellite pustules of toxic erythema of newborn; (D) Erythema toxicum neonatorum, note bright red erythema and pustular lesions.

etiology can be done. The smear in case of toxic erythema reveals cluster of eosinophils. This is in sharp contrast to bacterial infections where cluster of neutrophils are seen.

Treatment

As the condition is benign, self-limiting, and asymptomatic no treatment is required. It resolves spontaneously by 10–14 days.

Intertrigo (Figs. 8A to F)

Intertrigo is a term applied to an inflammatory dermatosis that is more or less confined to the major body folds and provoked by moisture and constant friction between opposing skin surfaces. Obesity, poor hygiene, overwarm clothing, hot and humid climatic conditions are the predisposing factors. Relative obesity of well-nourished infants accounts for the unusually high incidence during the early months of life. Intertrigo is likely to become colonized and secondarily infected by both bacteria and yeast, particularly *Candida albicans*. Clinically, it manifests as symmetrical areas of sharply marginated erythema confined to areas of skin apposition. In infants, the folds of the neck, the axillae, the genitocrural flexures, and the intergluteal cleft are the predilection sites. Miliarial lesions are readily apparent within the affected area. When *C. albicans* infection supervenes, erythema takes on a deep red hue along with maceration, oozing, and satellite pustules. Rarely it may become superinfected with group A streptococci and *Corynebacterium diphtheriae*.

Management

Management of intertrigo is mainly removal of predisposing factors, cool environment, loose cotton clothes, and topical antibacterial and antifungals. If bacterial

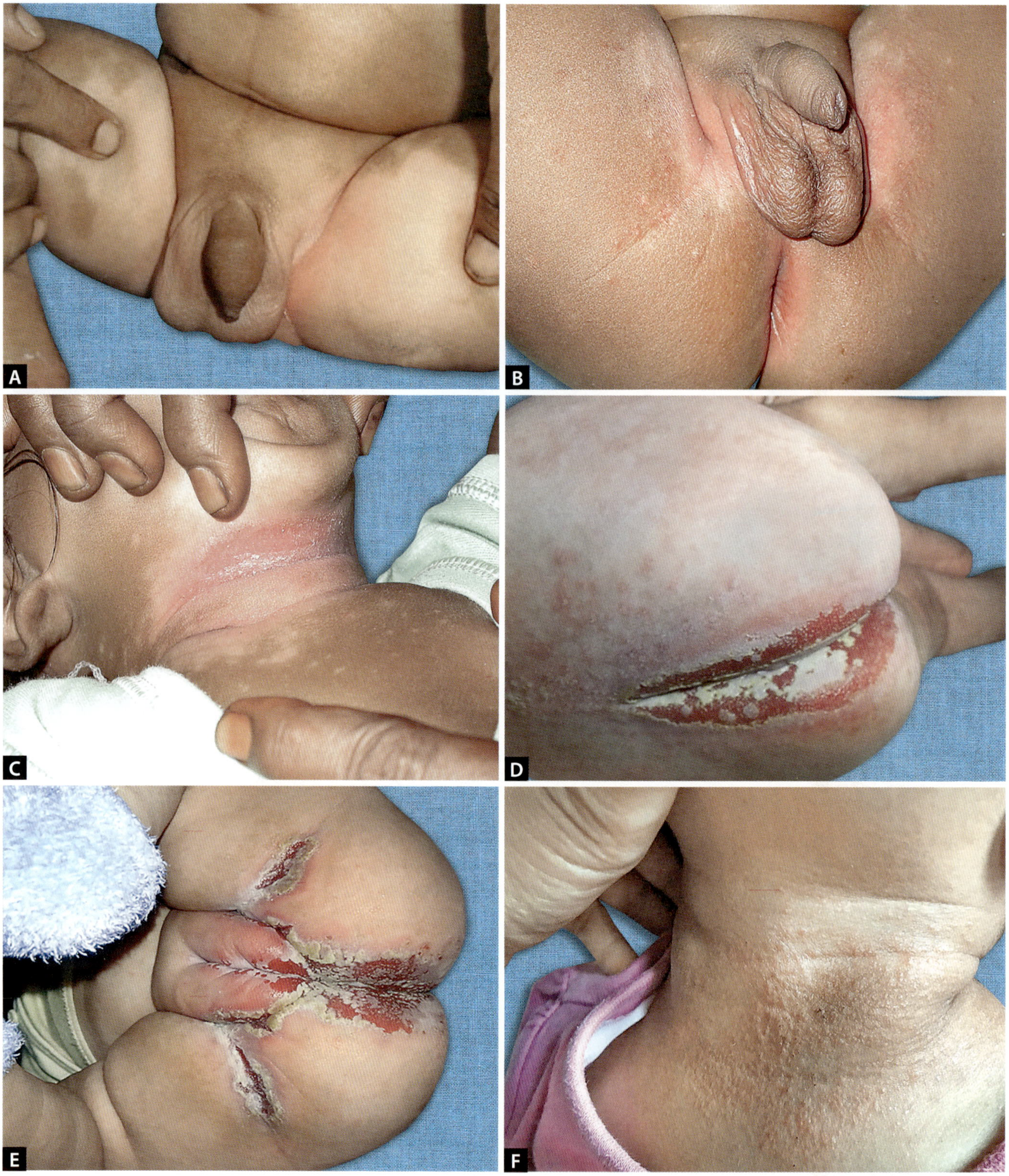

Figs. 8A to F: Intertrigo. (A) Intertrigo of inguinal folds; (B) Note erythema over inguinal and perianal area; (C) Note postinflammatory hypopigmentation surrounding erythema; (D) Intertrigo, severe perianal involvement; (E) Severe intertrigo; (F) Intertrigo seen in the neck fold.

"When one door of happiness closes, another opens; but often we look so long at the closed door that we do not see the other one that has been opened for us." —**Helen Keller**

superadded infection is evident, a topical antibacterial-like mupirocin may be useful. Topical antifungals such as clotrimazole and miconazole are effective for candidal intertrigo.

Miliaria (Figs. 9A to E)

Miliaria occurs when the flow of eccrine sweat is impeded by obstruction of the intraepidermal portion of the sweat duct. Miliaria crystallina appears to reflect obstruction of

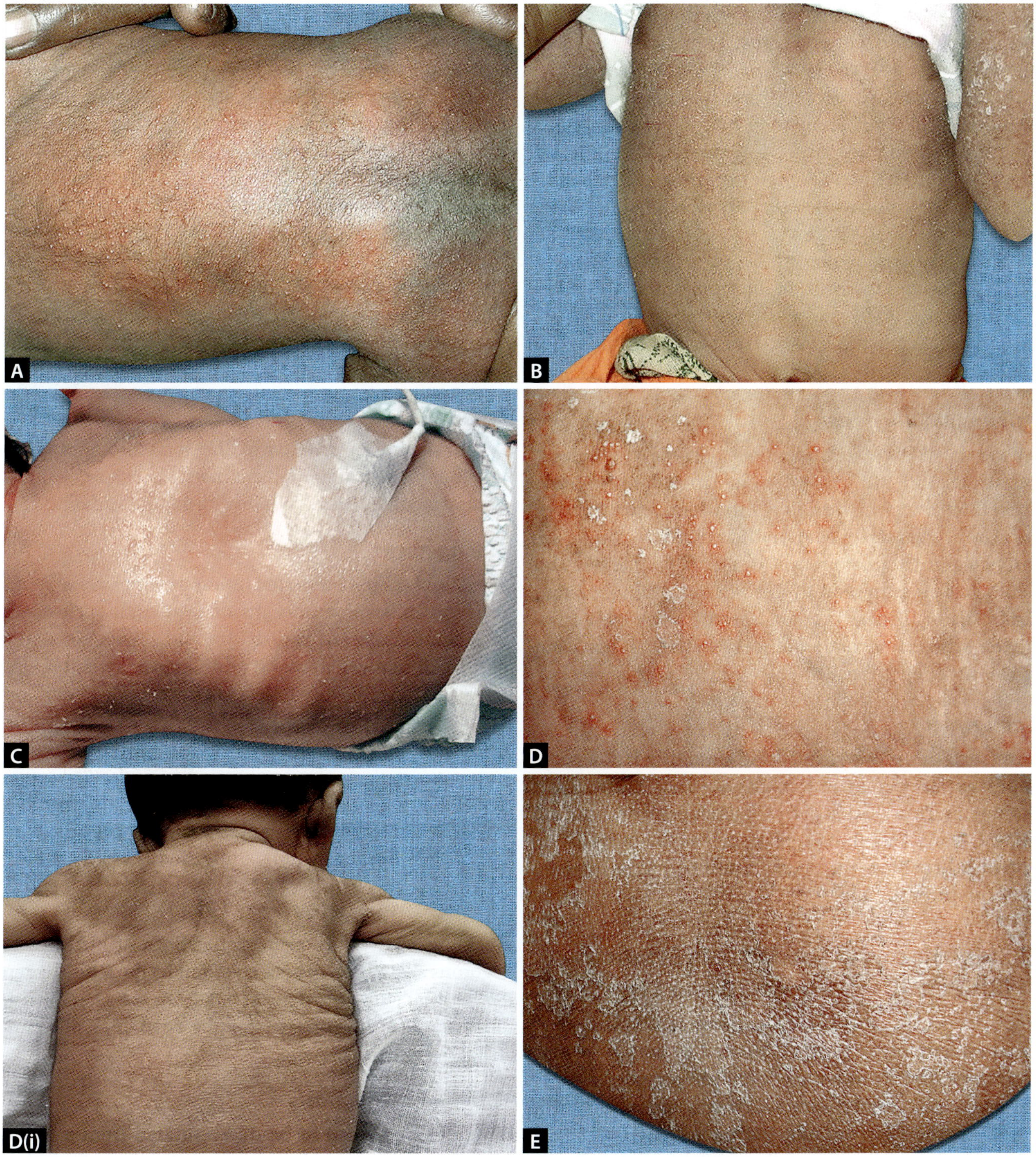

Figs. 9A to E: (A) Miliaria rubra and pustulosa in a newborn; (B) Exfoliating miliaria rubra; (C) Miliaria crystalline in newborn; (D) Miliaria pustulosa (D)(i) Miliaria pustulosa healing with postinflammatory hypopigmentation; (E) Subsiding miliaria, note fine branny scales.

"It is impossible to live without failing at something, unless you live so cautiously that you might as well not have lived at all—in which case you fail by default." —**JK Rowling**

the sweat duct within the stratum corneum. Miliaria rubra occurs when there is sweat duct obstruction deeper in the epidermis.

Miliaria crystallina presents as crops of clear thin-walled, superficial vesicles, 1–2 mm in diameter without associated erythema resembling water droplets on the scalp, forehead, neck, and upper trunk. They rupture within 24 hours followed by branny desquamation.

Miliaria rubra, seen most commonly in the neonatal period, comprises of grouped to discrete erythematous nonfollicular, papules, and papulovesicles, measuring about 1-4 mm in diameter on a background of macular erythema. Staphylococcal secondary infection of miliaria may lead to sweat gland abscesses. The symmetrical crops of miliaria rubra occur most often in flexural areas, especially around the neck, in the groins, and the axillae. The face, scalp, and upper trunk are frequently affected. These lesions subside in 2–3 days but recurrences are common.

Differential Diagnosis

Differential diagnosis includes neonatal acne, candidiasis, staphylococcal, and herpes simplex infections. Miliaria crystallina is distinguishable from viral infections of the skin by the lack of background erythema and by the absence of inflammatory cells or giant keratinocytes on cytological examination of the vesicles. Miliaria rubra can be distinguished from toxic erythema by its flexural predominance, frequent presence of vesicular lesions and by the tendency to recur.

Management

Avoidance of excessive heat and humidity is the most important aspect of management. Cool baths, light clothing, and installation of air conditioner in the room are helpful. Topical soothing agents such as calamine lotion help in most of the cases. Systemic antibiotics can be given for secondary infection.

Staphylococcal Scalded Skin Syndrome (Ritter's Disease) (Figs. 10 and 11)

Staphylococcal scalded skin syndrome (SSSS) is caused by an epidermolytic toxin elaborated by certain strains of *Staphylococcus aureus*, commonly phage group II. The condition is most commonly seen in the first 5 years of life. It is particularly common during the neonatal period occurring in association with purulent conjunctivitis or an upper respiratory tract infection. Sites of predilection are the central part of the face (periorificial), the axillae, and groins. The orange-red, scarlatiniform eruption spreads rapidly. Tenderness of the skin is an early and striking feature. The eruption gradually becomes extensive and turns to a confluent deep erythema and edema in the next 24–48 hours. The surface becomes wrinkled before starting to separate out leaving raw red erosions. Nikolsky's sign is positive. The child is pyrexial and distressed. Radial crusting and fissuring around the eyes, angles of mouth occurs. The only differential diagnosis which poses a problem is toxic epidermal necrolysis, which is however, relatively rare in young children and is characterized by marked mucosal involvement.

Diagnosis

The diagnosis of SSSS can be established by isolation of coagulase positive *Staphylococcus aureus* from the pyogenic skin lesions or from nostril and areas around eyes.

Prognosis

Prognosis is good with early diagnosis and appropriate treatment. The condition has a mortality of approximately 5% and fatalities occur mostly in debilitated infants.

Management

Treatment should be started promptly with a penicillinase resistant antistaphylococcal antibiotic such as cloxacillin or a combination of amoxicillin and clavulanic acid or cefadroxil orally. Parenteral antibiotics may be required in cases of extensive skin lesions or severely ill children. Local cleaning of the skin with distilled water or normal saline soaked cotton is sufficient. Antiseptic cleaning is better avoided, so also application of prolonged topical antibiotic for fear of emergence of resistant strains of *S. aureus*. Parenteral vancomycin is preferred for methicillin-resistant *S. aureus* infection.

Suckling Blister (Fig. 12)

Suckling blisters are seen in newborn at birth due to vigorous sucking on the affected part by the fetus in utero. Solitary bullae or erosions of 0.5–2 cm are seen over the dorsal aspect of the fingers, thumbs, wrists, lips, and radial aspect of forearms.

Differential Diagnosis

These lesions need to be differentiated from a host of conditions such as bullous impetigo, epidermolysis bullosa, and neonatal herpes simplex.

"Believe you can and you're halfway there." —**Theodore Roosevelt**

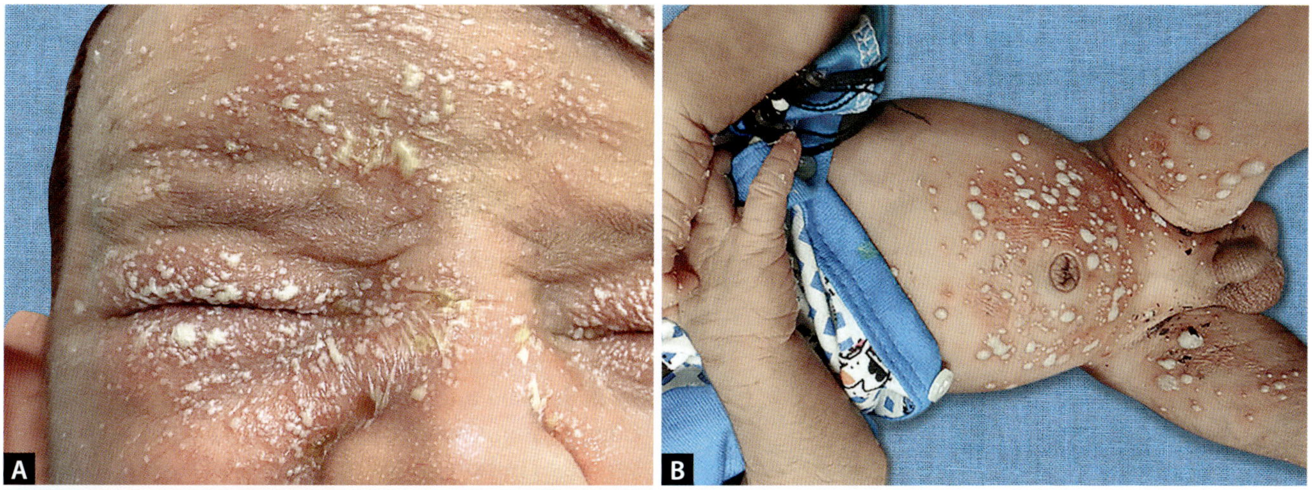

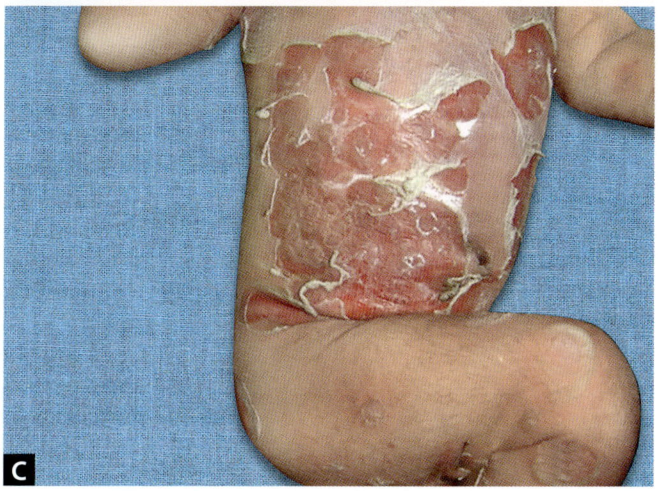

Figs. 10A to C: (A) Staphylococcal scalded skin syndrome (SSSS), early stage; (B) Impending SSSS, note extensive impetigo bullosa indicating impending SSSS; (C) Full blown SSSS.

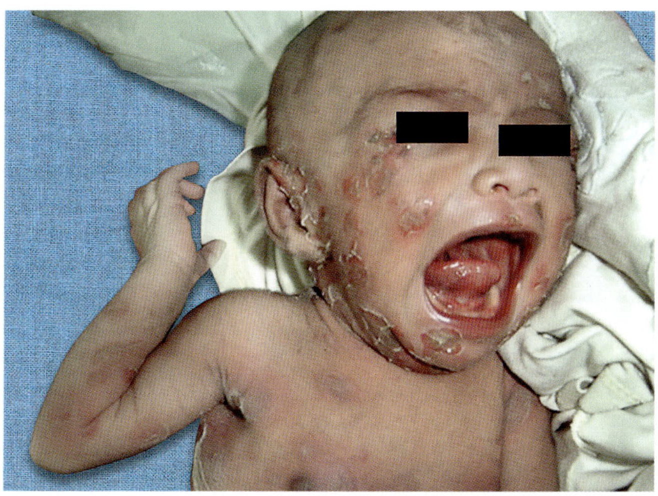

Fig. 11: Involvement of face and upper extremities in staphylococcal scalded skin syndrome.

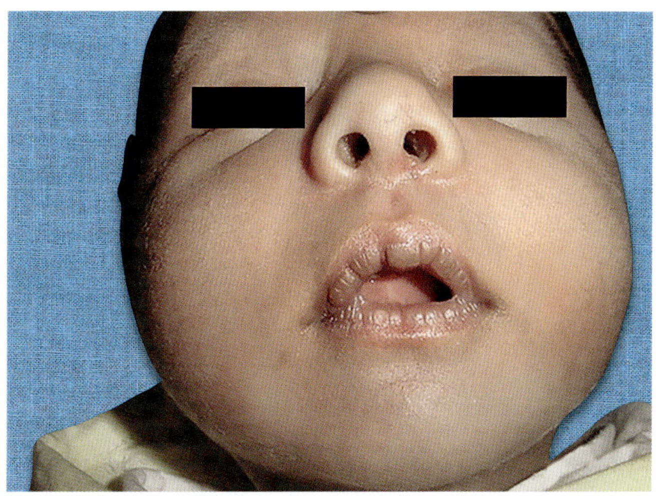

Fig. 12: Suckling blisters over upper lip in a newborn.

"Knowledge has a beginning but no end." —**Geeta Iyengar**

Treatment

Resolves rapidly without any treatment and sequelae.

Neonatal Herpes (Figs. 13 to 15)

Infection of the neonate by herpes simplex virus ranges from mild to potentially life-threatening condition with high mortality. The majority of these infections result from transmission of HSV-1 and HSV-2 from genital tract secretions during delivery. Transmission can occur during intrauterine, peripartum, and postpartum period. There is higher incidence of neonatal herpes (40–50%) during primary maternal infection than in recurrent infection (4–5%). Over 70% of the infection with neonatal HSV has skin or mucosal lesions. There are three distinct forms of neonatal herpes: Skin-eye-mouth (SEM), disseminated, and only nervous system involvement. Skin manifestations are in the form of multiple grouped vesicles on erythematous patches distributed over the scalp, face, trunk, and extremities. The vesicles have a tendency to localize over mucocutaneous junctions. Onset is between birth and 20 days. Oral lesions in the form of erosions of the tongue, palate, gingiva, and buccal mucosa are also common. Primary neonatal herpes simplex is a devastating life-threatening infection especially in the disseminated form involving multiple organs which must be diagnosed and treated with antiviral drugs promptly. Complications include pneumonia, seizures, encephalitis, keratitis, chorioretinitis, coagulopathy, and sepsis.

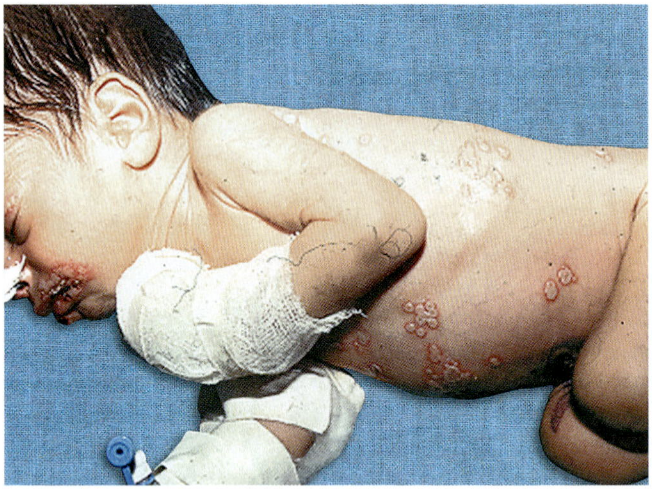

Fig. 13: Grouped vesicles of herpes simplex on erythematous base over the trunk.

Diagnosis

Diagnosis can be co-established with the help of Tzanck smear preparation, viral culture, use of monoclonal antibodies, and nucleic acid hybridization techniques.

Management

Intravenous (IV) acyclovir is the treatment of choice. It is given at a dose of 60 mg/kg/day in three divided doses for 14–21 days. There is no role of topical acyclovir ointment application over the lesions. Prophylactic ophthalmic topical preparations such as trifluridine or vidarabine are helpful.

Neonatal Varicella (Figs. 16A to D)

Neonatal varicella occurs in the first 28 days of life and is due to infection developed by mother during the last few weeks of pregnancy or first few days postpartum

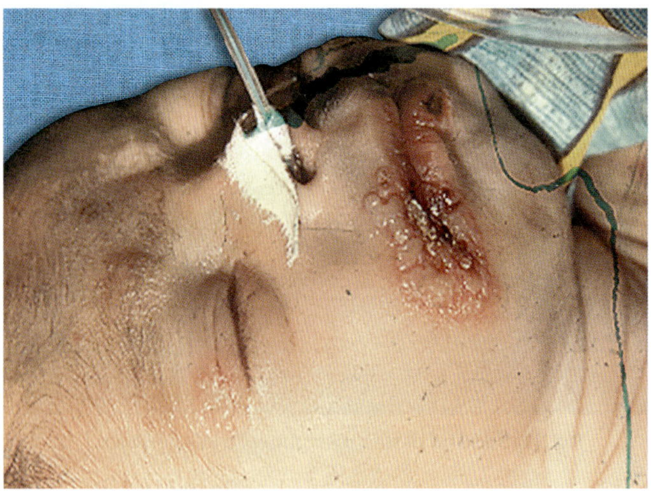

Fig. 14: Mucocutaneous localization of herpes lesions.

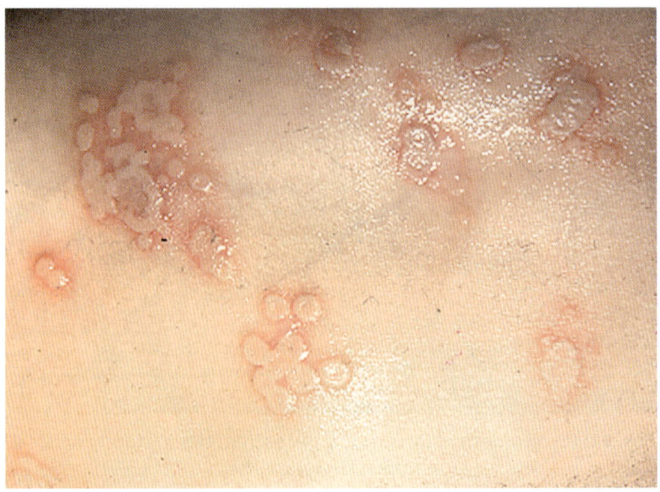

Fig. 15: Close-up view of herpetic lesions.

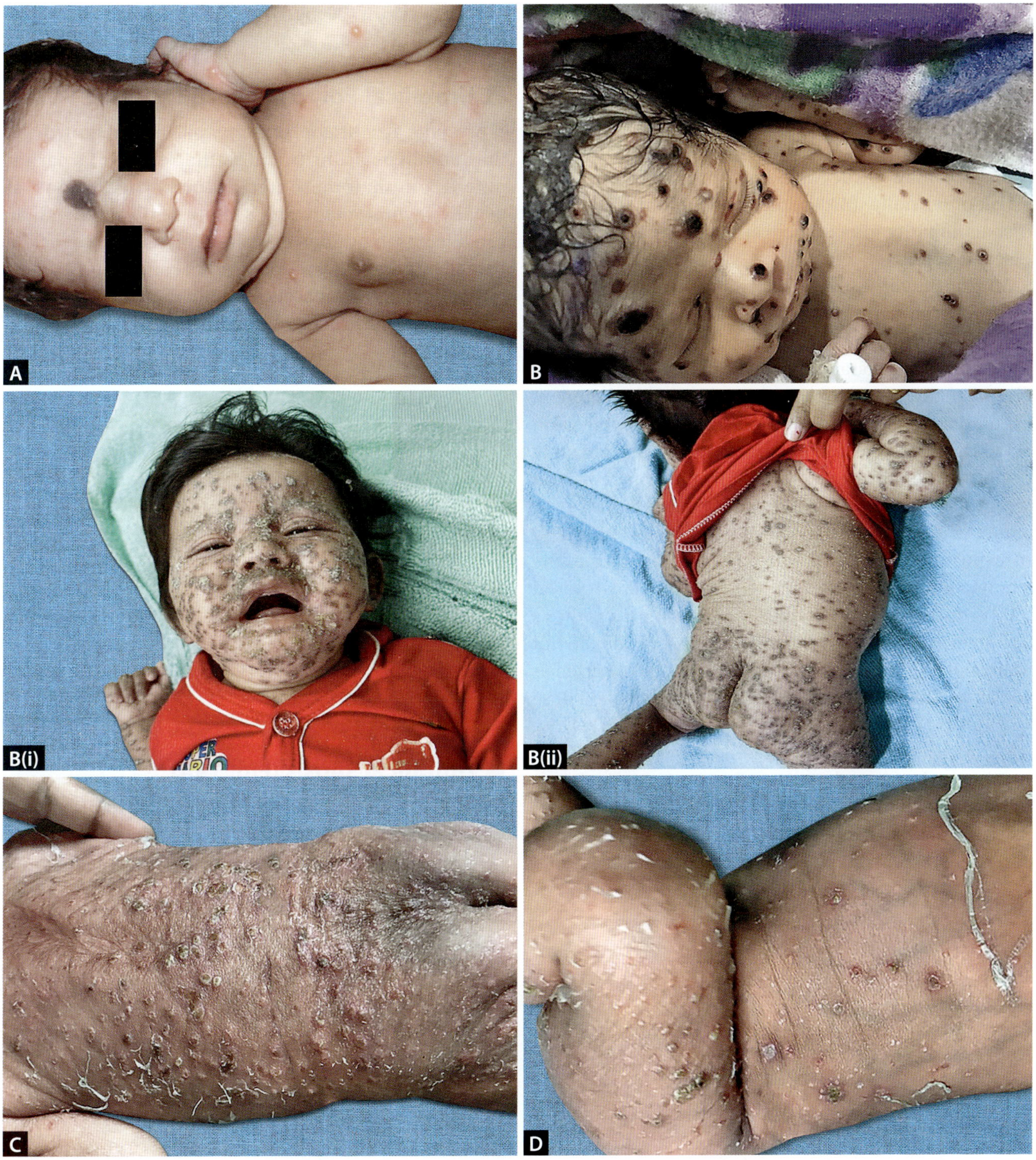

Figs. 16A to D: (A) Neonatal varicella; (B) Neonatal varicella, note polymorphous lesions; (B)(i) Neonatal varicella, note crusted lesions; (B)(ii) Neonatal varicella, crusted lesions; (C) Neonatal varicella, note subsiding lesions; (D) Neonatal varicella, note subsiding lesions.

or in case of similar infection acquired by other close contacts after birth. Premature infants are at increased risk for nosocomial acquisition of varicella-zoster virus (VZV) because active transfer of maternal IgG antibodies occurs primarily during the third trimester of pregnancy. Neonatal varicella is uncommon in Indian scenario, due to the presence of antibodies in the mother formed on prior exposure to illness.

"Happiness can be found, even in the darkest time, if one remembers to turn on the light". **—Albus Dumbledore**

Two types of varicella infection can occur in the newborn:

1. *Severe infection*: When the mother has been infected less than 5 days before birth or 2 days after delivery (as varicella-associated antibodies are not transmitted to the newborn) or the onset of infection in the newborn is between 5 and 10 days of birth. Disseminated disease may ensue with poor prognosis and high risk of mortality (30%) due to pneumonia, hepatitis, coagulopathy, meningoencephalitis, and secondary severe sepsis.
2. *Mild infection:* If the disease onset in the mother is 5 days prior to birth (antibodies are transmitted to the child) or in the newborn during the first 4 days of life.

Diagnosis of neonatal varicella can be made clinically from the pattern of rash and maternal history of infection. Definite diagnosis is made by virus isolation or amplification of viral DNA from the skin lesions by PCR. Management of newborns who are exposed to VZV by maternal infection (within 5 days before birth or 2 days after delivery) or contact with affected individuals includes isolation and postexposure prophylaxis with varicella-zoster immune globulin (VZIG). Healthy term neonates who are exposed to VZV postnatally (including infants whose mother's rash developed >48 hours after delivery) generally do not require postexposure prophylaxis. VZIG should be given as soon as possible and within 10 days of exposure at a dose of 125 units (1 vial) IM for neonates weighing >2.1–10 kg and 62.5 units (0.5 vial) IM for children weighing ≤2 kg. Intravenous immunoglobulin (IVIG) or IV acyclovir can be considered if VZIG is unavailable. Maternal treatment includes oral acyclovir within 24 hours of onset. Newborns with severe disseminated VZV infection should be treated with IV acyclovir (30 mg/kg/day in three divided doses) for 10 days.

Umbilical Polyp (Figs. 16E and 17)

It presents as a bright red shiny polypoidal growth over the umbilicus at birth and is the result of a partially patent omphalomesenteric duct. The lesions are usually asymptomatic and secrete serous, mucoid, and rarely serosanguinous exudate. Polyps may be accompanied by potentially serious internal omphalomesenteric remnant such as Meckel's diverticulum attached to the umbilicus by obstructing fibrous bands.

Treatment

The condition is treated by surgical excision. However, underlying intestinal and urinary tract abnormalities are to be ruled out.

Umbilical Granuloma (Fig. 18)

It is basically a granuloma pyogenicum of the umbilicus. It presents as a red raw granulomatous growth over the umbilicus with purulent discharge.

Treatment

Treatment is cauterization with 75% silver nitrate solution, 20% potassium hydroxide or phenol.

Umbilical Sepsis (Fig. 19A)

Umbilical sepsis, also known as omphalitis, is the inflammation of the umbilical stump of newborns. Most commonly it is attributed to bacterial infection. Normally

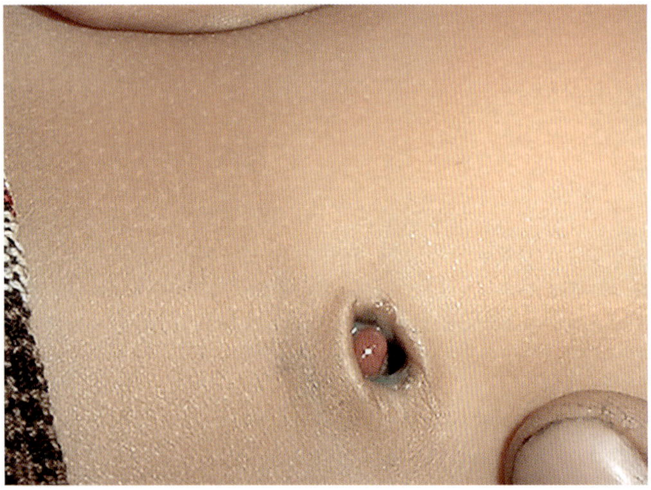

Fig. 16E: Shiny exudative lesion of umbilical polyp.

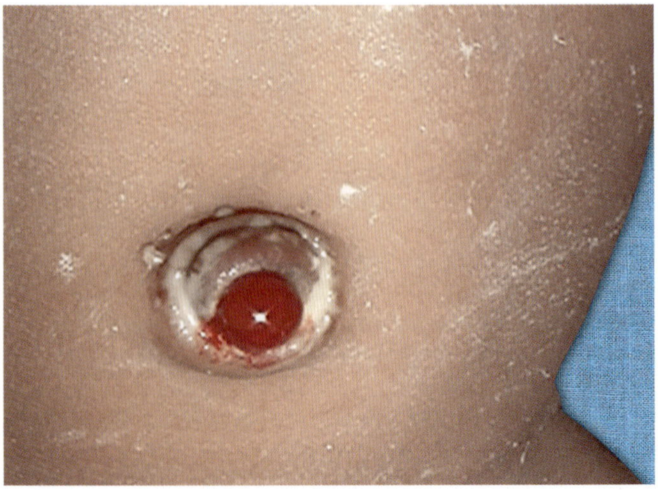

Fig. 17: Umbilical polyp, note cherry red color of the growth.

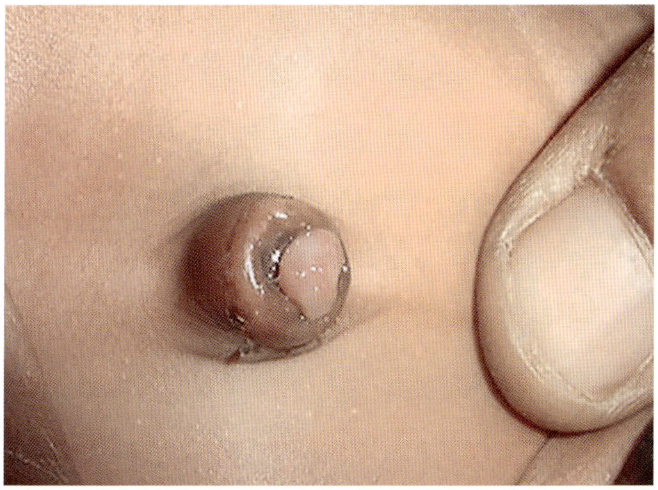

Fig. 18: Granulomatous lesion of umbilical granuloma.

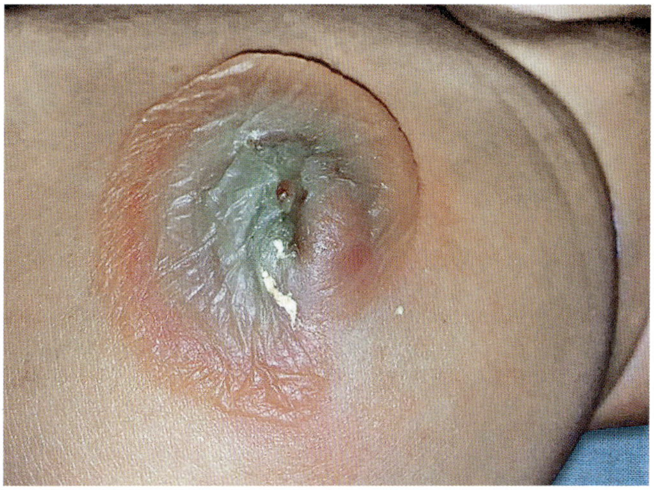

Fig. 19A: Umbilical sepsis.

the stump separates from the skin within 5–40 days after birth. A small amount of pus-like material is commonly seen at the base of the stump and can be controlled by keeping the stump open to air to dry. Certain bacteria can grow and infect the stump during this process and as a result significant redness and swelling may develop, and in some cases the infection can then spread through the umbilical vessels to the surrounding skin. Clinically, neonates with umbilical sepsis present with visible pus or grossly inflamed umbilical stump with history of high grade fever, vomiting, and poor feeding. It is an emergency and needs to be managed with promptness with oral/parenteral antibiotics and topical antibiotic cream/ointment. Cleaning of umbilical stump with antiseptics is also important.

Congenital Syphilis [Figs. 19B(i to vi)]

In congenital syphilis, the fetus becomes infected with the spirochete *Treponema pallidum* by way of placenta usually after 16th week of pregnancy. The clinical manifestations of early congenital syphilis (those occurring before 2 years of age) are anemia, fever, wasting, hepatosplenomegaly, lymphadenopathy, rhinitis, mucocutaneous eruptions, edema, desquamation, and pseudoparalysis. Of these, rhinitis or snuffles is the first sign to appear. It manifests between the 2nd and 6th week of life and is the result of an ulcerative lesion of the nasal mucosa. Deeper involvement of nasal cartilage can result in "saddle-nose deformity". The cutaneous lesions are seen in one-third to one-half of infants affected by this disorder and appear as maculopapular or papulosquamous lesions most prominent on the face, trunk and extremities, diaper area, and palms and soles. The eruption generally develops slowly, as bright pink or red macules and papules and gradually fades to copper brown. It disappears spontaneously over 1–3 months leaving hypo- or hyperpigmented areas. The rare vesiculobullous, hemorrhagic lesions, when seen on the palms and soles, are highly diagnostic of this disorder. The palms and soles may be fissured, erythematous, and indurated. Desquamation of the skin in large dry flakes may occur over the entire body. Mucous membrane lesions, seen in one-third of the infants, are seen as weeping lesions or fissures at mucocutaneous junctions extending out from the lips in a radiating fashion over the skin. When deep, they leave residual scars (rhagades) in the adjacent circumoral region. Raised, flat, moist, wart-like lesions of condylomata lata are seen commonly over the anogenital region, around the nares, and at the angles of the mouth. About 90% of the infants show radiological evidence of osteochondritis and periostitis after the first month of life, most frequently affecting the long bones.

In late congenital syphilis, the disease persists beyond 2 years of age. It includes various signs and stigmata of congenital syphilis in infants in whom the diagnosis was overlooked or those who were inadequately treated early in the course of the disease. These include frontal bossing, saddle nose, short maxillae, and dental changes manifested in the form of Hutchinson's teeth (peg-shaped upper incisors), Moon's mulberry molars, gummas affecting the bones in the skull or tibia, syphilitic arthritis, paroxysmal cold hemoglobinuria and ocular changes such

"A ship is always safe at shore but that is not what it's built for." —**Albert Einstein**

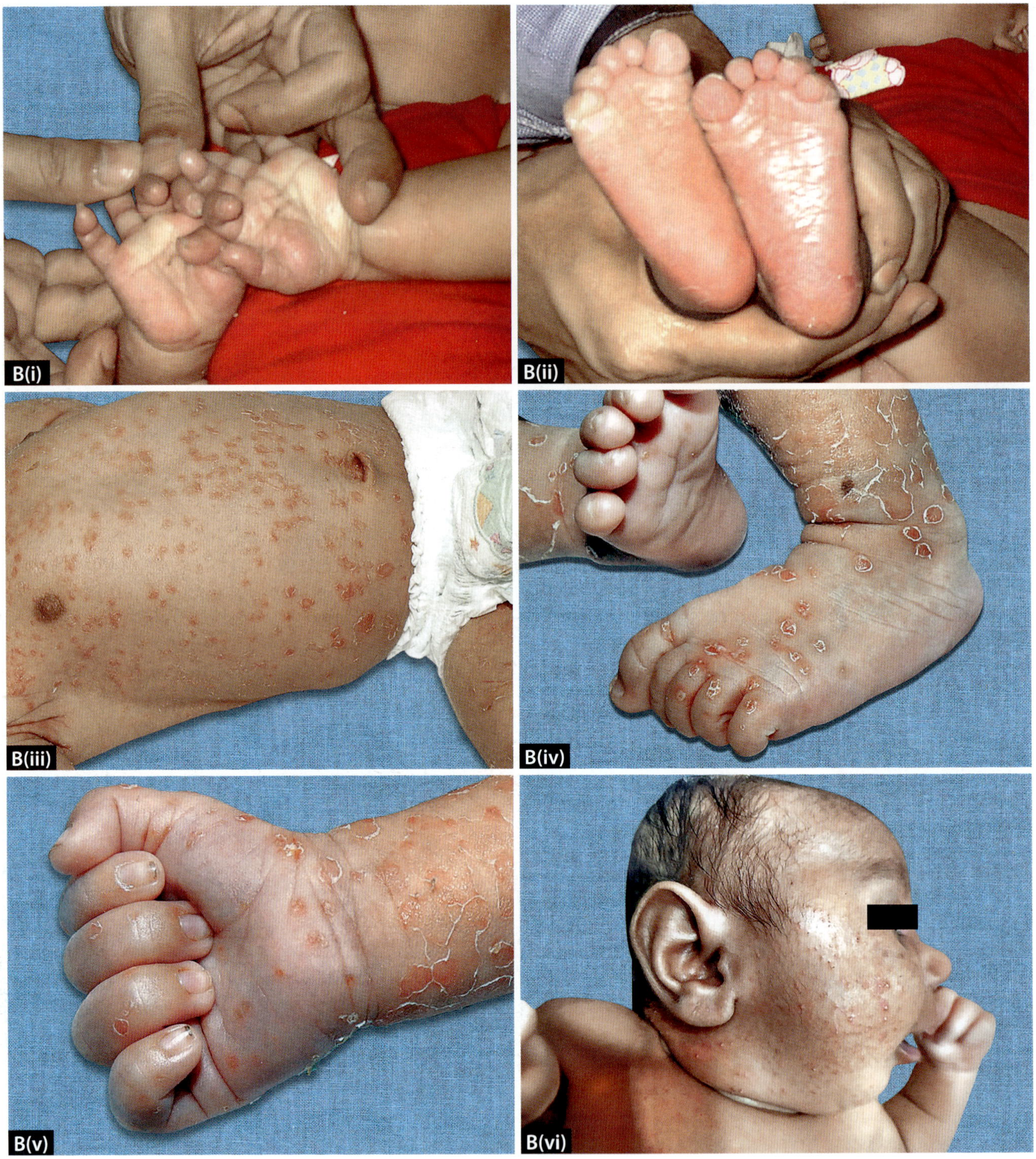

Figs. 19B(i to vi): B(i) Red shiny scaly lesions over palms of congenital syphilis; B(ii) Congenital syphilis, similar lesions over soles; B(iii) Congenital syphilis, trunk; B(iv) Congenital syphilis, note the scaly papules; B(v) Congenital syphilis, close-up view; B(vi) Congenital syphilis.

as retinitis and optic atrophy. Diagnosis is confirmed by serological testing and darkfield examination from the skin and mucous membranes.

Treatment

Penicillin is the treatment of choice for all forms of congenital as well as acquired syphilis. Treatment should

"Seek the wisdom of the ages, but look at the world through the eyes of a child." —**Ron Wild**

be started immediately after the diagnosis with aqueous crystalline penicillin G in a dosage of 100,000–150,000 units/kg administered intravenously every 8–12 hours or procaine penicillin G in dosage of 50,000 units/kg administered IM once daily for 10–14 days. Patients with congenital syphilis should have repeat quantitative, nontreponemal tests at 3, 6, and 12 months after treatment.

Subcutaneous Fat Necrosis (Figs. 20A to E)

It is a benign self-limiting dermatosis which affects apparently healthy full-term newborns and young infants. It presents as single to multiple sharply circumscribed areas of indurated and nodular plaques of skin over

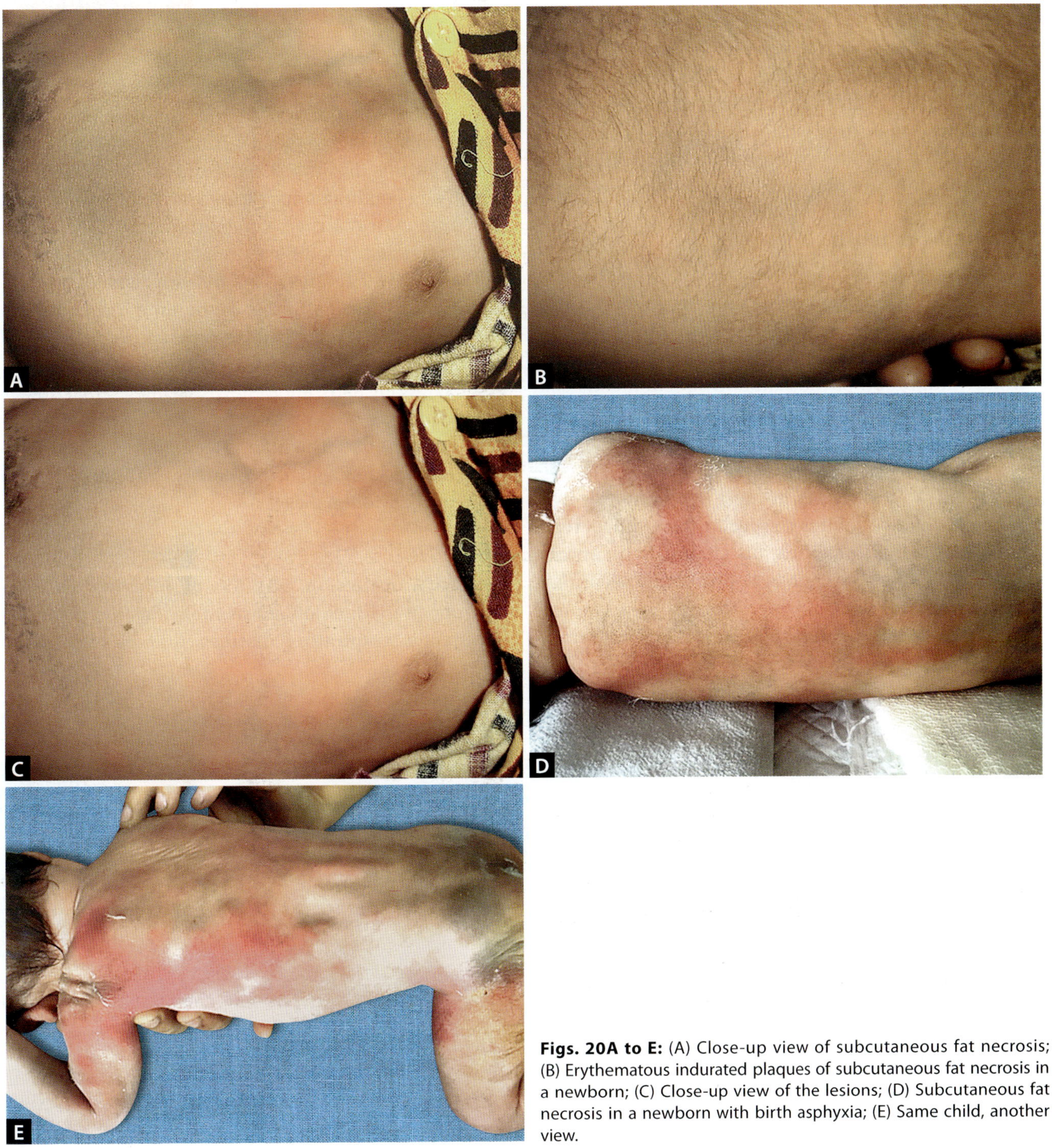

Figs. 20A to E: (A) Close-up view of subcutaneous fat necrosis; (B) Erythematous indurated plaques of subcutaneous fat necrosis in a newborn; (C) Close-up view of the lesions; (D) Subcutaneous fat necrosis in a newborn with birth asphyxia; (E) Same child, another view.

"Many of life's failures are people, who did not realize how close they were to success when they gave up." —**Thomas Edison**

back, buttocks, thighs and shoulders, arms, and trunk. Its exact etiology is not known but proposed hypotheses are pressure on bony prominences during delivery, pre-eclampsia, obstetric trauma, fetal asphyxia or hypothermia, and neonatal infections. The hypercalcemia in subcutaneous fat necrosis is thought to be secondary to uncontrolled production of 1,25(OH)2D by activated macrophages infiltrating the necrotic fat. It is also seen in infants delivered by cesarean section and infants born to diabetic mothers. The onset of fat necrosis usually occurs in the first few days to weeks of life. The lesions at times may get calcified. However, most of the lesions undergo spontaneous resolution within few weeks to months. Complications include hypercalcemia, hypoglycemia, anemia, and thrombocytopenia.

Differential Diagnosis

The condition needs to be differentiated from sclerema neonatorum which primarily occurs in newborns with sepsis, severe diarrhea, respiratory failure or dehydration and is a fatal condition with high mortality rate. There is woody induration of the skin and subcutaneous skin sparing palms, soles, and genitalia.

Management

Subcutaneous fat necrosis in most newborns resolves spontaneously and requires no specific therapy. Fluctuant lesions in cases of calcification should be aspirated to prevent their spontaneous rupture and secondary infection. In rare cases of hypercalcemia, restriction of calcium and vitamin D intake, systemic corticosteroids may be required. Use of furosemide diuretic, calcitonin and bisphosphonates may be required in severe cases.

Sclerema Neonatorum (Figs. 21 and 22)

It is a diffuse, progressive, wax-like hardening of the skin and subcutaneous tissue that occurs in premature or debilitated infants during the first few weeks of life. In around 25% of cases, the mothers are ill at the time of delivery. Exposure to cold, peripheral chilling with vascular collapse, hypothermia, and an increase in the ratio of saturated to unsaturated fatty acids in the triglyceride fraction of the subcutaneous tissue have been hypothesized, but lack confirmation as possible causes for this disorder. This disorder is associated with underlying conditions such as sepsis, respiratory distress, dehydration or diarrhea, congenital heart disease and it is characterized by a diffuse nonpitting woody induration of the involved tissues. This disease usually starts on buttocks and legs and most of the time it progresses to involve all areas except palms, soles, and genitalia. When the disease spreads, the skin becomes mottled, cadaver-like, cold, stony hard, and yellowish white. At that time the face acquires a fixed mask-like expression and the limbs become immobile. The infants feed poorly, show clinical signs of shock, sluggish movements and in majority of cases the baby often dies.

Prognosis

Mortality occurs in 50–75% of affected children. Complications include sepsis, dehydration, electrolyte imbalance, respiratory distress, and gastrointestinal

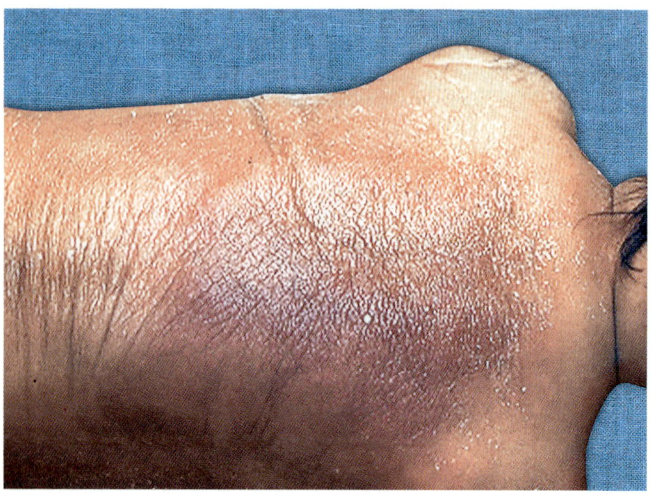

Fig. 21: Sclerema neonatorum.

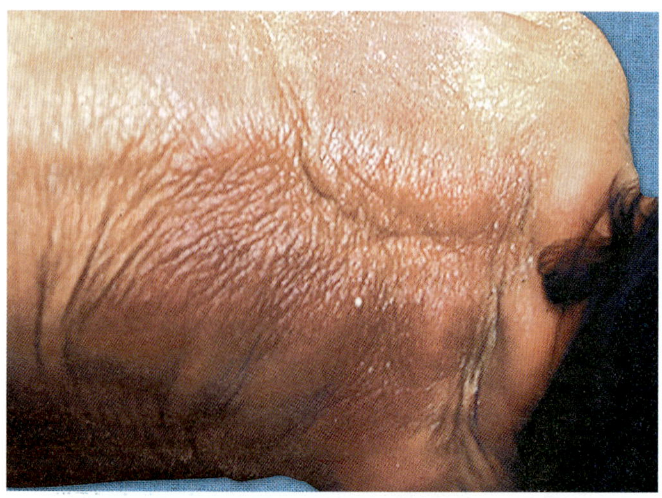

Fig. 22: Same infant (close-up view), sclerema neonatorum.

"Strive not to be having success, but rather to be of value." —**Albert Einstein**

disease. The infants, who survive this disease, resolve without residual sequelae.

Management

There is no specific therapy for treatment of sclerema neonatorum. Supportive care with rewarming and administration of oxygen, control of infection, treatment of the underlying disorder, and IV therapy for correction of fluid and electrolyte imbalance are essential. Although indications for their use are not clear and controlled studies fail to confirm their efficacy, systemic corticosteroids in addition to antimicrobial agents have been advocated for infants with this disorder. Exchange transfusion has shown decreased mortality.

Hairy Pinna (Fig. 23)

It is a Y-chromosome mediated trait. It is considered as a pathognomonic sign in infants born to diabetic mother.

Polythelia (Supernumerary Nipples) (Fig. 24)

Supernumerary nipples are the remnants of the embryological milk line which runs from the anterior axillary fold to the inner thigh. Most often they are distributed over the anterior chest wall and upper abdomen as pink, umbilicated or elevated papules surrounded by a pigmented areola. A nipple may also be seen without areola and vice-versa. Usually there is only a single lesion, but occasionally multiple or bilateral nipples are present. It has been shown to be more common in male gender and on the left side. Accessory nipples have been reported to be associated with malformations of the urinary tract, in particular the kidneys. The association has been questioned recently.

Treatment

The accessory breast tissue may underlay the nipple and enlarge at puberty or in pregnancy. In such cases, complete excision is recommended because of the risk of malignant change.

Physiological Exfoliation of Newborn (Figs. 25A to C)

Neonatal desquamation is seen in 72–83% of newborns. This is mostly seen in postmature neonates. The exact pathophysiology of it is not known. In full-term infants, there is fine desquamation at birth within 24–48 hours and is localized to hands, ankles, and feet. There is widespread desquamation and cracking in postmaturity. Neonatal desquamation should be differentiated from collodion baby. However, there is no ectropion, eclabium or gloved appearance. The scaling gradually subsides over a period of 4–6 weeks.

Treatment

Application of oil and emollient (white soft paraffin) helps to reduce scaling and moisturize the skin of the babies.

Cutis Marmorata (Figs. 26A to C)

Cutis marmorata presents as reticulated bluish mottling of the skin seen on the trunk and extremities of newborn and infants. This phenomenon is a physiologic response

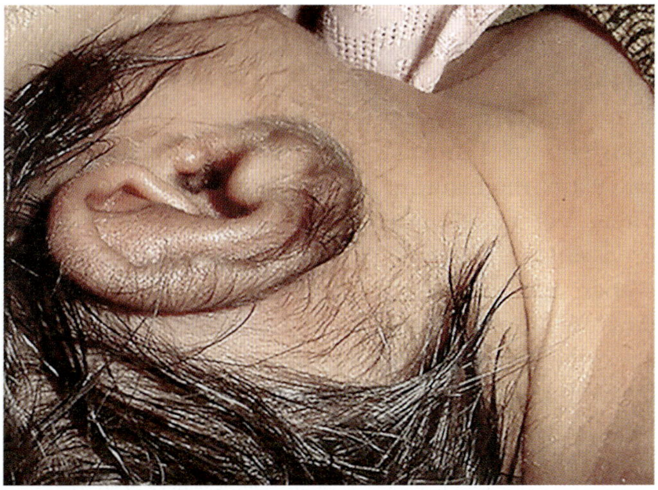

Fig. 23: Hairy tragus in a newborn.

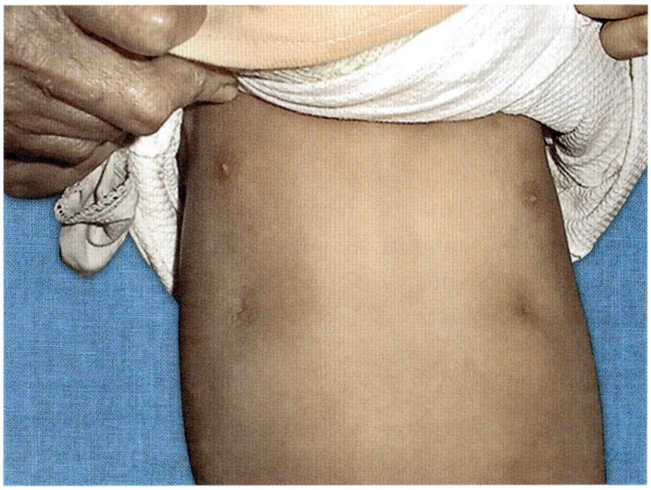

Fig. 24: Multiple accessory rudimentary nipples along the milk line.

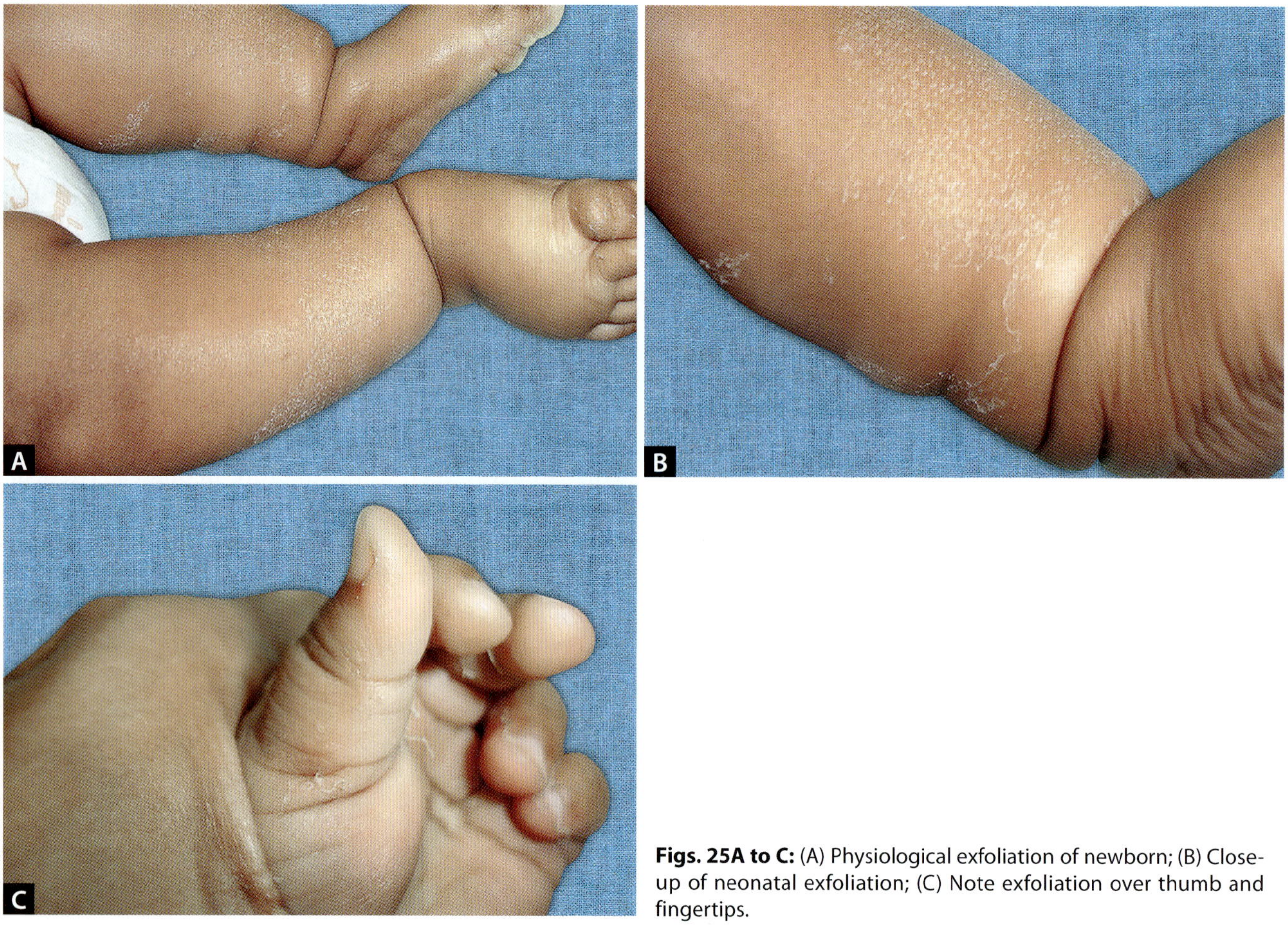

Figs. 25A to C: (A) Physiological exfoliation of newborn; (B) Close-up of neonatal exfoliation; (C) Note exfoliation over thumb and fingertips.

to chilling with resultant dilatation of capillaries and small venules. It usually disappears as the infant is rewarmed. Although a tendency to cutis marmorata may persist for several weeks or months, this disorder bears no medical significance and no treatment is usually required. In some children, cutis marmorata may tend to recur until early childhood. In patients with Down syndrome, trisomy 18, and Cornelia de Lange syndrome, this reticulated marbling pattern may be persistent. In some infants, a white negative pattern of this phenomenon (cutis marmorata alba) may be created by a transient hypertonia of the deep vasculature. It is known as cutis marmorata alba. It is a transitory disorder and appears to have no clinical significance.

Treatment

No treatment is required for this physiological condition in newborns and infants. Reassurance and counseling of the parents is important.

Cutis Marmorata Telangiectatica Congenita (Fig. 26D)

It is a condition which closely simulates cutis marmorata but does not disappear on rewarming. The condition presents at or shortly after birth. The pigmentation presents as red marbled mottled patches. The changes may be limited to a localized part of the body. The skin changes get accentuated by decrease in ambient temperature. Contrary to cutis marmorata or livedo reticularis, there may be atrophy or ulceration of the skin. There may be associated limb hypoplasia, hyperplasia or vascular abnormalities, e.g., port-wine stain, Sturge-Weber syndrome, etc. Various associated neurological disorders include seizures, hydrocephalus, and ocular abnormalities such as glaucoma, retinal pigmentation, and retinal detachment. A condition named Adams-Oliver syndrome is characterized by cutis marmorata telangiectatica congenita (CMTC) with aplasia cutis congenita (ACC) and distal transverse limb defects.

"If you cannot fly, then run; if you cannot run, then walk; if you cannot walk, then crawl but whatever you do, you have to keep moving forward."
—Martin Luther King JR

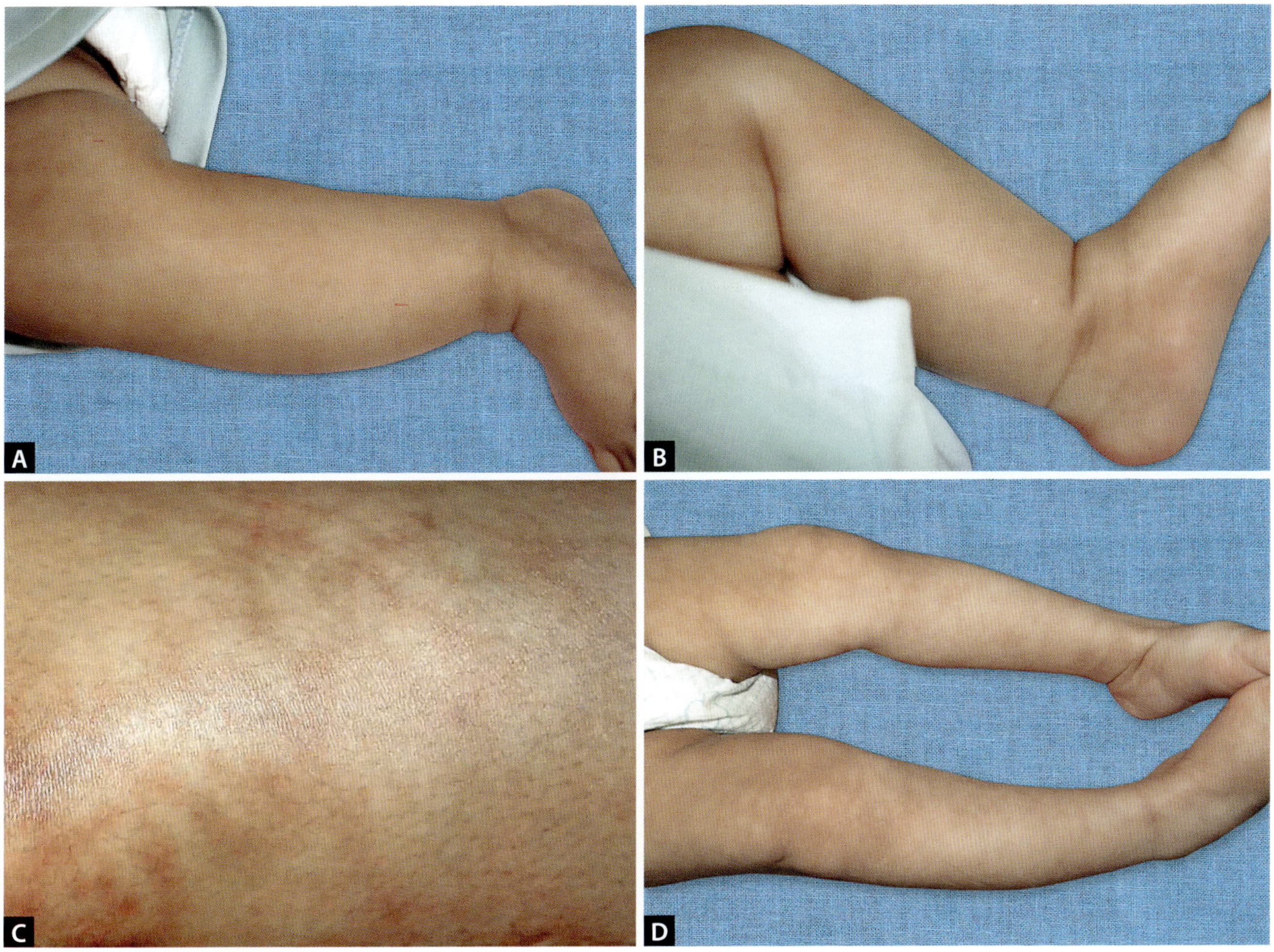

Figs. 26A to D: (A) Cutis marmorata telangiectasia in a newborn baby; (B) Same baby, note net-like telangiectasia; (C) Cutis marmorata, close-up view; (D) Cutis marmorata telangiectatica congenita.

Within first 2–3 years of life, CMTC gradually improves on its own. When the lesions are present over face, ophthalmological evaluation is necessary. When there are neurological symptoms, referral to a neurologist is necessary.

Neonatal Irritant Dermatitis (Figs. 27A and B)

Irritant dermatitis can develop within 24–48 hours of exposure to irritant chemicals. In newborn babies often various antiseptic cleansers and lotions cause dermatitis of the soft and sensitive skin. A severe form of irritant dermatitis can result in burn in neonatal intensive care unit (NICU) setup either from phototherapy, heater, or undiluted antiseptics.

Diagnosis

Intense erythema with formation of papules and vesicles over the areas of contact with the offending agents is seen. The newborn baby becomes restless and irritable.

Treatment

Avoidance of offending agent should be prompt. Cleansing of skin with distilled water or normal saline is to be done. Application of emollients such as white soft paraffin 2–3 times a day for 7–10 days clears the dermatitis in most of the newborn babies. Occasionally mild topical steroids, e.g., 1% hydrocortisone or clobetasone butyrate may be required.

"Opportunity is missed by most people because it is dressed in overalls and looks like work." **—Thomas Alva Edison**

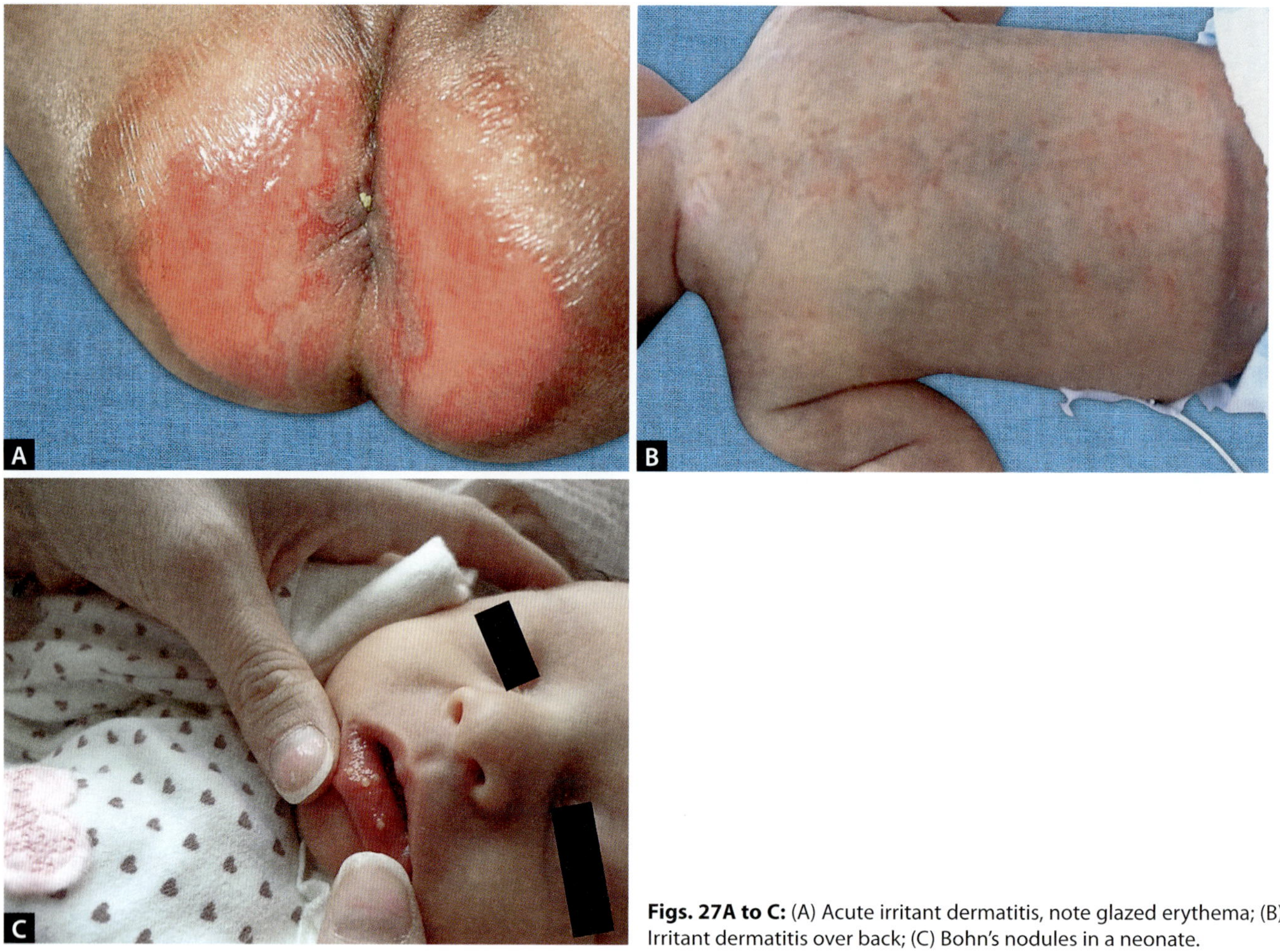

Figs. 27A to C: (A) Acute irritant dermatitis, note glazed erythema; (B) Irritant dermatitis over back; (C) Bohn's nodules in a neonate.

Epstein's Pearls and Bohn's Nodules (Fig. 27C)

Clinically these are counterpart of facial milia. These appear as multiple, discrete 2–3 mm pearly white or yellowish papules over midline of hard palate (Epstein's pearls) or gum margins (Bohn's nodules). They are seen in 64–94% of normal neonates, but less commonly affects the premature neonates.

Diagnosis

The characteristic appearance and location clinch the diagnosis.

Treatment

It is a physiological condition in newborns and usually disappears in 4–6 weeks time is to be explained to the parents.

Sebaceous Gland Hyperplasia (Fig. 28)

It manifests as multiple, tiny, pin-point yellowish papules distributed on the nose, upper lips, malar region, and chin. It is due to influence of maternal androgens. They are rarely seen in premature infants.

Diagnosis

Diagnosis is based on its characteristic appearance and site.

Treatment

Reassurance of anxious mother.

Transient Neonatal Pustular Melanosis [Figs. 29A to C(ii)]

It is a benign self-limiting disease of unknown etiology. This rare condition is mostly seen in darker skin. It is seen in less than 1% infants.

Diagnosis

Small sterile superficial vesiculopustules develop which rupture easily within 24–48 hours and evolve in to hyperpigmentation. The commonly affected areas are forehead, area below chin, neck, lower back and shins, but can become generalized. There is no systemic involvement. Though the lesions usually disappear within 2–3 days, hyperpigmentation lasts for 3 months.

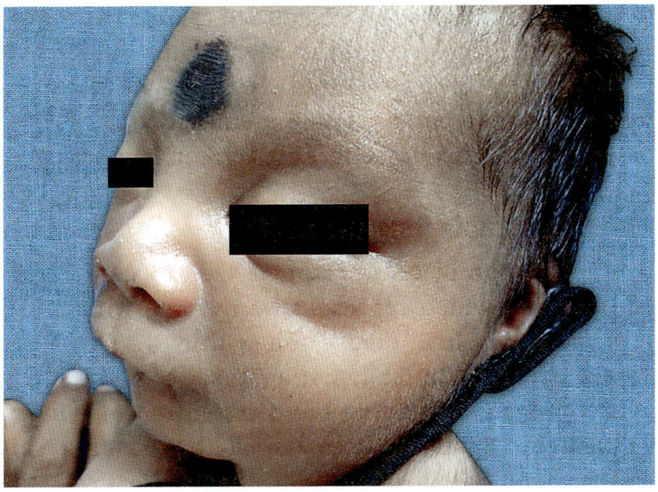

Fig. 28: Sebaceous hyperplasia.

Treatment

No treatment is required as it is a self-limiting condition.

Acropustulosis of Infancy

Acropustulosis of infancy is an idiopathic noninfective pustulosis affecting infants and small babies. Usually, it occurs between 2 months and 3 years of age. The lesions appear as recurrent crops for few weeks to months and subside by 3–4 years of age. Though the exact etiology is not known, a possible association with preceding scabies has been implicated.

Diagnosis

The lesions typically appear as pinpoint erythematous papules which transform into pustules within 24–48 hours.

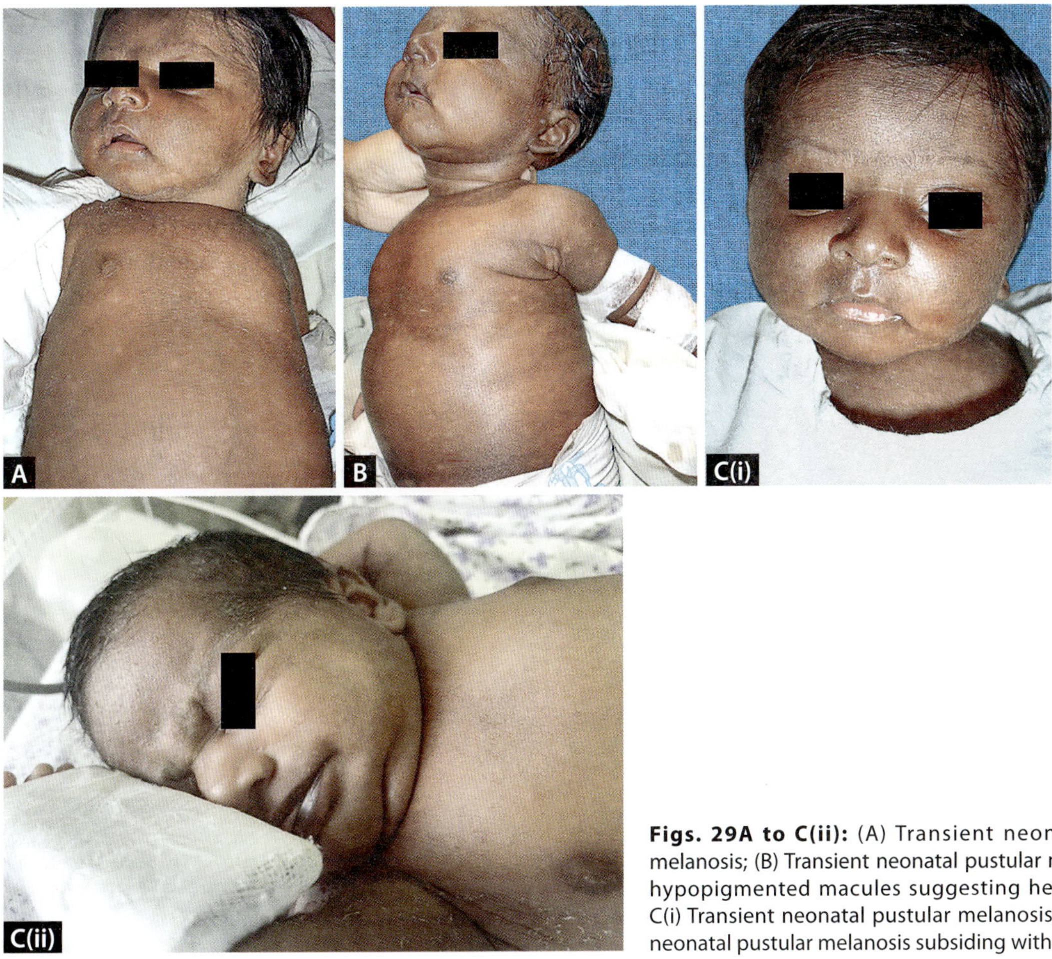

Figs. 29A to C(ii): (A) Transient neonatal pustular melanosis; (B) Transient neonatal pustular melanosis, note hypopigmented macules suggesting healed pustules; C(i) Transient neonatal pustular melanosis; C(ii) Transient neonatal pustular melanosis subsiding with scaling.

"The good life is one inspired by love and guided by knowledge." —**Bertrand Russell**

Palms, soles, dorsa of hands, and feet are the common sites affected. Usually it is associated with moderate-to-severe pruritus.

Differential Diagnosis

Various closely simulating conditions are scabies with secondary infection, impetigo, dyshidrotic eczema, erythema toxicum neonatorum, neonatal pustular melanosis, etc.

Treatment

Moderately potent topical corticosteroids such as mometasone or fluticasone may be used for 2–3 weeks. In severe cases, dapsone (2 mg/kg body weight in two divided doses) has also been used. Systemic antihistamines can be given for pruritus. Recently topical maxacalcitol has shown to improve the symptoms.

Infantile Gluteal Granuloma (Figs. 29D and E)

Infantile gluteal granuloma, also known as granuloma gluteale infantum, is a rare, benign nodular complication of irritant diaper dermatitis in infancy due to use of potent topical corticosteroid, prolonged occlusion from diapers resulting in increased exposure to feces and urine and secondary infection with candidiasis. It is seen more commonly in the age group of 4–9 months.

Diagnosis

The disease characteristically presents as multiple erythematous to violaceous papulonodules over the gluteal region, external genitalia, inner thighs, and lower abdomen in infants.

Treatment

Stoppage of topical steroid application is the first thing to be done. If there is any evidence of candidal infection, topical ketoconazole or clotrimazole should be prescribed. Otherwise, the lesions subside very slowly without any treatment over a period of 3–13 months. Reassurance of parents and their counseling is of paramount importance.

Trichostasis Spinulosa (Fig. 29F)

It is a common disorder characterized by comedone-like papules which represent horny plug with 25–50 telogen vellus hair embedded within it. The basic defect is infundibular hyperkeratosis of hair follicle which prevents shedding hence retention of telogen vellus hair originating from a single hair matrix. This entity can be classified into two variants. Classically the disease presents as comedone-like papules resembling black head distributed mainly over nose and forehead in elderly individuals. Other variant characterized by pruritic follicular papule resembling keratosis pilaris is distributed over the trunk and extremities of young individuals or newborns. Pathological condition commonly associated with this entity is renal failure. Diagnosis can be established with the use of dermoscope and microscope. Various treatment modalities are depilation, keratolytic, topical and systemic retinoids, and hydroactive adhesive pads. Pulsed diode laser shows encouraging result.

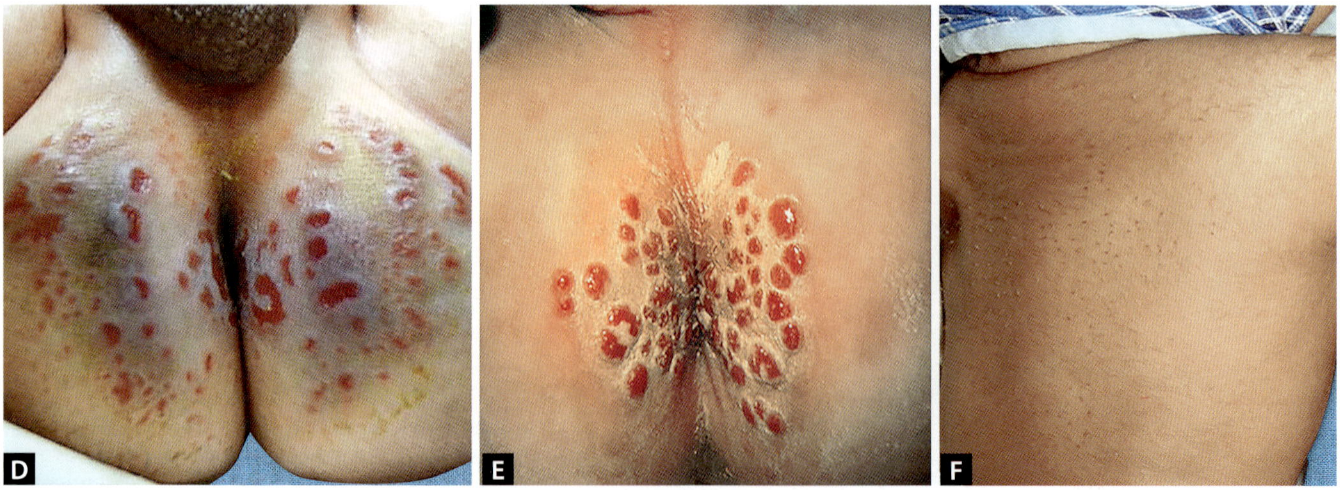

Figs. 29D to F: (D and E) Infantile gluteal granuloma; (F) Trichostasis spinulosa.

"Failure is simply the opportunity to begin again, this time more intelligently." —**Henry Ford**

Aplasia Cutis Congenita [Figs. 30 and 31A(i and ii)]

Aplasia cutis congenita is a congenital defect of unknown etiology characterized by congenital absence of skin in newborn babies. Histologically, there may be absence of either epidermis, dermis or subcutaneous tissue. It usually affects the scalp but face, trunk or extremities can also be involved. Most of the cases of ACC are sporadic. Familial cases have been reported. Antithyroid drug methimazole given to a pregnant mother is likely to produce ACC in newborn babies. However, the issue is far from being conclusive.

Diagnosis

Aplasia cutis congenita classically presents as single or multiple, oval to circular sharply demarcated granulating ulcerations over scalp. The size of the lesions usually varies from 1 to 3 cm. Occasionally, lesions may look like either a membrane or keloid.

Associations

Although most infants with ACC are otherwise well, various associated anomalies reported are cleft lip, cleft palate, hemiatrophy of limbs, ocular abnormalities, gastrointestinal malformations, spinal dysraphism, hydrocephalus, seizures, mental retardation, trisomy 13, vascular anomalies, etc. ACC is associated with fetus papyraceus (vanishing twin syndrome).

Differential Diagnosis

Forcep injury and other types of birth injury need to be differentiated.

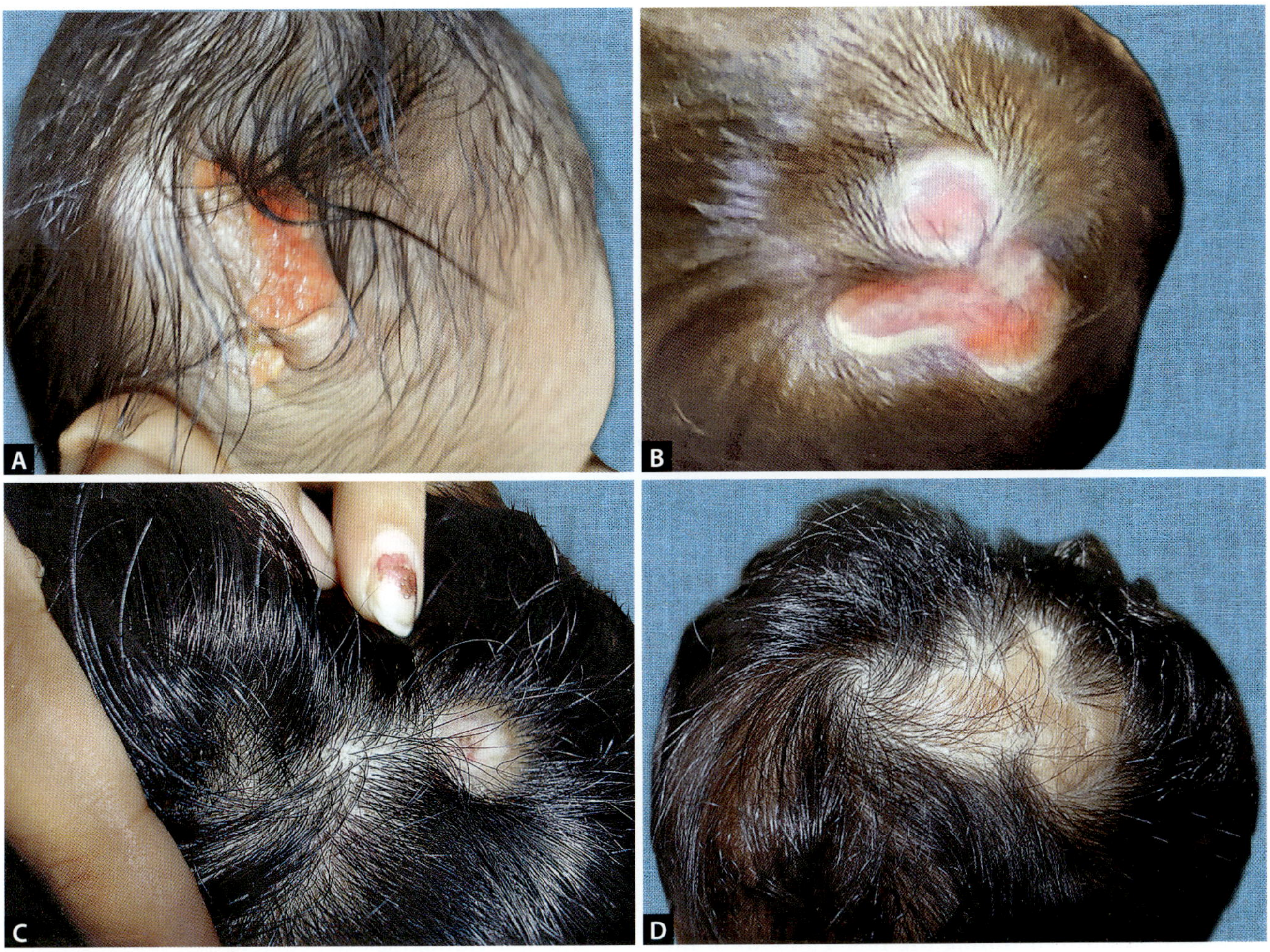

Figs. 30A to D: (A) Aplasia cutis congenita (ACC) at birth; (B) ACC in a newborn; (C) Close-up view of ACC, note prominent visible blood vessels; (D) Hairless patch of ACC over scalp.

"Everything that we ask about others can lead us to an understanding of ourselves." —**Carl Jung**

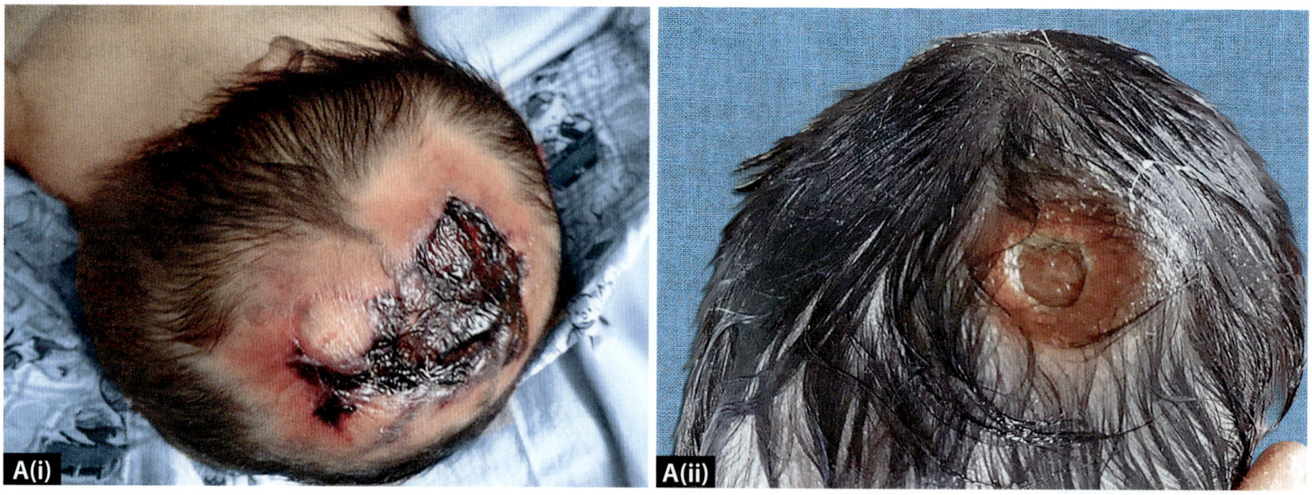

Figs. 31A(i and ii): A(i) Aplasia cutis congenita in a newborn; A(ii) Aplasia cutis congenita at birth in a mother on methimazole during pregnancy.

Treatment

By and large ACC with small defects (up to 3 cm) do not require any treatment. Proper cleansing of the area daily with betadine is required in cases of granulating lesions. Prevention of secondary infection is very important. Most of the lesions heal with scarring by 6 weeks to 6 months and occasionally by 12 months. The scars gradually become less conspicuous over next 4–5 years. However, for bigger defects (>3 cm), plastic surgery is advisable.

Venous Prominence Over Bridge of the Nose

This physiological condition is seen in 1 in 10,000 live births. A transverse superficial vein remains prominent over the bridge of the nose. This condition is usually seen in 3–9 months old babies. Subsequently it disappears. Similar prominent veins are seen over the chest of babies admitted in NICU with respiratory distress.

Treatment

Explaining the condition and its benign self-limiting nature to the anxious mother is all that is necessary.

Neonatal Erythroderma (Figs. 31B to F and 32)

Erythroderma is defined as any inflammatory condition involving >90% of body surface area. Neonatal erythroderma, also called as "red scaly baby," is a life-threatening entity seen at birth or during the first 1 month of life. Neonatal erythroderma can be part of genodermatosis, immune deficiency, inflammatory disorder, metabolic diseases, and infections. Atopic dermatitis presenting as erythroderma is usually observed later and hence not a common differential for neonatal exfoliative dermatitis. Various causes of neonatal erythroderma are:

Cutaneous disorders:
- Infantile seborrheic dermatitis
- Atopic dermatitis
- Psoriasis
- Pityriasis rubra pilaris
- Diffuse cutaneous mastocytosis
- Ectodermal dysplasia (hypohidrotic/anhidrotic)

Ichthyosis:
- Lamellar ichthyosis
- Nonbullous ichthyosiform erythroderma
- Conradi–Hünermann syndrome
- Bullous ichthyosiform erythroderma
- Netherton syndrome

Infections:
- Staphylococcal scalded skin syndrome
- Toxic shock syndrome
- Congenital cutaneous candidiasis

Immunodeficiency:
- Omenn syndrome
- Graft-versus-host reaction

Metabolic disorders:
- Disorders of biotin metabolism
- Essential fatty acid deficiency
- Multiple carboxylase deficiency
- Acrodermatitis enteropathica
- Leiner's disease

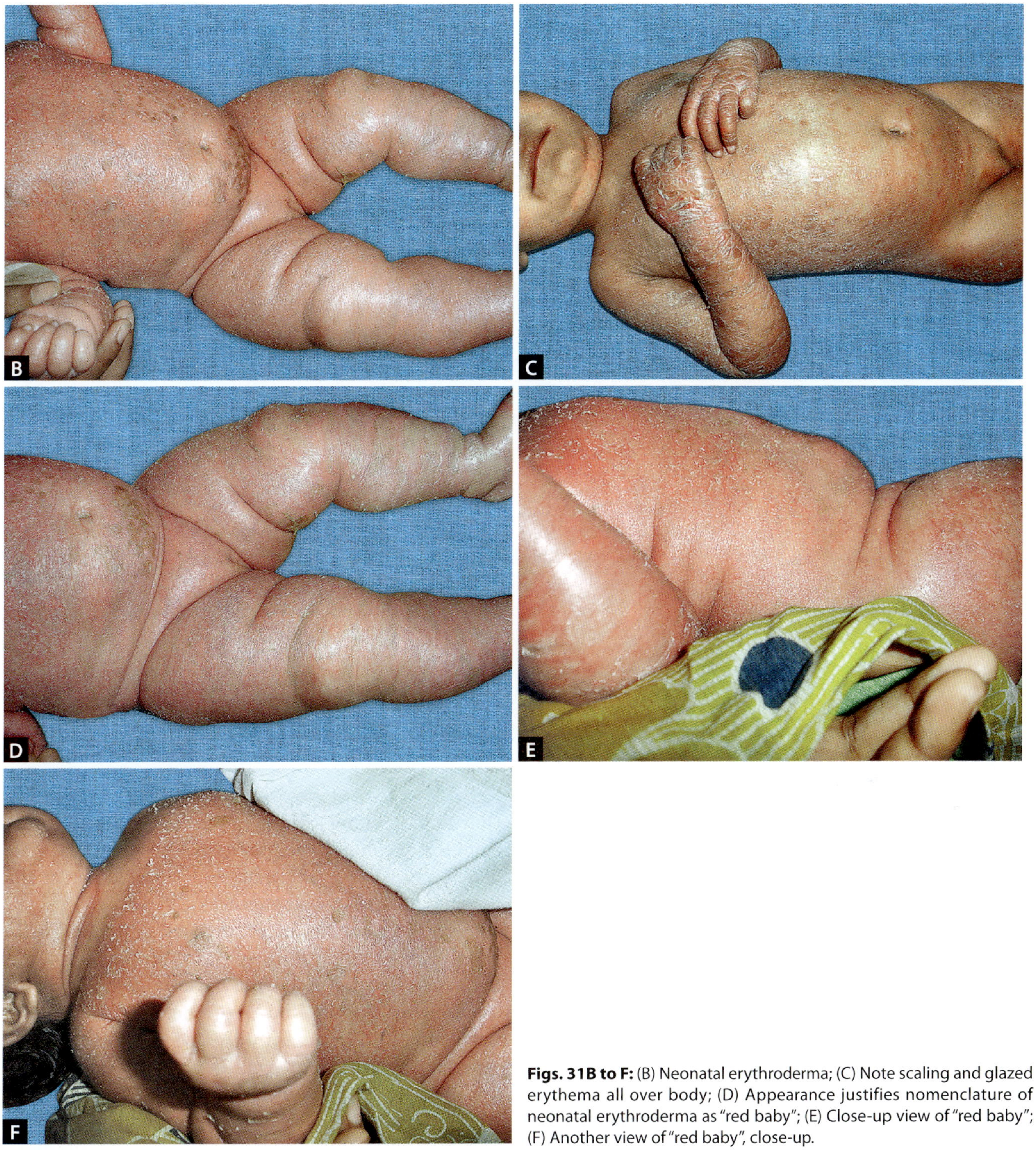

Figs. 31B to F: (B) Neonatal erythroderma; (C) Note scaling and glazed erythema all over body; (D) Appearance justifies nomenclature of neonatal erythroderma as "red baby"; (E) Close-up view of "red baby"; (F) Another view of "red baby", close-up.

Drugs:
- Ceftriaxone
- Vancomycin

Diagnosis

Infantile seborrheic dermatitis (ISD) which manifests in the neonatal period, usually presents with greasy scales

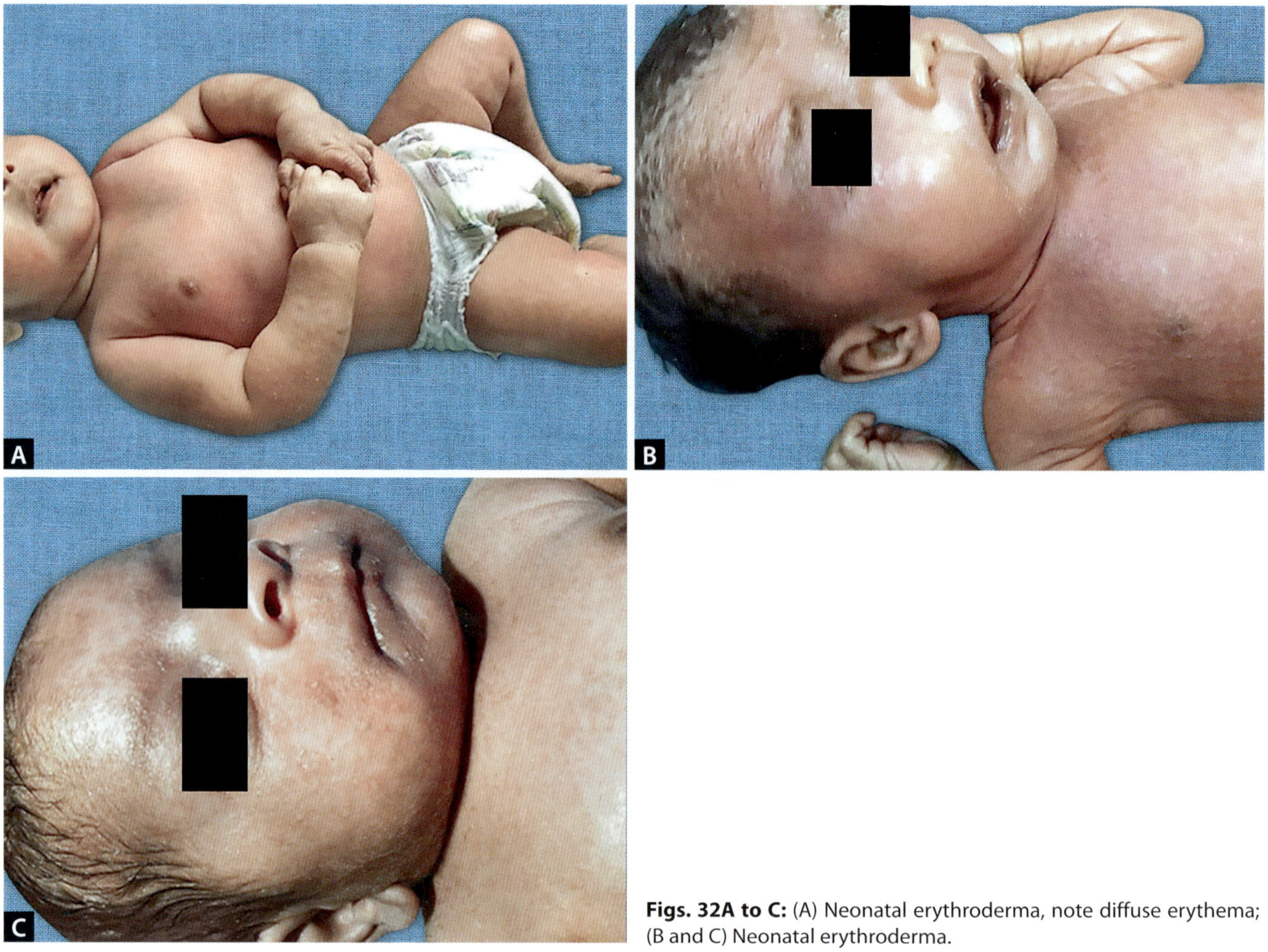

Figs. 32A to C: (A) Neonatal erythroderma, note diffuse erythema; (B and C) Neonatal erythroderma.

on the scalp (cradle cap), skin folds such as the axilla, neck, retroauricular, and diaper areas. Atopic dermatitis may have its onset in the first month; however, it is rarely erythrodermic in neonates. The lesions usually are vesicular and exudative in nature. Sometimes there is a significant overlap between ISD and atopic dermatitis.

Neonatal psoriatic erythroderma is a rare entity and it commonly presents as recalcitrant diaper dermatitis which may become generalized with a widespread pustular form of the disease. This is accompanied by periodic high fever, and the child becomes very toxic with recurrent crops of superficial pustules appearing on erythematous plaques. Psoriasis and pityriasis rubra pilaris may look similar with erythematous scaly plaques which may enlarge and become generalized to produce erythroderma. Heavy infiltration of the entire skin with mast cells results in diffuse cutaneous mastocytosis. The skin undergoes lichenification and is erythematous, producing urtication and hemorrhagic bullae formation on mild trauma. Diarrhea, flushing, and respiratory symptoms are the common accompaniments. Darier's sign, a wheal which flares on stroking the skin, is often positive. Although a life-threatening condition, it improves with age.

Several varieties of ichthyoses can manifest as erythroderma. Patients of nonbullous congenital ichthyosiform erythroderma have finer scales and are more inclined to develop erythroderma. The newborns have a collodion membrane which desquamates, revealing the erythroderma. It fades in mild disease but in the severe classic form, large plate-like scales with erythema persists. Harlequin ichthyosis infants with hyperkeratotic fissured plates often die due to respiratory problems; if they survive with treatment, they manifest generalized erythroderma. Epidermolytic hyperkeratosis or bullous ichthyosis has widespread denuded areas which resolve slowly, manifesting underlying erythroderma. Netherton syndrome presents with features of generalized erythroderma, fragile hair with trichorrhexis invaginata ("bamboo hair"), and atopic diathesis such as severe rhinorrhea, asthma, anaphylaxis due to food, and increased serum IgE levels. Erythroderma at birth is often the onset and it is a diagnostic dilemma where sparse hair with shaft defects may take several microscopic examinations, especially of eyebrows and lashes, before clinching the diagnosis. These patients are atopic and often have intercurrent infective episodes with high rates of mortality. The serum IgE levels are markedly raised and are even more than seen normally in atopic subjects.

Because of the protective effect of maternal immunity, congenital immunodeficiency syndromes are rarely symptomatic at birth. Graft-versus-host reaction from maternal engraftment can, however, occur even during intrauterine development. Omenn syndrome is a familial reticuloendotheliosis with eosinophilia having erythroderma, failure to thrive, lymphadenopathy, and recurrent infections. Marked leukocytosis, eosinophilia, anemia, and hypogammaglobulinemia are some of the findings in this histiocytic disorder. Hypogammaglobulinemia can start with diarrhea and periodic fever together with erythroderma. Dermatitis begins by 4 weeks of age and rapidly generalizes. DiGeorge syndrome and severe combined immunodeficiency may also present with eczematous dermatitis leading to erythroderma.

Graft-versus-host reaction may occur in T-cell immunodeficiency or as a result of transplacental transfer of maternal lymphocytes as a sequela of exchange transfusion. An erythematous nonspecific morbilliform rash may lead to erythroderma and epidermal sloughing. Neonatal cutaneous T-cell lymphoma can present with congenital ichthyosis with atypical Sezary-like lymphoid cells in skin and lymph nodes and other immunological abnormalities.

Metabolic and nutritional disorders are suspected when the infant has failure to thrive and the dermatitis manifests periorificially at the onset before it generalizes. Severe protein malnutrition during infancy can present with widespread erythema, edema, erosion, and desquamation of the skin. Deficiency of zinc due to malabsorption as in acrodermatitis enteropathica or low concentration of zinc in breast milk can begin with psoriasiform dermatitis in circumoral or periorificial areas which may crust and spread to involve other areas; this has also been reported in children with acquired immunodeficiency syndrome. Diarrhea, failure to thrive, irritability, and photophobia can accompany such dermatitis. Essential fatty acids, mostly found in dairy products and vegetable oils, are supplemented in the diet. Diffuse desquamation, lichenification, and intertriginous dermatitis can develop in such situations. Cystic fibrosis dermatitis presents with psoriasiform diaper rash not responsive to topical steroids or antifungals. This dermatitis may spread and is associated with growth failure and irritability. Deficiency of holocarboxylase synthetase manifests with neonatal erythroderma. The children have alopecia, secondary cutaneous candidiasis, dehydration, and ketoacidosis which can lead to a fatal outcome. Deficiency of holocarboxylase synthetase in skin fibroblasts clinches the diagnosis. Deficiency of biotinidase presents with patchy alopecia and acrodermatitis enteropathica-like skin lesions. These conditions encompass the group of "multiple carboxylase deficiency" disorders. Penicillins, aminoglycosides, and cephalosporins often produce erythematous maculopapular skin lesions, but rarely erythroderma. Ceftriaxone and vancomycin in neonates may produce erythroderma, and vancomycin may also induce hypotension on account of histamine release.

Leiner's disease is literally a clinical phenotype of acquired erythroderma, diarrhea, and failure to thrive. Desquamative generalized erythema and dermatitis with weight loss was thought to be common in breast-fed infants due to the deficiency of biotin. Cases of generalized dermatitis in seborrheic pattern due to immunodeficiencies were also included in this category.

Laboratory investigations are supportive to clinical diagnosis in neonatal erythroderma. Histopathology is not diagnostic in all conditions.

Treatment

Managing neonatal erythroderma is a therapeutic challenge as it is very difficult to treat this potentially life-threatening situation. Careful monitoring of the vital signs, maintenance of fluid and electrolyte balance, and prevention of hyperpyrexia are mandatory in the management. Application of emollients, wet dressings, topical steroids, and systemic antibiotics are the other modalities. Maintaining the skin barrier and proper hydration is the key to managing most of the conditions. Oral retinoids (acitretin) in dose of 0.5–1 mg/kg is indicated in congenital ichthyosis. Regular follow-up and prevention of complications reduce mortality in neonatal erythroderma.

"The whole problem with the world is that fools and fanatics are always so certain of themselves, and wiser people so full of doubts." —**Bertrand Russell**

Amniotic Band Syndrome (Figs. 33A and B)

Amniotic constriction bands are congenital anomalies characterized by constriction rings and digital amputation of one or more digits or limbs. The amniotic bands are confined to the skin, soft tissue and may extend deep into the tissue. It results from intrauterine rupture of amnion with formation of fibrous bands encircling the fetal parts resulting in constriction of the underlying tissue. The inheritance is sporadic. Constrictions can occur on limbs giving rise to swelling on the distal part, loss of distal part of one or more fingers, toes, contractures, and fracture. They can be associated with craniofacial and spinal defects. Rarely deformation of internal organs can occur.

Congenital Erosive and Vesicular Dermatosis (Figs. 34A to D)

The condition presents as vesicles and ulceration in newborns, almost exclusively in premature babies. The exact cause is not known but intrauterine infection and amniotic membrane adhesion are proposed hypothesis. Essentially it is a nonhereditary condition.

Diagnosis

Extensive vesicles and erosions in a reticulate pattern over extremities, trunk involving up to 75% of body surface during first month of life in premature babies is the usual presentation. The lesions soon get crusted and subsequently heal with distinctive supple and reticulate scarring. The scars over the trunk have a cobblestone-like appearance. There may be associated scarring alopecia and ulceration over the tongue. Nails may be either absent or hypoplastic. Sweating is absent over the scarred areas and the baby may present with hyperthermia. Rarely neurological and ocular abnormalities may be seen.

Differential Diagnosis

The condition needs to be differentiated from epidermolysis bullosa. Lack of involvement of face, hands and feet, characteristic rippled scar on healing and progress of lesions characterize the condition and differentiates it from epidermolysis bullosa.

Treatment

It is symptomatic and essentially care of the wound. Reassurance of parents is extremely important.

Harlequin Color Changes (Fig. 35)

Harlequin color change is a rare physiological phenomenon seen more commonly in preterm, low birth weight, sick infants, and with severe intracranial injury. It can affect 10% full-term infants. It is probably related to immaturity of the hypothalamic centers and autonomic control of vascular tone leading to capillary bed dysregulation. The color change occurs when the child is lying on one side; the dependent side becomes strikingly red with simultaneously blanching on the upper half of the body with a sharp line of demarcation. The mucosa and genitalia are spared. These episodes may persist for few seconds to minutes (30 s to 20 min). The color change is rapidly reversible with a change in position,

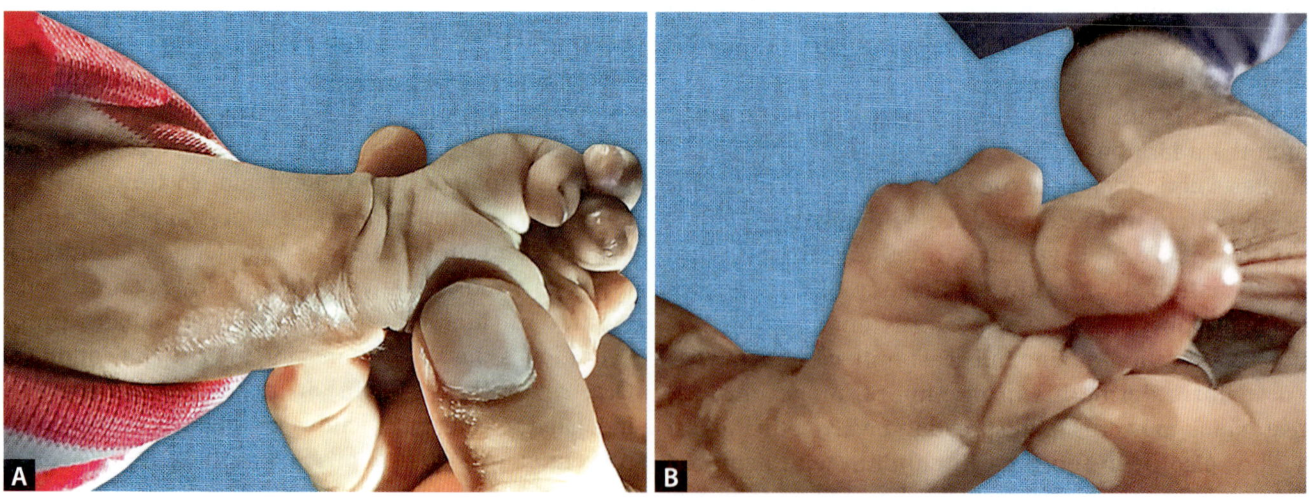

Figs. 33A and B: (A) Amniotic band syndrome; (B) Close-up view of amniotic band syndrome.

"It's amazing what you can get, if you quietly, clearly and authoritatively demand it." —**Meryl Streep**

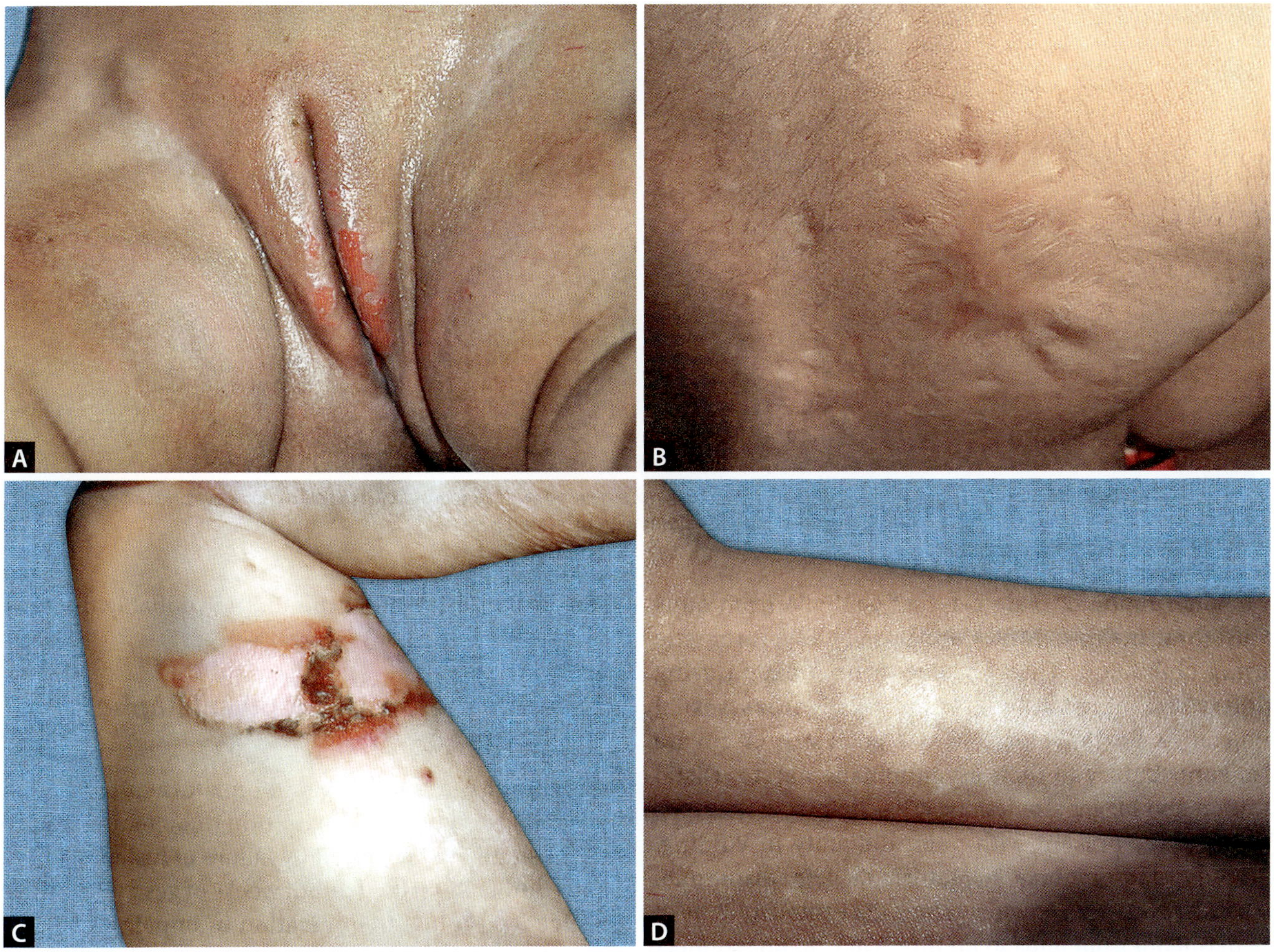

Figs. 34A to D: (A) Congenital erosive and vesicular dermatitis; (B) Congenital erosive and vesicular rash on healing; (C) Congenital erosive and vesicular dermatitis; (D) Healed pigmentary changes in congenital erosive and vesicular dermatitis, note the soft supple and reticulate scarring.

crying, and increased muscular activity. The onset of this phenomenon is seen at 2–5 days of age and may last up to 3 weeks, but can present within first few hours of birth. Repeated episodes can be present in 50% of the affected neonates. Other associated conditions that can trigger this phenomenon are meningitis, seizures, and tricuspid atresia.

Treatment

The condition needs to be explained to the parents and reassured.

Median Raphe Cyst (Figs. 36A to C)

Median raphe cyst (MRC) is a rare, congenital, benign lesion that can occur anywhere along the ventral side

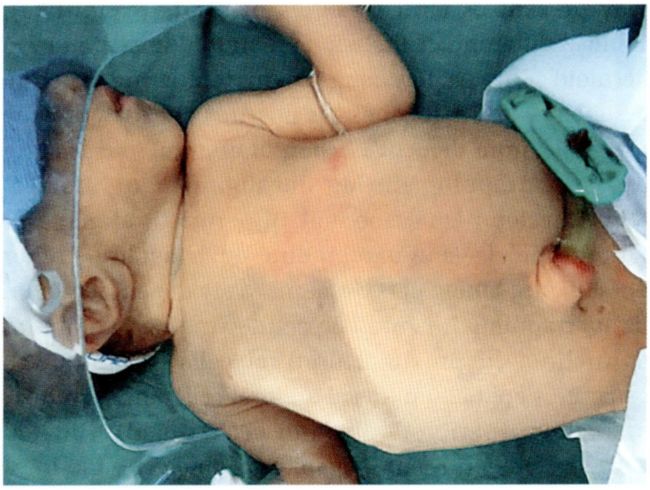

Fig. 35: Harlequin color change in newborn.

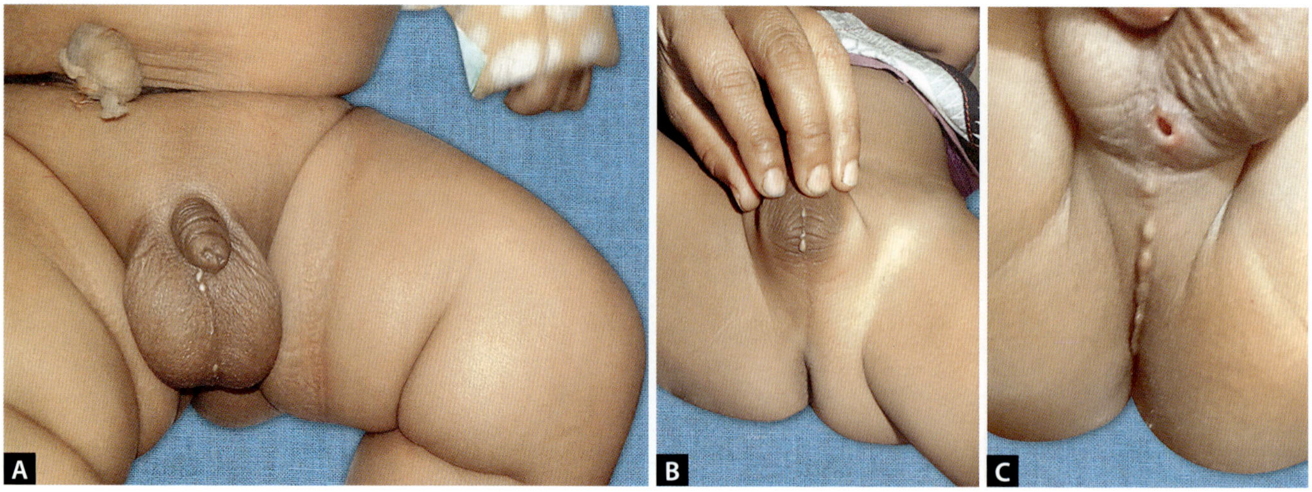

Figs. 36A to C: (A) Median raphe cyst; (B) Median raphe cyst, note beaded whitish papules; (C) Median raphe cyst, note beaded whitish papules along with ulcerated papule.

of median raphe of male external genitalia from anus to urethral meatus. MRCs are usually asymptomatic during childhood. They become symptomatic during adolescence or adulthood following vigorous sexual intercourse. Proximal location and small size, <2 cm are also contributory to their asymptomatic nature. Distal location and bigger size lesions are usually symptomatic. Patients may present with pain, difficulty in voiding, difficulty in intercourse, hematuria or hematospermia. Location of MRC varies widely along the ventral midline of the perineum from anus to urethra. They do not connect with urethra. The most common location is distal penile shaft and parameatal position. Rarely do they present at scrotum, glans penis, and prepuce. Sometimes they may present as cord or series of beads (canal-like). Clinical differentials include epidermoid inclusion cyst, dermoid cyst, steatocystoma, glomus tumor, and apocrine cystadenoma. Pathogenesis is not fully elucidated. They may arise from defective fusion of urethral fold leading to tissue trapping during development of urethral fold. Developmental anomaly of periurethral gland of Littre or blockage of paraurethral ducts could be other possibilities. Lining of the cyst may vary depending upon tissue trapping. It could be pseudo stratified columnar epithelium (if proximal urethral cells get trapped), squamous epithelium (distal urethral cell), and glandular epithelium (periurethral gland get trapped). Ciliated cells are rarely present. Metaplastic change due to local irritation is the most probable explanation. Treatment is surgical excision for cosmetic reason or for symptomatic lesion. Simple aspiration may lead to recurrence therefore wide local excision and aspiration is probably the better way to approach.

Sternal Cleft with Umbilical Raphe (Figs. 37A to C)

Sternal cleft is a rare congenital malformation that can be isolated or combined with other congenital defects. It is presumed to be caused by failure of fusion of sternal bands during the sixth to ninth weeks of gestation. Studies in mice lead to the identification of impairment in the expression of *Hoxb* genes as a possible cause of sternal defects. The malformation is usually sporadic, but there are reports of familial inheritance (autosomal dominant). They can be classified as superior, subtotal, total, and inferior. Superior sternal clefts are usually isolated but may be associated with vascular abnormalities such as craniofacial hemangioma (seen almost exclusively in females) and supraumbilical midline raphe extending from the umbilicus to the lower part of the sternal defect, first described by Leiber. Coarctation of the aorta with a right aortic arch and congenital aortic aneurysm has also been described in association with cleft sternum and supraumbilical raphe. PHACE syndrome (*p*osterior fossa anomalies, *h*emangioma, *a*rterial anomalies, *c*ardiac anomalies, and *e*ye anomalies) is sometimes associated with ventral developmental defects (sternal cleft, supraumbilical raphe, or both) and is then called as PHACE(S) syndrome.

It may be an abortive form of Pentalogy of Cantrell. Pentalogy of Cantrell is a condition characterized by a combination of midline birth defects that can potentially

"Change will not come if we wait for some other person or some other time. We are the ones we have been waiting for. We are the change that we seek." **—Barack Obama**

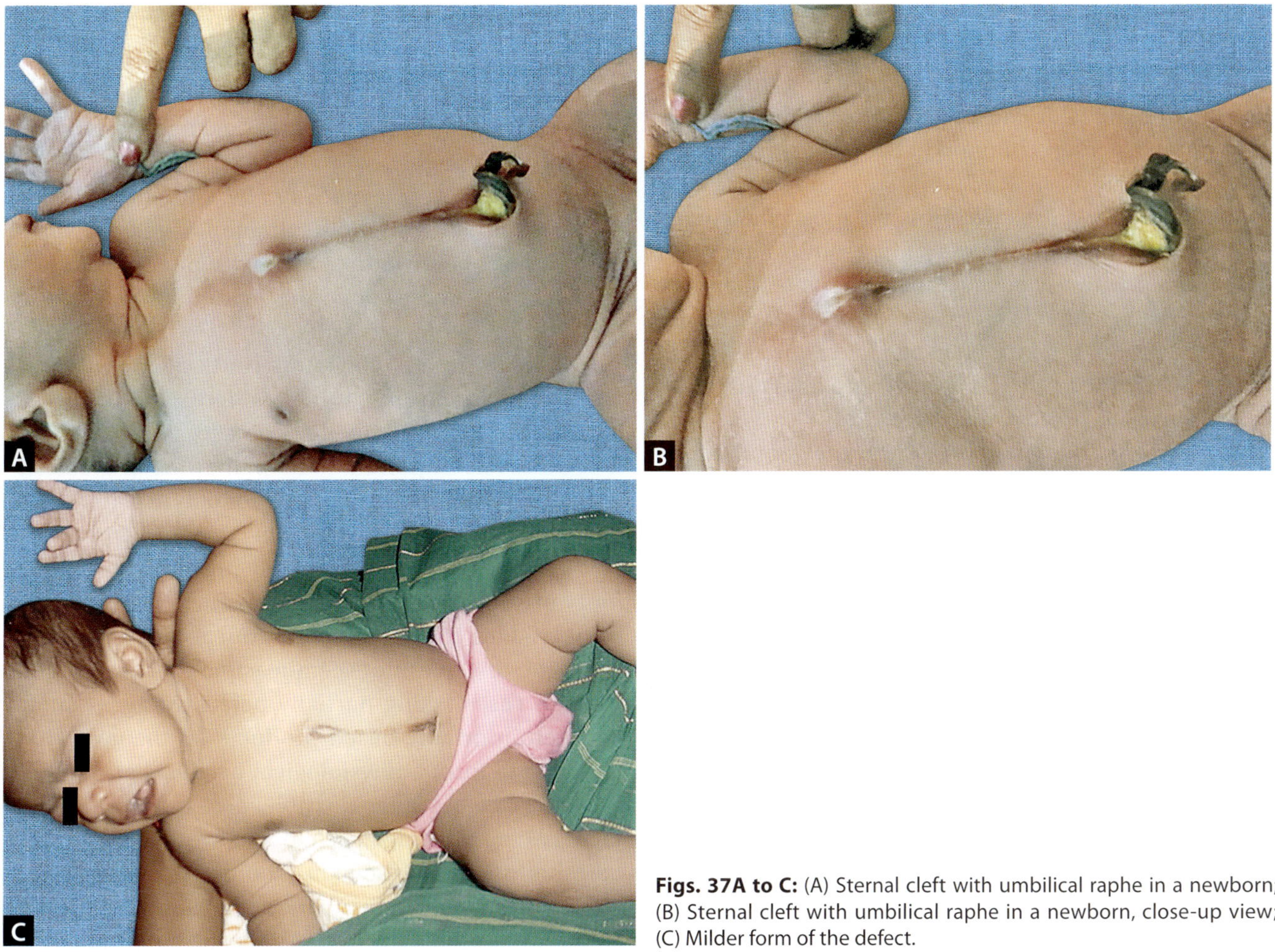

Figs. 37A to C: (A) Sternal cleft with umbilical raphe in a newborn; (B) Sternal cleft with umbilical raphe in a newborn, close-up view; (C) Milder form of the defect.

involve the breastbone (sternum); the muscle that separates the chest cavity from the abdomen and aids in breathing (diaphragm); the thin membrane that lines the heart (pericardium); the abdominal wall; and other vital organs.

Prenatal high-resolution ultrasonography may diagnose the condition and helps to accurately evaluate cartilaginous parts of the sternum and possible cardiovascular malformations postnatally. Surgical correction during the neonatal period is recommended as the compliant thorax allows direct approximation of the sternal halves.

CARE OF THE NEWBORN SKIN

The skin is the first barrier of the newborns to counter various noxious factors/agents of the environment once the baby comes out of the safe and secured intrauterine life to the external world. Various aspects of newborn skin care will be discussed under different headings.

Need for Special Skin Care for Babies

Baby's protective but delicate cover needs to be kept in a healthy condition and it should be disturbed as little as possible. Topical agents are more rapidly absorbed into infant skin due to deficient intercellular bridges. Besides, greater body surface area to weight ratio than adults also facilitates easy absorption and toxicity of topically applied substances. Infant skin cannot withstand the toxicity of most substances as they make this delicate skin more susceptible to electrolyte imbalance, fluid imbalance, and thermal instability. Infant skin is particularly very sensitive to cleansing agents as they contain stronger chemicals and may be drying. Hence, the product should be guaranteed of safety for use on babies.

"Don't chase people, be yourself, do your own things and work hard. The right people, the ones who really belong in your life, will come to you and stay." **—Will Smith**

Skin problems pertaining to dryness are common in babies due to inadequacies in the epidermal barrier. The skin irritation potential toward topical applicants is also more. Maintaining skin integrity and preventing exposure to toxic substances in childhood assures healthy skin for several years ahead.

Skin of the newborns performs the most challenging task as it is the outermost cover of the body. Moreover, it is confronted with various factors, namely, temperature changes, friction, microbes, etc., of the external world once the baby is born. As the structure and functions of the skin depend on whether a child is born at term or prematurely, skin care is related to gestational age.

At birth, microbial colonization of newborn skin is almost nil. But over a few hours, aerobic flora occupies skin at different concentrations at different sites, e.g., mostly over groins, axillae, and scalp. Coagulase negative *staphylococci* (*Staphylococcus epidermidis*) are the most commonly found microorganisms. *Staphylococcus aureus* appears only as contamination, usually from mother or nursing staff.

Skin Care at Birth

Removal of Vernix Caseosa

At birth the baby's skin is coated with vernix caseosa, blood, meconium, and cellular debris. Vernix caseosa has a protective function, contains both epidermal (triglycerides and cholesterol) and sebaceous (squalene and waxes) fat. Premature infants tend to have less of vernix than term babies and postmature babies have little vernix. There is considerable interindividual variation in the quality of vernix caseosa. Vernix caseosa should not be rubbed or removed as it dries and falls itself by 5–7 days.

Washing and Bathing

A bath is an ideal means of cleaning an infant completely. A bath in infant should not last for more than 5 minutes. The bath of approximately 5 minutes increases the hydration of skin and, thereby, reduces the threshold for friction. Newborn temperature should be stabilized before the first bath is given. Bathing should be deferred till fifth or seventh day. Sponge bathing can be given till the cord falls. Blood and meconium can be wiped with soft cotton dipped in warm water. Temperature of bath water should be equal to skin temperature (34–36°C).

A solid or liquid cleanser or a syndet can be used to clean baby skin. After bath, infants must be dried thoroughly, particularly over skin creases, groins, and axillae.

Diaper Care

Napkin should be changed frequently every 2 hours, at least at each nursing and feeding time. Cloth diaper should be carefully washed in lukewarm water and then rinsed off and dried thoroughly.

The diaper area is specifically vulnerable because it is a closed environment suitable for microorganisms and with frequent wetting, it is more often moist; hence the skin becomes prone to maceration and increases its permeability to other irritants.

The skin here is constantly in contact with strong alkalinizing agents, e.g., urine and feces and the pH here is prone to high alkalinity that damages the skin integrity. It is, thus, very important to be well-aware of the need to change nappies and the range of products that are available to prevent any rash or irritation in the nappy area.

Nappy rash can be reasonably prevented by reducing moisture by the frequent changing of nappies. This would reduce contact between urine, feces, and the skin. However, this does not seem feasible at most instances. In such cases, using partially occlusive agent such as petrolatum or zinc-based products on the genital area can help to form a physiological barrier that minimizes this interface. As far as possible, air exposure should be increased by allowing the child to move around the house bare-bottomed. Plastic pants should be avoided as they reduce the air circulation to the skin. Warm water and soft cotton wool should be used to wipe the nappy area. Feces have a tendency to stick and scrubbing only worsens the status of the delicate skin. Here, the use of an emulsion such as baby lotion can ease the removal by reducing the surface tension and cleaning the debris. Skin should then be thoroughly dried each time the diaper is changed by exposing it for a few minutes. The bottom should be wiped from front to back to avoid fecal matter from reaching the genitals. Soaps should be mild and should be used very rarely if a rash has developed. Use of powders in diaper areas is not recommended.

In general, the nappies should be made of cotton cloth and should be home laundered with mild detergents. Recent advances in diaper technology have led to decrease in frequency and severity of diaper rash. Diapers with highly superabsorbent acrylate gel can be used.

Scalp

Regular cleansing of scalp is necessary. Shampoo helps to remove scales and crust from the scalp (cradle cap). Coconut oil or mineral oil application softens the scales.

"A friend is one soul abiding in two souls." **—Aristotle**

Nails

Nail should be regularly trimmed and kept short and clean.

The Ears

Outer aspect of ear should be cleansed. Cotton swabs soaked in boiled water should be used to clean ears. Special care should be taken not to hurt auditory canals.

Umbilicus

After birth umbilical cord dries out and drops off within 5–10 days. No topical agents should be used on umbilical cord. Dry cord care is recommended. Prophylactic use of chlorhexidine reduces the colonization and prevents sepsis.

Skin Care in the Premature Infants

After birth, skin maturation proceeds rapidly in preterm infants. These infants are kept warm and nursed in closed incubators. Environmental conditions in these units are potentially harmful for infant skin, which is subject to scarring. Cosmetically or functionally, significant lesions may be caused by needle marks, central venous catheters, transcutaneous oxygen monitoring, chest drain insertion, extravasation of IV fluid **(Fig. 38)** or skin stripping due to adhesive tape. To reduce the frequency and severity of skin damage, neonatal staff need to know that many routine procedures can lead to long-term scarring and atrophy. Heaters should be kept at a safe distance in NICU as there is a risk of burn injury **(Fig. 39)**.

Preventive Measures

- *Disinfection:* The most common infective agents causing septicemia are coagulase-negative staphylococci in relation to catheter placement. For prevention, maintain hygiene by hand washing of the staff and parents. Cleaning with chlorhexidine-alcohol and povidone-iodine, two consecutive 10-second cleaning destroys more than a single 10-second wipe.
- *The incubator:* Frequent change of infants' position in the incubator reduces the risk of skin erosion and impending bed sore. Fingers and toes must be kept visible. Catheters or needles should be secured with a transparent tape to allow easy detection of fluid extravasation. Scarring alopecia can develop following pressure ulcer. The occurrence of nonblanchable erythema and disruption of epidermis indicate impending ulcer. The occurrence of scarring alopecia has been reported in infants from pressure necrosis.
- *Transcutaneous oxygen monitors:* Transcutaneous oxygen monitors should not be left in place for more than 1 hour without surveillance. Nonblanchable erythema has been reported with keeping such electrodes for prolonged period. The use of karaya electrodes has been demonstrated to be effective in cardiorespiratory monitoring with decreased trauma to the neonatal skin. Placement of electrodes on the limbs, especially in very low birth weight infants, can eliminate the need to frequently remove these pads to facilitate auscultation or other assessment of the chest wall.

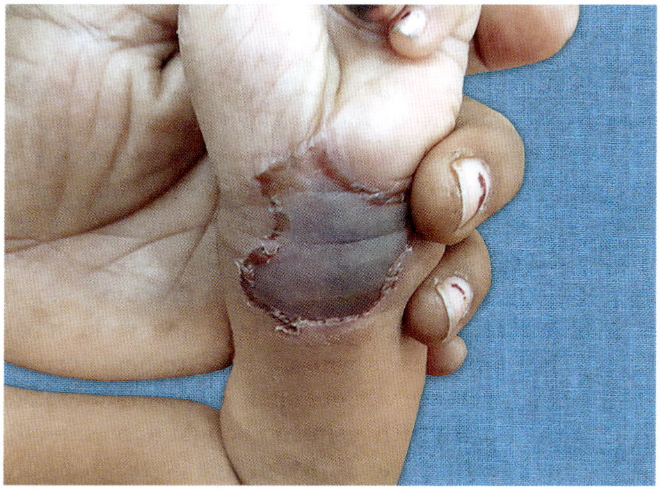

Fig. 38: Extravasation injuries.

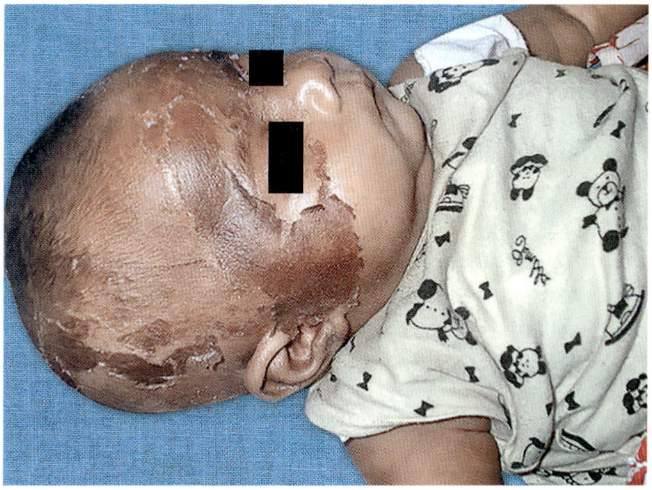

Fig. 39: Thermal burn of skin in a neonate in NICU from room heater.

"If you smile when you are alone, then you really mean it." —**Andy Rooney**

- *Minimal use of tape and adhesive:* The skin of the premature infants may be damaged by repeated attachment and removal of adhesive tapes to secure electrodes, IV cannulas, drains, etc. Adhesives should be used on small areas of skin and removed gently with warm water soaked gauze and diluted soap, but not alcohol, which may be irritant for baby's skin.
- *Emollients:* Application of emollient is a safe and effective way to decrease neonatal peeling and scaling dermatitis. Coconut oil or vegetable oil applied gently to the skin, reduce scaling and fissuring as well as increase skin hydration.

Skin Care of the Term Baby and Infant

The large number of infant skin-care products available over the counter is at times confusing for the average consumers. These have been the gifts of media and so-called health magazines for the lay people with all rosy advertisements. By and large the principle followed by a doctor should be to advice the parents to go for a product marketed by a multinational company or a company of good repute and stature or a product, which has been in the market for a considerable period of time and thus has stood "the test of time". Several types of products are used, namely soaps, shampoos, antiseptics, moisturizers, etc.

Detergents

The term "detergent" designates a substance capable of cleaning the skin, i.e., of removing impurities (dust, grease organic secretions, microorganisms). Washing with water alone does not remove all the impurities on the skin surface. Some are only fat soluble, thus requiring the use of products capable of emulsifying the fatty substance into fine droplets, which can then, be carried away by rinsing. These products are known as surfactants, act by suppressing the surface tension, which allows fatty substances to remain on the skin surface. Detergents act by reducing the surface tension between water and air, creating a foaming effect not directly correlated with the cleaning properties of the product. As a rule, a higher foaming power increases the risk of damage to the skin. Detergents are classified as ionic or nonionic products. In infants detergents should be used cautiously, followed by a thorough rinsing. Too much removal of lipids from the stratum corneum would eliminate those essential to the surface ecosystem.

Soaps are the products of saponification, i.e., the action of alkali on a fatty substance. In hard water, soaps tend to precipitate.

Syndets or synthetic detergents do not have the theoretical disadvantages of soap but are subject to rapid disintegration. They can produce excessive dryness of skin, if moisturizers are not added to it. Antiseptic soaps are useful in preparation of an operative field, but are unsuitable for daily use in infants as they can cause irritation to infants' skin. Moreover, antiseptic soaps remove the commensal organisms from the skin surface, thereby, making the skin prone to attack by virulent pathogenic organisms from outside.

Bubble bath products attract the infants and their parents because of its colorings and perfumes and, thereby, mask the risk of prolonging a bath and irritating the genital mucosa.

Most baby shampoos in the market contain anionic surfactant which ensures adequate cleansing. The pH should be close to that of tears and, thereby, would not cause irritation to the eyes. Special ingredients, e.g., selenium sulfide, ketoconazole or zinc pyrithione may be added to the shampoos for seborrheic dermatitis or seborrhea scalp. The basic principles of use of various antiseptics and emollients in term babies and infants are essentially the same as in preterm babies.

Protective creams: These are basically prepared to reduce the risk of irritation, particularly napkin rash, by isolating skin from numerous irritants for baby's skin. The creams contain a fatty phase, an aqueous phase, a surfactant, additives (zinc oxide), scents, and preservatives. These creams can paradoxically cause increased occlusion and irritant dermatitis to its ingredients.

Powders: Application of powders over the skin folds is not recommended.

Role of Massage

The act of touch fulfils the basic need to feel safe, comfortable and loved. Touch is also an intrinsic factor in child development. Touch is proposed to play a role in growth, development, and overall well-being. Massage is one of the most beautiful and gentle methods of touch. It is practiced in most countries and has recently been researched extensively in western countries. Indian form of infant massage is appreciated all over the world. It has been seen that massage with oil is more beneficial as compared to massage without oil. It is important to note that the oil used in such a situation ought to be smooth, of optimum viscosity, and friction free or else it would lead to abrasions on the skin surface. The oil should be nonocclusive so that it does not block the skin pores and allows the skin to breathe. It ought to be safe and mild to suit the baby's delicate skin and the ingredients should be thoroughly tested for their potential to cause contact sensitivity. Mineral oil is one of the best-known moisturizing ingredients ever found. It spreads easily and has a long-lasting tactile effect, making it an extremely efficacious emollient. Omission of low molecular weight hydrocarbons alleviates risks of carcinogenicity while the large particle size renders it incapable of blocking pores making it noncomedogenic.

Massage should be started after 1 month and can easily continue till 10 years and over. Benefits of massage are numerous. Appropriate knowledge of correct massage techniques is important in order to attain maximum therapeutic benefits from it. Complete head-to-toe massage should be a daily routine. But massage should be gentle and judicious. However, massage should be withheld for a few days in case either the baby has got any contagious infection of skin or the person offering massage has any infection over hands. Massage given by the mother increases the bondage between the mother and her baby. It helps in the physiological and psychological development of the babies.

Table 3: Approach to neonatal erythroderma.

Step 1	Medical history—family history, consanguinity, pregnancy, drugs Physical examination—alopecia (PID), collodion/ scaling (Ichthyoses), vesicles/bullae/pustules (congenital candidiasis, SSSS, DCM, EI)
Step 2	Routine investigations—CBC, LFT, RFT, CRP, ESR
Step 3	Extended investigations—skin biopsy (± IF), dermoscopy, trichoscopy, serum immunoglobulin assay, molecular genetic analysis
Step 4	Multi-speciality consultation (neurology, otorhinolaryngology, ophthalmology, cardiology, immunology) to rule out extracutaneous and/or systemic symptoms
Step 5	Consider rare diseases (AD, psoriasis, seborrheic dermatitis) in neonatal period when syndromic ichthyoses, PIDs and metabolic disorders ruled out
Step 6	Treatment of working diagnosis and follow up

WHAT'S NEW

A clinical approach to diagnosis of neonatal erythroderma **(Table 3)**.

SUGGESTED READINGS

1. Bayliss SJ, Colven R. Disorders of subcutaneous tissue in newborn. In: Irvine AD, Hoeger PH, Yan AC (Eds). Harper's Textbook of Dermatology, 3rd edition. Wiley-Blackwell; 2011. pp. 7.1-7.5.
2. Eichenfield LF, Frieden IJ, Esterly NB. Neonatal Dermatology, 3rd edition. Philadelphia PA: Saunders Elsevier; 2015.
3. Gorur DK, Murthy SC, Tamraparni S. Early neonatal dermatoses: a study among 1260 babies delivered at a tertiary care center in South India. Indian J Paediatr Dermatol. 2016;17:190-5.
4. Pandit VS, Udaya K. A study of neonatal dermatoses in a tertiary care center. Indian J Paediatr Dermatol. 2019;20:36-40.
5. Reginatto FP, Muller FM, Peruzzo J, Cestari TF. Epidemiology and predisposing factors for erythema toxicum neonatorum and transient neonatal pustular: a multicenter study. Pediatr Dermatol. 2017;34:422-6.
6. Cuperus E, Bygum A, Boeckmann L, Bodemer C, Bolling MC, Capron M, et al. Proposal for a 6-step approach for differential diagnosis of neonatal erythroderma. JEADV 2022;36:973-86.
7. Kuti BP, Ogunlesi TA, Oduwole O, Oringanje CCMO, Udoh EE, Bello S, et al. Hand hygiene for the prevention of infections in neonates. Cochrane Database of Systematic Reviews 2023, Issue 6. Art. No.: CD013326.

"Don't be pushed around by the fears in your mind. Be led by the dreams in your heart." —**Roy T Bennett**

CHAPTER

2 Vascular, Melanocytic, and Other Nevi

SALMON PATCH (FIGS. 1A AND B)

Salmon patch are extremely common anomalies which have been observed in the neonatal period in 20–60% of children of all races. They take the form of irregular, dull, pinkish-red, macular areas often with fine linear telangiectasia. The posterior neck followed by the face (forehead, glabella, upper eyelids) are the common sites of distribution. It is termed as *stork bite* when seen on the nape of neck and *angel kiss* when present on forehead or glabella.

Natural History

Most of these lesions fade rapidly and disappear within a year. However, nuchal lesions may persist up to adult life. It should be noted that slight erythematous color may persist or reappear over subsided salmon patches during episodes of crying, coughing, physical exertion, etc. Nuchal lesions, although, tend to persist up to adult life in some cases do not pose cosmetic problem as they are usually covered by scalp hair.

Management

Maintenance of serial photographs of the lesions, and counseling form the essential aspects of management.

HEMANGIOMA (FIGS. 2 TO 6P)

Infantile hemangiomas are benign developmental vascular tumors that appear during the first few months of life and which characteristically have an initial proliferative and a later involutional phase. The incidence is estimated to be 4–5% in infants. They have a high incidence in premature and low birth weight infants. Infantile hemangiomas become apparent during the first month of life in about 90% of cases and virtually 100% by the ninth month. Approximately 65% of infantile hemangiomas are superficial, 15% deep, and 20% mixed. Superficial infantile hemangioma presents as sharply circumscribed oval or round, soft, domed-shaped papules, and plaques of intense scarlet-red color. Deep hemangioma appears as flesh colored to blue mass in the deep dermis and subcutaneous

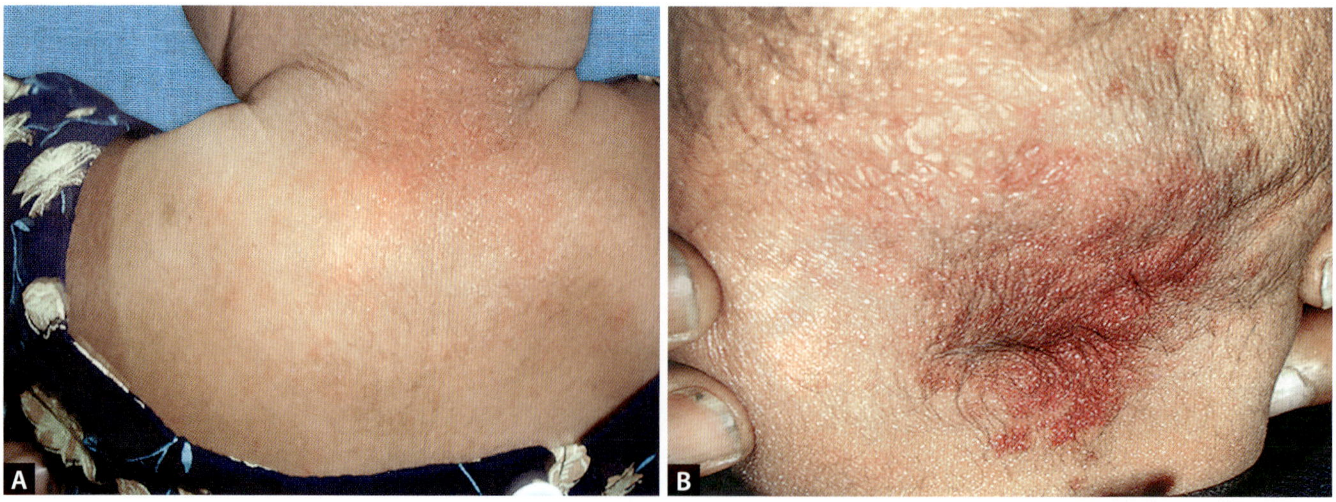

Figs. 1A and B: (A) Salmon patch over nape of the neck in a 2-year-old girl; (B) Salmon patch in a newborn.

"A person without the knowledge of their past history, origin and culture is like a tree without roots." —**Marcus Garvey**

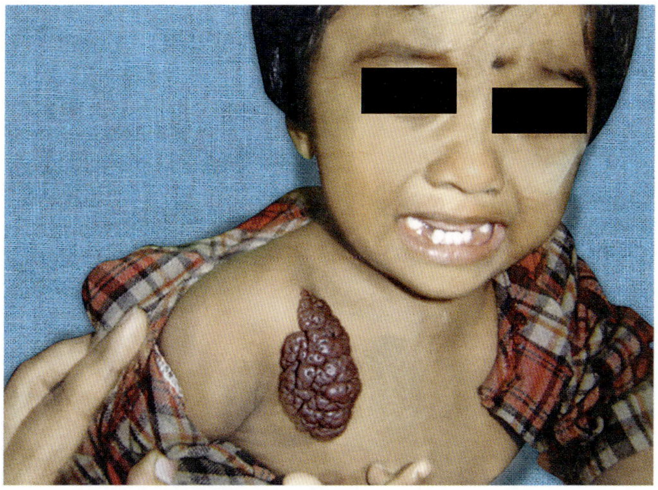

Fig. 2: Infantile hemangioma over front of the chest in a 3-year-old girl.

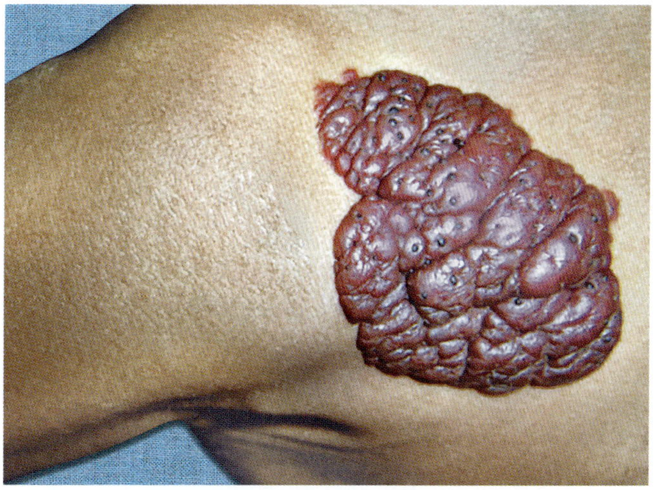

Fig. 3: Close-up view of the lesion, note black comedone-like lesions on the surface.

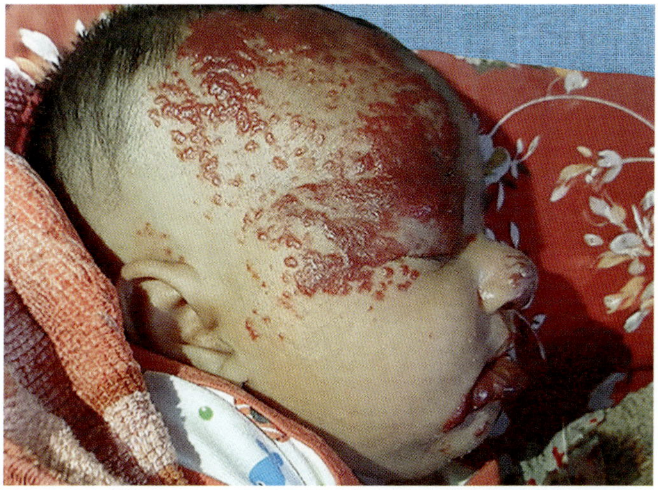

Fig. 4: Hemangioma over face.

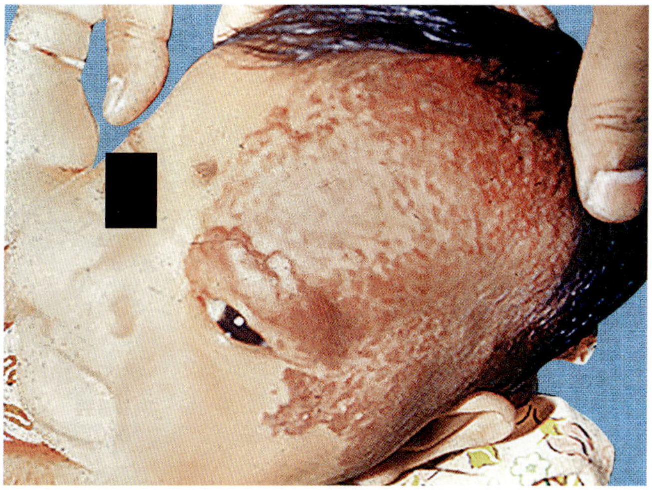

Fig. 5: Resolving hemangioma with oral corticosteroid.

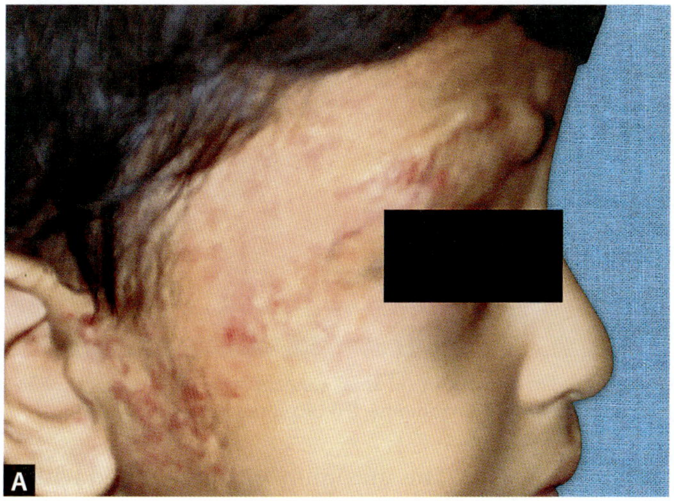

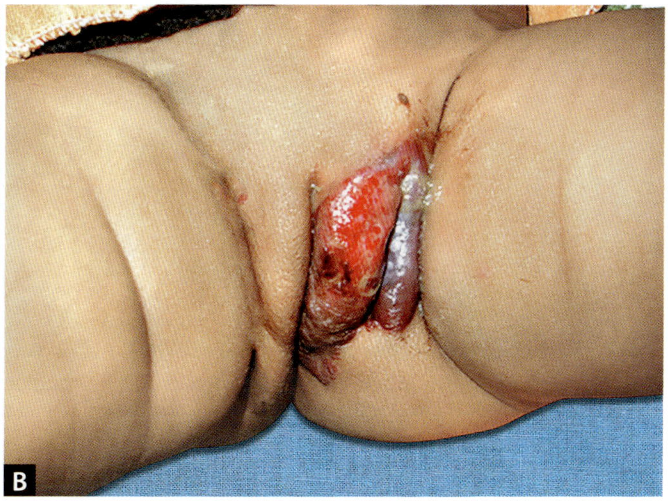

Figs. 6A and B: (A) The same boy at 5 years, note residual erythema and atrophy of skin at the healed site; (B) Ulcerated hemangioma in an infant.

"If you only walk on sunny days, you will never reach your destination." —**Paulo Coelho**

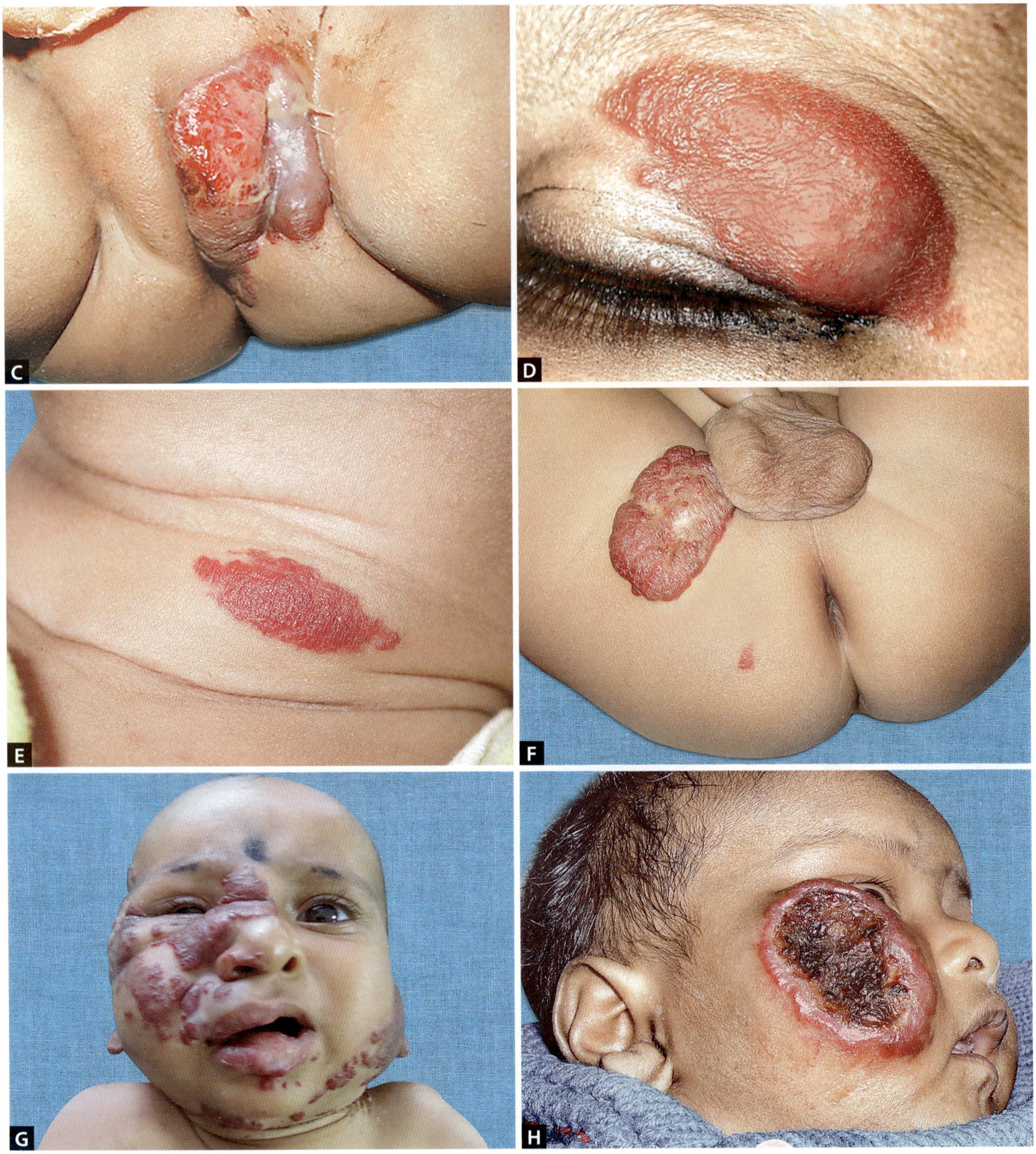

Figs. 6C to H: (C) Close-up view of the lesion; (D) Hemangioma over eyelid in a newborn; (E) Small hemangioma over neck; (F) Perianal hemangioma, susceptible to ulceration and infection; (G) Segmental hemangioma; (H) Ulcerated hemangioma.

tissue. Mixed type has both superficial and deeper components. The most common site is the head and neck region followed by the trunk. In 80% of cases, a single lesion is present. The maximum size is reached within 3–6 months of their first appearance, the final diameter vary from 1 to 25 cm, and spontaneously involute by

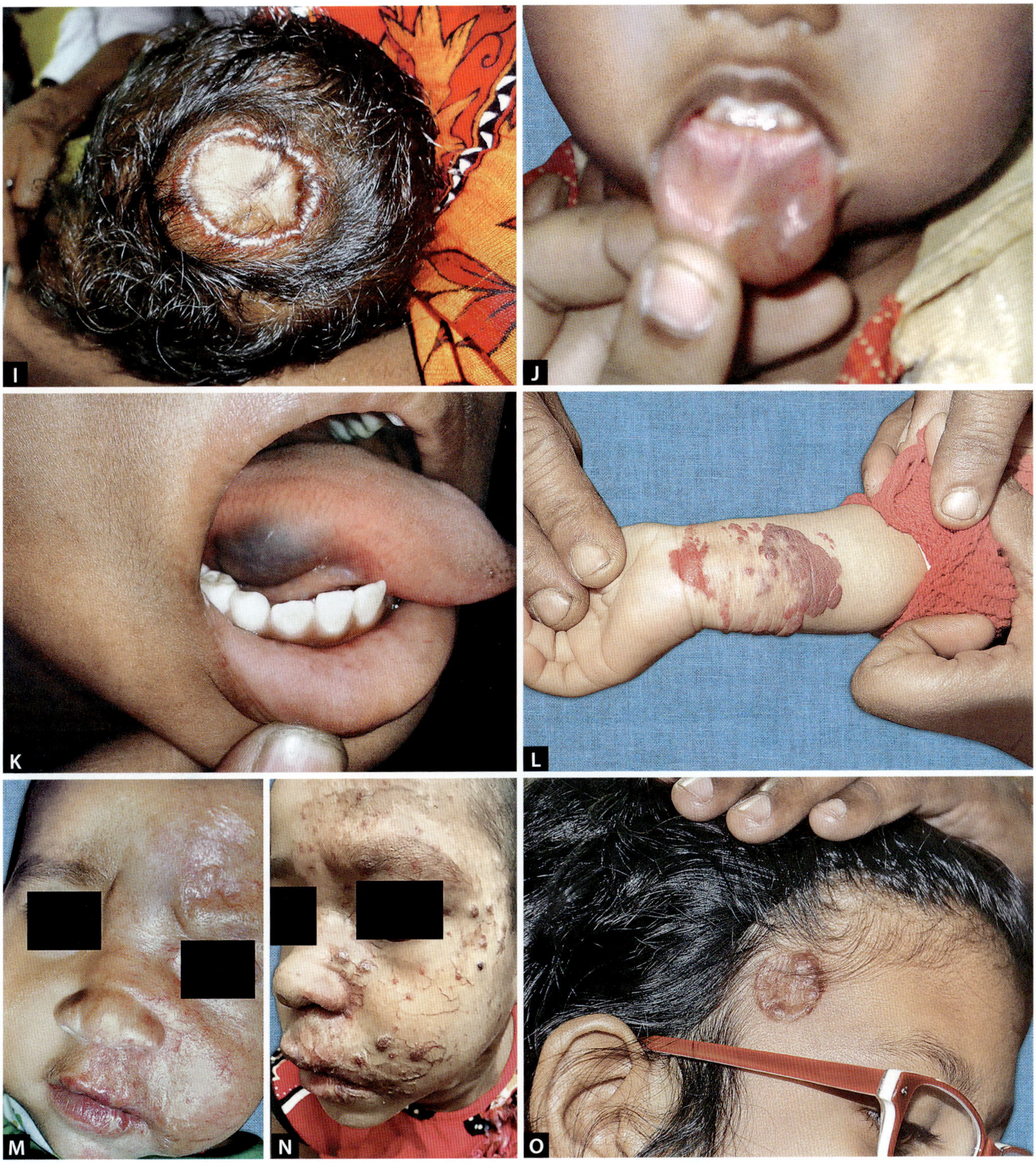

Figs. 6I to O: (I) Ulcerated hemangioma over scalp; (J) Hemangioma of lip; (K) Hemangioma of tongue; (L) Rapidly involuting congenital hemangioma (RICH); (M) Hemangioma over face treated with oral propranolol; (N) Hemangioma on propranolol for 6 months; (O) Hemangioma on topical timolol.

12 months. Most of the regression is seen by 4 years, leaving behind residual fibrofatty tissue and scarring. Multiple hemangiomas may be a marker of systemic involvement most commonly the liver. Segmental hemangioma has been associated with posterior fossa malformations, hemangioma, arterial anomalies, cardiac

"Our deepest fear is not that we are inadequate, our deepest fear is that we are powerful beyond measure. It is our light, not our darkness, that most frightens us." —**Marianne Williamson**

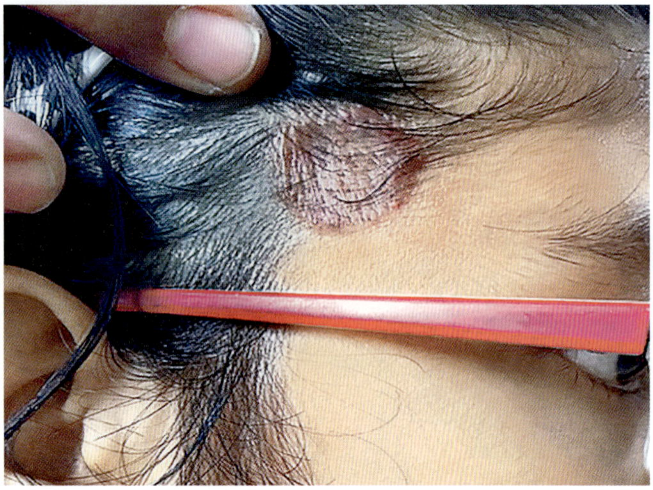

Figs. 6P: Hemangioma on topical timolol for 6 months.

defects, eye anomalies, and sternal defects (PHACES) and LUMBAR syndrome (lower body hemangioma, urogenital abnormalities/ulceration, myelopathy, bony deformities, arterial, and anorectal anomalies, renal anomalies). Based on the growth pattern, subtypes include infantile hemangioma with minimal or arrested growth (IH-MAG) which appears as telangiectatic patches and congenital hemangioma (NICH: non-involuting congenital hemangioma, RICH: rapidly involuting congenital hemangioma, and PICH: partially involuting congenital hemangioma).

Natural History

Most of the infantile hemangiomas undergo spontaneous regression which is complete or almost complete in about 95% of cases by 8–10 years of age. Most cases require no therapy because of the tendency of the hemangiomas to regress completely or almost completely. One must remember that the final results in untreated lesions are far superior to that obtained from any kind of therapeutic intervention.

Management

Intervention is indicated for lesions which are rapidly growing, compromising function of vital structures (viz., eyes, nares, auditory canals, pharynx, larynx), lumbosacral, segmental, multiple hemangiomas, large cavernous hemangioma with associated thrombocytopenia and consumption coagulopathy, lesions susceptible to trauma, hemorrhage, ulceration, and secondary infection. Propranolol, a nonselective beta-blocker is the first line of therapy. It is initially started at a dose of 0.5–1 mg/kg and slowly increased to 2–3 mg/kg/day in two to three divided doses. Potential side effects include hypotension, bradycardia, hypoglycemia, hypothermia, bronchospasm, and night mares. Before prescribing oral propranolol, baseline evaluation should be performed at initiation and during dose escalation, and these include blood pressure, heart rate, blood sugars, and electrocardiogram. Hypoglycemia can be avoided by giving propranolol along with feeding and avoiding long fasting periods. Child should be admitted and monitored while initiating the therapy. Other systemic beta-blockers that have been found useful are atenolol and nadolol. For small, superficial, uncomplicated hemangioma topical timolol 0.5% solution/gel has been used and tolerated well. It is applied as 1–2 drops twice per day. For ulcerated hemangioma wound care with antibacterials, systemic beta-blockers or intralesional or systemic corticosteroids, pulsed dye laser, and surgical excision are useful. Segmental hemangioma warrants thorough imaging and MRI before initiation of therapy.

Oral prednisolone is given at a dose of 2–4 mg/kg/day for 4 weeks followed by on alternate days for 4–6 weeks. Triamcinolone acetonide intralesional injection is given at a dose of 1–3 mg/kg, 2–3 injections at 2–3 weeks intervals.

Various other therapeutic modalities are light applications of dry ice or liquid nitrogen, tunable pulse dye laser therapy or Grenz ray therapy. Even compression with a pressure dressing and frequent massage often help in resolution of hemangiomas.

BLUE RUBBER BLEB NEVUS SYNDROME (FIGS. 6Q TO S)

Blue rubber bleb nevus syndrome (BRBNS, Bean syndrome) is a rare disorder characterized by multiple widely distributed venous malformations in the skin and gastrointestinal (GI) tract and, less often, in other organ systems. The cause of this syndrome is unknown. Most patients with BRBNS are diagnosed at birth or during early infancy. Most cases are sporadic, but autosomal dominant inheritance has also been reported. A new somatic double (cis) mutation in the *TEK* gene encoding for TIE2, also known as an angiopoietin-1 receptor expressed in the endothelial cells, has been discovered.

Cutaneous lesions, which are the first clinically visible manifestations, appear as asymptomatic, multiple, small, well circumscribed, dark-blue, soft, rubbery, compressible blebs that can appear anywhere on the body but are usually present on the neck, limbs, and oral or perianal

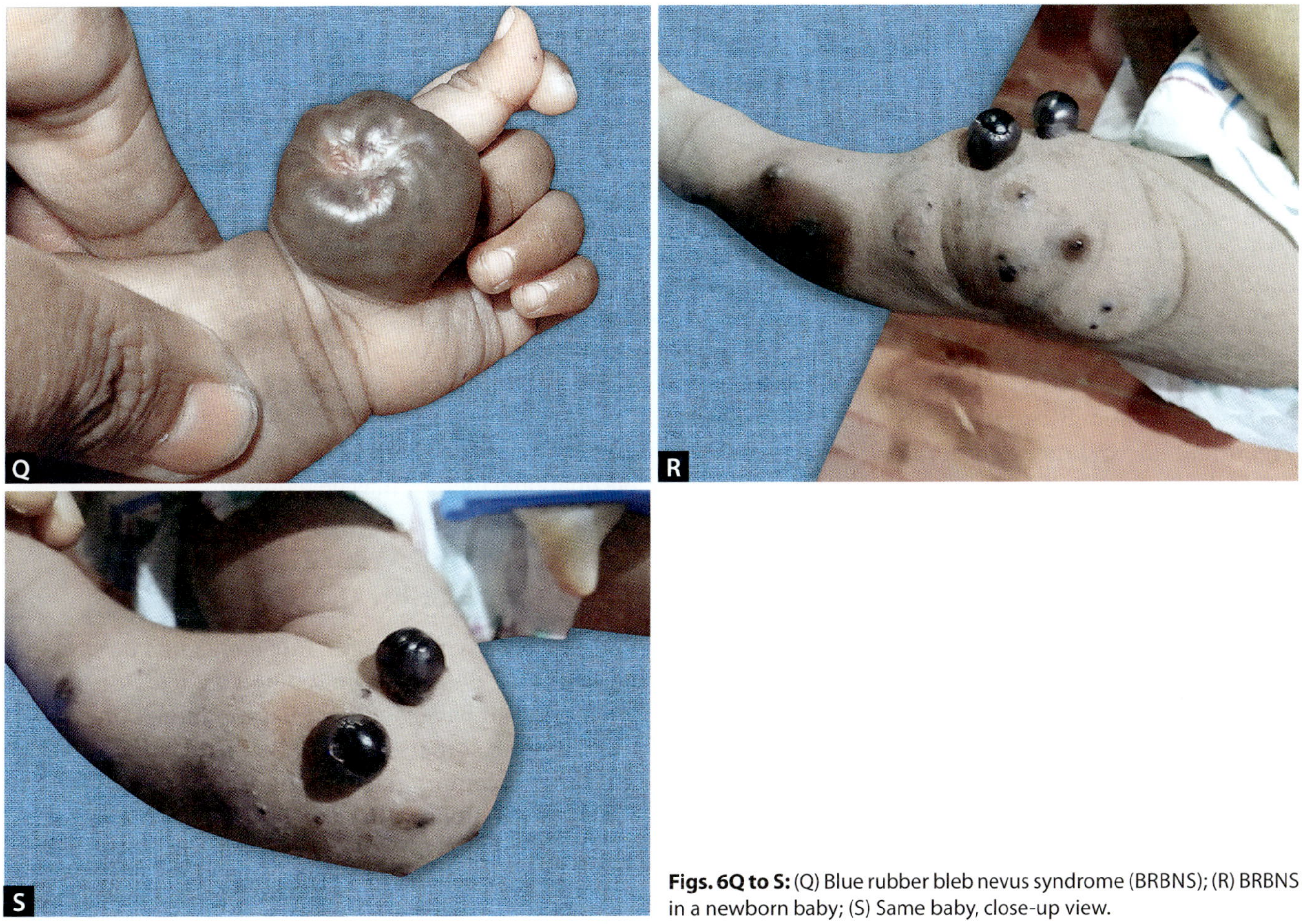

Figs. 6Q to S: (Q) Blue rubber bleb nevus syndrome (BRBNS); (R) BRBNS in a newborn baby; (S) Same baby, close-up view.

mucosa. New lesions continue to appear until puberty after which the incidence of new lesions decreases. Rarely, patients might complain of pain and sweating. No malignant transformation has been reported. Three types of cutaneous lesions have been described by Bean:

Type I: Major, obscure, red-to-purple venous malformations of 10 cm or more that may be disfiguring or obstruct vital organ systems (large cavernous lesions).

Type II: "Rubber bluish nipple" lesions, characterized by nodular and rubber lesions, are easily compressed by touch, followed by slow reconstitution. They are usually asymptomatic.

Type III: Blue to black punctiform macules and papules, which can be adjacent to, or over, a blue macule. They do not disappear with light pressure.

Gastrointestinal manifestations involve bleeding and iron deficiency anemia, followed by abdominal pain due to intussusception, intestinal torsion, and rupture. Malformations appear most commonly in the small bowel and distal colon. CNS manifestations (seizures, subarachnoid hemorrhage, and focal neurological deficits) are infrequent and occur late in the disease. Other findings based on the organ involved include menorrhagia, intermittent proptosis, hematuria, epistaxis, hemoptysis, hemothorax, hemopericardium, and thrombotic complications. Skeletal involvement in BRBNS is uncommon and may present with pain, decreased range of joint movement, and, occasionally, deformity. Morbidity and mortality depend on the extent of visceral organ involvement and in most cases are associated with severe bowel bleeding and coagulopathy.

Diagnosis is suspected based on characteristic cutaneous lesions. Histologically, vascular lesions are characterized by a cluster of dilated irregular capillary spaces lined by a thin layer of endothelial cells in the dermis or subcutaneous fat. Recently, lymphatic component has also been identified in lesions of BRBNS.

"You drown not by falling into a river, but by staying submerged in it." —**Paulo Coelho**

No immunohistochemical marker has yet been identified. Differential diagnosis of BRBNS includes hereditary hemorrhagic telangiectasia, Klippel–Trenaunay syndrome, and Maffucci syndrome. Basic evaluation includes complete blood count, coagulation tests, stool guaiac test and a urinary sample for the detection of occult bleeding, evaluation of the bleeding site, depending on the location (e.g., abdominal radiography, barium studies, endoscopy, colonoscopy, and angiography). Computed tomography and MRI can be helpful in visualizing internal lesions in patients and in evaluating asymptomatic family members.

There is no curative therapy for BRBNS at present. Treatment for cutaneous lesions is indicated when cosmetically unacceptable or when function is compromised. Laser ablation (Ruby, argon, CO_2, PDL), electrodessication, scalpel excision, and injection sclerotherapy can be used for the cutaneous lesions. Oral iron supplementation, steroids, interferon alpha-2, and octreotide have been used for GI manifestations. Sirolimus has shown to be safe and efficient for the treatment of BRBNS, when other therapies have been ineffective.

KLIPPEL–TRENAUNAY SYNDROME (FIGS. 7 AND 8)

Klippel–Trenaunay syndrome/disease (KTD) is a triad of vascular malformation [port-wine stain (PWS)], venous varicosity, and hyperplasia of soft tissue and bone. All these three malformations are usually distributed on the same extremity. When there is arteriovenous malformation, it is called Parkes Weber syndrome. Parkes Weber syndrome may have associated lymphatic malformations also in the form of lymphoedema, lymphangiectasia, lymphangioma circumscriptum, etc. Varicosities often develop with aging.

Complications: Recurrent thrombophlebitis, coagulopathy, congestive heart failure, pulmonary embolism, stasis dermatitis, cutaneous ulceration, and bleeding. Various other complications are kyphoscoliosis, dislocation of hips, facial asymmetry, and dental malocclusion.

Treatment: It is basically supportive. Compression bandages and laser therapy for cutaneous vascular malformations. Orthopedic and surgical interventions are required when there is limb discrepancy. Physical and occupational therapy may be required.

PARKES WEBER SYNDROME [FIGS. 9A TO B(iii)]

Parkes Weber syndrome is a rare congenital disease that is associated with abnormal blood vessels. It is mainly characterized by a capillary malformation, bony hypertrophy, and soft tissue growth in the affected limb and arteriovenous fistula. There may be discordant limb growth along with occasional pain. An abnormal mutation of the *RASA1* gene has been suspected in certain cases which has an autosomal dominant mode of inheritance.

Signs and associated symptoms of Parkes Weber syndrome may be the following:

- Birthmarks in the form of capillary malformation or PWS which are cosmetically disfiguring.

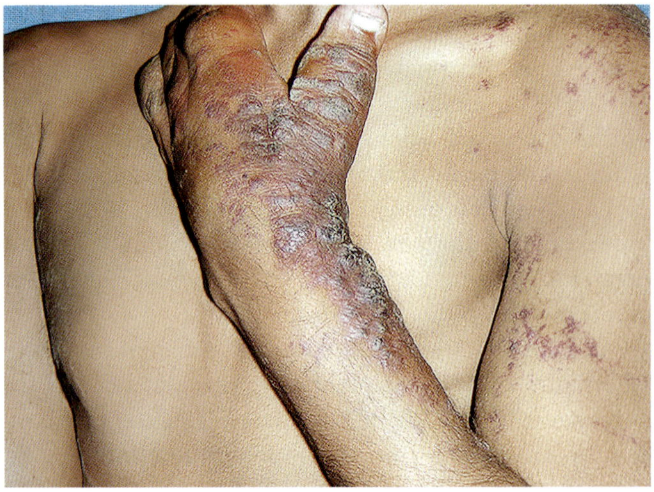

Fig. 7: Klippel–Trenaunay syndrome, note hypertrophy of forearm and hand.

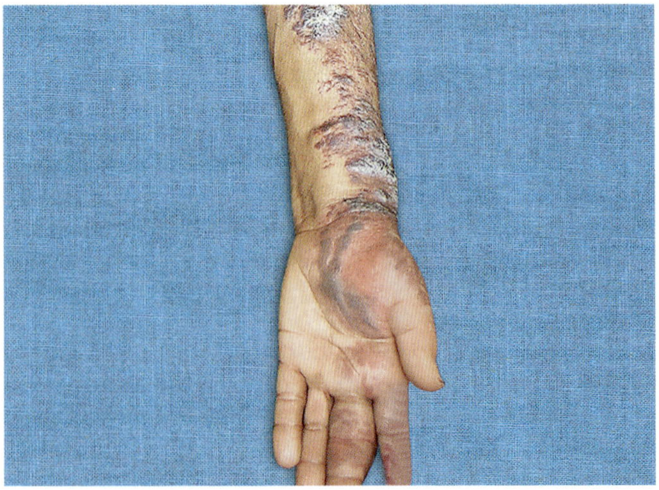

Fig. 8: Close-up view of same patient.

"Everything can be taken from a man but one thing: the last of the human freedoms – to choose one's attitude in any given set of circumstances, to choose one's own way." —**Viktor Frankl**

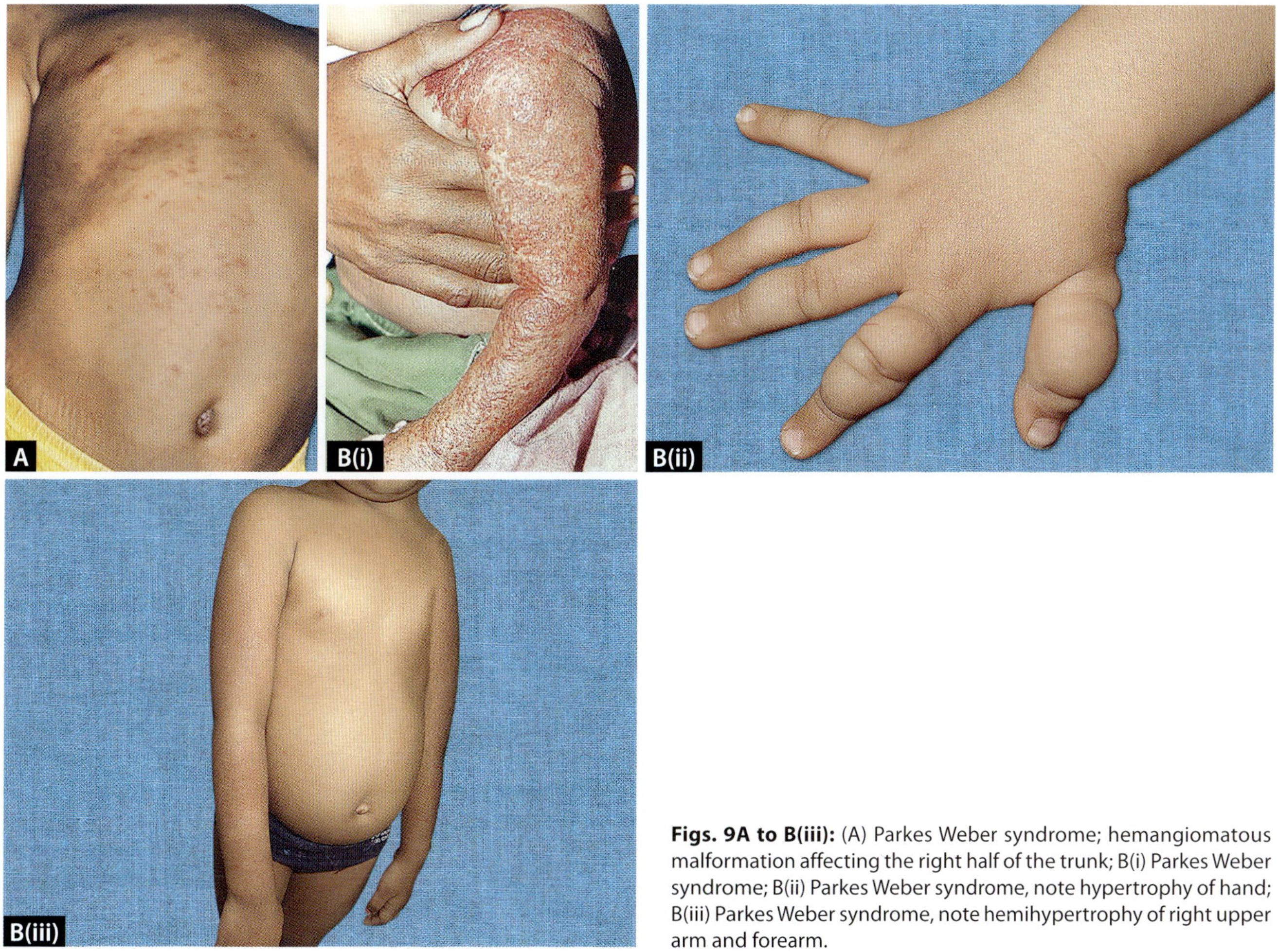

Figs. 9A to B(iii): (A) Parkes Weber syndrome; hemangiomatous malformation affecting the right half of the trunk; B(i) Parkes Weber syndrome; B(ii) Parkes Weber syndrome, note hypertrophy of hand; B(iii) Parkes Weber syndrome, note hemihypertrophy of right upper arm and forearm.

- Excessive growth of bones and soft tissue which may lead to limb length discordance and functional impairment.
- Arteriovenous malformations leading to fistulas which can cause hemorrhage and heart failure.

Diagnosis is based on typical clinical features along with a thorough physical examination and radiological and laboratory examinations. Genetic testing and counseling may be offered to parents as the disease, if caused due to gene mutation, has an autosomal dominant mode of inheritance.

The treatment of this condition is mainly symptomatic and needs an interdisciplinary approach involving dermatologists, radiologists, neurologists, and orthopedicians.

Supportive therapy can be given with compression garments, limb prosthesis, etc.

STURGE–WEBER SYNDROME [FIGS. 9C(i) AND (ii)]

Sturge–Weber syndrome (SWS), also called as encephalotrigeminal angiomatosis, clinically presents as triad of PWS over ophthalmic division of trigeminal (Vth) nerve, leptomeningeal hemangiomatosis manifesting as convulsion, and ocular involvement manifesting as glaucoma.

Seizures often are common features of SWS and may start below 1-year of age. PWS almost always affects ophthalmic division of Vth nerve. However, with V_1, V_2, and V_3 involvement the risk of SWS is more. Bilateral PWS involvement is associated with greater risk of central nervous system. PWS tends to darken and becomes hypertrophied with age and may develop multiple vascular nodules such as pyogenic granuloma. Other features are headache, neurocognitive, and

"Be a lifelong student. The more you learn, the more you earn and more self-confidence you will have." —**Brian Tracy**

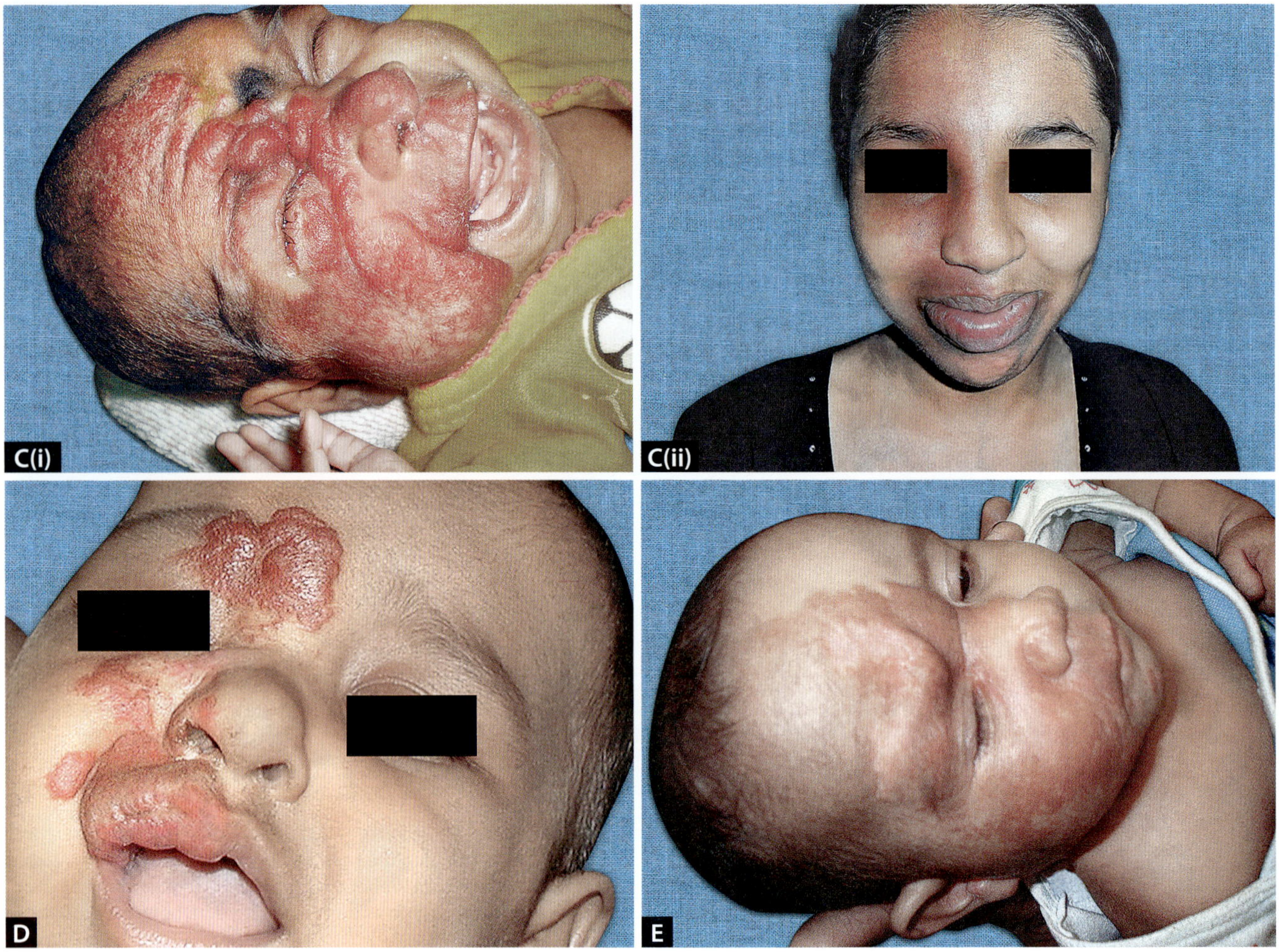

Figs. 9C(i) to E: C(i) Sturge–Weber syndrome; C(ii) Sturge–Weber syndrome; (D) Child with PHACES syndrome; (E) PHACES syndrome.

behavioral problems. Leptomeningeal involvement is very common and is present ipsilateral to the cutaneous vascular stain. Cerebral atrophy and intracranial calcification are usually picked up by MRI. Glaucoma is seen in 60% cases with SWS. Other ocular features include buphthalmos, blindness, and nevus of Ota.

Management is mainly multidisciplinary approach. Treatment of PWS is mainly for aesthetic reasons. Pulsed dye laser has been useful for treating PWS. Seizure is basically controlled with pharmacologic therapy. In intractable cases, hemispherectomy may be required.

PHACES SYNDROME (FIGS. 9D AND E)

The PHACES syndrome is an uncommon association with infantile hemangioma. It is a constellation of features that include central nervous system abnormalities (posterior fossa malformations), hemangioma, arterial anomalies, cardiac abnormalities (coarctation of aorta), eye abnormalities and sternal defect; 90% of the affected children are females. PHACES syndrome is commonly seen with large facial hemangioma, although not always. CNS abnormalities include Dandy-Walker malformation, cerebellar hypoplasia and dysplasia. Seizures and developmental delay have been associated. Coarctation of aorta involves transverse aorta. Most common eye abnormalities seen are 'morning glory anomaly', increased vascularity, micropthalmia, congenital cataract and optic nerve hypoplasia. A child presenting with extensive facial hemangioma should be thoroughly examined and investigated for PHACES syndrome. Echocardiogram, MRI of brain and periodic ophthalmological and neurological assessment should be considered. Regular follow-up of the child will prevent morbidities.

"Who looks outside, dreams; who looks inside, awakes." —**Carl Jung**

DIFFUSE NEONATAL HEMANGIOMATOSIS (FIGS. 9F TO I)

Cutaneous hemangiomas are common benign tumors found in infants either as single lesion or multiple ones. They are mostly cosmetically deforming if present on exposed parts of the body, but if present over major underlying structures, they can cause certain difficulties.

Cutaneous hemangiomas, if present along with visceral hemangiomas, lead to an uncommon condition known as diffuse neonatal hemangiomatosis (DNH). Hemangiomatosis is said to occur when more than 5 lesions are present on the body. Mostly this condition is benign, but it can be associated with a mortality risk varying between 50 and 90%. While visceral hemangiomas can affect any organ in the body, the sites where these are most found are liver, central nervous system, GI tract, and lungs. There are many reports of sporadic occurence in bones. Skin lesions can be extensive and range from 50 to 500 in number with size 5–15 mm in diameter.

The most common cause of mortality depends upon the system affected; thus, it may be due to massive hemorrhage if present in the liver or GI tract, or high-output cardiac failure if there exists an arteriovenous shunt in the liver.

What leads to the development of DNH is unknown although a genetic factor is thought to be associated with their formation. These vascular lesions have a proliferating endothelial lining. Caucasian babies are more prone to developing DNH with a female preponderance. As the visceral hemangiomas enlarge, they steal blood from the heart and can progress to heart failure.

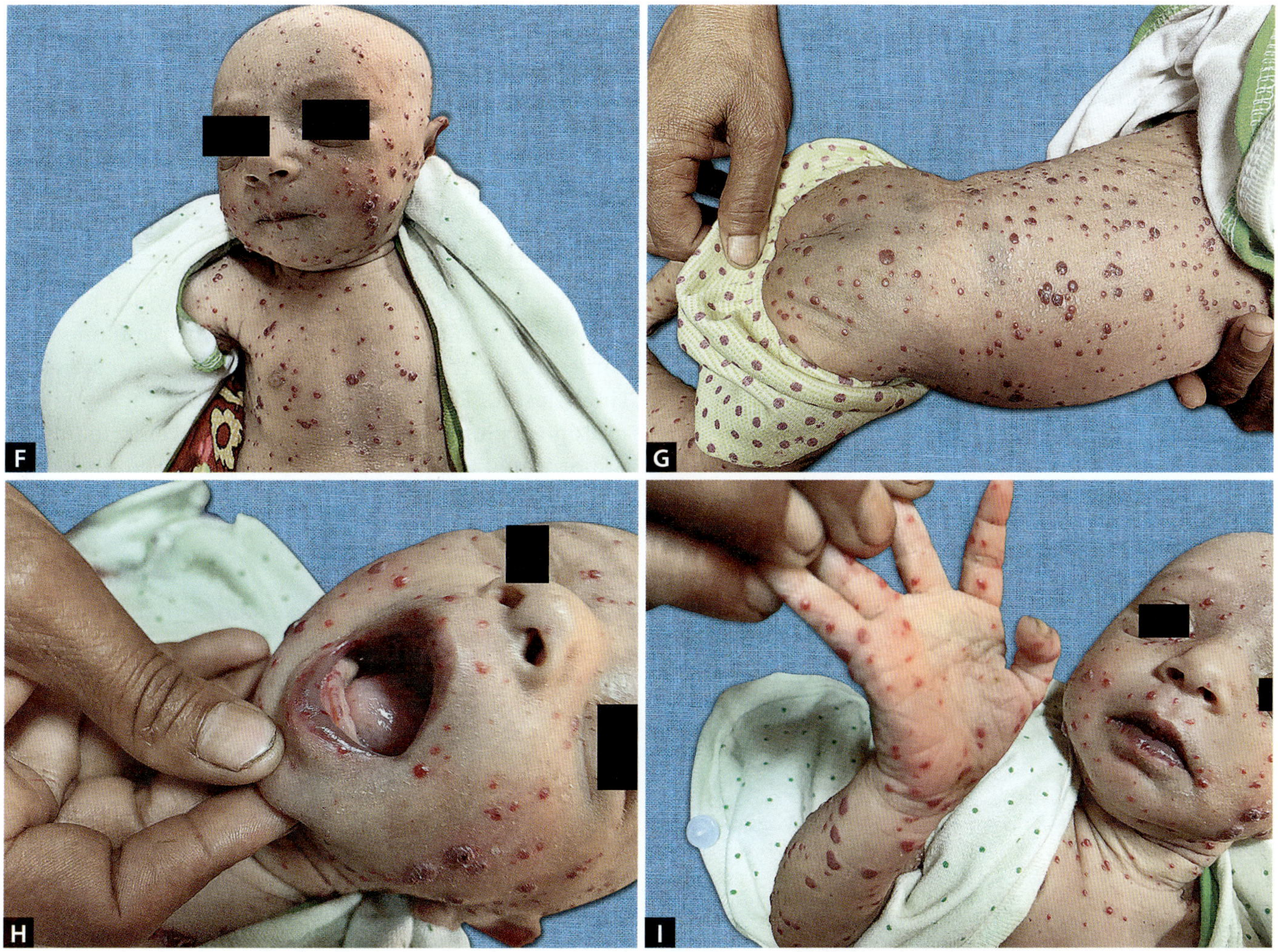

Figs. 9F to I: (F) Diffuse neonatal hemangiomatosis (DNH); (G) Same baby, look at back lesions; (H) DNH with mucosal involvement; (I) DNH with palmar lesions.

"Should you find yourself in a chronically leaking boat, energy devoted to changing vessels is likely to be more productive than energy devoted to patching leaks." —**Warren Buffett**

Diagnosis of these visceral hemangiomas is done using color flow Doppler sonography. Features include hypo- or hyper-echoic areas with acoustic enhancement. Hypervascular flow can be seen on Doppler. Sonographically, it can be distinguished from metastases, lymphomas, adenomas, etc.

So, when an infant presents with multiple cutaneous hemangiomas, a thorough physical examination must be undertaken along with a skin biopsy, complete blood counts, imaging of internal organs with sonography, and magnetic resonance imaging.

Once a diagnosis of DNH has been made, the main aim of treatment is to hasten the rate of involution of the hemangiomas while preventing the occurrence of the life-threatening complications. The treatment of choice involves the use of systemic steroids which can cause vasoconstriction and accelerate the involution of the hemangiomas. Oral propranolol therapy has also met with considerable success in DNH.

Radiation therapy was used in the past but has been abandoned due to the risk of development of other neoplasm. Other treatment options include interferon alpha 2a or 2b, partial liver resection, and hepatic artery embolization. An early and aggressive management protocol is essential for infants with DNH to ensure optimal survival.

ANGIOKERATOMA CIRCUMSCRIPTUM (FIGS. 10 AND 11A)

This condition is rare and characteristically takes the form of a fairly extensive hyperkeratotic vascular plaque usually present at birth. They are situated unilaterally on a lower leg or foot but can also occur on the thigh, buttock or any part of the body. They are deep red to blue-black in color and tend to take on a streaky banded or zosteriform appearance. The lesions become increasingly studded with warty, keratotic papules or nodules and may bleed easily on trauma. Clinically these lesions may be confused with arteriovenous malformation and lymphangioma circumscriptum. Angiokeratoma circumscriptum has been associated with Klippel–Trenaunay–Weber syndrome (KTWS), Cobb syndrome, nevus flammeus, and traumatic arteriovenous fistula.

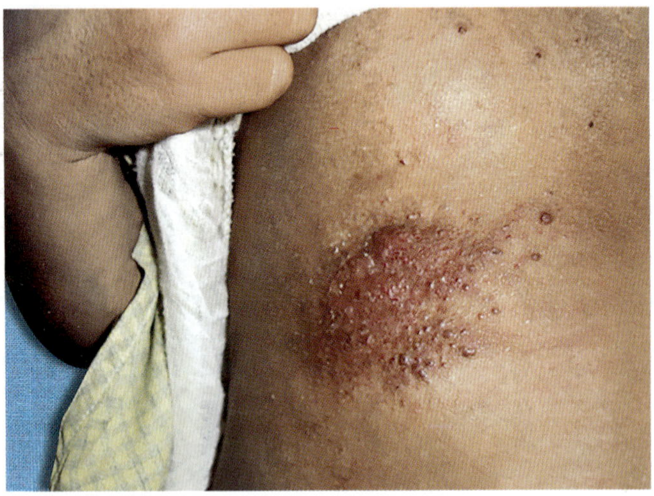

Fig. 10: Angiokeratoma lesions over the trunk, note clustering of lesions.

Natural History

Angiokeratoma circumscriptum does not show a tendency to spontaneous resolution.

Treatment

For small lesions excision, cryotherapy, electrodessication or pulse dye laser are the therapeutic options. For large lesions, extensive excision surgery has to be done. Lesions over lips, tongue, and oral mucosa may be treated with either electrodessication or laser therapy.

PYOGENIC GRANULOMA [FIGS. 11B TO C(ii)]

It is a common, acquired vascular lesion which presents as a smooth, lobulated, small papule or papulonodule, sometimes with a peduncle. Usually it presents as single lesion. However, on rare occasions there may be multiple lesions. The lesions mostly develop following minor trauma and have a tendency to bleed profusely. The common sites are fingers, hands, feet, toes, and lips.

Treatment

The treatment of choice is excision. Other modalities include cryotherapy, electrocautery, curettage, sclerotherapy, and laser therapy. Topical timolol 0.5% has been useful in managing small lesions.

ANGIOLYMPHOID HYPERPLASIA WITH EOSINOPHILIA [FIG. 11C(iii)]

Angiolymphoid hyperplasia with eosinophilia is a rare benign, disfiguring vascular proliferation rarely seen in children. Initially angiolymphoid hyperplasia was considered as part of Kimura's disease, but recently it is described as a distinct entity. It presents as erythematous

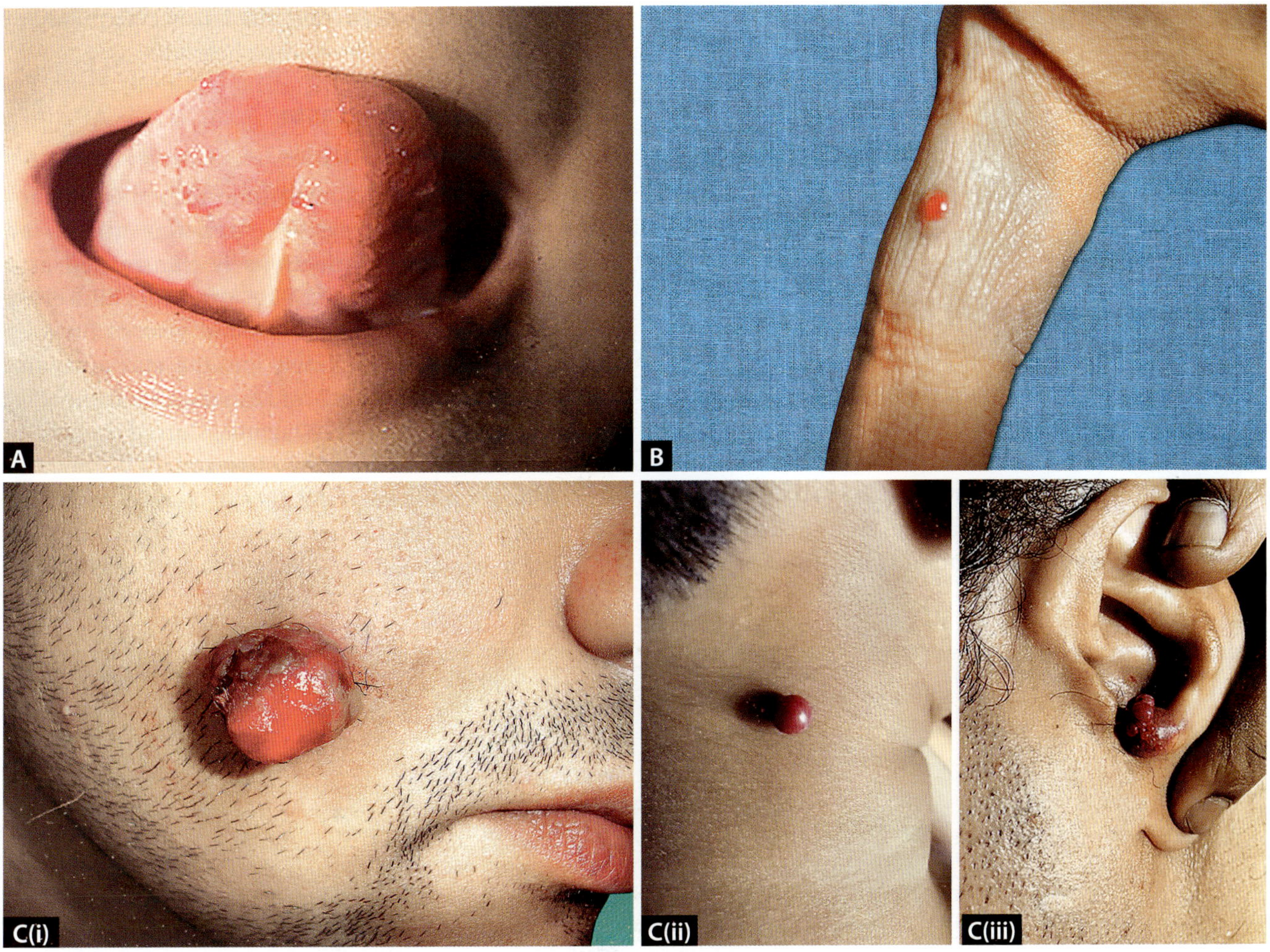

Figs. 11A to C(iii): (A) Angiokeratoma circumscriptum over tongue (a rare presentation); (B) Granuloma pyogenicum (GP); C(i) Close-up view of GP; C(ii) GP over neck; C(iii) Angiolymphoid hyperplasia.

or skin colored papules and nodules on head and neck region especially around the ears. It can be associated with pain, spontaneous bleeding, pulsation, pruritus, and hypertrophy. Eosinophilia can be seen in 20% cases. Lymphadenopathy is uncommon. Rarely lower lip and lower back in zosteriform distribution has been reported. Histopathological findings include proliferation of small to medium sized blood vessels lined by endothelial cells along with perivascular inflammatory infiltrate of lymphocytes and eosinophils. Extracutaneous involvement is rarely seen. The treatment of choice is surgical excision. Other modalities of treatment include cryotherapy, laser ablation, steroids, radiation, and chemotherapy.

GLOMUS TUMOR

It is a benign growth or hamartoma of "glomus body". Glomus body is the temperature regulating arteriovenous shunt (AV shunt). The "glomus cells" which proliferate in this disorder are modified smooth muscle cells.

Glomus tumor presents as solitary or multiple bluish papules or nodules and look like venous prominences. Glomus tumors are painful and associated with cold sensitivity.

Differential Diagnoses

- Blue rubber bleb nevus syndrome
- Leiomyoma
- Blue nevus
- Melanoma

Treatment

Surgical excision is the main treatment for solitary glomus tumor. For multiple lesions, sclerotherapy, carbon dioxide laser are effective. Subungual glomus tumor is treated surgically.

"You can do anything if you have enthusiasm." —**Henry Ford**

TELANGIECTASIA (FIGS. 11D AND E)

These are permanent dilatation of capillaries, venules or arterioles in the skin. On pressure with a glass slide the telangiectases blanch completely. This is called positive "diascopy" test. The cause of telangiectases may be either primary defect or secondary to prolonged sun exposure, collagen vascular disorders, chronic liver disease, etc.

Generalized (Benign) Essential Telangiectasia [Fig. 11F(i)]

It is a disorder of multiple cutaneous telangiectases without bleeding diathesis. The condition is usually widespread, progressive and permanent, and girls are more commonly affected than boys. The lower limbs are usually affected. Involvement of oral mucosa and conjunctiva is very uncommon. The etiology is unknown. The treatment of this condition is usually not required. However, pulsed dye or Nd:YAG laser treatment may be helpful.

Ataxia Telangiectasia [Figs. 11F(ii) and (iii)]

Ataxia telangiectasia, a syndrome of oculocutaneous telangiectasias, progressive cerebellar ataxia, and recurrent respiratory infections is transmitted as an autosomal recessive trait. The affected children are apparently normal until the second year of life when they are noticed to be clumsy and the ataxia becomes progressive so that by the age of 12 years, they are unable to walk without assistance. Nystagmus, slurred speech, and mental deterioration may be observed. Telangiectasias usually develop between the ages of 3 and 5 years. They first appear on the bulbar conjunctiva and gradually involve the ear, eyelids, butterfly area of the cheeks, and

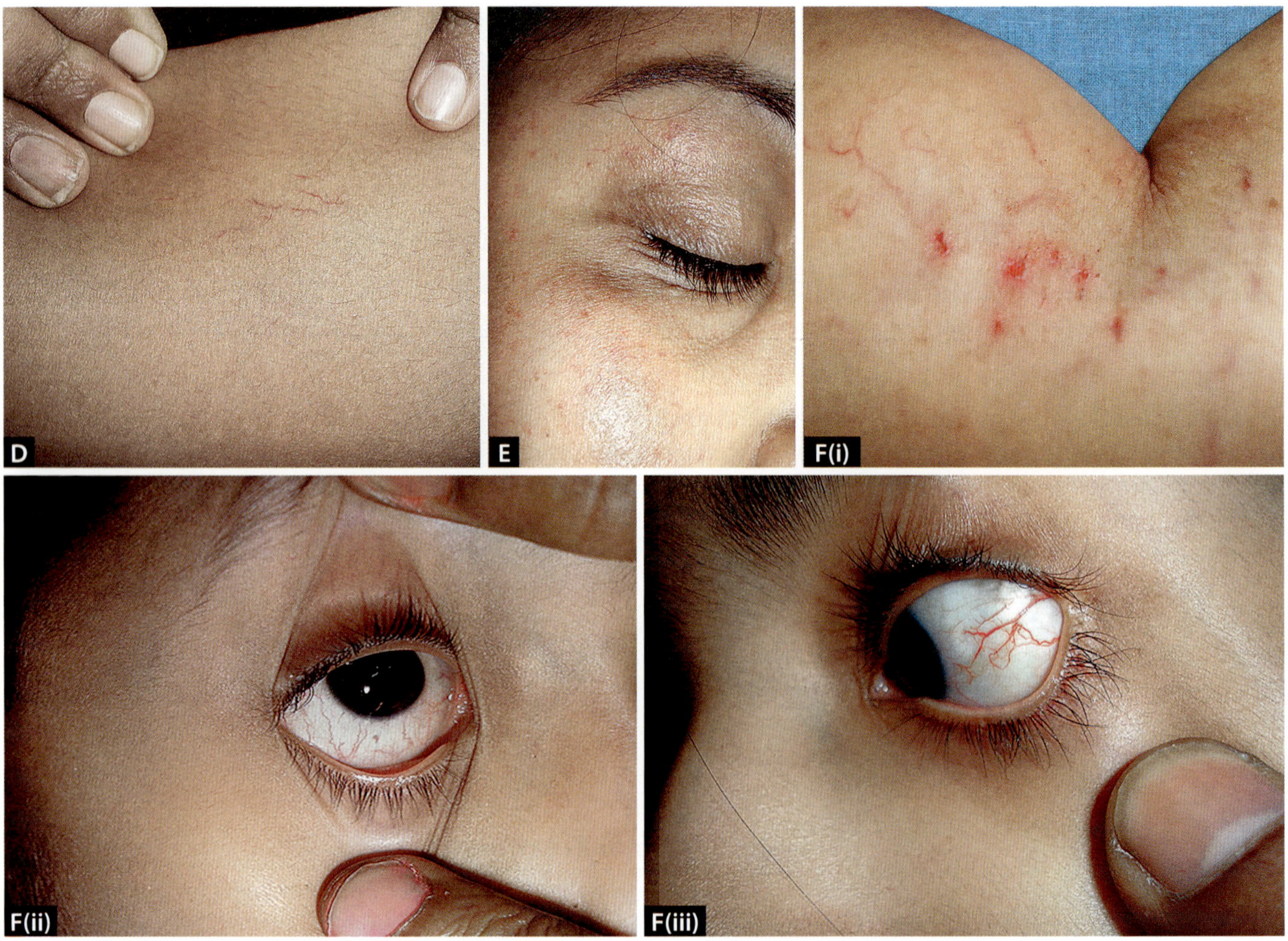

Figs. 11D to F(iii): (D) Telangiectasia; (E) Telangiectasia over face in an adolescent girl; F(i) Benign essential telangiectasia; F(ii) Telangiectasia over conjunctiva in ataxia telangiectasia; F(iii) Same child, close-up view.

"I am not what happened to me, I am what I chose to become." —**Carl Jung**

limbs. There may be some atrophy, dryness of skin, and premature aging. Disturbances of pigmentation and eczematous lesions may also occur. Mortality is due to chronic bronchiectasis, pulmonary insufficiency, pneumonia, and hematological malignancies.

PHAKOMATOSIS PIGMENTOVASCULARIS [FIGS. 11G(i) TO (iii)]

Phakomatosis pigmentovascularis is a term used to describe association of capillary malformation with pigmented nevi. It is a clinical diagnosis and classified into five types **(Table 1)**. Type II is more commonly seen. Type IIa is seen without extracutaneous involvement and type IIb is associated with extracutaneous involvement. Extracutaneous features include neurological abnormalities such as seizures, psychomotor retardation, cerebral atrophy, hydrocephalus and ophthalmic abnormalities such as conjunctival melanocytosis, glaucoma, and episcleral vascular malformation.

PIGMENTED PURPURIC DERMATOSES (FIGS. 11H TO K)

Pigmented purpuric dermatosis is a type of capillaritis and comprise a group of diseases which present as petechiae, purpura, and brownish hyperpigmentation around ankles and legs. These conditions, although occur mostly in adults, may affect children. Rarely, it may affect infants.

Schamberg's disease is the prototype for pigmented purpuric dermatoses (PPD) in which there are red brown punctate macules and many of them coalesce to form red-brown patches. There are no symptoms such as itching, pain or burning sensation. Various other types are Majocchi disease or annular pigmented purpura, lichen aureus where lichenoid golden brown lesions are seen, eczematid-like purpura of Doucas and Kapetanakis, and lichenoid lesions of Gougerot and Blum.

Various treatment options are topical steroid, short course of oral steroid for rapidly spreading lesions, and phototherapy. Oral pentoxifylline can be given to children above 12 years of age.

PURPURA FULMINANS (FIGS. 11L TO P)

Purpura fulminans is an acute condition which is characterized by development of hemorrhagic necrosis of skin with disseminated intravascular coagulation. It is more common in infants and children than adults and usually follows meningococcal infections, rickettsial infections, post-scarlet fever, varicella or pneumococcal infection.

Table 1: Classification of phakomatosis pigmentovascularis.

Type	Vascular lesion	Cutaneous lesion
I	Nevus flammeus	Epidermal nevus
II	Nevus flammeus ± nevus anemicus	Dermal melanocytosis
III	Nevus flammeus ± nevus anemicus	Nevus spilus
IV	Nevus flammeus ± nevus anemicus	Dermal melanocytosis ± nevus spilus
V	Cutis marmorata telangiectatica congenita	Dermal melanocytosis

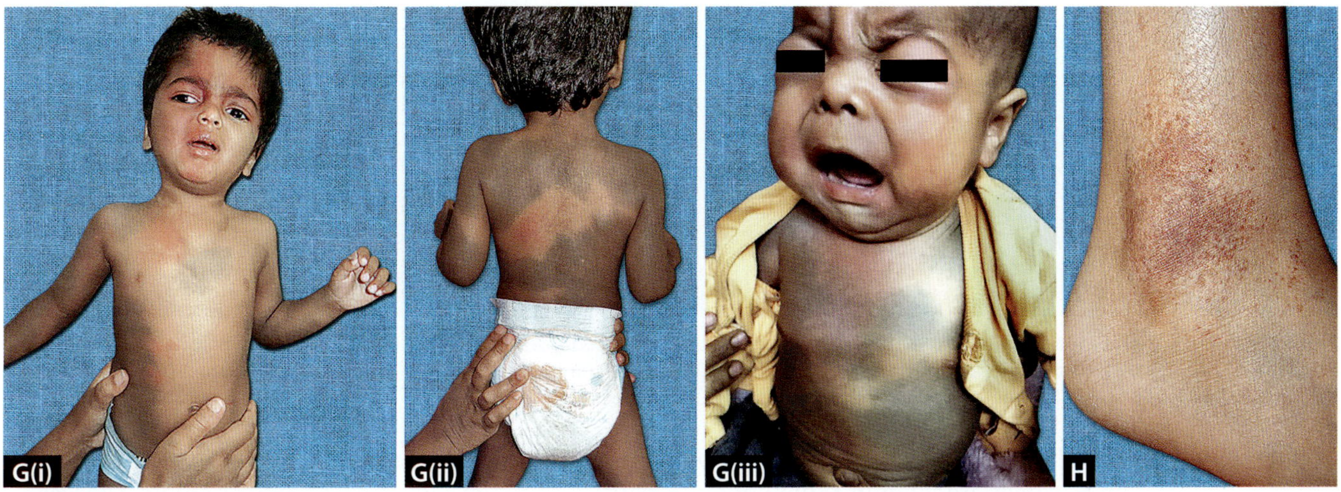

Figs. 11G(i) to H: G(i) Phakomatosis pigmentovascularis; G(ii) Same child, close-up view of back; G(iii) Phakomatosis pigmentovascularis, close-up view of face and trunk; (H) Pigmented purpuric dermatoses lesions around ankle.

"Knowledge is learning something every day. Wisdom is letting go of something every day." **—Zen Proverb**

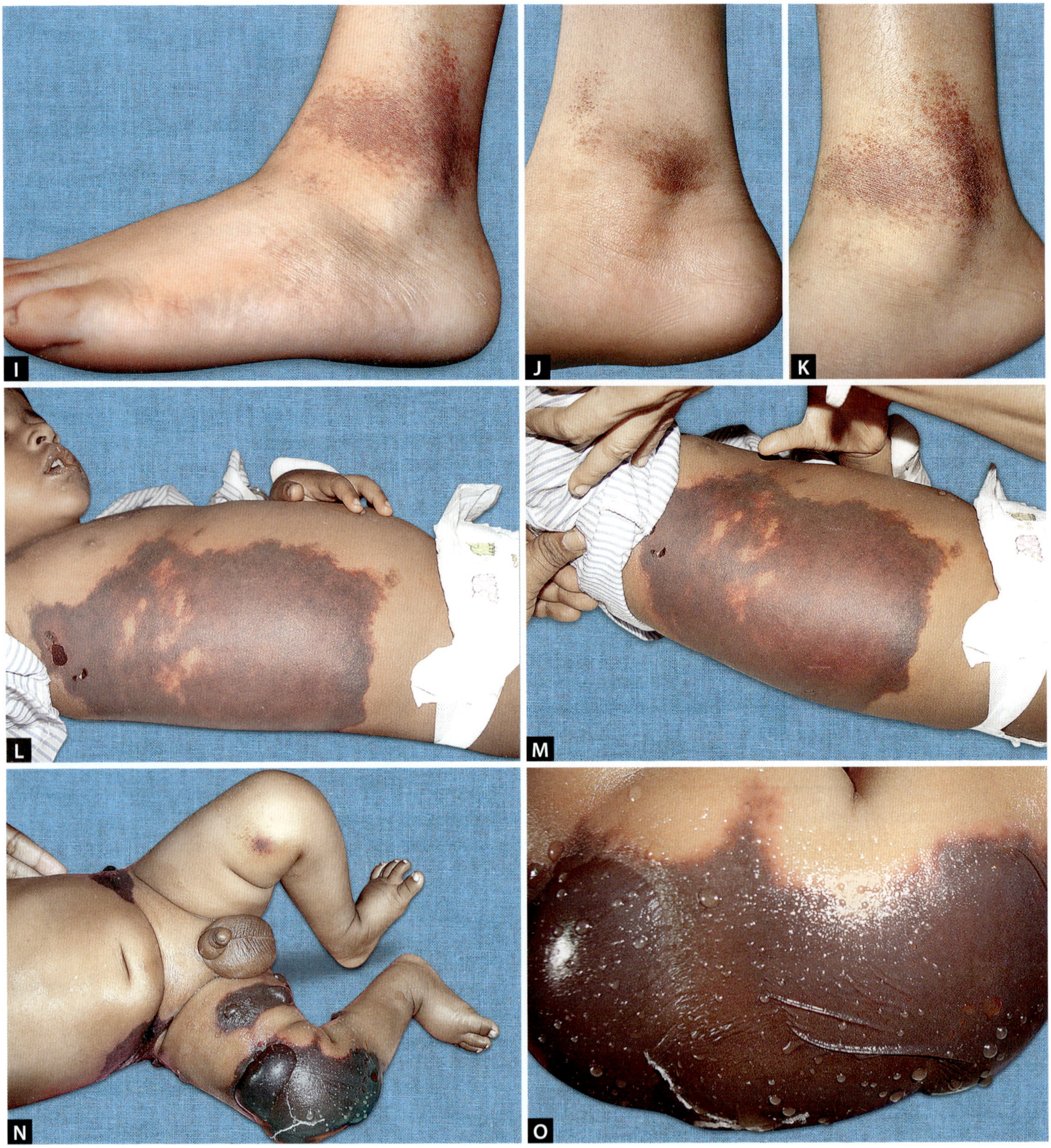

Figs. 11I to O: (I) Pigmented purpuric dermatitis around ankle; (J) Pigmented purpuric dermatitis, note golden color and hemorrhagic appearance; (K) Pigmented purpuric dermatitis, close-up view; (L) Purpura fulminans; (M) Close-up view, note jagged border of lesions; (N) Purpura fulminans in an infant, note large hemorrhagic blisters; (O) Same baby, close-up view.

The condition is related to the deficiency or absence of protein C or protein S, which are vitamin K-dependent glycoproteins with antithrombotic properties.

The condition presents as tender, ecchymoses particularly often with sharp irregular borders. The lesions are mostly located over legs and spread rapidly over thigh,

"Some people come in our life as blessings, some come in your life as lessons." —**Mother Teresa**

buttocks, and trunk. The condition is usually associated with high fever, prostration, and features of toxicities.

Laboratory investigation shows thrombocytopenia and decreased fibrinogen. The prothrombin time and partial thromboplastin time are prolonged and fibrin degradation products are increased. Protein C, protein S, and thrombin III levels are decreased.

Management of purpura fulminans depends on treatment of associated infection. Initial management includes fluid resuscitation, ventilator support, and parenteral antibiotics. Administration of protein C or S, wound care, debridement, amputation, and skin grafting may be necessary.

LYMPHANGIOMA CIRCUMSCRIPTUM (FIGS. 12 TO 14C)

The term describes a lymphatic malformation which is localized to an area of skin, subcutaneous tissue, and sometimes muscle. The lesions are usually noted at birth or appear during childhood. The common sites being axillary folds, shoulders, flanks, proximal parts of limbs, and perineum. They present as fluid-filled vesicles which bulge on the skin surface. The vesicles may be well defined and discrete or grouped into structures resembling "frog spawn". The lymphangiomas may be translucent when the over lying epidermis is very thin or they may vary in color from red to blue-black when containing blood. The

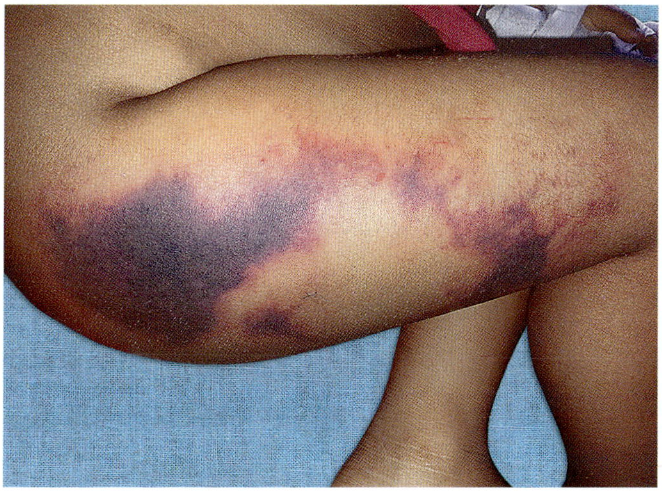

Fig. 11P: Purpura fulminans (early lesion).

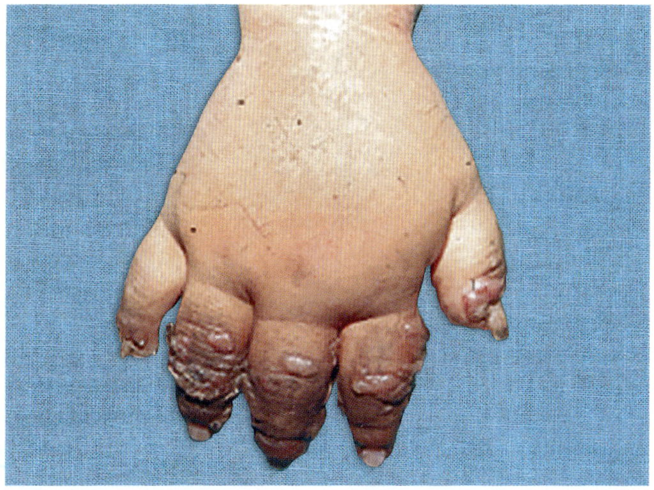

Fig. 12: Involvement of multiple fingers with gross swelling of hand in lymphangioma circumscriptum.

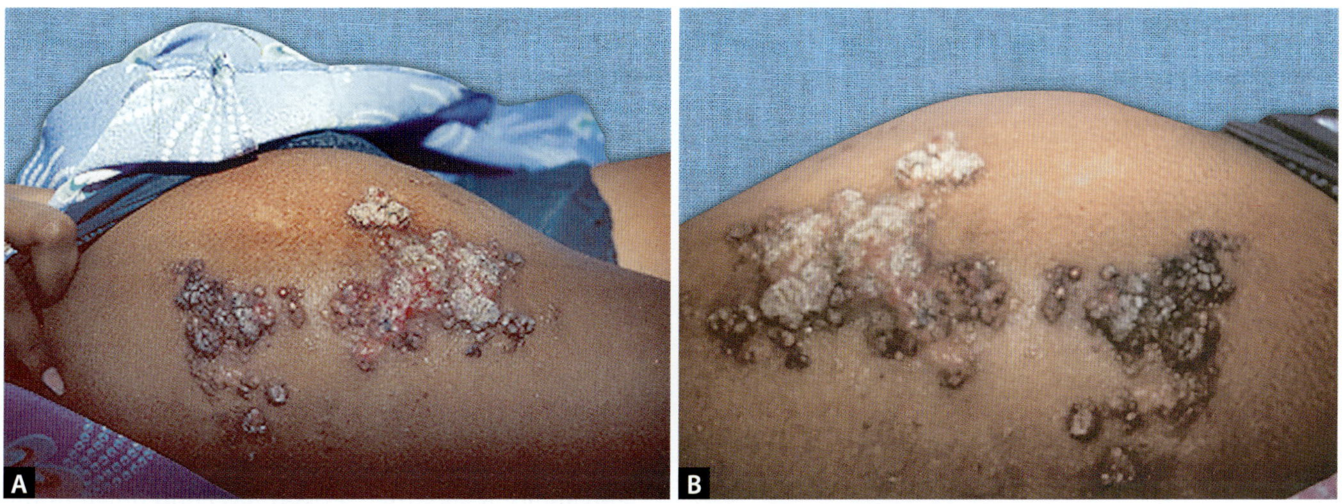

Figs. 13A and B: (A) Lymphangioma circumscriptum over buttock, note hemorrhagic lesions; (B) Close-up view.

"There is only one thing that makes a dream impossible to achieve, the fear of failure." —**Paulo Coelho**

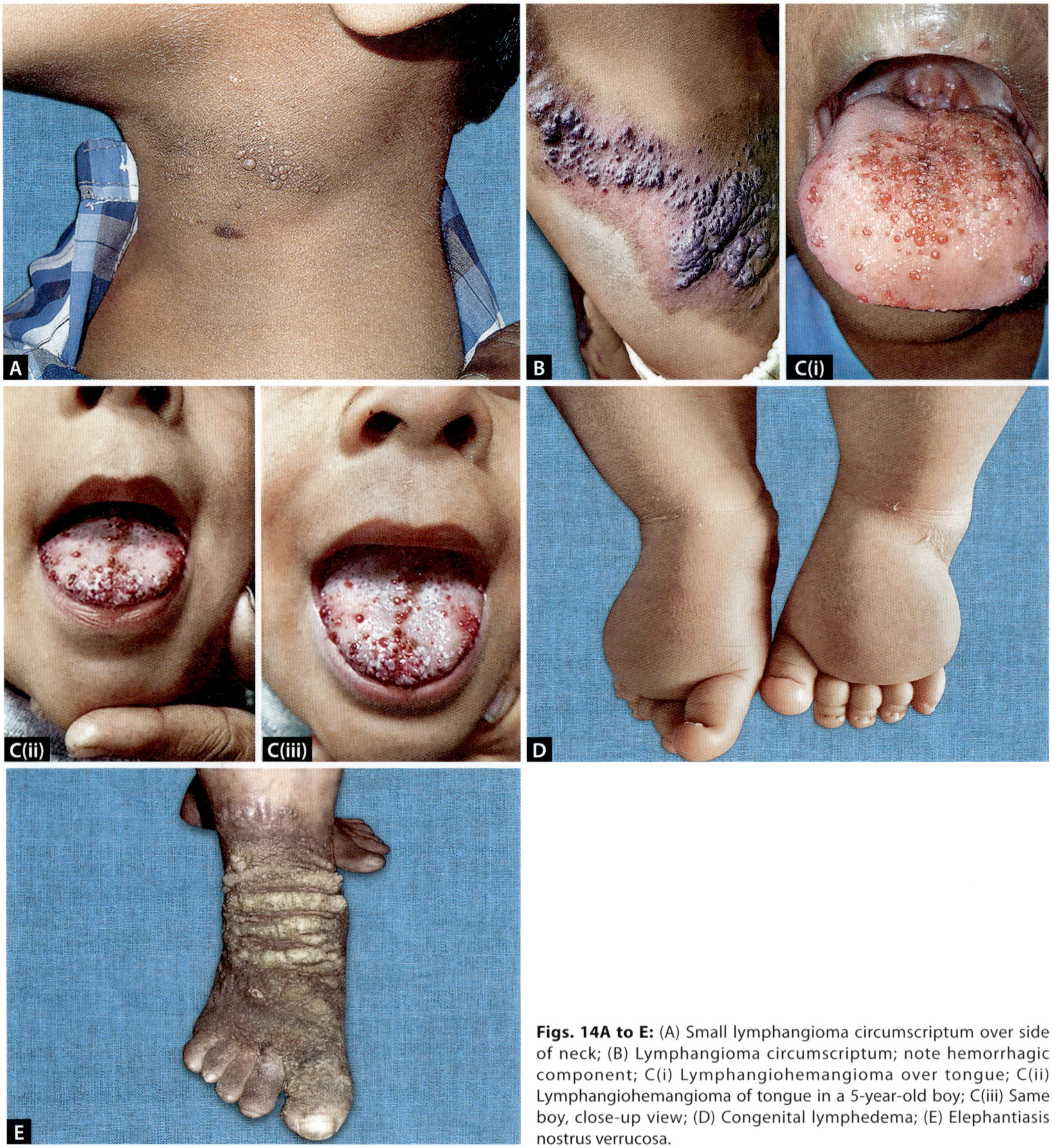

Figs. 14A to E: (A) Small lymphangioma circumscriptum over side of neck; (B) Lymphangioma circumscriptum; note hemorrhagic component; C(i) Lymphangiohemangioma over tongue; C(ii) Lymphangiohemangioma of tongue in a 5-year-old boy; C(iii) Same boy, close-up view; (D) Congenital lymphedema; (E) Elephantiasis nostrus verrucosa.

presence of limb swelling suggests extensive underlying lymphatic abnormality. There may be associated hemangiomatous component in a good number of cases (Lymphangiohemangioma). In such cases the lesions may suddenly increase in size because of sudden bleeding into lymphatic spaces.

Treatment

Electrosurgery or cryosurgery is of little help in cases of lymphangioma circumscriptum.

If surgery is required, a deep resection down to the fascial plane with extensive, excision repair has to be done.

"Don't let the noise of others' opinions drown out your own inner voice. Have the courage to follow your own heart and intuition." —**Steve Jobs**

Since lymphatic channels are innumerable and highly ramifying, recurrences are not uncommon. Recently, topical rapamycin has shown good results in management of small lymphangioma.

LYMPHEDEMA (FIG. 14D)

Lymphedema is characterized by soft tissue swelling due to accumulation of excess amount of protein rich lymph due to output failure. In chronic cases edema becomes nonpitting. Lymphedema can be classified as below:

Primary lymphedema (intrinsic defects in lymphatic channels):

- Congenital lymphedema (Milroy's disease)
- Lymphedema praecox
- Lymphedema tarda.

Syndromes associated with primary lymphedema: Turner syndrome, Noonan syndrome, Yellow nail syndrome, Proteus syndrome, Emberger syndrome, Distichiasis-lymphedema syndrome.

Cutaneous disorders associated with primary lymphedema: Hemangiomas, congenital absence of nail, xanthomatosis with chylous lymphedema.

Secondary lymphedema:

- *Iatrogenic*: Radiotherapy, radical lymph node dissection, postmastectomy
- *Infection*: Recurrent bacterial cellulitis/lymphangitis, filariasis, lymphogranuloma venereum
- *Inflammatory*: Rosacea, sarcoidosis, rheumatoid arthritis, lymphedema of upper limb due to recurrent eczema
- *Malignancy*: Hodgkin lymphoma, Kaposi sarcoma
- *Vascular*: Post phlebitis syndrome, venous ulcer
- *Factitial*: Repeated application of tourniquet to the wrist (Secretan's syndrome)
- *Others*: Bullous lymphedema due to congestive cardiac failure, podoconiosis, persistent hand edema of drivers.

Milroy's disease is characterized by unilateral/bilateral lymphedema of lower leg, predominantly affecting females and present since birth. Mode of inheritance is autosomal dominant with underlying inactivation of VEGFR-3, responsible for lymphangiogenesis. Genitalia, face, and arm can be involved.

Lymphedema praecox: It is the most common form of primary lymphedema predominantly affecting females and presents before 35 years of age. Underlying defect may be hypoplasia, aplasia or hyperplasia with varicose dilatation of lymphatic systems. Swelling starts from ankle and gradually moves upward to involve entire leg with a dull pain.

Lymphedema tarda accounts for <10% of cases and presents after 35 years of age.

The usual chief complaint of the patient suffering from lymphedema is heaviness and fatigue of the affected limb with gradual worsening of edema particularly toward evening which reduces on limb elevation. In chronic cases, edema becomes indurated and nonpitting. Squaring of the toe and difficulty in pinching the skin over second toe (Stemmer's sign) may be the presenting feature.

Alarming complications are recurrent cellulitis or lymphangitis. Ulceration, post-mastectomy lymphangiosarcoma (Stewart–Treves syndrome), elephantiasis verrucosa nostra cutis (thickening, hyperkeratosis, and pseudo papillary growth of overlying skin).

The investigation for confirmation of lymphedema is isotope lymphoscintigraphy. Many other investigations can be performed with their individual merits; duplex ultrasound to rule out venous pathology where CT scan to exclude any obstructing mass.

Permanent cure is impossible. Different modalities of treatment are used to offer the patient an acceptable quality of life starting from skin surface massage to improve lymphatic flow, limb elevation, graded compression stockings, pneumatic compression therapy, use of diuretics, antibiotic therapy to deal with episodes of cellulitis/lymphangitis, and long-term prophylaxis with ivermectin or diethylcarbamazine. Surgical therapy may aggravate the condition by obliterating lymphatic channels.

NEVUS OF OTA AND ITO (FIGS. 15 AND 16)

Nevus of Ota (nevus fusco-caeruleus ophthalmomaxillaris) presents as an extensive, blue, patch like area of dermal melanocytic pigmentation of the sclera and the skin adjacent to the eye in the distribution of first and second division of trigeminal nerve. It is more common in Asian people. The pigmentation is often speckled and is composed of deeper bluish and more superficial brownish elements which do not always coincide. This is best appreciated in the eye where the affected sclera is blue and the conjunctiva brown. The areas involved are the eyelids, the bulbar and palpebral conjunctiva, the sclera, cheeks, forehead, scalp, alae nasi, and ears.

"Your time is limited, don't waste it living someone else's life." —**Steve Jobs**

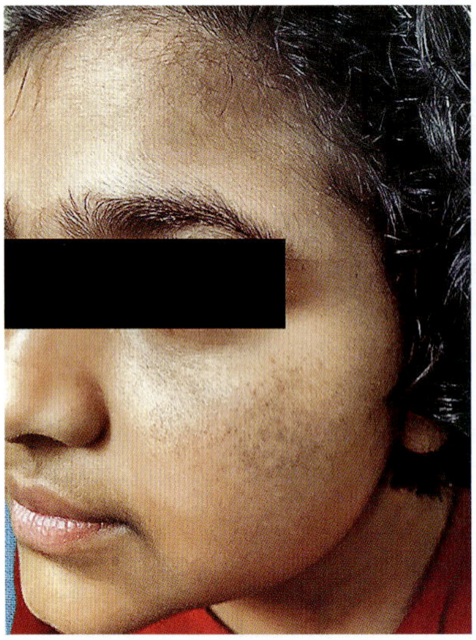

Fig. 15: Nevus of Ota.

The pigmented spots usually appear in childhood and increase in number and extent to become confluent in some areas. The nevus of Ito involves the acromioclavicular region and the upper chest and like Ota's, is largely confined to the Asian population. It can be associated with phakomatosis pigmentovascularis.

Management

The disorder is generally benign although it does not disappear spontaneously. Cosmetic camouflage can disguise the blemish. Recently Q-switched ruby laser or Argon laser has shown good results.

MELANOCYTIC NEVUS (FIGS. 17 TO 20H)

Melanocytic nevi are only rarely present at birth. Most nevi appear in adolescence or early childhood. However,

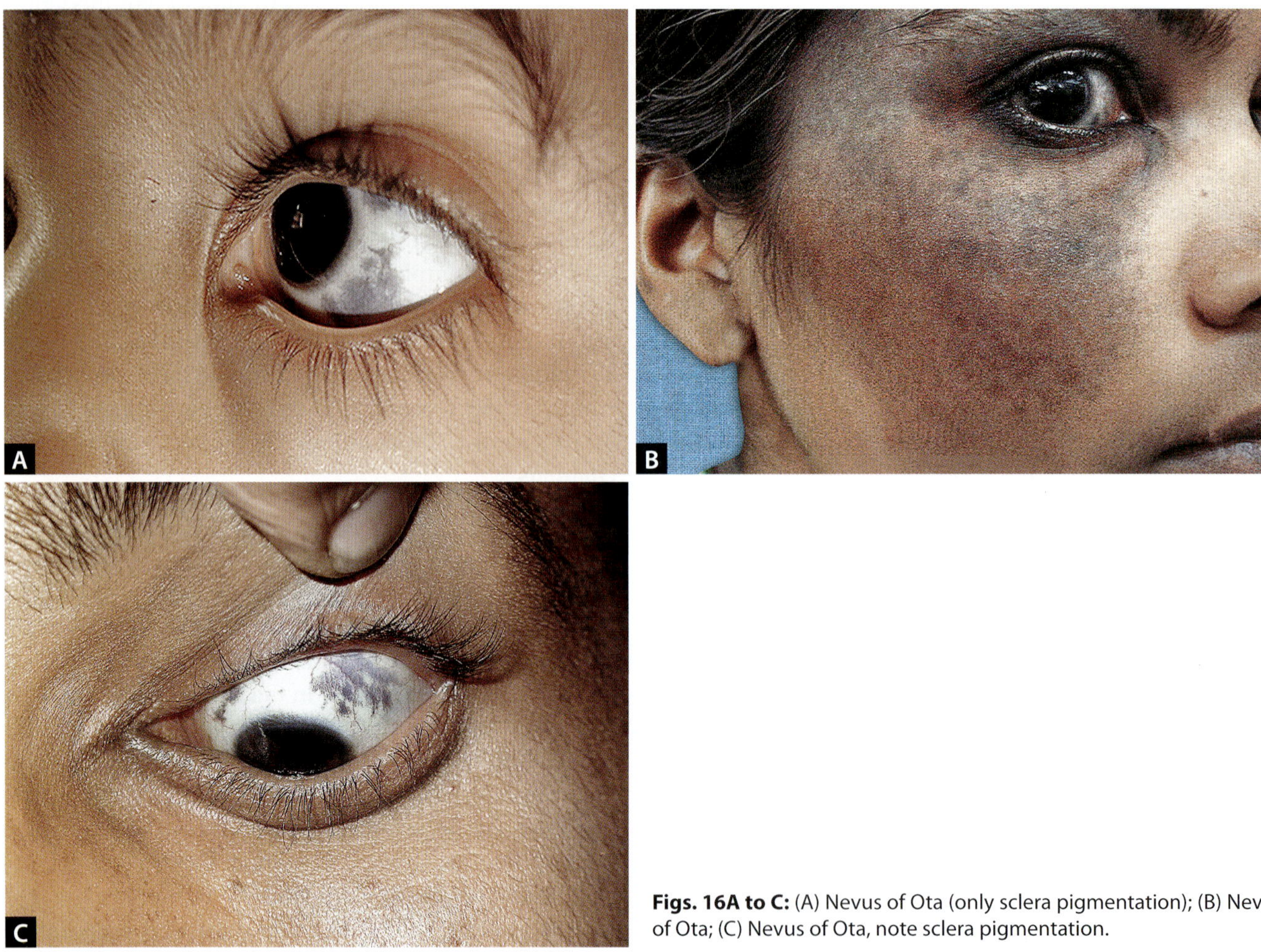

Figs. 16A to C: (A) Nevus of Ota (only sclera pigmentation); (B) Nevus of Ota; (C) Nevus of Ota, note sclera pigmentation.

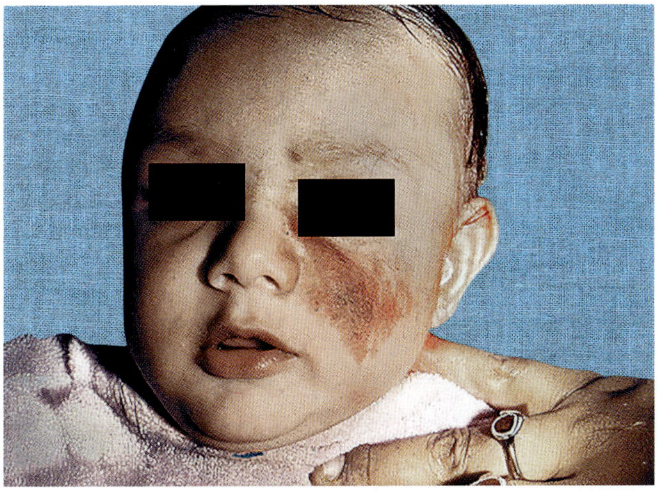

Fig. 17: Melanocytic nevus.

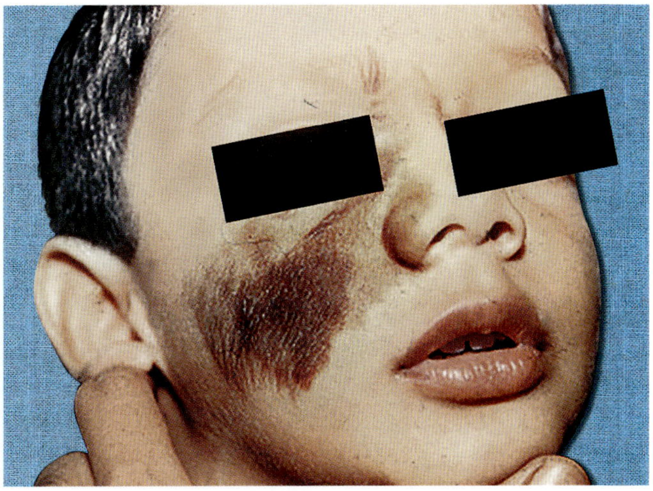

Fig. 18: Gradual growth of hair in a melanocytic nevus.

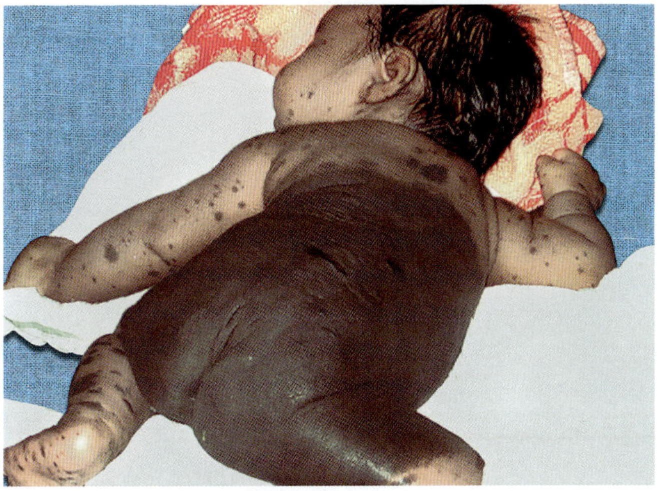

Fig. 19: Melanocytic nevus in a bathing trunk distribution in a newborn.

congenital nevi are found in about 1–2% of newborn infants. Congenital nevi are usually larger than acquired nevi, measuring from 1.5 to >20 cm in diameter. Giant congenital melanocytic nevus or bathing trunk nevus is present at birth. The common site is the lower back and thigh area and a very large proportion of the infant's surface area may be involved and often associated with hypertrichosis. Multiple satellite lesions may be seen along with giant congenital melanocytic nevi. Congenital melanocytic nevi with associated melanosis of central nervous system are termed as neurocutaneous melanosis.

Natural History

As the infant grows, the surface may become rugose or warty and nodules may develop on it. The hairy component present in 95% cases tends to become more prominent in late childhood but at this stage the nevus ceases to thicken and becomes paler. There is increased risk of transformation into malignancy especially malignant melanoma.

Systemic Association

There may be associated abnormalities such as meningeal involvement, spina bifida or meningocele when the nevus is over the vertebral column or club foot and hypertrophy or atrophy of the deeper structures of a limb. Congenital melanocytic nevi can be associated with neurological symptoms and leptomeningeal melanocytosis.

Management

For removal of small lesions, dermabrasion and Q-switched ruby laser therapy are recommended. In large congenital melanocytic nevi, advances in soft tissue expansion technique may add to cosmetic gain in surgical approaches.

BECKER'S NEVUS (FIGS. 20I AND J)

Also known as Becker's melanosis, it presents as an irregular macular hyperpigmentation with hypertrichosis characteristically seen on the shoulders, anterior chest, and scapular region of adolescent males.

Becker's nevus may begin in childhood, usually following exposure to sunlight in otherwise normal males (occasionally females), at or shortly after puberty. The first change generally appears as a grayish brown pigmentation on the chest, back or upper arm that spreads in an irregular

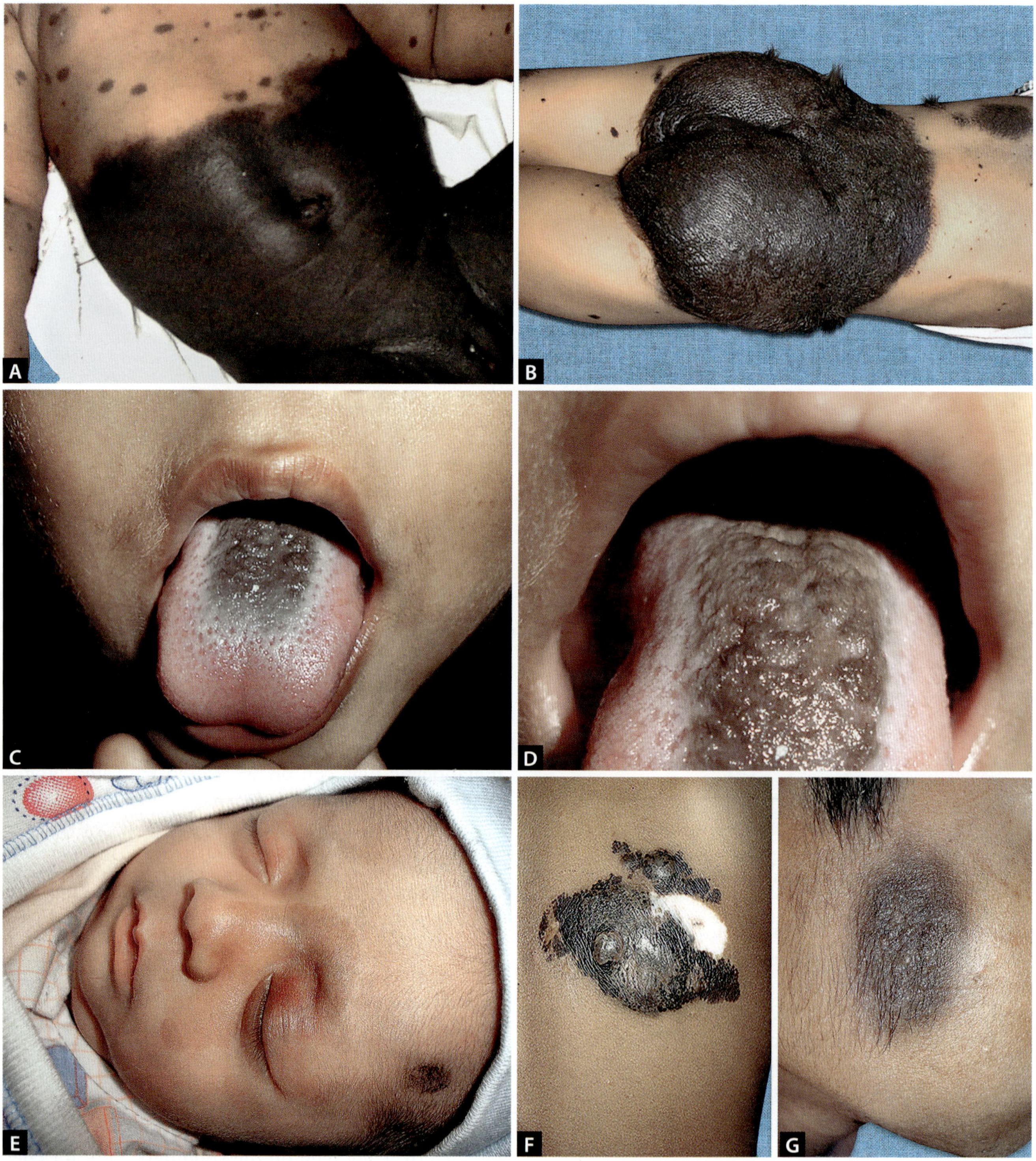

Figs. 20A to G: (A) Close-up view showing satellite lesions; (B) Giant hairy melanocytic nevus in a 5-year-old boy; (C) Melanocytic nevus over tongue in a 3-year-old boy; (D) Higher magnification; (E) Congenital melanocytic nevus at birth; (F) Melanocytic nevus, presence of depigmented patch is rare; (G) Melanocytic nevus over face in a school-going boy.

fashion until it reaches an area 10–15 cm in diameter (about the size of a hand or larger). The outline is sharply demarcated, irregular, and often surrounded by island of blotchy pigmentation. Although characteristically seen unilaterally on the upper half of the trunk, especially around the shoulder, it has also been reported in other

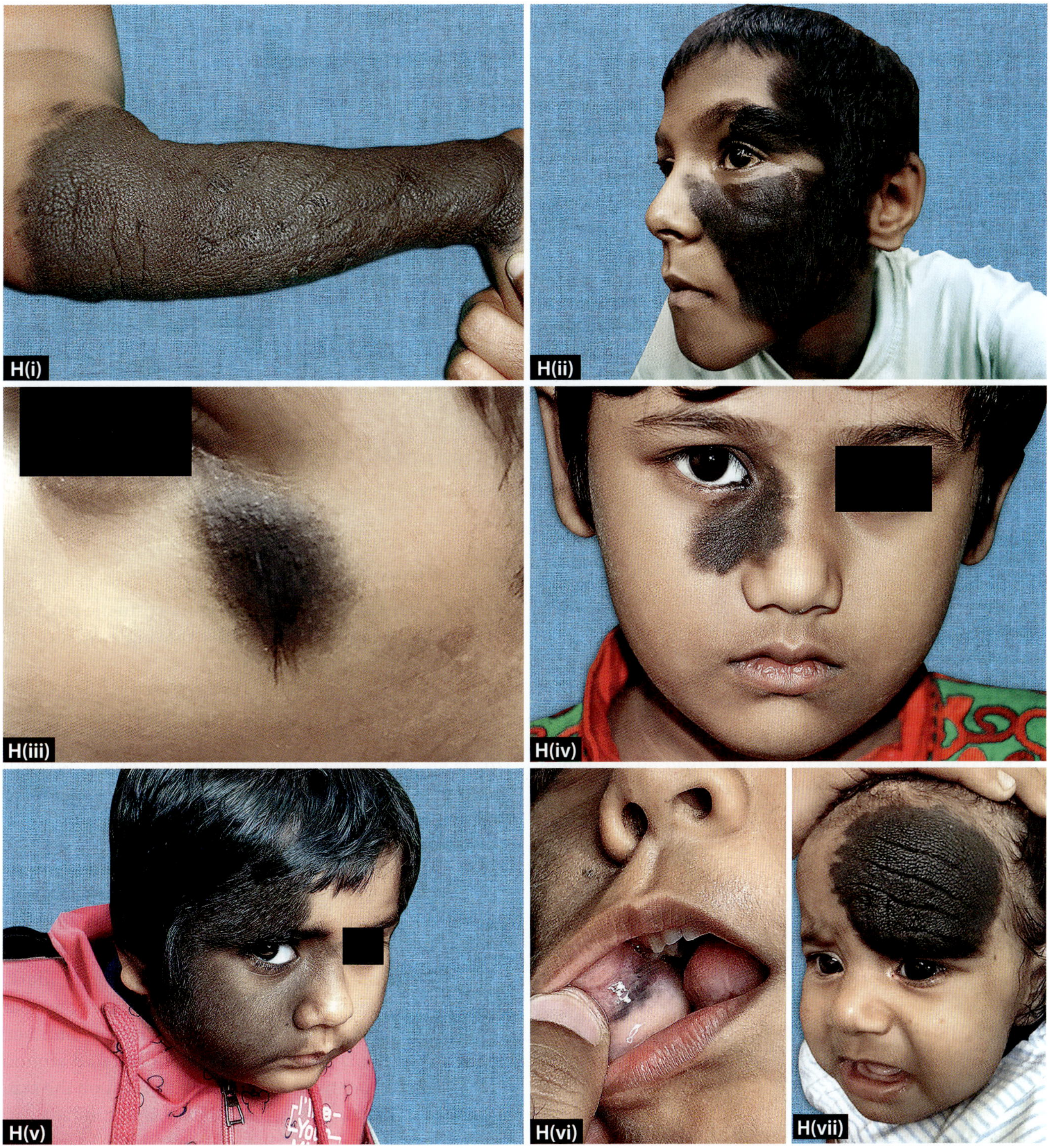

Figs. 20H(i) to (vii): H(i) Congenital hairy melanocytic nevus encircling whole leg; H(ii) Giant dermal melanocytic nevus, note terminal hair; H(iii) Small dermal melanocytic nevus, note terminal hair; H(iv) Dermal melanocytic nevus, hair yet to grow; H(v) Congenital melanocytic nevus in a 3-year-old girl; H(vi) Same child with mucosal involvement; H(vii) Congenital melanocytic nevus over forehead.

areas on the trunk, forehead, cheeks, supraclavicular region, abdomen, forearm, wrist, buttocks, and shins. Approximately after 1–2 years, coarse hair appear over the patch. The intensity of pigmentation may fade somewhat as the patient becomes older, but the hyperpigmentation and hypertrichosis tend to persist throughout life.

"Silence is the sleep that nourishes wisdom." —**Francis Bacon**

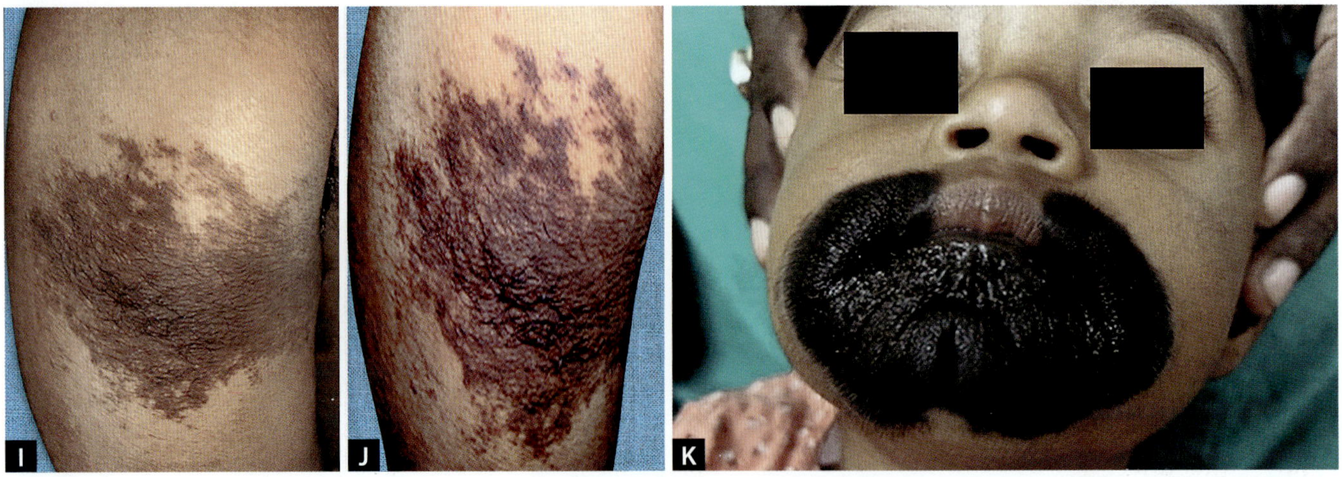

Figs. 20I to K: (I) Becker's nevus over side of trunk in a young adolescent boy; (J) Same boy, close-up view; (K) Congenital melanocytic nevus in a young boy

Associated features include unilateral breast hypoplasia, limb asymmetry, and spina bifida.

Etiology

The etiology of Becker's nevus is unknown, but androgen receptor assays suggest that a localized increase in the receptors seen in individuals with this disorder. In addition, reports of familial cases raise the question of a genetic influence in some patients and the occasional association of smooth muscle hamartoma and Becker's nevi occur without other pathologic findings. Some workers feel that Becker's melanosis may represent an organoid nevus and part of the spectrum of epidermal nevi and the epidermal nevus syndrome.

Treatment

Treatment of this disorder is purely cosmetic and consists of therapy with Q-switched ruby laser or excision with split thickness skin grafts. Unfortunately, these procedures usually yield results far from satisfactory.

LENTIGINES (FIGS. 21A TO D)

These are small, tan, dark brown or black, flat oval or circular macules that appear in childhood and increase in number with age. Their size varies from 3 to 15 mm, may occur on any mucocutaneous surface, show uniform pigmentation, and appear darker than freckles. It is seen on both exposed and unexposed part of the body. It can occur as an isolated form or part of an underlying syndrome. Syndromes associated with lentigines are Peutz-Jeghers syndrome, LEOPARD syndrome, Bannayan-Zonana syndrome, Cowden syndrome, and Carney complex.

Natural History

Lesions that appear in early childhood may fade or disappear.

Treatment

For permanent lesions, treatment is for cosmetic purpose. Excision by a small punch biopsy, shaving, cryosurgery, laser, etc. may be beneficial.

LEOPARD SYNDROME (FIG. 22A)

This is an autosomal dominant (AD) disorder with high penetrance and variable expressivity characterized by striking cutaneous pigmentation. The term LEOPARD syndrome is actually a mnemonic used to describe the many protean manifestations of this disorder viz., Lentigenes, Electrocardiographic conduction defects, Ocular hypertelorism, Pulmonary stenosis, Abnormalities of genitalia, Retardation of growth, and Deafness. The cutaneous pigmentation is in the form of small, dark, 1–5 mm lentigines which are usually congenital or appear soon after birth. With age, they increase in size, number, and depth of color. They tend to be concentrated around the neck and upper trunk but may also appear on the skin of the face and scalp, arms, palms, soles, and genitalia.

FRECKLES (EPHELIDES) (FIGS. 22B AND C)

Freckles are red or light brown well-defined circumscribed macules, usually <5 mm in diameter, which appear in childhood especially over exposed areas of skin. They often arise in early childhood, generally between 2 and 4 years of age but not in infancy. These appear to be

"I learned that courage was not the absence of fear, but the triumph over it. The brave man is not he who does not feel afraid, but he who conquers that fear."

—Nelson Mandela

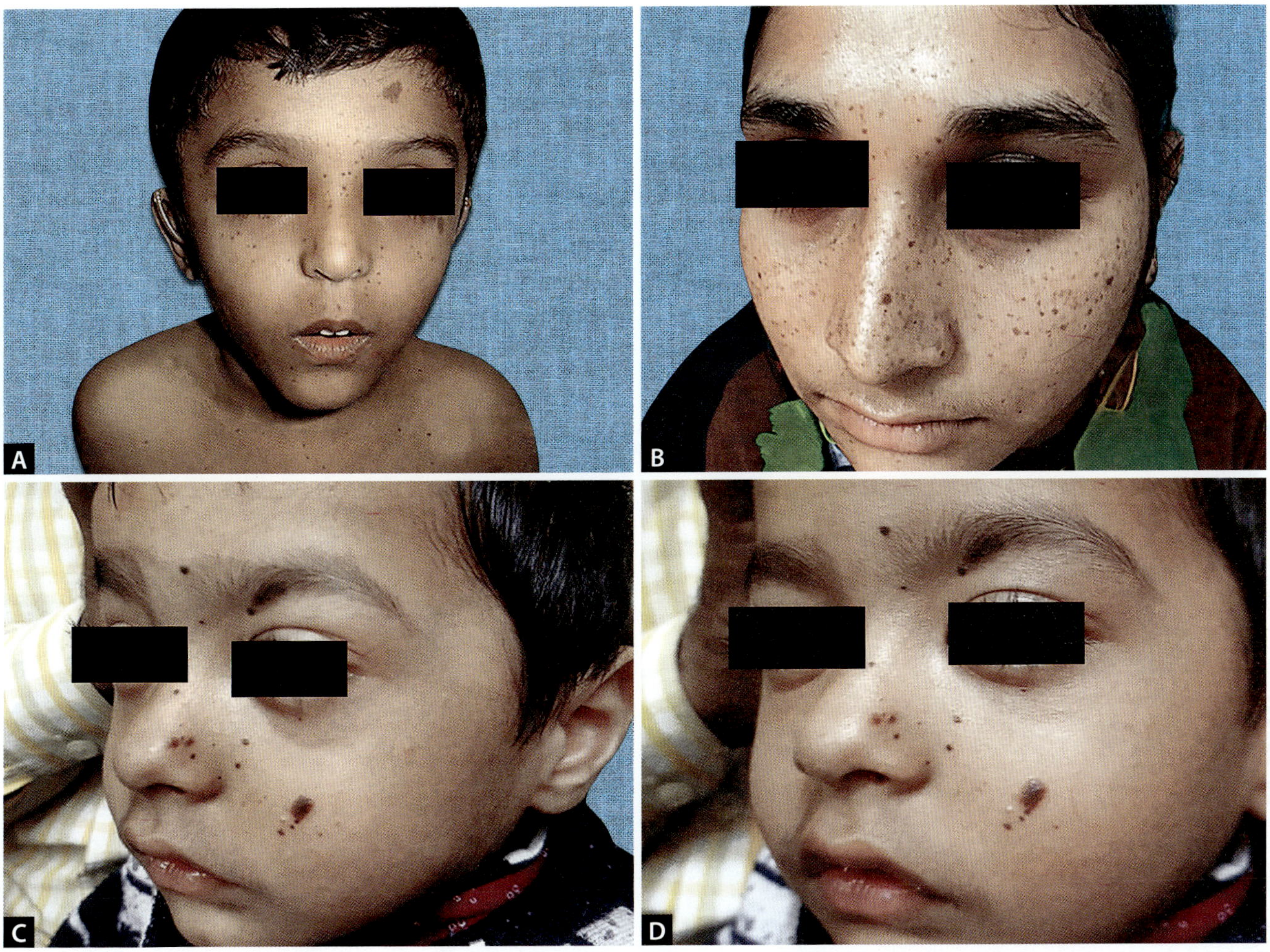

Figs. 21A to D: (A) Lentigines over face in a 6-year-old boy; (B) Lentigines over face in 17-year-old girl; (C) Unilateral lentiginosis over face in a 4-year-old boy; (D) Same boy, close-up view of lesions.

inherited as autosomal dominant trait and more common in individuals with fair skin and red hair. They have only cosmetic but no systemic connotations.

Lentigines are differentiated from freckles by their darker color, scattered distribution, comparative sparseness, and the fact they do not darken and increase in number on exposure to the sunlight.

Treatment

Regular application of sunscreens blocking both UVB and UVA are helpful. Extensive lesions, when seen in a young girl, various treatment options can be offered. These are chemical peeling (using 50% trichloroacetic acid, 10% glycolic acid, etc.,) cryotherapy, light electrofulguration, laser, etc. Avoidance of direct exposure to sun is of paramount importance.

NEVUS SPILUS (FIGS. 22D TO G)

It presents as a solitary, nonhairy, flat brown patch dotted by smaller dark brown to blackish brown freckle-like areas of pigmentation. This is a common disorder usually appearing at birth, infancy or childhood. It is estimated to occur in 2–3% of the adult population. Its size may vary from 1 to 20 cm in diameter and can appear on any area of the face, trunk, or extremities without relation to sun exposure. They often can be associated with phakomatosis pigmentovascularis.

Although there are reports of malignant melanoma developing within lesions of nevus spilus, it does not necessitate routine removal of uncomplicated lesions. It only needs a cosmetic camouflage.

"A loving heart is the truest wisdom." —**Charles Dickens**

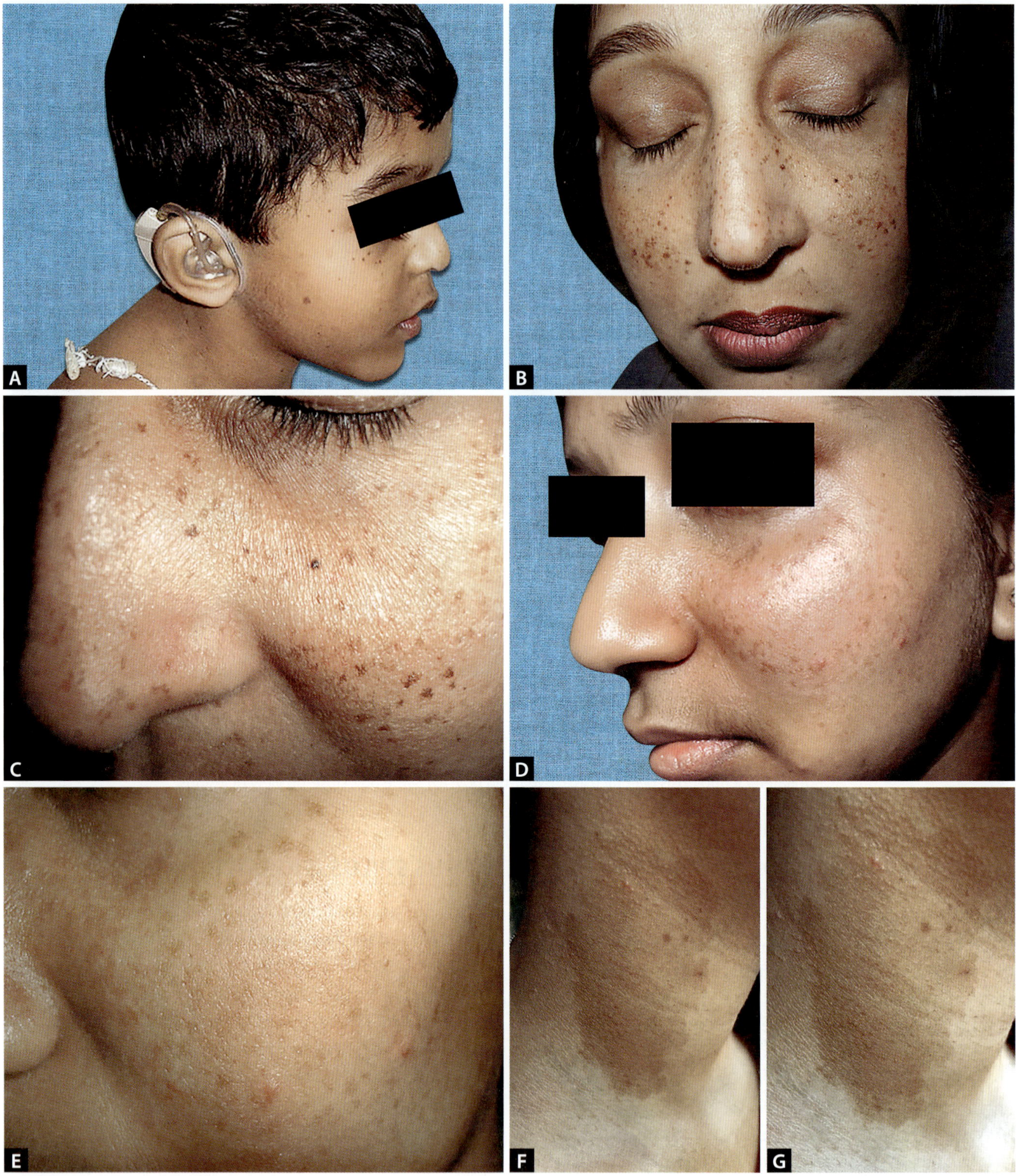

Figs. 22A to G: (A) LEOPARD syndrome, note the child having lentigines along with hearing aid (indicative of deafness); (B) Freckles over face; (C) Close-up view of freckles; (D) Nevus spilus over face in a 14-year-old girl; (E) Close-up view of nevus spilus; (F) Nevus spilus in an adolescent girl; (G) Same girl, close-up view.

"People never learn anything by being told, they have to find out for themselves." —**Paulo Coelho**

PEUTZ–JEGHERS SYNDROME [FIGS. 23 TO 26A(ii)]

This is an autosomal dominant disorder caused due to mutation in *STK11* gene, on chromosome 19p which codes for serine-threonine kinase. It is characterized by mucocutaneous pigmentation and generalized intestinal polyposis. The cutaneous lesions appear as flat, bluish brown to black irregularly oval spots <5 mm in diameter. They are seen most commonly on the lips, buccal mucosa, nasal and periorbital regions, elbows, dorsal aspects of the fingers and toes, palms, soles and periumbilical, perianal or labial regions. Occasionally the gums and hard palate and rarely the tongue may be affected. The spots on the skin and lip often fade after puberty whereas those on the buccal mucosa, palate, and tongue tend to persist. The GI polyps may be present anywhere between the gastroesophageal junction to the anal canal. Majority of the polyps are seen in jejunum. The polyps represent benign hamartomas and have a low malignant potential. Children frequently present with abdominal pain, melena or intussusception.

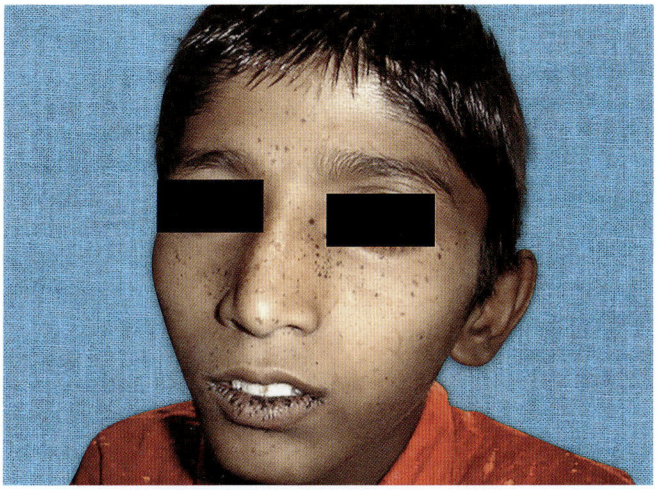

Fig. 23: Hyperpigmented macules over the face in Peutz–Jeghers syndrome.

Management

Management of cutaneous pigmentation mainly consists of reassurance of parents. Treatment of polyposis is limited to relief of symptoms as multiple resections may lead to malabsorption.

EPIDERMAL NEVI (FIGS. 26B TO P)

Epidermal nevi represent a benign congenital disorder that is characterized by circumscribed hyperkeratosis and hypertrophy of the epidermis. This disorder, usually apparent at birth or in early childhood, affects both sexes equally and is known by several descriptive names, nevus verrucosus, nevus unius lateris, and ichthyosis hystrix. The lesions may be deeply or slightly pigmented, have either a unilateral or a bilateral distribution and often favor the extremities in what appears to be a dermatomal distribution, but may occur anywhere on the cutaneous surface. Although single lesion may occur, the disorder generally consists of multiple lesions arranged in a linear distribution.

Usually present at birth, it may also appear in infancy, early childhood, and occasionally in adult life. Lesions

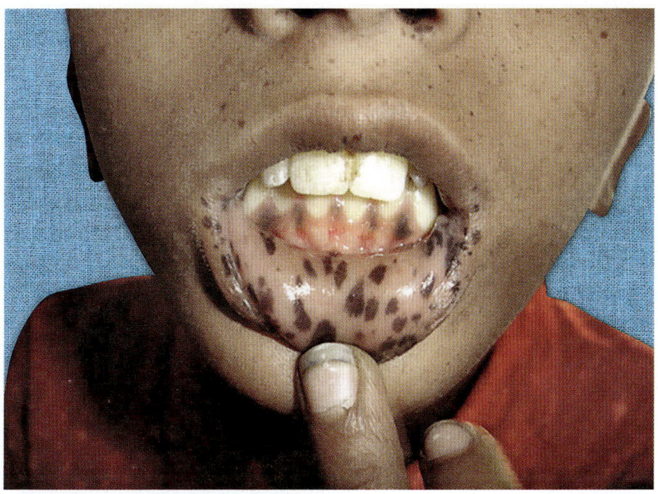

Fig. 24: Close-up view of hyperpigmented macules over the lips.

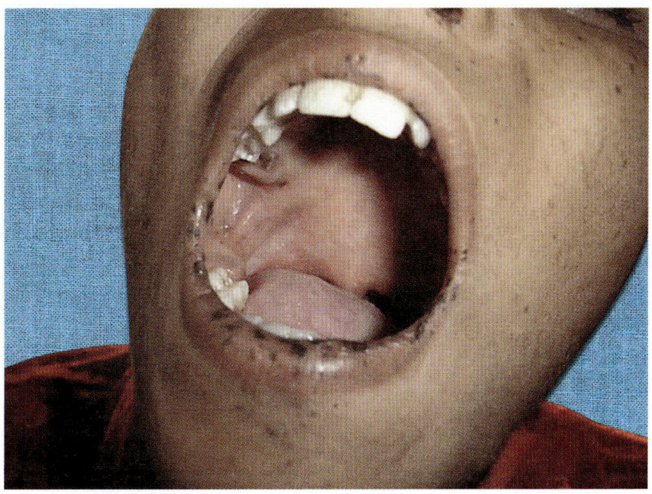

Fig. 25: Close-up view of hyperpigmented macules over the oral mucosa.

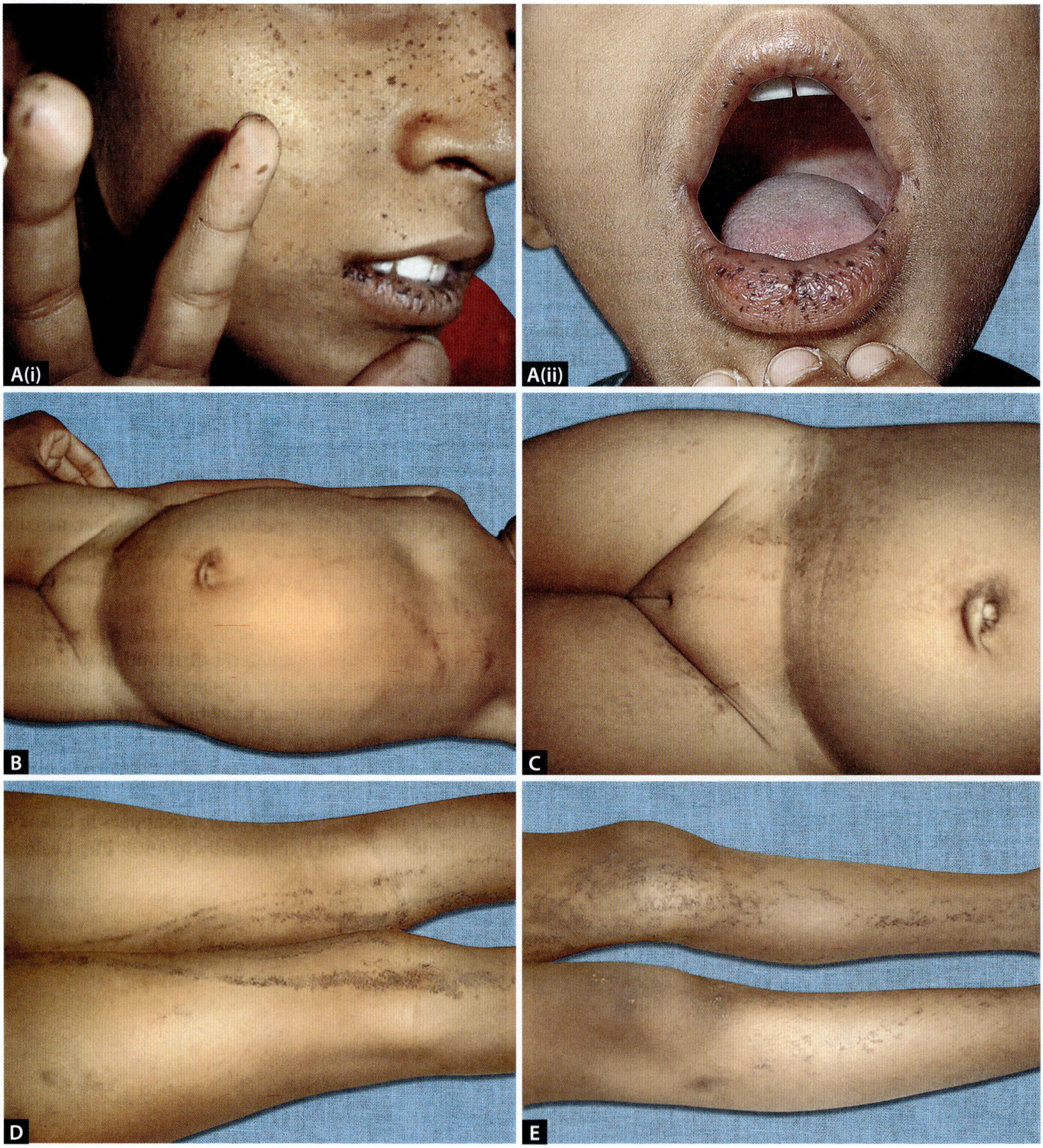

Figs. 26A(i) to E: A(i) Pigmented macules over the fingertips; A(ii) Pigmented macules over lips in a case of Peutz–Jeghers syndrome; (B) Verrucous epidermal nevus (VEN), note lesions along Blaschko's lines; (C) VEN in a 3-year-old girl; (D) Lesions of VEN along Blaschko's lines; (E) Same boy, lesions over legs.

may be grayish yellow-brown and velvety, granular, warty, or papillomatous. More often noted on the trunk or limb then on the head or neck, they may be single or multiple and round or oval. They vary from 2 to 3 cm or more in diameter and, when seen on the limbs, frequently appear in a linear distribution.

"Stay hungry. Stay foolish." —**Steve jobs**

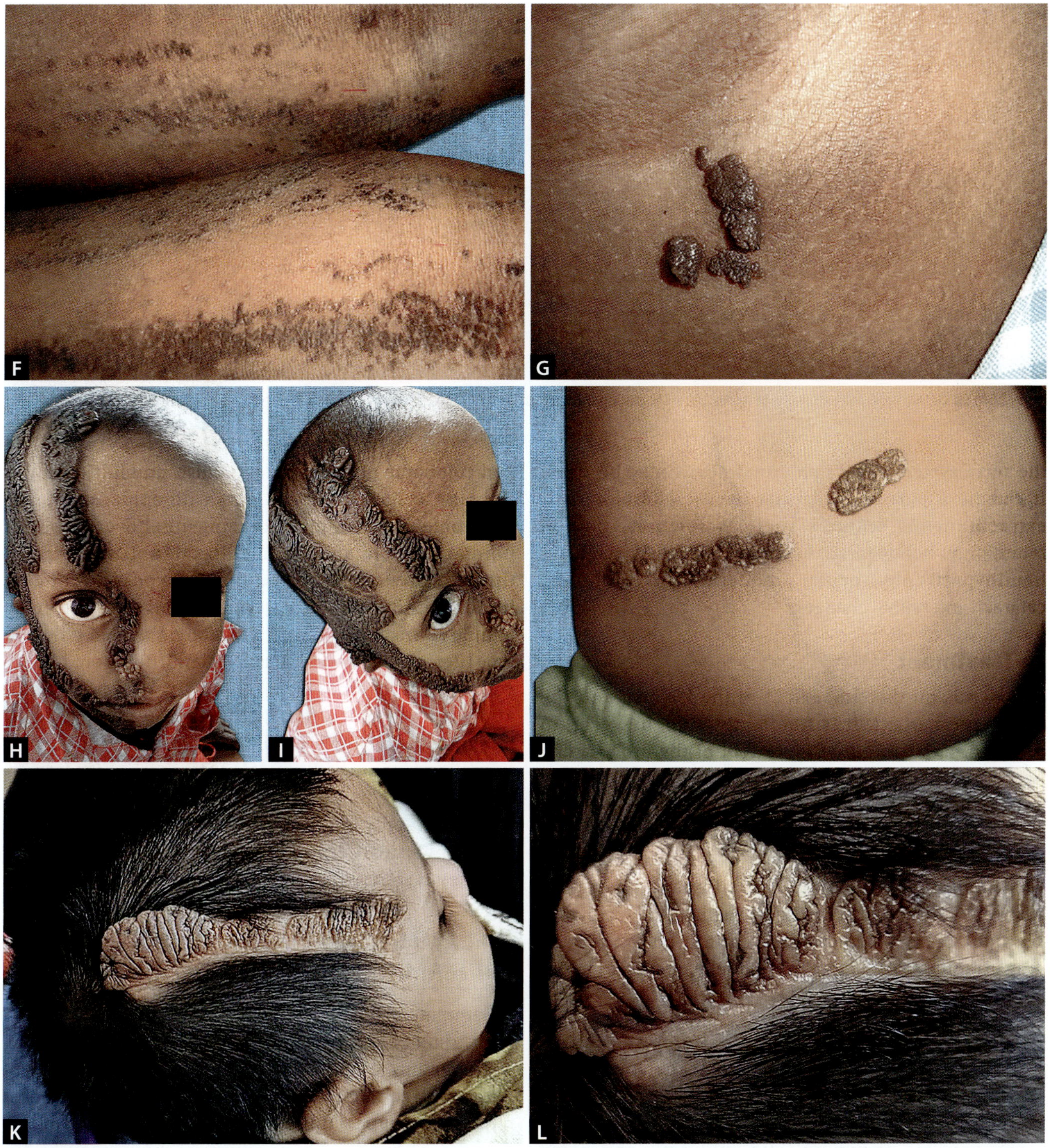

Figs. 26F to L: (F) Close-up view of verrucous epidermal nevus (VEN); (G) VEN over axilla in a 4-year-old girl; (H) VEN over face and scalp; (I) Same boy, another view; (J) VEN, close-up view; (K) VEN over scalp; (L) Same child, close-up view.

Nevus unius lateralis may present as a single linear or spiral warty lesions or at time as an elaborate continuous or interrupted pattern affecting multiple sites, usually on one half of the body. On the extremities, lesions usually follow the long axis, and on the trunk, they may be arranged in groups or as spiral streaks. On the trunk, the lesions frequently tend to have a transverse orientation. If a large area of the body is affected,

"I can understand wanting to have a million dollars but once you get beyond that, I have to tell you, it's the same hamburger." **—Bill gates**

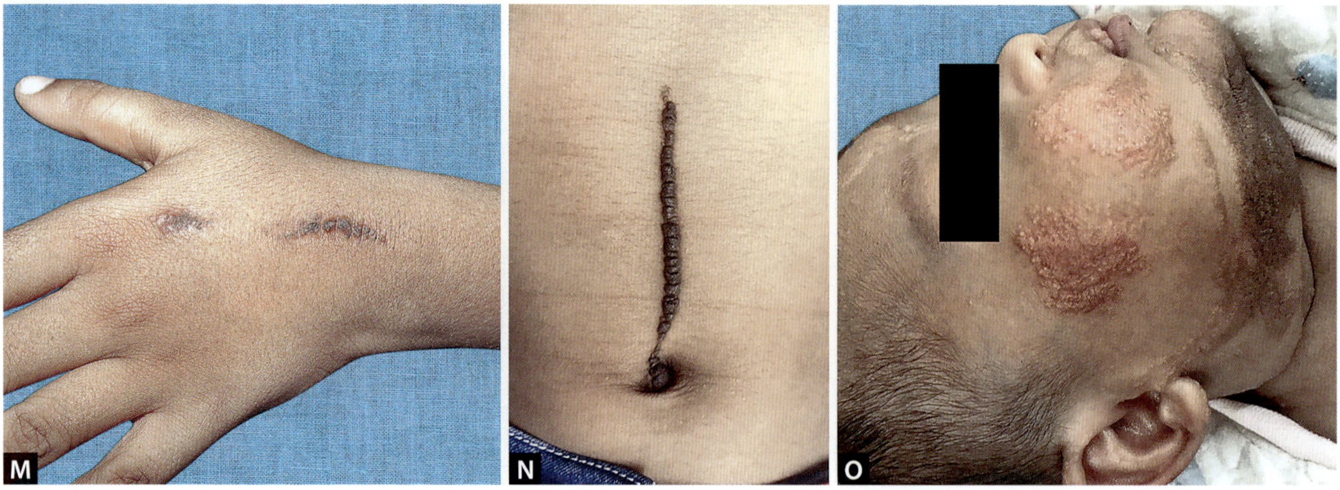

Figs. 26M to O: (M) VEN, over dorsum of hand; (N) VEN, peculiar distribution; (O) Epidermal nevus syndrome in a 3-month-old infant.

the term systematized epidermal nevus may be used. It can be a part of epidermal nevus syndrome with extracutaneous features such as seizures, mental retardation, hemiparesis, hypotonia, kyphosis, scoliosis, hemihypertrophy, ocular lipodermoids, coloboma, cataract, and retinal changes.

Treatment

It depends on the site, extent of the lesions, and the age of the patient. It is frequently wise, however, to delay surgery until the final extent of the process can be determined since early excision may result in the appearance of new lesions in or adjacent to the region of previously treated areas. Excision by a plastic surgeon is the treatment of choice for lesions that are unsightly or uncomfortable, or when malignant change is suspected. Although cryosurgery (with liquid nitrogen), dermabrasion, or electrodesiccation, and curettage may produce gratifying results initially, recurrences are common.

VERRUCOUS EPIDERMAL NEVUS WITH OCULAR CHORISTOMA (FIGS. 26Q TO S)

Verrucous epidermal nevus (VEN), a keratinocyte hamartoma, consists of hyperplastic epidermis appearing clinically as skin-colored to brown verrucous papules or well-demarcated papillomatous plaques located anywhere, but less commonly on the head and neck, face, and oral mucosa. It presents as vertical, linear or S-shaped lesion, and does not normally cross the midline. Ocular abnormalities (choristomas, epibulbar dermoids, and coloboma of the uvea, optic disc, and lids) occur in as many as 50% of the patients with epidermal nevus syndrome. Choristomas are congenital overgrowth of normal tissue in an abnormal location. Histologically, they are divided into four main types—dermoids, lipodermoids, simple, and complex choristomas. Simple choristomas consist of ectopic tissue of only one type (dermis-like tissue, lacrimal gland, bone, etc.), while complex choristomas have ectopic tissue of ectodermal and mesodermal origin, and may be comprised of lacrimal gland, bone, cartilage, adipose tissue, neural tissue, and/or smooth muscle interspersed in dermis-like connective tissue. Mixed (complex) choristomas are most commonly found in ENS and are usually bilateral and symmetrical. It has been described in association with nevus sebaceous more commonly than with VEN.

INFLAMMATORY LINEAR VERRUCOUS EPIDERMAL NEVUS (FIGS. 27A TO C)

Inflammatory linear verrucous epidermal nevi (ILVEN) is a variant of epidermal nevus characterized by pruritic, erythematous scaly, verrucous papules along the lines of Blaschko. It commonly affects females. It is often present at birth or may appear during the childhood and distributed over the extremities. Lesions improve spontaneously, but eventually reappear. Their extent varies from unilateral to bilateral involvement. They run a chronic course and are often resistant to treatment. The linear epidermal nevus in its systematized form may be associated with skeletal deformities and central nervous system defects. Differential diagnosis includes epidermal nevi, Darier's

"If people are not laughing at your goals, your goals are too small." —**Azim Premji**

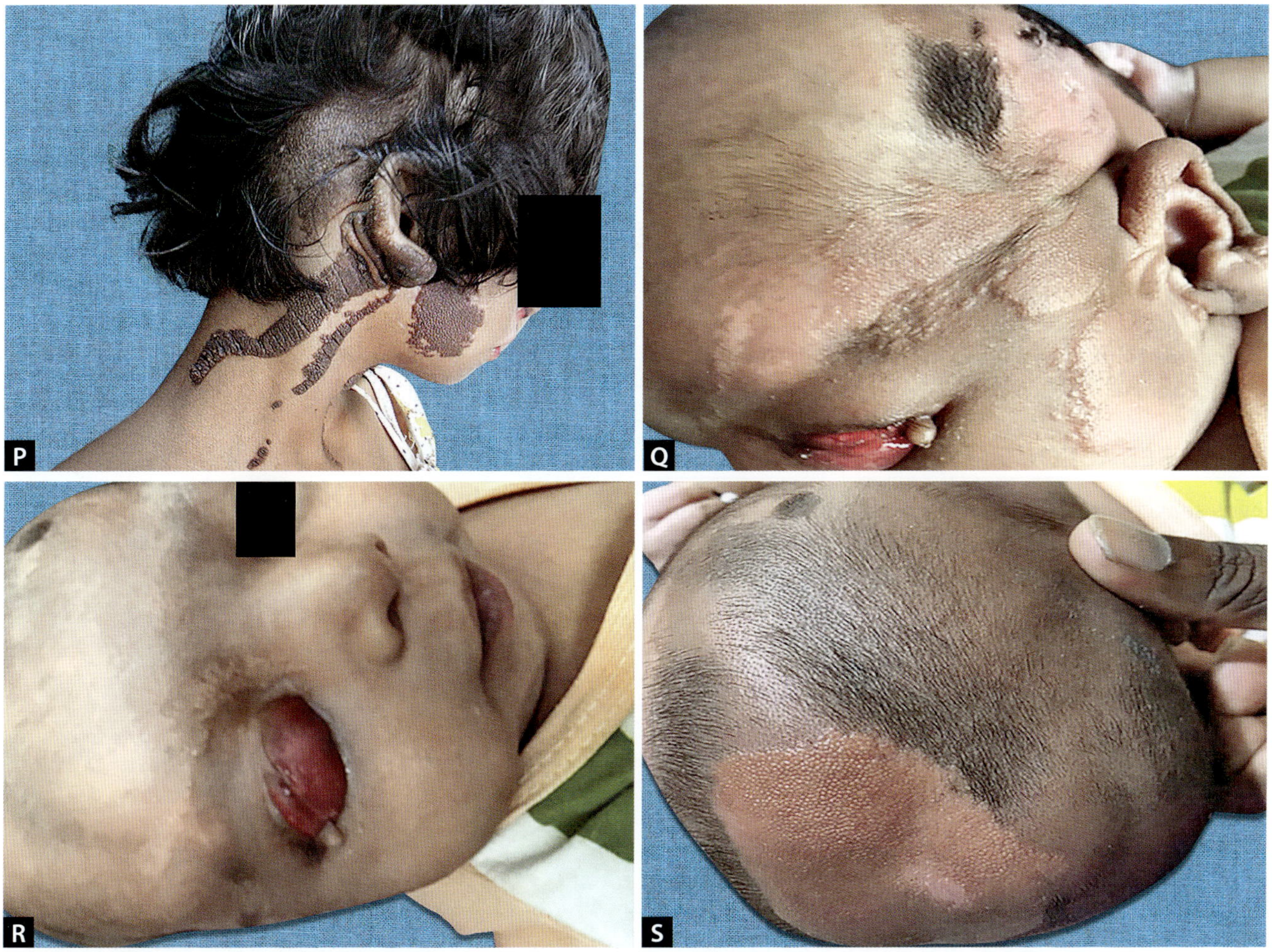

Figs. 26P to S: (P) Epidermal nevus syndrome in an 5-year-old girl; (Q) Verrucous epidermal nevus (VEN) with ocular choristoma in a 1-month-old baby; (R) Close-up view of choristoma; (S) Close-up view of VEN over scalp.

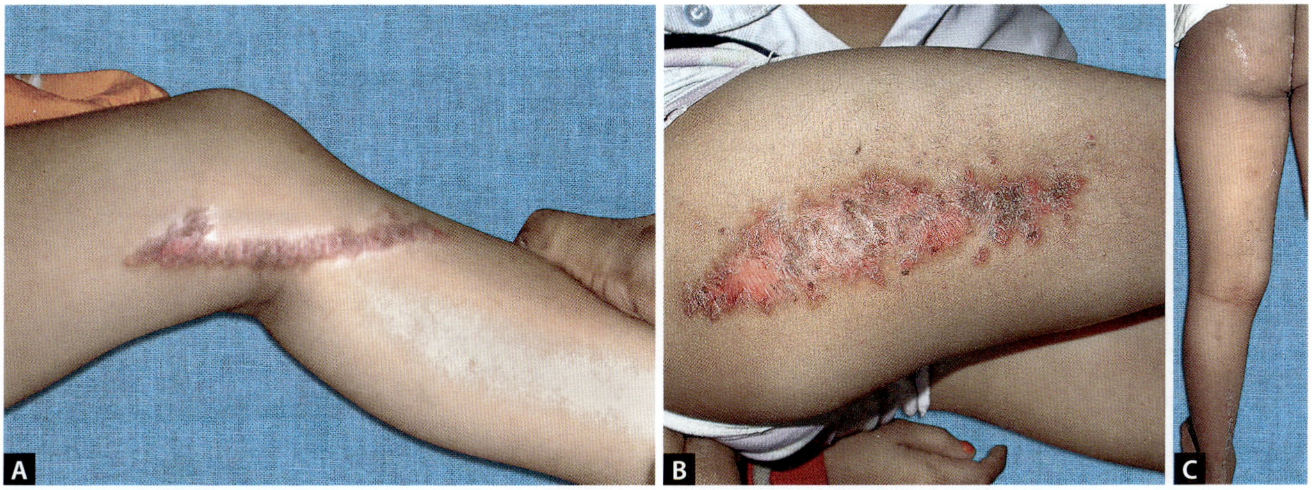

Figs. 27A to C: (A) Linear verrucous band-like lesion with erythema; (B) Inflammatory linear verrucous epidermal nevus (ILVEN) over thigh; (C) ILVEN over thigh and leg.

"When you take risks you learn that, there will be times when you succeed and there will be times when you fail, and both are equally important."

—Ellen DeGeneres

disease, nevoid psoriasis, linear porokeratosis, linear lichen planus and lichen striatus.

Management

Moderate to potent topical corticosteroids for 2–4 weeks may help subsidence of inflammation. Intralesional triamcinolone acetonide injection every 3 weekly for 2–3 months may give similar results. However, the remission is temporary and lesions tend to recur with wearing off of the action of injected/applied steroid. Surgical excision, deep-shave excision or dermabrasion may be curative.

NEVUS SEBACEOUS (FIGS. 28A TO H)

Nevus sebaceous of Jadassohn presents as well circumscribed hairless plaque at birth or early childhood. In the young, they are yellow or yellowish brown with a flat and velvety appearance. With puberty the lesions become raised, thickened, and nodular with closely set papillomatous projections. The lesion is round, oval or linear and varies from few millimeters to several centimeters in diameter. During adolescence and adult life, 10–15% of the lesions undergo secondary neoplastic changes most commonly trichoblastoma and syringocystadenoma papilliferum. Malignant change is usually heralded by ulceration or rapid enlargement in size. Other neoplasms that can arise from nevus sebaceous are leiomyoma, piloleiomyoma, hidradenoma, apocrine cystadenoma, basal cell carcinoma (BCC), and squamous cell carcinoma.

Systemic Associations

Large lesions may be associated with ophthalmic, skeletal, neurologic, and pigmentary abnormalities.

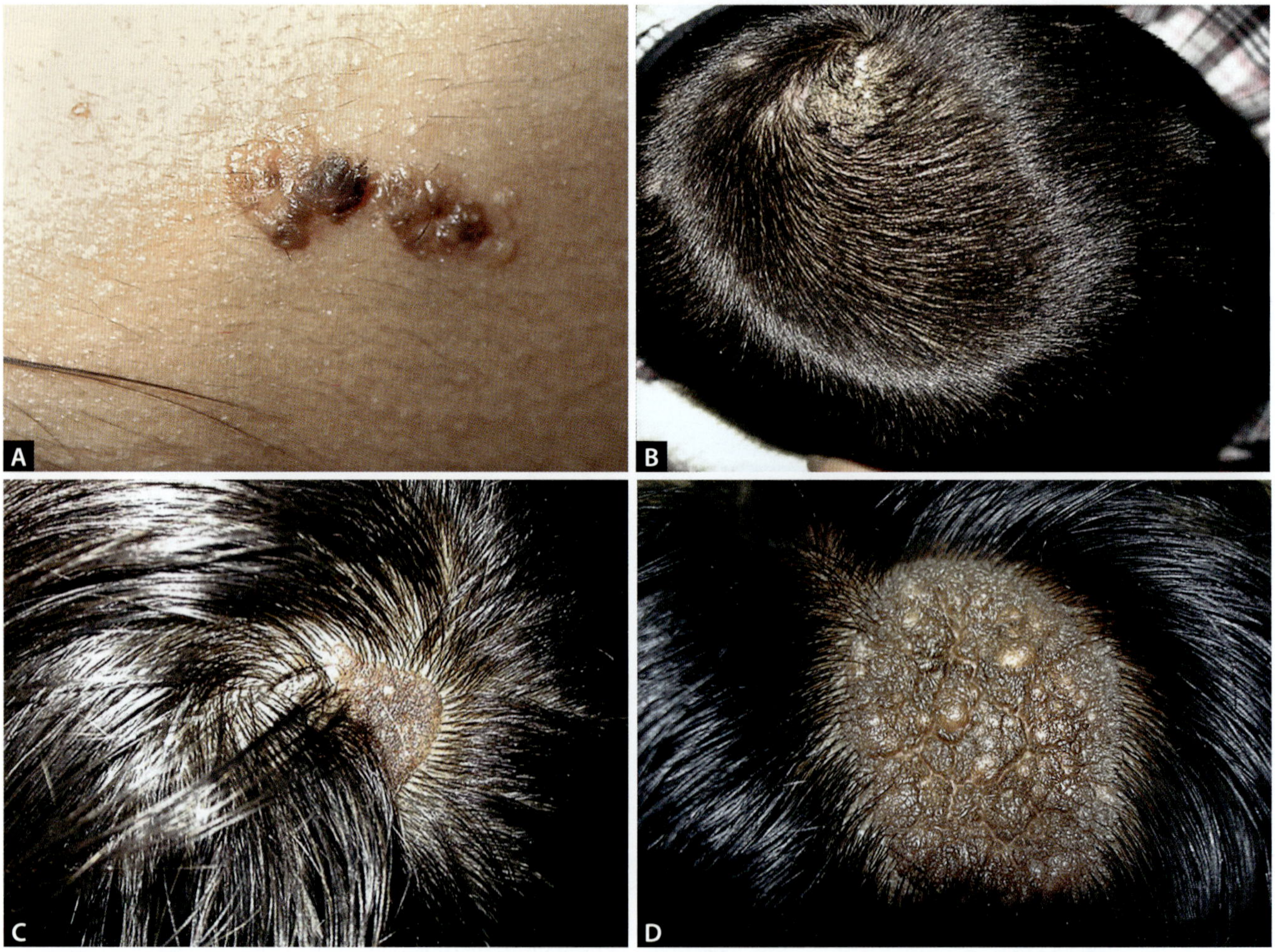

Figs. 28A to D: (A) Greasy papulonodular lesions of nevus sebaceous in clusters; (B) Nevus sebaceous in 6-year-old boy; (C) Same boy, close-up view of the lesion; (D) Nevus sebaceous, note huge size and nodularity of the lesion.

"What makes you different or weird—that's your strength." **—Meryl Streep**

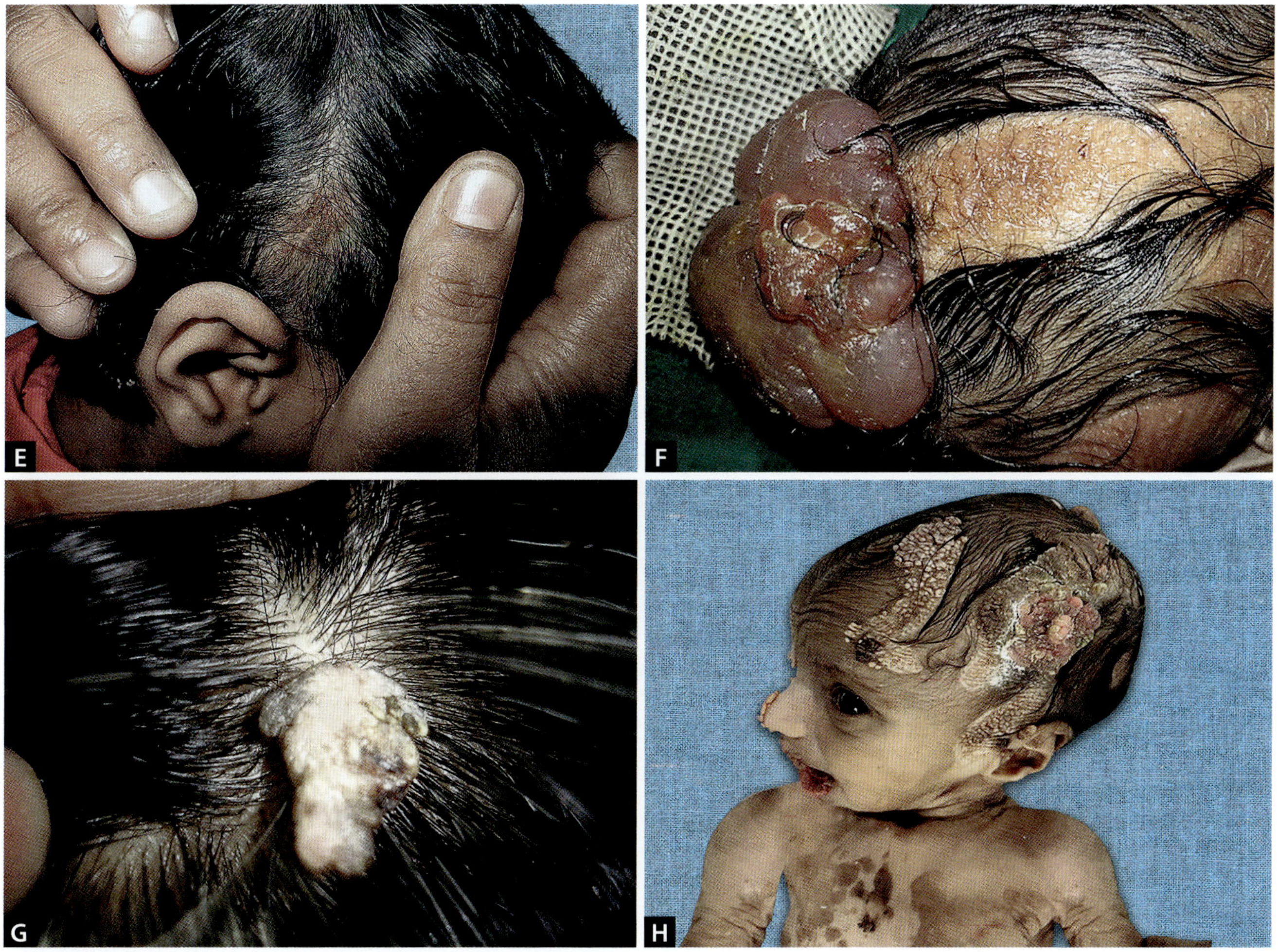

Figs. 28E to H: (E) Nevus sebaceous over scalp; (F) Nevus sebaceous with syringocystadenoma papilliferum; (G) Syringocystadenoma papilliferum; (H) nevus sebaceous (Schimmelpenning syndrome).

Schimmelpenning syndrome (Schimmelpenning-Feuerstein-Mims syndrome) is a rare epidermal nevus syndrome characterized by the hallmark nevus sebaceous associated with extracutaneous anomalies. The various extracutaneous features described are mainly neurological (mental retardation, seizures, hemiparesis, lateral ventricle enlargement, complete or partial hemimegalencephaly) along with ophthalmological (colobomas and choristomas), genitourinary (horseshoe kidney and duplicated urinary collecting system), cardiovascular (ventricular septal defect, coarctation of the aorta, aortic hypoplasia), endocrine (hypophosphatemic rickets), dental alterations (hemi-hyperplasia of the tongue, bone cysts, aplasia of the teeth, hypoplastic enamel), and neoplasms (BCC). The cause is hypothesized to be genomic mosaicism.

Treatment

Early diagnosis and treatment is important because of its potential malignant transformation. Local deep full thickness surgical excision by a pediatric/plastic surgeon is ideally recommended.

NEVUS COMEDONICUS (FIGS. 29A TO D)

This developmental disorder is believed to result from a failure in development of the mesodermal component of the pilosebaceous complex. It occurs with equal frequency in males and females and half the cases present at birth. The lesions manifest as groups of closely set, slightly elevated papules that have in their center a dark firm hyperkeratotic plug resembling a comedo in a linear or band-like distribution on the body particularly on the face, neck, upper arm, chest, and abdomen.

"I find that the harder I work, the more luck I seem to have." —**Thomas Jefferson**

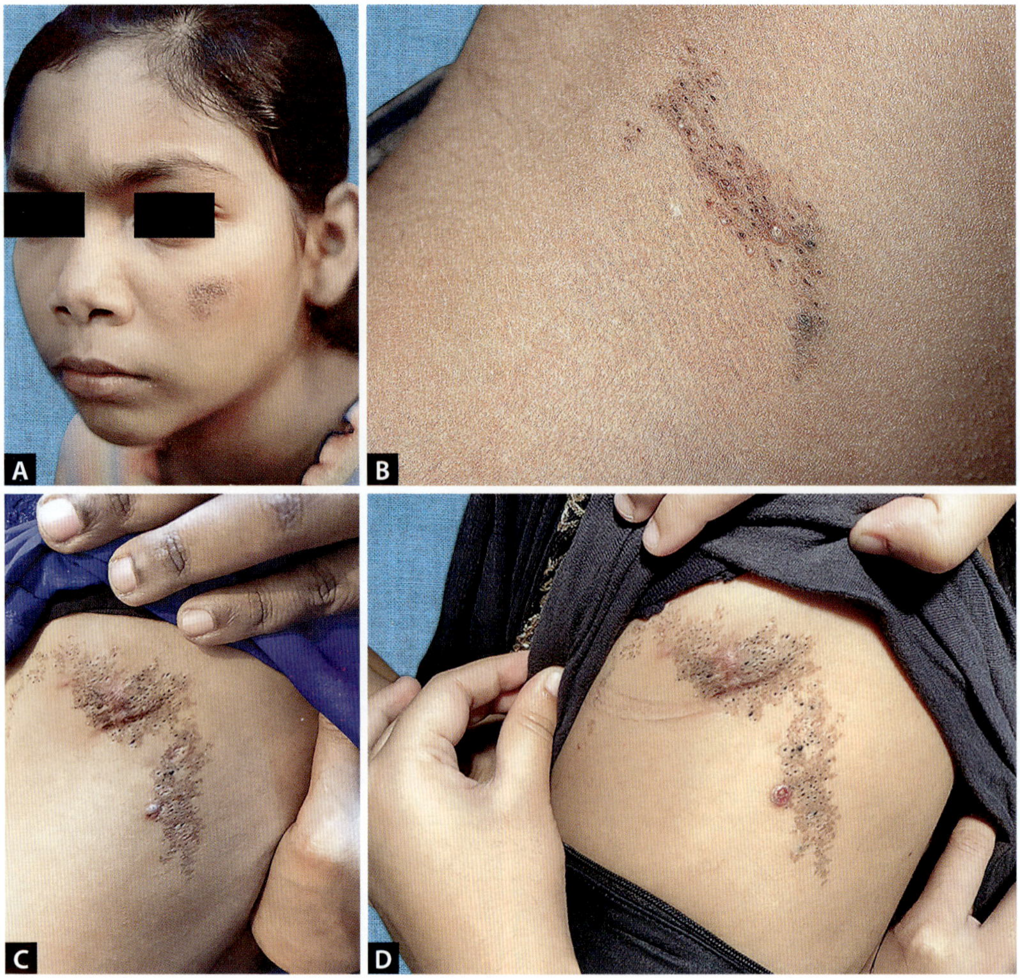

Figs. 29A to D: (A) Clustered black comedo-like lesions of nevus comedonicus over cheek; (B) Nevus comedonicus; (C) Nevus comedonicus over back in an 11-year-old girl; (D) Same girl with nevus comedonicus.

Natural History

The lesions increase in size with age and extend above the cutaneous surface giving a nutmeg grater-like feeling to the skin. The lesions may get complicated by secondary infection and abscess formation.

Management

Management includes treatment of secondary infection and surgical excision of the entire lesion.

NEVUS LIPOMATOSUS SUPERFICIALIS (FIG. 30)

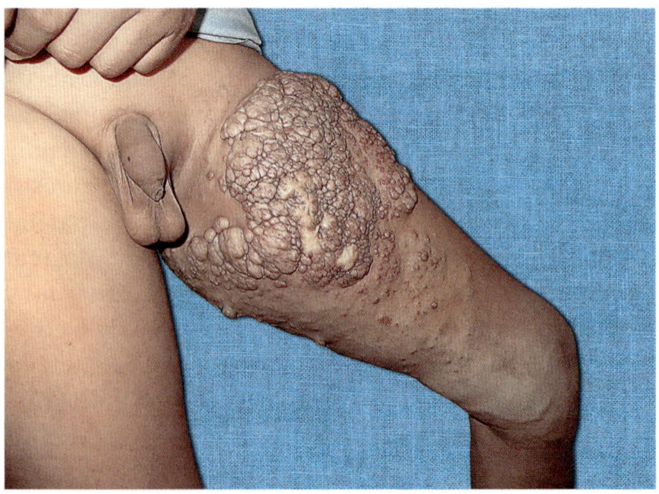

Fig. 30: Nevus Lipomatosus superficialis.

Nevus lipomatosus superficialis is a rare benign cutaneous tumor characterized by dermal deposition of mature ectopic adipose tissue. It presents at birth or in childhood

"Beware of advice, even this." —**Carl Sandburg**

with no familial tendency. There are two variants: Classical form and solitary form. The classical form presents as multiple, clustered, soft, flesh-colored to yellowish pedunculated papules and nodules with a smooth and wrinkled appearance distributed on the lower back, pelvic girdle, buttocks, and upper thighs in a zosteriform pattern. Solitary form presents as dome-shaped sessile papule or nodule seen in third to fourth decade of life distributed on scalp, face, eyelids, and clitoris. Rarely ulceration can be seen. It can co-exist with café-au-lait macules, leukoderma, overlying hypertrichosis, and comedo-like alterations. Differential diagnosis includes connective tissue nevus, nevus sebaceous, neurofibroma, lymphangioma, hemangioma, and focal dermal hypoplasia. Surgical excision is the treatment of choice.

FIBROUS PAPULE OF NOSE (FIGS. 31A AND B)

Fibrous papule of nose is classically described as solitary, sessile, skin colored or reddish, dome-shaped papule of 3–6 mm in diameter commonly appears on face of late adolescent or adults; more precisely over nose. It may contain central hair. Lesions may be multiple. Close differentials are intradermal melanocytic nevus, neurofibroma, BCC, and adnexal tumor. In comparison with melanocytic nevus, fibrous papule is firmer in consistency. BCC usually appear late in life and has tendency of bleeding and ulceration. Fibrous papule comes under broader term cutaneous angiofibroma which include other angiofibroma including pearly penile papule. Multiple fibrous papule should alert the clinicians about possibilities such as neurofibromatosis type 2, tuberous sclerosis (TS), Birt-Hogg-Dube syndrome, and multiple endocrine neoplasia type 1. Histopathology is characterized by concentric band of collagenous fibrous stroma surrounding blood vessels and hair follicles. Proliferation of plump or satellite fibroblasts is the finding. Other variants which have been described are clear cell, granular cell, and epithelioid variety. Superficial shave biopsy may be misleading due to junctional melanocytes. It usually requires no treatment and persists for life. Complete excision of the lesion is the treatment of choice. Electrosurgery can be done.

CUTANEOUS LEIOMYOMA (FIGS. 32A AND B)

Cutaneous leiomyomas, rare benign tumors arising from the smooth muscles of the skin represent only 3–5% of leiomyomas. Skin is the second most common location for leiomyoma after uterus. They are more likely to occur in adults than in children and are rarely encountered at birth. There are few reports of cutaneous leiomyomas presenting in infants. These may be hereditary or sporadic.

Cutaneous leiomyomas are classified into three main types:

1. Piloleiomyoma—derived from the arrector pili muscle of hair follicles
2. Angioleiomyoma—originate from the vascular smooth muscle
3. Solitary genital and mammary leiomyomas—originate from the smooth muscle of genital skin (dartoic type) and nipples.

Piloleiomyoma is the most common type of cutaneous leiomyoma. They present clinically as either solitary or multiple lesions ranging from 2 to 20 mm in diameter as skin-colored, red or dusky brown firm papules and

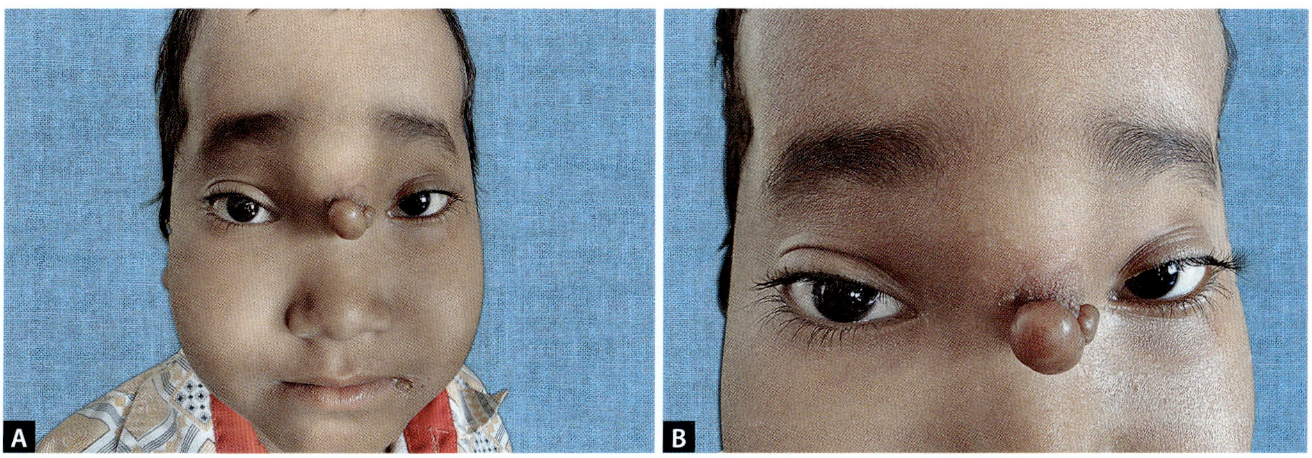

Figs. 31A and B: (A) Fibrous papule of nose; (B) Fibrous papule of nose, close-up view.

"If you can change your mind, you can change your life." —**William James**

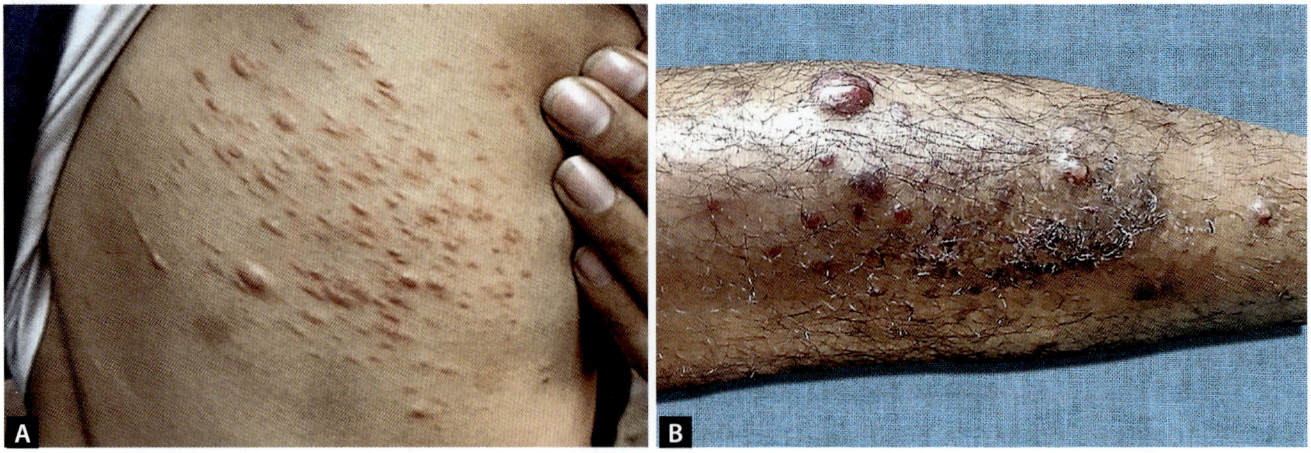

Figs. 32A and B: (A) Leiomyoma cutis in zosteriform distribution; (B) Cutaneous leiomyoma in an 18-year-old boy.

nodules, most commonly located in the extremities. They may be asymptomatic, but are typically extremely painful due to compression of cutaneous nerves or contraction of fibers within the tumor in case of cold weather or emotional stress. Multiple leiomyomas typically consist of grouped red-brown to blue, firm intradermal nodules with a translucent or waxy appearance, commonly located on the trunk or the extremities, but may occur on the face and neck and rarely in the mouth. They form a component of the autosomal dominant syndromes, multiple cutaneous and uterine leiomyomatosis syndrome and the hereditary leiomyomatosis and renal cell cancer syndrome, both of which are caused by heterozygous mutations in the fumarate hydratase (*FH*) gene.

Solitary angioleiomyoma presents as subcutaneous lesions derived from vascular smooth muscles occurring most commonly on the lower extremities of men and not exceeding 4 cm in diameter. Dartoic leiomyomas are nearly always solitary and rarely cause significant pain.

Histopathologically, pilar leiomyomas appear as noncapsulated, circumscribed dermal tumors composed of interlacing and whorled bundles of smooth muscle cells in the upper dermis without atypia and mitotic activity. There is presence of increased nerve density within the lesional skin compared with the surrounding dermis. Histopathological examination, special stain, and immunohistochemistry help to confirm the diagnosis of leiomyoma. Leiomyomas have a high recurrence rate. Total surgical excision is the treatment of choice and is curative for smaller, localized lesions. Multiple lesions are usually difficult to treat and laser ablation has been used with some success.

WHAT'S NEW?

- High frequency cutaneous USG represents a promising non-invasive diagnostic tool in pediatric vascular anomalies. It has also been used as an objective tool to assess the efficacy of treatment in IH.
- Topical beta blockers like atenolol, timolol, carteolol and topical sirolimus have been found effective in localized hemangiomas. The basis of use of Sirolimus in vascular anomalies relies on its antiangiogenic properties.
- Cutaneous hemangioma has been described in two patients with congenital portosystemic venous shunts and may be a pointer to Abernethy syndrome.

SUGGESTED READINGS

1. Asch S, Sugarman JL. Epidermal nevus syndromes: new insights into whorls and swirls. Pediatr Dermatol. 2018;35(1):21-9.
2. Hamm H, Emmerich K, Olk J. Pigmentierte Flecken als mögliche Frühzeichen genetischer Syndrome (Pigmented macules as possible early signs of genetic syndromes). Hautarzt. 2019;70(7):506-13.
3. Perera TB, Murphy-Lavoie HM. Purpura Fulminans. In: Stat Pearls. Treasure Island (FL): Stat Pearls Publishing; 2020.
4. Slaughter KA, Chen T, Williams E 3rd. Vascular lesions. Facial Plast Surg Clin North Am. 2016;24(4):559-71.
5. Vivar KL, Mancini AJ. Infantile hemangioma: an update on pathogenesis, associations and management. Indian J Paediatr Dermatol. 2018;19:293-303.
6. Bandera AIR, Sebaratnam DK, Rodriguez MF, Laguna RL. Cutaneous ultrasound and its utility in Pediatric Dermatology: Part II - Developmental anomalies and vascular lesions. Pediatric Dermatology. 2019;00:1-12.
7. Jahnke MN, O'Haver J, Gupta D, Hawryluk EB, Finelt N, Kruse L, et al. Care of Congenital Melanocytic Nevi in Newborns and Infants: Review and Management Recommendations. Pediatrics. 2021;148(6):e2021051536.

"Home is the nicest word there is." —**Laura Wilder**

CHAPTER

3

Genodermatoses

ECTODERMAL DYSPLASIA (FIGS. 1 TO 4A)

Ectodermal dysplasias are heterogeneous group of disorders involving both ectodermal and nonectodermal features mainly involving skin, hair, nail, teeth, and sweat glands. There are approximately 200 different types of ectodermal dysplasia. The most common ectodermal dysplasias are of two types—hypohidrotic/anhidrotic and hidrotic.

- *Hypohidrotic/anhidrotic ectodermal dysplasia*: It is essentially X-linked recessive disorder but autosomal dominant and recessive form can occur. It commonly affects male children and is caused by mutations in ectodysplasin-A1 (*EDA1*), ectodysplasin A receptor (*EDAR*) and EDAR-associated death domain (*EDARADD*). It is characterized by partial or complete absence of sweat glands, hypotrichosis and hypodontia. The essential features of this disease are absence or reduction of sweating, hypotrichosis and total or partial anodontia. Face has a characteristic appearance with prominent frontal ridge and chin, saddle nose, sunken cheeks, thick everted lips, large ears and sparse hair. They often appear like each other than their own unaffected siblings. The skin is smooth, soft, dry and appears prematurely aged. Heat intolerance is a regular feature. Hair is thin, light colored and sparse with almost total absence of eyebrows and eyelashes. Fine wrinkling along with pigmentation is seen on the periocular and perioral region. Nails are brittle, thin and ridged. Teeth may be conical or peg-shaped. Other features include atopic dermatitis, asthma and recurrent bacterial and fungal infections. Osteopetrosis, lymphedema, autoimmune disorders and immunodeficiency can be seen in anhidrotic ectodermal dysplasia.
- *Hidrotic ectodermal dysplasia*: The most common form is the Clouston syndrome. It is an autosomal dominant condition with mutation in *GJB6* gene, characterized by generalized hypotrichosis, palmoplantar keratoderma (PPK) and nail dystrophy. Dystrophy of the nails is the key feature of this syndrome. They have normal facies with no abnormalities in sweating. Skin thickening is seen beneath the free edges of the

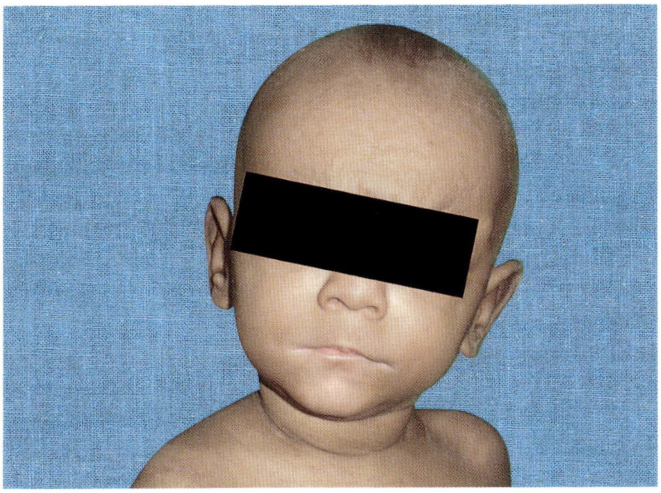

Fig. 1: Hypohidrotic ectodermal dysplasia in a 4-year-old boy.

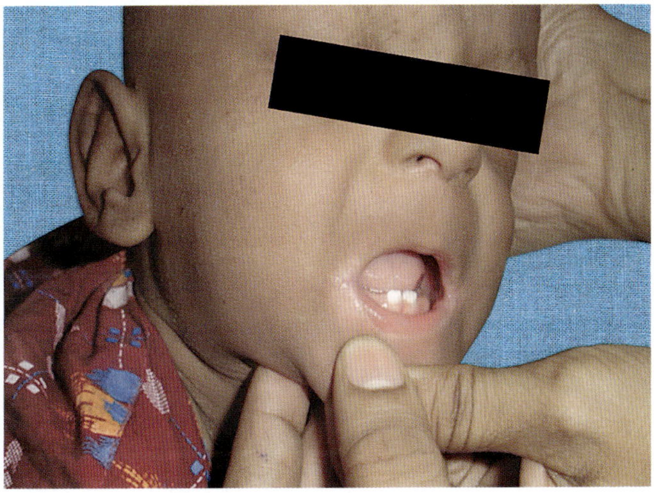

Fig. 2: Same boy, lack of dentition.

"Strength does not come from winning. Your struggles develop your strengths. When you go through hardship and decide not to surrender, that is strength." —**Arnold Schwarzenegger**

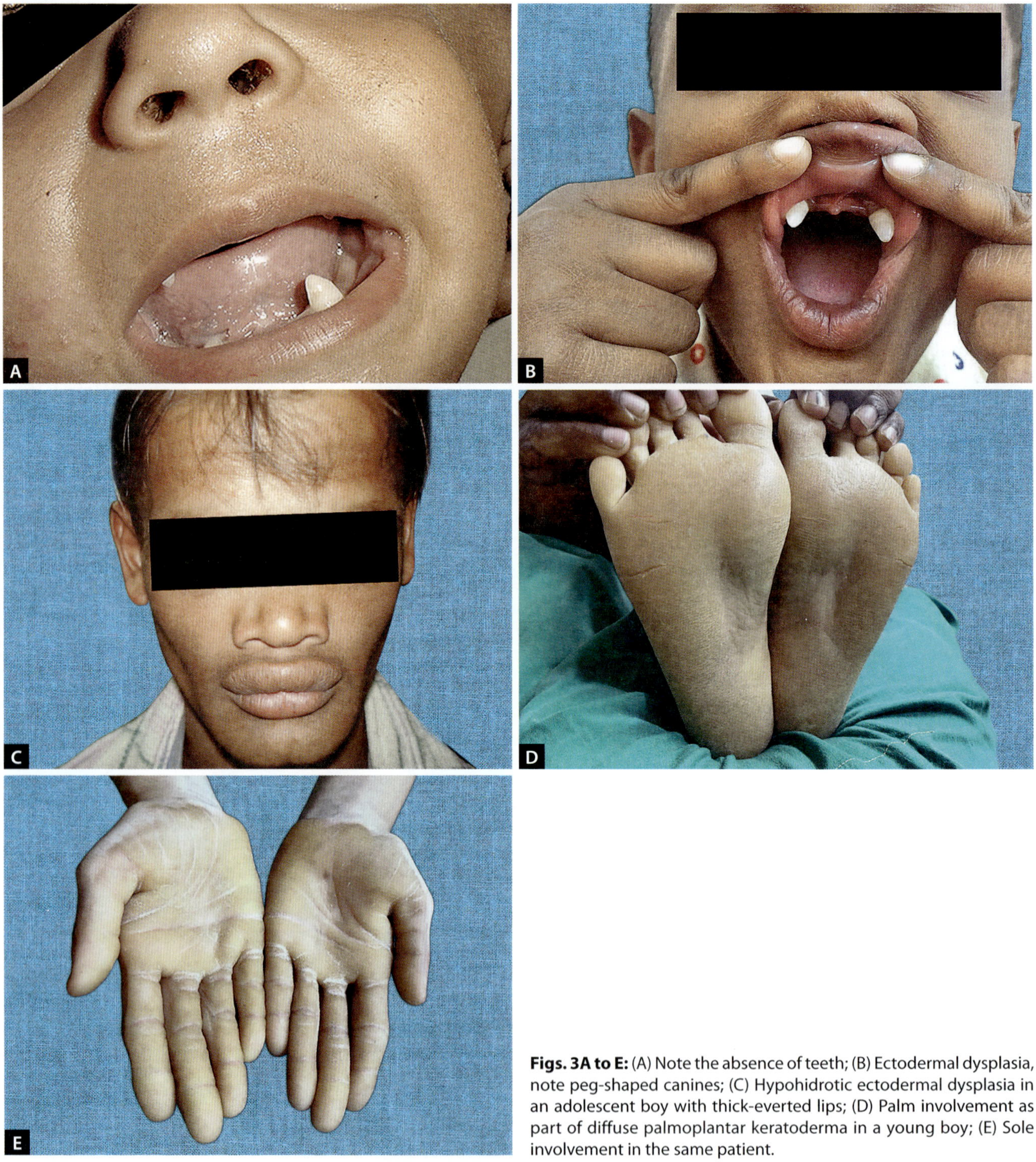

Figs. 3A to E: (A) Note the absence of teeth; (B) Ectodermal dysplasia, note peg-shaped canines; (C) Hypohidrotic ectodermal dysplasia in an adolescent boy with thick-everted lips; (D) Palm involvement as part of diffuse palmoplantar keratoderma in a young boy; (E) Sole involvement in the same patient.

nails, finger joints, knuckles, elbows and knees. Teeth may be normal. Other associated features include syndactyly, polydactyly, ocular abnormalities such as strabismus, conjunctivitis, cataract and sensorineural hearing loss.

Course and Prognosis

Chronic pyogenic infections and chronic pharyngitis can occur in hypohidrotic ectodermal dysplasia. In hidrotic form, persistent paronychia and onychomycosis are troublesome. The life expectancy is usually normal.

"Don't be too timid and squeamish about your actions. All life is an experiment. The more experiments you make the better." **—Ralph Waldo Emerson**

Management

Treatment of this condition is mainly multidisciplinary approach. Temperature regulation, cool baths, air conditioning environment, avoidance of sunlight, loose cotton clothes, cooling jackets to prevent hypothermia and encouraging children for water-related sports activities is useful. Emollients for dry skin and keratolytics for PPK are necessary. Dental interventions and regular ocular follow up should be done. Genetic counseling and prenatal diagnosis is the mainstay of management.

PALMOPLANTAR KERATODERMAS

Palmoplantar keratoderma refers to thickening of palms and soles either localized or diffuse because of genetic predisposition or inflammatory condition secondary to psoriasis, pityriasis rubra pilaris or Reiter's disease. Hereditary PPK involves genes encoding intracellular structural proteins, desmosomal proteins, gap junction components and enzymes. They occur as an isolated defect or may be associated with abnormalities in nails, teeth or with extracutaneous involvement.

DIFFUSE KERATODERMAS

Epidermolytic (Vorner Type) and Nonepidermolytic Palmoplantar Keratoderma (Unna Thost) (Figs. 4B to D)

It is an autosomal dominant disorder characterized by diffuse palmoplantar thickening caused by K9 and K1 mutations. The keratoderma usually begins in infancy and manifests as symmetric, diffuse, thick, yellowish hyperkeratosis with sharply demarcated erythematous margins with no transgrediens. This is often associated with hyperhidrosis, maceration and secondary dermatophyte infections. Epidermolytic hyperkeratosis is seen in epidermolytic PPK.

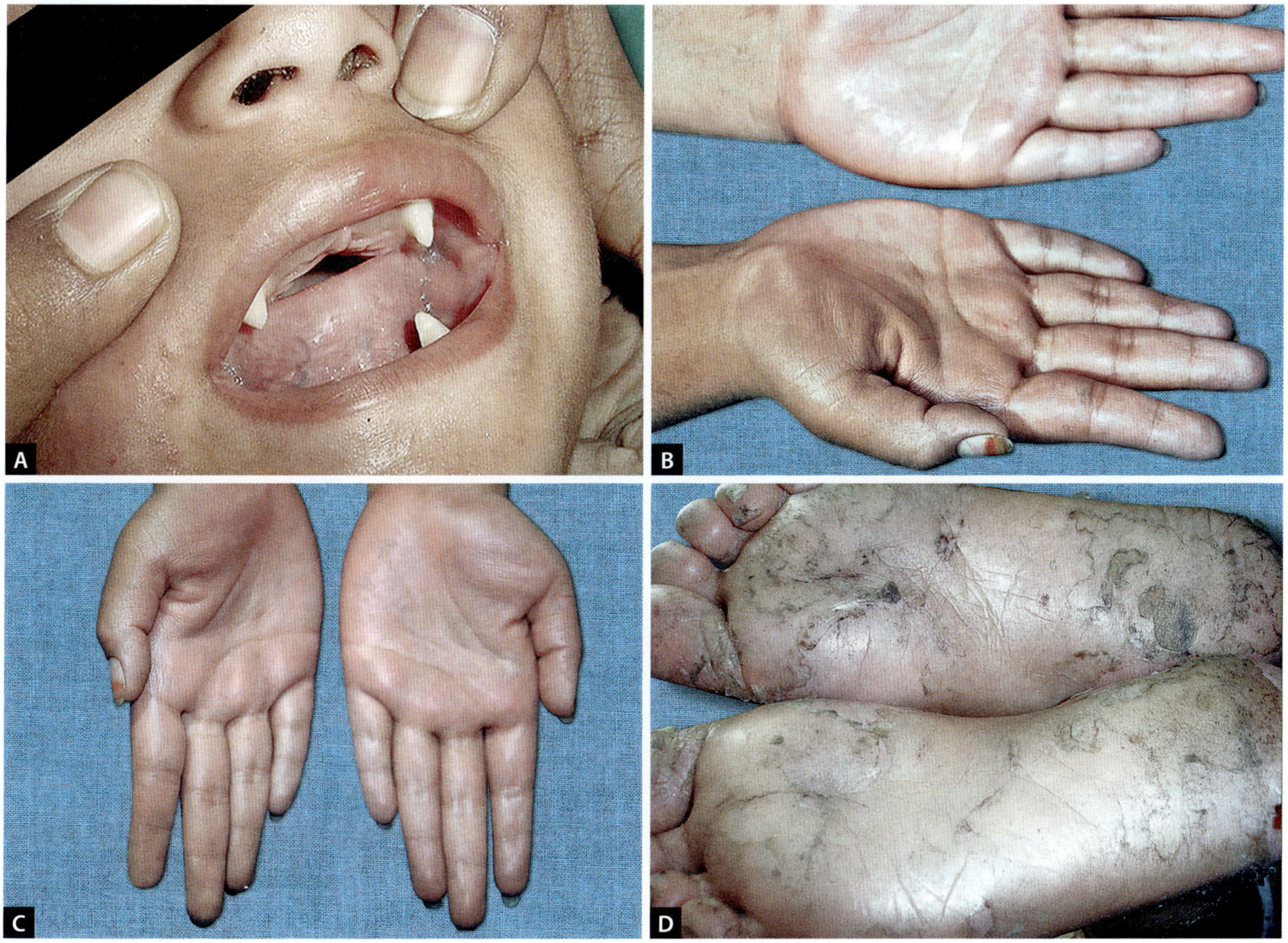

Figs. 4A to D: (A) Peg-shaped canines; (B) Palmar keratoderma, note the associated erythema; (C) Same patient with palmar keratoderma; (D) Diffuse plantar keratoderma.

"Knowledge is power. And you need power in this world. You need as many advantages as you can get." —**Ellen DeGeneres**

Vohwinkel Syndrome (Fig. 4E)

It is an autosomal dominant disorder caused by mutation in *GJB2* gene encoding connexin 26. It is a type of mutilating keratoderma characterized by extensive PPK with "honeycomb" pattern and constrictions (pseudoainhum) that may lead to amputation of distal digits. Other features

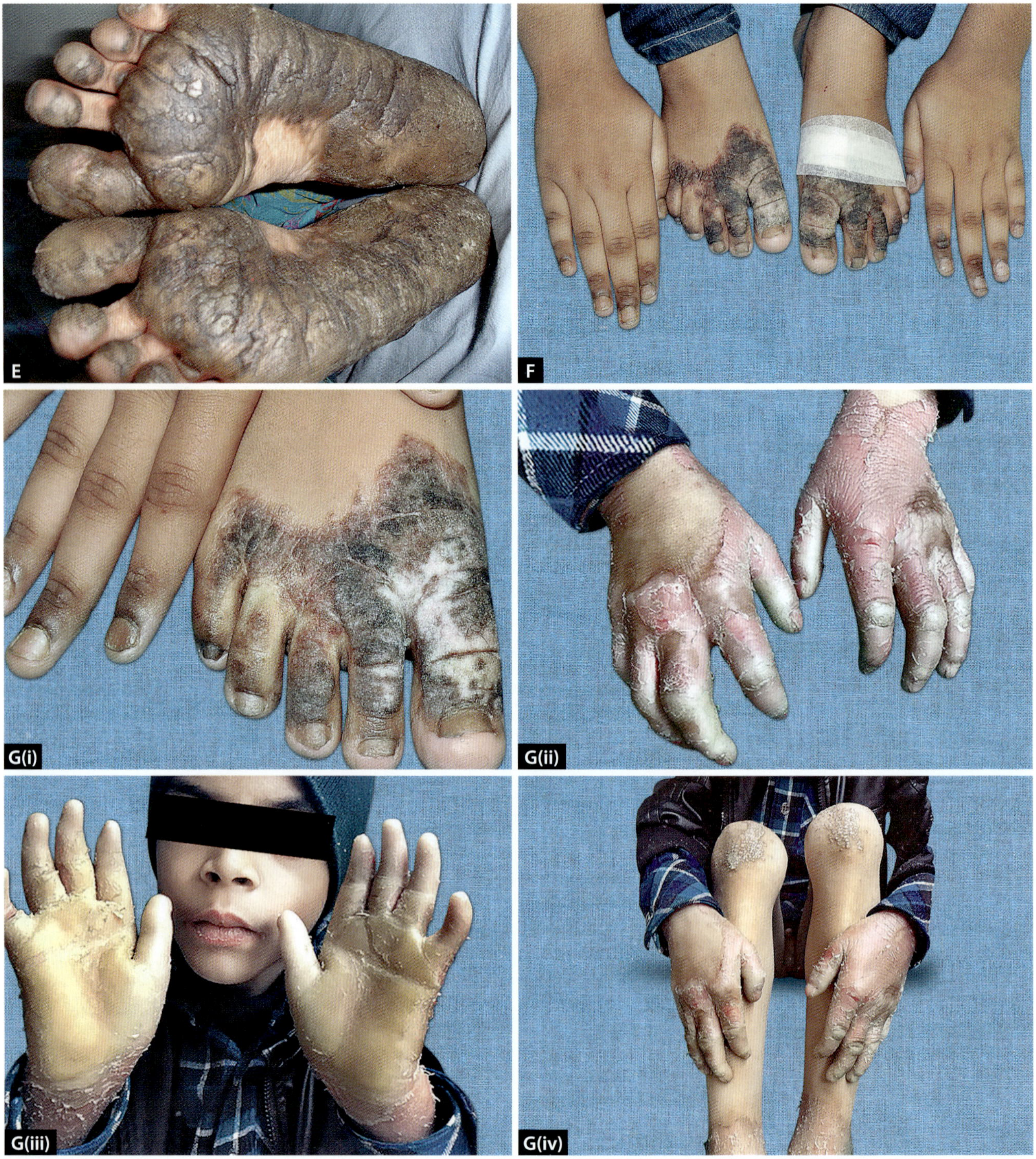

Figs. 4E to G(iv): (E) Honeycomb pattern of plantar keratoderma; (F) Palmoplantar keratoderma. Note that lesions are spreading over dorsal aspect of hand and feet; G(i) Palmoplantar keratoderma encroaching over dorsum of feet, close-up view; G(ii) Mal de Meleda, note diffuse keratoderma over dorsal aspect of hands; G(iii) Same boy showing thick yellowish palmar keratoderma along with perioral and lip erythema; G(iv) Same boy showing psoriasiform over knees and ankles.

"I have learnt over the years that when one's mind is made up, this diminishes fear; knowing what must be done does away with fear." —**Rosa Parks**

are presence of knuckle pads, leukonychia, myopathy, ichthyosiform dermatitis, alopecia and sensorineural deafness.

Mal De Meleda [Figs. 4F to G(iv)]

It is a rare form of autosomal recessive disorder characterized by diffuse, waxy, thick, yellowish hyperkeratosis of the palms and soles with transgrediens. Hyperhidrosis and candidal/fungal infection may be associated. There is occasional perioral erythema. Nail changes include subungual hyperkeratosis, Beau's lines, onycholysis, koilonychia, and onychogryphosis.

Olmsted Syndrome (Mutilating PPK with Periorificial Plaques) (Fig. 4H)

It is a rare autosomal dominant disorder presenting with progressive development of painful plaques of keratoderma over palms and soles that begins during infancy to early childhood. The borders of keratoderma tend to be erythematous. Autoamputation from progressive constriction of digits is common. Other features are periorificial thickening, fissuring, alopecia and nail dystrophy.

Papillon–Lefèvre Syndrome (Figs. 4I to K)

It is an autosomal recessive condition manifesting as a triad of diffuse PPK **(Fig. 4L)**, periodontitis and susceptibility to cutaneous and systemic infections. PPK often extends on the dorsal surface of the hands and feet. Rarely focal or punctate keratoderma can occur. Psoriasis-like lesions are seen over knees and elbows. As early as at 3 years of age, there may be development of periodontitis with loss of both permanent and deciduous teeth. Most of the patients may become edentulous by 15 years of age. They are more susceptible to pyogenic skin and liver infections (hepatic abscess).

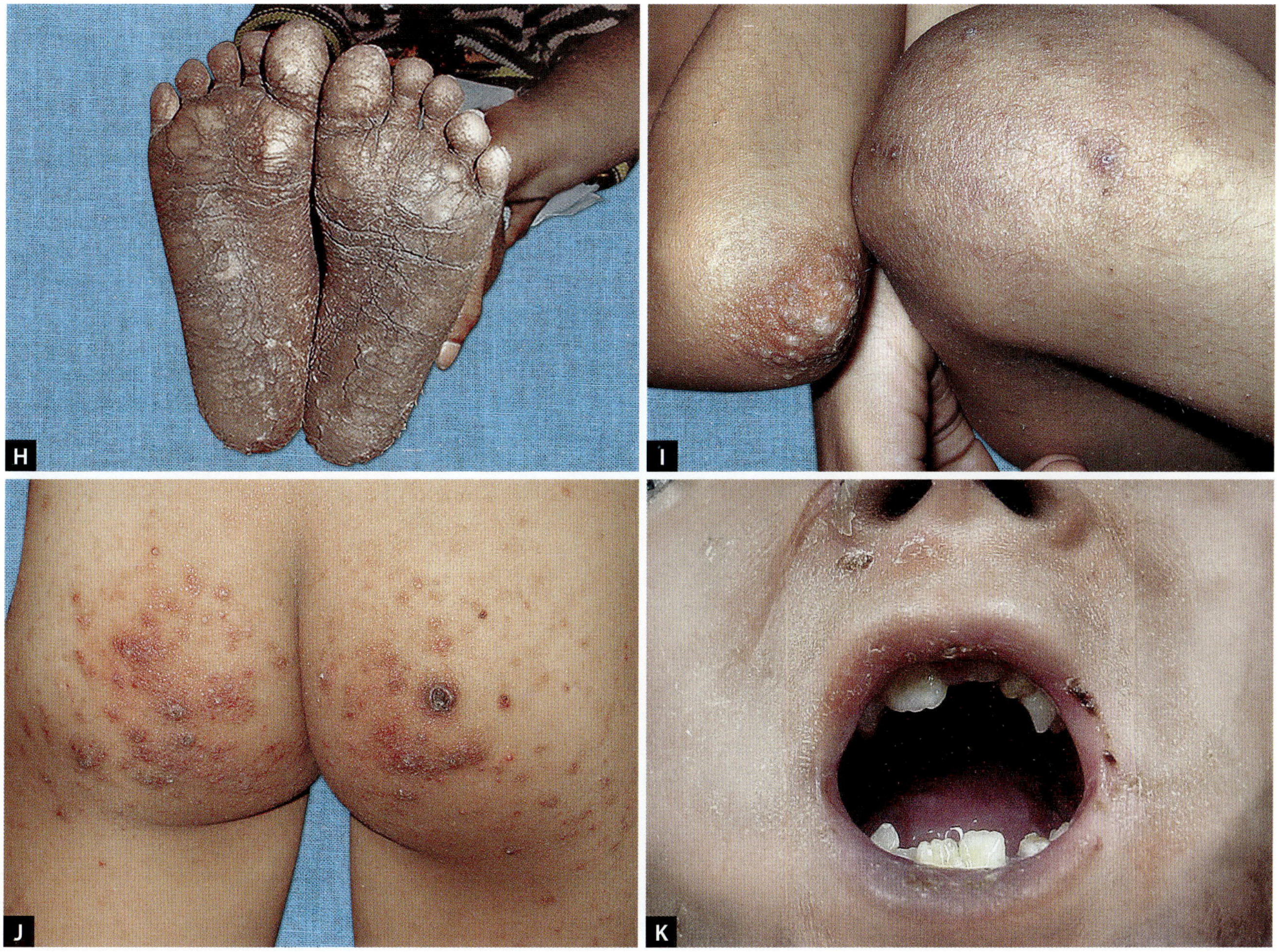

Figs. 4H to K: (H) Plantar keratoderma with mutilating toes; (I) Hyperkeratotic plaque over elbow in pachyonychia congenita type 2; (J) Follicular keratosis over buttocks in pachyonychia congenita type 2; (K) Papillon–Lefèvre syndrome; periodontitis.

"If you want to be successful you must respect one rule, never lie to yourself." **—Paulo Coelho**

FOCAL KERATODERMAS

It refers to localized keratodermas over palms and soles. Various conditions which present as focal keratodermas are:

- Pachyonychia congenita (PC)
- Richner–Hanhart syndrome
- Howel–Evans syndrome

Pachyonychia Congenita (Figs. 4L to O)

Pachyonychia congenita encompasses a group of autosomal dominant conditions which manifests as focal keratoderma and occurs due to mutations in one of the four keratin genes, *KRT6A, KRT6B, KRT16*, or *KRT17*. Based on the specific keratin mutation, it has been classified into PC-6a, PC-6b, PC-16, PC-17, and PC-unknown. PC-6a and PC-16 are most common. Clinical features include focal plantar keratoderma, fingernail and toenail dystrophy. At birth there is nail changes but as the child grows, PPK becomes evident. Periungual infection, fissuring, blisters and ulceration, follicular keratoses, hoarseness and oral leukoplakia are often associated features. Systemic and topical preparations of sirolimus are being tried for painful palmoplantar keratoderma in pachyonychia congenita.

Richner–Hanhart Syndrome

It is an autosomal recessive condition in which there is focal PPK with tyrosinemia because of deficiency of hepatic aminotransferase enzyme.

The early skin lesions are seen in first year of life as yellowish keratotic papules over palms and soles. But often they appear at teenage. The lesions become erythematous, erosive and painful with time. Associated features are photophobia and corneal erosions which usually develop by 6 months of life.

Treatment

Restriction of tyrosine with low phenylalanine and low tyrosine containing diet.

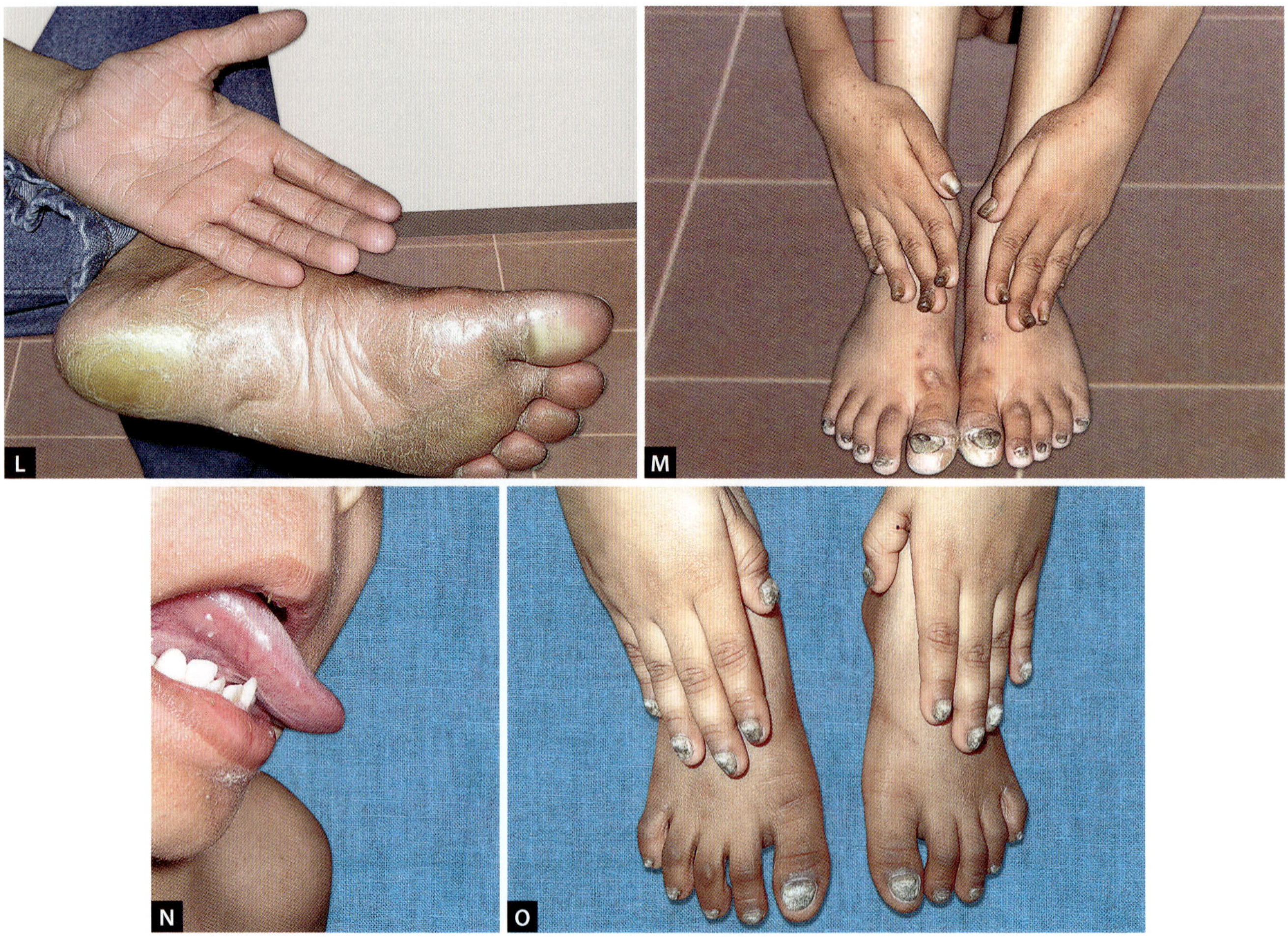

Figs. 4L to O: (L) Diffuse palmoplantar keratoderma; (M) Thickened nails in pachyonychia congenita type 1; (N) Oral leukokeratosis in pachyonychia congenita type 1; (O) Thickened nails in pachyonychia congenita type 2.

"There are two educations. One should teach us how to make a living and the other how to live." **—John Adams**

Howel–Evans Syndrome (Tylosis with Esophageal Cancer)

In this condition, there is late-onset dominant focal PPK with development of esophageal carcinoma at around sixth decade of life in most of the individuals.

PUNCTATE PALMOPLANTAR KERATODERMA (FIG. 4P)

This condition is characterized by development of discrete keratoses over palms and soles. The punctate keratodermas vary from 1 to 3 mm in size and are mostly

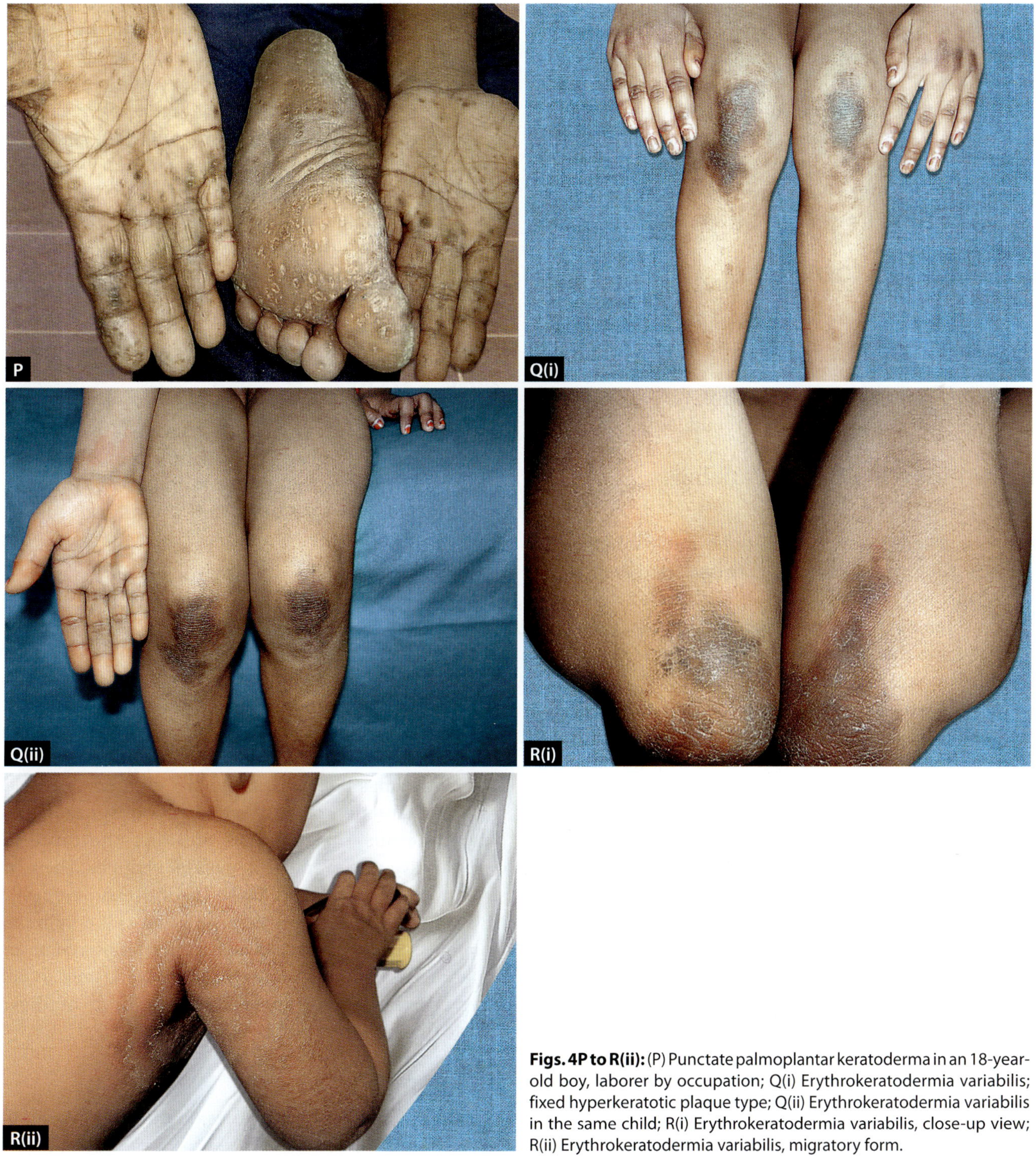

Figs. 4P to R(ii): (P) Punctate palmoplantar keratoderma in an 18-year-old boy, laborer by occupation; Q(i) Erythrokeratodermia variabilis; fixed hyperkeratotic plaque type; Q(ii) Erythrokeratodermia variabilis in the same child; R(i) Erythrokeratodermia variabilis, close-up view; R(ii) Erythrokeratodermia variabilis, migratory form.

distributed over palmar creases and volar aspect of fingers. The central keratinous plugs, if picked out, leaves a shallow depressed pit with a keratotic base. The lesions are usually asymptomatic but may be painful on walking.

Treatment

There is no curative treatment as hereditary PPK persists lifelong and affects the quality of life. Treatment of all forms of hyperkeratosis of palms and soles is done with emollients, mechanical debridement, keratolytics such as 10–20% salicylic acid and 20–40% urea either alone or in combination and treatment of underlying secondary infection. For severe discomfort or symptomatic PPK, oral retinoids may be used for short duration. Multidisciplinary approach along with genetic counseling is necessary.

ERYTHROKERATODERMAS

Erythrokeratodermas are a group of keratinizing disorders, which present as hyperkeratotic plaques over different parts of the body. Two types have been recognized:

1. Erythrokeratodermia variabilis (EKV)
2. Progressive symmetric erythrokeratoderma

Erythrokeratodermia Variabilis [Figs. 4Q(i) to R(ii)]

It is an autosomal dominant disorder rarely inherited as recessive pattern characterized by two distinct type of lesions:

1. Sharply marginated pruritic patches of erythema which are often figurate in configuration and undergo changes in size, shape and configuration over a period of days to weeks.
2. Fixed hyperkeratotic plaques with the thick yellow-brown scales that usually overlie erythema.

Lesions are most often distributed over limbs, trunk and buttocks. They are often distributed symmetrically. Face is relatively spared.

The lesions are mostly noted first at birth or during the first year of life. The condition exacerbates in winter and regress in summer spontaneously. In most, the lesions tend to improve at puberty.

Treatment

There is no specific therapy for erythrokeratodermia variabilis. Various topical therapies used are emollients, retinoic acid, keratolytics, tazarotene, alpha-hydroxy acid, and topical corticosteroids. Oral retinoids such as acitretin, etretinate, and isotretinoin have been found to be very effective. They can be given for long-term intermittently. Lesions reappear once the therapy is stopped. Counseling parents about the prognosis is necessary.

Progressive Symmetric Erythrokeratoderma [Figs. 4S(i) to T(ii)]

The condition has features almost identical to that of EKV. However, the absence of migrating red patches and higher incidence of PPK distinguishes it from EKV. The disorder tends to have its onset during infancy, is usually limited to extremities, buttocks and face. The condition tends to regress at puberty. It usually follows an autosomal dominant pattern with no confirmed candidate gene. The classical features of progressive symmetric erythrokeratoderma consist of symmetrically distributed, nonmigratory, large, well-defined, erythematous, hyperkeratotic plaques with marked peripheral erythema. It has to be differentiated from psoriasis, EKV and pityriasis rubra pilaris.

XERODERMA PIGMENTOSUM (FIGS. 5 TO 8)

Xeroderma pigmentosum (XP) is a severe rare autosomal recessive disorder characterized by cutaneous photosensitivity, a decreased ability to repair DNA damage by ultraviolet (UV) radiation and a tendency to early development of cutaneous malignancies. Symptoms appear between 6 months and 3 years of age; the tumor stage is reached by 20 years of age. The characteristic clinical features include erythema, freckling, both hyperpigmentation and depigmentation, premature aging, telangiectasia, hyperkeratosis, ulceration, keratoacanthomas, and after a relatively short period of time, skin cancer. In the acute form, the first manifestation appears early, sometimes shortly after birth after the first exposure to the sun. Initial clinical findings being photophobia, erythema, freckled hyperpigmentation of exposed parts, and subsequently, papillomatous or verrucous lesions, followed by degenerative and eventual malignant changes. There are seven types of XP (XPA to XPG). The most common XP is XPC. Malignant changes include basal cell carcinoma, squamous cell carcinoma, angiosarcoma, fibrosarcoma and melanoma. Neurological complications are seen in 30% cases, especially in XPA group. There may be an overlap of XP and Cockayne syndrome (CS).

Natural History

The severity of the disease varies; in the severe form, the disease is fatal by 10 years of age.

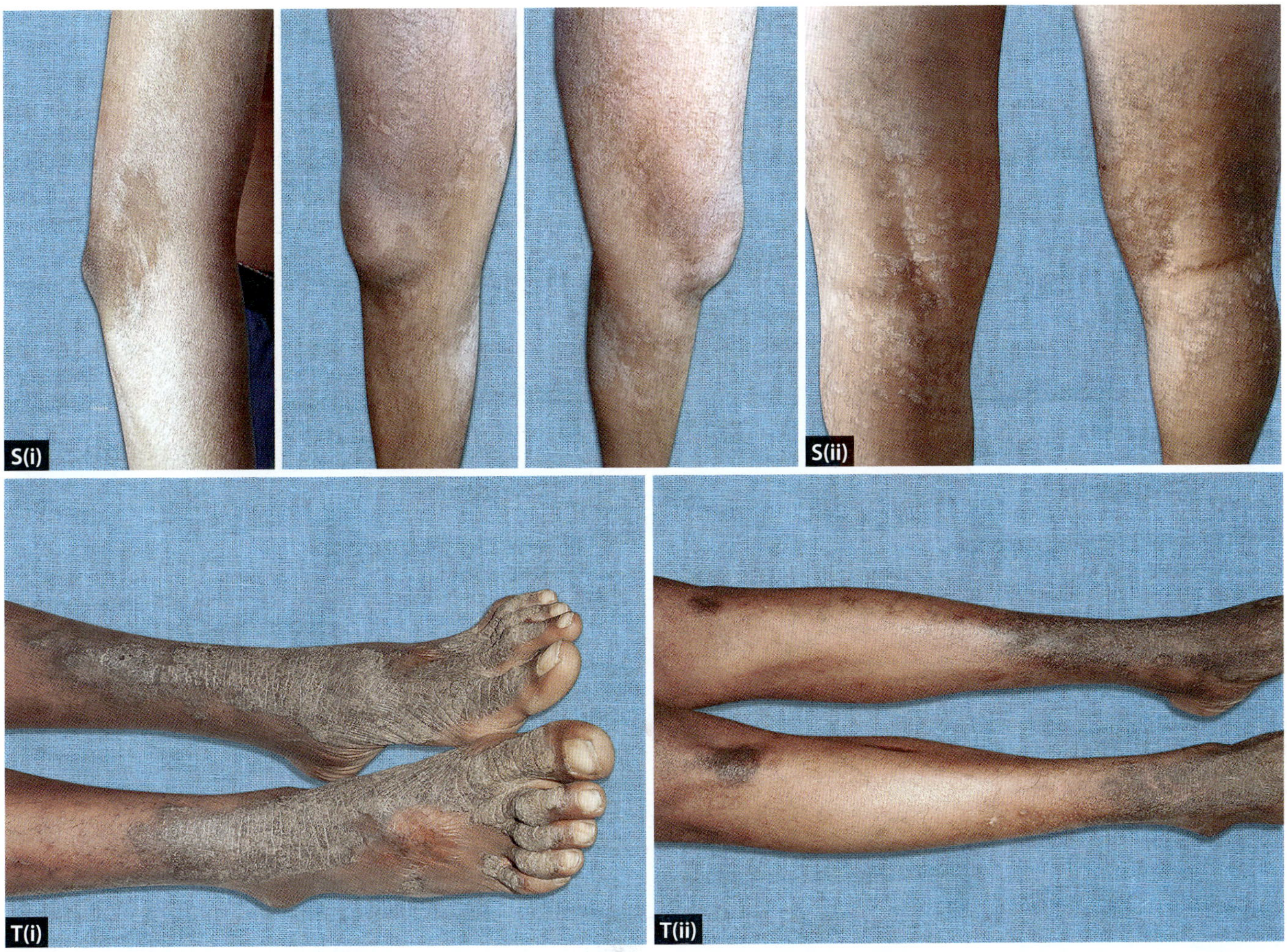

Figs. 4S(i) to T(ii): S(i) Progressive symmetric erythrokeratoderma; S(ii) Same child, close-up view; T(i) Progressive symmetric erythrokeratoderma in an 18-year-old boy; T(ii) Progressive symmetric erythrokeratoderma.

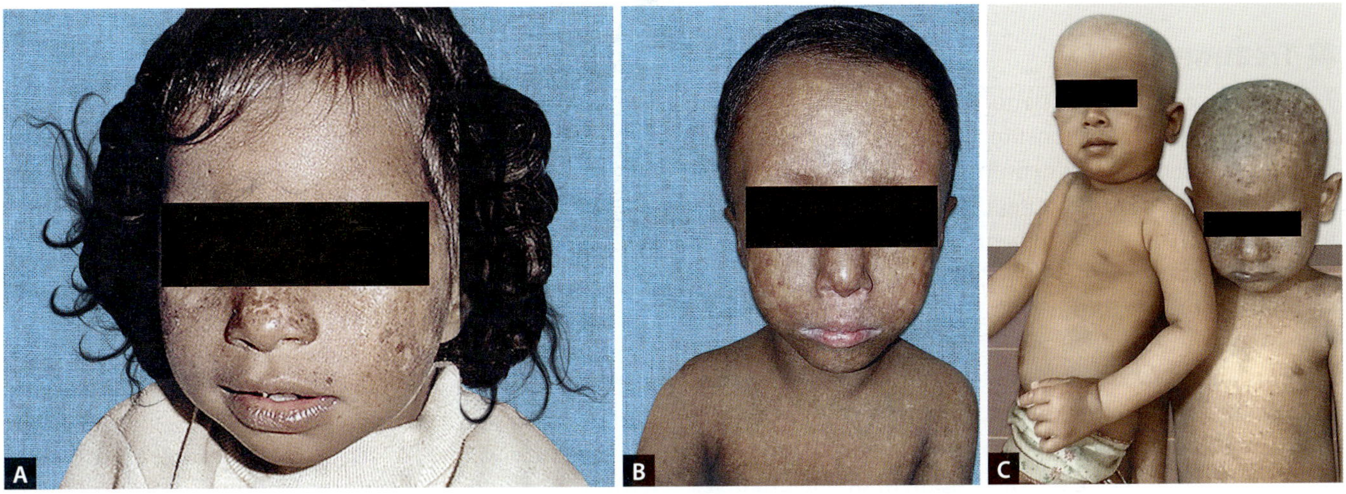

Figs. 5A to C: (A) Pigmented and depigmented macules over photosensitive distribution; (B) Xeroderma pigmentosum; (C) Xeroderma pigmentosum in two siblings; note difference in degree of involvement.

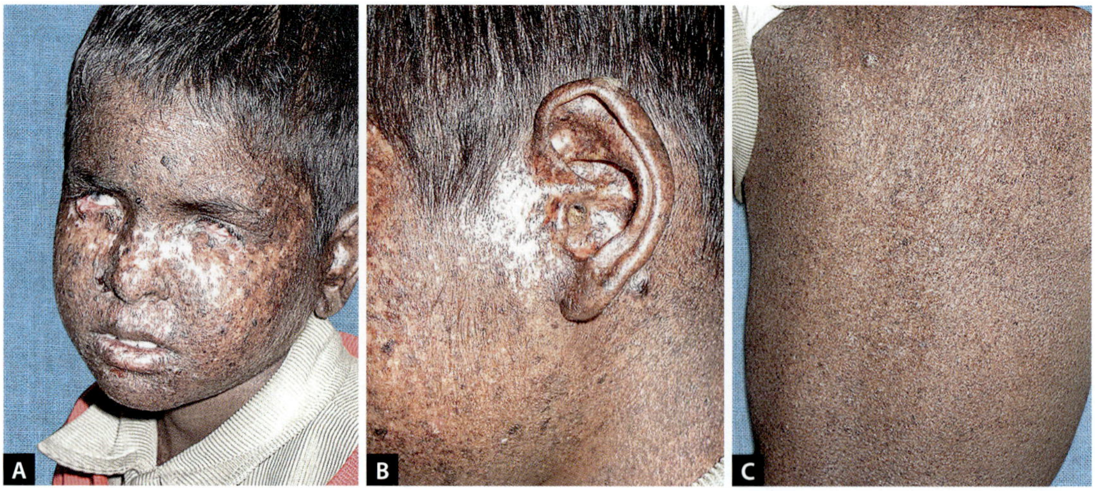

Figs. 6A to C: (A) Pigmented and depigmented macules, angiomas and telangiectasia over the entire face in a 5-year-old boy with xeroderma pigmentosum. (B) Xeroderma pigmentosum; same child, close-up view; (C) Same child, back.

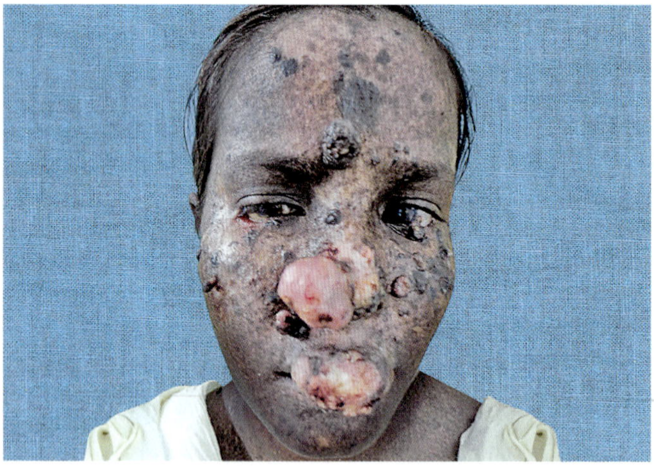

Fig. 7: Xeroderma pigmentosum (XP) in a 9-year-old girl with all three types of skin malignancy.

Treatment

Treatment consists of genetic counseling, vigorous avoidance of UV light exposure, UV protective glasses, full sleeved clothes, methyl cellulose eye drops to keep the cornea moist and soft contact lenses to protect against mechanical trauma. Children should be encouraged for indoor sports activities. Parents should be taught to palpate the lesions regularly for any changes like elevation to rule out premalignant conditions as early diagnosis can prevent mortality. The premalignant and malignant tumors are treated by topical application of antimetabolites and surgical removal. Oral retinoids have been useful in delaying the development of malignancies of the skin. Dermabrasion and skin grafting are tried for actinically damaged skin.

COCKAYNE SYNDROME (FIG. 8B)

Cockayne syndrome is a rare genodermatosis with autosomal recessive inheritance. The syndrome is characterized by profound growth retardation, microcephaly, neurodevelopmental impairment, photosensitive skin eruption, premature skin aging, disproportionately large hands, feet and ears, ocular defects, and extreme demyelination. This syndrome has been described in children from every race and affects males and females with almost equal frequency. Cultured fibroblasts from affected patients are hypersensitive to UV light-induced inhibition of growth and colony-forming abilities with a defective subpathway of nucleotide excision repair process. Mutation in genes *ERCC8* and *ERCC6* coding for protein in transcription-coupled repair is thought to be responsible for Cockayne phenotype in the majority of cases. The clinical symptoms of the multisystem involvement in CS are quite heterogeneous and can vary considerably in their severity. Although very early onset has been reported in a significant minority of cases, the child usually appears normal in the first year when facial erythema in the butterfly area distribution develops after exposure to sunlight without excess pigmentary abnormalities. There is a marked loss of subcutaneous fat resulting in a wizened appearance with typical "bird-headed" facies, prominent "mickey mouse" ears, sparse dry hair, and thin nose. Many patients exhibit a characteristic stooped appearance with kyphoscoliosis and flexion deformities of hips, knees, and ankles. Ocular findings include pigmentary retinal degeneration with a characteristic "salt and pepper" appearance of retina, cataracts, optic nerve atrophy, optic disc pallor, iris hypoplasia, and microphthalmus. Neurological abnormalities include deafness, peripheral neuropathy, normal pressure hydrocephalus, and microcephaly. Intellectual deterioration may be nonuniform with some preserved better than others. Dental caries, renal abnormalities with decreased creatinine clearance, hypertension, and retarded reproductive development are reported in few CS patients.

PIGMENTED XERODERMOID (FIGS. 8C TO E)

Pigmented xerodermoid is a variant of XP. It has a later age at onset in the third or fourth decade of life in comparison to XP which has an onset within 1–2 years after birth.

Pigmented xerodermoid or XP-variant patients have cutaneous and ocular manifestations similar to XP but

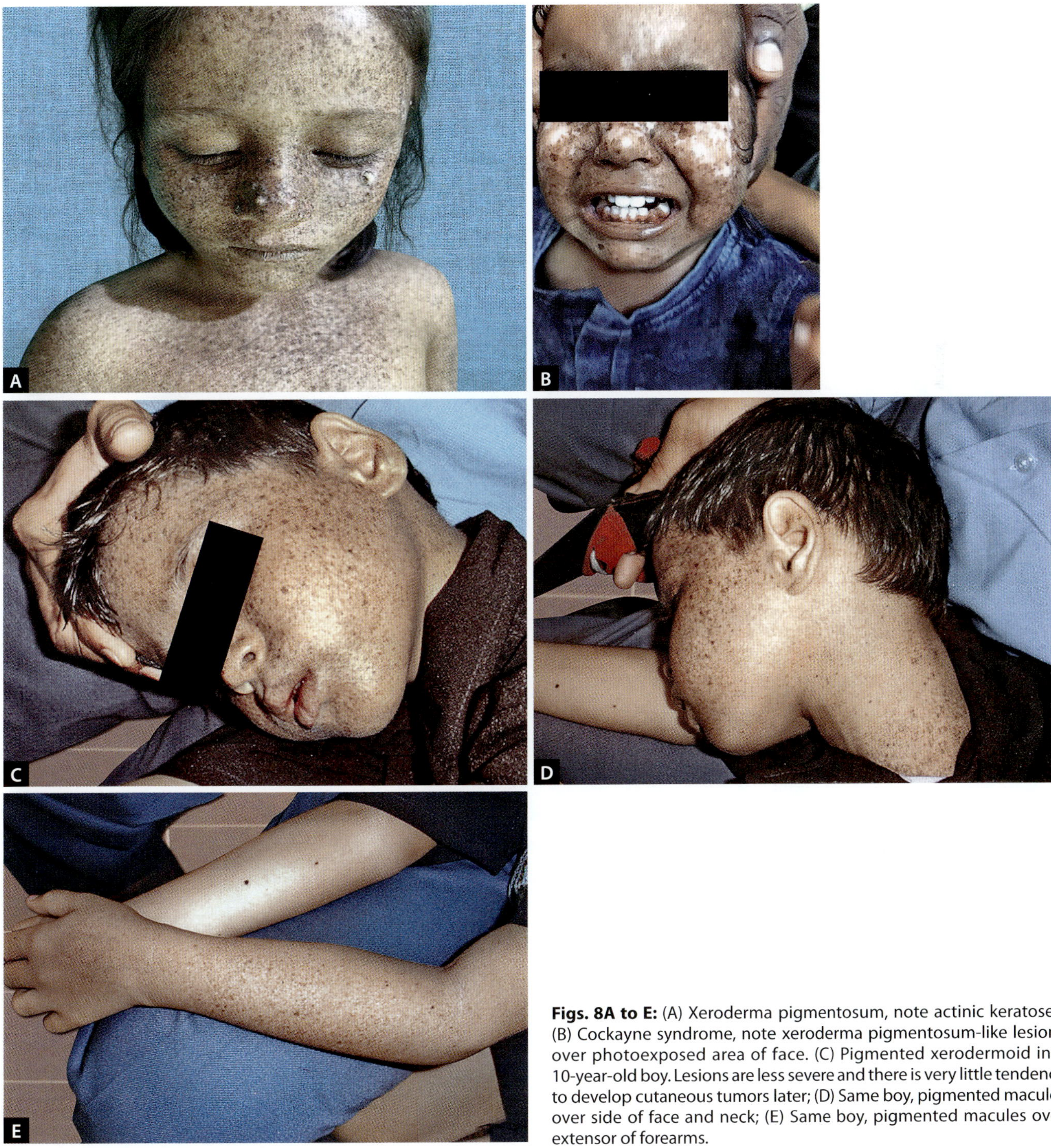

Figs. 8A to E: (A) Xeroderma pigmentosum, note actinic keratoses; (B) Cockayne syndrome, note xeroderma pigmentosum-like lesions over photoexposed area of face. (C) Pigmented xerodermoid in a 10-year-old boy. Lesions are less severe and there is very little tendency to develop cutaneous tumors later; (D) Same boy, pigmented macules over side of face and neck; (E) Same boy, pigmented macules over extensor of forearms.

"I have learnt that people will forget what you said, people will forget what you did, but people will never forget how you made them feel." —**Maya Angelou**

neurologic involvement is rare. Clinical features may be mild in some and severe in others.

Clinically it needs to be differentiated from other variants of XP, XP with neurologic abnormalities, CS, XP/CS complex, trichothiodystrophy (TTD), XP/TTD complex, cerebro-oculo-facio-skeletal (COFS) syndrome, COFS/TTD, CS/TTD complex, and UV-sensitive syndrome and other diseases with cutaneous photosensitivity such as Rothmund-Thomson syndrome and Hartnup disease.

Treatment consists of stringent photo protection of the skin and eyes. Lubricating eye drops must be used. Total body examination must be carried out at regular intervals for early identification of malignancies. Premalignant lesions such as actinic keratoses may be treated with cryotherapy and malignancies treated along same protocols as in patients without XP. Isotretinoin and acitretin may be tried to prevent cutaneous malignancies. Since exposure to sunlight is minimized, vitamin D may be given prophylactically to prevent bone fractures.

Affected parents can undergo genetic testing to find out the risk of having an offspring with the disease. Prenatal testing and genetic counseling have an important role to play in the diagnosis and management of the disease.

BLOOM'S SYNDROME (FIGS. 8F TO 8L)

Bloom's syndrome (BS) is a rare genetic disorder characterized by short stature, sun-sensitive skin changes, an increased risk of cancer, and other health issues. It is caused by mutations in the *BLM* gene, which encodes a DNA helicase enzyme involved in maintaining genomic stability.

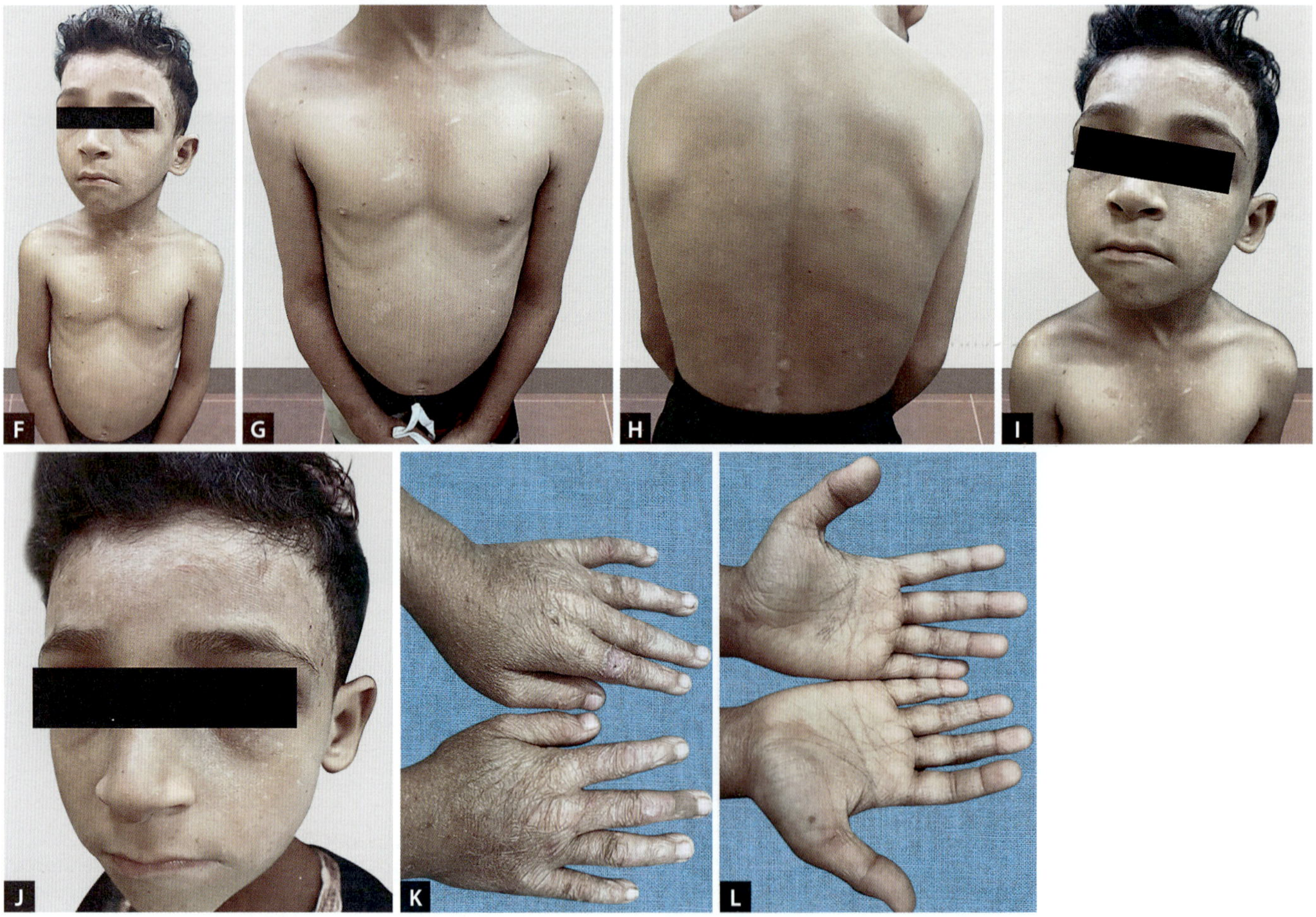

Figs. 8F to L: (F) Short stature of Bloom's syndrome. (G) Front of the trunk, note multiple café-au-lait macules and Ash-leaf macules. (H) Back showing similar lesions. (I) Elongated flattened face, beaked nose, micrognathia. (J) Close-up of face. (K) Wrinkled skin like progeria hands. (L) Wrinkled skin over palms, xerotic palms with increased palmar creases.

"Always do your best. What you plant now, you will harvest later." —**OG Mandino**

Here are some details about Bloom's syndrome and the genes involved:

- ***BLM* gene:** Mutations in the *BLM* gene are responsible for Bloom's syndrome. This gene is located on chromosome 15 and encodes the BLM protein, which is part of the RecQ family of DNA helicases. The BLM protein plays a critical role in DNA repair, particularly in resolving DNA structures that can arise during processes like DNA replication and recombination. Mutations in BLM lead to impaired DNA repair mechanisms, which results in genomic instability, a hallmark of Bloom's syndrome.
- **Type of inheritance:** Bloom's syndrome follows an autosomal recessive pattern of inheritance. This means that an individual must inherit two copies of the mutated *BLM* gene (one from each parent) to develop the disorder. Carriers, who have one mutated copy of the gene and one normal copy, typically do not show symptoms but can pass the mutated gene to their children.
- **Genetic instability and cancer risk:** Individuals with Bloom's syndrome have a significantly increased risk of developing various types of cancer, including leukemia, lymphoma, and cancers of the skin, breast, and gastrointestinal tract. The genomic instability caused by BLM mutations predisposes cells to accumulate mutations and chromosomal abnormalities, which can contribute to cancer development.
- **Other clinical features:** Apart from cancer predisposition, Bloom's syndrome is characterized by distinctive physical features such as short stature, a narrow face with a prominent nose, and a red rash on the face (often referred to as a "butterfly rash"). Affected individuals also tend to have recurrent infections, particularly of the respiratory tract.

Diagnosis and Management

Diagnosis of Bloom's syndrome involves genetic testing to identify mutations in the BLM gene. Management of Bloom's syndrome involves regular monitoring for cancer and other potential health issues, along with supportive care to manage symptoms. Genetic counseling is essential for families with a history of Bloom's syndrome to understand the risks and inheritance patterns associated with the condition.

In summary, Bloom's syndrome is a genetic disorder caused by mutations in the *BLM* gene, leading to genomic instability, increased cancer risk, and characteristic physical features. Understanding the role of the *BLM* gene helps in both diagnosing the condition and developing strategies for managing its associated health risks.

PSEUDOXANTHOMA ELASTICUM (FIGS. 9 AND 10A)

This genetic disorder of the elastic tissue involves the skin, eye and the cardiovascular system. Both autosomal dominant and autosomal recessive transmission may occur. Skin lesions that are hallmark of this disorder is characterized by yellowish xanthoma-like flat papules and linear plaques resembling plucked chicken skin, Morocco leather or orange skin (peau d'orange) distributed on neck, below the clavicles, flexures, perineum and thighs. As these lesions are tiny initially, diagnosis may be delayed till the 2nd or 3rd decade.

Systemic Associations

Eye changes are seen as slate gray to reddish brown linear bands (angioid streaks) which are uncommon in childhood. Loss of central vision is the most frequent disability. Significant cardiovascular changes include peripheral disease with easy fatigability, intermittent claudication, hypertension, mitral valve prolapse, coronary artery involvement, and cerebral, gastrointestinal or uterine hemorrhage.

Management

There is no specific treatment for this disorder. Genetic counseling should be provided and the patients should be advised to avoid strenuous activities and go for regular vascular survey and ophthalmologic examinations.

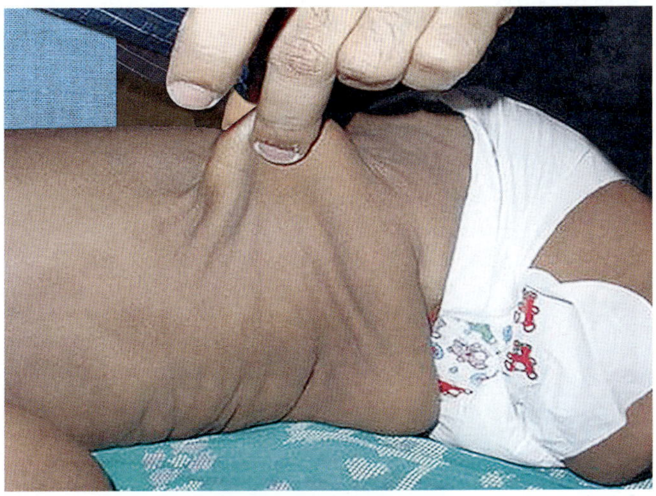

Fig. 9: Elasticity of lax skin.

CUTIS LAXA (FIGS. 10B TO F)

It is a heterogeneous group of disorder clinically characterized by loose, redundant, inelastic skin, and histologically, by loss of elastic tissue in the dermis. This entity may be inherited or acquired.

The condition, also known as dermatomegaly, dermatolysis, generalized elastolysis or chalazoderma, has three well-recognized genetic form; autosomal dominant, autosomal recessive and X-linked of which the autosomal recessive one is the most frequent and most severe. Frame shift or splicing mutation of elastin gene is responsible for autosomal dominant form; mutation in *fibulin-5* gene may cause either autosomal dominant or recessive cutis laxa whereas fibulin-4 mutation is solely associated with autosomal recessive variety with different system involvement. X-linked cutis laxa or occipital horn syndrome [previously type IX Ehlers-Danlos syndrome (EDS)] is due to defect in copper transporter ATP7A.

The benign, dominant form primarily restricted to the skin has good prognosis. Loose inelastic skin with reduced resilience produces aged appearance of the patients. Pendulous skin around eye, face and neck gives the appearance of bloodhound-like facies. Involvement of shoulder girdle simulates St Bernard dog.

Autosomal recessive form is associated with severe systemic involvements such as diverticula, pulmonary emphysema, hernia, cor pulmonale, osteoporosis, aortic aneurysm, large fontanelles with delayed closure, congenital dislocation of hip and lax joints. Congestive cardiac failure may be the presenting feature in infancy. Death usually occurs within 1st year of life.

X-linked cutis laxa is associated with parasagittal exostoses arising from occipital bone along with different system involvement including gastrointestinal tract.

Acquired form of cutis laxa resembles phenotypically milder variety of inherited cutis laxa with no positive family

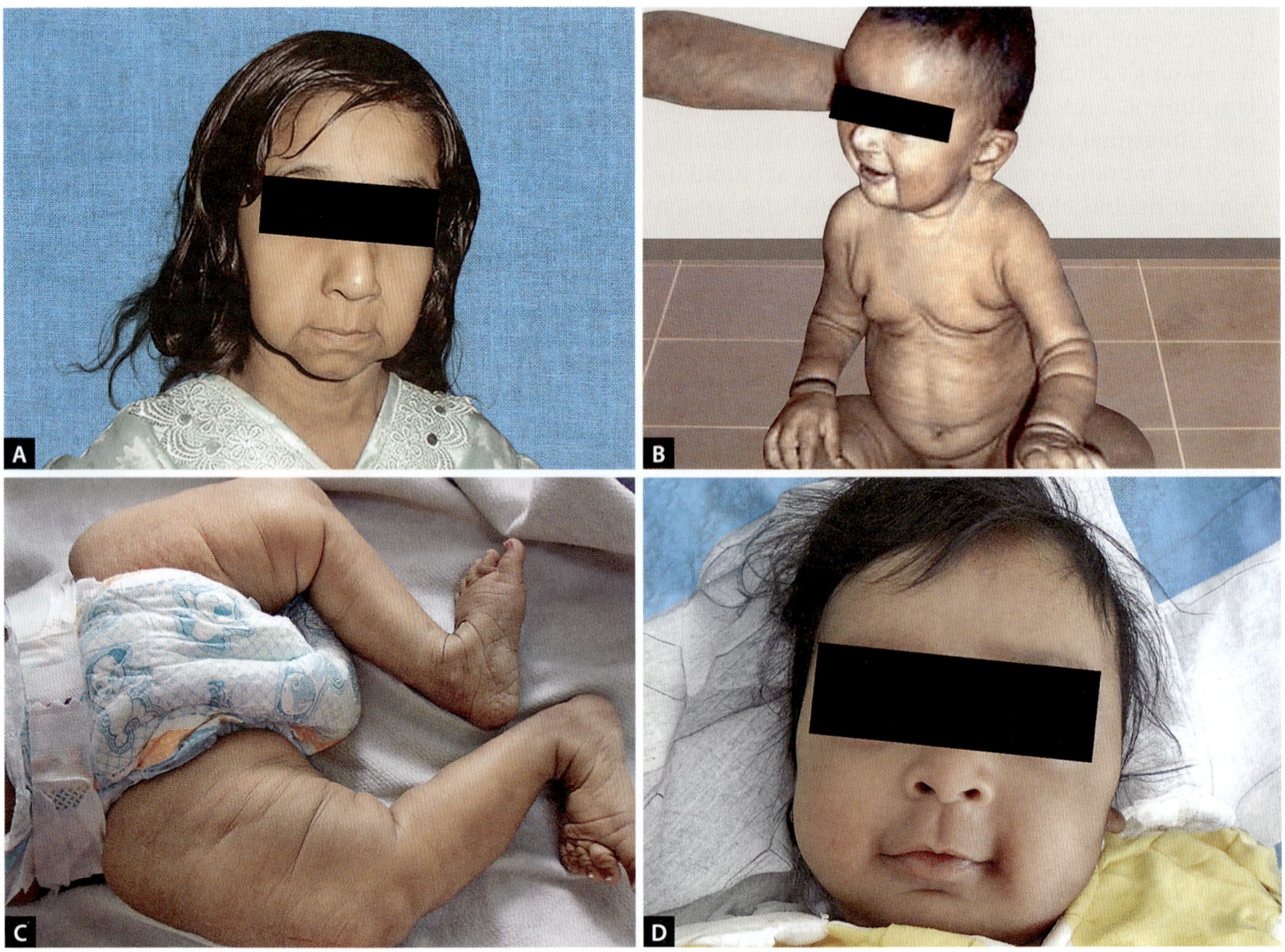

Figs. 10A to D: (A) Redundant skin over the face; (B) Cutis laxa, note laxity of skin; (C) Cutis laxa, thighs and legs; (D) Same child, face.

"A man who acquires the ability to take full possession of his own mind may take possession of anything else to which he is justly entitled." —**Andrew Carnegie**

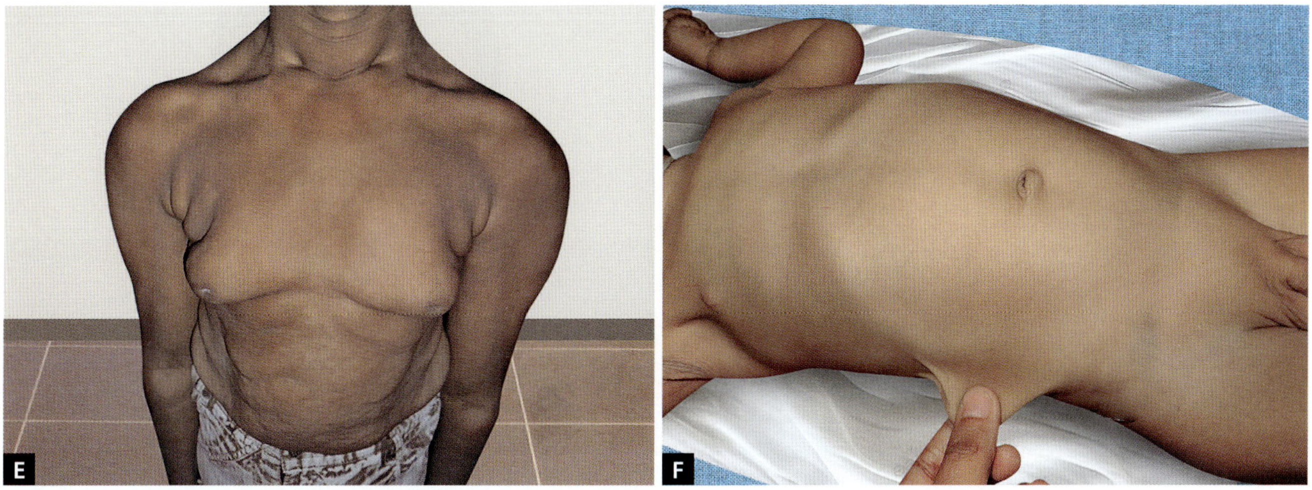

Figs. 10E and F: (E) Cutis laxa, note loose skin over chest and abdomen; (F) Cutis laxa.

history and has a late onset. Acquired variety may be idiopathic, paraneoplastic, postinflammatory (urticaria, erythema multiforme, systemic lupus erythematosus, angioedema, rheumatoid arthritis), drug induced (penicillin, penicillamine) and hematological (multiple myeloma). Acquired cutis laxa can be further classified into generalized and localized. Localized variety is usually restricted around eye, palms and soles.

Among the differentials, most important and confusing ones are EDS and pseudoxanthoma elasticum (PXE). In EDS, skin is hyperextensible but still elastic and recoil normally. Histopathology further supports the diagnosis of EDS where pathology is in collagen fibers in contrast to cutis laxa where pathology lies within elastic fibers. Though PXE skin is also loose and fails to recoil like that of cutis laxa, papules at the affected site (pebbly appearance) favors the diagnosis.

Though reconstructive surgery dramatically improves cosmetic appearance its role is only temporary as recurrence is common. Involvement of internal organs requires multidisciplinary approach.

EHLERS–DANLOS SYNDROME (FIGS. 10G TO L)

Ehlers-Danlos syndrome (EDS) is an inherited disorder of collagen metabolism characterized by hyperextensible, fragile skin and hypermobility of joints. There are six major types of EDS—four are autosomal dominant and two autosomal recessive in inheritance. The major features are hyperstretchable skin, fragile skin and hypermobility of joints. In general, the skin is thin, velvety and hyperelastic but not lax. Palms and soles may have loose skin simulating loose gloves. Wound healing is poor resulting in thin, wide, atrophic, cigarette paper-like scars over bony prominences. Approximately 50% of patients (as compared to 10% of normal individuals) can touch the tip of their nose with tongue tip (Gorlin's sign).

DARIER DISEASE (FIGS. 11 TO 13)

Darier disease, also known as keratosis follicularis, is an autosomal dominant disorder characterized by greasy crusted papules on the scalp, face, neck, seborrheic areas of the trunk and flexures of the extremities. The age at onset varies from early childhood through adulthood, though it typically appears between 8 and 15 years of age. The lesions start as pinhead to pea-sized flesh-colored papules. Most papules are perifollicular and as the disease progresses, they coalesce to form plaques covered with flesh-colored yellowish brown greasy crusts that tend to become purulent and malodorous. The lesions exacerbate in summer. Nail involvement beginning as a red streak with subungual hyperkeratosis accompanied by adjacent white streaks on the nail plate is often the first sign of the disorder and may be the only manifestation in early childhood. Subsequently, fragility, splitting, fissuring of the nails and subungual splinter hemorrhage occur. Lesions of the mucous membrane consist of small white papules resembling leukoplakia. Palmoplantar hyperkeratosis is present in 10% of the affected individuals. Palmar pits can be seen. Histopathological features are characteristic with acantholytic dyskeratosis which is characterized by intraepidermal suprabasal clefts and

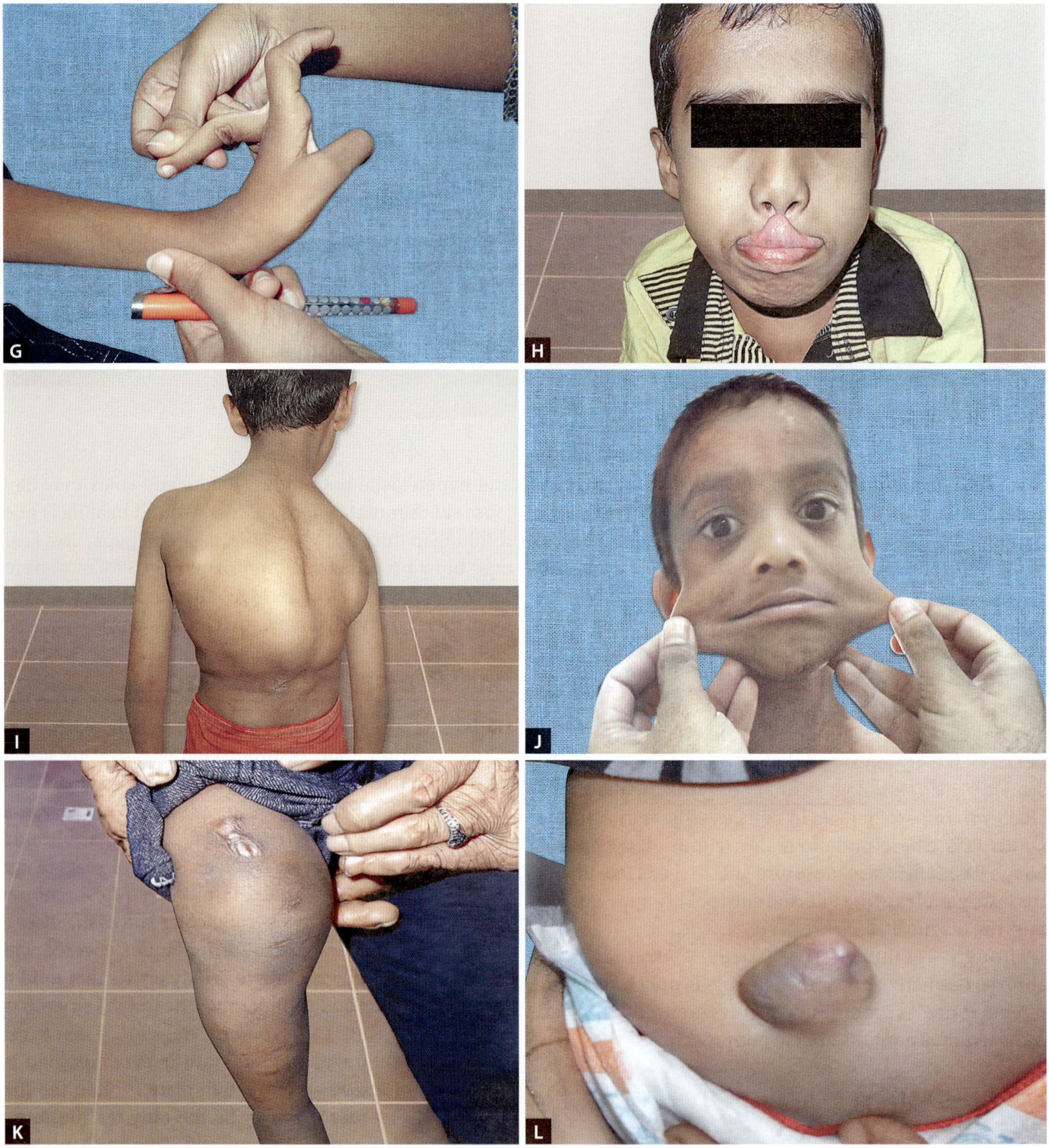

Figs. 10G to L: (G) Ehlers–Danlos syndrome (EDS), demonstration of hyperextensibility of finger; (H) EDS, demonstration of Gorlin's sign; (I) EDS; kyphoscoliosis; (J) EDS, note elasticity of cheek tissue; (K) EDS, note cigarette paper-like scar; (L) EDS, note umbilical prolapse.

"corps ronds" and "grains". Indolent papules resembling flat warts on the dorsal aspect of the hands and feet (a disorder termed "acrokeratosis verruciformis of Hopf") have been described in association with Darier disease.

Management

There is no specific therapy for Darier disease. Patients are instructed to avoid sun exposure, heat and humidity as the lesions are exacerbated in summer and aggravated by

"Do one thing you think you cannot do. Fail at it. Try again. Do better the second time. The only people who never tumble are those who never mount the high wire. This is your moment. Own it." —**Oprah Winfrey**

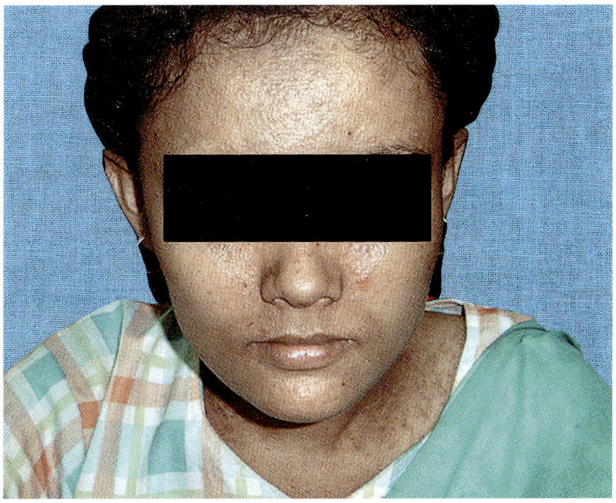

Fig. 11: Dirty warty papules of Darier disease over face and neck of an adolescent girl.

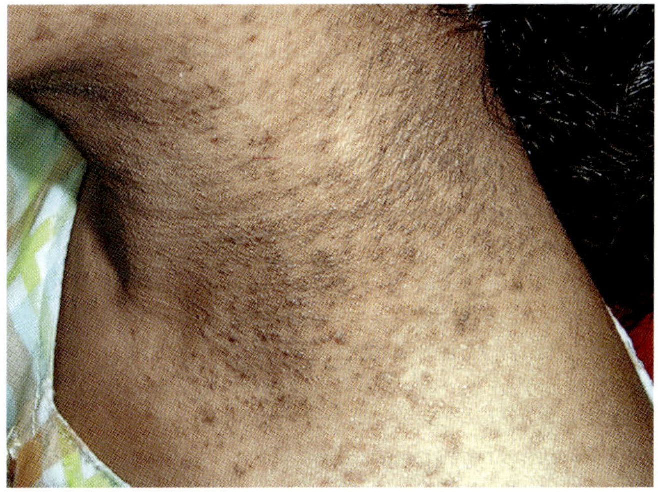

Fig. 12: Same girl, close-up view of neck lesions.

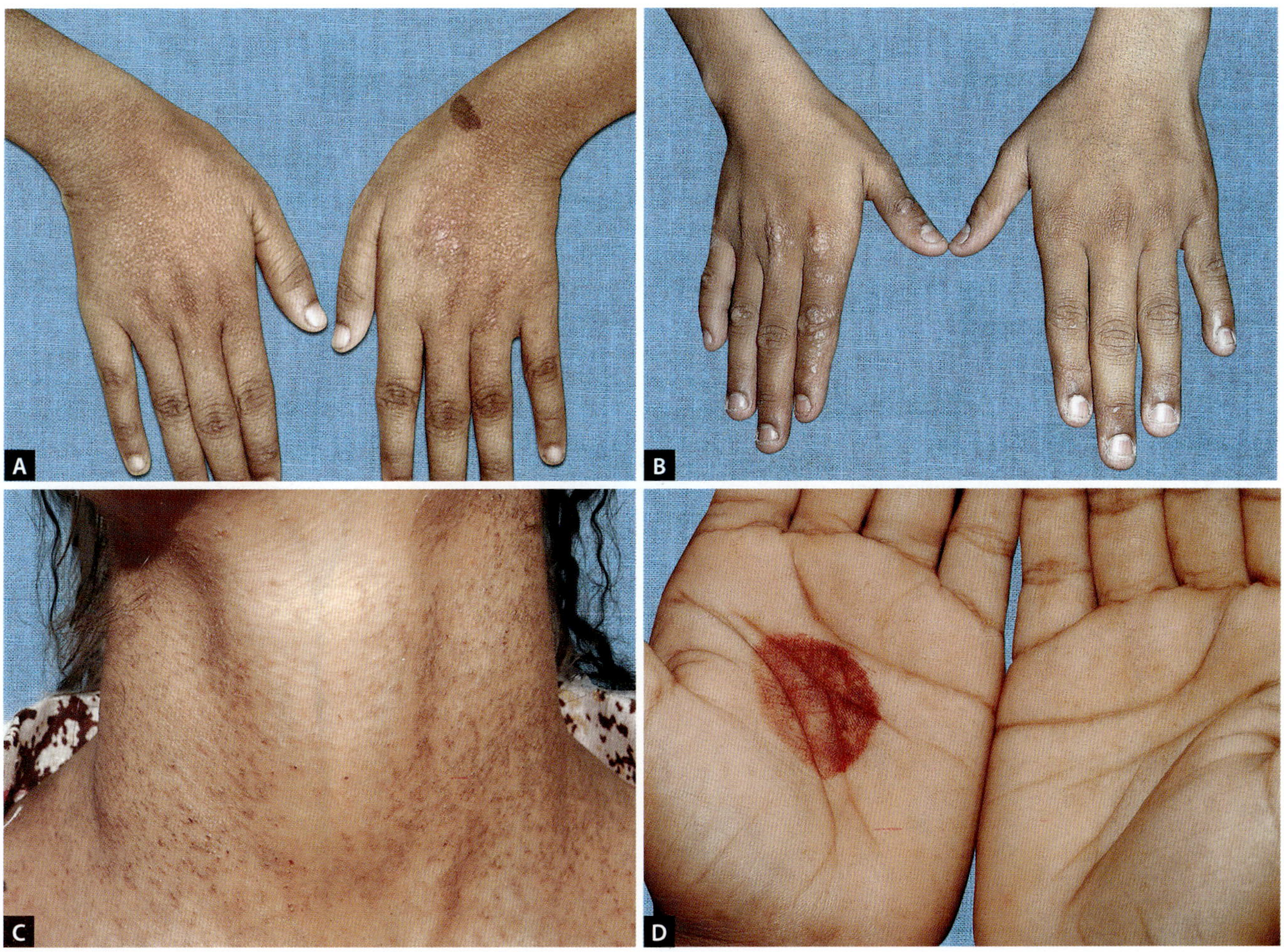

Figs. 13A to D: (A) Plane wart-like lesions over dorsa of hands in the same girl; (B) Acrokeratosis lesions over classical site, often present in children with Darier disease; (C) Darier disease, note dirty warty papules on neck; (D) Palmar pit in same girl.

"Any fool can know. The point is to understand." —**Albert Einstein**

sunlight, UV exposure and perspiration. Topical vitamin A acids are helpful in controlling the lesions; however, prolonged remissions are not seen.

PROGERIA (FIGS. 14 TO 18)

Progeria (Hutchinson-Gilford syndrome) is a rare disease characterized by a combination of dwarfism, generalized atrophy of the subcutaneous tissue and muscle, a high incidence of generalized atherosclerosis, and early onset of progressive senile degenerative changes. Usually there is a history of consanguineous marriage in the parents and the disease affects other siblings as well suggesting an autosomal recessive pattern. However, there are only a handful families with progeria that have been documented across the globe. There is no sex predilection. The classical

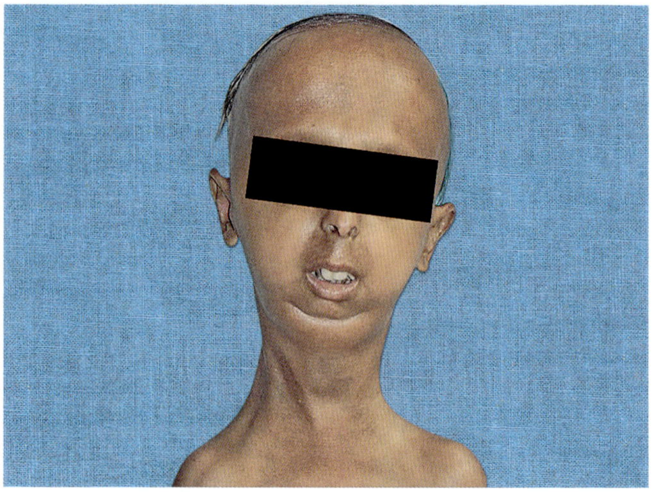

Fig. 14: Progeria in an 18-year-old boy.

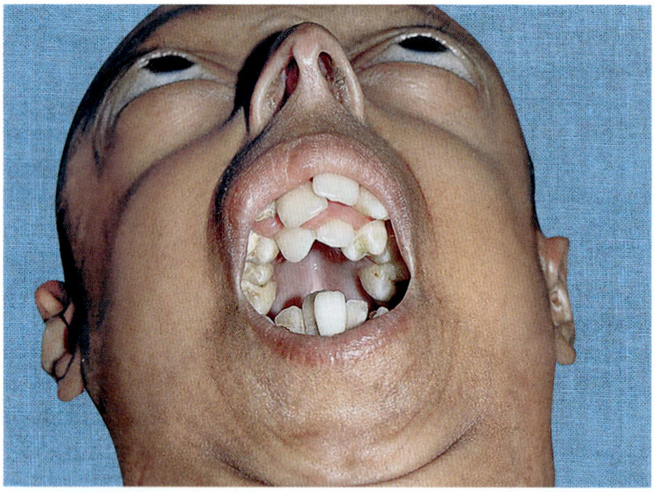

Fig. 15: Overcrowding of teeth causing dental malocclusion.

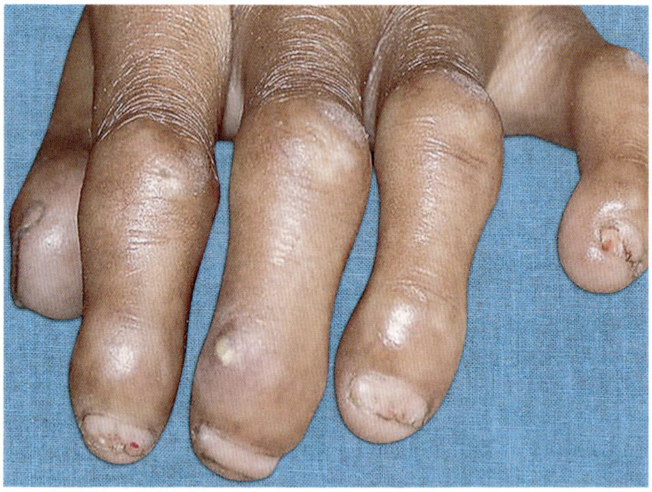

Fig. 16: Fingers showing acro-osteolysis and sclerodermoid changes.

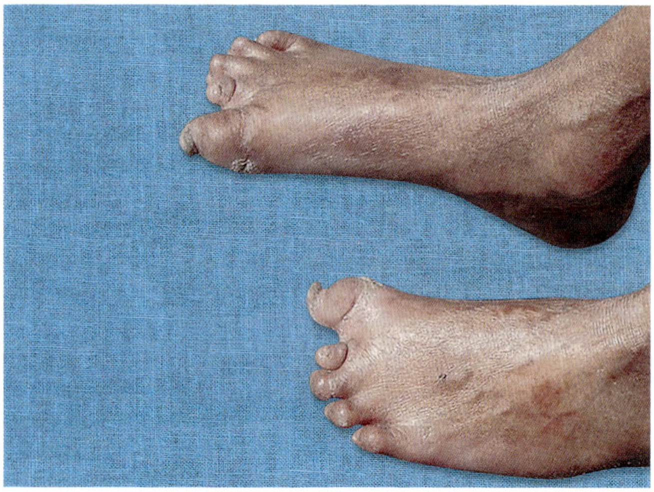

Fig. 17: Resorption of toes and repeated ulcerations.

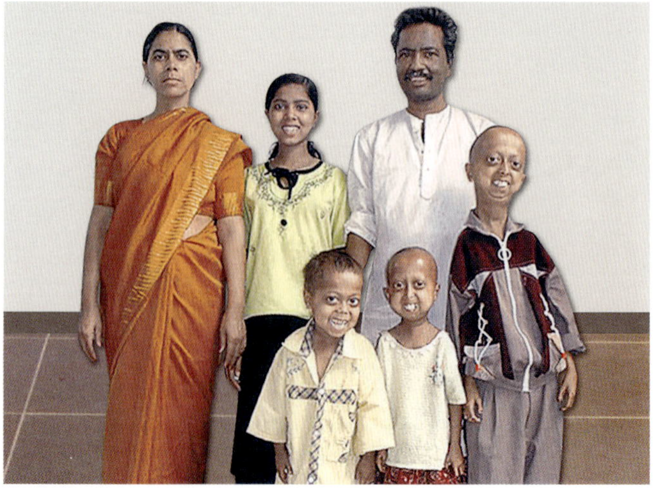

Fig. 18: Progeria family, consanguinity between parents.

"Those who deny freedom to others deserve it not for themselves." **—Abraham Lincoln**

clinical features consist of dwarfism, alopecia of the scalp, eyebrows and eyelashes, prominent scalp veins and generalized atrophy of muscle and subcutaneous tissue. The face is small with recession of the chin; a thin beaked nose gives a bird-like appearance. The head gives a hydrocephalic appearance. The skin is generally thin, dry, wrinkled with mottled brownish hyperpigmentation. The fingers and toes show sclerodermatous changes; there is terminal tuft resorption; and contractures may also be seen. The nails are thin, brittle and resorption of bones leads to osteoporosis and tendencies to frequent fractures. There is crowding of teeth as the deciduous teeth are often retained leading to a double chin appearance. The chest becomes narrow with a protuberant abdomen. Differential diagnosis includes scleroderma, Cockayne syndrome, Bloom syndrome and Rothmund-Thomson syndrome.

Prognosis

The overall prognosis is poor with development of early and extensive atherosclerosis after the age of 5 years. This may lead to hypertension, cardiomegaly, angina, myocardial infarction and congestive cardiac failure. Death usually occurs during the second decade of life.

KINDLER SYNDROME (FIGS. 19 TO 21)

It is a rare autosomal recessive condition characterized by skin fragility, acral blisters, photosensitivity, poikiloderma, cutaneous atrophy and mucosal inflammation. In the new classification, epidermolysis bullosa (EB) is divided into four types: (1) intraepidermal (EB simplex); (2) junctional; (3) dystrophic; and (4) mixed type (Kindler syndrome). The gene involved in Kindler syndrome is *FERMT1* (previously known as *KIND1*) which encodes a protein linking actin with the extracellular matrix, thus affecting skin integrity.

The major features of Kindler syndrome in infancy are skin fragility and photosensitivity. Blisters appear either immediately or shortly after birth. The blister formation may improve during childhood variably.

In early childhood, the atrophy and "cigarette paper-like" wrinkling of dorsum of hands and feet become more apparent. Photosensitivity is absent at birth but develops gradually. Webbing of fingers and toes have been reported. Other features are mild-to-moderate gingivitis, gingival fragility and periodontitis. Various other complications are esophageal stricture and stenosis, anal stenosis, urethral stricture, keratoconjunctivitis, ectropion and conjunctival scarring.

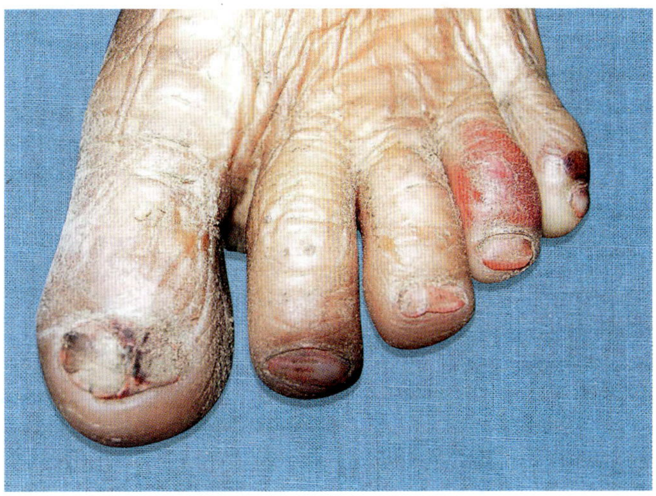

Fig. 20: Same child, note scarring on foot.

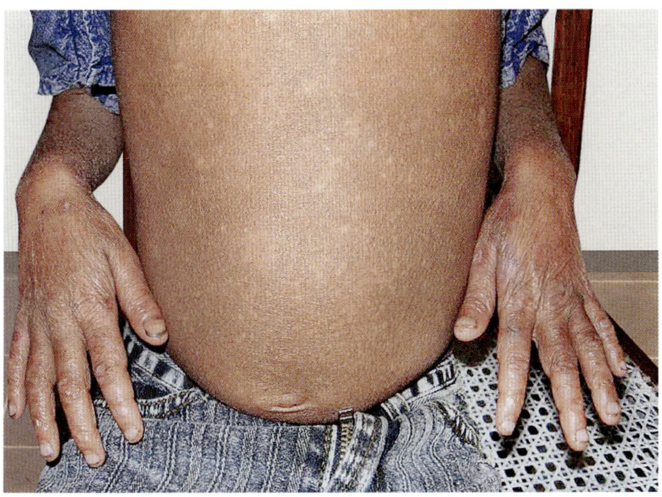

Fig. 19: Kindler syndrome, note scarring on dorsum of hands.

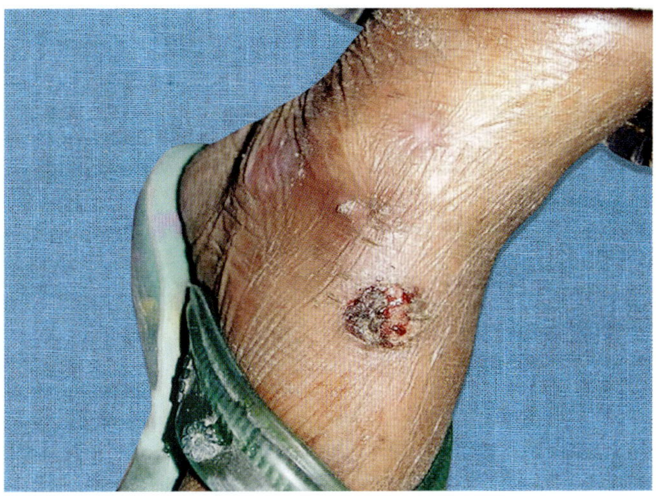

Fig. 21: Kindler syndrome.

"Spread love everywhere you go. Let no one ever come to you without leaving happier." —**Mother Teresa**

Prognosis

Normal life expectancy.

Treatment

These cases are best managed by multidisciplinary team comprising of dermatologists, pediatricians, specialist nurse, dietician, dentists and ophthalmologists. The most important thing is to emphasize regular use of sunscreen and sun-protective clothes.

LIPOID PROTEINOSIS (HYALINOSIS CUTIS ET MUCOSAE) (FIG. 22)

It is an autosomal recessive disorder characterized by hoarseness and yellowish beaded papules and nodules in the skin secondary to abnormal hyaline deposition in the skin and mucus membrane. There is loss of function mutation in the extracellular matrix protein 1 (ECAM1). Hoarseness secondary to vocal cord involvement begins in infancy. Linear and discrete varioliform scars are seen on face, trunk and upper extremities. The eyelid margins show string of bead-like papules followed by loss of cilia. The tongue becomes thick, firm and woody, bound to the floor of mouth. Yellowish-white infiltrating papules and nodules can be demonstrated on the skin and oral mucosa. Diagnosis is mostly clinical and histopathology of skin shows homogenous bands of eosinophilic, PAS positive, hyaline-like amorphous material in the upper dermis. It has a chronic and benign course with mainly symptomatic treatment consisting of surgical or laser removal of laryngeal nodules and laser resurfacing or dermabrasion for cutaneous lesions on face. Acitretin has shown improvement in hoarseness and skin lesions.

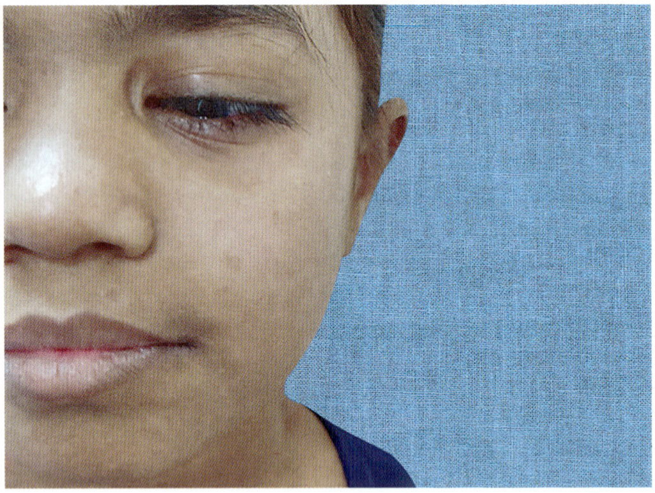

Fig. 22: Lipoid proteinosis, note bead-like papules on eyelid margin and varioliform scars on face.

PROTEUS SYNDROME (FIGS. 23A TO C)

Proteus syndrome (PS) is an extremely rare and sporadic disorder caused by a mosaic activating mutation in *AKT1* gene. It is characterized by postnatal segmental, disproportionate and progressive overgrowth of multiple tissues, especially the skin and subcutis, connective tissue, central nervous system and viscera. The condition is usually not evident until late infancy or early childhood.

Cutaneous findings include capillary, lymphatic, or venous malformations, epidermal nevi, connective tissue nevi (cerebriform connective tissue nevus of palms and soles is diagnostic), lipomas, and café-au-lait macules.

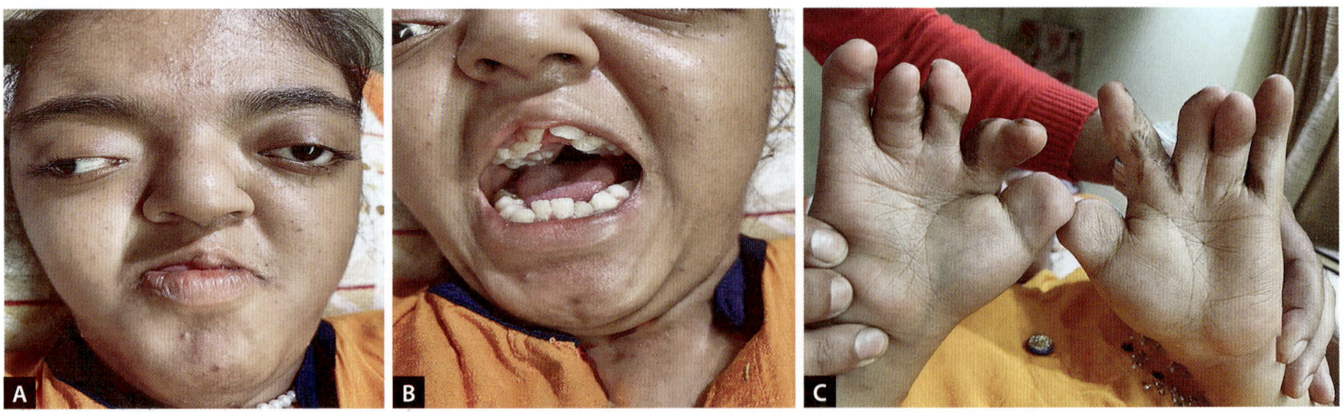

Figs. 23A to C: (A) Proteus syndrome, note dysmorphic facies; (B) Proteus syndrome, note crowding of teeth; (C) Same patient, note overgrowth of soft tissue hand.

"Always remember that you are absolutely unique. Just like everyone else." —**Margaret Mead**

Other features include dysmorphic facies (dolichocephaly, elongated facies, low nasal bridge, downslanting palpebral features, and wide or anteverted nares), macrocephaly, macrodactyly, visceral vascular malformations, adenomas of the ovaries or parotid glands, hemimegalencephaly (most common central nervous system finding) and ocular findings (strabismus, nystagmus, high myopia, cataracts and retinal pigmentary abnormalities).

Morbidity in these patients includes skeletal abnormalities, benign and malignant tumors, specific vesicular skin lesions, and life-threatening complications such as deep vein thrombosis and pulmonary embolism.

The most definitive method is molecular genetic testing for the *AKT1* gene (standard peripheral blood DNA samples are much less informative than samples from affected tissues and should be avoided) and *PTEN* and *GPC3* genes to evaluate for the possible mutation. Management includes a multidisciplinary approach involving the dermatologist, geneticist and orthopedic specialist whenever necessary. Miransertib (ARQ 092), an oral, selective pan-AKT inhibitor, is being evaluated for the treatment of PS.

GOLTZ SYNDROME

Focal dermal hypoplasia (Goltz syndrome) is a rare X-linked dominant multisystem disorder resulting from mutations to the *PORCN* gene on chromosome Xp11.23, responsible for the encoding of a protein involved in Wnt signaling embryogenesis. Only 10% of cases occur in males, and survival is thought to be due to either sporadic new mutation or somatic mosaicism. It is characterized by linear or reticular pattern of patchy dermal hypoplasia and multiple cutaneous and extracutaneous abnormalities. Clinical diagnostic criteria for focal dermal hypoplasia include at least three of the major characteristic skin findings (congenital patchy skin aplasia, congenital nodular fat herniation, congenital hyper- or hypopigmentation in Blaschko-linear distribution, telangiectasia, congenital ridged dysplastic nails) and one major limb malformation (split hand/foot, transverse limb defects, syndactyly, oligodactyly, marked long bone reduction). Other cutaneous manifestations include large cutaneous ulcers caused by complete absence of skin which heals with atrophy, pebble textured skin, papillomas, photosensitivity and thin and sparse hair. Extracutaneous manifestations apart from skeletal abnormalities include dental anomalies (dental crowding, hypodontia, supernumerary teeth, oligodontia, microdontia, enamel hypoplasia), ocular manifestations (microphthalmia, iris and chorioretinal colobomas, nystagmus, cataracts and strabismus), hernias (umbilical/inguinal), hearing defects, congenital heart disease, microcephaly, facial asymmetry, cleft lip/palate, central nervous system abnormalities (sensorineural hearing loss, hydrocephalus, agenesis of the corpus callosum, and Arnold-Chiari malformation), intellectual disability, urogenital anomalies (labia minora hypoplasia and short perineum body, asymmetry of the breast/nipples, bicornuate uterus, unilateral absent kidney, hypoplastic kidney, fused/horseshoe kidney, cystic renal dysplasia), giant cell tumor of the bone and multiple basal-cell carcinomas.

The differential diagnosis of focal dermal hypoplasia includes MIDAS (microphthalmia, dermal aplasia, and sclerocornea), incontinentia pigmenti, Rothmund-Thomson syndrome, nevus lipomatosus superficialis, Adams-Oliver syndrome and aplasia cutis. The clinical diagnosis can be supported by osteopathia striata (radiologically) and confirmed by detection of the *PORCN* gene mutation through gene sequence analysis. Management involves a multidisciplinary approach involving a pediatrician, pediatric dermatologist, otolaryngologist, dentist, plastic surgeon, ophthalmologist, neurologist, and geneticist. Genetic counseling needs to be done. Prognosis is excellent for females while, for males, it is lethal in utero or if a mutation is present, 10% may survive.

RESTRICTIVE DERMOPATHY (FIGS. 24A TO D)

Restrictive dermopathy is a rare autosomal recessive disorder characterized by taut, translucent rigid skin along with erosions, limb contractures, and restriction of respiratory movements. It is fatal in the neonatal period. It is caused by loss of function mutations in both alleles of *ZMPSTE24* gene. There is a primary defect in the synthesis and orientation of collagen and reduction in elastic tissue. Other clinical features include intrauterine growth retardation, prominent superficial vasculature, dysmorphic facies, low set ears, hypertelorism, micrognathia, persistently open fixed o-shaped mouth, prenatal teeth, sparse eyebrows and eyelashes, cleft palate, rocker bottom feet, and adrenal hypoplasia. Differential diagnosis includes scleroderma, stiff skin syndrome, infantile systemic hyalinosis, and cerebro-oculo-facio-skeletal syndrome. Genetic counseling is important.

"One day i will find the right words and they will be simple." **—Jack Kerovac**

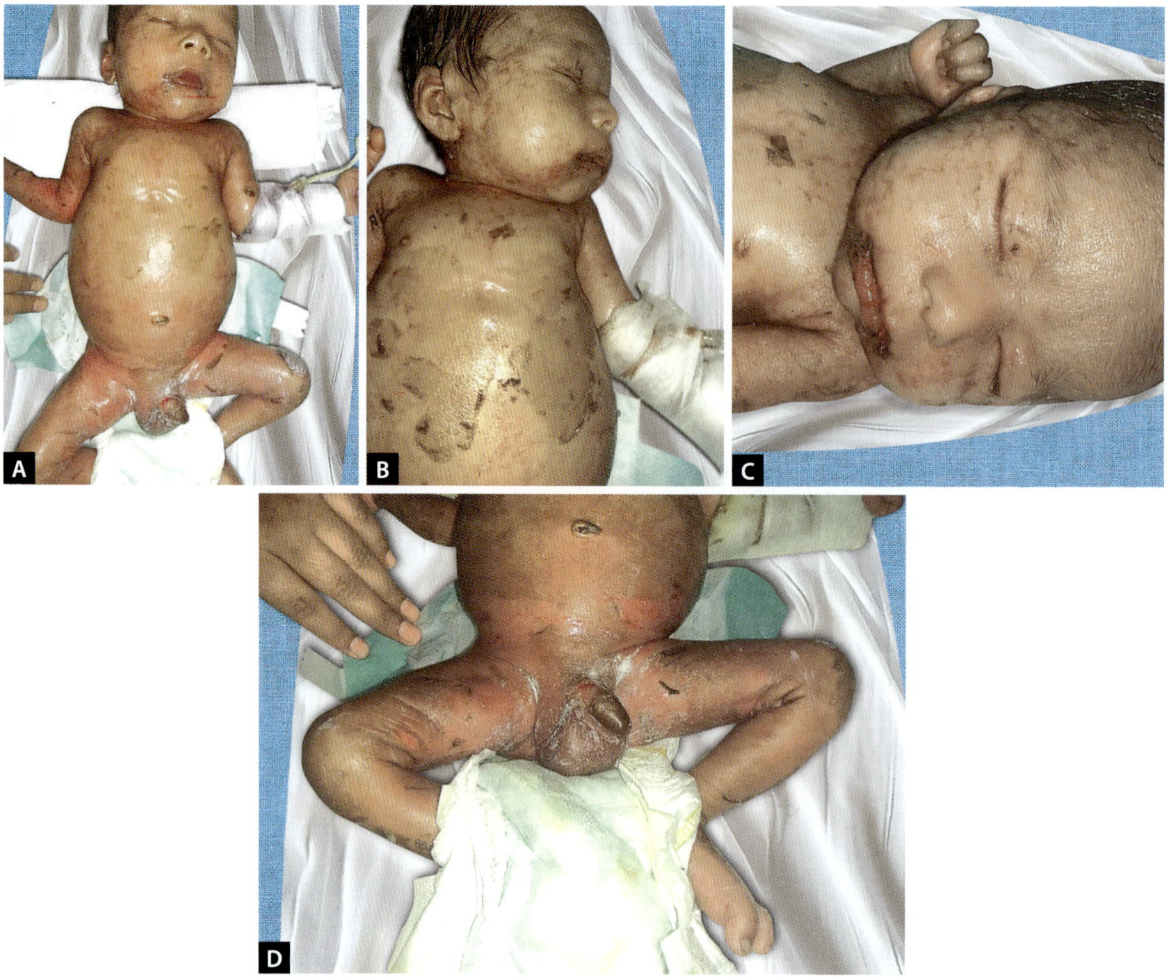

Figs. 24A to D: (A) Restrictive dermopathy, note tight appearance of skin with dysmorphic features; (B) Same child, close-up view showing prominent superficial vasculature; (C) Look at dysmorphic face with o-shaped mouth; (D) Same baby, groin, thighs and legs.

STIFF SKIN SYNDROME (FIGS. 25A TO D)

Stiff skin syndrome is a rare syndrome characterized by hard, thick skin, usually on the entire body. The thickening of the skin can limit joint mobility significantly and can lead to joint contracture. The signs and symptom of this condition can manifest for the first time at birth through childhood. Other features are loss of body fat, hypertrichosis, scoliosis.

Stiff skin syndrome is autosomal dominant in inheritance, caused by mutations in the Hyperlink *https://ghr.nlm.nih.gov/gene/FBN1 FBN1* gene. Diagnosis is based on a clinical evaluation that is consistent with stiff skin syndrome, and the diagnosis can be confirmed with genetic testing. Treatment is symptomatic and physiotherapy to increase joint mobility.

WHAT'S NEW

- XFEPS (XPF-ERCC1 Progeroid syndrome) — photosensitivity and progeroid features in multiple organs, but no predisposition to malignancy.
- Randomized clinical trials on T4N5 liposomes (Dimericine) has shown promising results in decreasing the incidence of actinic keratosis and basal cell carcinomas in XP.
- Darier's disease is considered to be a multiorgan disease manifesting extracutaneous involvement like diabetes, heart failure and CNS (epilepsy, psychiatric disorders) involvement.
- Low dose TGF-β1 and Octyl Itaconate, a novel nuclear factor E2-related factor 2 (NRF2) activator provide a wide spectrum of potential targets for effective therapeutic treatments of Vohwinkel syndrome by promoting the proliferation of keratinocytes.

"There is only one plot, things are not how they seem." —**Jim Thompson**

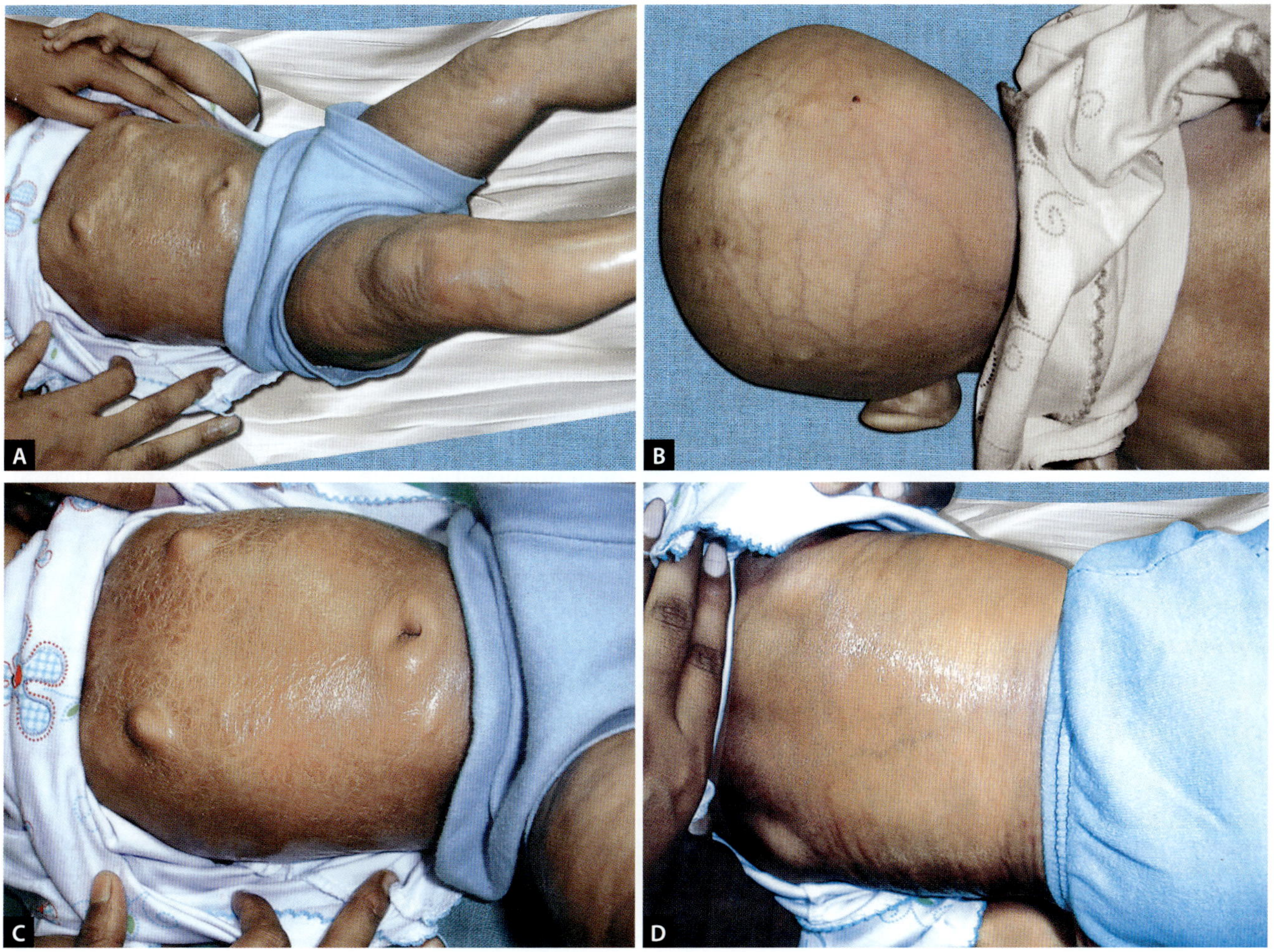

Figs. 25A and B: (A) Stiff skin syndrome in an infant; (B) Scalp showing prominence of superficial veins; (C) Close-up view of abdomen. Look at tight skin, protruded nipples and umbilicus; (D) Close-up view of back showing tight shinny skin.

SUGGESTED READINGS

1. Anbouba GM, Carmany EP, Natoli JL. The characterization of hypodontia, hypohidrosis, and hypotrichosis associated with X-linked hypohidrotic ectodermal dysplasia: a systematic review. Am J Med Genet A. 2020;182(4):831-41.
2. Dev T, Mahajan VK, Sethuraman G. Hereditary palmoplantar keratoderma: a practical approach to the diagnosis. Indian Dermatol Online J. 2019;10:365-79.
3. Hereditary disorders of the dermis. In: Paller AS, Mancini AJ (Eds). Hurwitz Clinical Pediatric Dermatology: A Textbook of Skin Disorders of Childhood and Adolescence, 5th edition. Edinburgh: Elsevier; 2016. pp. 119-35.
4. Ling X, Dong S, Zhang L. Low dose TGF-β1 can improve Vohwinkel syndrome by promoting the proliferation of keratinocytes. Acta Histochemica. 2023;125(2):152010.
5. Patro N, Sathishkumar D, Panda M, Mahajan R. Algorithmic approach toward diagnosis of patients with congenital photosensitivity disorders and review of literature. Int J Dermatol. 2023; DOI:10.1111/ijd.16965.
6. Srinivas SM, Dhar S. Erythrokeratodermia variabilis and erythrokeratoderma en cocardes: case series with review of literature. Indian J Paediatr Dermatol. 2016;17:202-5.

"The scariest moment is just before you start". —**Stephen King**

CHAPTER

4

Disorders of Keratinization

INHERITED ICHTHYOSIS

Inherited ichthyosis is classified based on the 2009 Ichthyosis Consensus Conference into nonsyndromic and syndromic forms **(Tables 1 and 2)**.

ICHTHYOSIS VULGARIS (FIGS. 1 AND 2)

This is an autosomal semidominant condition caused by loss of function mutation in *FLG* gene and is the most common form of ichthyosis. It is more common in temperate climates with an equal sex distribution. It shares a close relationship with atopic diseases. The skin may appear dry and scaly in the neonatal period; however, scaling becomes more prominent from 2 months onwards or in infancy. The scale is white or gray, small, flaky and semi-adherent with turned up edges. It is most pronounced on the extensor surfaces of the arms and lower legs and characteristically spares the flexural creases. The trunk is mildly affected and the napkin area is spared. Facial scaling, generally forehead and perioral, mild scaling on scalp and involvement of the pinnae is seen in some patients. The palms and soles are usually free of scales but palmoplantar

Table 1: Clinicogenetic classification of inherited ichthyoses—nonsyndromic forms.

Disease		Inheritance	Genetic defect
Common ichthyosis	Ichthyosis vulgaris (IV)	Autosomal semidominant	*FLG*
	Recessive X-linked ichthyosis (RXLI)	X-linked recessive	*STS*
ARCI (major types)	Harlequin ichthyosis (HI)	Autosomal recessive	*ABCA12*
	Lamellar ichthyosis (LI)	Autosomal recessive	*TGM1/NIPAL4/ALOX12B/ABCA12/PNPLA1/CERS3/LIPH*/loci on *12p11.2-q13*
	Congenital ichthyosiform erythroderma (CIE)	Autosomal recessive	*ALOXE3/ALOX12B/ABCA12/CYP4F22/NIPAL4/TGM1/PNPLA1/CERS3/LIPH*/loci on *12p11.2-q13*
ARCI (minor subtypes)	Self-improving collodion ichthyosis (SICI)	Autosomal recessive	*TGM1, ALOX12B, ALOXE3*
	Acral self-healing collodion baby (ASHCB)	Autosomal recessive	*TGM1*
	Bathing suit ichthyosis (BSI)	Autosomal recessive	*TGM1*
Keratinopathic ichthyosis (major types)	Epidermolytic ichthyosis (EI)	Autosomal dominant	*KRT1/KRT10*
	Superficial epidermolytic ichthyosis (SEI)	Autosomal dominant	*KRT2E*
Keratinopathic ichthyosis (minor types)	Annular epidermolytic ichthyosis (AEI)	Autosomal dominant	*KRT1/KRT10*
	Congenital reticular ichthyosiform erythroderma (CRIE)	Autosomal dominant	*KRT10*
	Ichthyosis Curth–Macklin (ICM)	Autosomal dominant	*KRT1*
	Autosomal recessive epidermolytic ichthyosis (AREI)	Autosomal recessive	*KRT10*
	Epidermolytic nevi	Somatic mutations	*KRT1/KRT10*

Continued

"I believe every human has a finite number of heartbeats. I don't intend to waste any of mine." **—Neil Armstrong**

Continued

Disease		Inheritance	Genetic defect
Other forms	Loricrin keratoderma (LK)	Autosomal dominant	*LOR*
	Erythrokeratodermia variabilis (EKV)	Autosomal dominant	*GJB3/GJB4*
	Inflammatory peeling skin disease (IPSD)	Autosomal recessive	*CDSN*
	Keratosis linearis-ichthyosis congenita-keratoderma (KLICK)	Autosomal recessive	*POMP*

(*ABCA12*: ATP-binding cassette subfamily A12; *ARCI*: autosomal recessive congenital ichthyosis; *FLG*: filaggrin; *GJB*: gap junction protein-beta; *KRT*: keratin; *LOR*: loricrin; *STS*: steroid sulfatase; *TGM1*: transglutaminase 1; *CDSN*: corneodesmosin; *POMP*: proteasome maturation protein)

Source: Adapted from Oji V, Tadini G, Akiyama M, Blanchet Bardon C, Bodemer C, Bourrat E, et al. Revised nomenclature and classification of inherited ichthyoses: results of the First Ichthyosis Consensus Conference in Sorèze 2009. J Am Acad Dermatol. 2010;63(4):607-41.

Table 2: Clinicogenetic classification of inherited ichthyoses—syndromic forms.

Disease		Inheritance	Gene
X-linked ichthyosis syndromes	Recessive X-linked ichthyosis syndrome	X-linked recessive	*STS* (and others in context of contiguous gene syndromes)
	Ichthyosis follicularis/atrichia/photophobia (IFAP) syndrome	X-linked recessive	*MBTPS2*
	Conradi–Hünermann–Happle syndrome	X-linked dominant	*EBP (CDPX2)*
	Congenital hemidysplasia/ichthyosiform nevus/limb defects syndrome (CHILD) syndrome	X-linked dominant	*NSDHL*
Autosomal syndromes			
Prominent hair abnormalities	Netherton syndrome	Autosomal recessive	*SPINK5*
	Trichothiodystrophy (congenital)	Autosomal recessive	*ERCC2/XPD* *ERCC3/XPB* *GTF2H5/TTDA*
	Trichothiodystrophy (noncongenital)	Autosomal recessive	*C7orf11/TTDN1*
	Ichthyosis/hypotrichosis syndrome	Autosomal recessive	*ST14*
	Ichthyosis/hypotrichosis/sclerosing cholangitis syndrome	Autosomal recessive	*CLDN1*
Prominent neurologic signs	Sjögren–Larsson syndrome	Autosomal recessive	*ALDH3A2*
	Refsum syndrome	Autosomal recessive	*PHYH/PEX7*
	Mental retardation/enteropathy/deafness/neuropathy/ichthyosis/keratoderma (MEDNIK) syndrome	Autosomal recessive	*AP1S1*
Fatal diseases course	Gaucher syndrome type 2	Autosomal recessive	*GBA*
	Multiple sulfatase deficiency	Autosomal recessive	*SUMF1*
	Cerebral dysgenesis/neuropathy/ichthyosis/ palmoplantar keratoderma (CEDNIK) syndrome	Autosomal recessive	*SNAP29*
	Arthrogryposis/renal dysfunction/cholestasis (ARC) syndrome	Autosomal recessive	*VPS33B*
Others	Keratitis/ichthyosis/deafness (KID) syndrome	Autosomal dominant	*GJB2 (GJB6)*
	Neutral lipid storage disease with ichthyosis	Autosomal recessive	*ABHD5*
	Ichthyosis prematurity syndrome	Autosomal recessive	*SLC27A4*

(*ABHD5*: α/β-hydrolase domain containing protein 5; *EBP*: emopamil binding protein; *GJB2*: gap junction beta-2 protein; *MBTPS2*: membrane bound transcription factor peptidase, site 2; *NSDHL*: NAD (P) dependent steroid dehydrogenase-like; *SLC27A4*: solute carrier family 27 member 4; *SNAP29*: synaptosomal-associated protein 29; *SPINK5*: serine protease inhibitor Kazal-type 5 protein; *STS*: steroid sulfatase; *SUMF1*: sulfatase modifying factor 1; *VPS33B*: vacuolar protein sorting 33B; *XPD*: xeroderma pigmentosum group D)

Source: Adapted from Oji V, Tadini G, Akiyama M, Blanchet Bardon C, Bodemer C, Bourrat E, et al. Revised nomenclature and classification of inherited ichthyoses: results of the First Ichthyosis Consensus Conference in Sorèze 2009. J Am Acad Dermatol. 2010;63(4):607-41.

"Do not look for approval except for the consciousness of doing your best." —**Andrew Carnegie**

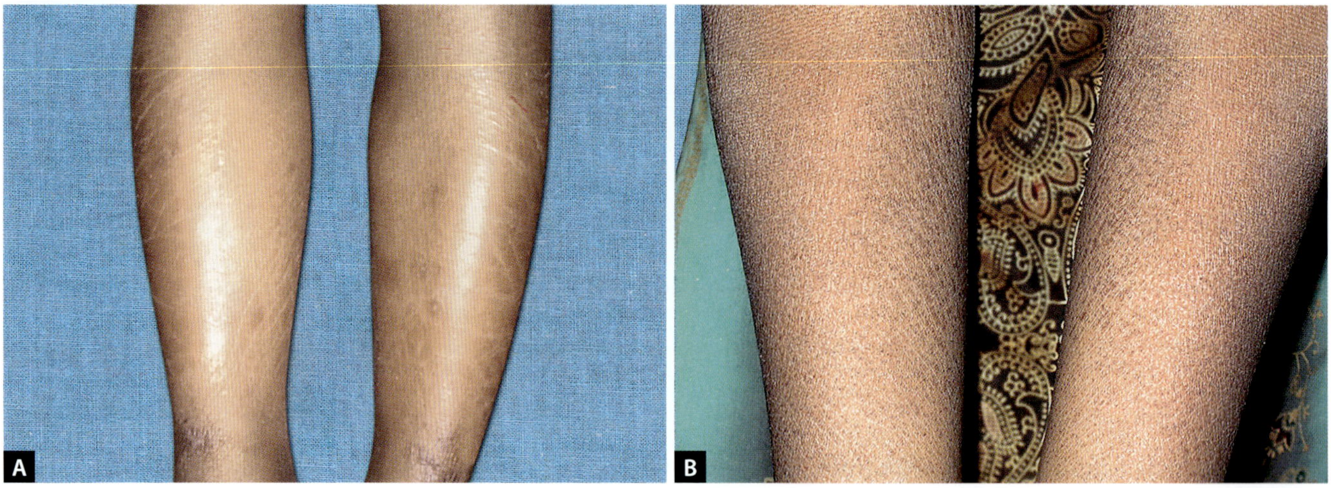

Figs. 1A and B: (A) Brown small scales of ichthyosis vulgaris distributed in a bilaterally symmetrical pattern; (B) Ichthyosis vulgaris, note fine scales.

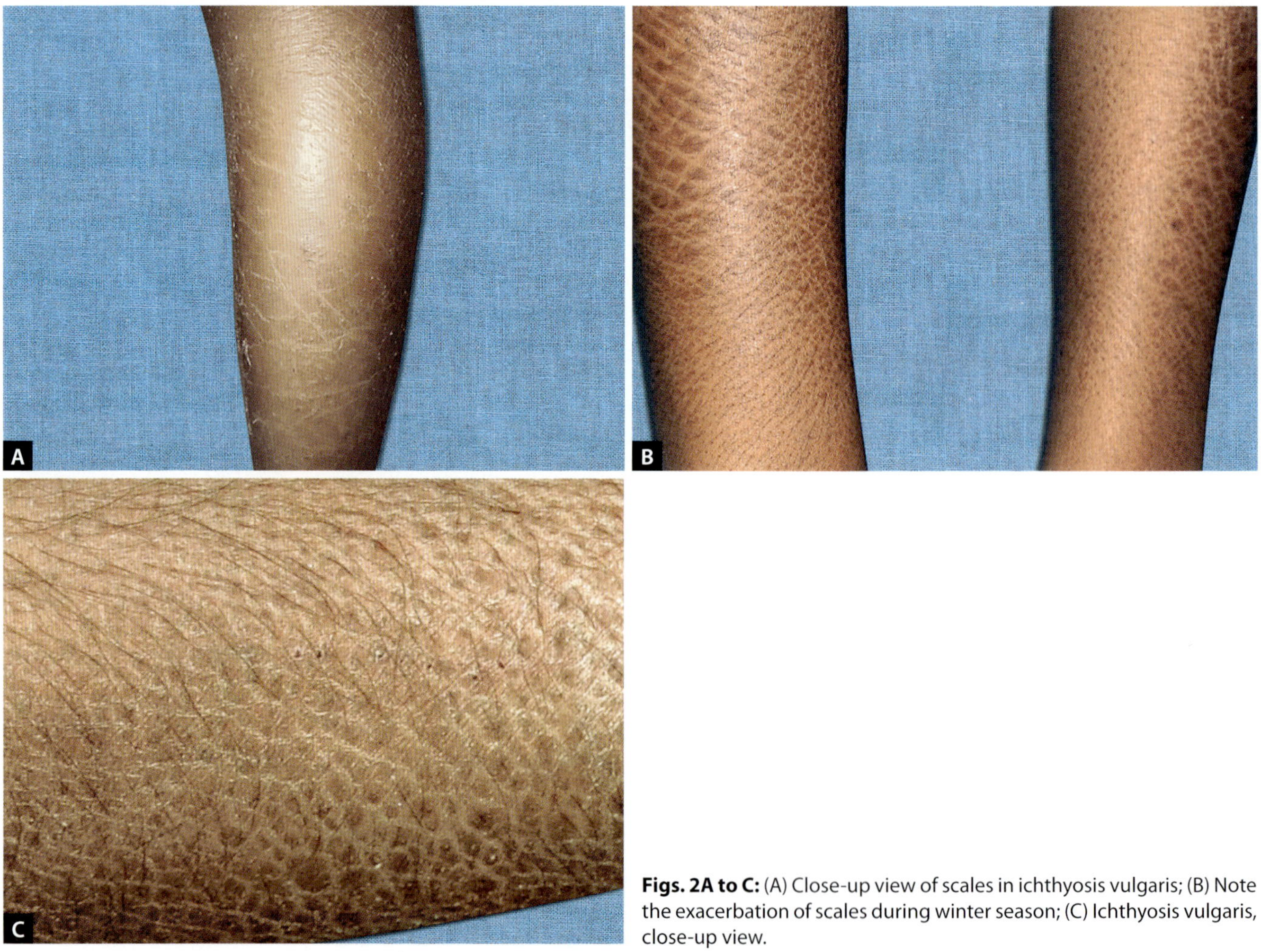

Figs. 2A to C: (A) Close-up view of scales in ichthyosis vulgaris; (B) Note the exacerbation of scales during winter season; (C) Ichthyosis vulgaris, close-up view.

hyperlinearity is a helpful feature to assess whether they have coexistent atopic dermatitis. Other features include keratosis pilaris and hypohidrosis. Symptoms of ichthyosis are few and limited to complaints of dryness and roughness. In patients with coexistent eczema, flexural lichenification and pruritus with excoriation are additional features.

Natural History

There is improvement of the condition in warm to sunny weather. Many sufferers have a gradual improvement in adolescence.

Management

Increasing the humidity in the environment is a beneficial measure in all patients with ichthyosis. Regular emollient application is necessary. The emollient may be in the form of aqueous cream for mild-to-moderate ichthyosis vulgaris or in the form of paraffin based or cetyl and stearyl alcohol containing emollients for severely affected ones. Bath oils and emollient soap substitutes are useful. Keratolytic agents, such as 1–5% salicylic acid may be added to emollient cream bases to encourage shedding of the scales but their widespread usage should be avoided in children because of their systemic toxicity. Urea containing emollient base improves epidermal hydration, cause lysis of keratin and are bacteriostatic. Patients with atopic dermatitis having ichthyosis will need treatment of atopic dermatitis along with treatment of ichthyosis.

X-LINKED RECESSIVE ICHTHYOSIS (FIGS. 3A TO D)

X-linked recessive ichthyosis (XLRI) caused by deficiency of steroid sulfatase enzyme (STS), due to mutations in *STS* gene affects male offspring of female carriers who are asymptomatic. In 75% of cases, scaling is evident within the first week of life although parents may not become aware of persistent scaling until some months later. A prominent peeling episode takes place by 6 months. The scaling of XLRI tends to increase throughout childhood, often spreading up from the lower legs to the trunk. Scaling is most prominent on the extensor surfaces of the upper

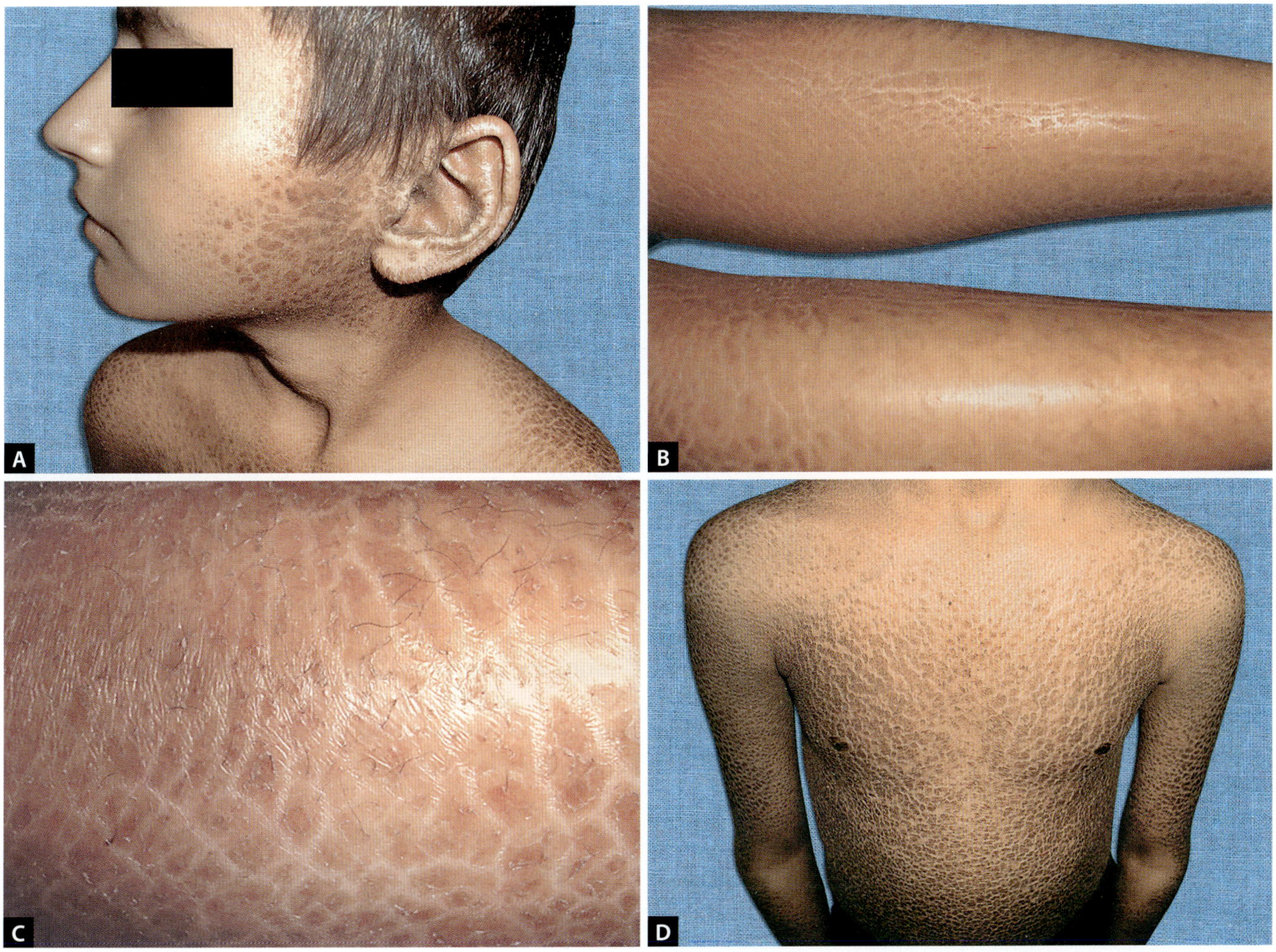

Figs. 3A to D: (A) Involvement of face and neck in X-linked recessive ichthyosis (XLRI); (B) Large, thick, brown scales of XLRI; (C) Close-up view of scales of XLRI; (D) XLRI, involvement of trunk and upper limbs.

"There is no use whatever trying to help people who do not help themselves. You cannot push anyone up a ladder unless he is willing to climb himself."

—Andrew Carnegie

arms, the outer thighs and around the lower legs. Typically, the scale is medium to large polygonal, adherent, dull and light brown or muddy in color. In contrast to ichthyosis vulgaris, the flexures may be involved. Palms and soles are spared.

Systemic Associations

X-linked recessive ichthyosis is often associated with contiguous gene syndromes, maldescended testes, cryptorchidism, abnormalities of sperm count or motility leading to infertility and testicular cancer, inguinal hernia and unilateral renal agenesis. Corneal dots, thread-like or comma-shaped opacities, detected with slit-lamp microscope, occur in 50–100% of adult patients and in 25% of female carriers.

Natural History

Spontaneous improvement to some extent occurs during summer and daily application of emollient is helpful. Unlike ichthyosis vulgaris, XLRI do not improve with age.

Treatment

Keratolytics and urea-containing preparations are beneficial and are found to be less irritant than in cases of ichthyosis vulgaris. In severe cases of XLRI, intermittent short courses of oral retinoids is beneficial.

LAMELLAR ICHTHYOSIS (FIGS. 4 AND 5)

It belongs to the group of autosomal recessive congenital ichthyosis which includes a spectrum of harlequin ichthyosis, nonbullous congenital ichthyosiform erythroderma (NBCIE) and classical lamellar ichthyosis (LI). The most common mutated gene involved is *TGM1* and *ABCA12*. It is characterized by the presence of large, quadrangular, hyperkeratotic, pigmented scales in the absence of erythema. At birth, most present as a collodion baby and after shedding show a less intense erythroderma than nonbullous ichthyosiform erythroderma (NBIE), an important distinguishing feature. Scaling occurs within the first month of life and may affect the whole skin surface or localize to the scalp, abdomen and lower legs. Associated features include palmoplantar keratoderma, scarring alopecia, eclabium, ectropion, heat intolerance, sclerodactyly and contractures. Bathing suit ichthyosis is a rare variant of LI where the lamellar scaling is confined to bathing suit areas such as axillae, trunk, scalp, neck, and forehead and this is due to temperature sensitive mutations in *TGM1* gene. Most of the children with LI have vitamin D deficiency rickets and growth retardation.

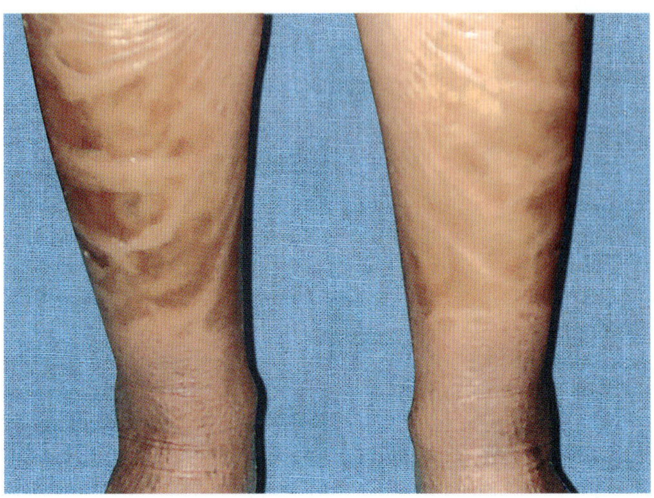

Fig. 4: Large, thick, quadrangular, dark scales of lamellar ichthyosis.

Management

Treatment is more or less same as other forms of ichthyosis. Keratolytics such as urea, lactic acid and hydrophilic petrolatum are useful.

Hydroxy acid or propylene glycol are also effective. Regular use of antiseptic washes and appropriate systemic antibiotics may be required in severe cases with repeated cutaneous bacterial and fungal infection and associated body odor. Topical calcipotriol, a vitamin D_3 analog, produces slight reduction in scaling. Oral retinoid therapy is beneficial in some patients. Acitretin and isotretinoin have been used to treat severe cases. There is no standard guidelines as there is paucity of clinical trials. Acitretin can be started at the dose of 0.5–1 mg/kg/day and can be given for several months intermittently. Regular monitoring of blood counts and lipid profile is necessary while treating with retinoids. To prevent the toxicity of acitretin, oral isotretinoin (1 mg/kg/day) have been used but the results are not that satisfactory as compared to acitretin. Newer therapies that have been used are liarozole, a retinoic acid-metabolism blocking agent, secukinumab and apremilast. Vitamin D_3 supplementation is necessary.

NONBULLOUS ICHTHYOSIFORM ERYTHRODERMA (FIGS. 6 TO 9)

Nonbullous ichthyosiform erythroderma is a rare and usually severe autosomal recessive inflammatory ichthyosis. In over 90% of cases, it presents at birth with a

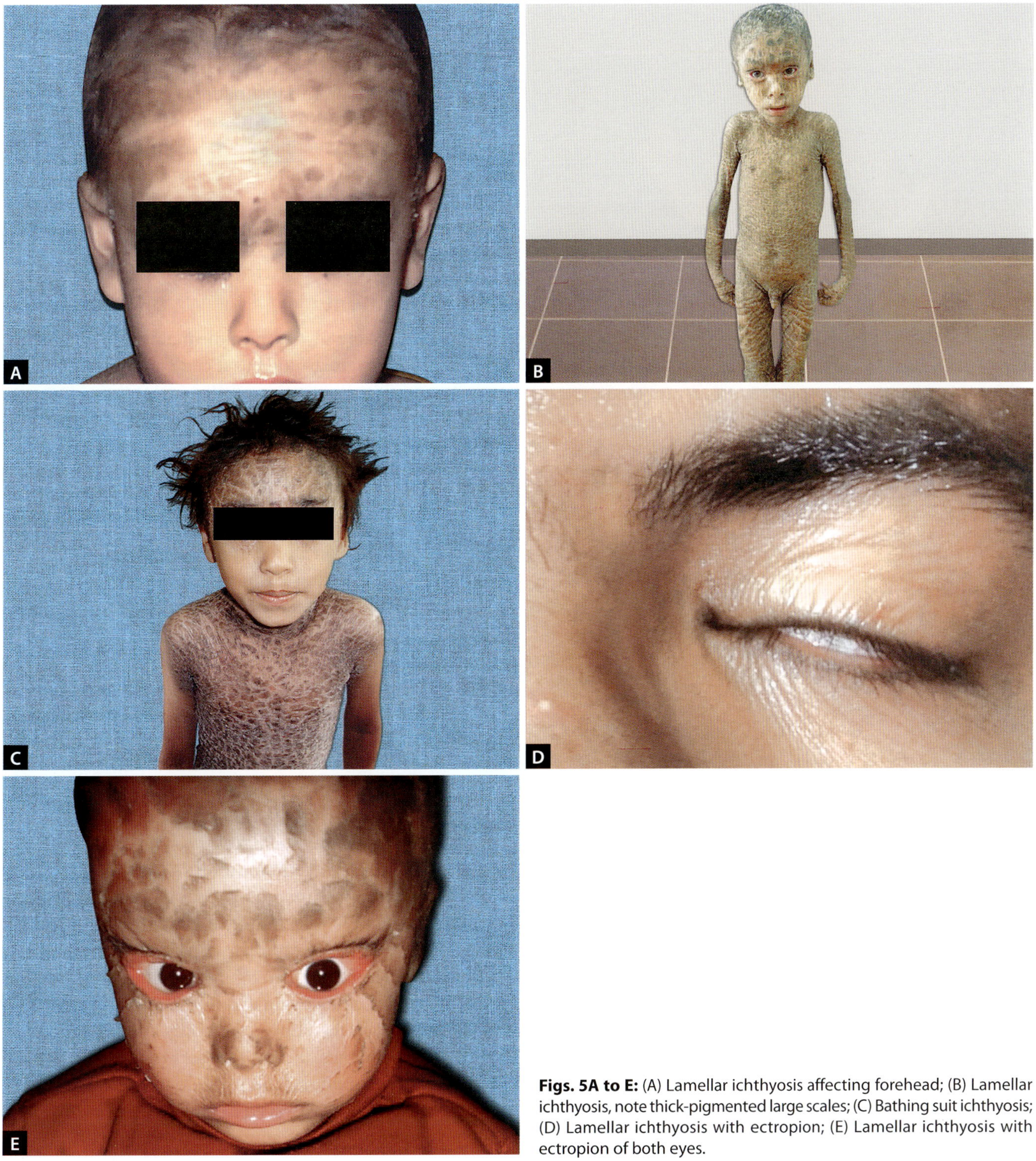

Figs. 5A to E: (A) Lamellar ichthyosis affecting forehead; (B) Lamellar ichthyosis, note thick-pigmented large scales; (C) Bathing suit ichthyosis; (D) Lamellar ichthyosis with ectropion; (E) Lamellar ichthyosis with ectropion of both eyes.

collodion baby appearance. After shedding of the collodion membrane, generalized scaly erythroderma is apparent and, in severe cases, persistent. Erythroderma, generally, lessens in childhood. Scaling can affect all areas including the scalp, ears, face, flexures, palms and soles. The scale of NBIE is white or gray, light superficial and semi-adherent. Palmoplantar hyperkeratosis occurs in 70% of patients. Ectropion with loss of eyebrows and lashes compound the ocular problem. Scalp involvement often causes pityriasis amiantacea and may lead to patchy cicatricial alopecia,

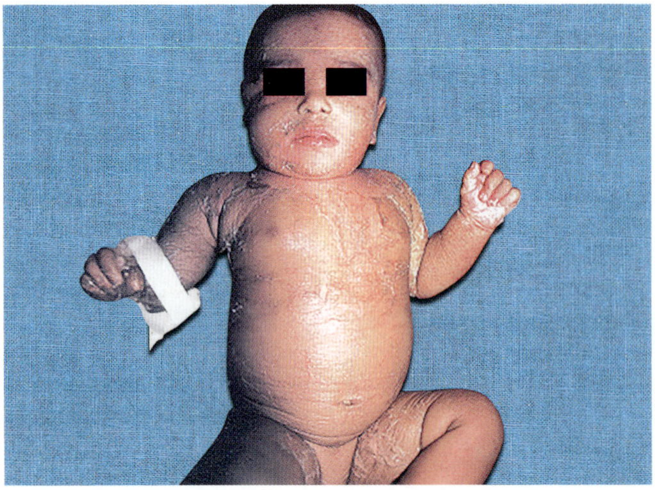

Fig. 6: Large, thick pigmented scales of nonbullous ichthyosiform erythroderma.

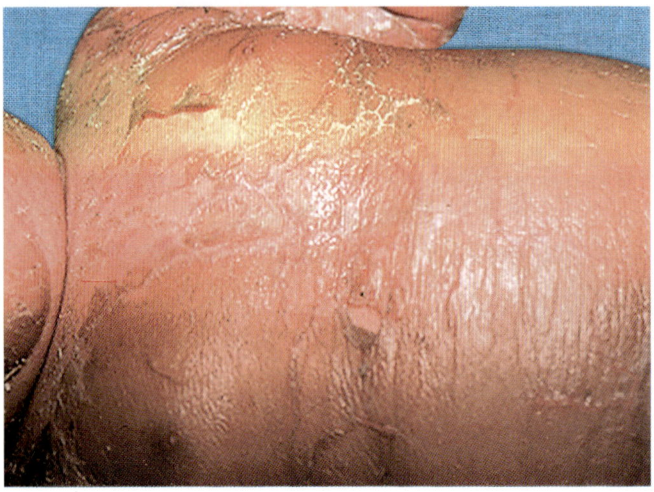

Fig. 7: Severe involvement of trunk in nonbullous ichthyosiform erythroderma.

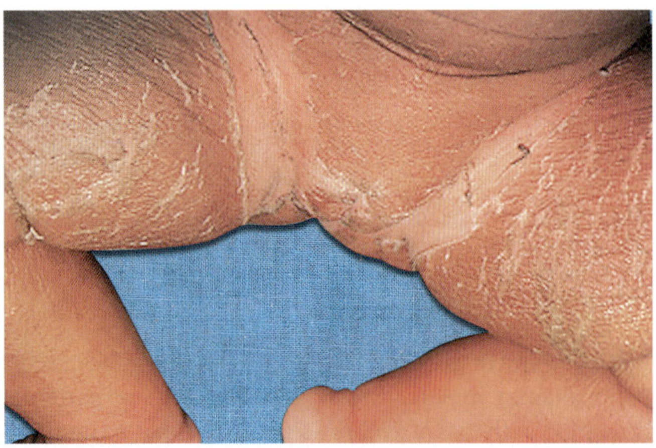

Fig. 8: Involvement of thighs in nonbullous ichthyosiform erythroderma.

hypoplasia of the nasal and aural cartilages may occur as a result of compression and scarring. A mild nail dystrophy occurs in up to 50% of cases but hair, teeth and mucosal surfaces are normal. In most patients, sweating is absent or markedly reduced from infancy onwards. Pruritus is common but skin infections are rare. NBIE differs from LI in having finer scaling and more pronounced erythema. There may be fine scaling on trunk and lamellar type of scales on extremities. NBIE is associated with vitamin D deficiency rickets.

Management

Emollients and keratolytics form the mainstay of treatment. Topical retinoids are avoided as it can cause irritation over an inflamed skin. Prevention of sunburn and sun-induced damage is mandatory. Systemic retinoids may be helpful. Acitretin is given at a starting dose of 0.5–0.75 mg/kg/day and continued till 2–3 weeks when good response is usually seen. The dose of acitretin is then brought down to a minimum effective dose of 0.1–0.25 mg/kg/day and may be continued for many months to years intermittently. The first author has experience of giving oral retinoids to children for 12–16 years intermittently.

EPIDERMOLYTIC HYPERKERATOSIS (BULLOUS ICHTHYOSIFORM ERYTHRODERMA) (FIGS. 10 TO 13)

This is a rare autosomal dominant disorder of keratinization which, in its early phase, is associated with blistering. Epidermolytic ichthyosis (EI) is caused by heterozygous mutations in the genes encoding *keratin 1* and *keratin 10* (*KRT1* and *KRT10*), located on chromosomes 17q12-21 and 12q11-13. Patients present with a mild generalized erythroderma at birth. The skin is very fragile leading to flaccid blisters and peeling at sites of minor trauma within the first few hours of life. Frequent misdiagnosis at this stage includes staphylococcal scalded skin syndrome and epidermolysis bullosa. However, the baby is generally apyrexic and well. Many of these babies succumb to severe infection, severe dehydration and malnutrition subsequently leading to very high mortality. With improved neonatal intensive care, the prognosis has improved to some extent. Erythroderma fades in infancy but the characteristic gray, waxy scale progresses. Increasing hyperkeratosis is obvious from early childhood and is most prominent around joint flexures, scalp, anterior neck, abdominal wall and infragluteal folds (porcupine appearance). At these sites, yellow-brown waxy and ridged scales build up in skin creases. Cobblestone keratoses and

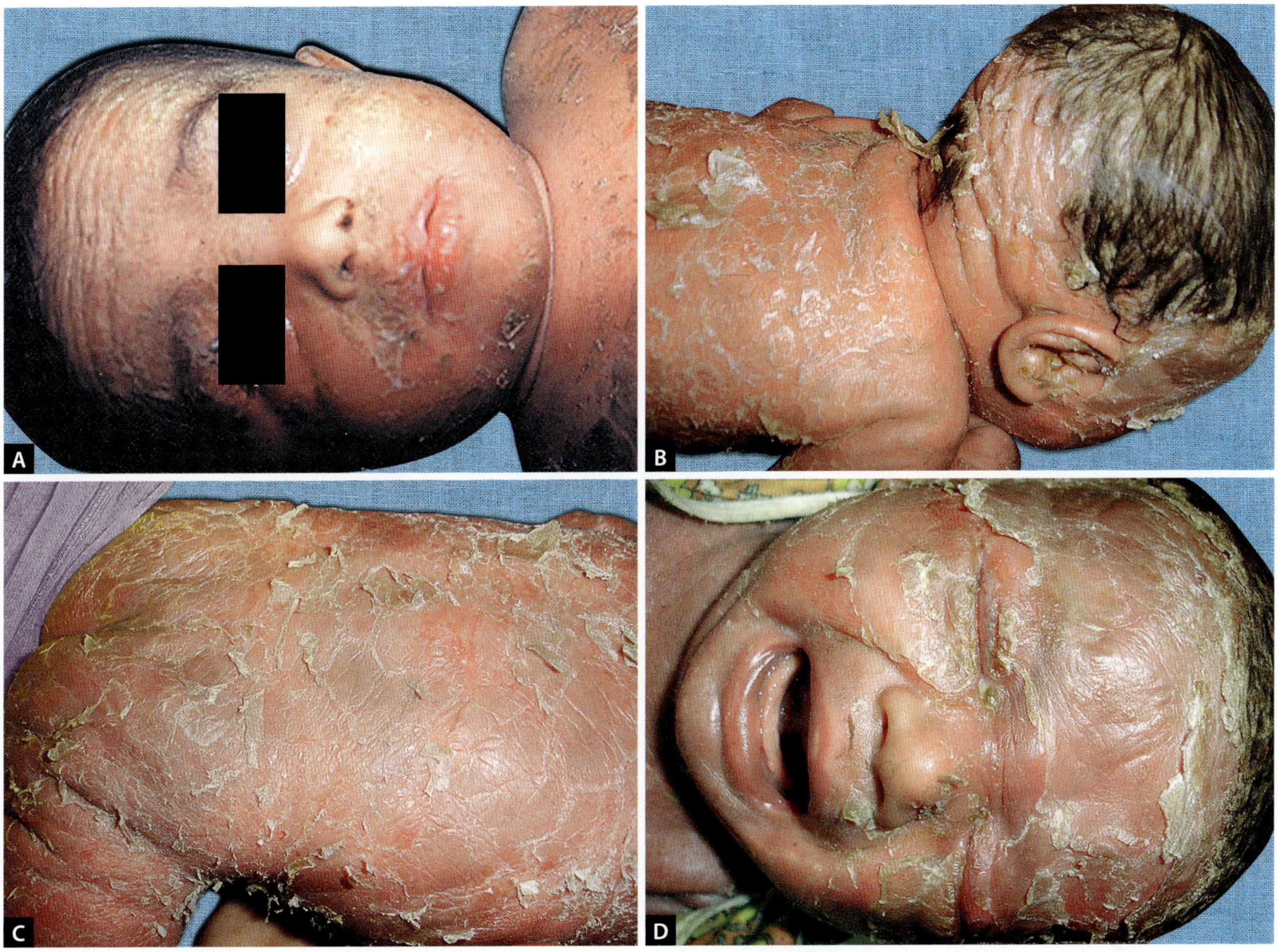

Figs. 9A to D: (A) Same child showing involvement of face; (B) Nonbullous ichthyosiform erythroderma (NBIE) baby; (C) NBIE, note skin over back; (D) NBIE, close-up view of face.

verrucous plaques may develop at other sites. Repeated skin infections and cellulitis are troublesome complications in these children. Palmoplantar hyperkeratosis develops in approximately 60% of these patients. Epidermolytic hyperkeratosis is a characteristic feature on histopathology. Severely affected patients suffer significant physical and psychological morbidity.

Differential Diagnosis

In the neonatal period, other blistering disorders such as epidermolysis bullosa, staphylococcal scalded skin syndrome, herpetic infection and incontinentia pigmenti must be excluded by clinical, histopathological and microbiological assessment.

Management

Emollients are of limited value in BIE as the scales are often hyperkeratotic and the skin remains sodden and macerated. Keratolytic preparations like salicylic acid, alpha-hydroxy acids, or propylene glycol are effective. Regular use of antiseptic baths/washes, rotational systemic antibiotics, and anticandidal preparations may be required in severe cases with repeated bacterial or fungal (candidal) infections and associated body odor. For localized lesions at puberty or late childhood, topical calcipotriol is found to be effective. For extensive lesions, oral retinoid is beneficial in such patients but it should be used cautiously as it can worsen skin fragility. Low-dose acitretin (0.25–0.5 mg/kg/day) is useful.

"If you truly love life, don't waste time because time is what life is made of." —**Bruce Lee**

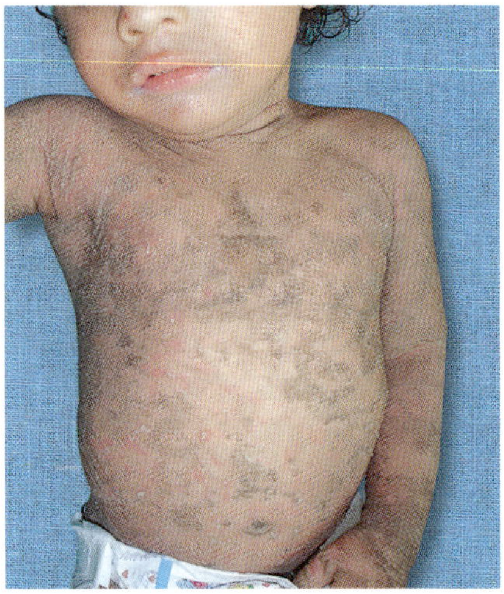

Fig. 10: Epidermolytic hyperkeratosis.

COLLODION BABY (FIGS. 14 TO 19)

The term "collodion baby" is used to describe infants who are born with a membrane-like covering resembling collodion or oiled parchment. The collodion baby is not a disease entity but is a phenotype common to several disorders. Majority of the cases are due to underlying autosomal recessive congenital ichthyosis mostly being LI and NBIE. Other causes are Netherton syndrome, Conradi–Hünermann–Happle disease, trichothiodystrophy, Sjögren–Larsson syndrome and rarely recessive X-linked ichthyosis and ichthyosis vulgaris. In 10–25% infants, collodion baby evolves into normal child with mild scaling called "self-improving congenital ichthyosis" previously called as self-healing collodion baby.

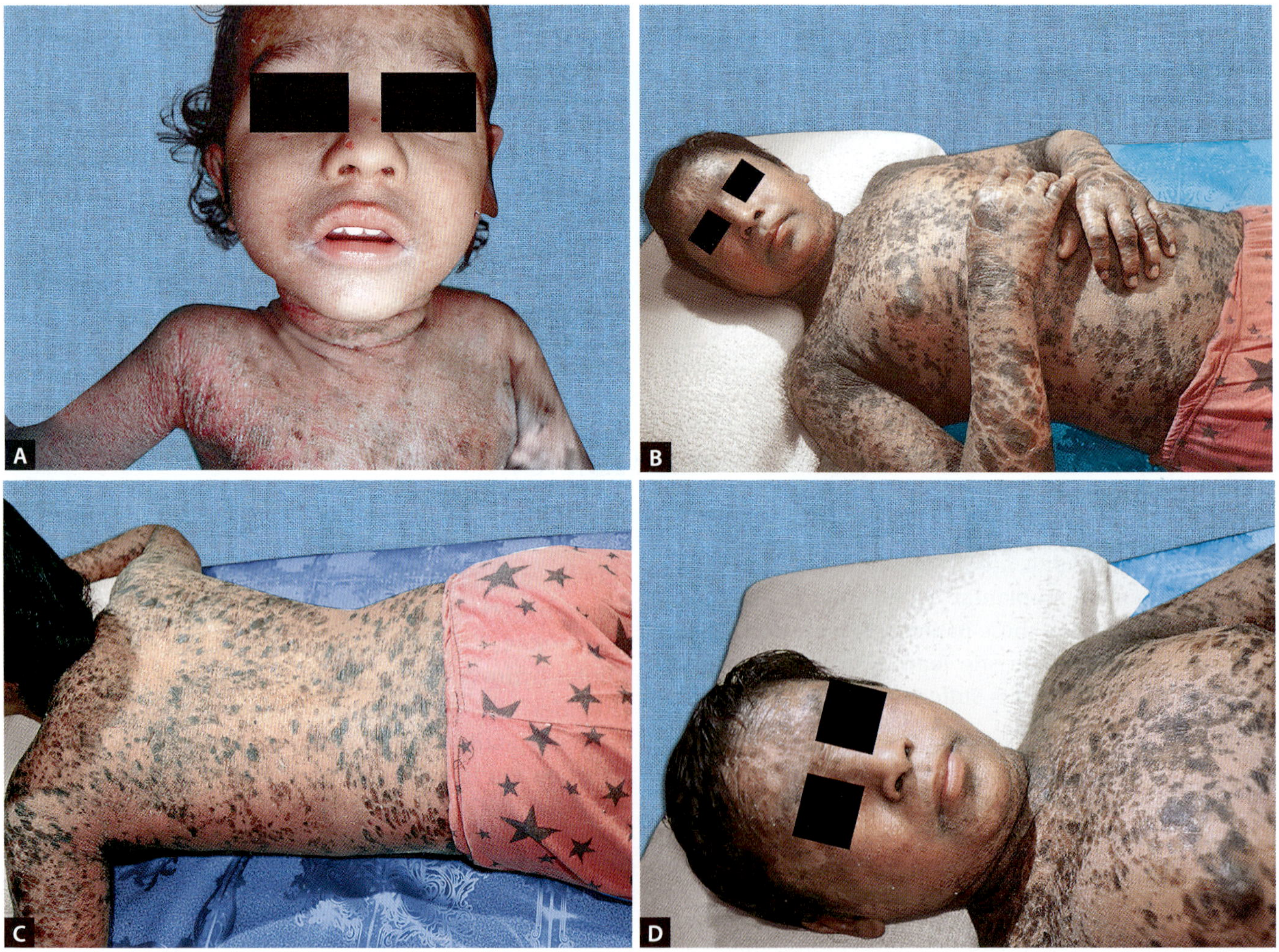

Figs. 11A to D: (A) Epidermolytic hyperkeratosis showing thick scales on face and neck; (B) Epidermolytic hyperkeratosis; note large, thick and dark scales; (C) Same boy, note the dark, thick scales on back; (D) Close-up view of scales.

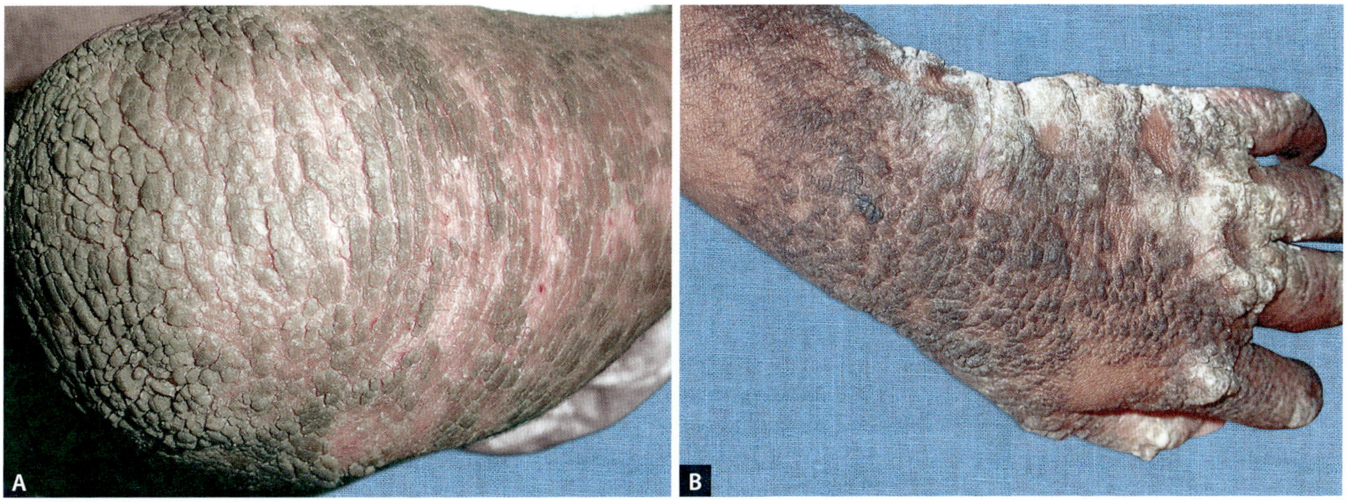

Figs. 12A and B: (A) Thick scales giving a fissured appearance; (B) Epidermolytic hyperkeratosis, note porcupine-like appearance of skin.

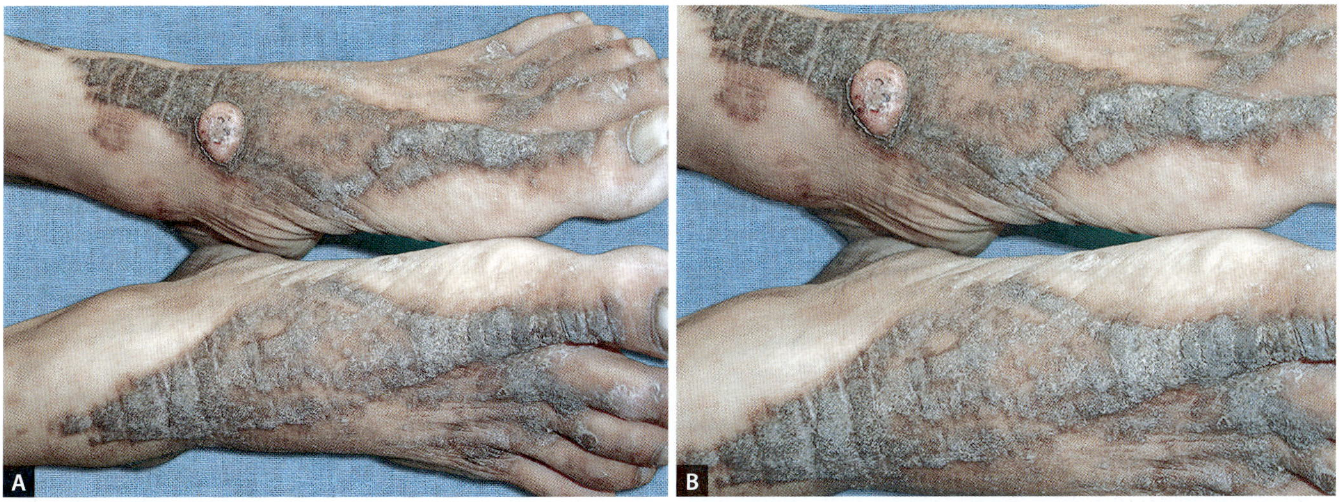

Figs. 13A and B: (A) Epidermolytic hyperkeratosis over dorsum of feet, bilateral in a 17-year-old boy; (B) Same boy, close-up view of lesions.

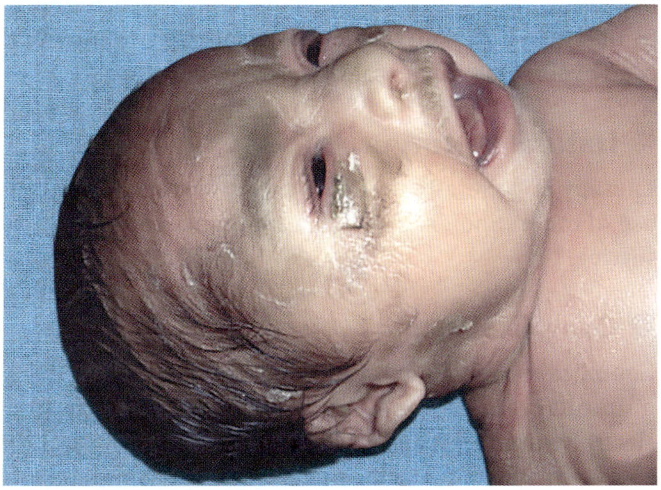

Fig. 14: Collodion baby, note parchment-like membrane along with peeling on the face.

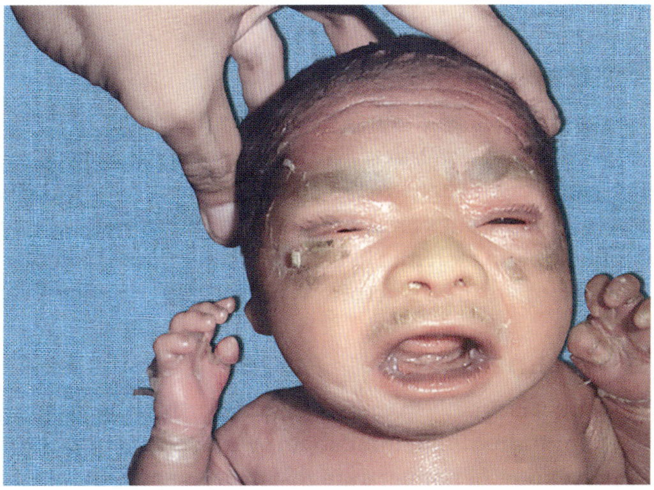

Fig. 15: Same baby showing ectropion and eclabium.

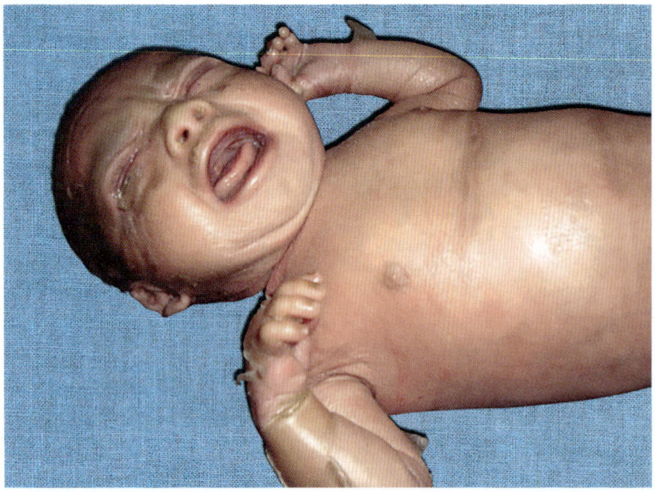

Fig. 16: Membrane-like thick sheets of scales peeling from different parts of the body.

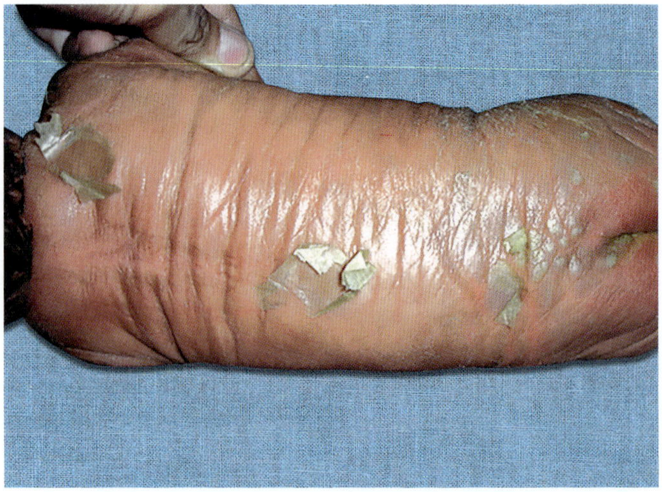

Fig. 17: Membrane-like thick sheets of scales peeling from different parts of the body, back view.

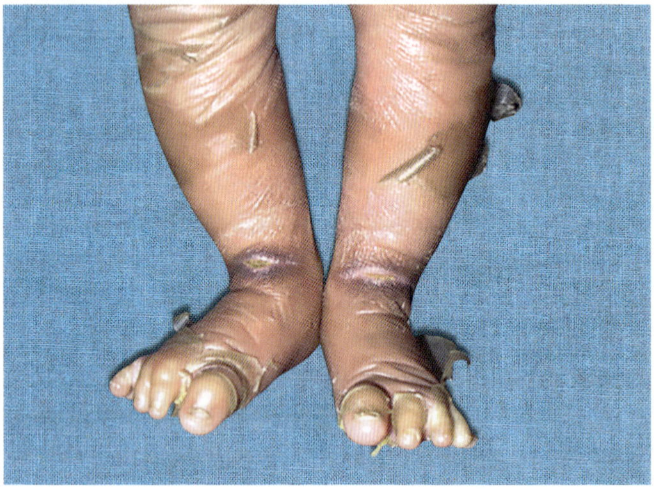

Fig. 18: Membrane-like thick sheets of scales peeling over the lower legs.

Complications

The membrane, by its tautness, causes distortion of facial features and extremities. There is associated ectropion, eclabium, digital constrictions, and tethered ears. Infants are unable to suck and breathe properly, suffer from cutaneous and systemic infection, temperature instability and electrolyte imbalance.

Treatment

Treatment is mainly in the form of supportive care. Infants are kept in humidified incubator with special attention to prevention of temperature instability, sepsis, fluid and electrolyte imbalance. Topical therapy can be provided in the form of light emollient preparations. Genetic counseling is necessary.

HARLEQUIN FETUS (FIGS. 20A TO E)

The term harlequin fetus refers to the most severe form of congenital ichthyosis inherited as an autosomal recessive trait. Clinically presents as thickened gray- or yellow-colored skin divided into polygonal, triangular or diamond-shaped plaques by deep reddish brown fissures resulting from severe keratosis, resembling the traditional costume of a "harlequin". Rigidity of the skin results in ectropion, fish mouth deformity of lips, and distorted nose and ears. Nails are hypoplastic or absent. There is difficulty in sucking, breathing and swallowing with flexion deformity of all joints of the limbs. Massive thickening results in "coat of armor" appearance. It should be differentiated from restrictive dermopathy where there is no hyperkeratosis or scaling.

Natural History

Therapy is generally ineffective, but currently with the use of oral retinoids, a significant proportion of children survive.

Complications

Complications include breathing and feeding difficulties, pulmonary infections, temperature dysregulation, electrolyte imbalance and dehydration, hearing difficulties and ophthalmologic complications such as recurrent conjunctivitis, exposure keratitis, squint and nystagmus.

"You will never change your life until you change something you do daily." —**Mike Murdock**

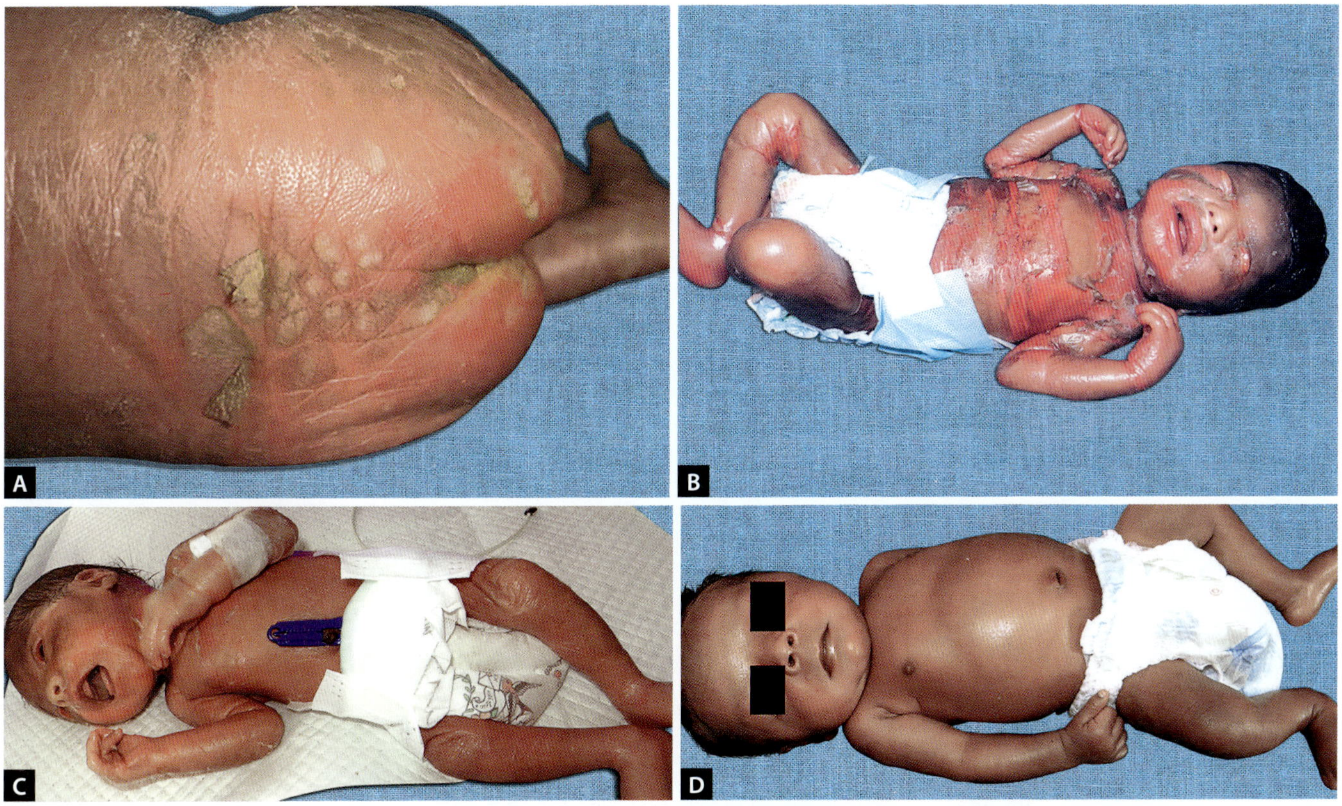

Figs. 19A to D: (A) Membrane-like thick sheets of scales peeling on the lower back and gluteal region; (B) Collodion baby, very severe form; (C) Self-healing collodion baby; (D) Same baby at 1 month of age.

Treatment

Multidisciplinary approach is necessary. Treatment with oral retinoids like acitretin and etretinate and intensive skincare can prolong survival but at the cost of quality of life. Acitretin and isotretinoin can be started from the first day of life. Etretinate (1 mg/kg/day, no longer available), acitretin (0.5–1 mg/kg/day) and isotretinoin (0.5–1 mg/kg/day) have shown beneficial effects. Liver function and serum lipid levels should be monitored during retinoid therapy. Monitoring for skeletal adverse effects should be done periodically. Genetic counseling should be offered to parents.

The consensus recommendations on the use of long term systemic retinoids in children with ichthyosis suggest, starting with a lower dose, lower dose in warmer, humid weathers, considering drug holidays, serum lipid profile and liver function test to be done at baseline, repeated after 1–2 months of retinoid initiation and thereafter every 6–12 months (children with persistent abnormal lipid profile may continue treatment with effective lipid management), annual growth assessment (height, weight, BMI, growth curve), ophthalmologic evaluation recommended after 4–6 months of starting systemic retinoid and thereafter every 6–12 months.

PITYRIASIS RUBRA PILARIS (FIGS. 21 TO 24)

This disorder is characterized by circumscribed follicular keratoses, palmoplantar keratoderma and erythroderma, affecting both sexes equally. In the classical adult onset pityriasis rubra pilaris (PRP), the eruption starts most often on the head, neck or upper trunk as an erythematous slightly scaly macule. Erythematous perifollicular papules with a central follicular plug appear few weeks later. These coalesce to form orange, red scaly plaques that frequently contain islands of normal appearing skin. The classical juvenile PRP has early onset, between 5 and 10 years of age. In the circumscribed juvenile PRP which affects children, sharply demarcated areas of follicular hyperkeratosis and erythema are seen over the knees and elbows.

"I can accept failure, everyone fails at something. But I can't accept not trying." —**Michael Jordan**

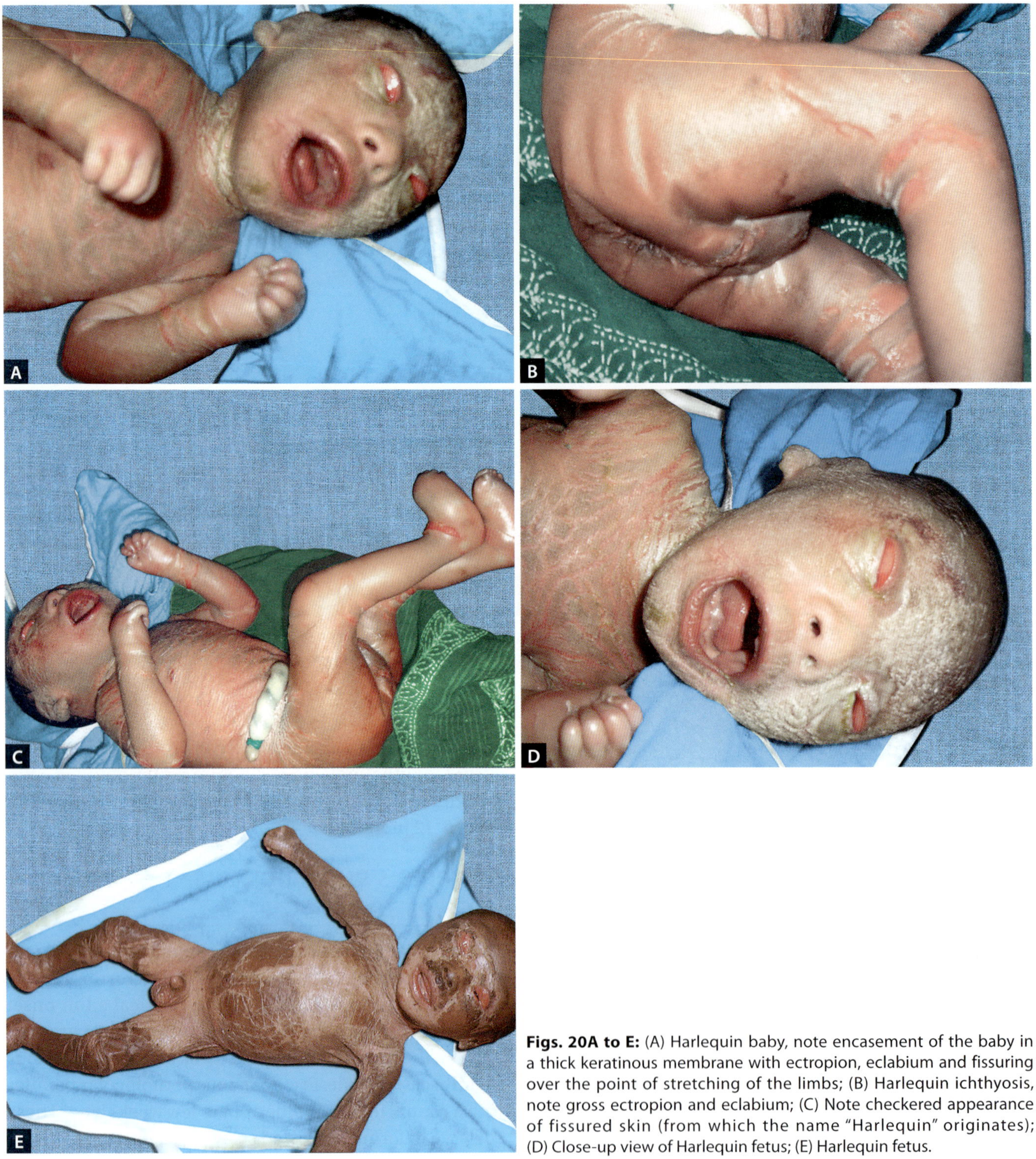

Figs. 20A to E: (A) Harlequin baby, note encasement of the baby in a thick keratinous membrane with ectropion, eclabium and fissuring over the point of stretching of the limbs; (B) Harlequin ichthyosis, note gross ectropion and eclabium; (C) Note checkered appearance of fissured skin (from which the name "Harlequin" originates); (D) Close-up view of Harlequin fetus; (E) Harlequin fetus.

Treatment

Bland emollient applications are of immense help. Equal parts of liquid paraffin and soft white paraffin applied frequently reduce the exfoliation. In the active erythrodermic phase, acitretin can be used at a dosage of 0.75 mg/kg/day or isotretinoin at a dosage of 1.0–1.5 mg/kg/day.

"While it may seem small, the ripple effect of small things is extraordinary." **—Mat Bevin**

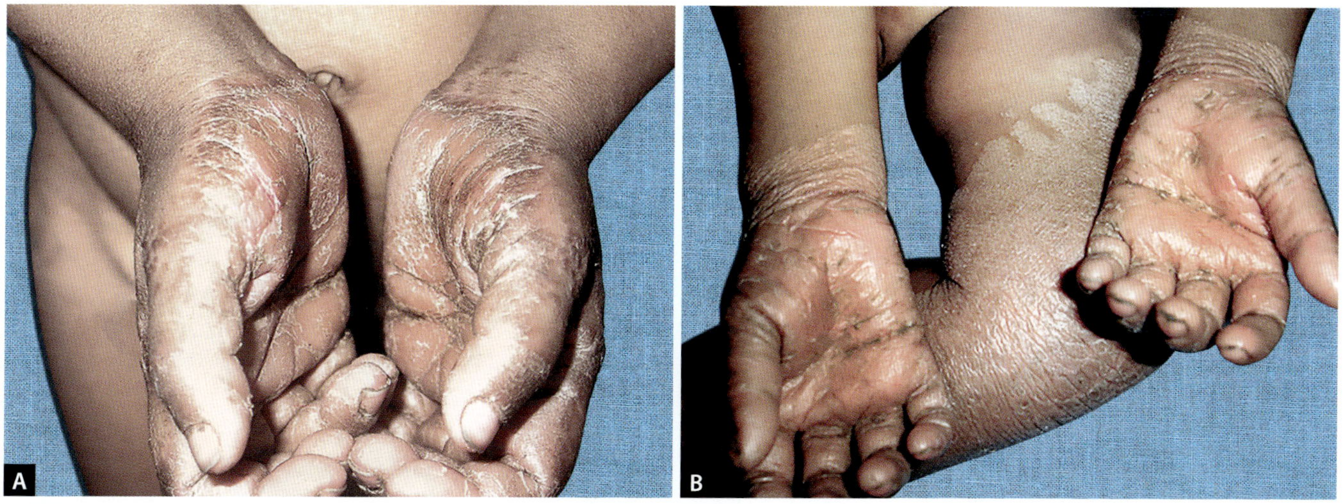

Figs. 21A and B: (A) Diffuse hyperkeratosis over the palms in a 10-year-old boy with pityriasis rubra pilaris (PRP); (B) PRP palms, note thickening and fissuring.

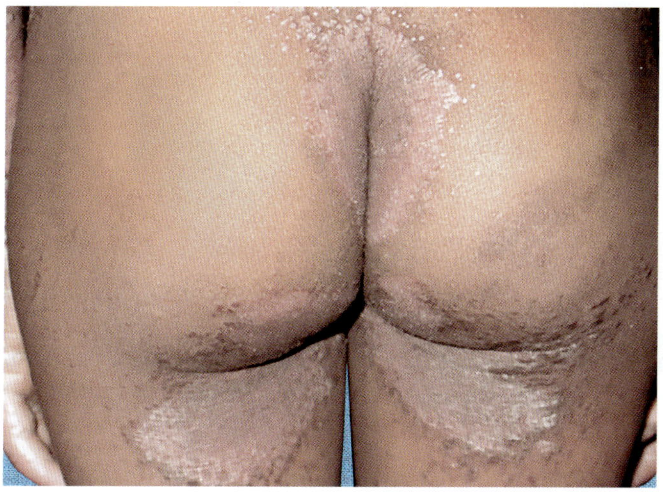

Fig. 22: Hyperkeratotic lesions over the buttocks and thighs.

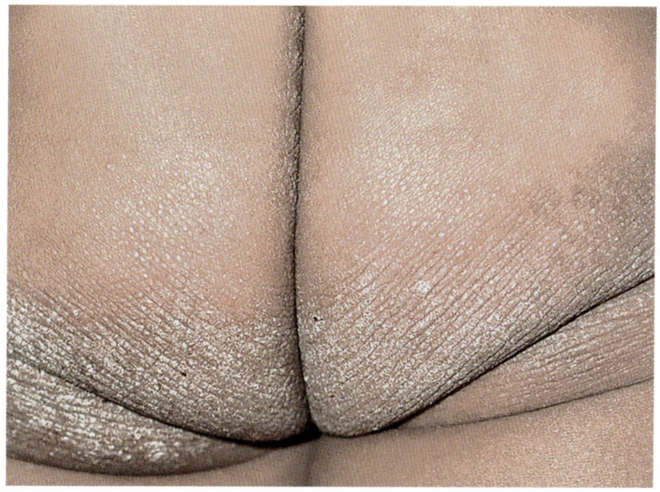

Fig. 23: Hyperkeratotic lesions over the buttocks.

KERATITIS–ICHTHYOSIS–DEAFNESS (KID) SYNDROME (FIGS. 25A TO C)

It is an autosomal dominant disorder characterized by keratitis (with progressive corneal opacification), ichthyosis and sensorineural deafness. It results from mutation of *GJB2* encoding for connexin 26. It presents with erythematous, symmetric plaques on face with verrucous appearance and furrowing around mouth (perioral rugae). Generalized tiny stippled papules are characteristic. Leather-like palmar and plantar keratoderma is almost always present. Nail changes manifest in the form of rough cuticles, subungual hyperkeratosis with leukonychia. Follicular hyperkeratosis leading to scarring alopecia may be present. Affected individuals have increased susceptibility to infections. Squamous cell carcinoma of the tongue and skin have been reported in 10–20% cases. They are more prone for recurrent bacterial and candidal infections.

Treatment

In contrast to other ichthyotic conditions, treatment of these patients with oral retinoids has been reported to be of little benefit and to exacerbate the corneal neovascularization. Multidisciplinary approach and genetic counseling are necessary.

"It's amazing. Life changes very quickly, in a very positive way, if you let it." —**Lindsey Vonn**

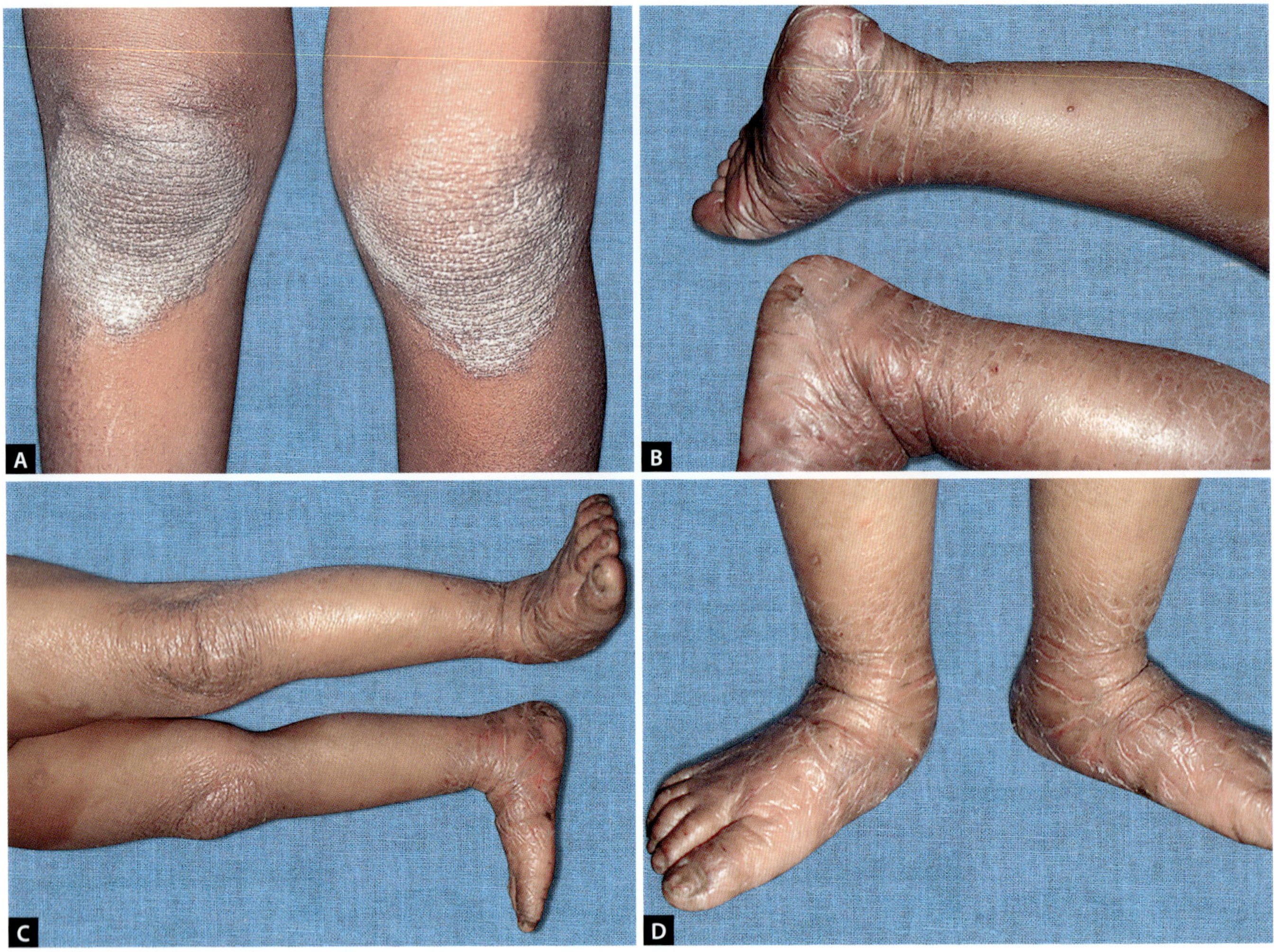

Figs. 24A to D: (A) Hyperkeratotic spiny lesions over the knees; (B) Lower legs and soles in pityriasis rubra pilaris (PRP); (C) Legs and soles in PRP; (D) Bilateral thickening, scaling and fissuring of feet in PRP.

NETHERTON SYNDROME [FIGS. 26A TO D(iv)]

It is an autosomal recessive disorder characterized by ichthyosis, atopy and a structural hair shaft defect. It occurs due to mutation in *SPINK5* gene encoding for serine protease inhibitor LEKTI (lymphoepithelial Kazal-type-related inhibitor) in the epithelial cell. At birth, it presents as neonatal erythroderma. It presents with ichthyosis linearis circumflexa (polycyclic serpiginous and erythematous plaques with migratory double-edged scales at the margins) after 2 years and atopic dermatitis manifesting as food allergy, asthma or dry itchy skin leading to lichenification over flexures at later stages. Hair shaft abnormality in the form of trichorrhexis invaginata, in which the distal hair segment is telescoped into the proximal one leading to a ball and socket deformity is found on microscopy and is diagnostic of Netherton syndrome. Multiple hairs should be examined as it affects only 20–50% hairs. Other hair shaft abnormalities include trichorrhexis nodosa and pili torti. Hair abnormalities improve with age. Other features include recurrent infections, epilepsy and growth hormone deficiency.

Prenatal diagnosis using molecular assay is possible. As Netherton syndrome is complicated by an impaired skin barrier, a caution should be exercised while using topical steroids and calcineurin inhibitors. Oral retinoids are contraindicated in Netherton syndrome as it can exacerbate the condition. Narrow band ultraviolet B (UVB) therapy, intravenous immunoglobulin therapy and infliximab have shown promising results.

"It is a characteristic of wisdom not to do desperate things." —**Henry David Thoreau**

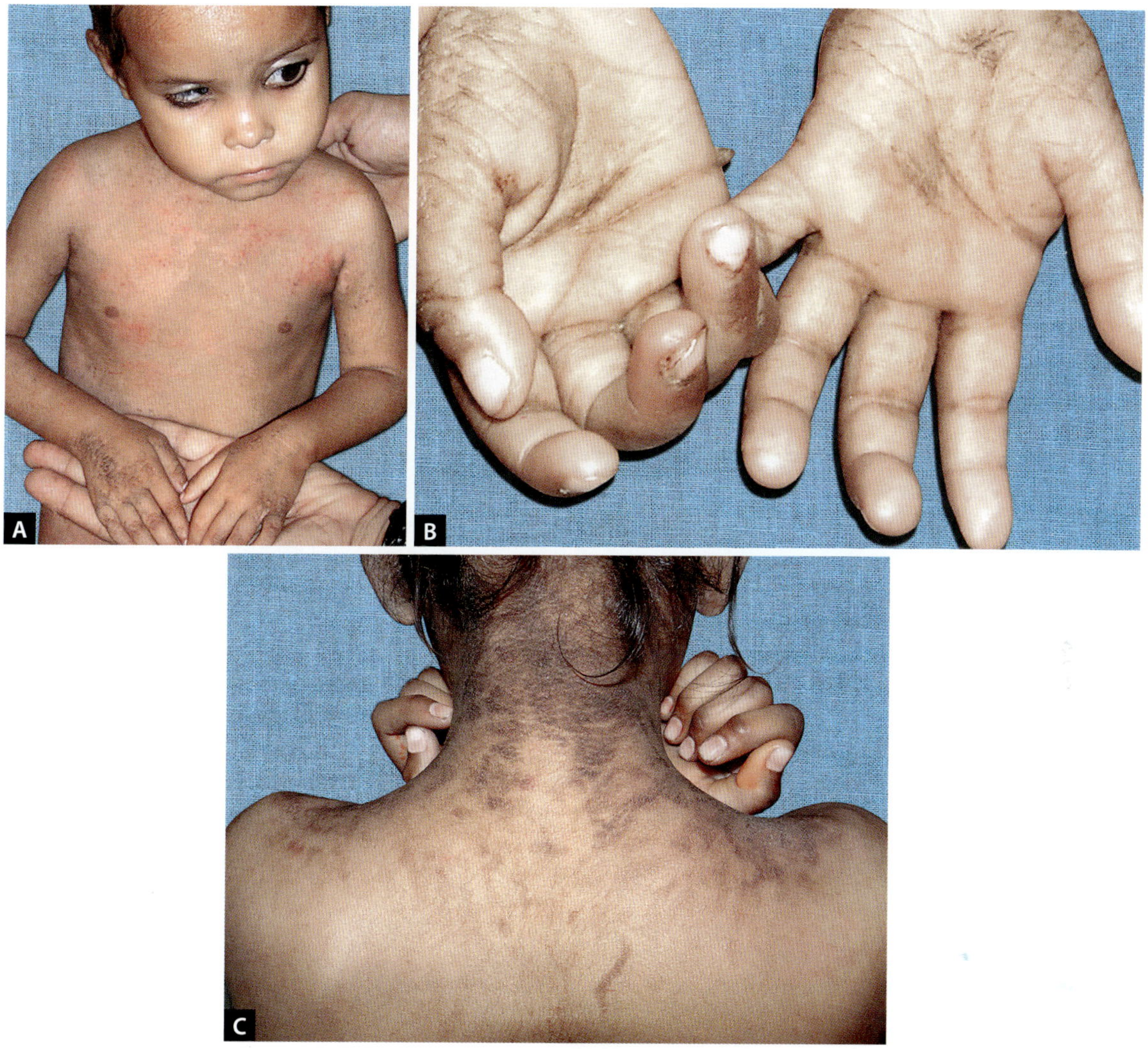

Figs. 25A to C: (A) Keratitis–ichthyosis–deafness (KID) syndrome, note keratitis and ichthyosis; (B) Involvement of palms in KID syndrome; (C) Close-up view of neck lesions in KID syndrome.

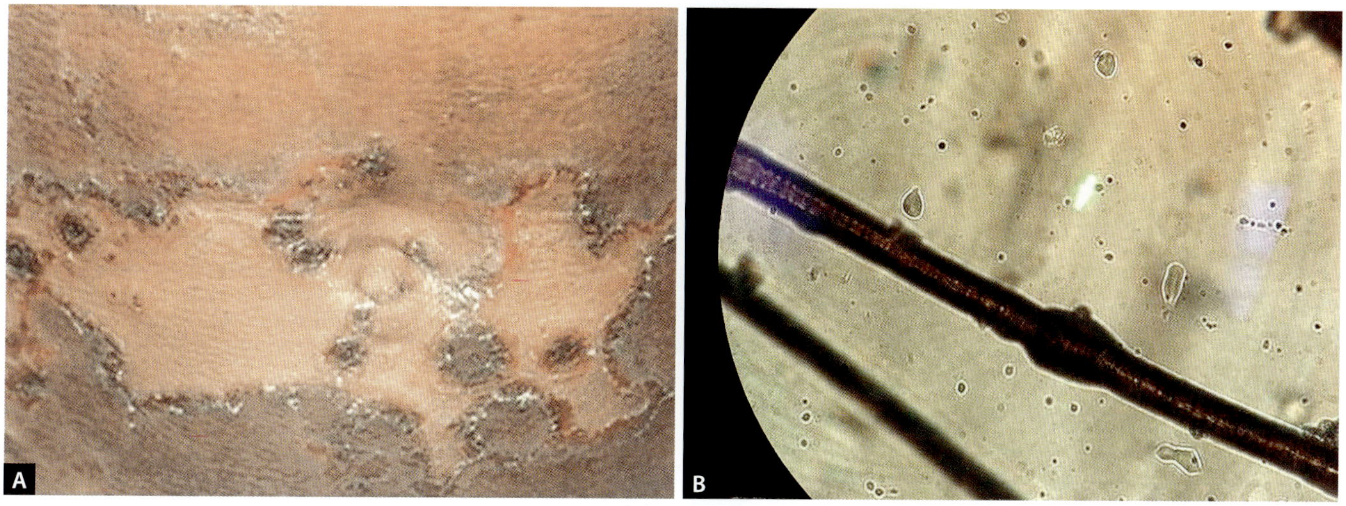

Figs. 26A and B: (A) Classical skin lesions of Netherton syndrome, ichthyosis linearis circumflexa. Note double-edged scales; (B) Light microscopy of hair showing trichorrhexis invaginata.

"Happiness is not something you postpone for the future; it is something you design for the present." —**Jim Rohn**

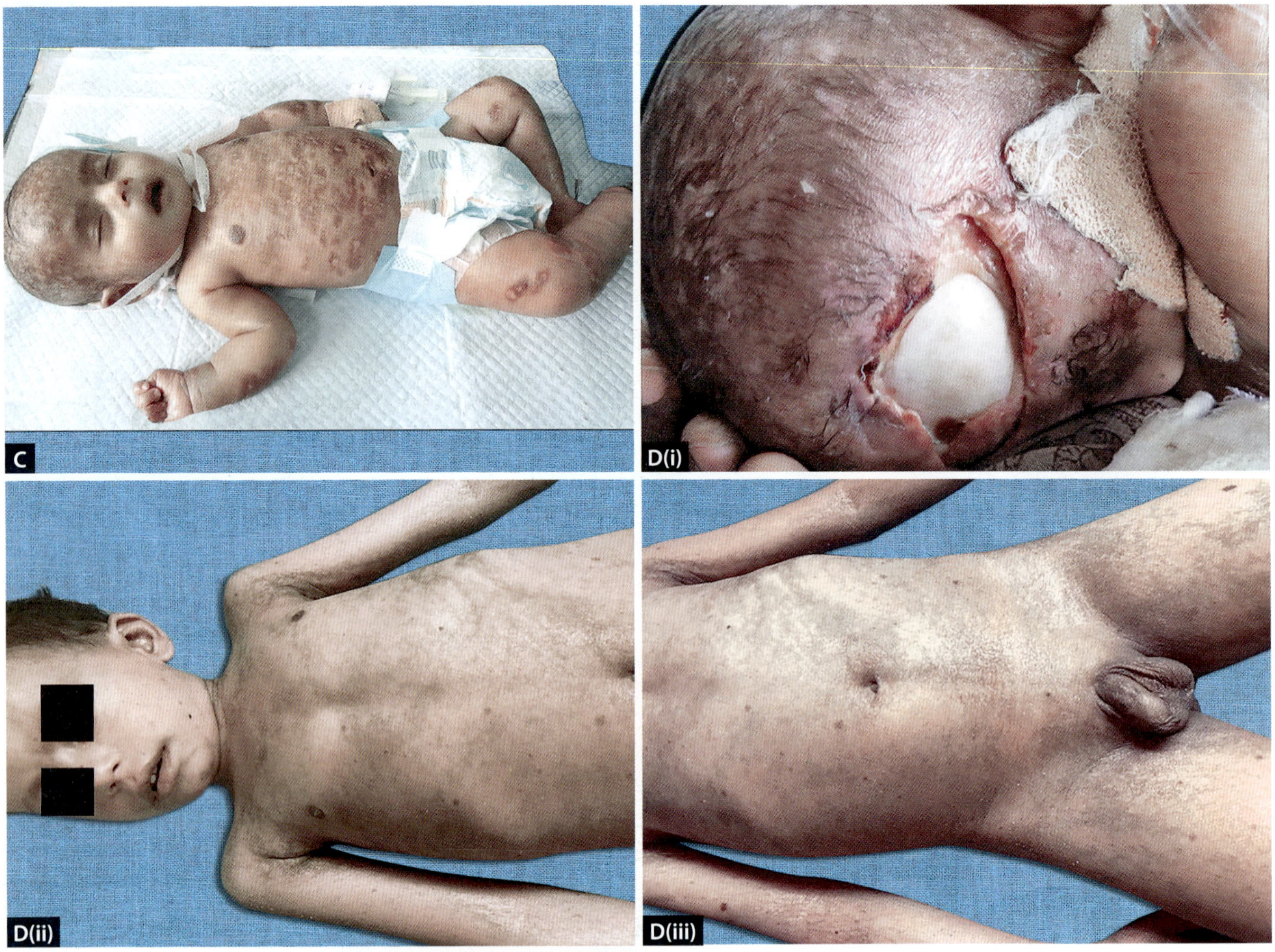

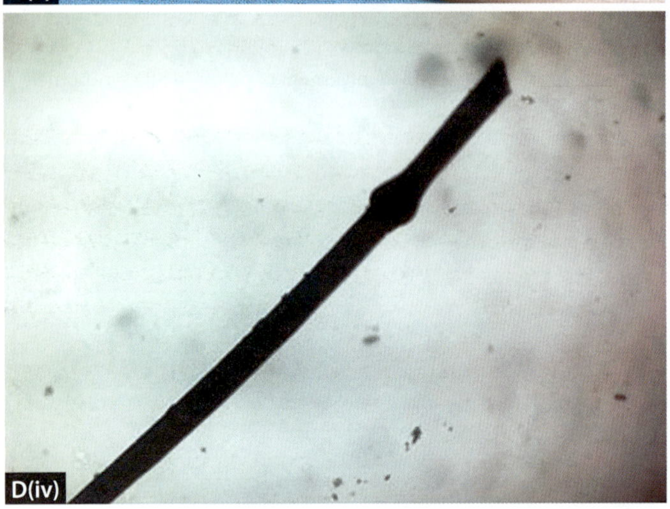

Figs. 26C to D(iv): (C) Netherton syndrome presenting with atypical ichthyosis; D(i) Netherton syndrome with atypical presentation, scalp abscess; D(ii) Netherton syndrome; D(iii) Same boy with Netherton syndrome; D(iv) Hair in Netherton syndrome, note "bamboo hair defect" in shaft.

SJÖGREN–LARSSON SYNDROME [FIGS. 26D(v) TO (viii)]

This is an autosomal recessive condition characterized by congenital ichthyosis, spastic paralysis and mental retardation. It occurs due to mutation in the fatty aldehyde dehydrogenase (*FALDH*) gene. The ichthyosis may manifest at birth with fine-to-thick scales giving a yellowish hue to the thickened hyperkeratotic areas and accentuated skin markings. The

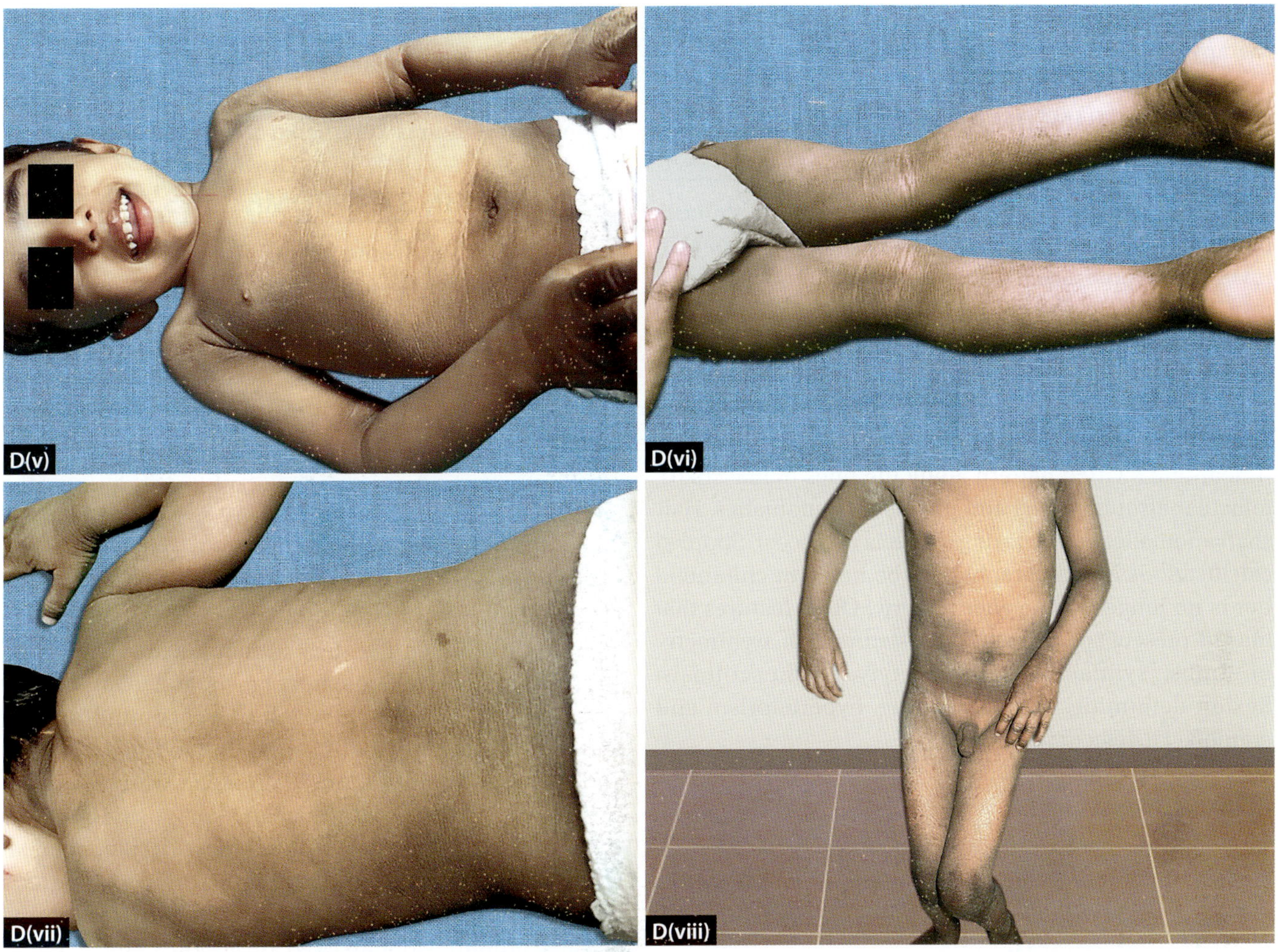

Figs. 26D(v) to (viii): D(v) Sjögren–Larsson syndrome; D(vi) Same boy, lower extremity; D(vii) Close-up view of back; D(viii) Sjögren–Larsson syndrome with neurological deficit (spastic paraplegia).

commonly affected sites include neck, lower abdomen and flexures. During the first 2–3 years, spastic diplegia or tetraplegia develops with mental retardation, seizures and speech delay. A characteristic finding that manifests after one year of age is the glistening white dots in the macula of the retina. Photophobia is common.

Treatment

Topical emollients, keratolytics and systemic retinoids are useful. Recently, bezafibrate, a lipid-lowering agent and zileuton, a 5-lipoxygenase inhibitor have been in trials.

REFSUM DISEASE

It is an autosomal recessive condition occurring due to the impaired breakdown of dietary phytanic acid caused by a deficiency of phytanoyl-coenzyme A hydroxylase (*PHYH*), leading to its accumulation in the tissues. Clinical manifestations include retinitis pigmentosa, peripheral neuropathy, cerebellar ataxia, cranial nerve dysfunction, miosis, electrocardiographic changes, cardiomyopathy, renal tubular dysfunction and skeletal abnormalities. Ichthyosis manifesting as small white scales generally manifests in late childhood and adolescence.

Diagnosis

The diagnosis is made by elevated levels of plasma phytanic acid.

Treatment

It includes dietary restriction of foods containing phytanic acid and its precursors, plasmapheresis and lipapheresis. This disease should be considered in a clinical setting of

"Share your knowledge. It is a way to achieve immortality." —**Dalai Lama**

delayed onset ichthyosis with neurologic impairment as therapy can arrest the progression.

CONRADI–HÜNERMANN–HAPPLE SYNDROME

It is also known as X-linked dominant chondrodysplasia punctata type 2 characterized by mosaic pattern of skin involvement and occurs only in females. It occurs due to a mutation in the emopamil binding protein (*EBP*) gene. It is lethal to males. Affected females have normal life expectancy. It presents at birth with congenital ichthyosiform erythroderma which clears over months and is replaced within 3–6 months by linear hyperkeratosis (linear and swirled pattern along the lines of blaschko), follicular atrophoderma and pigmentary anomalies. Hair shaft anomalies with scarring alopecia can occur. Stippled calcifications in radiographs may be noted in childhood but is no longer visible after puberty. Other features that may be present are cataract, short stature with asymmetry of limbs, syndactyly, clinodactyly, kyphoscoliosis, flexion deformities, frontal bossing, hypertelorism and craniofacial defects.

Treatment

Treatment in the form of correction surgeries for limb length may be offered. Emollients are helpful for ichthyosis.

CHILD SYNDROME

CHILD syndrome is a rare, X-linked dominant disorder present since birth. The acronym is self-explanatory, congenital hemidysplasia, ichthyosiform erythroderma and limb defects. Ichthyosiform erythroderma usually has a unilateral involvement with ipsilateral hypoplasia of different systems including musculoskeletal, central nervous system and cardiovascular system. It is caused by mutations in NAD(P)-dependent steroid dehydrogenase-like (*NSDHL*) gene, encoding the enzyme 3β-hydroxysteroid dehydrogenase. Defects in intermediate steps of cholesterol biosynthesis are responsible for this condition. Ichthyosiform erythroderma presents at birth as yellow and waxy scaling along with erythema and hyperkeratosis distributed on one-half of the body or in a blaschkoid distribution. Extent of limb defect varies from digital hypoplasia to complete absence of extremity. Biopsy may demonstrate abnormal lamellar granules in stratum spinosum.

Treatment

Recently, topical cholesterol 2% along with a topical statin (lovastatin 2% or simvastatin 2%) has been used showing complete resolution in erythema and hyperkeratosis.

PEELING SKIN SYNDROME (FIGS. 26E TO H)

Peeling skin syndrome (PSS) is a rare, autosomal recessive disorder clinically characterized by continuous shedding of stratum corneum throughout life and histopathologically by separation of epidermis in between stratum corneum and stratum granulosum. It may be associated with pruritus, easily pluckable hair, growth retardation, shedding of nail, hypogonadism and anosmia. This entity is also known as "idiopathic deciduous skin" or "keratolysis exfoliativa congenita." Two subtypes of peeling skin syndrome: acral PSS and generalized PSS have been proposed. A mutation in transglutaminase 5 is identified to give rise to acral PSS, characterized by peeling restricted to hands and feet. Generalized type is sub-classified into noninflammatory type A and inflammatory type B. Type A is characterized by year-round peeling of stratum corneum without inflammatory changes and is due to mutation of *CHST8* gene which encodes a Golgi transmembrane N-acetylgalactosamine-4-O-sulfotransferase. The main features of type B is congenital ichthyosiform erythroderma characterized by patchy migratory peeling of skin along with pruritus, atopy, elevated immunoglobulin E (IgE) level and aminoaciduria. Type B is caused by homozygous mutation of *CSDN* gene encoding corneodesmosin. Usually, there is no seasonal variation but summer aggravation may be seen in some of the patients. Therapies such as emollients, salicylic acid and oral retinoids may be effective.

HAILEY–HAILEY DISEASE (FIGS. 27A TO D)

Hailey–Hailey disease is a rare, autosomal dominant disease characterized by recurrent bullous and vesicular dermatitis of intertriginous area, though intact blisters are rarely seen. The disease is prevalent in second and third decade with equal sex involvement. Rarely reported in infants. Occasionally, adolescent boys or girls can also get affected. The disease gets aggravated typically during summer, may be due to excessive sun exposure, sweating and maceration. Other precipitating factors are trauma, heat, friction, bacterial and fungal infection. The basic defect is due to loss of function

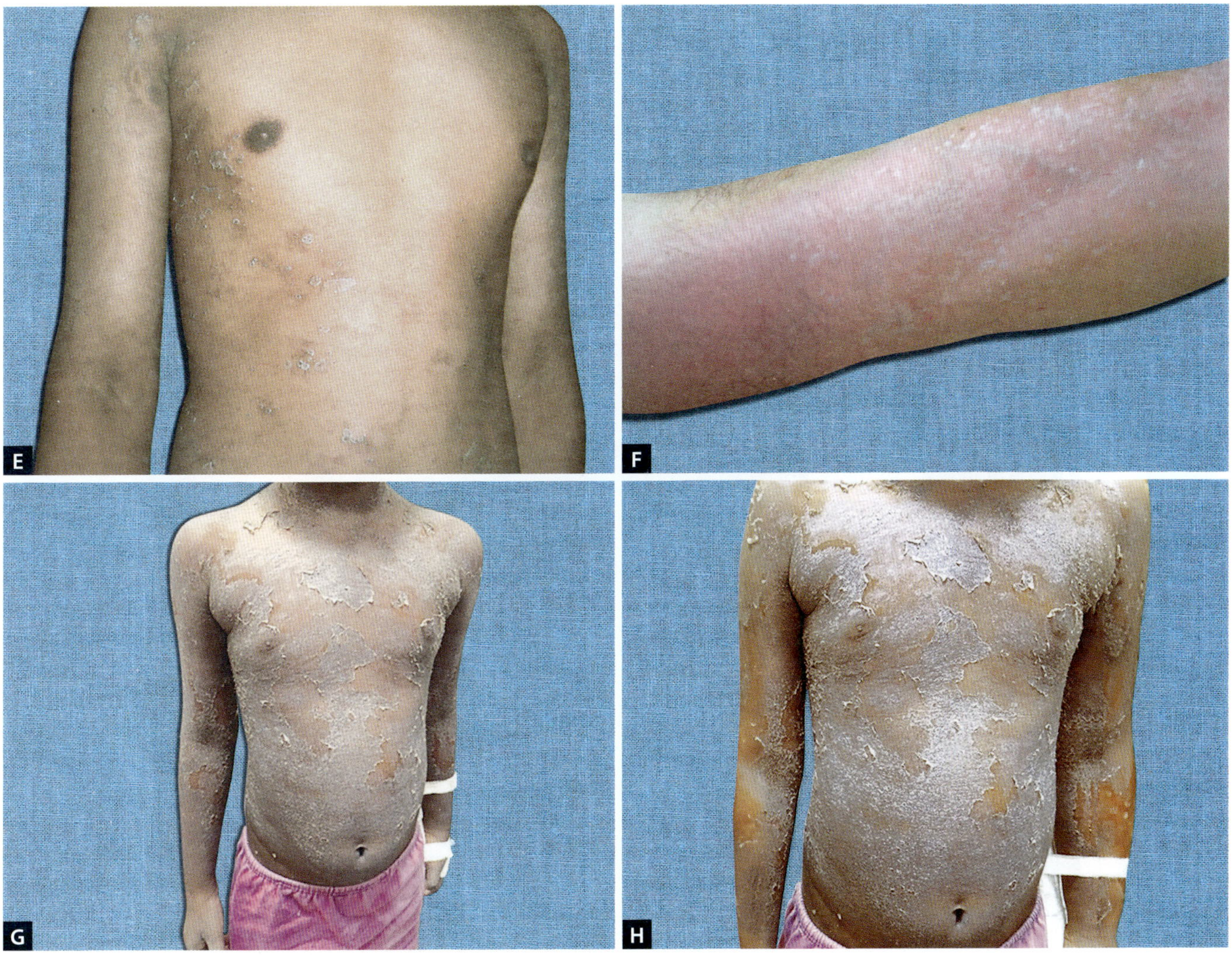

Figs. 26E to H: (E) Peeling skin syndrome over trunk; (F) Peeling skin syndrome over forearm; (G) Peeling skin syndrome; (H) Same boy, close-up view.

mutation of *ATP2C1* gene encoding the human secretory pathway calcium/magnesium adenosine triphosphatase (hSPCA1) which transports calcium within Golgi apparatus, thus maintaining calcium homeostasis within keratinocytes.

Clinical Features

Clinically presents with painful erosions covered with impetiginous crust. Sometimes the lesions assume circinate pattern with spreading active inflammatory border and dry crusted center. Mucosal involvement is rare. Some patients present with longitudinal white lines in nail and palmar pits. Classical histopathological finding is full thickness incomplete acantholysis giving rise to a "dilapidated brick wall appearance". Disease is characterized by frequent exacerbations and remissions.

Differential Diagnoses

Close differentials are Darier disease, candidal intertrigo, eczema and pemphigus vegetans.

Treatment

Different modalities of treatment have been tried including oral antibiotics, dapsone, oral retinoids, and systemic and topical steroids. Treatment with topical tacrolimus and topical calcipotriol is also effective.

"Science is organized knowledge. Wisdom is organized life." —**Immanuel Kant**

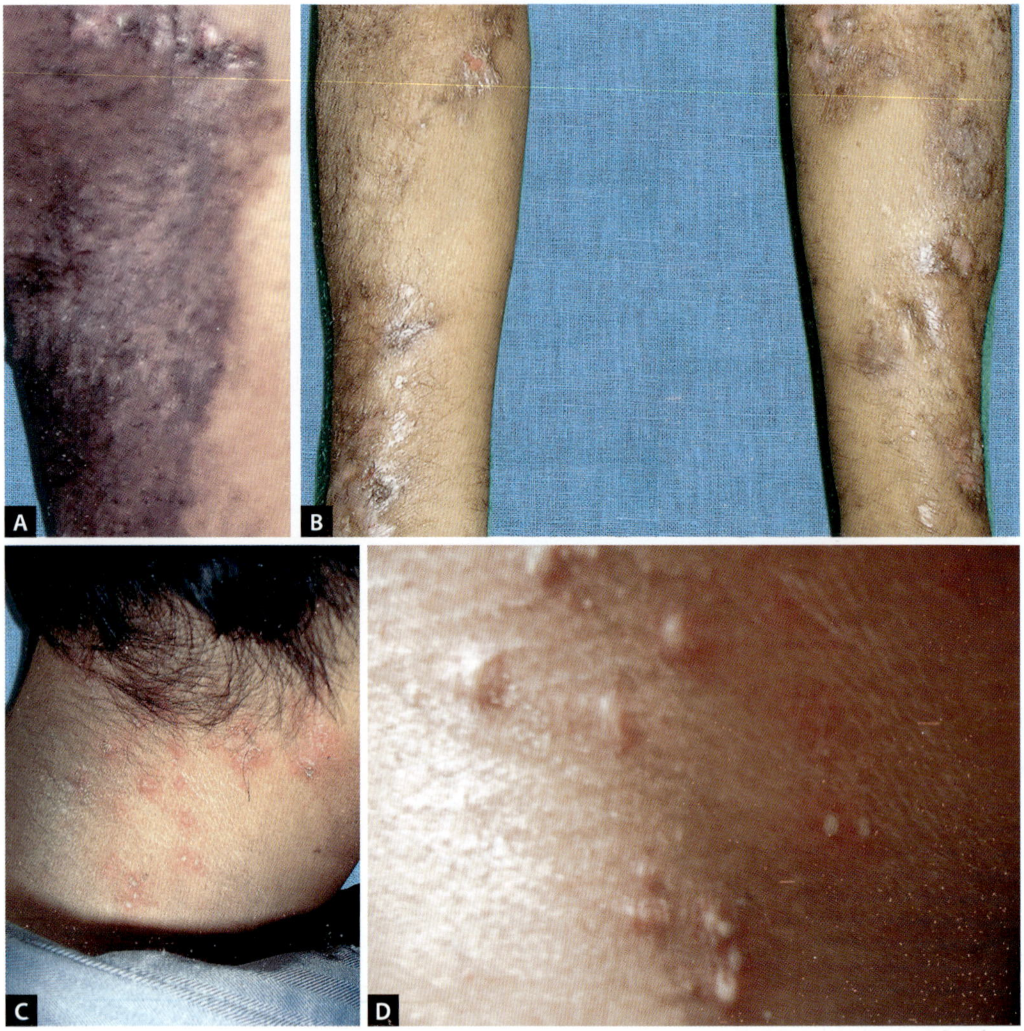

Figs. 27A to D: (A) Axilla, a common site in Hailey–Hailey disease; (B) Hailey–Hailey disease aggravated during summer; (C) Lesions of Hailey–Hailey disease over neck in an adolescent boy; (D) Classical lesions of benign chronic familial pemphigus (Hailey–Hailey disease).

POROKERATOSIS (FIGS. 28 TO 32)

Porokeratosis is a clonal disorder of keratinization characterized clinically by hyperkeratotic papules and plaques with thread-like elevated border and histopathologically by cornoid lamella with absent granular layer beneath it. Keratotic ridge can be accentuated by application of gentian violet followed by removal with alcohol.

Etiopathogenesis

It is a genetically heterogeneous disorder where the mode of inheritance is autosomal dominant. Various pathomechanisms have been described including overexpression of *p53* and *pRB* gene, abnormal expression of involucrin, loricrin, and mutation of *SART3* gene especially in disseminated superficial actinic porokeratosis (DSAP). Various triggers of malignant transformation are immunosuppression, ultraviolet exposure and radiation therapy which promote dysplastic changes of affected keratinocytes. Different clinical types have been described including porokeratosis of Mibelli, DSAP, disseminated superficial porokeratosis (DSP), DSP of immunosuppression including human immunodeficiency virus infection, linear porokeratosis, punctate porokeratosis, hypertrophic variant mimicking hypertrophic lichen planus, porokeratosis palmaris et plantaris disseminata and associated syndromes.

"The Highest education is that which does not merely give us information but makes our life in harmony with all existence." —**Rabindranath Tagore**

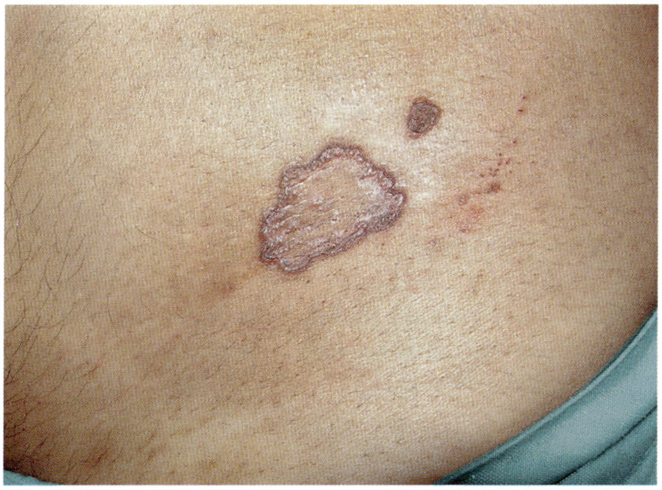

Fig. 28: Porokeratosis of Mibelli, note keratotic ridge at the border.

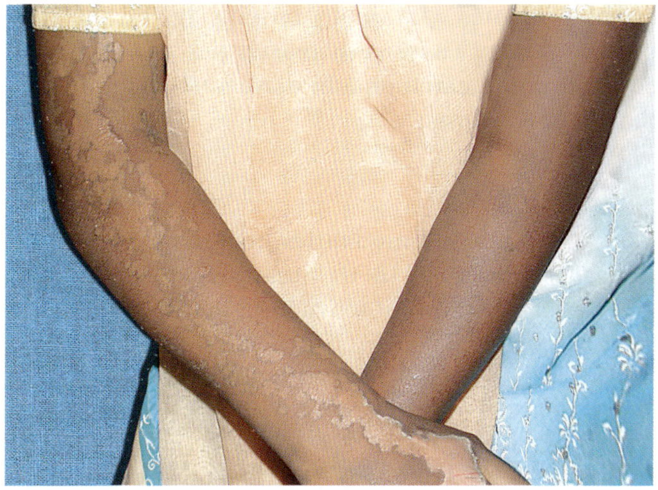

Fig. 29: Linear porokeratosis.

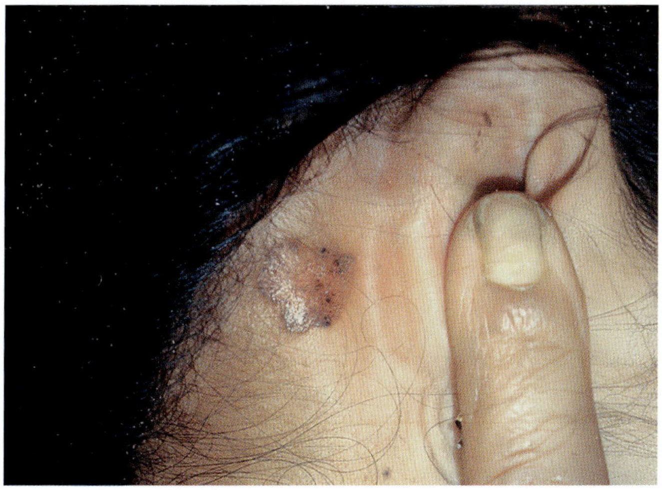

Fig. 30: Porokeratosis behind ear.

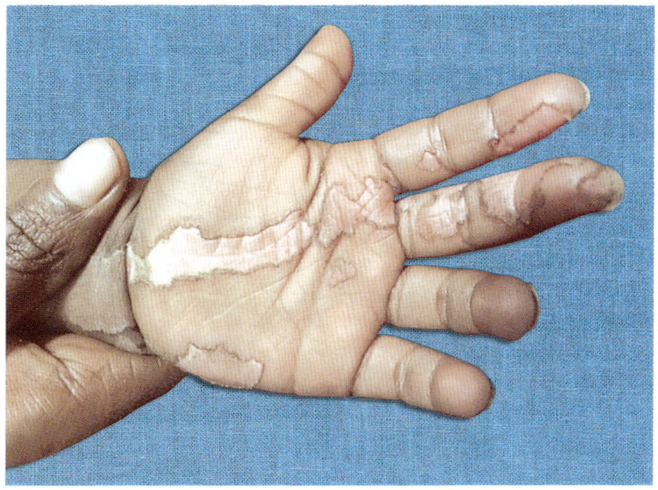

Fig. 31: Porokeratosis over palm.

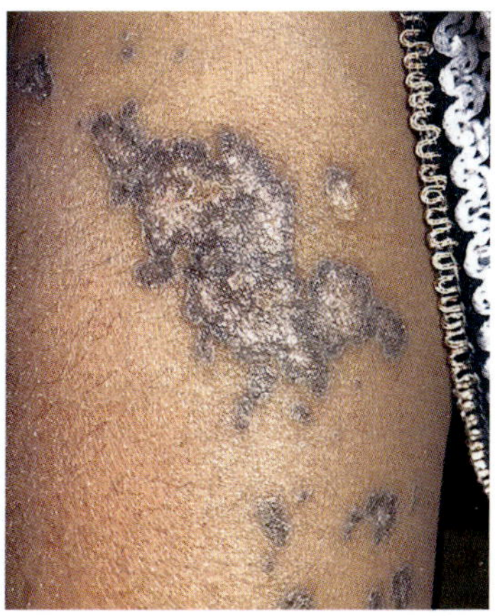

Fig. 32: Porokeratosis, close-up view of lesion.

Clinical Features

Porokeratosis of Mibelli usually appears in childhood as a small crateriform hyperkeratotic plaque which slowly enlarges to form annular plaques with hyperkeratotic peripheral ridge distributed over the face, neck and extremities. Linear porokeratosis occurs as two forms: localized type which is unilateral affecting the distal portion and generalized form affecting trunk and extremities. Punctate type is seen in adolescent age group, presents as 1–2 mm punctate papules on the palms and soles. Disseminated superficial actinic type is very rare in childhood; presents as multiple, superficial

"To succeed in life you need two things, ignorance and confidence." —**Mark Twain**

annular plaques with mildly raised ridge on the sun-exposed areas. There is increased risk of developing squamous cell carcinoma in disseminated, giant and linear porokeratosis.

Treatment

Various treatment modalities include keratolytics, topical 5-fluorouracil (5FU), oral retinoid, cryotherapy, electrodessication, photodynamic therapy, and laser therapy.

WHAT'S NEW

- Novel topical isotretinoin ointment formulation (PAT-001/TMB-001) for congenital ichthyosis found safe and effective in phase 2 trials.
- Trifarotene FDA approved for treatment of LI.
- Dermoscopic findings of Hailey–Hailey disease (white clouds separated by pink furrows and crumbled fabric pattern) and Darier disease (star-like/oval-shaped yellow areas surrounded by whitish halo and pinkish homogenous structureless background) have been described.

SUGGESTED READINGS

1. Kurzeja M, Rakowska A, Jasinska M, Warszawik-Hendzel O, Olszewska M, Rudnicka L. Dermoscopy as a Noninvasive Diagnostic Tool for Hailey-Hailey Disease and Darier Disease. Dermatol Ther 2023;13:2345-5.
2. Roenneberg S, Biedermann T. Pityriasis rubra pilaris: algorithms for diagnosis and treatment. J Eur Acad Dermatol Venereol. 2018;32(6):889-98.
3. Sarri CA, Roussaki-Schulze A, Vasilopoulos Y, Zafiriou E, Patsatsi A, Stamatis C, et al. Netherton syndrome: a genotype-phenotype review. Mol Diagn Ther. 2017;21(2):137-52.
4. Sood S, Akuffo-Addo E, Yeung J, Mufti A. Biologic treatment options for pityriasis rubra pilaris: An evidence-based systematic review. J Am Acad Dermatol. 2023;89(6):1306-8.
5. Swarnkar B, Sarkar R. Neonatal and infantile erythroderma revisited. Indian J Paediatr Dermatol. 2020;21:15-21.
6. Vega Almendra N, Aranibar Duran L. Ictiosis hereditaria: desafío diagnóstico y terapéutico [Hereditary ichthyosis: a diagnostic and therapeutic challenge]. Rev Chil Pediatr. 2016;87(3): 213-23.

"A book is a gift you can open again, and again and again." **—Garrison Keillor**

CHAPTER

5

Infections and Infestations

SCABIES (FIGS. 1 TO 3F)

Scabies is a common, itchy condition caused by the mite *Sarcoptes scabiei* var. *hominis*. The itching is worst at night when the patient is warm. The onset occurs 3–4 weeks after the infection is acquired and it coincides with a widespread eruption of inflammatory papules. The pathognomonic lesions of scabies are burrows which appear as slightly raised, brownish tortuous lesions. They occur commonly on the wrists, borders of the hands, the sides of the fingers and the finger web spaces, the feet particularly the instep and, the genitalia. In infants the head and neck may be involved. With the development of hypersensitivity, pruritic papules develop. Secondary changes may frequently confuse the clinical picture. Eczematous changes are common and may be widespread and severe. Secondary infection, manifests as folliculitis or impetigo, may also be severe and extensive.

In infants in addition to the more extensive burrows seen in older children and adults, vesicular and vesiculopustular lesions on the hands and feet are frequent. Extensive eczematization is often present and there may be multiple crusted nodules on the trunk and limbs. Many children with scabies develop persistent skin colored to reddish nodules over axillae, shoulders, groin, buttocks, and scrotum. These lesions result from the hypersensitivity reaction to scabies mite and tend to persist for months together even after treatment of scabies. Crusted scabies also called as Norwegian scabies though uncommon in children is extremely contagious, can be seen in immunocompromised, human immunodeficiency virus (HIV) infection and neurological manifestations such as mental retardation. Along with eczematous lesions, there is diffuse crusting and hyperkeratosis.

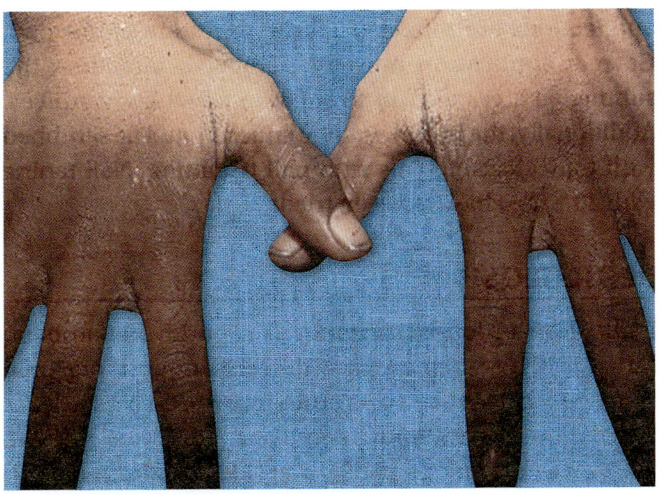

Fig. 1: Inflammatory papules and burrows over finger web spaces in scabies.

Complications

Secondary infections of scabies lead to pustule formation and impetiginization. Nephritogenic strain of *Streptococcus* may rarely cause glomerulonephritis.

Treatment

Permethrin (5%) cream is the treatment of choice in infants and children. It can be used safely in infants as young as 2 months of age. It is to be applied in adults and young children from neck to toes and in infants from head to toes including palms and soles. It is to be left on for 8–14 hours. If necessary, it may be repeated after 1 week. Treatment of close contacts and all family members is necessary.

Gamma-benzene hexachloride (1%) is the most widely used antiscabietic because of its efficacy and cheaper cost than permethrin. There are occasional reports of neurotoxicities which are almost exclusively due to its inappropriate, prolonged or repetitive use or accidental ingestion by infants/young children. It is not recommended in infants and small children and cannot be applied over head and face. Systemic treatment includes oral ivermectin. It is considered to be safe in children above 2 years of age. Two doses of 200 µg/kg of body weight at 1-week interval have been recommended.

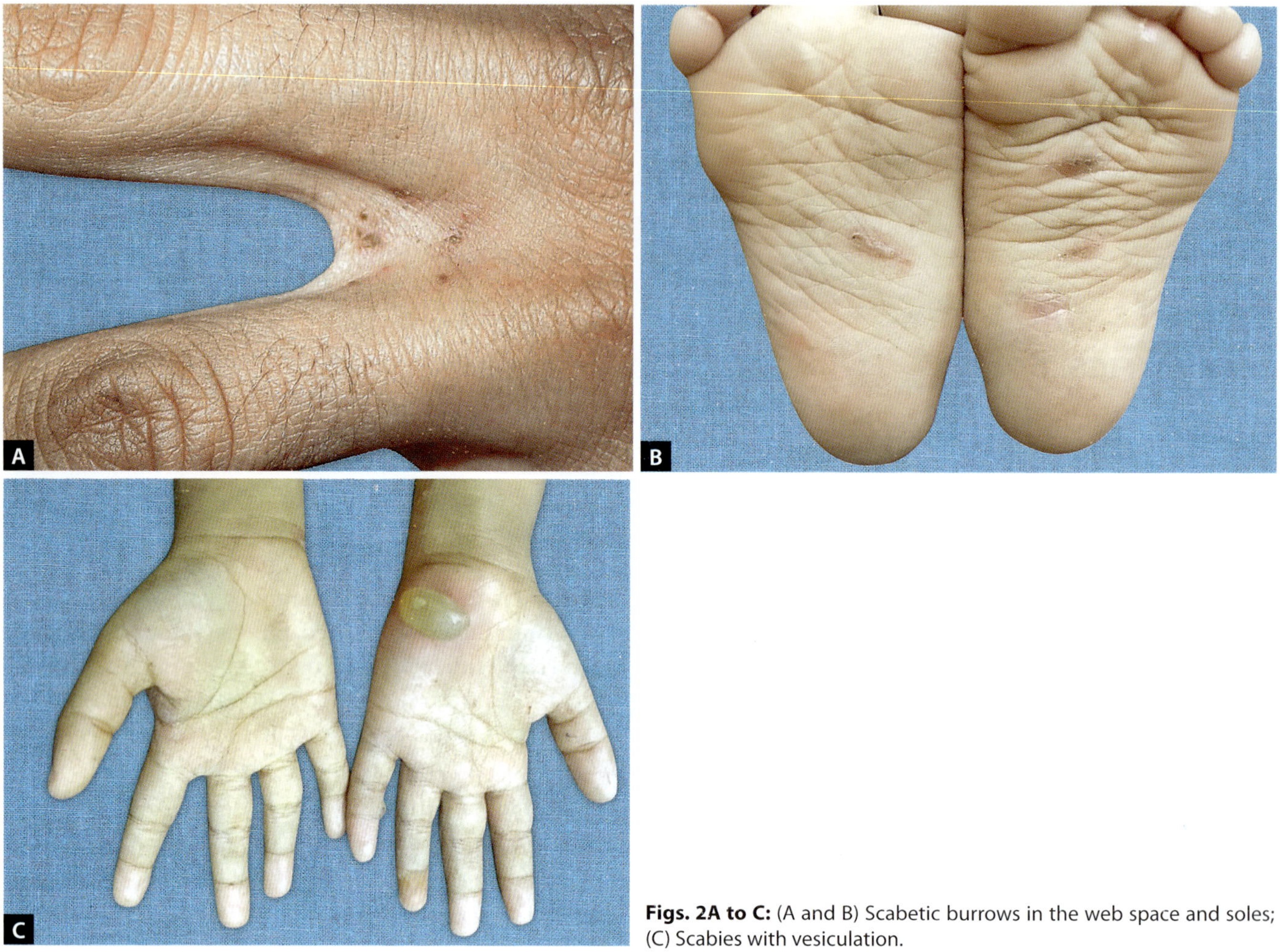

Figs. 2A to C: (A and B) Scabetic burrows in the web space and soles; (C) Scabies with vesiculation.

Decontamination of the environment and systemic antibiotics for secondary infection are necessary.

NORWEGIAN SCABIES (FIGS. 3G TO K)

It is also known as crusted scabies. It occurs usually in immunocompromised individuals, but may occur rarely in immunocompetent persons and in Down's syndrome. It presents with crusting, scaling and psoriasiform changes. It may be localized to scalp, face, fingers including nails, toenails, palms, and soles. As compared to 10–12 mites in classical scabies in Norwegian scabies, there may be millions of mites. Hence, it is extremely contagious and often results in outbreak of scabies in families, crèches, schools, swimming pools, and hospitals. Treatment failure is common. Concomitant oral and topical treatment is useful in patients with crusted scabies. This avoids repeated dosing and ensures early cure. Combination treatment regimens used include use of topical agents such as permethrin 5% cream with oral ivermectin. It was found that topical benzyl benzoate emulsion with oral ivermectin was successful in severe crusted scabies. These applications are repeated till the mites are eradicated. Correct application must be achieved, including the subungual areas and up to edges of lower body orifices. Additionally, the hyperkeratotic crusts should be scrubbed with topical scabicidals with nail trimming. Nail taping with 40% urea has also been tried.

PEDICULOSIS

Pediculosis or louse infestation is a worldwide problem but poor living conditions with resultant poor personal hygiene contribute to epidemic proportions of the infestation in developing countries. The three types of lice that infest human beings are: (1) *Pediculus humanus capitis* (head louse), (2) *Pediculus humanus corporis* (body louse), and (3) *Pthirus pubis* (crab louse).

"It's not hard to make decisions when you know what your values are." —**Roy E Disney**

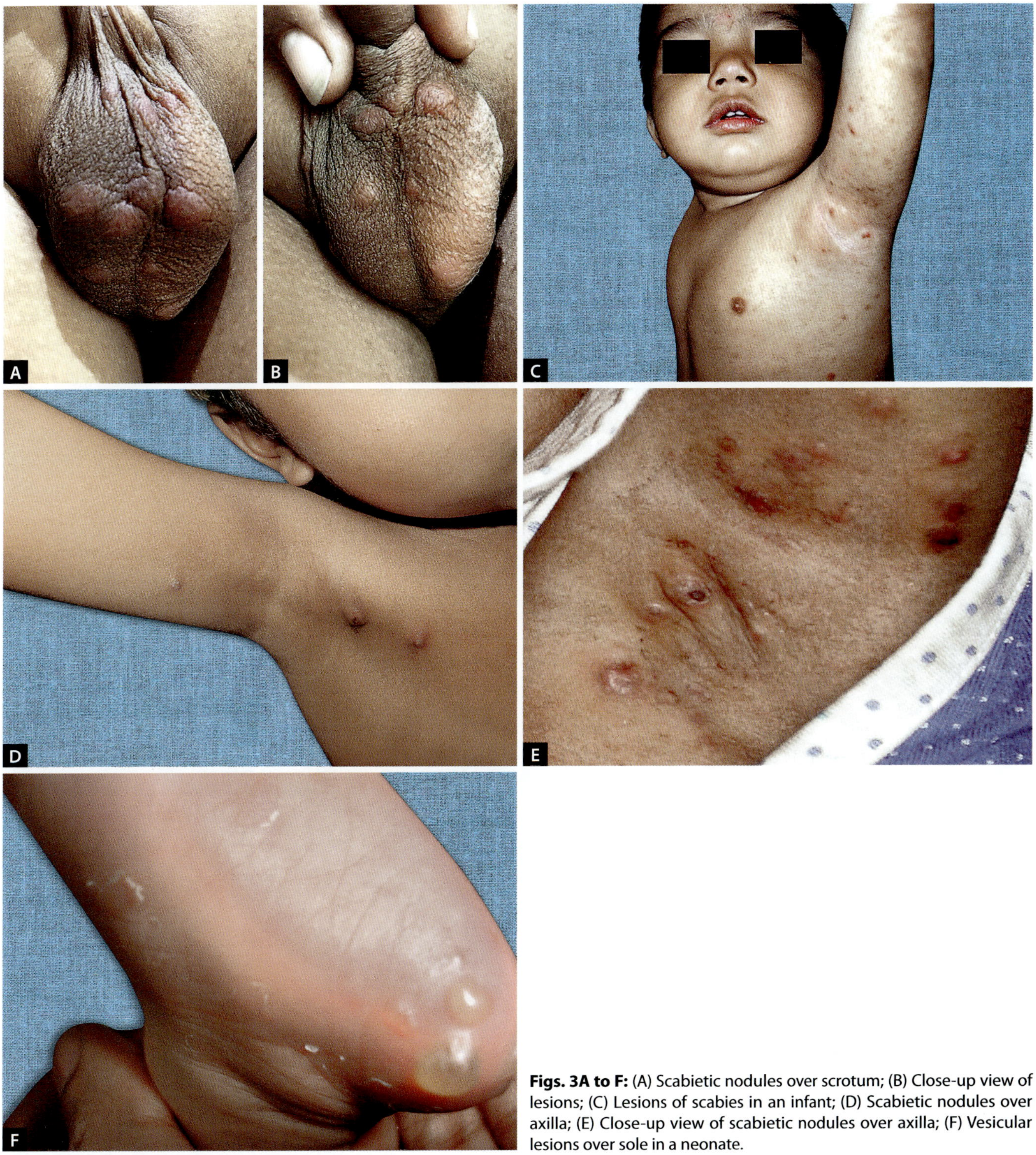

Figs. 3A to F: (A) Scabietic nodules over scrotum; (B) Close-up view of lesions; (C) Lesions of scabies in an infant; (D) Scabietic nodules over axilla; (E) Close-up view of scabietic nodules over axilla; (F) Vesicular lesions over sole in a neonate.

Pediculosis Capitis (Head Louse Infestation) (Figs. 3L to N)

It is caused by infestation of the scalp with *Pediculus humanus capitis*. Head louse is brown in color and lays about 50–150 ova (nits) during an average adult life of approximately 16 days and it measures 1–2 mm in length. They molt three times to develop into an adult over a period of almost 2 weeks. Head louse infestation

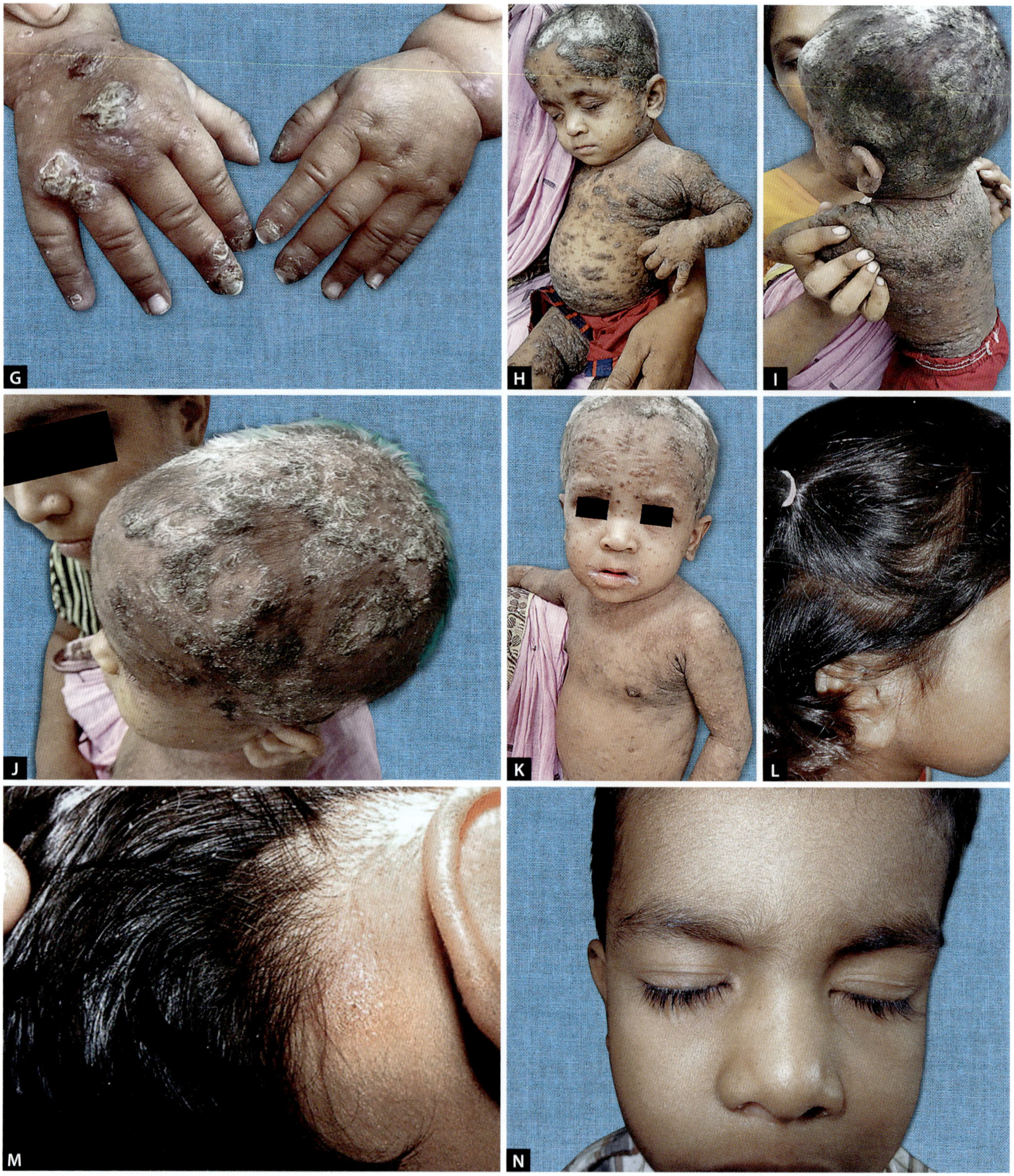

Figs. 3G to N: (G) Hyperkeratotic lesions over hands in Norwegian scabies; (H) Norwegian scabies, note extensive crusted lesions and scabietic papules in finger web spaces of accompanying lady; (I) Same child, close-up view of back lesions; (J) Close-up view of scalp lesions, showing extensive crusted plaques; (K) After 3 weeks' treatment; (L) Pediculosis capitis; (M) Pediculosis capitis, note nits attached to scalp hairs; (N) Pediculosis of eyelids.

"You have to take risks. We will only understand the miracle of life fully when we allow the unexpected to happen." **—Paulo Coelho**

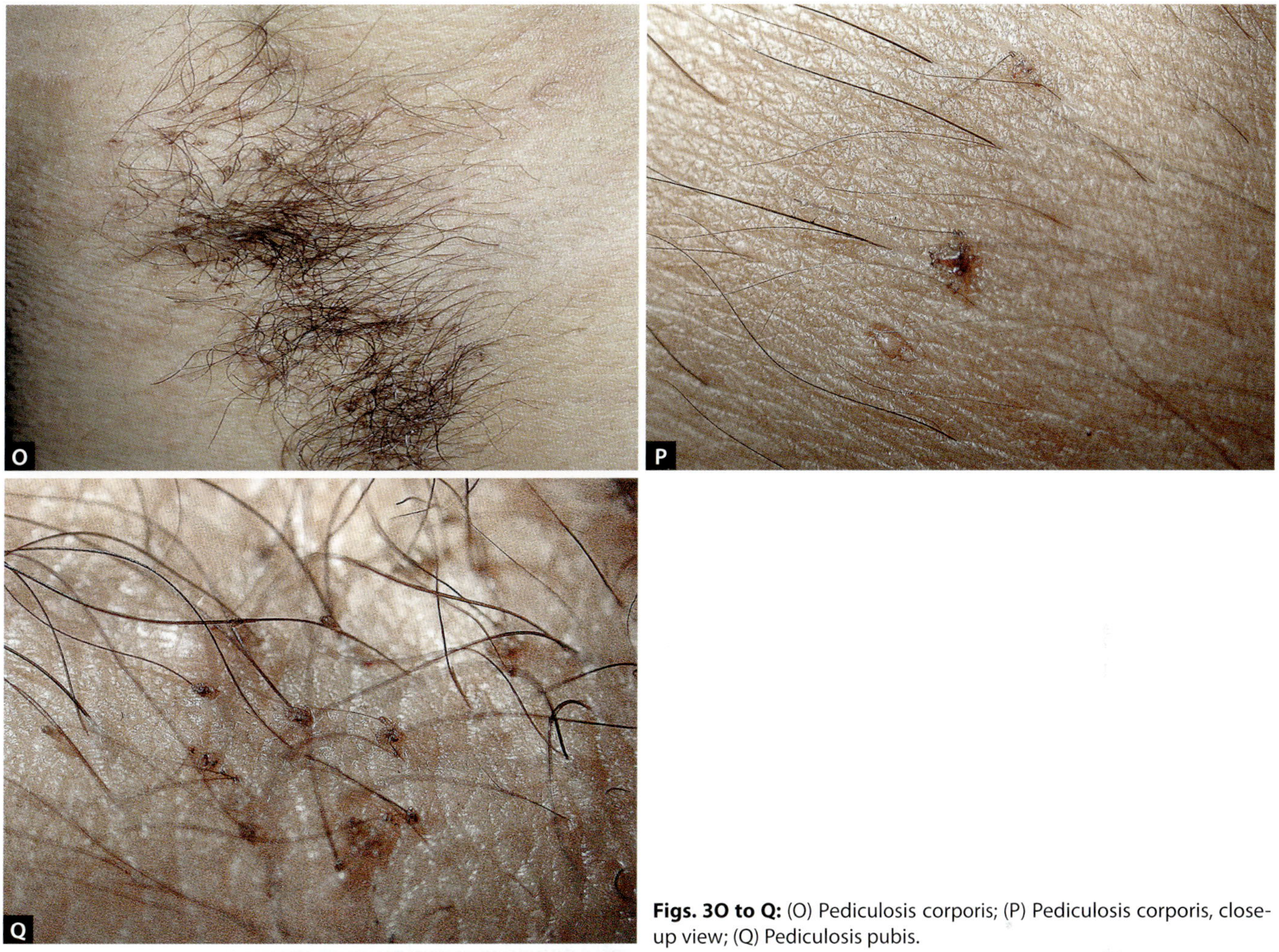

Figs. 3O to Q: (O) Pediculosis corporis; (P) Pediculosis corporis, close-up view; (Q) Pediculosis pubis.

commonly affects females with long hair. The nits are firmly attached to the hair and can slide along the hair but cannot be shed off like scales and the nits are grayish white, oval in shape and about 0.5 mm in length. The transmission is through close contact, sharing of headgear, combs and hairbrushes. In head louse, itching is the predominant symptom and secondary infection with enlargement of occipital lymph glands is the common presentation. Diagnosis is definitive when crawling lice can be seen on a naked eye but microscopic identification of the louse or the stuck on nits on the hair shafts is confirmatory. Exudation, crusting, excoriations and erythematous papules on the neck in females should arouse suspicion of pediculosis capitis.

Manual removal of nits and lice has been practiced from ages but it is a tedious job. Treatment of choice for pediculosis capitis is 1% permethrin. It is applied on slightly damp hair for 5–10 minutes and rinsed off. Second application is necessary after 1 week. Other modalities of treatment that have been used include gamma benzene hexachloride 1%, malathion 0.5%, and spinosad 0.9%. For severe cases, off-labelly oral ivermectin and trimethoprim-sulfamethoxazole have been used. Careful examination of all family members and close contacts is necessary and those with evidence of lice should be treated.

Pediculosis Corporis (Figs. 3O and P) (Body Louse Infestation)

It is generally seen among the poor, homeless or mentally retarded subjects. Body lice generally thrive in conditions of poverty, war, and natural disaster. It is rarely seen in children.

The body louse is about 4 mm in length and lives in the seams of clothes and lays about 270–300 ova during an average 18 days of adult life. Nits incubate for 8–10 days and nymphs mature into adults over about 2 weeks.

"A dream doesn't become reality through magic; it takes sweat, determination and hard work." —**Colin Powell**

Severe itching, excoriations, hemorrhagic crusts and blood-stained clothes are the presentation of body louse infestation. In chronic cases, hyperpigmentation and lichenification can also be seen. The diagnosis can be made by high degree of suspicion and demonstration of lice or nits from the seams of clothing. Treatment consists of proper hygiene, laundering and ironing of clothes and application of insecticides to clothing. Application of permethrin or gamma benzene hexachloride to body hair may be helpful.

Pediculosis Pubis (Fig. 3Q)

Pediculosis pubis is caused by crab louse. It is commonly spread by sexual contact but can be transmitted by clothing or towels. An adult female can lay about 25 eggs during its life span. It mainly attaches to the pubic hair but can be spread occasionally to axillary hair, eyebrows, and eyelashes. The patient complains of itching and on examination bluish gray macules (maculae ceruleae) can be seen on the lower abdomen and thighs. The lice look-like brownish spots attached to the hair.

Therapy consists of single application of pediculicides that is gamma benzene hexachloride 1% or permethrin 1%. In case of eyelash involvement, petrolatum can be applied three to four times a day for 7 days. Manual removal, shaving of hair and even oral ivermectin can be employed as measures for eradication. Sexual partners should also be treated.

BURROWING BUG PIGMENTATION (FIGS. 3R TO U)

Burrowing bugs, also called as *Cydnidae* bugs, are arthropods of the order *Hemiptera* causing exogenous pigmentation of the skin due to release of an odorous substance from special glands that serve as self-defense rather than a bite. It forms pigmented macules when it comes in contact with the human skin. This pigmentation is seen in children especially in rainy season during outdoor activities. Clinically presents as sudden onset of pin-point to few millimeters size, discrete to grouped asymptomatic pigmented (brownish-orange hue) macules distributed mainly on palms, soles and rarely chest and neck. These pigmented macules are bizarre, streaky in shape with tapering edges. The pigmentation could be rubbed off by acetone. Differential diagnoses include acral melanocytic nevi, lentiginous nevi, petechiae, dengue-induced purpura, dermatitis neglecta, postinflammatory pigmentation, postviral exanthem, and pigmentation due to contact with chemicals. Dermoscopy helps in ruling out other differential diagnosis. Dermoscopy of burrowing bug pigmentation shows cluster of oval to bizarre-shaped brown and shiny globules and clods with a superficial "stuck on" appearance. Lesions resolve spontaneously in few days without any residual changes.

LARVA MIGRANS (FIG. 3V TO X)

Cutaneous larva migrans or creeping eruption is a serpiginous cutaneous eruption resulting from penetration of human skin by various animal worms.Common worms are *Ancylostoma braziliense* (cat hookworm) and *Ancylostoma caninum* (dog hookworm). Humans acquire it from an environment contaminated with animal feces containing eggs of worms. There may be two modes of spread: (1) Cutaneous (cutaneous larva migrans); and (2) Oral (visceral larva migrans). Clinically, lesions of cutaneous larva migrans present as itchy serpiginous lesions, sometimes erythematous most commonly over hands, wrist, feet, ankle or lower legs. The diameter of the thread-like line is usually 3 mm. The larvae usually migrate at the rate of few millimeters daily, rarely few centimeters per day, when the line spreads quite rapidly. If cutaneous larva migrans remains unrecognized, it usually dies in 2–8 weeks' time. The condition is treated with a single dose of ivermectin 200 mg/kg of body weight. Other option is albendazole 400 mg/day for 3–7 days. The lesion stops progression after 5–7 days' treatment and itching also subsides completely.

FURUNCULOSIS (FIG. 4)

This is an acute, painful and deep necrotic infection of a hair follicle with *Staphylococcus aureus.* A furuncle presents initially as a small, follicular, inflammatory nodule, soon becoming pustular and then necrotic and healing after discharge of a necrotic core to leave a violaceous macule and ultimately a permanent scar. Tenderness is a constant feature. Lesions may be single or multiple and tend to appear in crops. The sites involved are the face and neck, the arms, wrists and fingers, the buttocks and the anogenital region. In some individuals, crops continue to develop for many months or even years. Associated features include fever and lymphadenopathy. Recurrent furunculosis refers to three or more episodes of furuncles within a 12-month period. Colonization of *S. aureus* in anterior nares can lead to chronic or recurrent furunculosis. Other predisposing factors for recurrent furunculosis are anemia, previous antibiotic therapy,

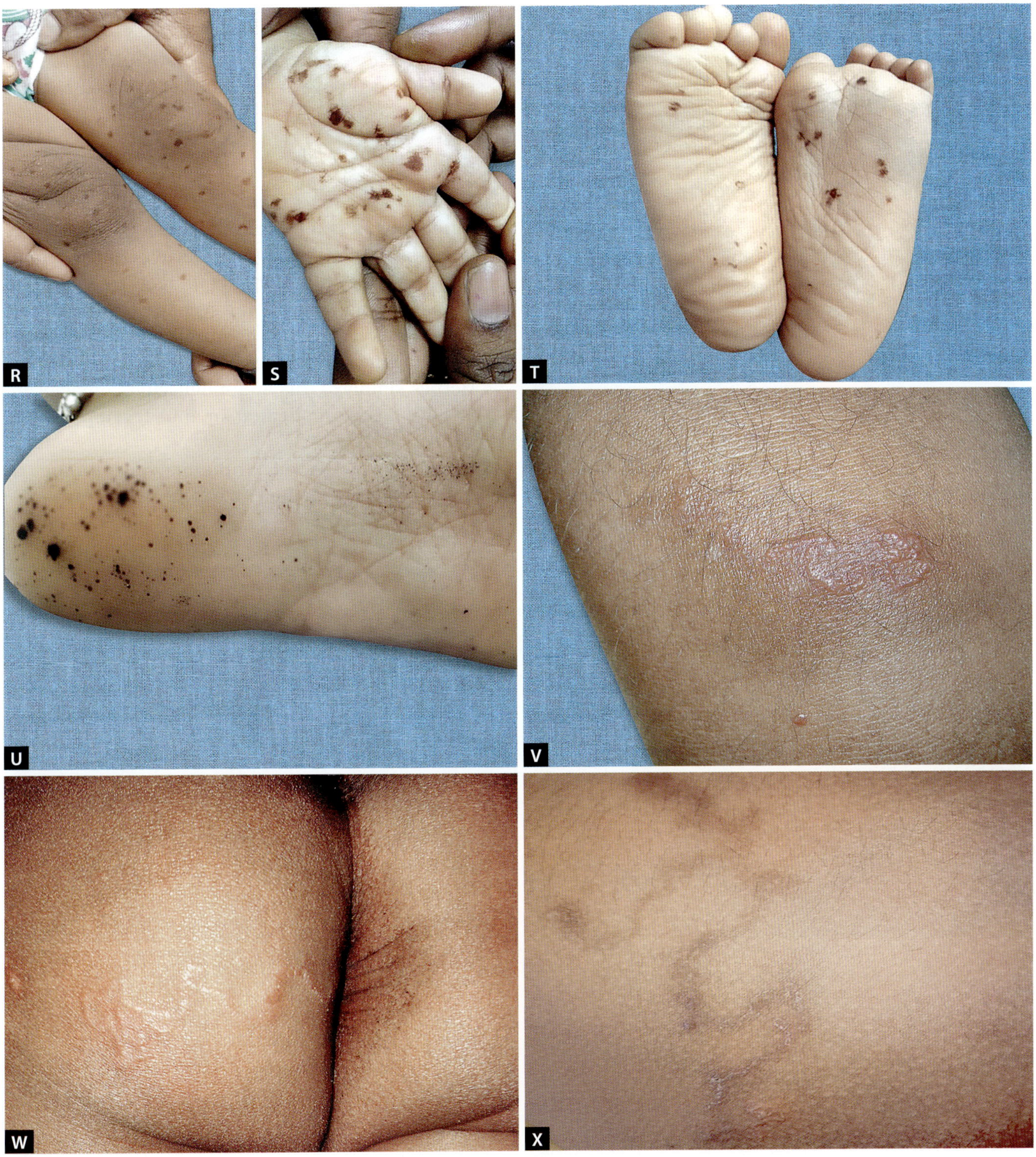

Figs. 3R to X: (R) Burrowing bug pigmentation, multiple discrete hyperpigmented macules on knee joint; (S) Burrowing bug pigmentation lesions over palms; (T) Same child, lesions over soles; (U) Blackish macules of burrowing bug pigmentation over sole; (V) Larva migrans; (W) Creeping eruption over buttocks; (X) Creeping eruption over trunk.

methicillin-resistant *S. aureus* (MRSA) infection, poor personal hygiene, and underlying systemic disorders.

The mainstay of therapy is topical and systemic antibiotics along with incision and drainage. For recurrent

"Why should I be unhappy? Every parcel of my being is in full bloom." —**Rumi**

furunculosis, decolonization with topical mupirocin ointment to anterior nares, behind the ears and groin are important.

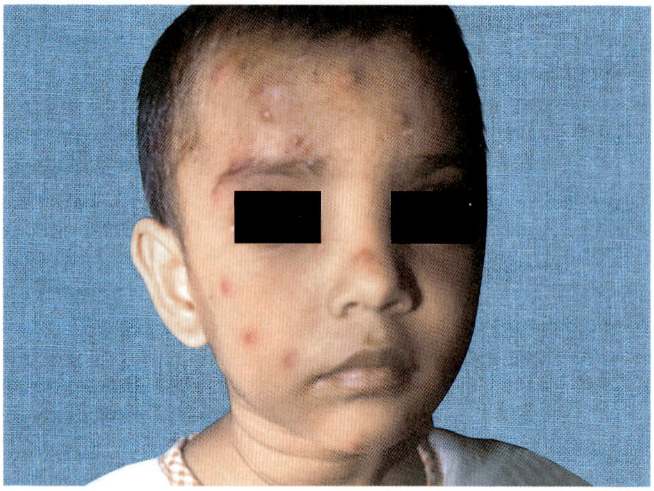

Fig. 4: Inflammatory papulopustules of furuncle over forehead.

FOLLICULITIS (FIGS. 5A TO E)

Folliculitis refers to pyoderma of the hair follicles and is classified according to the depth of involvement and microbial etiology.

Etiology

Staphylococcus aureus is the most common cause of bacterial folliculitis; however, the other causes include *Pseudomonas aeruginosa* (hot tub folliculitis), gram-negative folliculitis (in patients of acne on long-term topical and oral antibiotics), and syphilitic folliculitis.

Fungi implicated include dermatophytes, *Pityrosporum ovale*, and candidal species.

Herpes simplex virus and molluscum contagiosum virus have been implicated in the development of folliculitis.

Infestation by demodex mite may also present as folliculitis lesions predominantly on the perioral area.

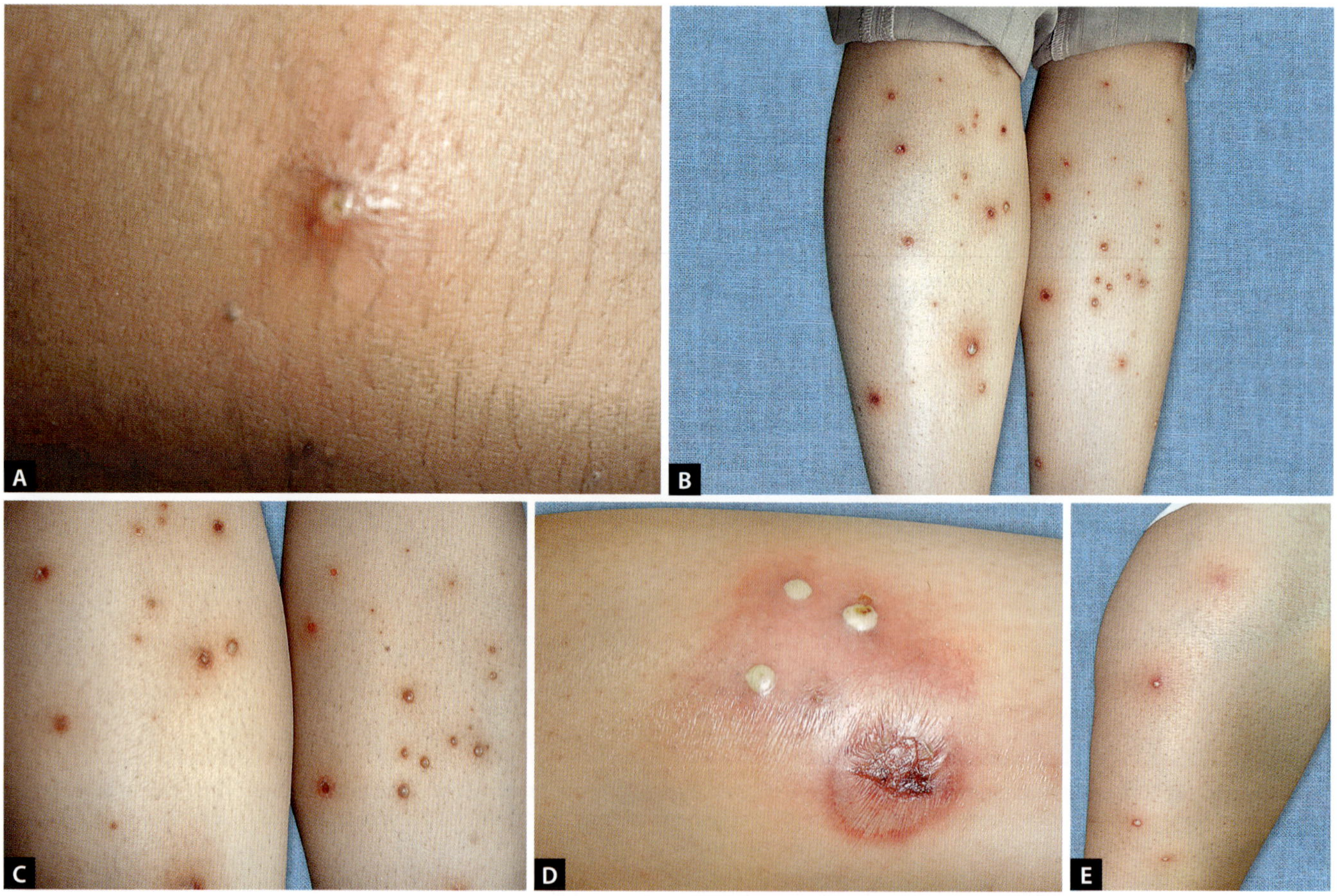

Figs. 5A to E: (A) Close-up view of furuncle; (B) Folliculitis over leg; (C) Folliculitis, note erythematous papulopustular lesions; (D) Folliculitis lesions, close-up view; (E) Folliculitis over leg, very common after hair removal in young adolescent girls.

"Hard work beats talent when talent doesn't work hard." **—Tim Notke**

Clinical Features

Superficial Folliculitis

It is also known as Bockhart's impetigo and presents with a fragile pustule at the infundibulum of a hair follicle often on the scalp of children, beard area, buttocks and axillae of adults.

Sycosis barbae is a deep folliculitis of the beard region which if untreated can become more deep seated and chronic.

In fungal infections, there are more often suppurative or granulomatous nodules rather than frank pustules and it may be commonly noted on the shins of women using razor for shaving also known as Majocchi's granuloma. Tinea capitis of the inflammatory type may also present with follicular pustular lesions of the scalp in children which heals with scarring alopecia.

Differential Diagnosis

Most common differential diagnosis to be considered in neonatal age group include candidiasis, erythema toxicum neonatorum, occlusional folliculitis, allergic contact dermatitis, and impetigo.

The differentials considered would also include acne, miliaria pustulosa, and papular urticaria with secondary infection.

Laboratory Diagnosis

Gram stain from the lesion to determine the etiology should be done followed by pus culture and sensitivity to isolate the organism.

Treatment

Folliculitis responds to topical antibiotics and for severe cases systemic antibiotics should be given depending on the culture sensitivity.

PERIPORITIS (FIGS. 5F TO J)

Periporitis is a complication of sweat gland obstruction when it gets secondarily infected by *S. aureus*. Usually, it presents as complication of miliaria rubra or profunda. It is seen in newborns, infants, and young children. It is seen more in summer seasons. Clinically, it presents with multiple erythematous papules surmounted by pus in the middle, resembling folliculitis. It is easily misdiagnosed as furuncle or impetigo. Treatment is mainly systemic antibiotics.

IMPETIGO (FIGS. 6 TO 8)

Impetigo is a contagious superficial pyogenic infection of the skin. Two main clinical forms are recognized: (1) nonbullous and (2) bullous impetigo. Bullous impetigo is caused by staphylococci, the nonbullous form may be caused by staphylococci or streptococci or both organisms together. The nonbullous form presents initially as an erythematous papule or pustule or as a thin-walled vesicle on an erythematous base. However, the vesicle ruptures rapidly and so may be missed. The exuding serum dries to form yellowish-brown, honey-colored crusts. The lesions extend peripherally and multiple satellite lesions may appear. The crusts eventually dry and separate to leave erythema which heals without scarring. The face and the limbs are commonly involved. Spontaneous recovery may occur in 2–3 weeks. In bullous impetigo, the bullae are less rapidly ruptured and become much large; a diameter of 1–2 cm is common but they may be of very considerable size and persist for 2 or 3 days. After rupture, thin, flat and brownish crusts are formed. The face is most commonly involved; however, the lesions may occur anywhere and may be widely and irregularly distributed. Topical antibiotics (mupirocin) are useful for mild, localized lesions and systemic antibiotics are warranted for widespread lesions.

ECTHYMA (FIGS. 9 AND 10)

Ecthyma is a pyogenic infection of the skin caused by group A beta-hemolytic streptococci, characterized by the formation of adherent crusts beneath which ulceration occurs. It begins as small bullae or pustules on an erythematous base which is soon surrounded by a hard crust of dried exudate. The base may become indurated and a red edematous areola is often present. The crust is removed with difficulty, to reveal a purulent irregular ulcer. Healing occurs after a few weeks, with scarring. The buttocks, thighs, and legs are most commonly affected. The lesions are usually few but new lesions may develop by autoinoculation over a long period. Appropriate systemic antibiotics are necessary. Ecthyma gangrenosum is a gangrenous or necrotizing ecthyma usually caused by *Pseudomonas aeruginosa*.

CELLULITIS AND ERYSIPELAS (FIGS. 11A TO E)

The term cellulitis is applied to inflammation of subcutaneous tissue. Erysipelas is a bacterial infection

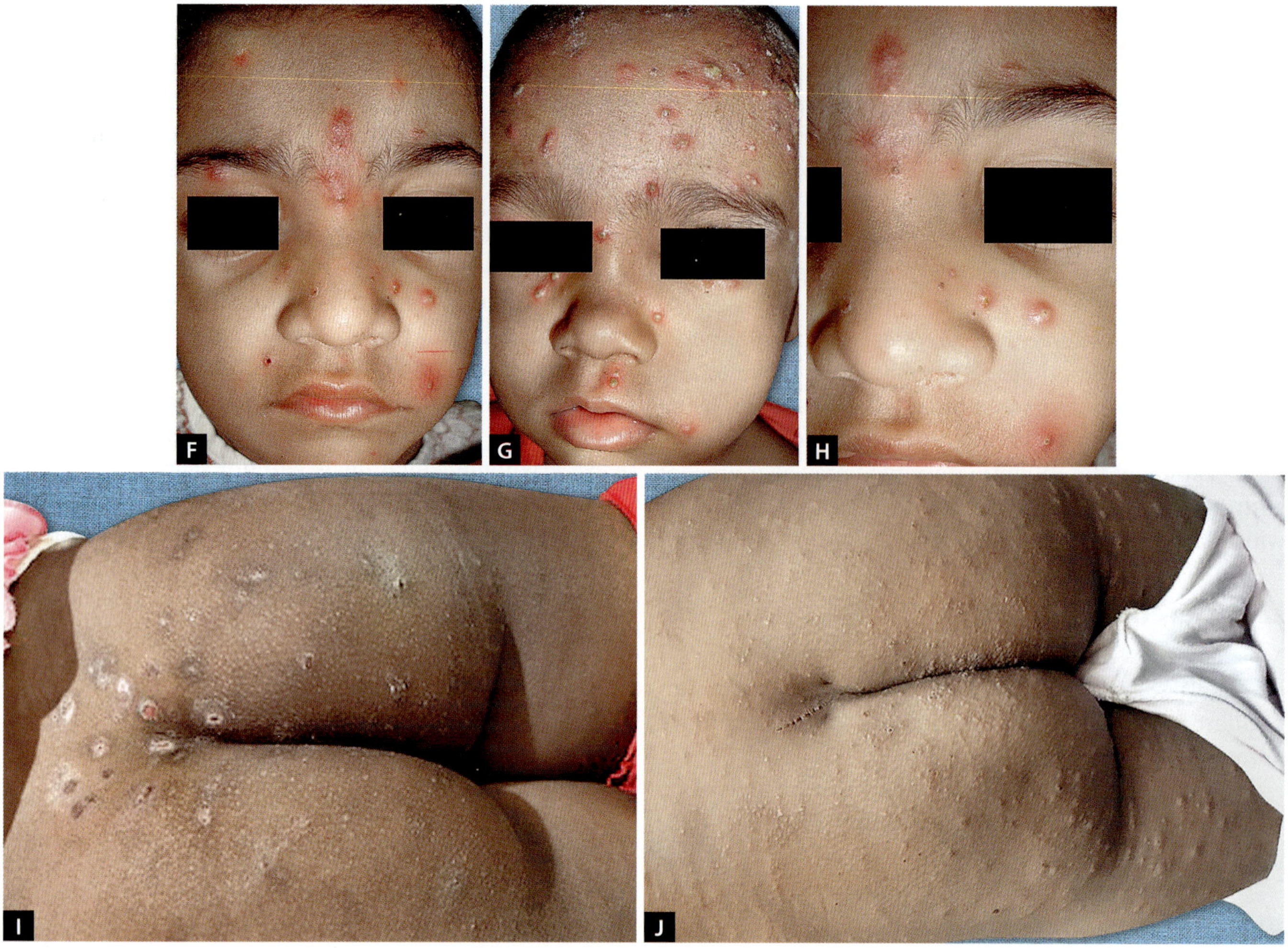

Figs. 5F to J: (F) Periporitis over face; (G) Note small red papules topped by pustules; (H) Close-up view of lesions; (I) Periporitis over buttock; (J) Buttock, a very common site of periporitis.

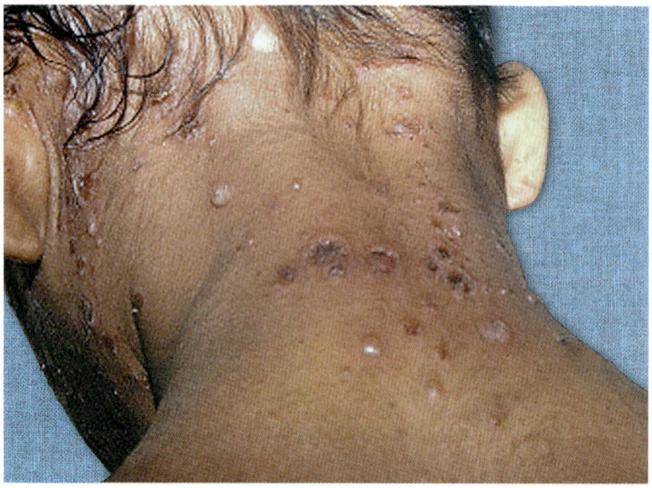

Fig. 6: Bullous impetigo over nape of the neck.

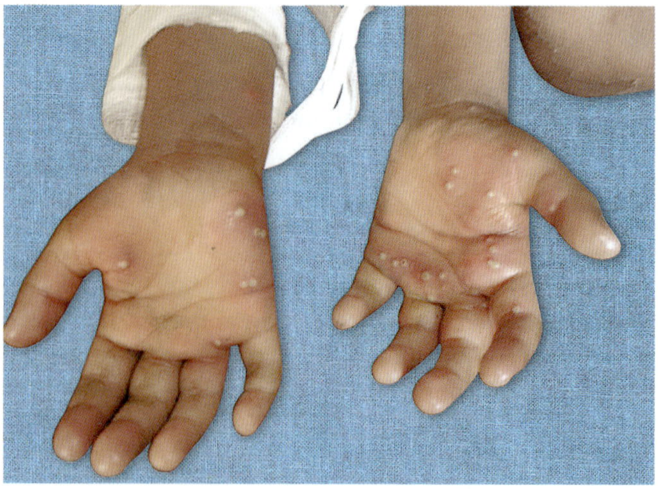

Fig. 7: Bullous impetigo over palms.

"The power of intention is the power to manifest, to create, to live a life of unlimited abundance, and to attract into your life the right people at the right moments." —**Wayne Dyer**

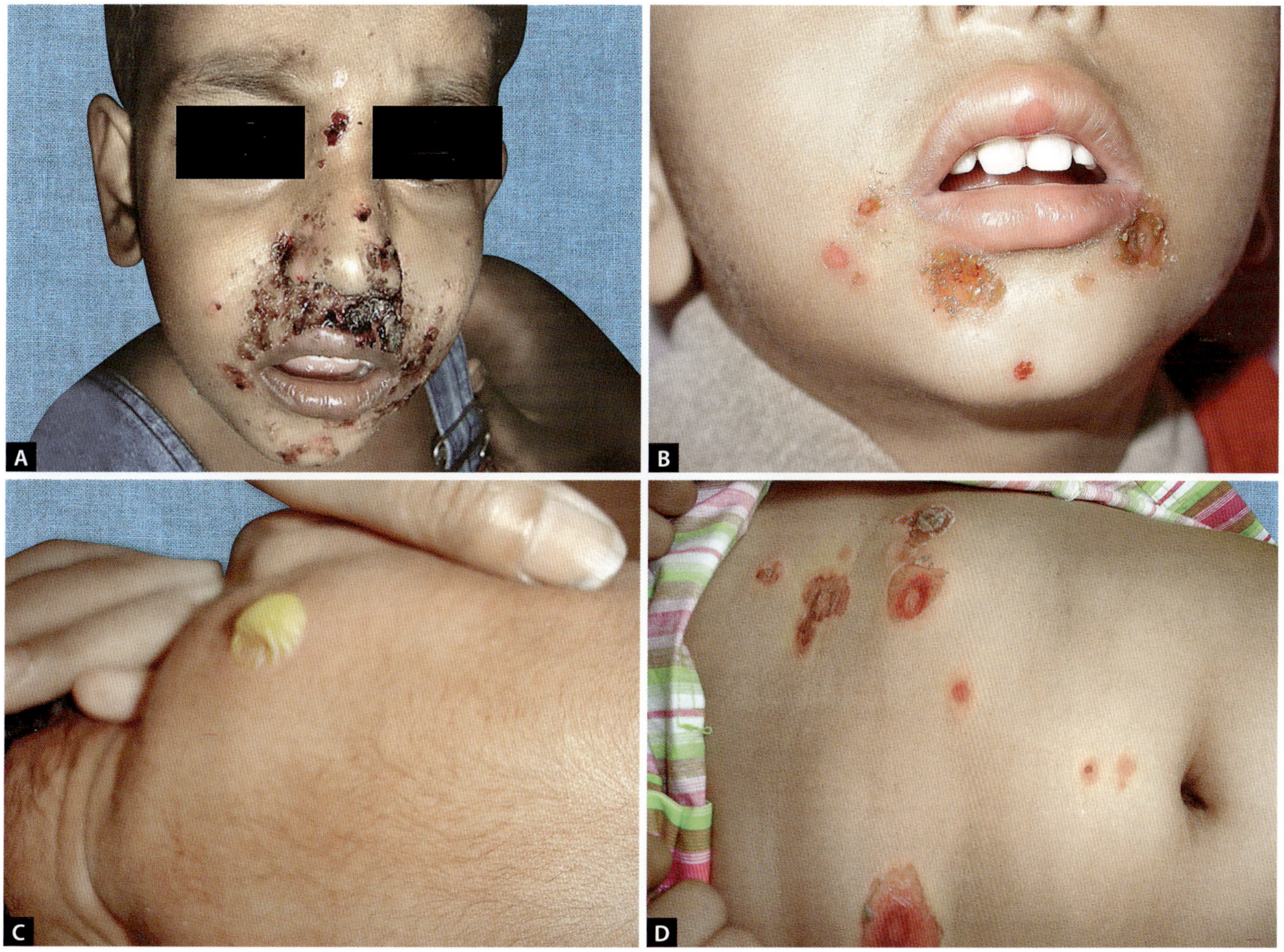

Figs. 8A to D: (A) Adherent scab and crust of impetigo contagiosa; (B) Impetigo contagiosa, note honey-colored crust; (C) Bullous impetigo in a newborn; (D) Impetigo bullosa, ruptured bullae with erythematous raw areas.

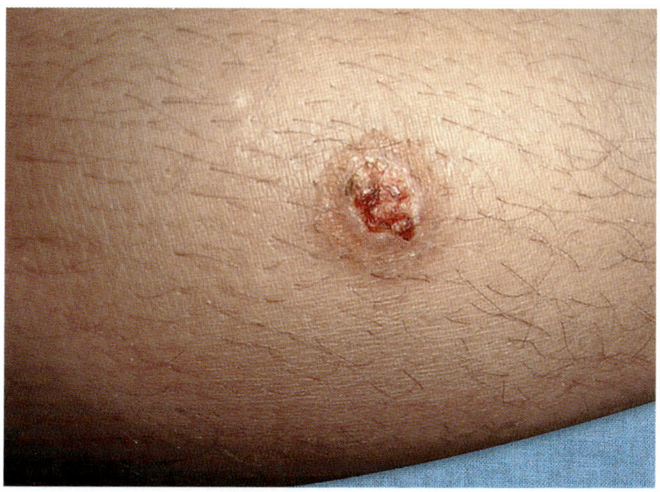

Fig. 9: Ecthyma over leg.

of the dermis and upper subcutaneous tissue. The two have similar bacteriology with streptococcal antigens being demonstrated in both lesions. Erythema, warm swelling, and pain or tenderness are constant features. In erysipelas, the edge of the lesion is well-demarcated and raised, but in cellulitis it is diffuse with blister formation or with hemorrhagic blister at the periphery is seen. Erysipelas and severe cellulitis can give rise to bullae formation with progression to dermal necrosis. Fasciitis and myositis are uncommon; however, lymphangitis and lymphadenopathy are frequent. The leg is most commonly involved followed by the face.

Complications

Complications are common with formation of subcutaneous abscesses, septicemia and in some streptococcal induced nephritis.

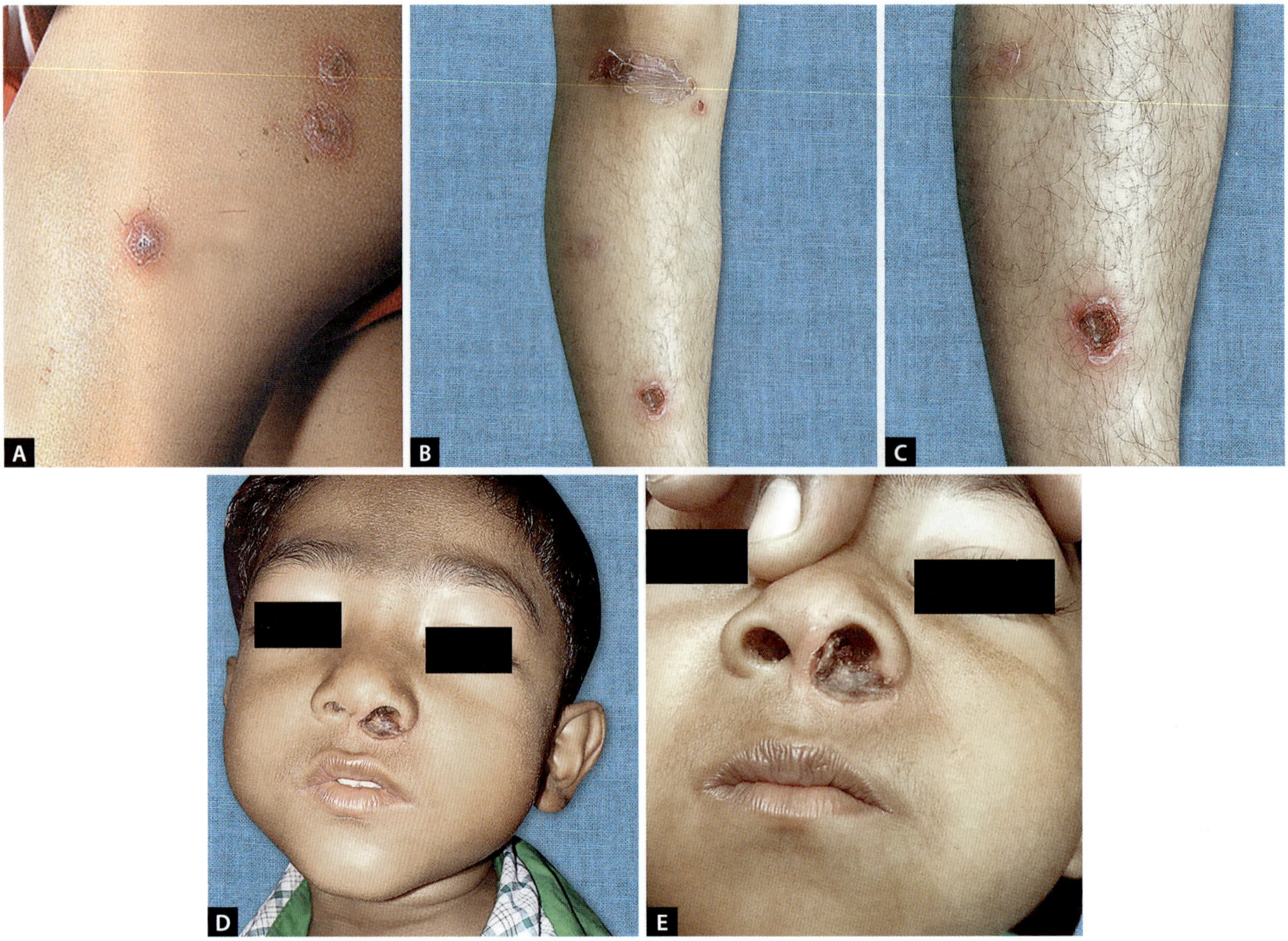

Figs. 10A to E: (A) Hard crust on an erythematous base in case of ecthyma over buttock and upper thigh; (B) Ecthyma over leg; (C) Same patient, close-up view; (D) Ecthyma gangrenosum at anterior nares; (E) Same child with ecthyma gangrenosum, close-up view.

Treatment

For furunculosis, impetigo, ecthyma either oral cloxacillin, amoxicillin and clavulanic acid combination or erythromycin is to be given for 7–10 days. Topical mupirocin or fusidic acid cream can be applied over surrounding skin to prevent contamination.

For erysipelas and cellulitis either cefadroxil, cefixime, erythromycin may be chosen. In severe cases, intravenous (IV) benzylpenicillin at a dose of 600–1,200 mg 6 hourly is preferred and continued for 10 days to combat long-term carriage state of *S. aureus* (particularly in atopics). Twice daily application of mupirocin cream inside nostrils, external auditory meatus and perianal area for 1 week each month for at least 6 months has been found to be very effective for recurrent lesions.

ACUTE LYMPHANGITIS (FIGS. 12A TO C)

It is a streptococcal infection of lymphatic vessels of the subcutaneous tissue, seen as erythematous, linear streaks of varying width, extending from the local lesion toward the regional lymph nodes. The latter are tender and enlarged.

Differential Diagnosis

Lymphangitis needs to be differentiated from thrombophlebitis. In cases of thrombophlebitis, the red streak of inflamed vein corresponds to the course of a superficial vein and often a part of vein is visible as bluish line as continuation of the red line.

"The simple things are also the most extraordinary things, and only the wise can see them." —**Paulo Coelho**

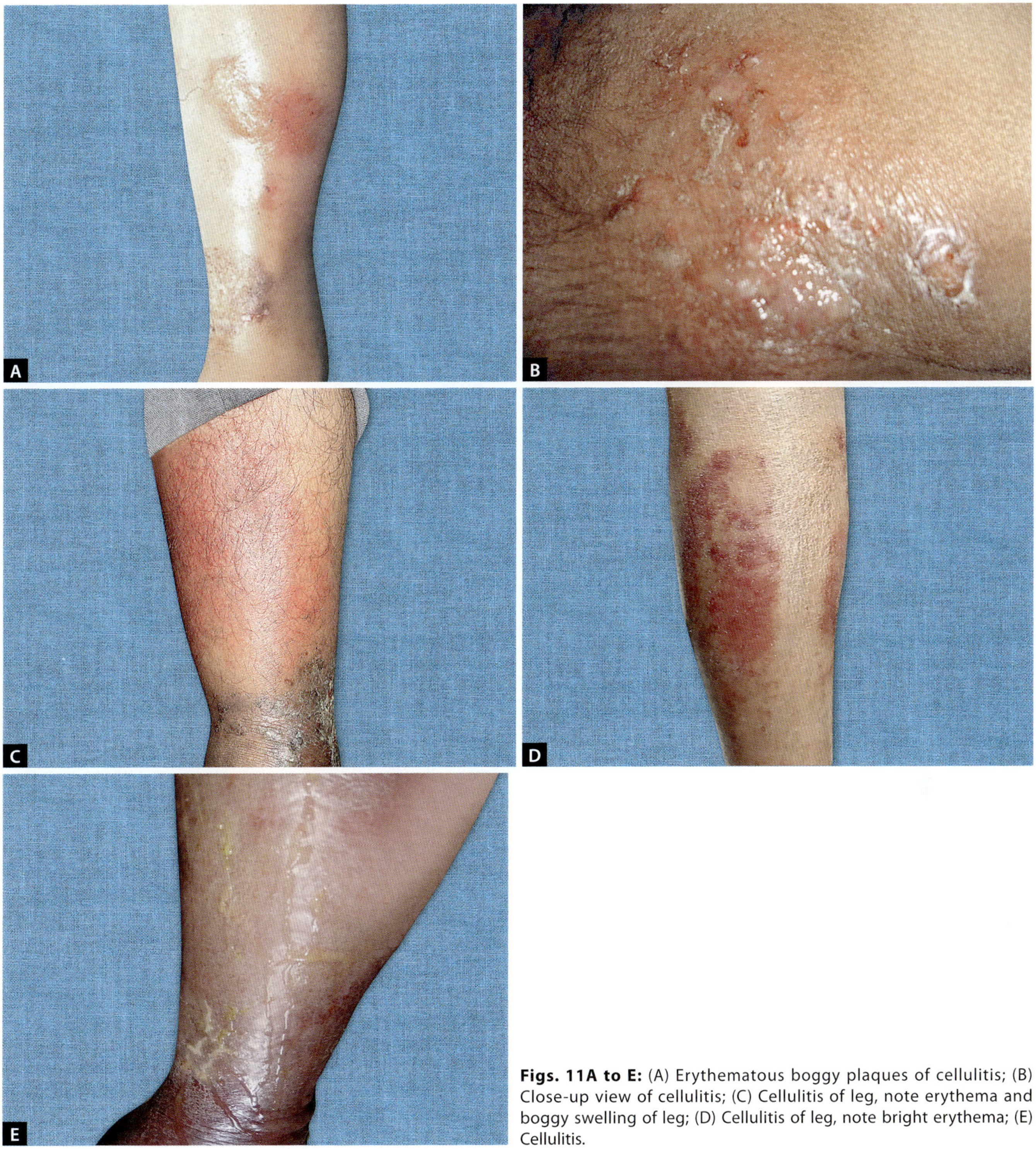

Figs. 11A to E: (A) Erythematous boggy plaques of cellulitis; (B) Close-up view of cellulitis; (C) Cellulitis of leg, note erythema and boggy swelling of leg; (D) Cellulitis of leg, note bright erythema; (E) Cellulitis.

SYCOSIS BARBAE (FIGS. 12D AND E)

Sycosis barbae is a subacute or chronic pyogenic infection involving the whole depth of hair follicle of the beard. It is most commonly seen in young adults and adolescent boys.

The essential lesion is an erythematous, edematous papule and pustule with a hair at the center. The individual papule/pustule usually remains discrete. However, there is a tendency to coalesce at times and boggy plaques or noduloplaque lesions studded with pustules may be seen.

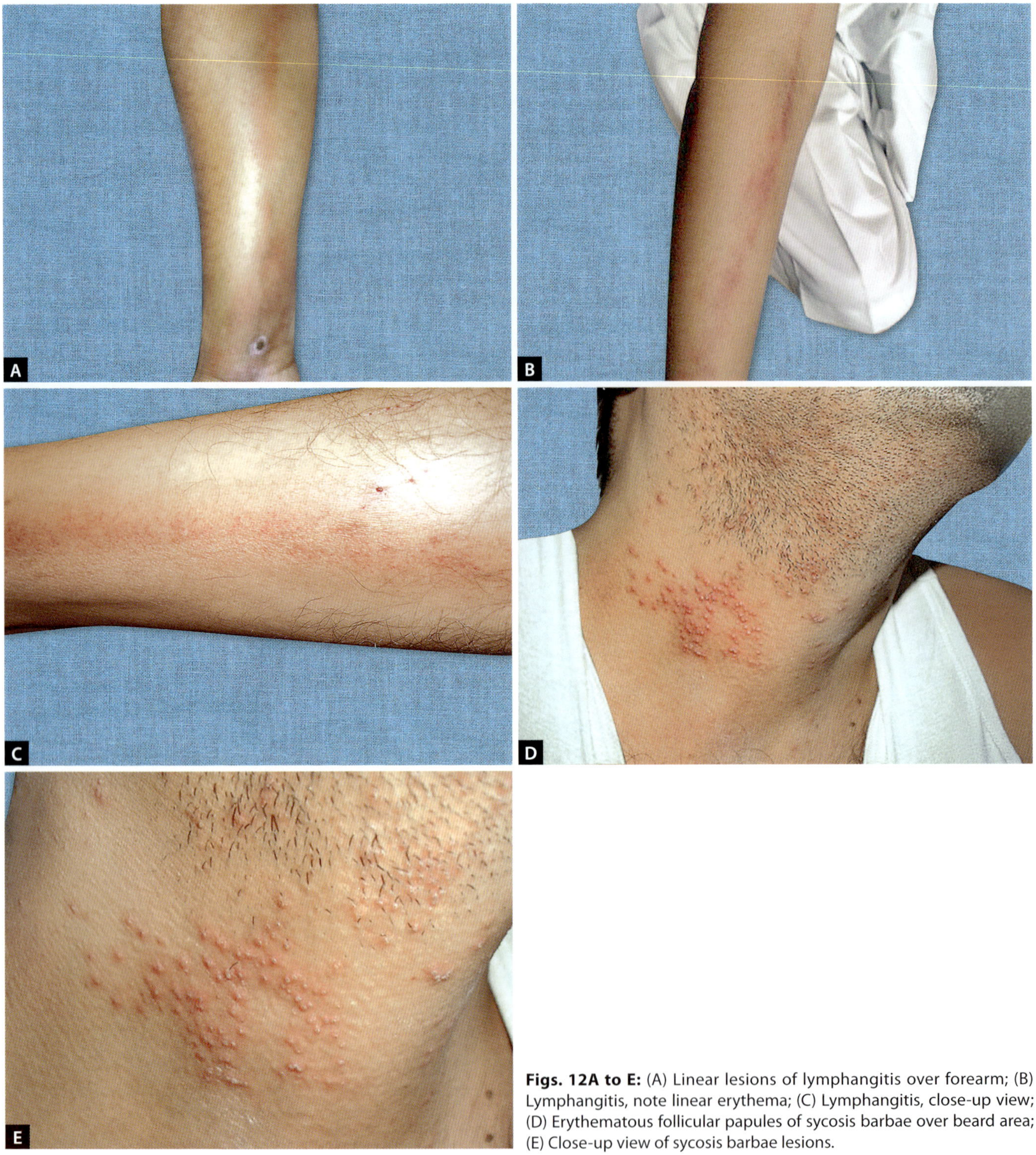

Figs. 12A to E: (A) Linear lesions of lymphangitis over forearm; (B) Lymphangitis, note linear erythema; (C) Lymphangitis, close-up view; (D) Erythematous follicular papules of sycosis barbae over beard area; (E) Close-up view of sycosis barbae lesions.

Etiology

The causative organism is *S. aureus*. The bacteria are thought to be either coming from its nasal carriage sites or inoculated from shaving, mostly from salon/parlour.

Management

The diagnosis is made in most of the cases going by its typical morphology. However, one may carry out culture of pus for documentation.

"The power of Intention is critical factor in all areas of life. Simply by intending to create synchronicity in your life, you can nurture that result."

—Deepak Chopra

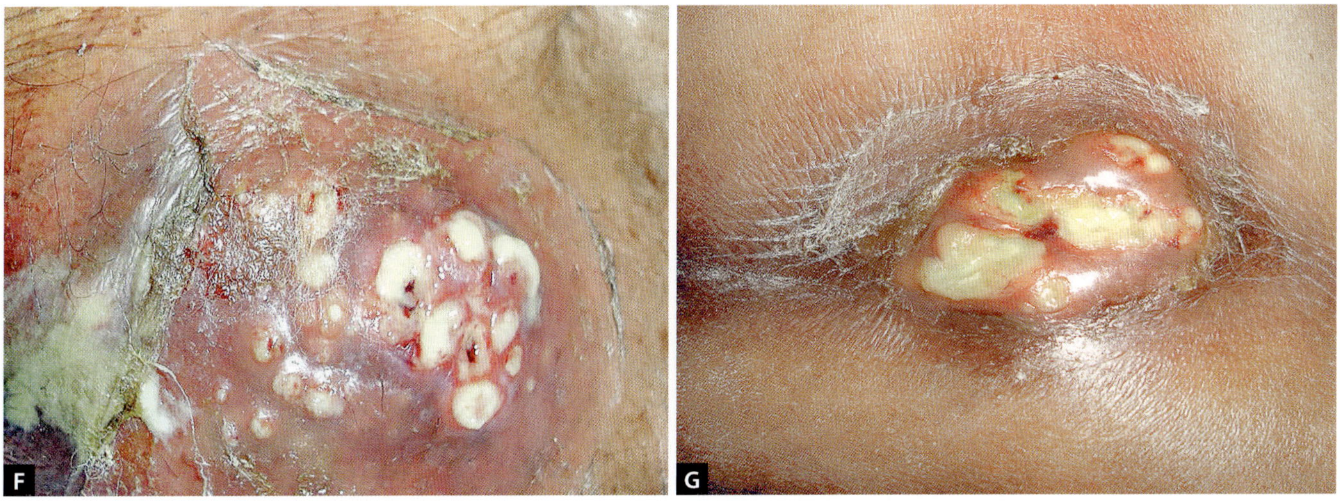

Figs. 12F and G: (F) Carbuncle, note multiple opening with pus discharge; (G) Carbuncle, close-up view.

The subacute forms can be controlled by topical antibiotics, e.g., mupirocin, fusidic acid, etc. However, in severe cases, several courses of antistaphylococcal antibiotics may be required. Regular cleaning of the beard with soap and water is a must. During acute/subacute stage, it is better to avoid shaving for 7–10 days. Nasal carriage of *S. aureus* can be controlled by application of mupirocin cream twice daily for 1 week each month for 6 months. Application of aftershave lotions is usually allowed.

CARBUNCLE (FIGS. 12F AND G)

Carbuncle is a collection of interconnected furuncles that extend deep into the subcutaneous tissue. Predisposing factors include diabetes, obesity, immunodeficiency, chemotherapy and malnutrition.

Clinical Features

The sites commonly affected include neck, back or thighs. The surface usually demonstrates multiple draining sinus tracts and sometimes ulceration. The affected area is red and indurated. The overlying area soon develops a yellow-gray irregular crater at the center which may heal slowly by granulating although the site may remain deeply violaceous for prolonged periods. Fever and malaise are often present and the patient may appear sick. Carbuncles result in dense and evident permanent scars on healing.

Differential Diagnosis

Various differential diagnoses are hidradenitis suppurativa, kerion, ruptured epidermal inclusion cyst, furuncular myiasis and osteomyelitis.

Laboratory Diagnosis

Gram stain and pus culture sensitivity of the purulent discharge helps in isolating the organism. There may be leukocytosis with elevation of blood levels of acute phase reactants.

Treatment

- General skin care to reduce the number of *Staphylococcus* on the skin includes regular usage of chlorhexidine baths and alcohol hand sanitizers.
- Use of loose nonocclusive clothings.
- Regular change of dressings.
- Cleansing using dilute chlorhexidine compresses or dilute potassium permanganate soaks.
- Topical application of fusidic acid or mupirocin ointment.
- Oral antibiotics such as penicillin in case of methicillin-sensitive *S. aureus* (MSSA) infections and linezolid in case of MRSA infections. IV antibiotics may be instituted in case the patient is sick with systemic symptoms.

NECROTIZING FASCIITIS (FIGS. 12H TO K)

It is a rapidly progressing necrotizing infection of the skin and subcutaneous tissue. This is usually associated with systemic toxicities and can be fatal if not diagnosed and treated at the earliest. Various other names for the condition are staphylococcal gangrene, gangrenous erysipelas and flesh-eating bacterial disease, etc. In neonates, it is associated with balanitis, omphalitis, and septicemia. The condition is caused by group A

"Good intentions are useless, until they are expressed in appropriate action!" —**Napoleon Hill**

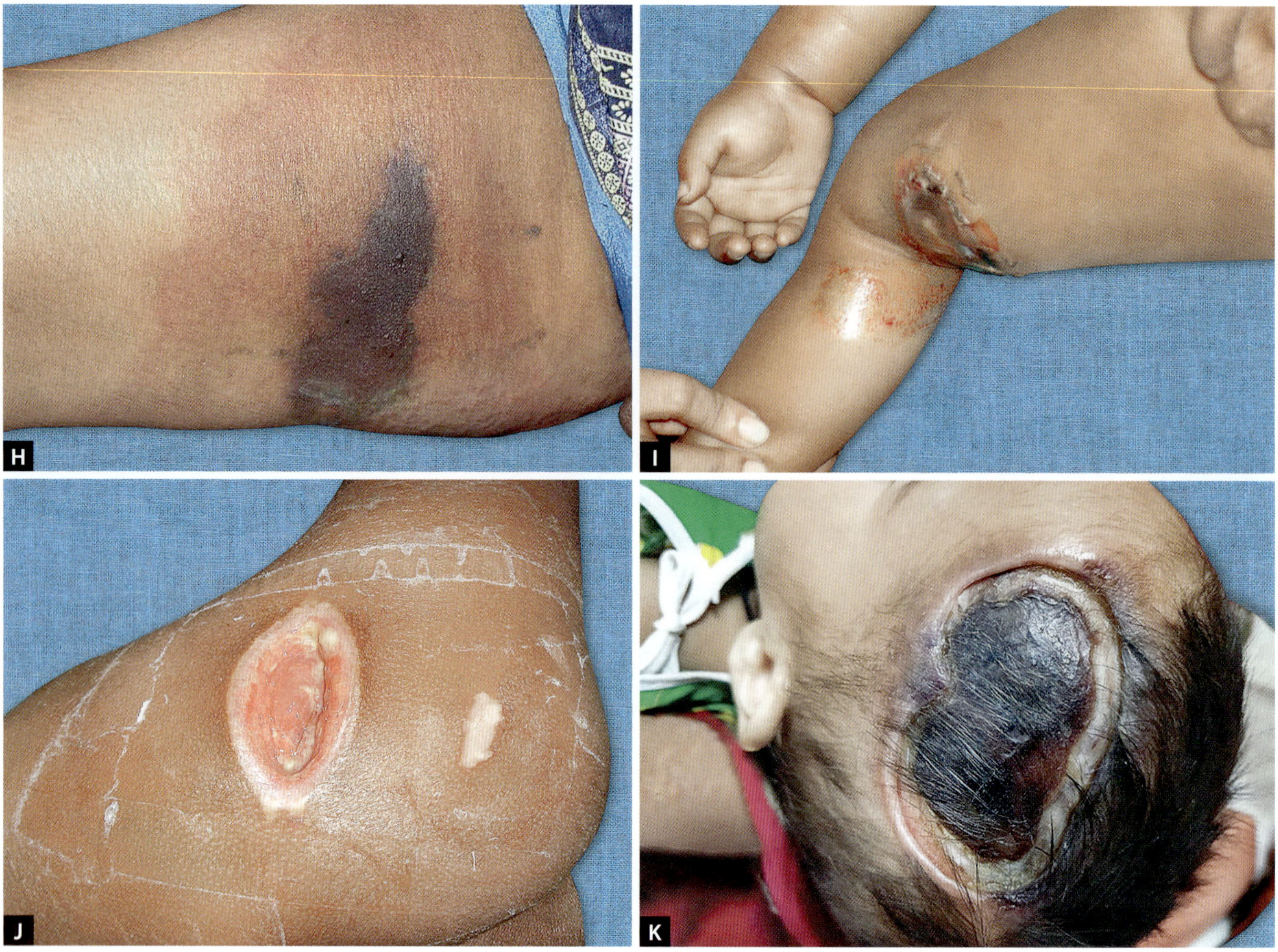

Figs. 12H to K: (H) Early lesions of necrotizing fasciitis; (I) Necrotizing fasciitis in 4-year-old girl; (J) Necrotizing fasciitis, close-up view; (K) Necrotizing fasciitis over scalp of an infant.

beta-hemolytic *Streptococcus* and polymicrobial in nature. Most of the times they have associated comorbid conditions like diabetes, HIV, renal failure, and autoimmune disorders.

Diagnosis

It usually affects extremities with erythema, edema, and excruciating pain over localized areas. Subsequently, bulla formation and necrosis develop and extend to fascial planes and hence the condition is known as necrotizing fasciitis. There may be associated streptococcal toxic shock syndrome. Routine examination of blood reveals a very high erythrocyte sedimentation rate (ESR) and leukocytosis. The serum creatine phosphokinase (CPK) is highly raised and blood culture grows either only group A beta-hemolytic streptococci or polymicrobes. Smear from necrotic area should be sent for Gram-stain and culture sensitivity tests.

Treatment

Early diagnosis of the condition and surgical debridement of necrotic tissue are of paramount importance. On admission, IV antibiotics should be started promptly. Subsequently, the antibiotic may be changed according to culture sensitivity report. Other essential measures are resuscitation of the newborn and maintenance of fluid and electrolyte balance.

NOMA (FIGS. 12L TO N)

Noma, also known as necrotizing ulcerative stomatitis or cancrum oris, is a gangrenous condition affecting mainly

"The only limits you have are limits you believe." —**Wayne Dyer**

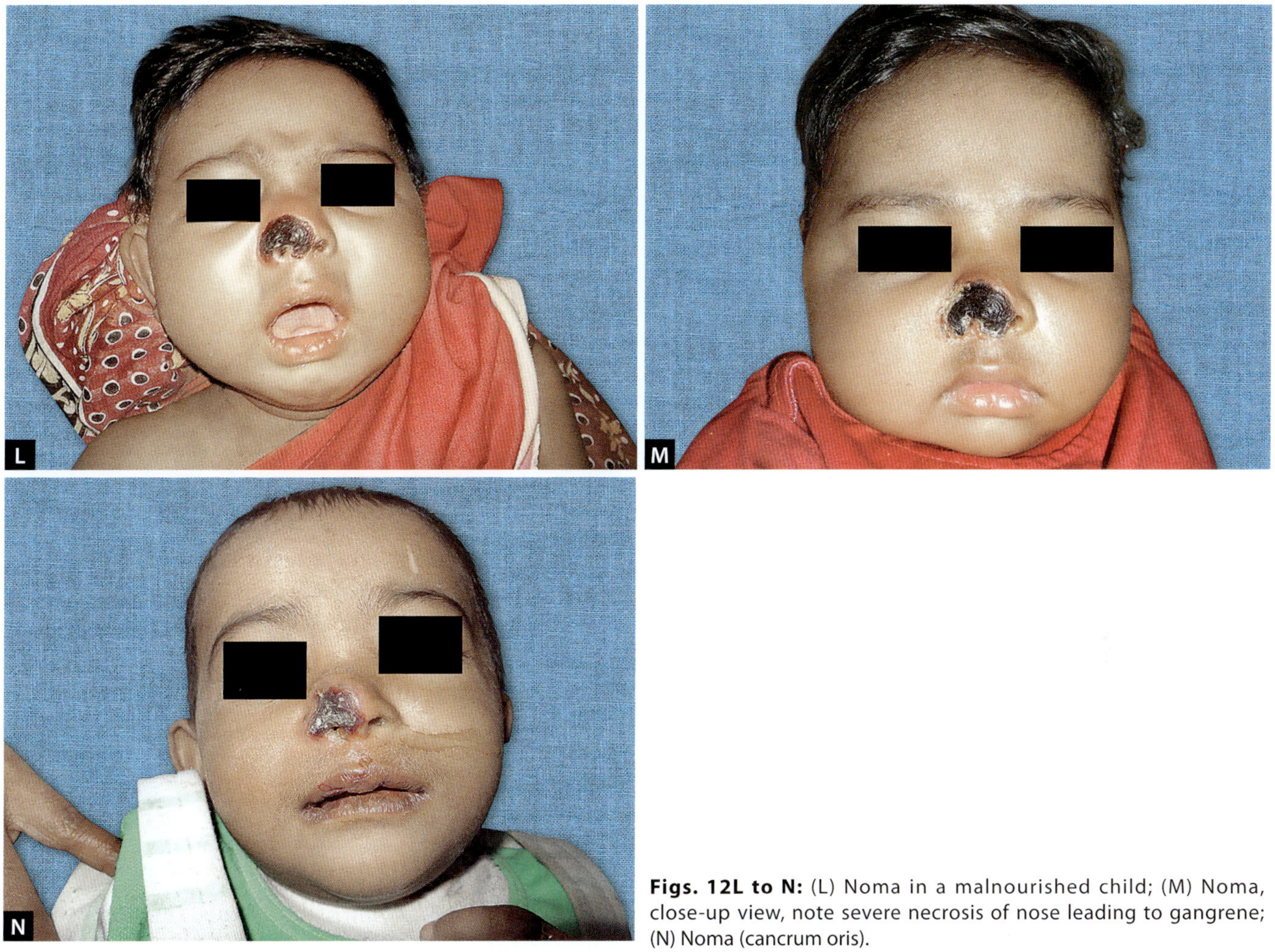

Figs. 12L to N: (L) Noma in a malnourished child; (M) Noma, close-up view, note severe necrosis of nose leading to gangrene; (N) Noma (cancrum oris).

children between the ages of 1 and 4 years that destroys the soft and hard tissue of the face.

Etiopathogenesis

It has been postulated that there is an immune dysfunction that occurs due to the following:

- Malnutrition and deficiencies of vitamin A, B6, C, and E; trace elements such as iron and zinc and certain amino acids
- Adrenal hyperfunction in protein energy malnutrition
- Early weaning leading to malnutrition and chronic infections

It is a polymicrobial infection with *Prevotella intermedia* and *Fusobacterium necrophorum*. Other frequently found organisms include *Tannerella, Peptostreptococcus, Campylobacter,* streptococci, and enteric gram-negative rods.

Clinical Features

It starts with initial fever and apathy. Acute noma presents with soreness of mouth, halitosis, tenderness of the orofacial area, cervical lymphadenopathy, and purulent oral discharge.

The intraoral lesion starts as necrotizing stomatitis starting on the alveolar margin and extending to mucosal surface of the cheeks in 24–48 hours. The overlying area develops a blackish blue discoloration. As the lesions expand, it forms a classic cone shape, cone gangreneux, with internal destruction greater than external involvement.

Acute necrotizing gingivitis occurs in patients with poor oral hygiene and dental caries is a precursor to noma.

Noma neonatorum is thought to be related but a separate entity from noma. It is caused by *P. aeruginosa* and gangrenous lesions appear on the nose, eyelid oral

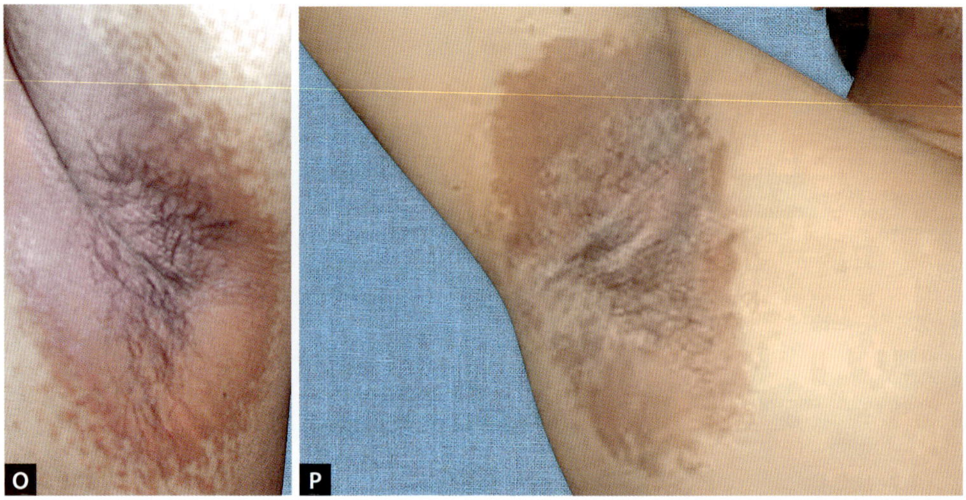

Figs. 12O and P: (O) Erythrasma over axilla in an adolescent obese boy; (P) Erythrasma of axilla.

cavity, and anogenital area. The course is almost always fatal.

The lesions heal with extensive scarring, fibrosis, strictures, dental malpositioning and sometimes complete closure of mouth.

Treatment

- Correction of dehydration and electrolyte imbalance
- Treatment of predisposing conditions
- *Antibiotics:* Broad-spectrum along with metronidazole
- Oral hygiene with regular chlorhexidine rinsing
- Local wound care
- Reconstructive surgeries with physiotherapy.

ERYTHRASMA (FIGS. 12O AND P)

It is a common superficial bacterial infection of the skin characterized by irregular red brown patches occurring predominantly in the intertriginous areas associated with maceration or fissuring.

Etiology

Corynebacterium minutissimum is a short gram-positive rod which is the etiologic agent of erythrasma.

Clinical Features

Symptoms vary from a completely asymptomatic form to an intensely pruritic genitocrural form and a generalized form with scaly plaques on trunk, inguinal area, and web spaces. The most common areas affected are the web spaces between the fourth and the fifth toe where it presents with a macerated hyperkeratotic white plaque. The other sites affected include genitocrural, axillary, and submammary areas where it presents with hyperpigmented velvety patches with finely wrinkled surface.

Differential Diagnosis

- Tinea versicolor
- Tinea cruris et corporis
- Inverse psoriasis

Laboratory Diagnosis

Wood's lamp examination of the affected site reveals coral-red fluorescence. Gram-stain shows rod-like gram-positive organisms in large numbers. Culture of the organism may also be done however in most cases it is not necessary.

Treatment

Systemic Therapy

For widespread involvement and recurrent lesions systemic therapy with oral erythromycin, roxithromycin or clarithromycin may be used.

Topical Therapy

Benzoyl peroxide washes and gels are found to be effective. Clindamycin 2% or miconazole 2% gels may also give similar results. Prophylactic use of benzoyl peroxide bar may be helpful.

PITTED KERATOLYSIS (FIGS. 12Q TO S)

Pitted keratolysis involves the stratum corneum of the palms and soles along with web space involvement.

"Don't you know yet? It is your light that lights the worlds." —**Rumi**

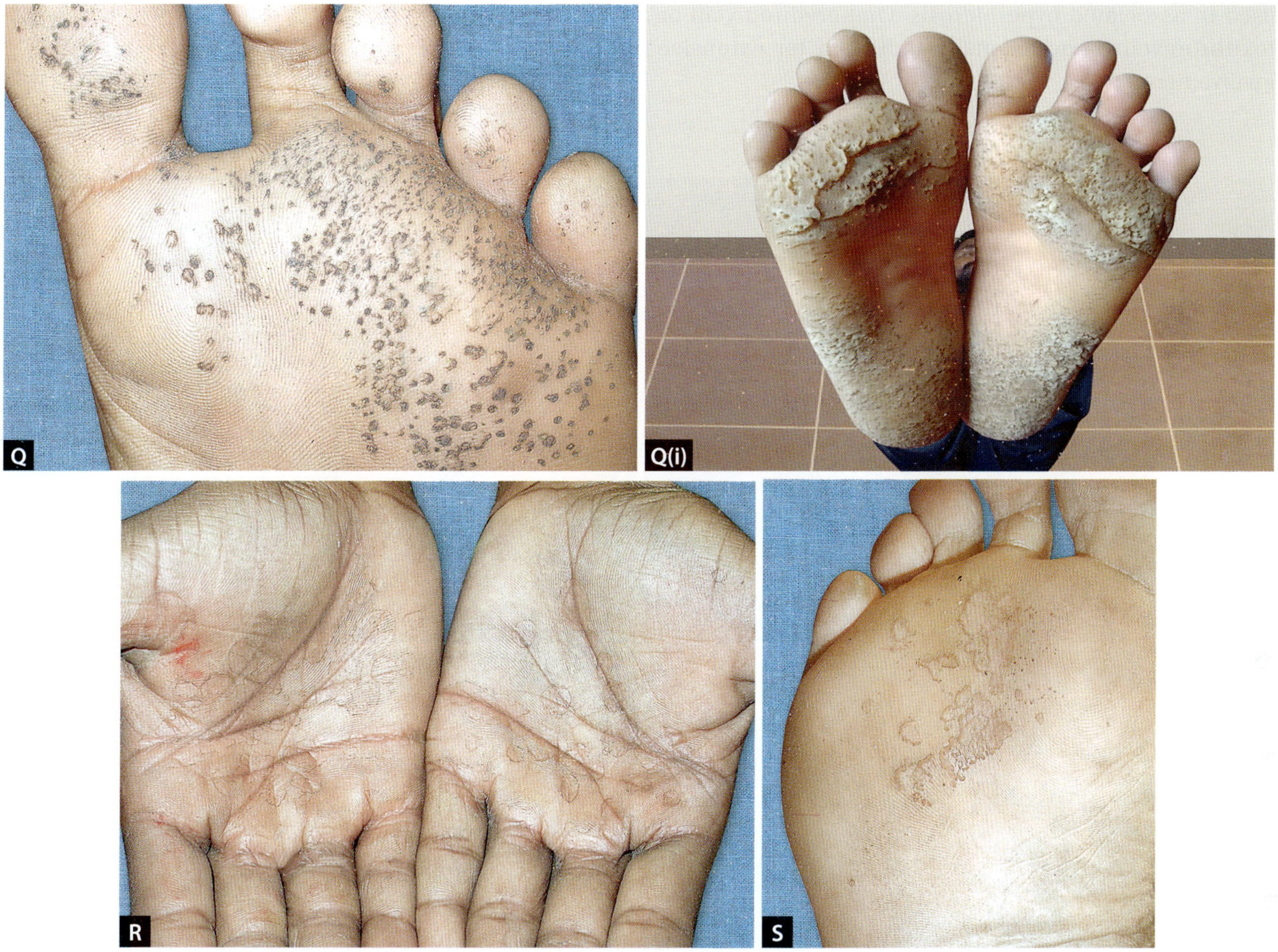

Figs. 12Q to S: (Q) Pitted keratolysis, crateriform pits on the plantar aspect of foot; Q(i) Pitted keratolysis, extensive involvement of feet; (R) Pitted keratolysis over palms; (S) Pitted keratolysis.

Etiology

It is caused by *Kytococcus sedentarius* (formerly *Micrococcus sedentarius*) which is a *Staphylococcus*-related gram-positive organism, that invades the stratum corneum softened by sweat production. The predisposing factors include sweating, prolonged occlusion and increased skin surface pH.

Clinical Features

It presents as small 1–7 mm crateriform pits coalescing to form a large discrete defect with serpiginous borders on the plantar aspect of the foot. It generally affects the pressure bearing areas; however, the instep of the sole may also be involved. The web space involvement may be the only manifestation in early stages.

Differential Diagnosis

- Palmoplantar punctate keratoderma
- Palmoplantar warts
- Pits of nevoid basal cell carcinoma syndrome
- Tinea pedis

Laboratory Diagnosis

The diagnosis is mainly clinical. Gram-stain from the lesions may detect the microorganism. There is no fluorescence on Wood's lamp examination.

Treatment

Topical mupirocin, clindamycin, erythromycin, tetracycline and azole antifungals have all been reported to be useful. Aluminum chloride 20% solution may be

"Education is the key to unlocking the world a passport to freedom." —**Oprah Winfrey**

used in associated hyperhidrosis. Oral erythromycin or roxithromycin is occasionally indicated for extensive involvement.

PERIANAL STREPTOCOCCAL DERMATITIS [FIGS. 12T(i) TO (iv)]

It is also known as perianal cellulitis.

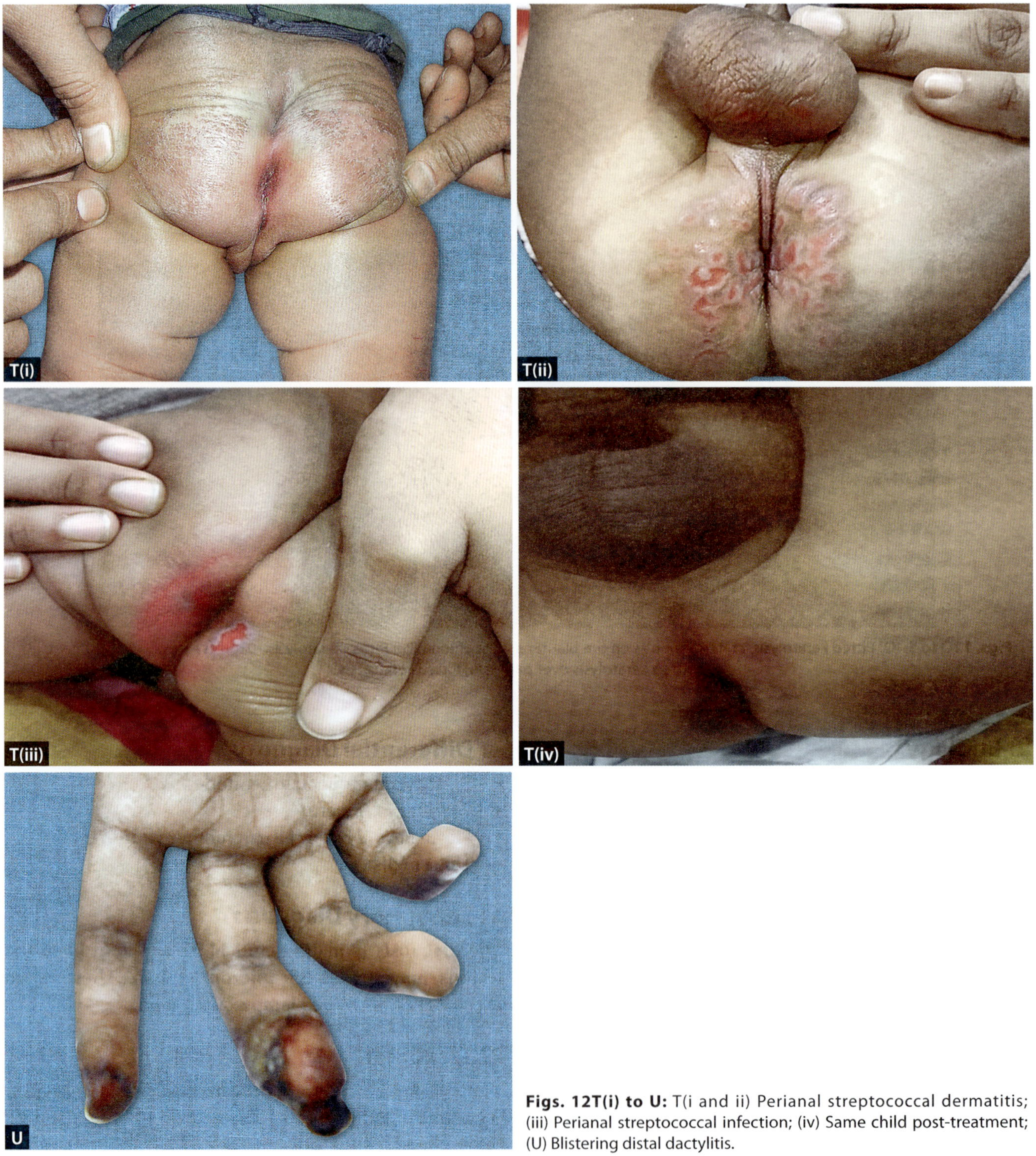

Figs. 12T(i) to U: T(i and ii) Perianal streptococcal dermatitis; (iii) Perianal streptococcal infection; (iv) Same child post-treatment; (U) Blistering distal dactylitis.

"The secret of life, though, is to fall seven times and to get up eight times." —**Paulo Coelho**

Etiology

It is caused by infection with group A *Streptococcus*.

Clinical Features

Children, most commonly boys under 4 years of age, are most commonly affected. It presents with sharply demarcated bright erythema extending 2–3 cm around the anal verge. Patients may complain of perianal pruritus, irritation, painful defecation, soiling of undergarments, and blood-streaked stools. Systemic symptoms are absent. It can be preceded by pharyngitis and should be considered in patients with an outbreak of guttate psoriasis.

Differential Diagnosis

Various mimickers are *S. aureus* infection, candidiasis, seborrheic dermatitis, pinworm infestation, inflammatory bowel disease, child abuse, early phase of Kawasaki disease.

Laboratory Diagnosis

It can be diagnosed by skin swab culture.

Treatment

A 7- to 10-day course of cefuroxime leads to resolution.

BLISTERING DISTAL DACTYLITIS (FIG. 12U)

It is also known as bulla repens and commonly affects children and adolescents.

Etiology

Majority of the cases is caused by group A *Streptococcus*; however, group B *Streptococcus* also can cause this infection.

Clinical Features

It presents with a large tense blister filled with seropurulent fluid over the volar skin pad of distal fingers or toes. The blisters are surrounded by an erythematous base. The lesion may be more proximally located on the finger or extend to the nailfold. It is seen more commonly between the age group of 2–16 years.

Differential Diagnosis

Various mimickers are staphylococcal blistering distal dactylitis and herpetic whitlow.

Laboratory Diagnosis

Gram-stain from the lesional fluid reveals organisms in chains. Confirmation of the diagnosis is done by culture of the seropurulent fluid.

Treatment

This condition may be treated using penicillins or erythromycin. Drainage of subungual pus may be required.

LUPUS VULGARIS (FIGS. 13A TO E)

Lupus vulgaris is a progressive form of cutaneous tuberculosis (TB) which occurs usually on the head or neck. The skin of and around the nose is frequently involved. In children, lupus vulgaris predominantly affects the lower half of the body like lower trunk, buttocks, thighs, lower legs, and feet. It presents as asymptomatic papules, nodules or plaque, progresses in one area and heals at another area with atrophy and scarring.

These multiple papules and nodules which on diascopy test stand out clearly as yellow-brown macules, referred to as apple jelly nodules, because of their color. The disease is very chronic, with slow peripheral extension of the lesions. In the course of time, the affected areas become atrophic, with contraction of the tissue. Characteristically, new lesions may appear in areas of atrophy. Superficial ulceration or verrucous thickening of the skin occurs occasionally. Rarely, mutilation of ears and nose may occur. Other morphological variants include keratotic, hyperkeratotic, ulcerative, sclerotic, and sporotrichoid form.

SCROFULODERMA [FIGS. 14A TO D(ii)]

Scrofuloderma is the most common form of childhood TB and represents a direct extension to the skin from an underlying tuberculous infection, present most commonly in a lymph node or a bone. The lesion first manifests itself as a blue-red, painless swelling that breaks open and then forms an ulcer with irregular, undermined blue borders. Numerous fistulae may intercommunicate beneath ridges of a bluish skin. Progression and scarring produce irregular adherent masses, densely fibrous plaques in some areas and fluctuant or discharging in others. After healing, characteristic puckered or cribriform scarring marks the site of the infection.

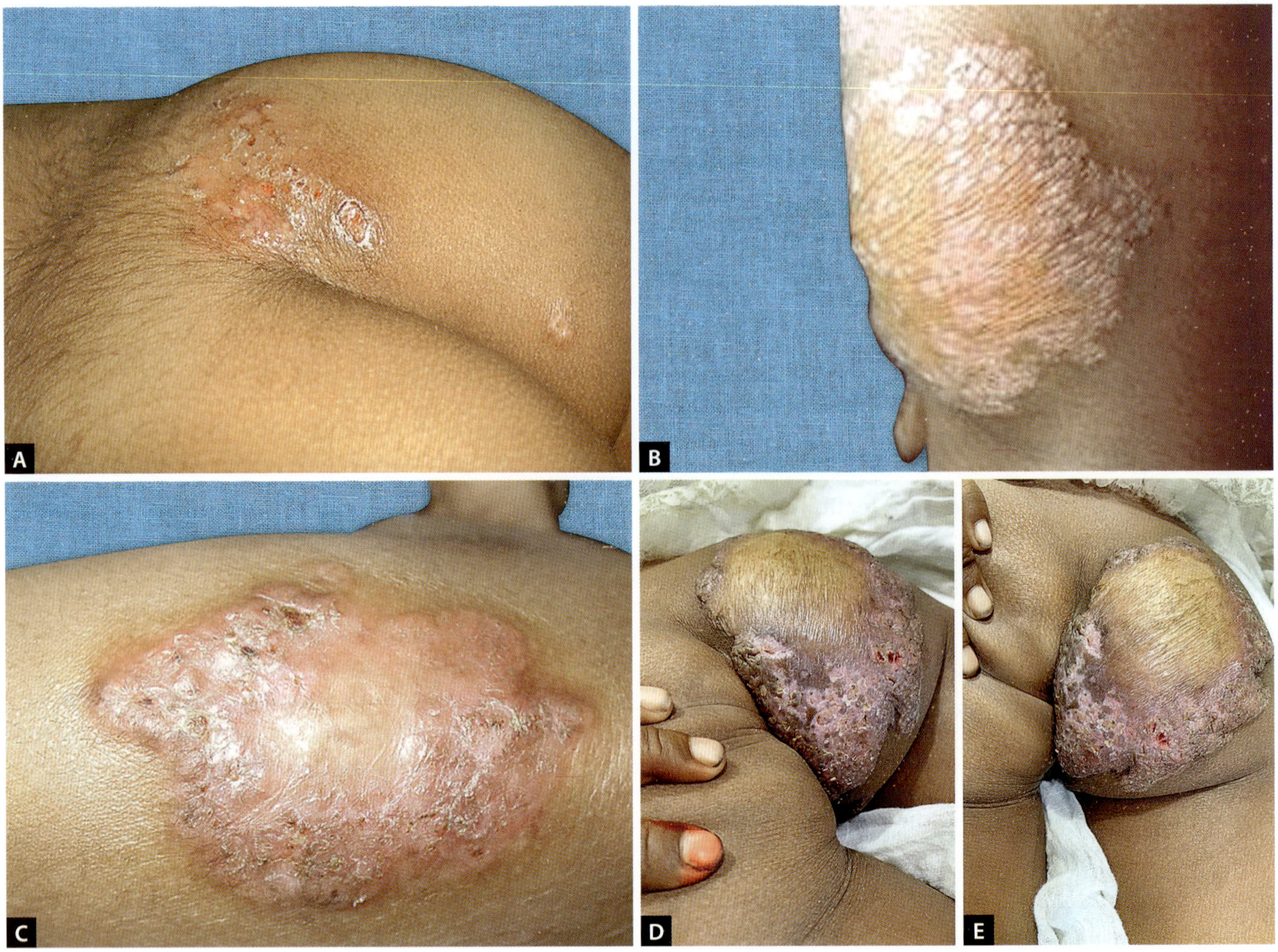

Figs. 13A to E: (A) Erythematous infiltrated mild scaly plaque with central clearing over buttock in 5-year-old boy with lupus vulgaris; (B) Lupus vulgaris lesion over knee in a 10-year-old boy; (C) Indurated scaly erythematous plaque of lupus vulgaris with central clearing; (D) Huge lupus vulgaris over buttock; (E) Same child, close-up view.

TUBERCULOSIS VERRUCOSA CUTIS (FIGS. 14E TO H)

This type of cutaneous TB results from inoculation in a person who has moderate or high degree of immunity. Laborers and manual workers are often the victims and is secondary to trauma and lower limbs are commonly affected. It is an occupational hazard in veterinarians, pathologists, anatomists and butchers who handle the diseased tissue and hands are often affected (prosector's wart, butcher's wart). The prevalence in children is <4.5% in India.

The clinical features are variable but large warty lesions of long duration affecting the hands or feet should arouse suspicion. Initially, the lesions are dull red, deep-seated papule or nodule which slowly enlarge and become warty over the period. These lesions sometimes become worse during summer season and may become crusted. On healing, there are atrophic scars left behind.

Treatment

Multidrug therapy (MDT) has eased the treatment of cutaneous TB and the outcome is very good. The total duration of treatment is essentially 6 months, which is divided into initial 2 months intensive phase and continuation phase for 4–7 months. During intensive phase, various drugs used are isoniazid (5 mg/kg/day), rifampicin (10 mg/kg/day), pyrazinamide (30 mg/kg/day), and ethambutol (15 mg/kg/day). For cutaneous TB without any systemic involvement, 4 months' continuation phase is adequate. However, if there is underlying systemic involvement, the duration may need to be prolonged.

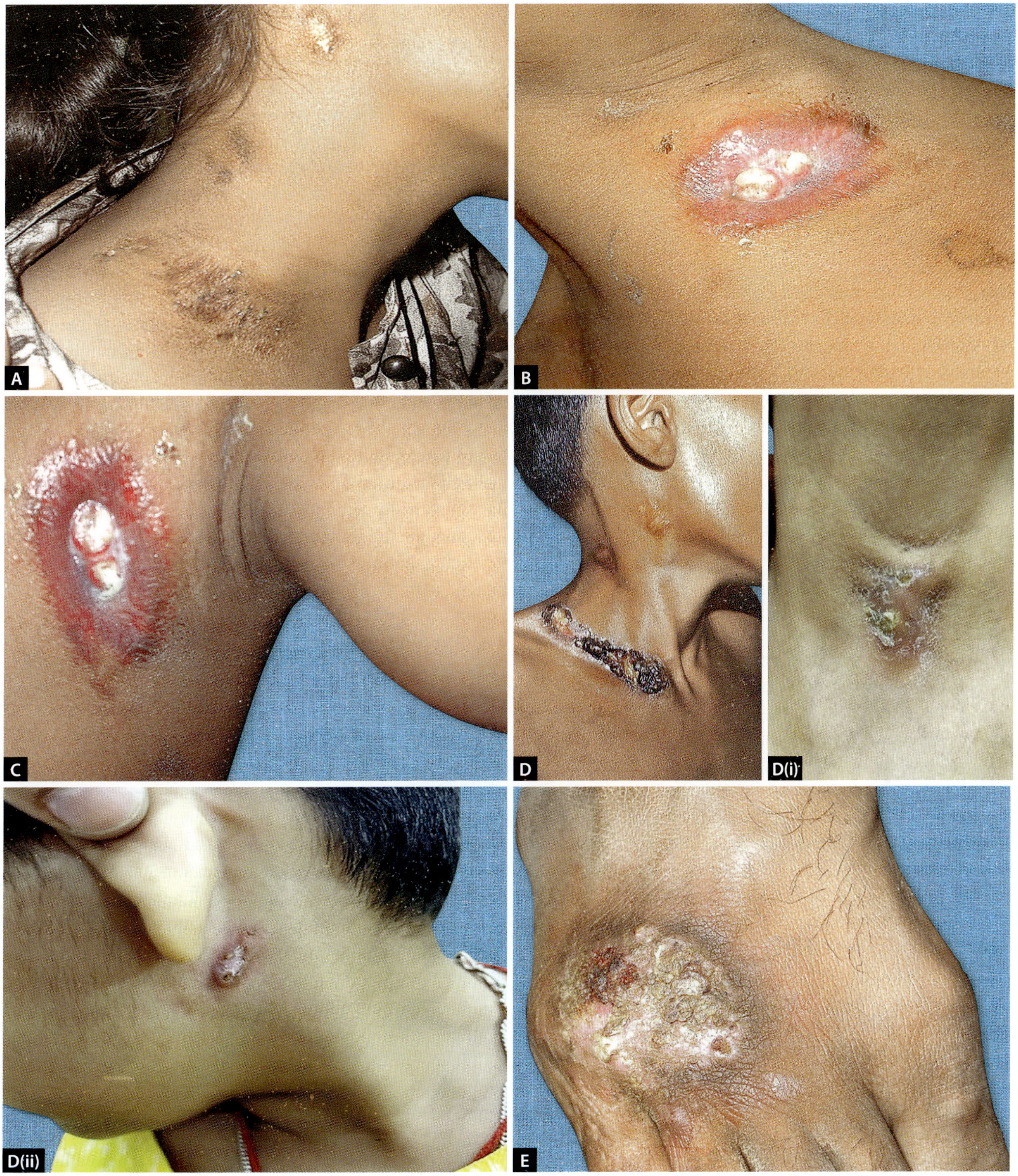

Figs. 14A to E: (A) Scrofuloderma over cervical region; (B) Close-up view, note cutaneous ulcer adherent to underlying lymph nodes; (C) Close-up view of ulcer; (D) Scrofuloderma over neck, a very common site; D(i) Scrofuloderma over neck; D(ii) Scrofuloderma over post auricular area; (E) Warty lesion of tuberculosis verrucosa cutis over dorsum of foot.

"The Struggle is not with others, but within us, to do what we are called to do." —**John Geddes**

During isoniazid therapy, pyridoxine supplementation is routinely given. Associated malnutrition, if any, needs to be treated simultaneously.

PAPULONECROTIC TUBERCULID (FIG. 14I)

Papulonecrotic tuberculid (PNT), the most common of the tuberculid disorders, is most frequently seen in children and young adults and may coexist with other tuberculids, lupus vulgaris, and scrofuloderma. It is typically characterized by recurrent eruption of symmetrically distributed firm and dusky-red, 2–8 mm papules with central depression that subsequently become pustular or necrotic, occurring most commonly on the face, ears, extensor extremities, and buttocks and rarely involving the palms. Constitutional symptoms may precede the appearance of skin lesions and associated lymphadenitis is common. The lesions heal over several weeks with pitted or varioliform scarring. It is considered to be a type III hypersensitivity reaction to a particular tuberculous antigen and living organism, mainly *Mycobacterium tuberculosis* infection elsewhere in the body. Rarely, it has been reported as a complication to bacillus Calmette-Guérin (BCG) vaccination. Phlyctenular conjunctivitis and associated TB are more common in childhood PNT compared to adults while scrofuloderma and concomitant erythema induratum are unusual, and vasculitis is not found. Presence of consistent clinical and histopathologic findings in a patient with risk factors for TB suggests the diagnosis of PNT. Typical histopathological findings include wedge-shaped necrosis along with nonspecific perivascular infiltrate or typical tuberculoid granulomatous inflammation, along with leukocytoclastic vasculitis, and perivascular edema or follicular necrosis with suppuration. Acid-fast bacillus (AFB) is not usually demonstrable; however, *M. tuberculosis* DNA can be detected by polymerase chain reaction (PCR). It has been suggested to use the term "papulonecrotic TB" over papulonecrotic tuberculid in cases where *M. tuberculosis* DNA can be confirmed by PCR. An extracutaneous focus of TB (e.g., cervical lymph nodes, lungs, or other sites) is usually detectable. Clinically, it has to be differentiated from pityriasis lichenoides et varioliformis acuta (PLEVA), prurigo, secondary syphilis, varicella, lymphomatoid papulosis and perforating disorders while histological differentials include PLEVA, inflammatory palisading granulomas, necrotizing vasculitis, and Churg-Strauss granuloma. Patients typically respond promptly within days to weeks of initiation of anti-TB therapy.

ATYPICAL MYCOBACTERIAL INFECTION (FIG. 14J)

Atypical mycobacteria are common in the environment and can be found in water (including tap water), soil, food, and on animals. Occasionally, atypical mycobacteria cause disease in humans. Examples of atypical mycobacteria include: *M. abscessus*, *M. marinum*, *M. avium-intracellulare* complex (MAC). The method of spread of atypical mycobacteria is uncertain but it is likely spread is through—contamination of broken skin, such as cuts or insect bites, injection of contaminated fluids, contamination of surgical wounds, medical equipment or implants, ingestion of contaminated food or drink, breathing in tiny particles containing the infectious organisms. Skin and soft tissue infection with ulcers (e.g., Buruli ulcer) or nodules, which can progress to involve tendons or bone. Diagnosis is confirmed by laboratory testing (culture or PCR) on clinical specimens such as abscess fluid or ulcer biopsy. Several specimens may be needed to confirm the diagnosis as detection can be difficult. Laboratory results need to be interpreted with care and in conjunction with clinical findings as colonization or specimen contamination may occur.

Antibiotic treatment may or may not be needed and courses may be complex; in some cases, several antibiotics may be needed for up to 2 years. Surgical removal of the infected area may be needed.

LEPROSY

Three cardinal features of leprosy are: (1) hypopigmented or erythematous hypoesthetic patch, (2) thickened peripheral nerves with sensory and/or motor deficit, and (3) presence of AFB in the skin lesions. The presence of at least one of them is sufficient to make a diagnosis of leprosy. As per Ridley-Jopling classification, leprosy is divided into five clinical types: (1) lepromatous, (2) borderline lepromatous (BL), (3) mid-borderline, (4) borderline tuberculoid (BT), and (5) tuberculoid types. Other clinical forms of leprosy seen in India are indeterminate, pure neuritic, and histoid leprosy. Leprosy in children is seen most commonly between the age group of 5 and 14 years.

Two types of lepra reactions are seen in clinical practice. Type I lepra reaction occurs usually within first 6 months of treatment of BT leprosy with MDT and may last for few months. There may be erythema, edema, and tenderness over the lesions and the affected limbs may become tender. Tender nerves or neuritis is a constant

"It is never too late to be who you might have been." —**George Eliot**

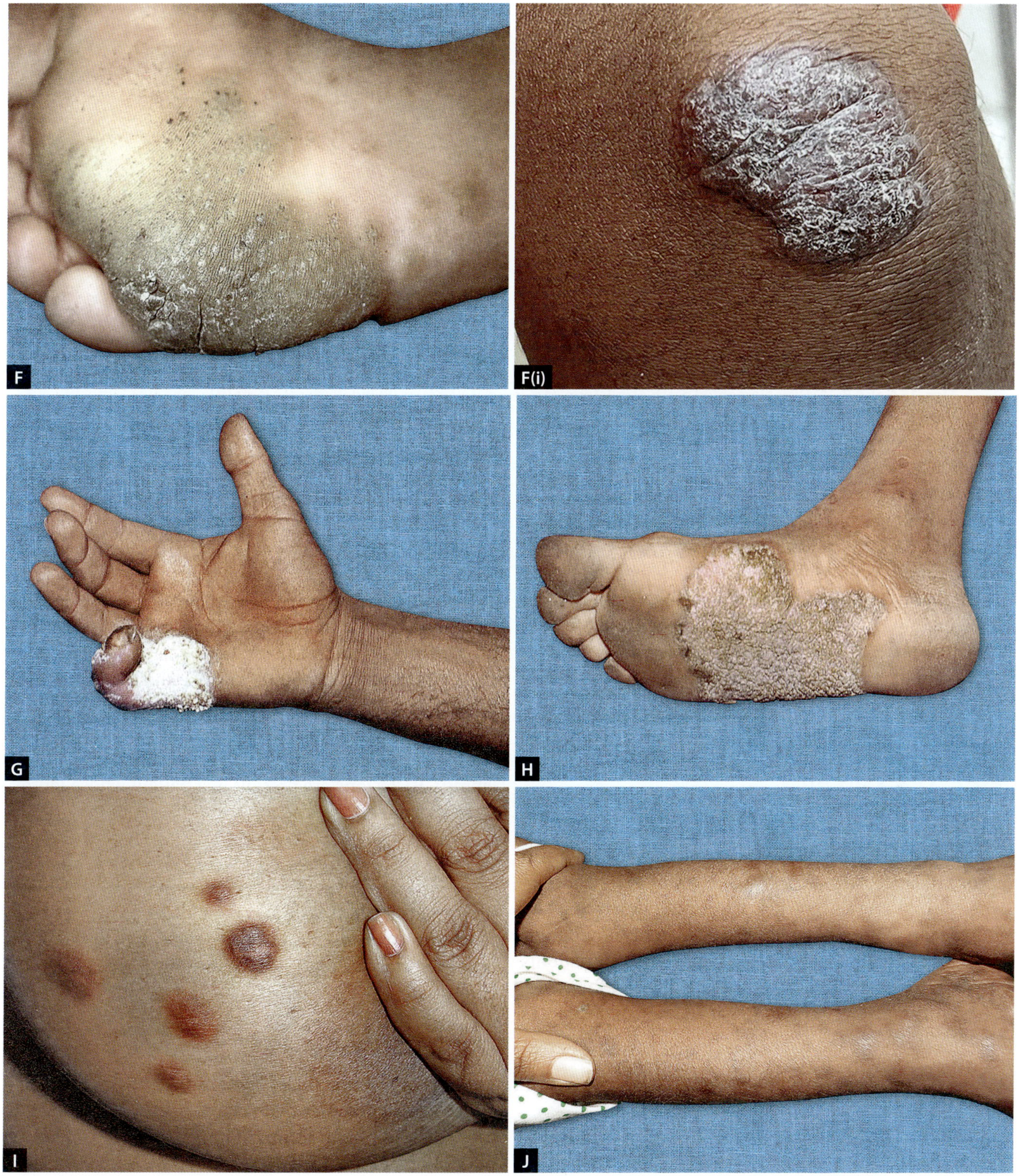

Figs. 14F to J: (F) Tuberculosis verrucosa cutis lesions over sole; F(i) Tubeculosis verrucosa cutis over knee joint; (G) Tuberculosis verrucosa cutis over palm in a 5-year-old boy; (H) Tuberculosis verrucosa cutis over sole; (I) Papulonecrotic tuberculid over breast of an adolescent girl; (J) Atypical mycobacterial infection.

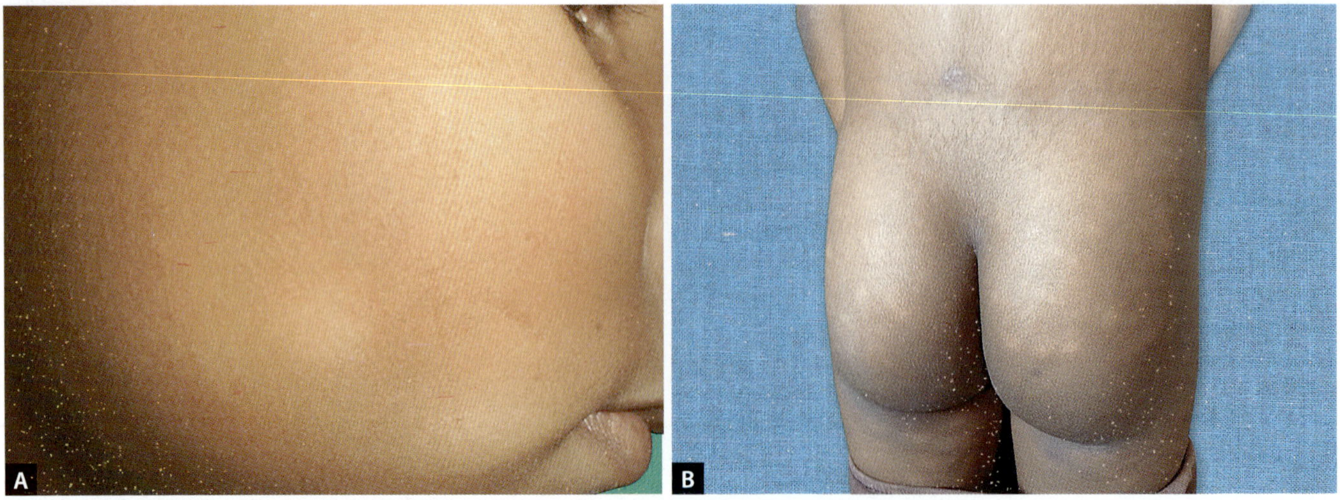

Figs. 15A and B: (A) Hypopigmented patch of indeterminate leprosy over face; (B) Indeterminate leprosy lesions over buttocks.

feature. In severe cases, associated constitutional features such as fever, malaise, arthralgia may develop.

Type II lepra reaction or erythema nodosum leprosum (ENL) reaction occurs in BL or lepromatous cases mostly within first 6 months of treatment, with MDT, sometimes in untreated cases. Erythematous tender evanescent papules and nodules develop over extremities, face, and sometimes back. It is associated with high fever and constitutional symptoms. There may be associated neuritis, inflammation of eyes, testes, liver, kidneys, spleen, and lymph nodes.

INDETERMINATE LEPROSY (FIGS. 15A AND B)

It presents as hypopigmented ill-defined macules or patches over the face, trunk, and extremities. This type of leprosy is mostly seen in children. There is very negligible hypoesthesia over the patches, if at all. Slit skin smears do not reveal presence of any AFB, and skin histopathology does not show any granuloma. Therefore, the patients are always kept under observation. In >80% of the cases, the lesions subside spontaneously as their immunity is supposed to be good.

BORDERLINE TUBERCULOID LEPROSY (FIGS. 16 TO 17E)

It presents as hypopigmented patch or plaque with variable degree of hypoesthesia. The border of a lesion is irregular with breakage of the lesion to form satellite lesions. The lesions may be distributed over the trunk or extremities. The feeding nerve to the patch may be palpable. The nerve proximal to the lesions is usually thickened. There may be redness and scaling over the lesion(s) because of type I reaction and the lesion(s) may be tender.

BORDERLINE LEPROMATOUS LEPROSY (FIGS. 17F AND G)

It starts as macular lesions which become infiltrated plaques and nodules. The infiltration begins in the center rise to a margin into normal skin. Lesions are numerous, more symmetrical and bilateral. Many large peripheral nerves are symmetrically thickened. The thickening occurs earlier in the course of the disease than lepromatous leprosy. BT lesions are present in a patient whose leprosy has downgraded.

LEPROMATOUS LEPROSY (FIGS. 17H TO M)

Lepromatous leprosy rates in children are very low ranging from 1.6 to 4.9%. The course of leprosy in childhood is unpredictable. Progression and regression of lesions are common.

Clinical Features

The early lesions of lepromatous leprosy are small innumerable macules distributed symmetrically may or may not have slight infiltration. As the lesions progress infiltration of the skin results in the following presentation pattern:

- *Diffuse lepromatous leprosy*: It results from gradual coalescing of the macules. The skin has a stretched shiny look with mild infiltration.

"Obstacles are the cost of greatness." —**Robin Sharma**

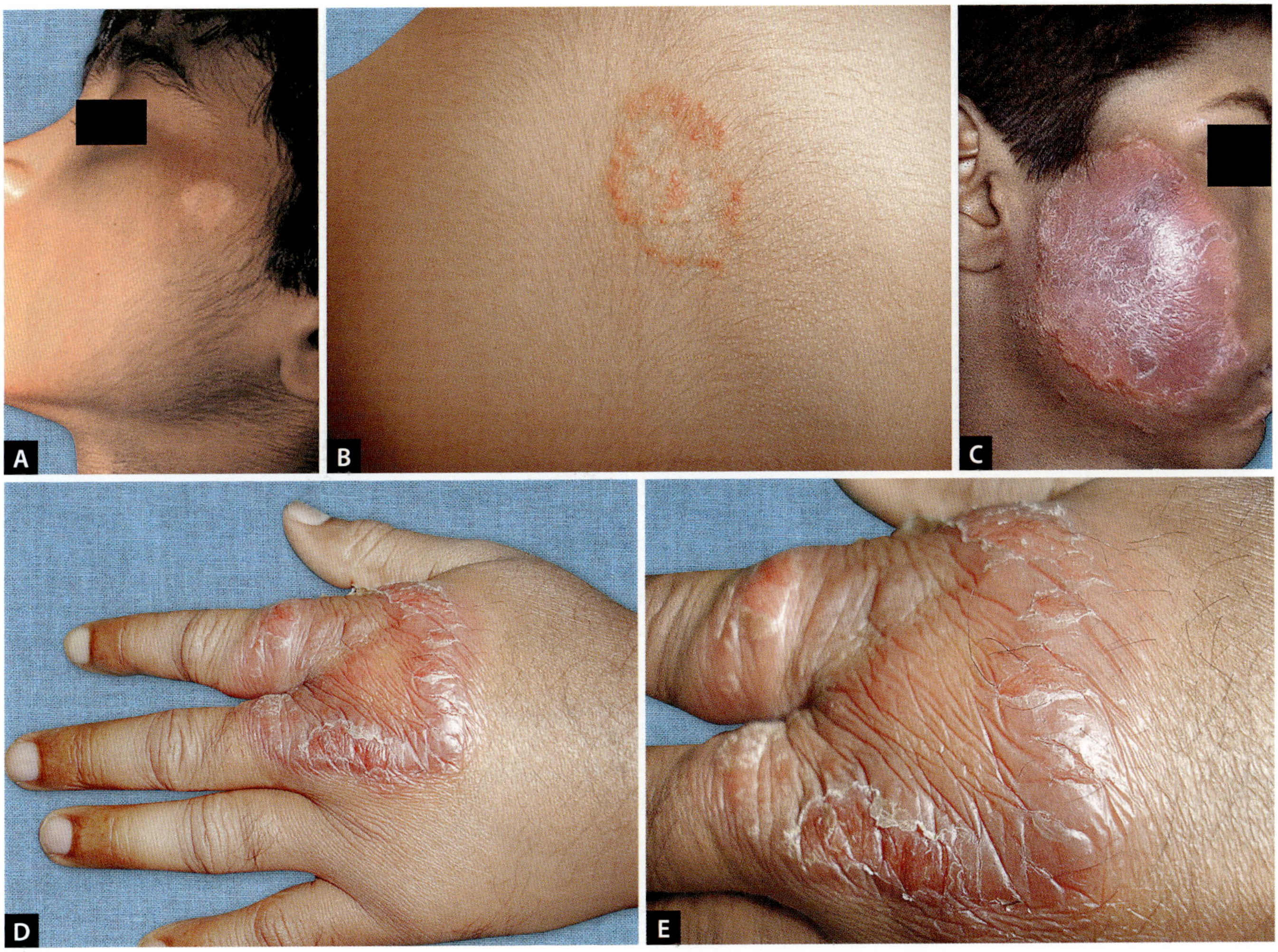

Figs. 16A to E: (A) Well-defined hypoesthetic hypopigmented patch of borderline tuberculoid (BT) leprosy; (B) Classical lesion of BT Hansen's disease, note beaded margin; (C) BT Hansen's disease over face with type 1 reaction; (D) BT Hansen's disease with type 1 reaction; (E) Same patient, close-up view.

- *Infiltrated lepromatous leprosy*: It is an advanced stage of the macular lepromatous leprosy with easily visible infiltration. Lesions are often shiny and succulent in consistency.
- *Nodular lepromatous leprosy*: It occurs from the deterioration of the above-mentioned two forms of leprosy. It occurs most commonly over the elbows, fingers, joints, and buttocks. The infiltrated plaque accentuates the skinfolds giving rise to leonine facies.
- Other features include anhidrosis with compensatory hyperhidrosis of face, axilla, and trunk. The sensory loss being symmetrical gives rise to the glove and stocking anesthesia. There may be fusiform swelling of the digits with resorption. Involvement of the upper respiratory tract results in stuffy nose along with epistaxis. Ocular manifestation in the form of lagophthalmos, uveitis and corneal opacity and perforation may also occur.

Differential Diagnosis of Facial Infiltration

- Post-kala-azar dermal leishmaniasis
- Rosacea
- Reticulohistiocytosis
- Sarcoidosis
- Disseminated cutaneous leishmaniasis
- Lipoid proteinosis

Laboratory Diagnosis

Slit skin smear with smear positivity and high bacillary index. Biopsy done from the skin lesions show a

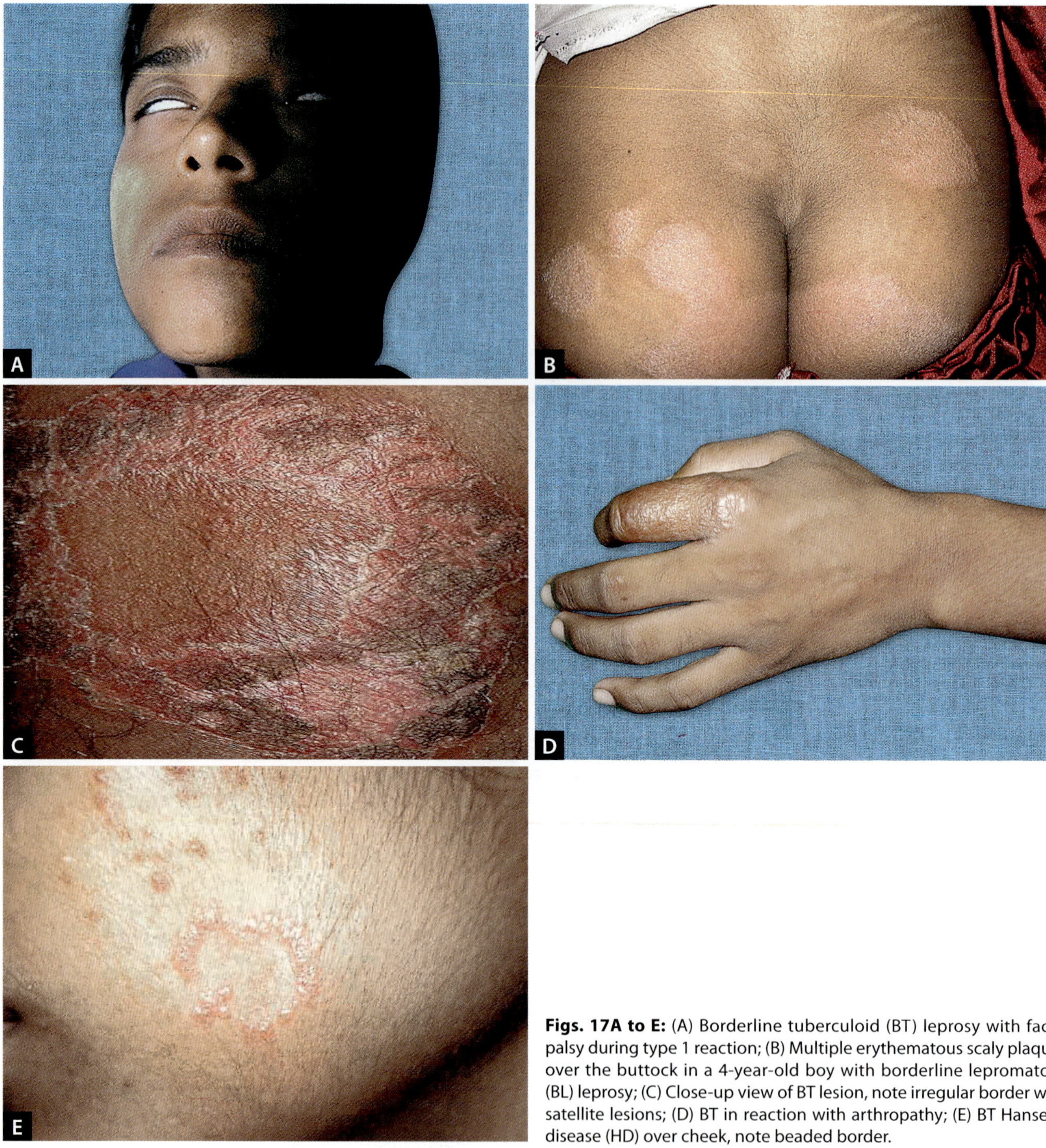

Figs. 17A to E: (A) Borderline tuberculoid (BT) leprosy with facial palsy during type 1 reaction; (B) Multiple erythematous scaly plaques over the buttock in a 4-year-old boy with borderline lepromatous (BL) leprosy; (C) Close-up view of BT lesion, note irregular border with satellite lesions; (D) BT in reaction with arthropathy; (E) BT Hansen's disease (HD) over cheek, note beaded border.

granuloma without caseation necrosis and numerous foamy macrophages. AFB stain is generally positive.

HISTOID LEPROSY (FIGS. 17N AND O)

Histoid leprosy is an expression of multibacillary (MB) leprosy characterized by typical cutaneous features with unique histopathology and bacterial morphology. It has rarely been reported in children; however, the lowest age of occurrence has been recorded as 10 years. It generally manifests in patients treated with dapsone monotherapy. Development of drug resistance to dapsone and mutant organisms are the other two hypotheses for the development of histoid leprosy.

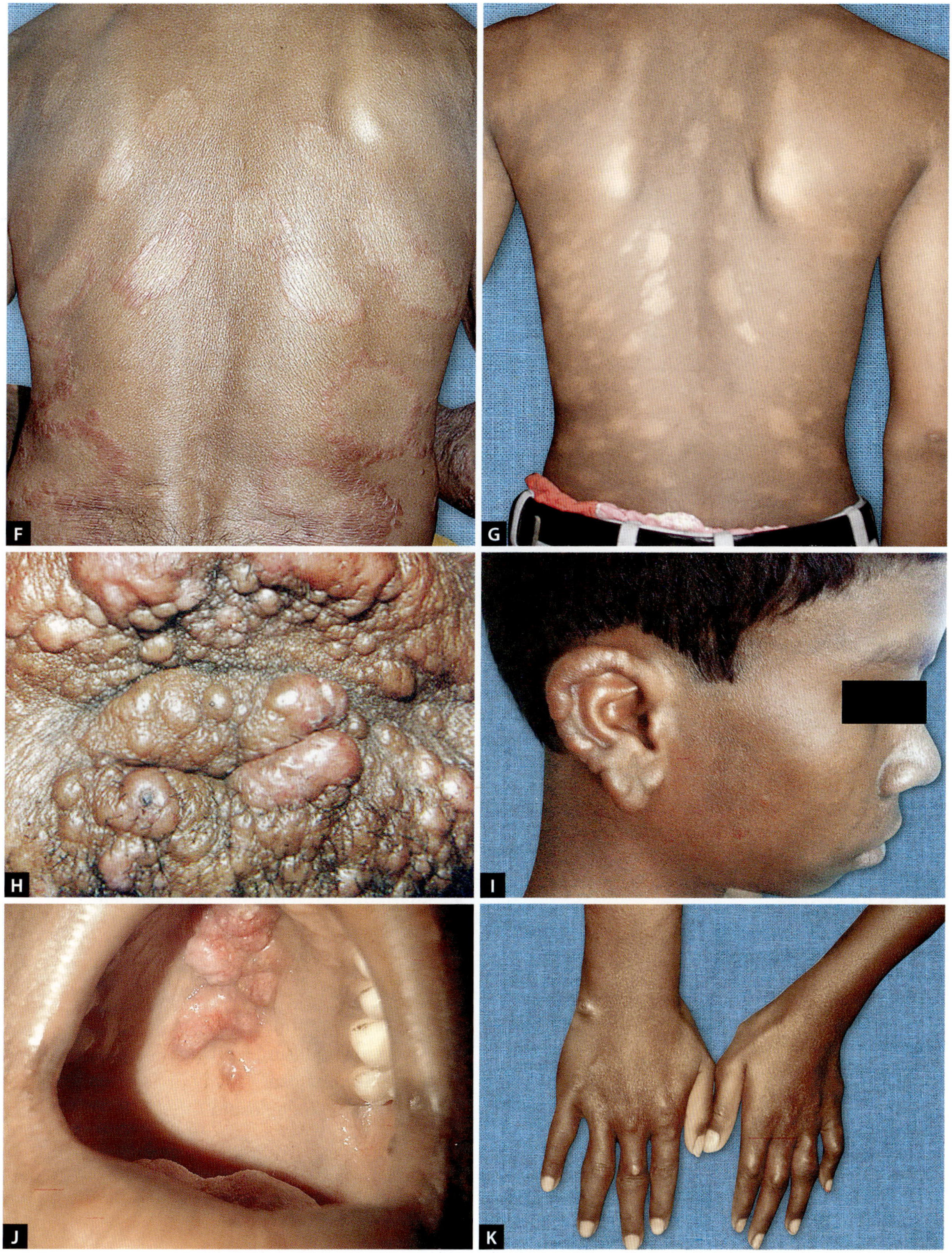

Figs. 17F to K: (F) Borderline lepromatous (BL) Hansen's disease (HD), note multiple annular infiltrated plaques of variable size and shape; (G) BL lesions over back; (H) Lepromatous leprosy (LL) nodules and infiltration of skin, close-up view; (I) LL, note nodules over pinna and earlobe; (J) Leprous nodules over palate, a rare observation; (K) Dactylitis in LL.

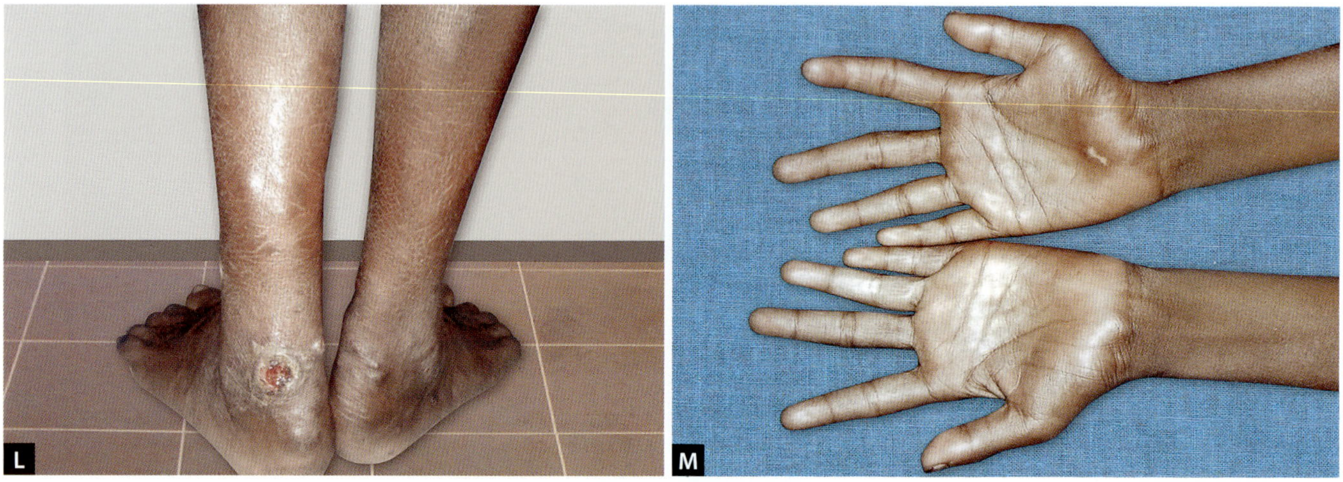

Figs. 17L and M: (L) Lepromatous leprosy (LL) patient with trophic ulcer of foot; (M) LL patient with claw hand. Note atrophy of thenar and hypothenar eminences.

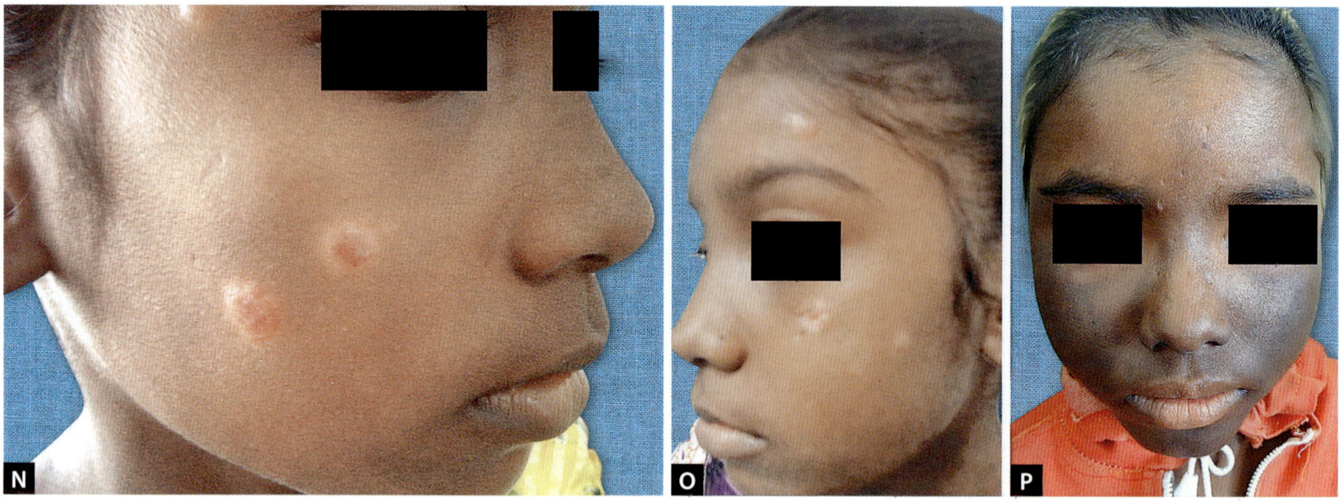

Figs. 17N to P: (N) Histoid lesions; (O) Histoid leprosy; (P) Clofazimine-induced slate-gray hyperpigmentation.

Clinical Features

Histoid leprosy can present with cutaneous nodules that may be superficial, subcutaneous or deep and also can present as plaques or pads. The number of lesions vary from 3 to 50 located generally on the limbs, back, buttocks, face, and bony prominences.

The typical lesions have been described as dome-shaped, reddish to skin-colored papules with shiny smooth surface and a stretched overlying skin. The plaques and pad type of lesions are more common over the bony prominences.

Two types of facies have been described:

1. Resembling relics of a burnt-out leprosy
2. Normal facies.

The noticeable features of histoid leprosy include:

- Persistence of the eyebrow
- Sparing of nasal mucosa and cartilage
- Good general health of the patient.

Differential Diagnosis

- Lepromatous nodules
- Erythema nodosum leprosum
- Neurofibromatosis
- Molluscum contagiosum
- Sarcoidosis

Laboratory Diagnosis

Slit skin smears show smear positivity with a high bacillary index. Biopsy done from the lesion shows a well-circumscribed granuloma with lepra bacilli in a histoid habitus.

"The greatest discovery of all time is that a person can change his future by merely changing his attitude." —**Oprah Winfrey**

Treatment

Multidrug therapy is the mainstay of leprosy treatment. The World Health Organization (WHO) recommended fixed duration multidrug treatment for 6 months in paucibacillary (PB) leprosy and 12 months in cases of MB leprosy.

Paucibacillary-MDT (10–14 Years)

Rifampicin 450 mg once/month supervised dose along with dapsone 50 mg daily unsupervised dose.

Multibacillary-MDT for Children

Multibacillary child treatment (10–14 years):

Once a month:
Day 1—

- 2 capsules of rifampicin (300 mg + 150 mg)
- 3 capsules of clofazimine (50 mg × 3)
- 1 tablet of dapsone (50 mg)

Once a day:
Days 2–28—

- 1 capsule of clofazimine every other day (50 mg)
- 1 tablet of dapsone (50 mg)

Full course:
12 blister packs.

Adverse effects of MDT are varied. Side effects of dapsone include dapsone hypersensitivity reactions (dapsone syndrome), exfoliative dermatitis, hemolytic anemia, agranulocytosis, methemoglobinemia and peripheral neuropathy. Clofazamine can cause diffuse pigmentation over the photoexposed areas and gastro-intestinal side effects **(Fig. 17P)**.

COMMON WARTS (VERRUCA VULGARIS) (FIGS. 18 TO 19P)

Common warts are caused by human papillomavirus (HPV) 1, 2, 4, 7. They can occur anywhere on the body but more commonly on trauma prone areas. Being firm papules with a rough, horny surface, they range in size from 1 mm to over 1 cm in diameter and by confluence may form large masses. About 65% of warts disappear spontaneously.

Natural History

Warts are known to regress spontaneously over a period of 6 months to 2 years. However, treatment is required to stop their spread as well as transmission to others.

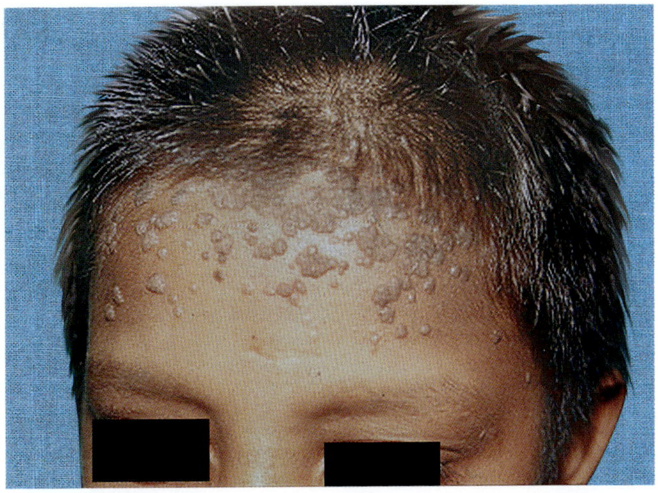

Fig. 18: Classical warty lesions of verruca vulgaris over forehead.

Treatment

Treatment of warts is essentially done either by cauterization with 50–60% trichloroacetic acid, phenol, etc., or by electrodesiccation, cryotherapy or CO_2 laser treatment.

VERRUCA PLANA (FIGS. 19Q TO S)

Plane warts occur primarily on the face, neck, arms and legs, and are present as skin-colored, grayish-brown, smooth, flat and slightly elevated papules, 2–5 mm in diameter with a round or polygonal base. Young children are mostly affected. Koebner's phenomenon is seen frequently. Plane warts spread in the beard area of men and in the legs of women. It may spread along the microtrauma caused by shaving. Contiguous warts often coalesce to form firm, papular or plaque-like lesions; slightly elevated lesions in areas of scratch marks are characteristic of this disorder. Spontaneous regression after a few months is seen quite often.

Treatment

Treatment is more or less same as that of common warts described above.

MOLLUSCUM CONTAGIOSUM (FIGS. 20 TO 24)

This condition caused by *Poxviridae* (*molluscum contagiosum virus*) is characterized by the appearance of umbilicated skin papules or nodules. The incubation period varies from 14 days to 6 months. The individual

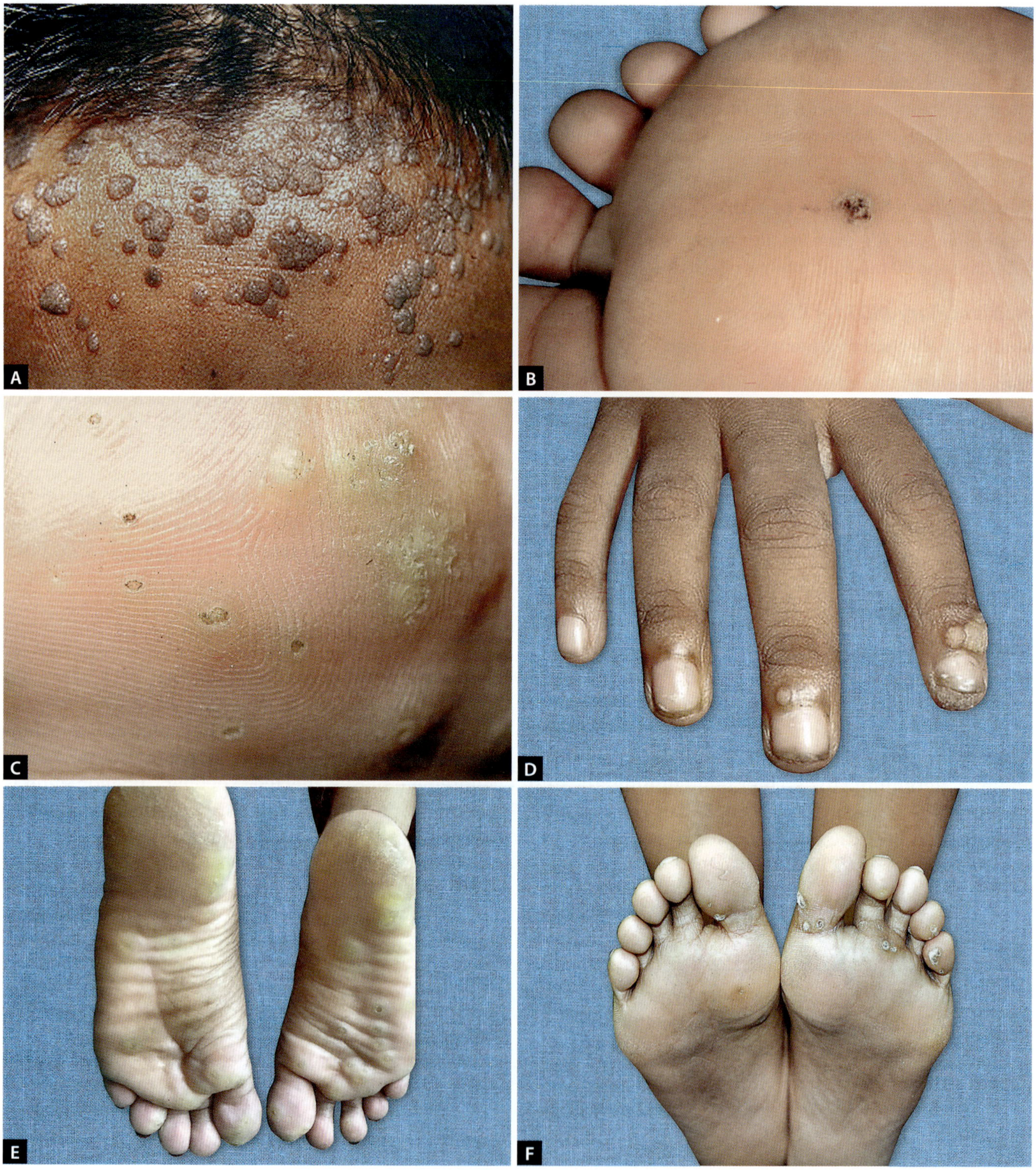

Figs. 19A to F: (A) Close-up view of same child (Fig. 18), verruca vulgaris; (B) Plantar wart, note black hemorrhagic dots on scraping with a scalpel blade; (C) Multiple warts over sole; (D) Warts over anterior, posterior, and lateral nail-folds of index finger; (E) Plantar warts; (F) Plantar warts, another view.

lesion is a shiny, pearly, white hemispherical, umbilicated papule which may show a central pore. It grows to a diameter of 5–10 mm in 6–12 weeks. The lesions spread frequently and are sometimes present in large number.

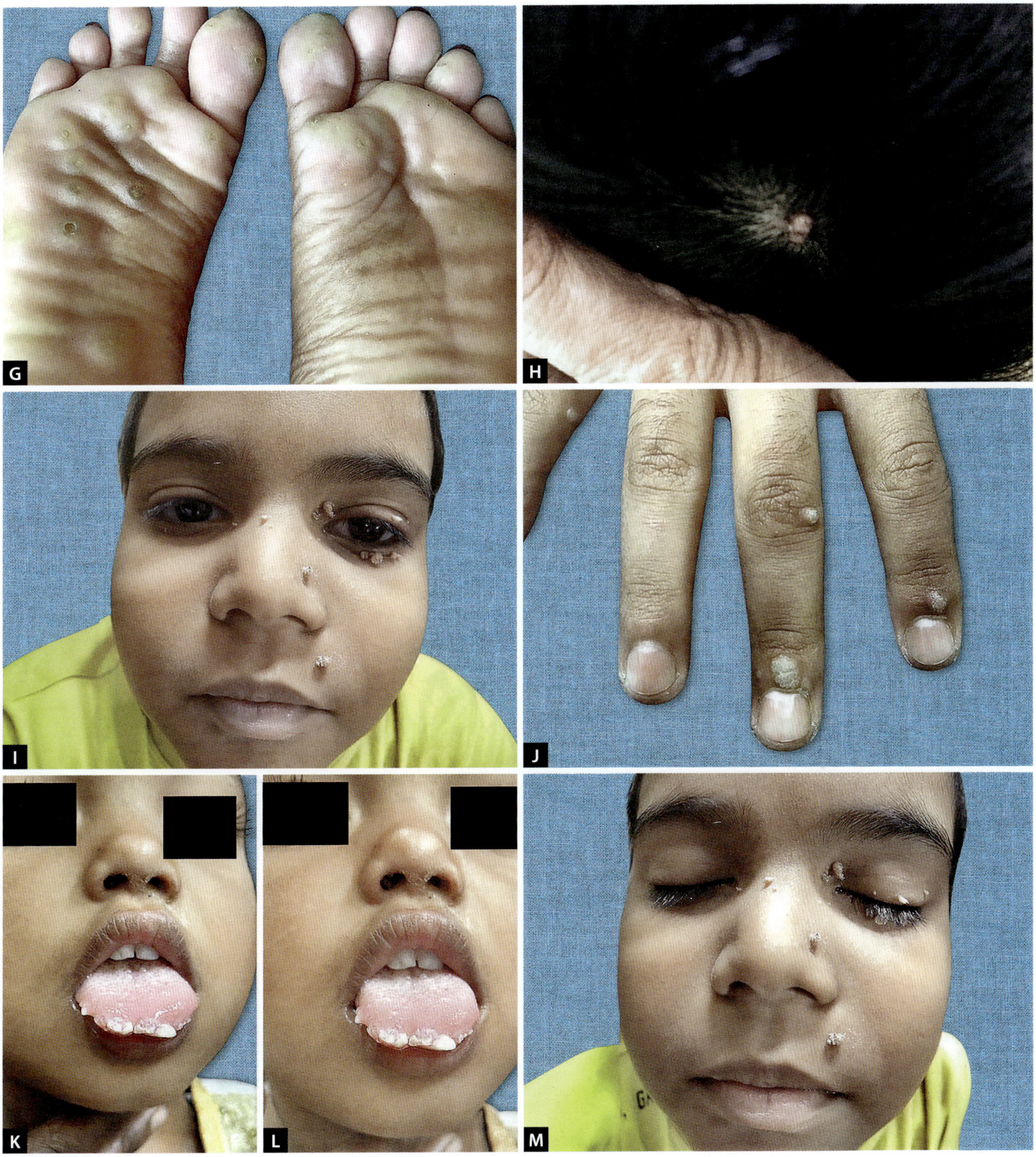

Figs. 19G to M: (G) Plantar warts (close-up view); (H) Scalp wart; (I) Warts over face; (J) Verruca vulgaris over fingers; (K) Verruca vulgaris over tongue; (L) Same child, close-up view; (M) Verruca vulgaris over eyelids and face.

After trauma or spontaneously after several months, inflammatory changes result in suppuration, crusting, and destruction of the base. Eczematous lesions can occur surrounding molluscum contagiosum called as "molluscum dermatitis" and indicates resolving lesion. The most common site affected is the face. But it may

"The wound is the place where the light enters you." —**Rumi**

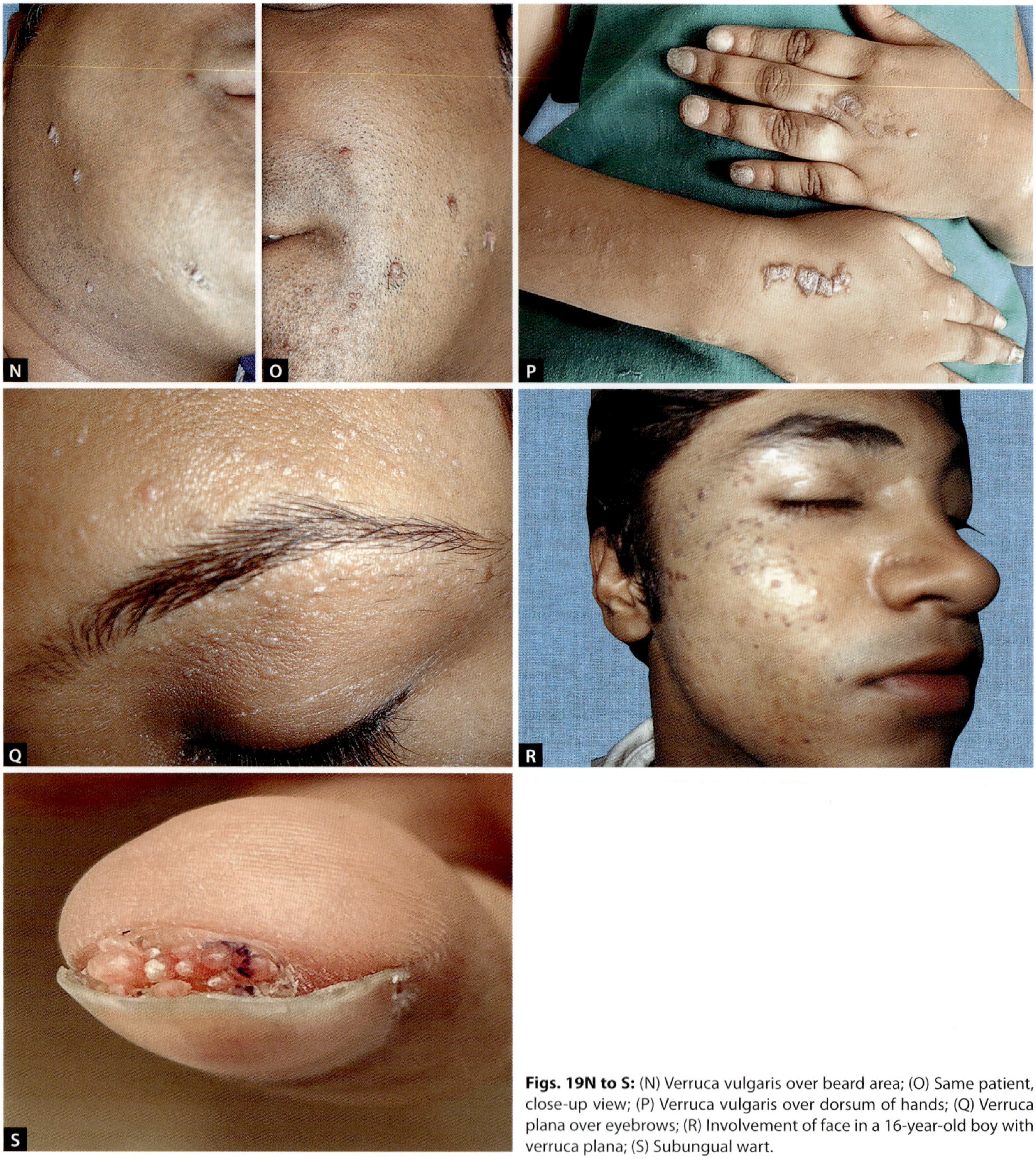

Figs. 19N to S: (N) Verruca vulgaris over beard area; (O) Same patient, close-up view; (P) Verruca vulgaris over dorsum of hands; (Q) Verruca plana over eyebrows; (R) Involvement of face in a 16-year-old boy with verruca plana; (S) Subungual wart.

also affect the scalp, trunk, mucous membrane or any other part of the body. Most cases are self-limiting in 6–9 months. In immunocompromised patients and underlying lymphoma, the lesions may be huge in size and number.

Treatment

Lesions are treated by chemical cautery using 50–60% trichloroacetic acid, phenol, cantharidin or silver nitrate. The caustic is applied with either a sterile

"Don't let rejection create self-doubt. The founder of Starbucks was turned down by 217 of the 242 investors he initially spoke with." —**Elizabeth Galbut**

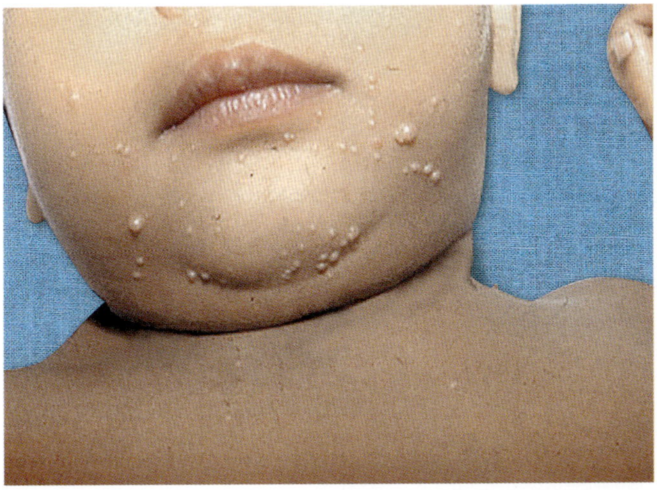

Fig. 20: Pearly white umbilicated papules of molluscum contagiosum.

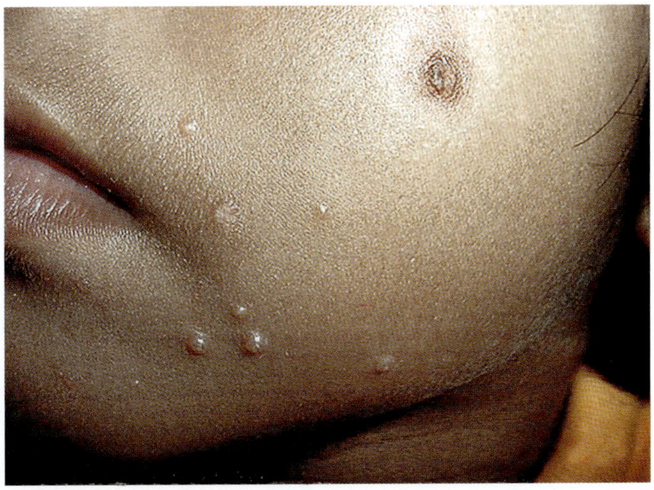

Fig. 21: Multiple umbilicated papules of molluscum contagiosum.

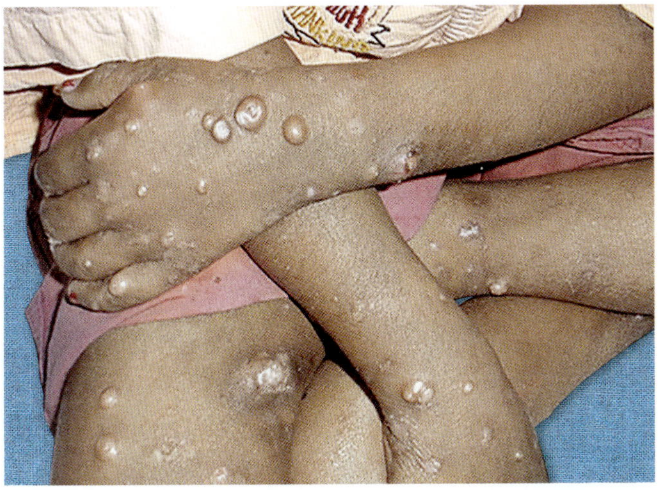

Fig. 22: Extensive and giant molluscum contagiosum in an immunocompromised child.

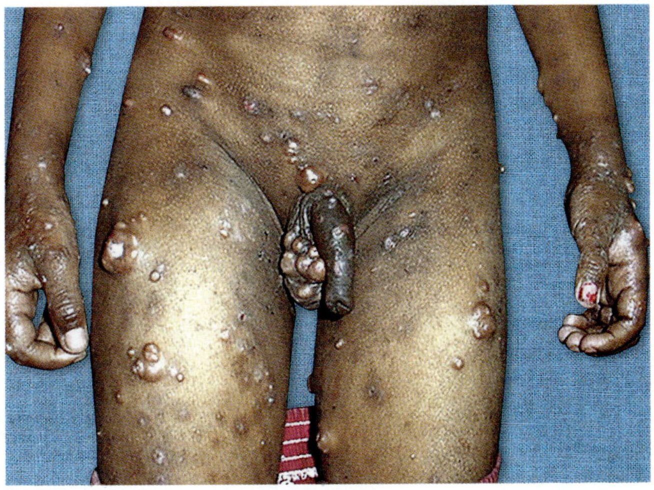

Fig. 23: Same child, note giant lesions.

needle or a toothpick. Other options are electrodesiccation, cryotherapy or application of imiquimod, an immunomodulator.

PITYRIASIS ROSEA (FIGS. 25 AND 26)

Pityriasis rosea is an acute, self-limiting disease caused by human herpesvirus 6 (HHV-6) and/or HHV-7, characterized by a distinctive skin eruption and minimal constitutional symptoms. The etiology is considered to be infective with the appearance of the herald patch, which is larger and more conspicuous than the lesions of the later eruption, usually situated on the thigh, upper arm, the trunk or the neck. It is a sharply defined, bright-red, round or oval plaque covered by a fine scale which reaches a size of 2–5 cm. After an interval of 5–15 days, the general eruption begins to appear in crops at 2–3 days interval over a week or 10 days. They appear in the forms of discrete medallions, dull pink in color covered by fine dry, gray scales. The center tends to clear, assumes a wrinkled, atrophic appearance and a tawny color with a marginal collarette of scales attached peripherally, with the free edge of the scales internally. The medallions are commonly associated with pink macules of varying sizes. The lesions are usually confined to the trunk, the base of the neck and the upper third of the arms and legs. Involvement of the face and scalp is common in children. The skin lesions commonly fades spontaneously after 3–6 weeks with postinflammatory hypopigmentation.

"Play to your strengths. If you aren't great at something, do more of what you're great at." **—Jason Lemkin**

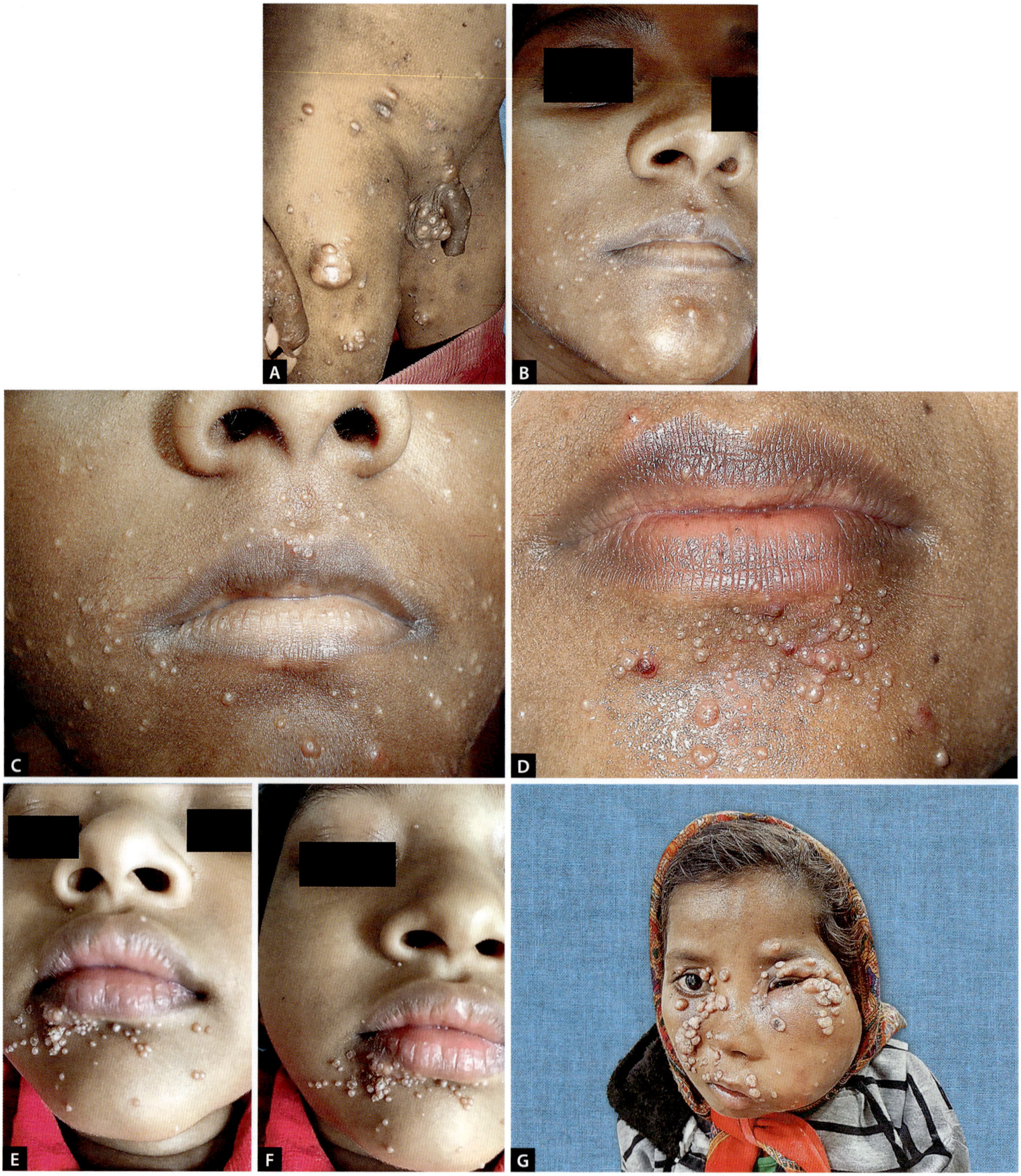

Figs. 24A to G: (A) Close-up view of giant molluscum contagiosum (MC) lesions; (B) Multiple micropapules of MC; (C) Same patient, close-up view; (D) Close-up view of MC lesions; (E) Clustered lesions of molluscum contagiosum at the angle of mouth; (F) Same child, another view; (G) Florid and giant molluscum contagiosum lesions in an adolescent girl suffering from Burkitt's lymphoma.

"If people are doubting how far you can go, go so far that you can't hear them anymore." —**Michele Ruiz**

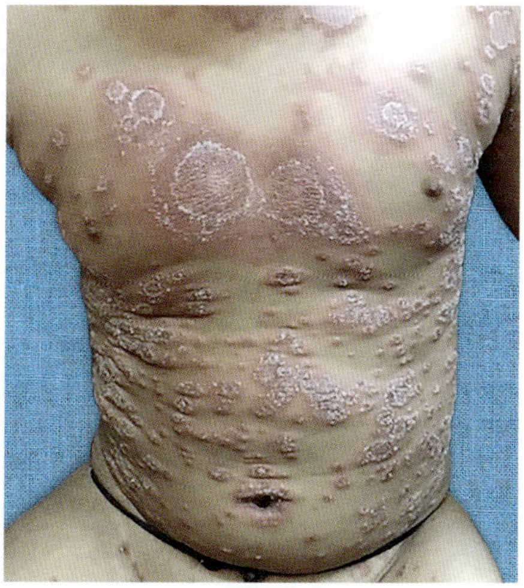

Fig. 25: Pityriasis rosea in a 4-year-old boy.

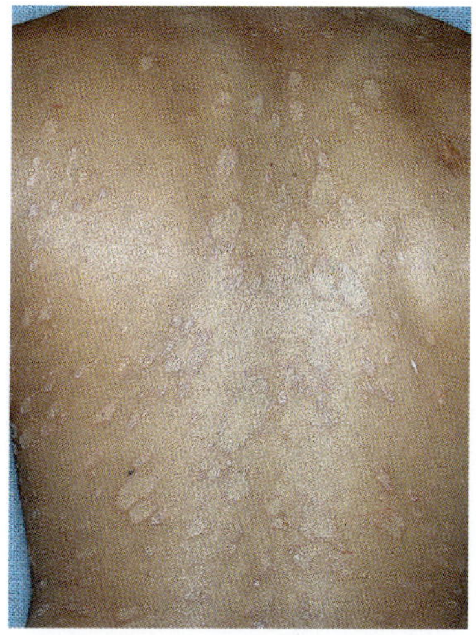

Fig. 26: Multiple ringworm-like lesions in pityriasis rosea with peripheral collarette of scales.

Natural History

It is a self-limiting condition and resolves spontaneously by 4–6 weeks, although rarely it may persist up to 3 months or even longer.

Treatment

Treatment is mainly symptomatic and requires only reassurance. Topical emollients, calamine lotion and mild topical steroids can be given to decrease the pruritus. Oral antihistamines are indicated for severe itching. Narrowband ultraviolet B (NB-UVB) therapy can be given to improve the postinflammatory hypopigmentation and persistent lesions.

HERPES SIMPLEX INFECTION (FIGS. 27 TO 30)

Herpes simplex is one of the most common viral infection occurring throughout the world and is caused by herpes simplex virus type 1 (HSV-1) and HSV-2. Primary infection may be subclinical but when clinical lesions develop, the severity is generally greater than that in recurrences.

Herpetic Gingivostomatitis

This is the most common clinical manifestation of primary infection by HSV-1. Children between 1 and 5 years are usually affected. After an incubation period of approximately 5 days, the stomatitis begins with fever, malaise, restlessness, and excessive dribbling. Drinking and eating become painful and the breath is foul.

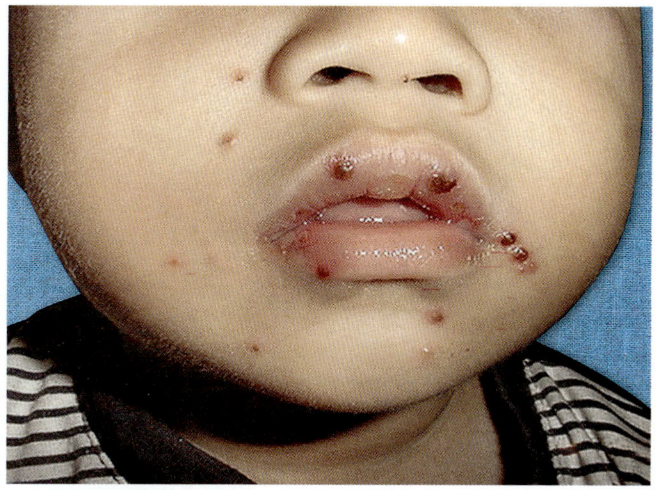

Fig. 27: Vesicular lesions of herpes labialis.

Gums are swollen, painful and bleed easily. Vesicles presenting as white plaques appear on the tongue, pharynx, palate, and buccal mucous membrane. Regional lymph nodes are enlarged and tender. The fever subsides in 3–5 days and recovery is complete in 1 week. Symptomatic treatment along with oral acyclovir is the mainstay of management.

Herpes Genitalis

Infection with HSV-2 occurs after the onset of sexual activity. Penile ulceration from herpetic infection is the most frequent type of genital ulceration. The ulcers which may be preceded by a general malaise, are most frequent on the glans, prepuce, and shaft of the penis. They are

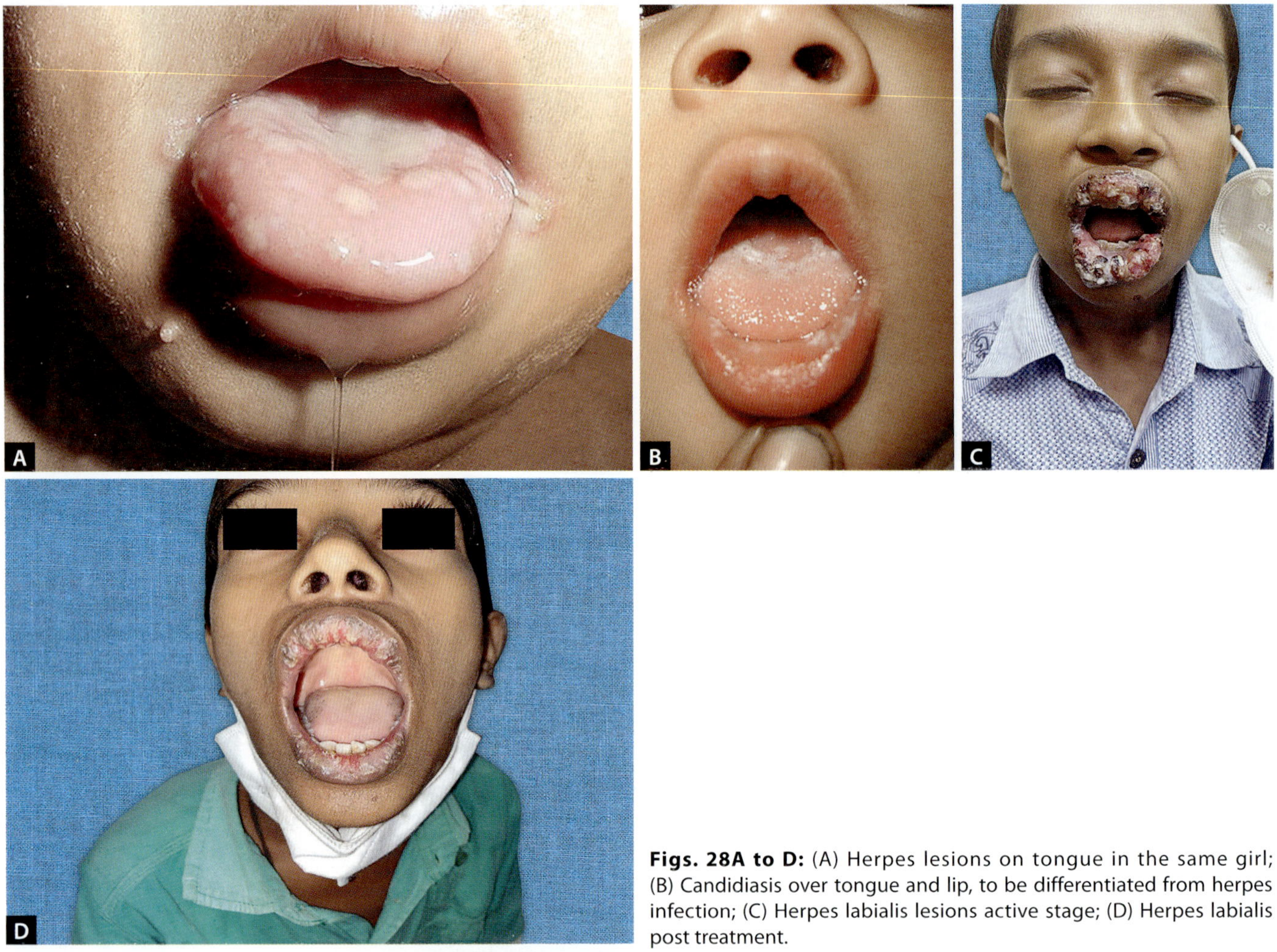

Figs. 28A to D: (A) Herpes lesions on tongue in the same girl; (B) Candidiasis over tongue and lip, to be differentiated from herpes infection; (C) Herpes labialis lesions active stage; (D) Herpes labialis post treatment.

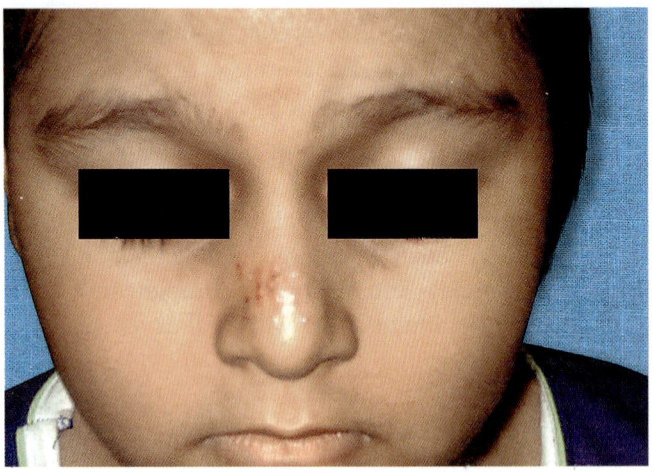

Fig. 29: Herpes simplex lesions over nose.

small and painful with serpiginous border and last for 2–3 weeks if untreated. In females, similar ulcerations occur on the external genitalia and mucosae of the vulva, vagina, and cervix. Pain and dysuria are common. Tender inguinal lymphadenopathy is present. Maternal-fetal transmission may result in neonatal herpes. Diagnosis of herpes genitalis in a child should raise the suspicion of child abuse. Diagnosis is mainly by Tzanck smear and viral culture. Oral acyclovir is the treatment of choice.

Keratoconjunctivitis

Primary herpes infection of the eye causes a severe and often purulent conjunctivitis with opacity and superficial ulceration of the cornea.

HERPES ZOSTER (FIGS. 31 TO 33)

Varicella and zoster are caused by the same virus, varicella zoster virus. Pediatric herpes zoster is not only seen in immunocompromised but also in immunocompetent children. Recently, the increased incidence can be attributed to the varicella vaccination. Varicella is the

"I learned this, at least, by my experiment: that if one advances confidently in the direction of his dreams, and endeavours to live the life which he has imagined, he will meet with a success unexpected in common hours." —**Henry David Thoreau**

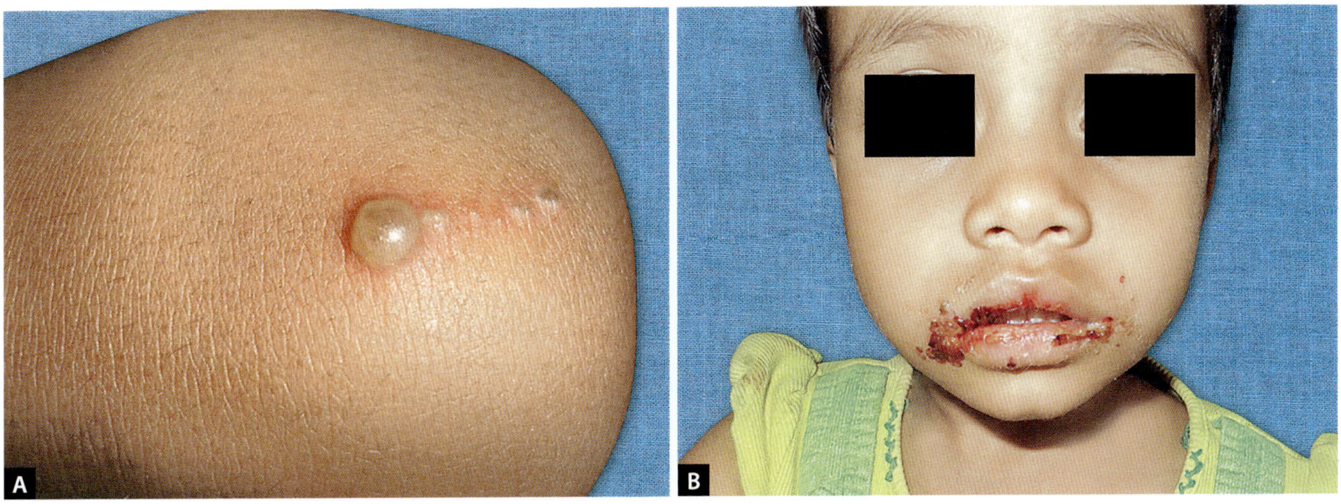

Figs. 30A and B: (A) Insect bite reaction in a 3-year-old boy, simulating herpes; (B) Herpes labialis.

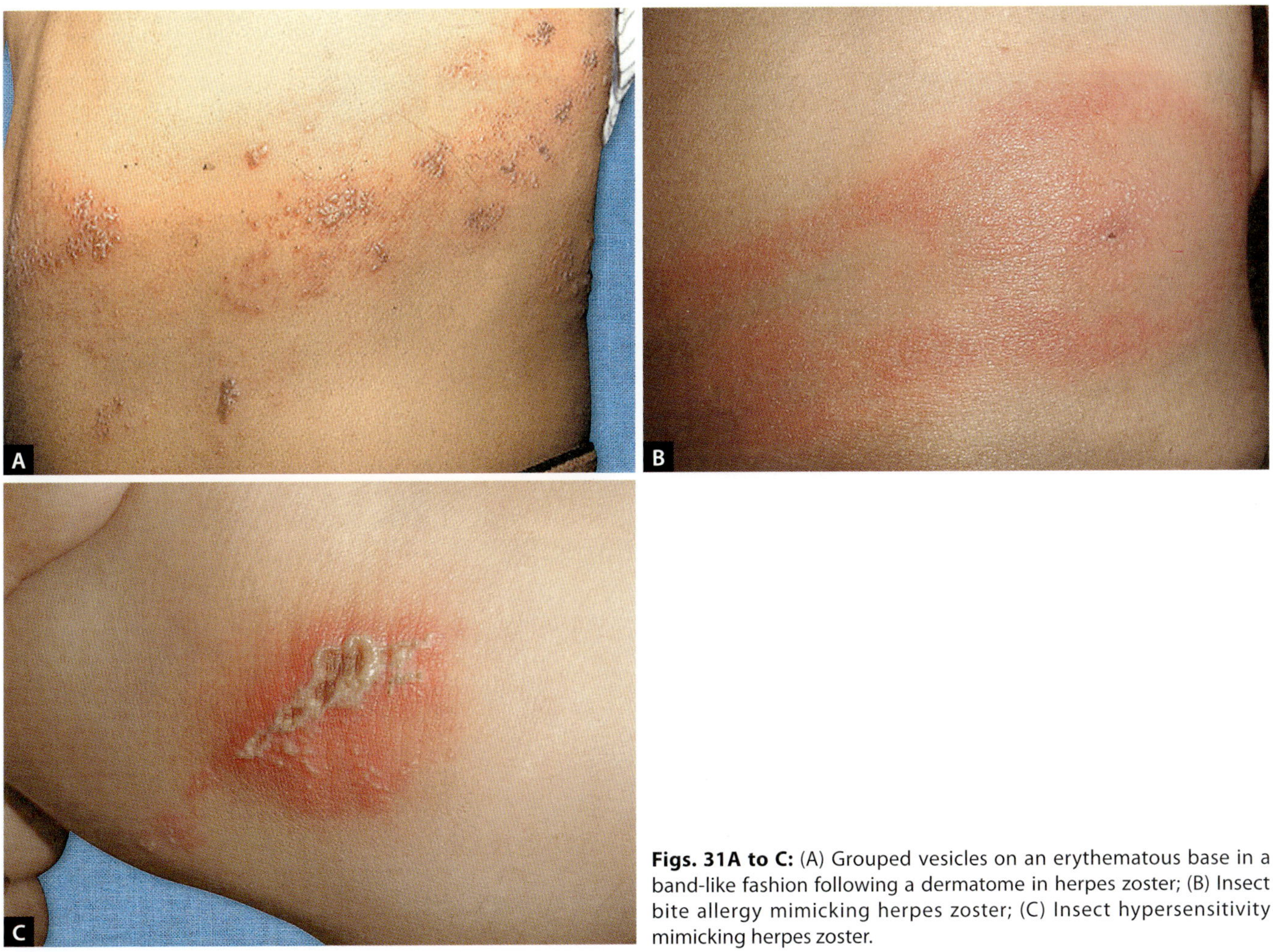

Figs. 31A to C: (A) Grouped vesicles on an erythematous base in a band-like fashion following a dermatome in herpes zoster; (B) Insect bite allergy mimicking herpes zoster; (C) Insect hypersensitivity mimicking herpes zoster.

primary infection with a viremic stage, after which the virus persists in nerve ganglion cells, usually sensory. Zoster is the result of reactivation of the residual latent virus. The first manifestation of zoster is usually pain which may be severe and may be accompanied by fever, headache, malaise, and tenderness localized to areas of one or more

"And so it is, that both the devil and the angelic spirits present us with objects of desire to awaken our power of choice." —**Rumi**

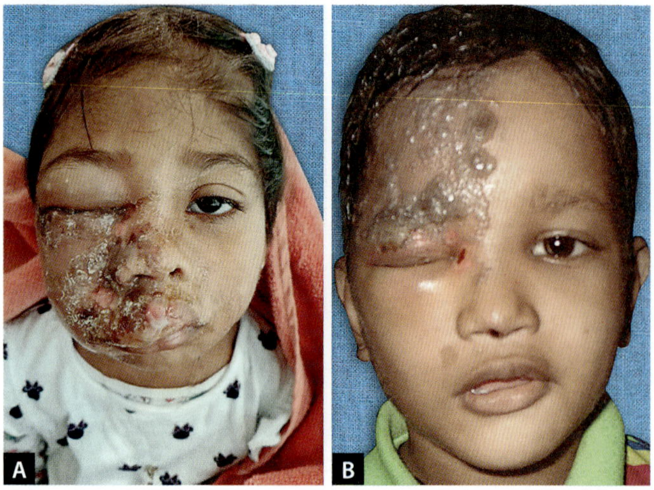

Figs. 32A and B: (A) Herpes zoster involving maxillary division of trigeminal nerve; (B) Herpes zoster ophthalmicus in a 5-year-old boy.

dorsal roots. Within 2–4 days, closely grouped red papules rapidly becoming vesicular and then pustular develop in a continuous or interrupted band in the area of one, occasionally two and rarely more contiguous dermatomes. Mucous membranes within the affected dermatomes are also involved. New vesicles continue to appear for several days. The lymph nodes draining the affected area are enlarged and tender. The pain and the constitutional symptoms subside gradually as the eruption heals. In uncomplicated cases, recovery is complete in 2–3 weeks in children and young adults. Rare complications include pneumonia, encephalitis, hepatitis, and septicemia.

Treatment

Acyclovir is the drug of choice for oral, genital and other herpes infections. For primary herpes simplex, the dose

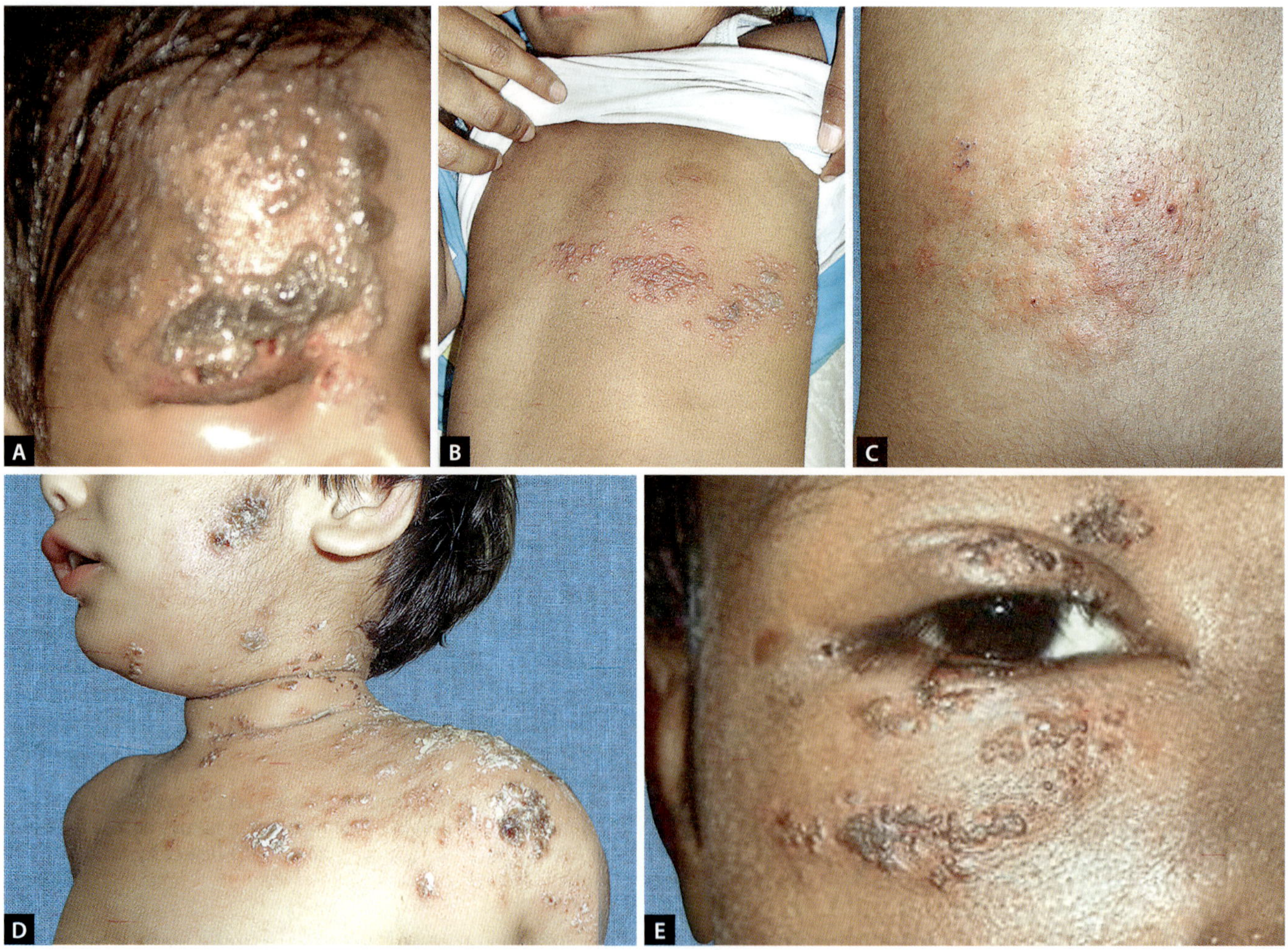

Figs. 33A to E: (A) Same boy, note lesions do not cross midline; (B) Herpes zoster in a 3-year-old girl; (C) Herpes zoster; (D) Herpes zoster over shoulder in a 4-year-old boy; (E) Herpes zoster ophthalmicus.

"If you're brave enough to say goodbye, life will reward you with new hello." —**Paulo Coelho**

is 200–400 mg three times/day for 10 days. To prevent frequent attacks, long-term prophylaxis with 200–400 mg two times/day for 6–18 months has been recommended. Valacyclovir and famciclovir need to undergo adequate trials before being prescribed in pediatric age group.

In milder cases of herpes zoster, topical calamine lotion and nonsteroidal anti-inflammatory drugs (NSAIDs) suffice. In severe and symptomatic cases, oral acyclovir 400–800 mg five times/day or famciclovir 250–500 mg three times/day for 7–10 days is advised. Supportive measures related to the local organ involvement (i.e., ocular involvement) are to be provided. Incidence of postherpetic neuralgia is fairly uncommon in cases of herpes zoster in children.

TINEA CORPORIS AND TINEA FACIEI (FIGS. 34 TO 36K)

Tinea corporis is a dermatophyte infection of the glabrous skin typically occurring on exposed areas. The causative organism in young children is usually *Microsporum canis* and in older children it is *Trichophyton rubrum*, *Trichophyton verrucosum*, *Trichophyton mentagrophytes*,

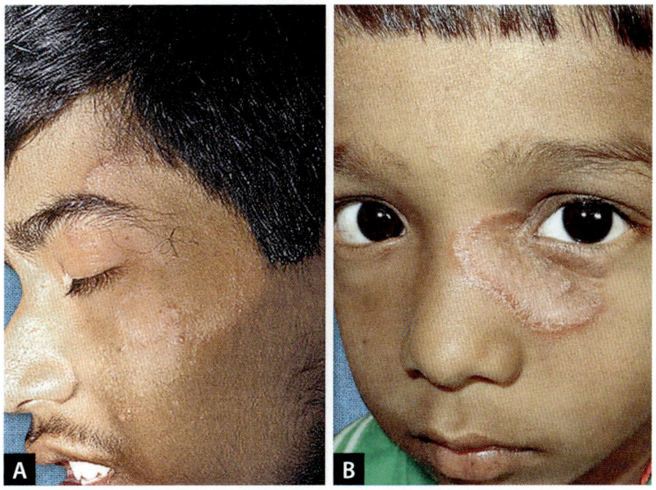

Figs. 34A and B: (A) Itchy papulovesicular ring of tinea faciei; (B) Tinea faciei in a 4-year-old boy.

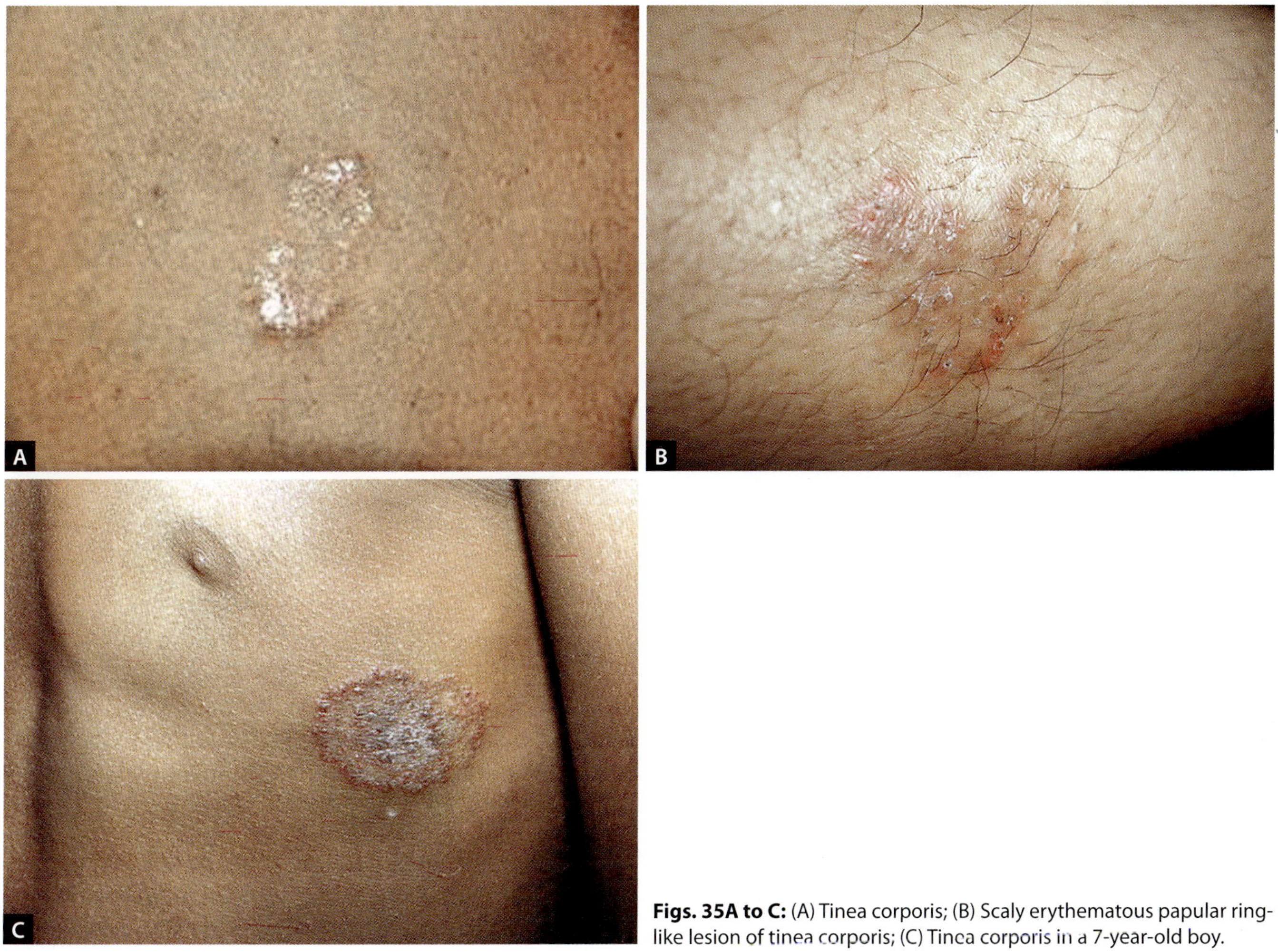

Figs. 35A to C: (A) Tinea corporis; (B) Scaly erythematous papular ring-like lesion of tinea corporis; (C) Tinea corporis in a 7-year-old boy.

"Why do they always teach us that it's easy and evil to do what we want and that we need discipline to restrain ourselves? It's the hardest thing in the world–to do what we want. And it takes the greatest kind of courage. I mean, what we really want." —**Ayn Rand**

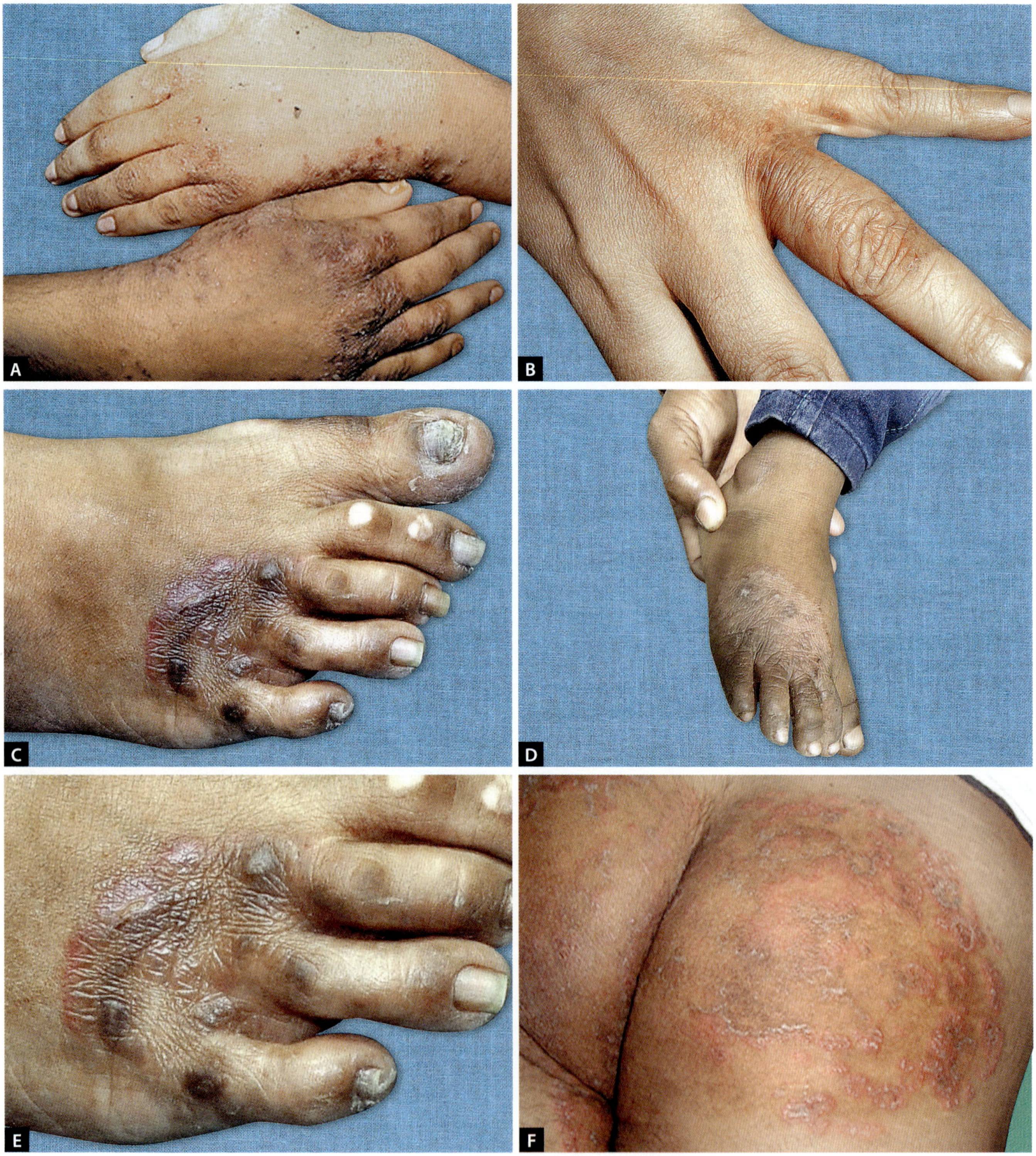

Figs. 36A to F: (A) Tinea corporis over hands; (B) Tinea manuum; (C) Tinea pedis; (D) Tinea pedis, note lichenified skin; (E) Same patient, close-up view; (F) Extensive tinea corporis over the gluteal region.

Trichophyton tonsurans or *Epidermophyton floccosum*. Transmission is by direct contact with infected peer groups and contact with pets such as puppies and kittens. Source of infection in children could be affected parents with tinea pedis, tinea unguium or onychomycosis. Lesions are circular, sharply marginated with a raised edge.

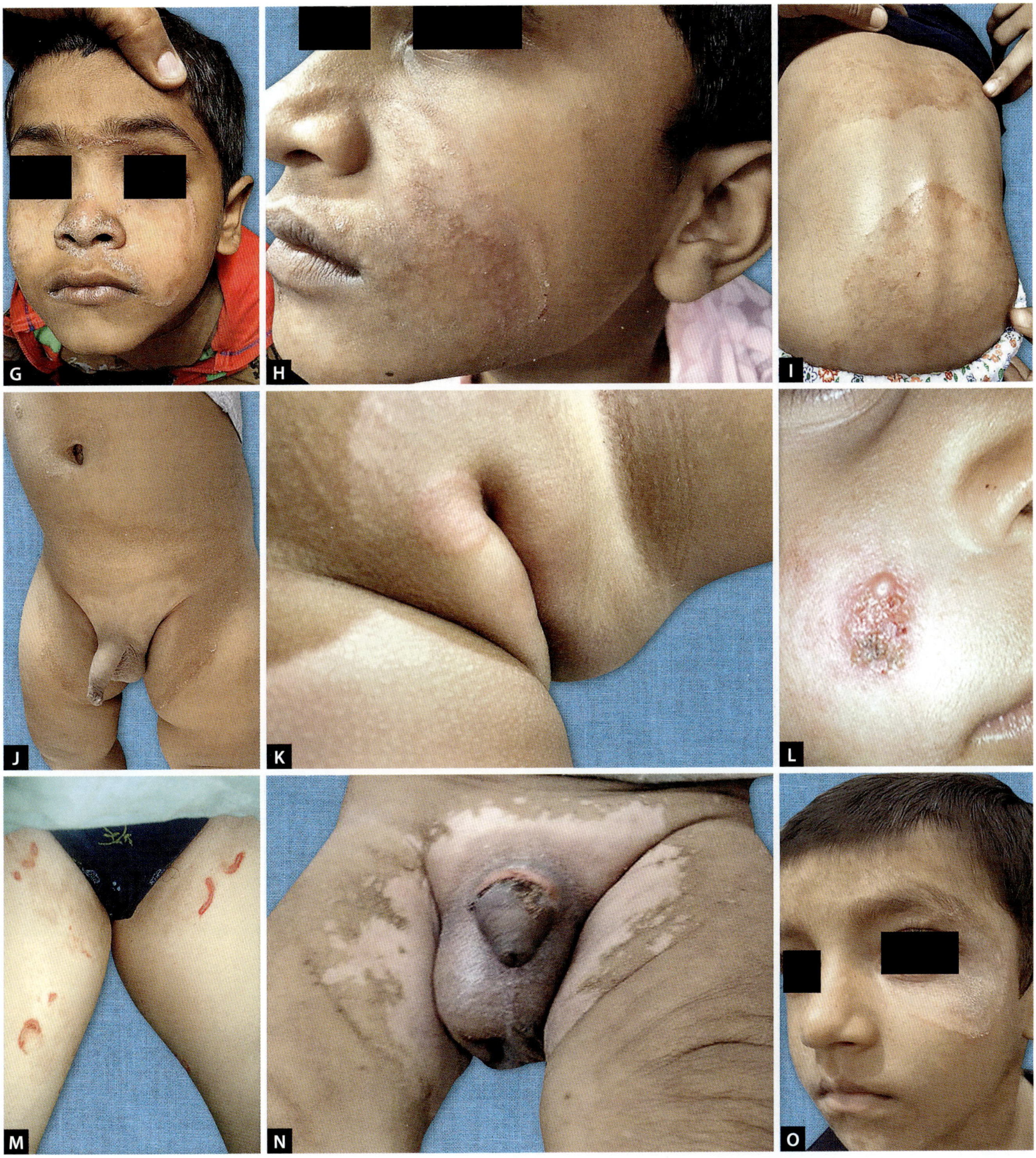

Figs. 36G to O: (G) Tinea faciei, note huge lesion; (H) Tinea faciei; (I) Extensive and giant tinea lesions; (J) Giant and extensive tinea corporis in a young boy; (K) Tinea lesion over vulva in a neonate; (L) Tinea incognito over face, note pustule; (M) Classical tinea incognito following abuse of potent steroid locally; (N) Steroid-modified tinea, note poststeroid hypopigmentation; (O) Steroid-modified tinea over face.

Single lesions occur or there may be multiple plaques. The degree of inflammation is variable. In inflammatory lesions, pustules or vesicles may dominate. Central resolution is common but not complete and the central skin may show postinflammatory pigmentation, a change of texture or residual erythematous dermal nodules.

"To improve is to change; to be perfect is to change often." —**Winston Churchill**

Tinea faciei is infection of the glabrous skin of the face with a dermatophyte fungus. Common symptoms include itching, burning, and exacerbation after sun exposure. Lesions may be simple papular lesions or flat patches of erythema. Sometimes annular or circinate lesions, indurated lesions with raised margins may be seen.

Management

For a single lesion, topical antifungals are sufficient. Various topical antifungals used are clotrimazole (1%), miconazole (2%), oxiconazole (1%), ketoconazole (2%), terbinafine (1%), butenafine (1%), and ciclopirox olamine (1%). Once or twice a day application for 2–3 weeks is recommended.

Systemic antifungals are required for extensive and/or persistent infection, associated infection over scalp and nails. Griseofulvin which is the drug of choice for tinea capitis is also fairly effective for other types of dermatophytosis. Ultramicronized form of griseofulvin has enhanced bioavailability and lower dosage schedule. It is given in a dose of 10–15 mg/kg of body weight/day for 4-6 weeks.

In case of intolerance to griseofulvin, other drugs which can be given are terbinafine 250 mg/day for older children (>40 kg) and adolescents for 14 days. Ketoconazole 4–7 mg/kg/day for 2–4 weeks, fluconazole 50 mg weekly for 4–6 weeks, itraconazole 100 mg daily for 10–14 days are alternative drugs.

TINEA INCOGNITO (FIGS. 36L TO R)

Tinea incognito refers to a dermatophytosis that has lost its usual clinical appearance, attributed to prior use of steroids or calcineurin inhibitors. It may present as irregular, poorly defined, erythematous desquamative plaques lacking the typical scale and elevated margin typical of cutaneous

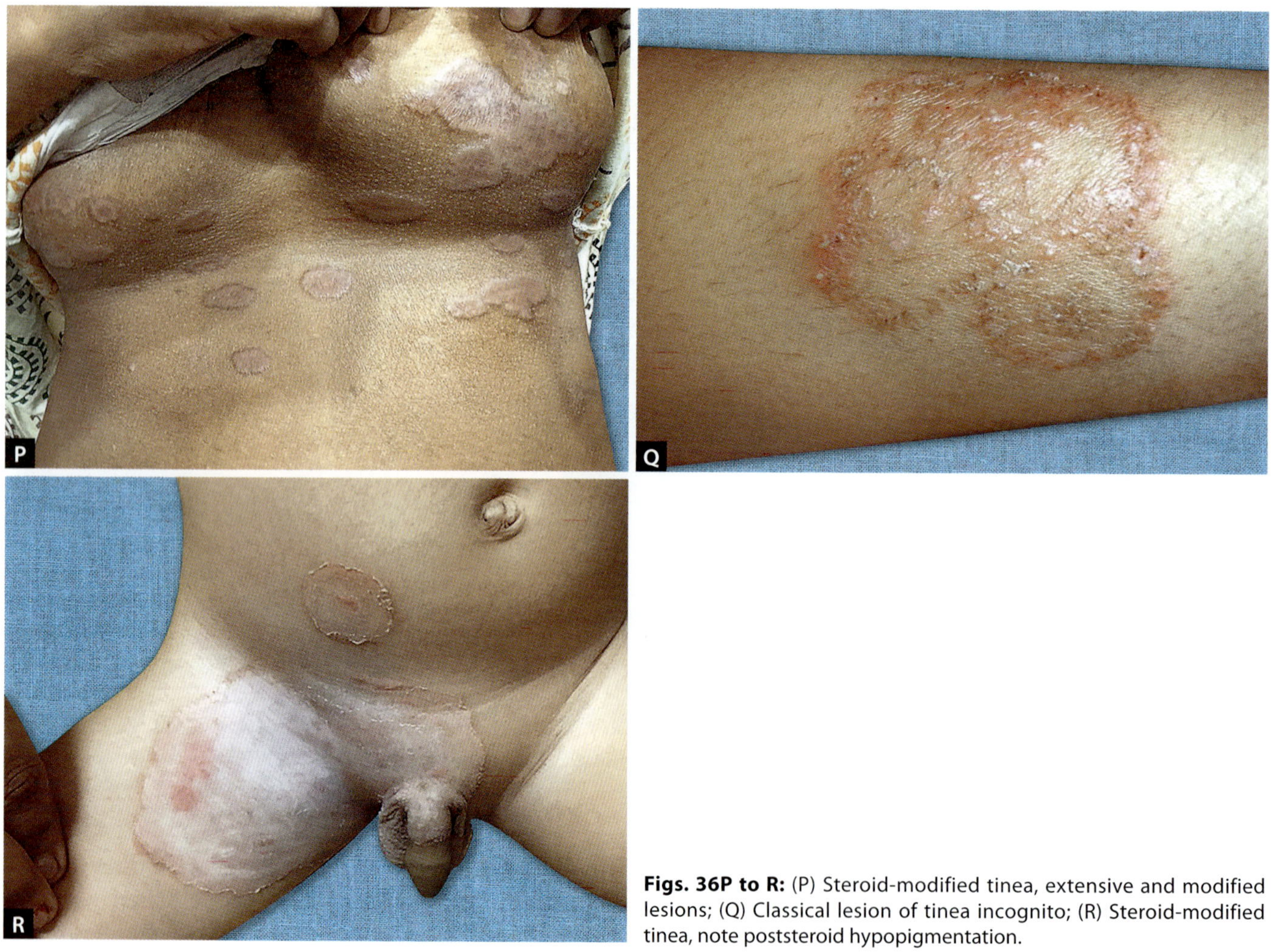

Figs. 36P to R: (P) Steroid-modified tinea, extensive and modified lesions; (Q) Classical lesion of tinea incognito; (R) Steroid-modified tinea, note poststeroid hypopigmentation.

"I can't change the direction of the wind, but I can adjust my sails to always reach my destination." **—Jimmy Dean**

dermatophytosis and can be mistaken for other pediatric cutaneous diseases, particularly atopic dermatitis. The atypical manifestations of tinea infection because of topical corticosteroid (TCS) abuse include a variety of skin presentations like lichenoid, pustular, rosacea-like, eczema-like, psoriasis-like, pityriasis rosea-like, purpura, etc. Pustular psoriasis-like presentation has also been reported in a child. Tinea pseudoimbricata or tinea indecisiva, "ring-within-a-ring" appearance has also been described recently as secondary to TCS misuse or some form of immunosuppression. Facial lesions modified by steroid use may raise suspicion of contact dermatitis and blepharitis due to *Demodex* mites (rosacea like dermatitis, folliculitis, and blepharitis). Tinea incognito is usually seen more in older children without any gender predilection. A high prevalence of clinical forms of tinea faciei and tinea corporis among cases of tinea incognito has been reported, while tinea capitis is unusual. *T. mentagrophytes* and *T. rubrum* are commonly isolated from lesions of tinea incognito. Local immunosuppression, barrier dysfunction, and increased multiplication of the dermatophytes result in atypical and persistent infections caused by TCS use. Intermittent use of TCS leads to suppression of inflammation and promotes survival of the dermatophyte which spreads centrifugally but also remains in the center due to inadequate clearance, resulting in the formation of multiple concentric rings with active borders.

Atypical presentations with history of topical steroid or topical calcineurin inhibitor (TCI) use, self-treatment or treatment by a quack or a nondermatologist, presence of other cutaneous adverse effects of steroid abuse such as striae, atrophy of skin and acneiform eruptions, and presence of satellite pustules and active borders in some case should raise the suspicion of tinea incognito. Suppression of steroid therapy usually makes the lesions more easily identifiable, although a mycological study [potassium hydroxide (KOH) examination and culture] can be performed to confirm the diagnosis. Stopping the use of topical steroids with proper use of antifungals is the mainstay of treatment.

Dermatophyte infection has been on a steep rise since a few years along with increased incidence of treatment-resistant cases. The unregulated over-the-counter sale of TCSs has been the main culprit for such atypical, chronic, and resistant cases. Steps need to be taken to educate the public and nonspecialist practitioners regarding the adverse effects of using topical steroids.

TINEA CAPITIS (FIGS. 37 TO 40J)

It is a dermatophytosis of the scalp caused by the *Trichophyton* and *Microsporum* species. It is the most common form of dermatophyte infection in children.

Etiology

Microsporum canis and *T. tonsurans* are the most common species. Other organisms include *Microsporum audouinii, Microsporum gypseum, Microsporum nanum, Microsporum ferrugineum, T. mentagrophytes, T. schoenleinii, T. tonsurans, T. verrucosum, and T. violaceum*. It is transmitted by close contact with affected children, shared brushes, combs, clothing, bed linen,

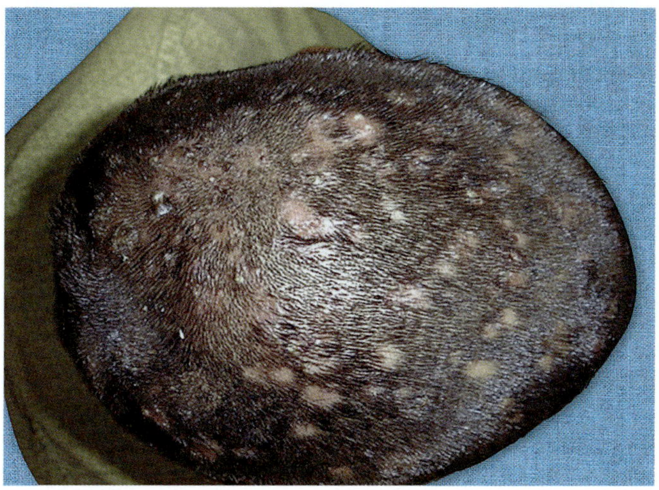

Fig. 37: Multiple alopecia patches with pustules in tinea capitis in an 11-year-old boy.

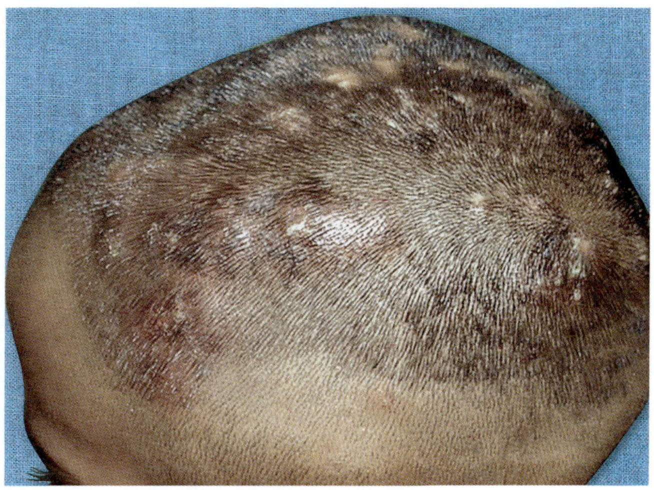

Fig. 38: Close-up view of scalp showing inflammatory papules and pustules.

"I want to sing like the birds sing, not worrying about who hears or what they think." **—Rumi**

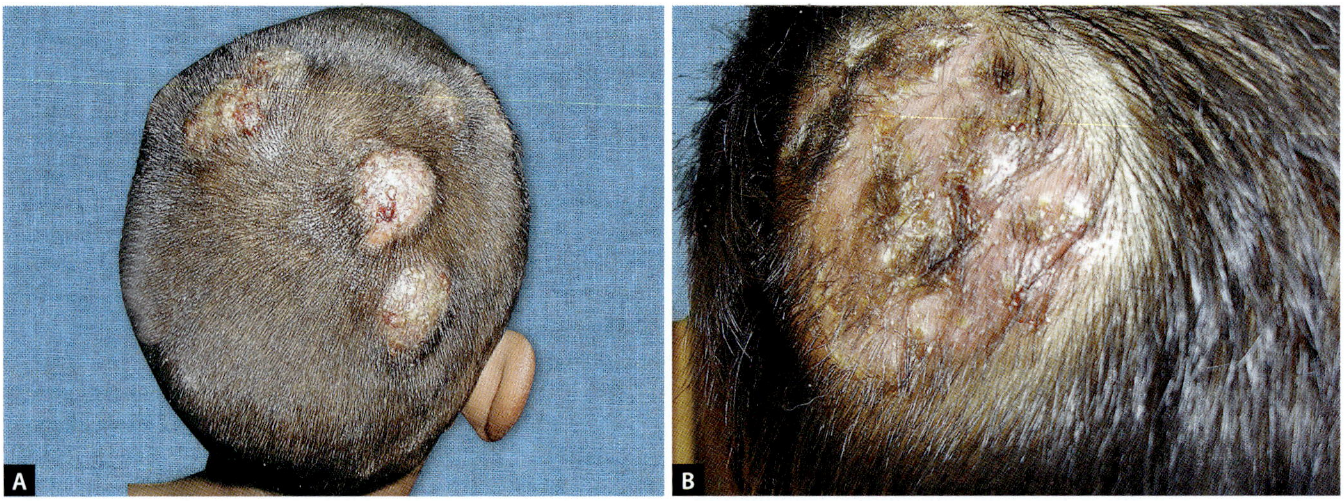

Figs. 39A and B: (A) Multiple lesions of kerion; (B) Kerion, close-up view.

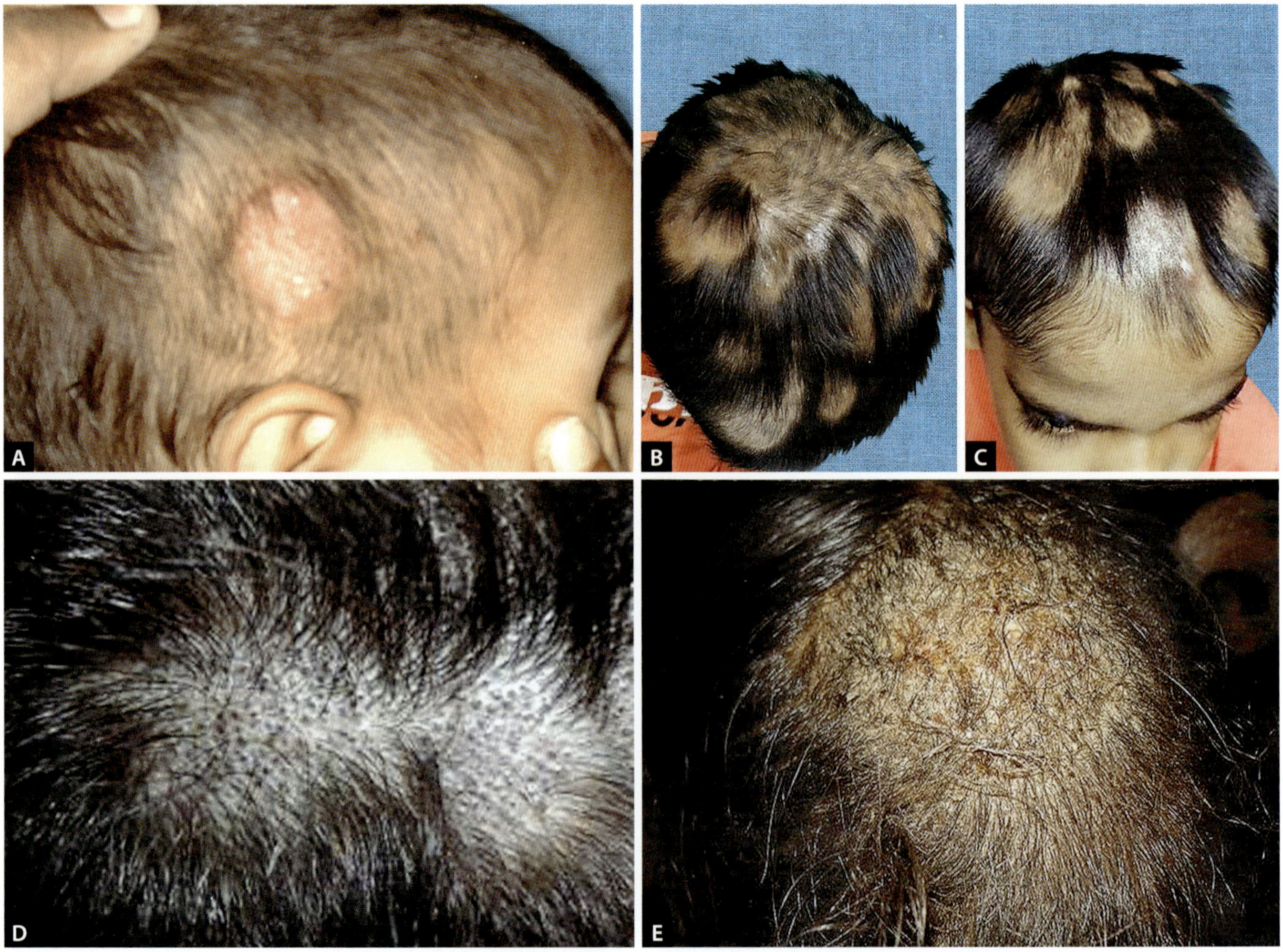

Figs. 40A to E: (A) Kerion in a 2-year-old girl; (B and C) Scarring alopecia secondary to extensive tinea with secondary infection; (D) Black dot tinea; (E) Favus, note scutula.

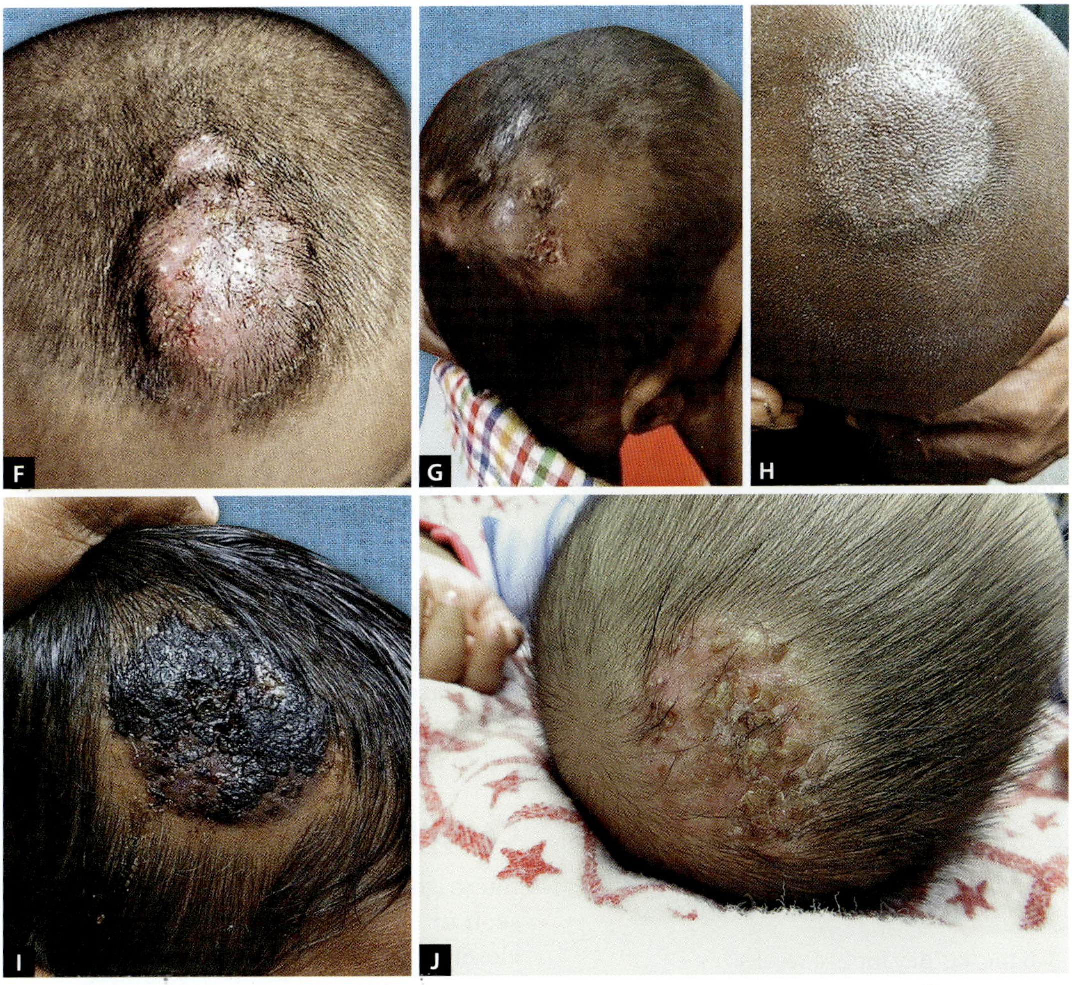

Figs. 40F to J: (F) Kerion, note boggy swelling studded with pustules; (G) Kerion on treatment; (H) Gray patch tinea; (I) Kerion; (J) Kerion in a neonate.

used hats and fomites. Reservoir of infection has been demonstrated in asymptomatic children contributing to the epidemiological factors.

Pathogenesis

Ectothrix dermatophytes establish in the perifollicular stratum corneum spreading around and into the hair shaft. In endothrix infection, the arthroconidia produced remain within the hair shaft replacing the intrapilar keratin.

Clinical Features

The non-inflammatory pattern is the most common occurring due to ectothrix organisms. This form is also called the seborrheic or gray patch type of tinea capitis. Hair in the affected area are dry and lusterless, break off easily just above the level of the scalp. They also can present as areas of well-defined round, hyperkeratotic scaly areas of alopecia.

Black dot tinea capitis is caused by the endothrix organisms. When hair loss occurs, it is broken off at the level of the scalp giving rise to the grouped black dots with diffuse scaling.

Inflammatory type of tinea capitis is seen by the geophilic or zoophilic fungi. It is a result of hypersensitivity reaction to the infection. It presents as an inflamed boggy swelling with studded pustules and purulent discharge. It generally heals with scarring alopecia. It is often associated with pain, pruritus, and cervical lymphadenopathy.

Tinea favosa is a chronic dermatophytic infection of the scalp characterized by thick yellow crusts called scutula within the hair follicles which leads to scarring alopecia.

"The secret of change is to focus all of your energy not on fighting the old, but on building the new." —**Socrates**

Differential Diagnosis

- Seborrheic dermatitis
- Scalp psoriasis
- Pyodermas
- Perifolliculitis capitis
- Alopecia areata
- Trichotillomania

Laboratory Diagnosis

The diagnosis can be made by a KOH mount of the hair and scales on the scalp. Fungal culture is warranted in view of strong suspicion of a negative KOH or a partially treated case. Sabouraud's dextrose agar is the most commonly used culture medium.

Treatment

Griseofulvin: 10–15 mg/kg/day of the ultramicronized form for 6–8 weeks taken with a fatty meal, 20–25 mg/kg/day of the micronized form for 6–8 weeks. The disadvantages include poor compliance, bitter taste, photosensitivity, and gastrointestinal side effects.

Fluconazole: 6 mg/kg/day for a total of 2–3 weeks.

Itraconazole: 5 mg/kg/day for 4–6 weeks have been effective. Pulse therapy at 5 mg/kg/day for 1 week/month for three pulses has also been used successfully.

Terbinafine: 3–6 mg/kg/day for 2–4 weeks.

Adjuvant therapies include shampoos consisting of selenium sulfide, zinc pyrithione, povidone-iodine or ketoconazole.

Ketoconazole shampoos may be used to prevent household transmission.

General management includes good hygiene, wearing loose cotton clothes, washing clothes separately and drying them in sunlight. Sharing of clothes, hats, jackets, hair brushes and toys should be discouraged in children. Treatment of affected family members and close contacts is necessary. Education of parents and school staff is necessary in children.

TINEA PEDIS AND TINEA MANUUM (FIGS. 40K TO M)

Tinea pedis is a fungal infection of the soles of feet with predilection for toe web space. It is commonly seen in adolescents and sometimes in prepubertal children. Use of occlusive footwear for prolonged period, increased sweating, and source of infection in the family can be predisposing factors in children. *T. tonsurans* is commonly associated with tinea pedis in children. Scaling and fissuring predominate.

In others vesiculopustular lesions, erythema and maceration are found. The infection starts and may remain in between and along toes. However, the lesions can spread over the dorsal and plantar surfaces as well. Patients complain of intense itching and at times burning sensation. Similarly, involvement of palms and web spaces is known as tinea manuum. Tinea manuum of one hand with tinea pedis of both feet is termed as "two feet-one hand syndrome".

Diagnosis

Diagnosis is confirmed by KOH preparation and culture of fungus.

Treatment

Treatment includes topical antifungals like clotrimazole, miconazole, ketoconazole or terbinafine creams along with oral antifungals like griseofulvin, fluconazole and terbinafine preparations.

CANDIDAL INTERTRIGO (FIG. 40N)

Intertrigo is one of the most common forms of candidiasis seen in the pediatric population which occurs on two closely opposed skin surfaces such as the axillae, scrotum, inguinal folds, intergluteal folds, inframammary folds, neck creases in infants, posterior auricular region and web spaces between the toes and fingers, as well as abdominal folds, especially in obese children in response to friction, humidity, maceration, or reduced air circulation. It initially appears as a minimal erythema of the folds. The moisture and increased temperature on the surface of opposing skinfolds provide a suitable medium for the growth of *Candida* and bacteria. Infants are at an increased risk to develop intertrigo due to drooling and short neck structure with prominent skinfolds and a flexed position. Chronic occlusion of the skin by wet diapers is also a leading risk factor in infants. Older children are also affected frequently. Other risk factors include tight underclothes, poor hygiene, malnutrition, inflammatory skin conditions such as psoriasis, diabetes mellitus, obesity, use of corticosteroids or wide-spectrum antibiotics, and immunosuppression including HIV infection.

Clinically, candidal intertrigo presents with erythematous and macerated plaques and erosions with satellite papulopustules and peripheral scaling. These papules

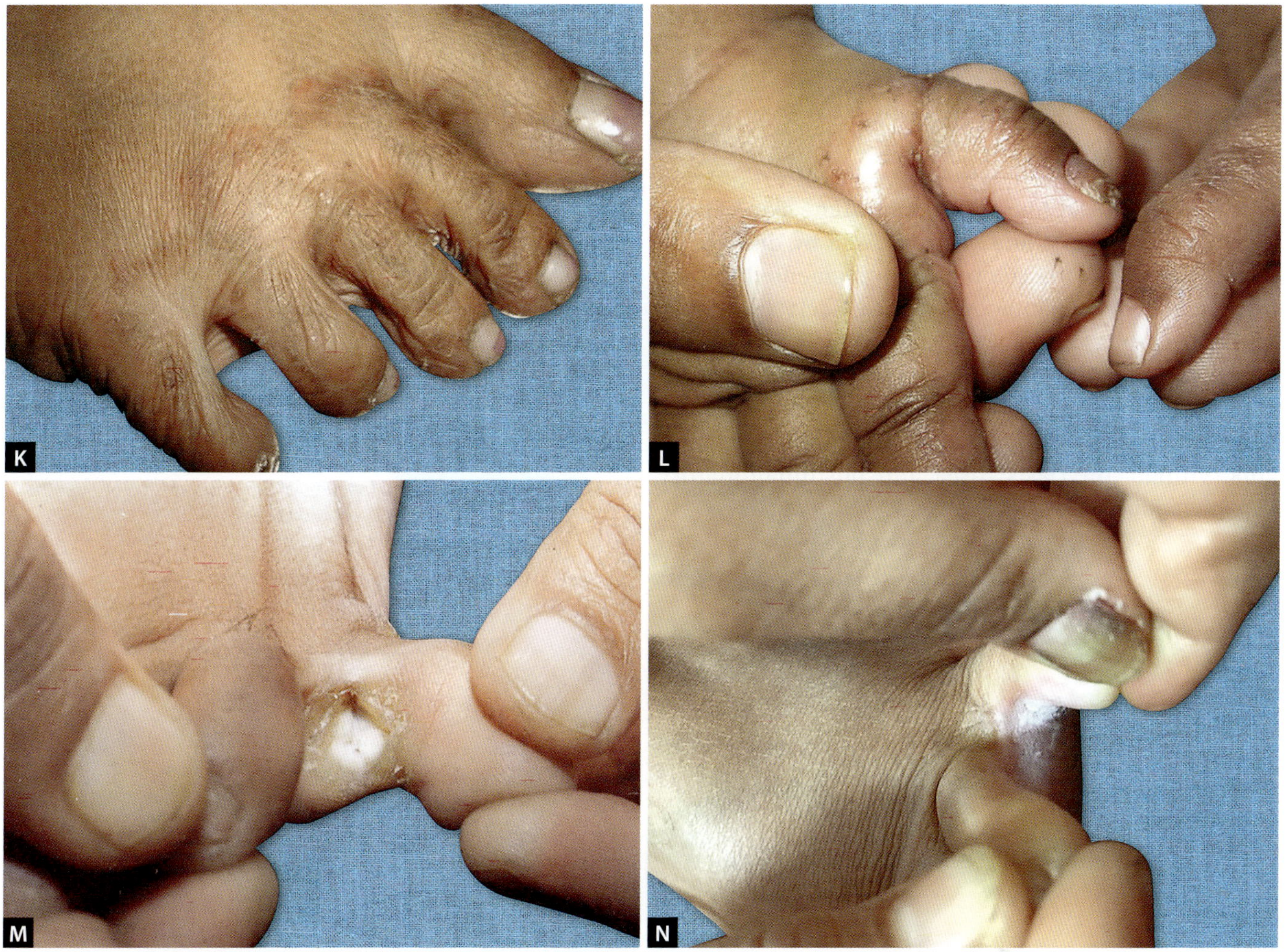

Figs. 40K to N: (K) Tinea pedis in a 15-year-old boy, note dorsal involvement; (L) Tinea manuum in an infant; (M) Tinea pedis; (N) Candidal intertrigo.

and pustules rapidly rupture, leading to the formation of a red base with a surrounding collarette of epidermis. Pruritus and pain may be associated. Differential diagnosis includes irritant diaper dermatitis, tinea cruris, contact dermatitis, atopic dermatitis, inverse psoriasis, seborrheic dermatitis, erythrasma, bacterial intertrigo, herpes simplex infection, and langerhans cell histiocytosis. Streptococcal intertrigo presents as well demarcated, intensely erythematous, weeping and superficially eroded areas lacking satellite pustules and associated with a foul odor.

Diagnosis is usually clinical. Laboratory investigations may be required in chronic, resistant, and recurrent cases. KOH preparation and calcofluor white staining of smears show presence of pseudohyphae or yeast forms under direct microscopic examination. Biopsy may be required to differentiate from psoriasis and other dermatoses of intertriginous areas. Identification of septa-free hyphae and yeast forms in periodic acid–Schiff (PAS)-stained histopathological samples is diagnostic for *Candida*. Management includes:

- Treatment of active infection by topical antifungals (clotrimazole, econazole, ketoconazole creams) applied two to three times daily
- Minimizing moisture and reducing friction, aeration of affected area, daily cleansing with a mild cleanser and use of barrier creams
- Addressing predisposing factors to reduce the risk of recurrence like weight loss in obese patients and treatment of coexisting diabetes mellitus.

Systemic treatment is required only in severe cases with widespread intertrigo with multiple site involvement, significant ulceration, and/or numerous areas of exudate and pustules. Low strength TCS in severe cases and oral

"Change will not come if we wait for some other person or some other time. We are the ones we've been waiting for. We are the change that we seek."

–Barack Obama

antibiotic in cases of secondary bacterial infections may be required.

PITYRIASIS VERSICOLOR (FIGS. 41 AND 42)

This is a superficial fungal infection of the skin caused by *Malassezia* yeasts and characterized by discrete or concrescent scaly discolored (hypopigmented/hyper-pigmented) areas mainly on the face, neck, and upper trunk. The primary lesion is a sharply demarcated macule characterized by a fine branny scaling. The eruption shows large confluent areas, scattered oval patches and outlying macules. Differential diagnosis includes pityriasis alba, vitiligo, pityriasis rosea and postinflammatory hypopigmentation.

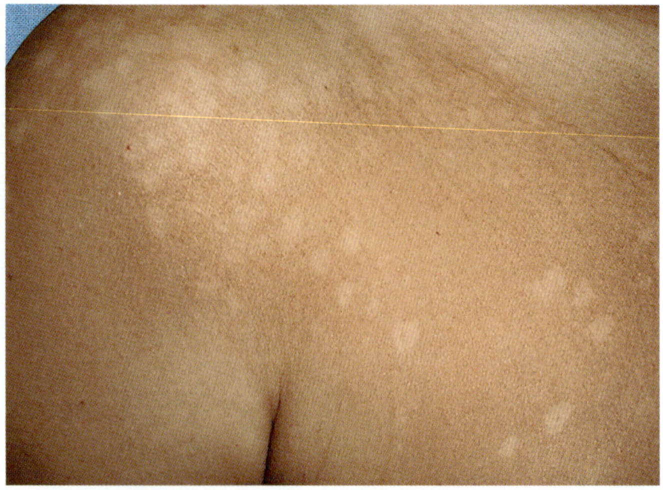

Fig. 41: Hypopigmented macules of pityriasis versicolor over the chest in an adolescent boy.

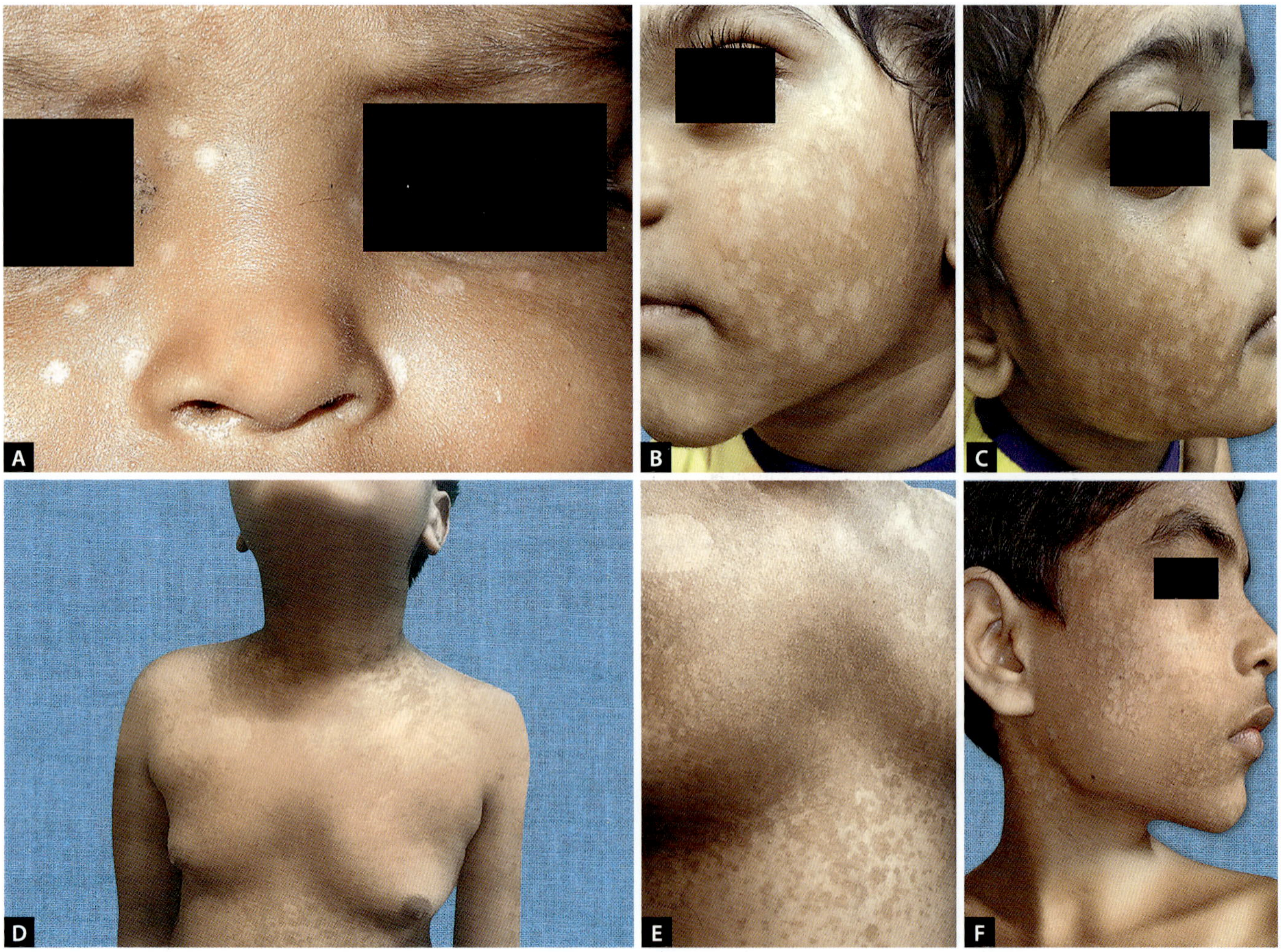

Figs. 42A to F: (A) Multiple hypopigmented scaly macules of pityriasis versicolor over face in a child; (B) Pityriasis versicolor; (C) Same child; (D) Brownish scales in pityriasis versicolor; (E) Brownish scales in pityriasis versicolor, another child; (F) Pityriasis versicolor over face and neck in a 7-year-old boy.

"The greatest discovery of all time is that a person can change his future by merely changing his attitude." —**Oprah Winfrey**

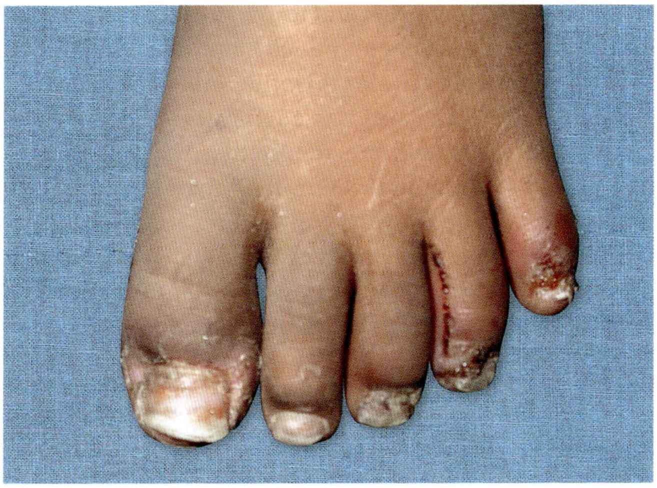

Fig. 43: Swelling and oozing from multiple nail folds in acute paronychia, nail plates are intact.

Treatment

Topical application of 2.5% selenium sulfide solution once a week for 3–4 weeks, then once a month for 3–4 months is effective. Other agents that are found effective are topical clotrimazole, ketoconazole, miconazole, terbinafine, and sertaconazole. For extensive and persistent lesions, various systemic antifungals which can be used are oral ketoconazole 200–400 mg/day for 5–7 days, fluconazole 50–100 mg single dose or itraconazole 100–200 mg/day for 5–7 days.

PARONYCHIA (FIGS. 43 AND 44A)

"Paronychia" means inflammation of the periungual skin. The etiology of paronychia can be acute or chronic. Chronic paronychia is mostly caused by candidal and other yeasts. Acute paronychia is predominantly a bacterial infection caused by *Staphylococcus*. Clinically, paronychia presents as swelling of the posterior and lateral nail folds. The swelling is associated with redness. In most of the cases, the cuticle is lost in acute or chronic paronychia. In acute paronychia, the nail fold swelling is associated with acute localized pain over the nail folds. In chronic paronychia, there is associated mild tenderness over the nail folds. The nail plates remain unaffected.

Treatment

For acute paronychia, a course of antistaphylococcal antibiotic for 5–7 days usually suffices. If there is collection of pus below the nail folds, an incision and drainage of the pus is mandatory. In cases of chronic paronychia, oral fluconazole, itraconazole or terbinafine on a long-term weekly basis for 3–6 months is often helpful. Local antifungal, although, has a limited role, is often helpful when applied over the nail folds regularly for few months.

CANDIDIASIS (FIG. 44B)

Candidiasis is an acute or chronic infection of the skin caused by *Candida* yeast. In infants, it usually presents as oral candidiasis, diaper candidiasis or intertrigo. Clinically, it presents as small satellite pustules, papulovesicles on the flexural areas along with maceration. Topical antifungals are the treatment of choice.

ORAL THRUSH (FIG. 44C)

Oral thrush, manifesting as pseudomembranous candidiasis is the most common form of oropharyngeal candidiasis caused by local overgrowth of *Candida albicans* and rarely by other species such as *Candida glabrata* and *Candida tropicalis*. It occurs in 20–40% of healthy children within the first year of life, most commonly encountered in the neonates either from passage through the vaginal canal or horizontally from the environment. The prevalence is much higher in bottle-fed versus breastfed infants. Predisposing factors that provoke oral thrush in infants and older children include cellular immune deficiency, treatment with antibiotics, inhaled glucocorticoids, chemotherapy or radiation therapy, impaired salivary gland function, diabetes, Cushing's syndrome, local trauma, poor denture hygiene, and malnutrition. Chronic or recurrent oral thrush in children suggests an underlying immunodeficiency. The common underlying link observed between all known host systemic conditions associated with oral *Candida* overgrowth is a functional immunodeficiency in the T-helper 17 (Th17) CD4+ cell subset. Fungal overgrowth results in accumulation of hyphae along with keratin, fibrin, necrotic tissue, and other products of epithelial cell desquamation resulting in the formation of confluent white plaques adherent on the hard and soft palate, tongue, buccal mucosa or oropharynx. Scraping of these plaques reveals an erythematous base with bleeding which aids in differentiating *Candida* infection from milk on the tongue. Patients are usually asymptomatic. Infants may present with poor feeding because of pain and older children may complain of a "cottony" feeling in the mouth, loss of taste, and sometimes pain on eating and swallowing. Oral thrush should be differentiated from viral tonsillar exudates,

"When the world pushes you to your knees, you're in the perfect position to pray." **—Rumi**

geographic tongue, recurrent aphthous stomatitis, burns, nutritional deficiency, as well as striated lichen planus in older children and oral hairy leukoplakia.

Diagnosis is primarily made clinically based on the characteristic white plaques. It can be confirmed by Gram stain or KOH preparation on the scrapings which demonstrates budding yeasts with or without pseudohyphae. Fungal culture is usually not required except in recalcitrant or recurrent cases. Evaluation for cellular immunodeficiency is recommended in children with recalcitrant, recurrent, or extensive oropharyngeal candidiasis and for children ≥12 months of age who develop oropharyngeal candidiasis in the absence of a predisposing factor.

In healthy term, asymptomatic infants at low risk of invasive candidiasis, treatment may not be required. Nystatin oral suspensions and topical azoles may be used for noninvasive mucocutaneous candidiasis. Systemic antifungal agents, preferably fluconazole (3 mg/kg, once a day for 7–14 days) is used only in refractory cases and if the child is immunocompromised. Decontamination of items that are placed in the infant's mouth (e.g., bottle nipples and pacifiers) by boiling and of mothers' breasts by application of an antifungal medication is important to prevent recurrences. Older children with mild thrush (<50% of the oral mucosa and absence of deep, erosive lesions), topical nystatin or clotrimazole is used. Systemic antifungal, fluconazole (3–6 mg/kg/day for 7–14 days) is recommended for moderate to severe thrush and for mild thrush in immunocompromised children. Intravenous antifungal therapy may be required if there is significant oropharyngeal pain and if there is

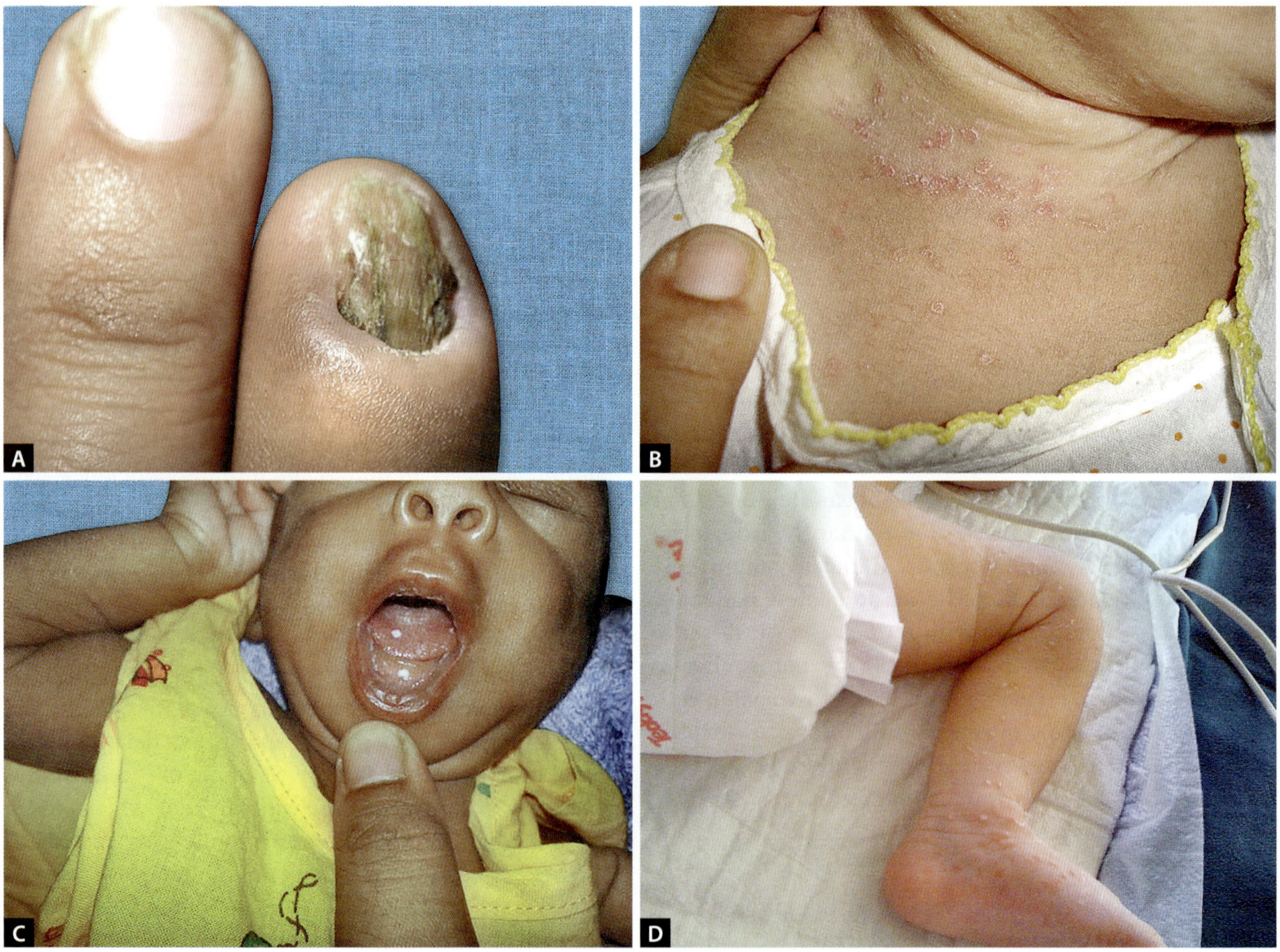

Figs. 44A to D: (A) Swelling of lateral and posterior nail folds in a single nail with destruction of nail plate in chronic paronychia; (B) Candidiasis over neck folds; (C) Oral thrush; (D) Congenital cutaneous candidiasis.

"You've done it before and you can do it now. See the positive possibilities. Redirect the substantial energy of your frustration and turn it into positive, effective, unstoppable determination." —**Ralph Marston**

no response to oral fluconazole in immunocompromised individuals.

CONGENITAL CUTANEOUS CANDIDIASIS (FIG. 44D)

Congenital cutaneous candidiasis (CCC) is a rare condition caused by exposure to *Candida* species through ascending infection in utero with around 100 cases being reported in the literature. It presents at birth or within the first 6 days of life presenting either as diffuse skin eruption without any systemic symptoms to severe systemic disease with or without cutaneous involvement. Vaginal colonization by *C. albicans* is usually seen in 20–30% of pregnant women, though only 1% of newborns develop CCC. However, it is suspected to have a greater prevalence since it can often go unnoticed due to its self-limiting and benign course in most cases. Non-*C. albicans* species such as *Candida parapsilosis* and *Candida ciferri* have been rarely reported to be the causative organism.

Candida species causes skin lesions by direct exposure to infected amniotic fluid as it can invade and penetrate intact membranes, while systemic infection occurs by placental invasion and/or the umbilical cord. Risk factors for CCC include prematurity, low birth weight, maternal vaginal candidiasis and presence of a foreign body in the cervix (intrauterine devices or sutures placed for cervical cerclage), chorioamnionitis, and amniocentesis. It is not associated with maternal age, parity, diabetes, type of delivery, prolonged labor, rupture of membranes, or maternal antibiotic or corticosteroid use. Congenital immunodeficiency should be suspected in case of systemic disease.

Congenital cutaneous candidiasis presents as generalized maculopapular and/or pustular rash on an erythematous base, as well as vesicles and blisters, most commonly located on the trunk, extensor surfaces, and intertriginous areas. Involvement of palms and soles with sparing of mucosae and napkin area is often characteristic of CCC. Paronychia and nail dystrophy can also be present. Skin lesions usually disappear within 1 or 2 weeks accompanied with peeling. Lesions on palms and soles may persist for a longer duration. In full-term neonates, the disease course is usually benign and self-limiting whereas prematurity and low birth weight are risk factors for developing systemic infection presenting as burn-like dermatitis, respiratory distress, hepatomegaly, hyperglycemia, glycosuria, sepsis or even early neonatal death. Funisitis and chorioamnionitis presenting as yellow-white plaques on the placenta and umbilical cord can occur.

Congenital cutaneous candidiasis should be differentiated from neonatal candidiasis which is acquired during passage through an infected birth canal and appears after the first week of life and commonly presents as thrush, perianal, and diaper dermatitis. Other diseases resembling CCC include impetigo, staphylococcal pustulosis, infection by *Listeria monocytogenes*, herpes simplex virus, varicella zoster virus and enterovirus, syphilis, erythema toxicum neonatorum, transient neonatal pustular melanosis, milia, miliaria, congenital ichthyosiform erythroderma, Ritter's disease, Leiner's disease, incontinentia pigmenti, epidermolysis bullosa, and Langerhans cell histiocytosis.

Diagnosis can be made clinically, but has to be confirmed by KOH preparation of the skin scrapings demonstrating budding yeast and pseudohyphae, skin biopsy with PAS staining, fungal culture from skin (two or more skin rash sites should be tested), mucous membrane, placenta and/or umbilical cord. Culture remains the gold standard method. Blood, urine, and cerebrospinal fluid (CSF) cultures are obtained to rule out systemic involvement, but they are not necessary for the diagnosis.

Full-term infants with CCC limited to the skin and without any risk factors for disseminated disease, topical antifungal therapy, preferably imidazoles is considered the first-line treatment and should be continued until the lesions have resolved. Presence of risk factors and systemic dissemination of infection requires parenteral antifungal therapy. Amphotericin B (0.5–1 mg/kg/day), lipid-associated amphotericin B preparations (3–5 mg/kg/day), and fluconazole (6–12 mg/kg/day) are the preferred agents, given for a minimum of 21–28 days. Echinocandins (caspofungin or micafungin) may also be used.

CHRONIC MUCOCUTANEOUS CANDIDIASIS (FIGS. 45 TO 49)

Chronic mucocutaneous candidiasis (CMC) represents a group of disorders characterized by progressive and recurrent infections of the nails, skin, and mucous membranes with *C. albicans*. Affected individuals have an ineffective immune response against this organism.

Etiopathogenesis

Affected individuals have a defective T cell-mediated immunity which hampers the clearance of the organism. Autoimmune polyendocrinopathy

"Just take any step, whether small or large. And then another and repeat day after day. It may take months, maybe years, but the path to success will become clear." —**Aaron Ross**

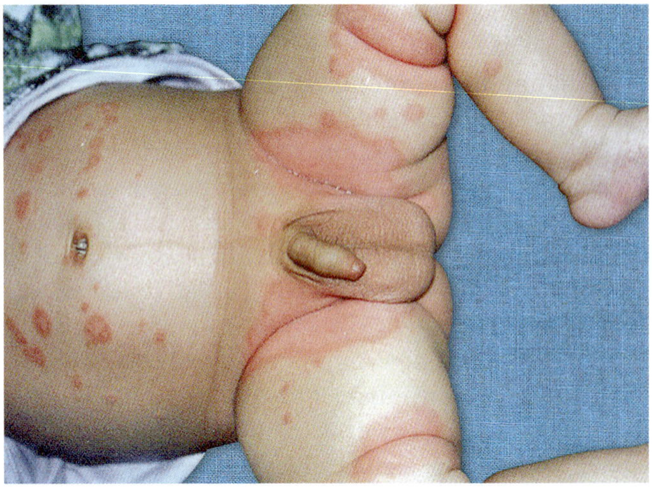

Fig. 45: Extensive involvement of folds in chronic mucocutaneous candidiasis (CMC).

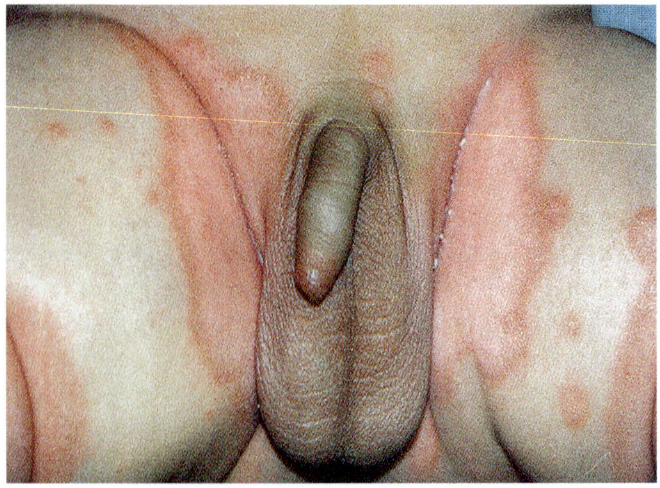

Fig. 46: Chronic mucocutaneous candidiasis, close-up view.

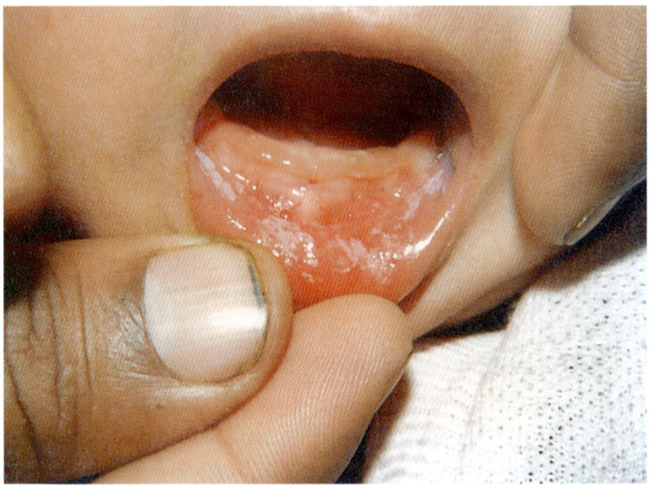

Fig. 47: Oral candidiasis in chronic mucocutaneous candidiasis.

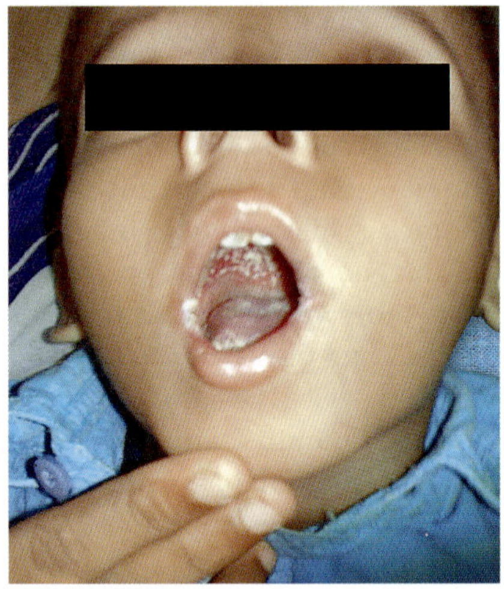

Fig. 48: Oral lesions of chronic mucocutaneous candidiasis.

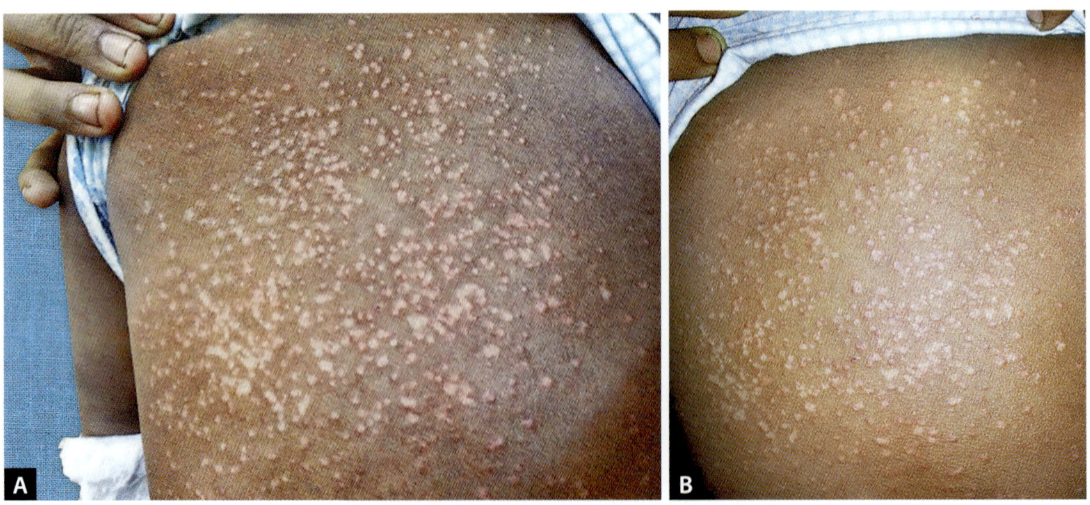

Figs. 49A and B: (A) Extensive skin involvement in chronic mucocutaneous candidiasis (CMC); (B) CMC, back view.

"Be brave. Take Risks. Nothing can substitute experience." —**Paulo Coelho**

candidiasis-ectodermal dystrophy syndrome (APECED) is a condition where there is failure to delete autoreactive T cells thus leading to an autoimmune response. CMC can be noted in the background of immunodeficiency associated with *DOCK8* and *STAT3* deficiency causing hyperimmunoglobulin E (IgE) syndrome. CMC can result due to interleukin (IL)-17F mutations, *Dectin-1* mutation, increased production of IL-6 or inadequate production of IL-23.

Clinical Features

The clinical severity ranges from recurrent treatment-resistant oral thrush or a few erythematous scaly plaques and dystrophic nails to severe generalized, crusted granulomatous plaques. These plaques mostly occur on the scalp, periorificial and intertriginous sites. Scalp infection may lead to scarring alopecia. The nails are thickened, brittle, and discolored with associated paronychia. Chronic lesions in the mouth, esophageal, genital and laryngeal mucosae can lead to stricture formation.

Subgroups of CMC described in children and adolescents are as follows:

- *Familial pure CMC*: It is an autosomal dominant condition. Oral candidiasis begins by the age of 2 years and nail and skin involvement occurs commonly.
- *Chronic localized candidiasis*: Majority have cutaneous lesions by 5 years with thick adherent crusts with concomitant oral candidiasis.
- *Autoimmune polyendocrinopathy candidiasis ectodermal dystrophy*: It is caused by mutations of the *AIRE* gene. In this condition, candidal infections begin by the age of 5 years and present with candidal granuloma of the scalp and face. Associated endocrinopathies include hypoparathyroidism, hypoadrenocorticism, hypogonadism, thyroid dysfunction, diabetes mellitus, and hypopituitarism. Cutaneous associations include alopecia areata, vitiligo, and lupus like panniculitis. Other disorders like pernicious anemia, chronic diarrhea, and malabsorption with dental anomalies may be present.
- *CARD9-associated CMC*: Chronic oral and vulvovaginal candidiasis is present. Fatal candidal infections of the brain in the second decade of life may occur in some individuals.
- *Dectin-1 deficiency*: It presents with chronic or recurrent vulvovaginal candidiasis and onychomycosis.
- *Late-onset CMC*: Infections present during early adolescence and is milder than other subgroups.
- *Familial chronic nail candidiasis*: The onset is in infancy and is limited to the nails of the hands and feet.
- *CMC-associated with keratitis*: CMC can occur with alopecia and keratitis. It has also been described with APECED syndrome and keratitis-ichthyosis-deafness (KID) syndrome.
- CMC-associated with other immunodeficiency disorders like severe combined immunodeficiency, DiGeorge syndrome, hyper-IgE syndrome and acrodermatitis enteropathica.

Differential Diagnosis

- Candidal infections
- Consideration for HIV infection
- Immunodysregulation polyendocrinopathy enteropathy X-linked (IPEX) syndrome

Laboratory Diagnosis

Demonstration of *Candida* repeatedly from the lesional site in spite of treatment. Gene mutation analysis study may be done.

Treatment

Patients may benefit from long-term therapy with systemic antifungals like itraconazole, fluconazole, and terbinafine.

Hematopoietic stem cell transplantation, fetal thymus grafts and leukocyte infusion have also been tried.

Annual evaluation of patients for the development of endocrinopathies needs to be done in cases with family history of CMC or APECED syndrome.

NOCARDIOSIS (FIG. 50A)

Nocardiosis is caused by a group of aerobic, gram-positive and weakly acid-fast filamentous bacteria *Nocardia* species. They occur predominantly in soil, house dust and decaying organic plant material. Nocardiosis are of two types: (1) primary cutaneous and (2) disseminated. Primary cutaneous nocardiosis is seen mostly in immunocompetent individuals; source of infection is exogenous through trauma and most common causative organism is *Nocardia brasiliensis*. Skin involvement is seen in 10% of disseminated cases. Underlying common causes of immunosuppression seen in disseminated form are organ transplant, acquired immunodeficiency syndrome (AIDS), hematological malignancy, and prolonged steroid therapy. Immunocompromised patients mainly present with lung infection most commonly caused by *Nocardia asteroides.*

Clinical Features

Cutaneous lesions vary from cellulitis, nodulo-pustule, ulcero-bullous to lymphocutaneous nodules in sporotrichoid pattern. Cellulitis most commonly involves lower extremities whereas sporotrichoid form involves upper extremities. It is rarely seen in children.

Laboratory Investigations

Direct microscopic examination reveals gram-positive delicate filamentous bacteria branching at right angle. But filaments are short and fragmentary than those of *Actinomyces*. Sulfur granules is seen only in disseminated forms. Culture is difficult. Splendore–Hoeppli phenomenon reveals smooth eosinophilic deposits than club-shaped seen in *Actinomyces.*

Differential Diagnoses

Important differentials are sporotrichosis, atypical mycobacterial infection, leishmaniasis, and deep fungal infections.

Treatment

Appropriate antibiotics and surgical debridement are the two mainstays of treatment modalities. Trimethoprim-sulfamethoxazole and amikacin are highly effective.

ACTINOMYCOSIS (FIGS. 50B AND C)

Actinomycosis is caused by a group of anaerobic, gram-positive filamentous bacteria named *Actinomyces*, previously wrongly classified as fungi due to their branching filaments producing tendency. These are the part of normal flora of respiratory, gastrointestinal, and genitourinary tract. Several species have been implicated; few of them are *Actinomyces israelii, Actinomyces gerencseriae*, and *Propionibacterium propionicum.* Though *Actinomyces* are the main culprit but in most of the cases it is a polymicrobial infection with other members of normal flora acting synergistically.

Clinical Features

Middle-aged men are most commonly affected. Infection most commonly affects cervicofacial area followed by abdominal wall, pelvis, and thoracic region. Mode of infection is endogenous; organism gains entry through a breach in mucous membrane. For cervicofacial cases, source of infection is periapical abscess or following any dental procedure. Whereas extension of infection to the thoracic and pelvic wall occurs from lung infection and ascending infection of female genital tract using intrauterine device respectively. Abdominal actinomycosis is a consequence of ruptured appendix, diverticulitis or gastrointestinal surgery. Patients initially present with inflammatory infiltrative firm plaque or nodule ultimately turn into abscess and draining sinuses.

Investigations

Sulfur granules, a clump of filamentous bacteria may be present in exudates but not always and not specific. Direct examination of gram-stained material shows delicate branching filaments. Brown–Brenn or Giemsa staining of tissue sample may reveal Splendore–Hoeppli phenomenon, eosinophilic club of immunoglobulin around granules. Culture is difficult.

Differential Diagnoses

Differentials vary according to site. Few important differentials are TB, odontogenic abscess, neoplasms, inflammatory bowel disease, and hidradenitis suppurativa.

Treatment

Effective antibiotics are large dose of penicillin G, ampicillin, and erythromycin. Debulking surgery with removal of sinus tract and draining of sinuses are required in many cases.

SPOROTRICHOSIS (FIGS. 50D TO F)

Sporotrichosis is a subcutaneous mycosis which usually affects gardeners or laborers. Direct injury from contaminated rose thorn, wood or other minor penetrating injury is the usual mode of transmission. The infection is caused by dimorphic fungi of the genus *Sporothrix*. Animal to human transmission is rare except through scratching of cat's claw. Rose thorn, grass, sphagnum moss, and barberry shrubs are the common source of infection. Sporotrichosis does not respect any geographical boundary. Humidity and raised temperature favor the infection. Presentation and course of the infection depends upon host immunity and virulence of the organism. In naïve hosts, earliest lesion would be a small papule or nodule at the injury site which eventually heals with ulceration or disappears. This event is followed by appearance of dermal or

"If your startup builds a room full of pessimists and you have one optimist at the table, then I think you're in the wrong business. But the other way around is invaluable and necessary." —**David Cohen**

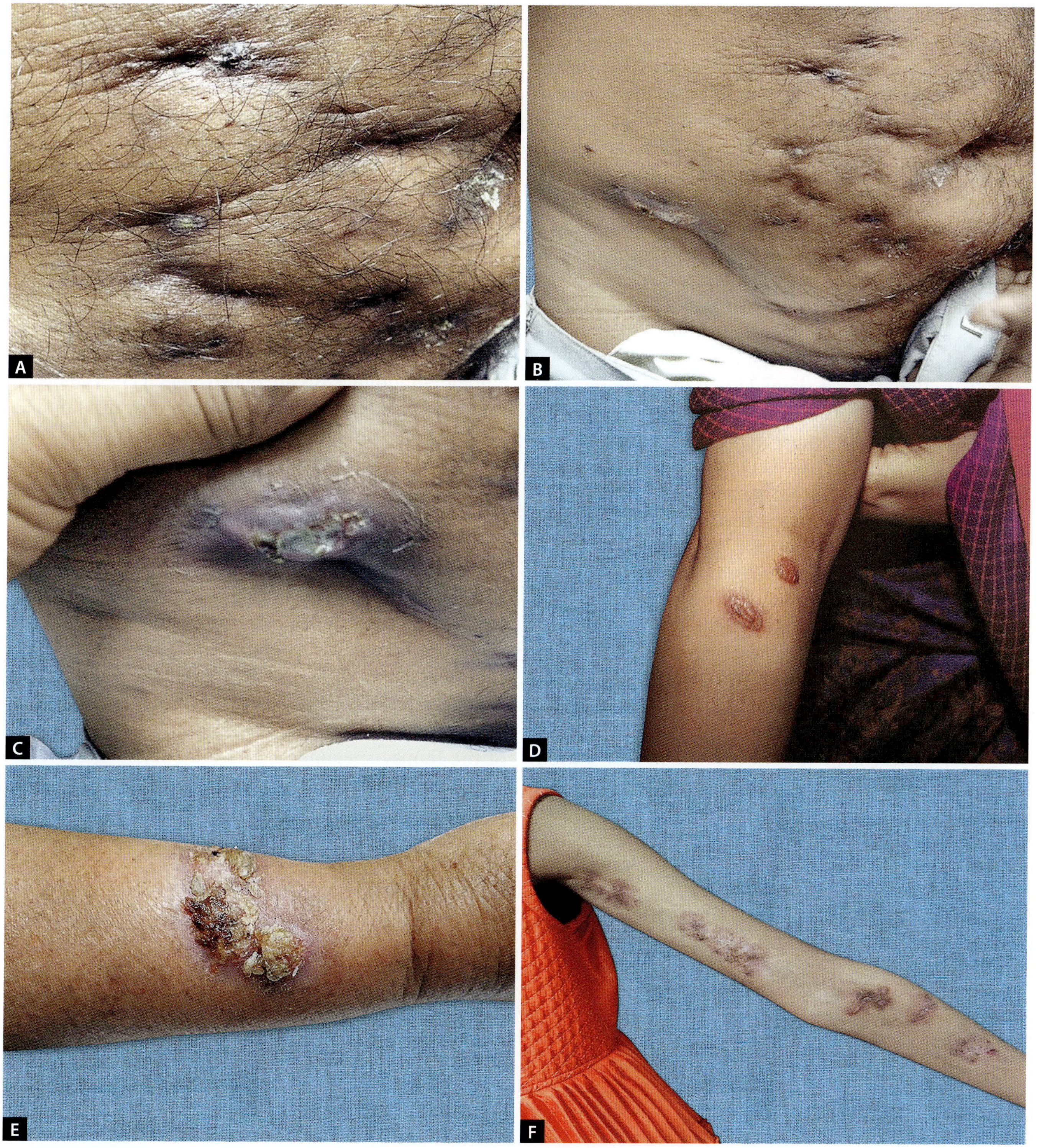

Figs. 50A to F: (A) Nocardiosis, note multiple discharging sinus; (B) Actinomycosis of anterior abdominal wall; (C) Actinomycosis, close-up view; (D) Lymphocutaneous sporotrichosis; (E) Fixed cutaneous sporotrichosis; (F) Sporotrichosis, note the scar post treatment.

subcutaneous nodule along the lymphatic within a few weeks' time. Initially the lesions are small, firm, painless nodule. Gradually, overlying skin of the lesion becomes fixed and lesion may ulcerate. This lymphocutaneous or sporotrichoid variety comprises 75% of cases. Lymphatic spread does not occur if there is previous exposure. Then

"Be full of sorrow, that you may become hill of joy; weep, that you may break into laughter." —**Rumi**

fixed cutaneous sporotrichosis develops at the site of inoculation and presents as solitary granulomatous plaque, nodule or ulcer. Sound host immunity, facial location in child, small inoculum and low virulence of the organism are contributory for the development of fixed cutaneous variety. Disseminated sporotrichosis develops in the setting of profound immunosuppression like diabetes, AIDS, biologic therapy, and hematological malignancy, etc. Reddish tender cutaneous lesions ultimately suppurate and turn into chronic ulcer and fistula. Arthritis or bone involvement is frequent. Other systems such as lung and gastrointestinal tract may get involved. Histopathology displays suppurative and granulomatous inflammation in dermis and subcutis. Organisms are rarely seen. Demonstration of cigar-shaped yeast in tissue requires special stain like PAS fluorescent antibody. Asteroid bodies and mycelia are more numerous in sporotrichoid form of sporotrichosis. Tissue culture is diagnostic. Being a dimorphic fungi *Sporothrix* species grows as moist white colony on Sabouraud's agar at 25°C which becomes ultimately black (due to melanin) and wrinkled. In slide culture preparation, septate mycelia can be seen. Conidia at the end of conidiospore are also seen. Culture at 37°C produces grayish yellow yeast-like colony. On microscopy, cigar-shaped budding yeasts are seen. Differentials are plenty starting from atypical mycobacteria, nocardiosis, leishmaniasis, anthrax, cutaneous TB, tularemia, glanders, and cat-scratch disease. Saturated solution of potassium iodide is quite cheap yet effective treatment option. It should be started at lower dose and gradual upward titration of dose is required. Itraconazole at a dose of 100–200 mg/day for 3–6 months is also effective.

SUBCUTANEOUS ZYGOMYCOSIS OR PHYCOMYCOSIS (FIGS. 51A TO C)

Subcutaneous zygomycosis presents as chronic infection of skin and subcutaneous tissue. It usually affects trunk and extremities without dissemination to internal organs. In India, the infection is more prevalent in south India. Zygomycosis or phycomycosis is a fungal infection caused by various organisms belonging to the class of Zygomycetes. Two medically important order Mucorales and Entomophthorales come under the class Zygomycetes. Mucorales are responsible for serious invasive disease involving pulmonary, brain, and gastrointestinal tract in immunocompromised hosts. Entomophthorales causing entomophthoromycosis are of two types: (1) *Basidiobolus ranarum* causing subcutaneous zygomycosis and (2) *Conidiobolus coronatus* causing rhinofacial zygomycosis. *B. ranarum* is a saprophyte fungus and survive on soil, gastrointestinal tract of frog and decaying vegetables. Initially, the lesion starts as nodule and gradually expands locally to form hard, nontender and painless swelling. Fingers can easily be insinuated below the lesion. Ulceration may occur. Certain important differentials such as mycobacterial infection, sporotrichosis, soft tissue tumor, synovial sarcoma, and Burkitt's lymphoma should be considered. Culture on Sabouraud's dextrose agar media from biopsy sample, abscess fluid is gold standard for diagnostic confirmation. Histopathology of the biopsy specimen could adequately suggest the disease. Histopathologically, subcutaneous zygomycosis is characterized by suppurative granuloma consisting of lymphocytes, histiocytes, plasma cell, multinucleated

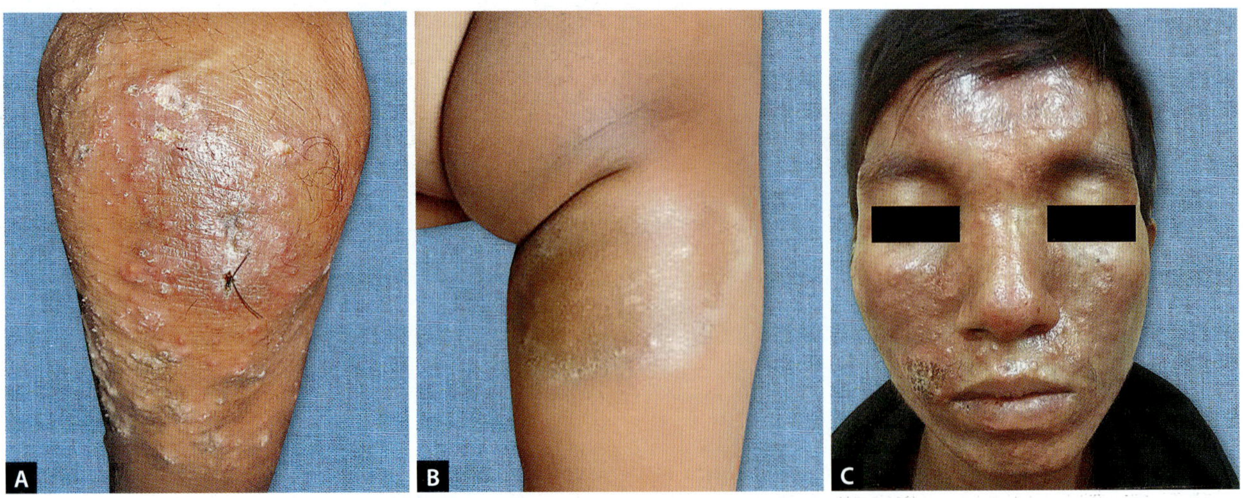

Figs. 51A to C: (A) Subcutaneous phycomycosis over knee in an 18-year-old boy; (B) Subcutaneous phycosis over back of thigh in a 3-year-old boy; (C) Subcutaneous phycomycosis over face, a rare site.

"You build on failure. You use it as a stepping stone. Close the door on the past. You don't try to forget the mistakes, but you don't dwell on it. You don't let it have any of your energy, or any of your time, or any of your space." —**Johnny Cash**

giant cells and eosinophils distributed all over the dermis and subcutis. The presence of eosinophilic infiltrate in the granuloma is so characteristic that it is also called eosinophilic granuloma. Degranulation of eosinophils leads to formation of eosinophilic sheath (Splendore–Hoeppli phenomenon) surrounding aseptate or infrequently septate thin-walled hyphae. Saturated solution of potassium iodide is the drug of choice. Azoles like itraconazole and amphotericin B also work effectively.

CHROMOMYCOSIS (FIGS. 52A TO C)

It is an infection of skin and subcutaneous tissue by dematiaceous fungi, e.g., *Phialophora verrucosa*, *Fonsecaea pedrosoi*, *Cladosporium carrionii*, etc. The lesions characteristically present as verrucous nodules and plaques, mostly over leg or foot. There is often bleeding on pressure or minor trauma. On the surface of the lesions, there are often visible "black dots" suggesting transepidermal migration of fungal spores. The diagnosis is established by and large by skin biopsy and histopathological examination. Special stains for fungus demonstrate Medlar bodies or "copper penny bodies".

For localized lesions, surgical excision, electrodesiccation, and cryotherapy are the treatment options offered. For extensive or large lesions, oral antifungals like itraconazole and terbinafine are effective.

LEISHMANIASIS (FIGS. 53 TO 55)

It is a protozoal disease caused by the *Leishmania* species. It can be divided into three types: (1) cutaneous, (2) mucocutaneous, and (3) visceral leishmaniasis. It has a characteristic geographic prevalence in the areas of Afghanistan, Iran, Brazil, Peru, and the northern belt of India extending eastward.

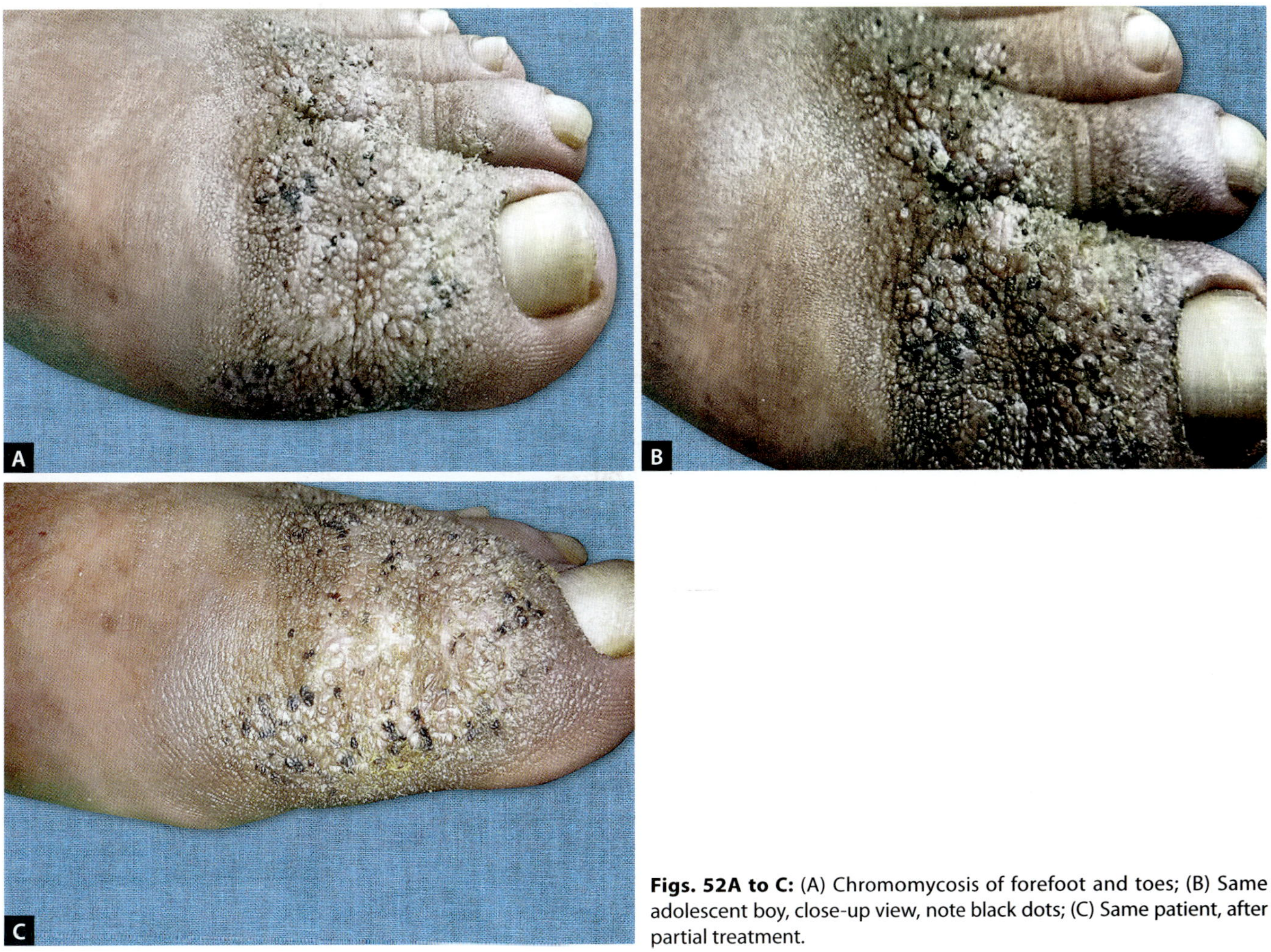

Figs. 52A to C: (A) Chromomycosis of forefoot and toes; (B) Same adolescent boy, close-up view, note black dots; (C) Same patient, after partial treatment.

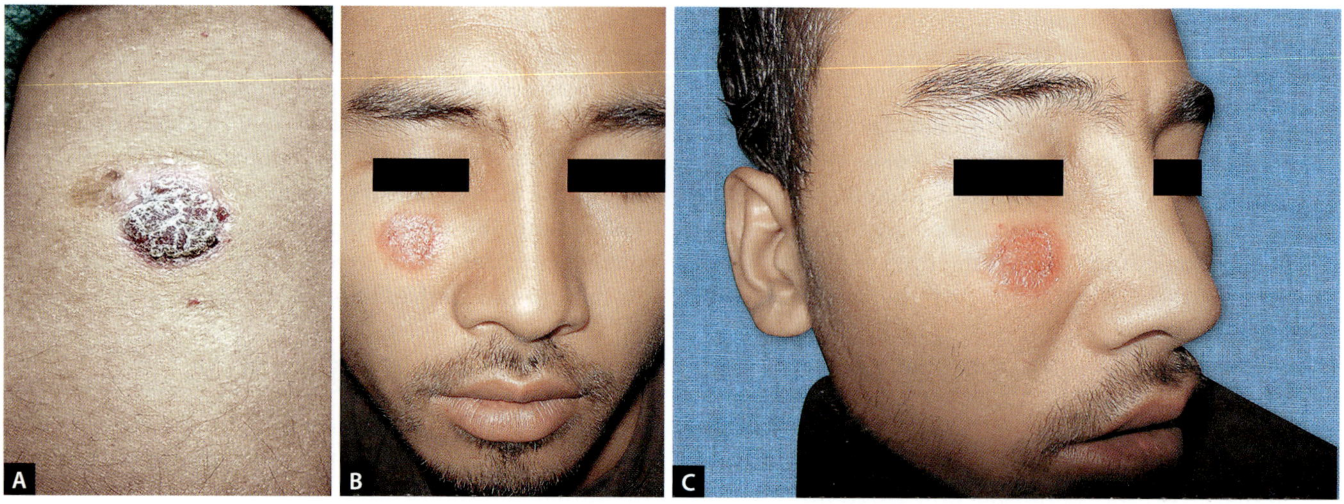

Figs. 53A to C: (A) Crusted plaque of cutaneous leishmaniasis; (B) Erythematous infiltrated asymptomatic plaque of leishmaniasis; (C) Close-up view of leishmaniasis.

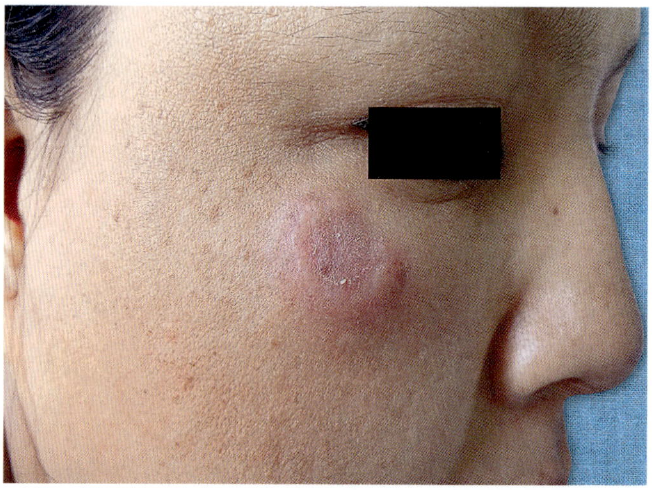

Fig. 54: Infiltrated asymptomatic plaque of leishmaniasis.

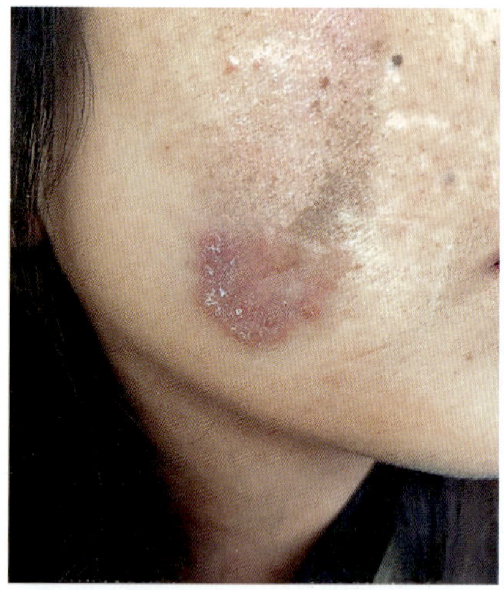

Fig. 55: Unusual presentation of cutaneous leishmaniasis.

Etiology

- *Cutaneous leishmaniasis*:
  - Old world disease is caused by *Leishmania tropica, Leishmania major*
  - New world disease is caused by *Leishmania braziliensis, Leishmania mexicana*
- *Mucocutaneous leishmaniasis:* Caused by *L. braziliensis*
- *Visceral leishmaniasis:* Caused by *Leishmania donovani*

Transmission is by the *Phlebotomus* species of sand fly. Recently, there has been a surge in leishmaniasis with the advent of HIV infection.

Clinical Features

Cutaneous leishmaniasis presents with an indolent skin ulcer with an incubation period of around 1–12 weeks. Sometimes there may be a subclinical infection. It starts as an erythematous papule which progresses to a painless ulcer with raised margin and a necrotic base. The lesions can vary from 1 to 2 in numbers to multiple. They may be distributed in a lymphatic distribution giving rise to a sporotrichoid appearance. There can be associated lymphadenopathy and secondary infection of the lesion giving rise to pain. It can also present as a dry ulcerative lesion which turns to a brown nodule that further ulcerates with an overlying adherent crust.

"True success is overcoming the fear of being unsuccessful." —**Paul Sweeney**

Leishmaniasis recidivans gives rise to red colored to yellowish hued papules in the old scars of a resolved cutaneous leishmaniasis lesion.

There can be nonulcerating generalized form resembling lepromatous leprosy and these patients are the reservoir of infection posing a threat to the community.

Differential Diagnosis

- Foreign body reaction
- Tropical or traumatic ulcer
- Infected insect bite reaction
- Myiasis
- Impetigo
- Fungal infection
- Sarcoidosis

Laboratory Diagnosis

The diagnosis generally can be made by the characteristic lesions and a history of travel to the endemic areas. However, it can be confirmed by doing a smear stained with Giemsa which shows the amastigotes within the cells. Culture of the tissue can be done along with isoenzyme analysis to confirm the diagnosis.

Treatment

Cutaneous leishmaniasis generally heals spontaneously however infection with *L. braziliensis* can progress to mucocutaneous disease.

The drugs which have been used and are effective include pentavalent antimonials, sodium stibogluconate, meglumine antimoniate, and amphotericin B.

Cryosurgery and intralesional sodium stibogluconate have also given good response in case of limited disease.

POST-KALA-AZAR DERMAL LEISHMANIASIS (FIGS. 56 TO 60)

Post-kala-azar dermal leishmaniasis (PKDL) is a complication of visceral leishmaniasis (VL) or kala-azar caused by *Leishmania donovani* which develops months to years after apparent cure from VL, and in some patients alongside VL. Younger patients (<15 years) tend to have significantly shorter intervals than the older age group. It is mostly confined to South Asia (India, Nepal, and Bangladesh) and East Africa, mainly Sudan. Clinically, it presents with hypopigmented macules, papules,

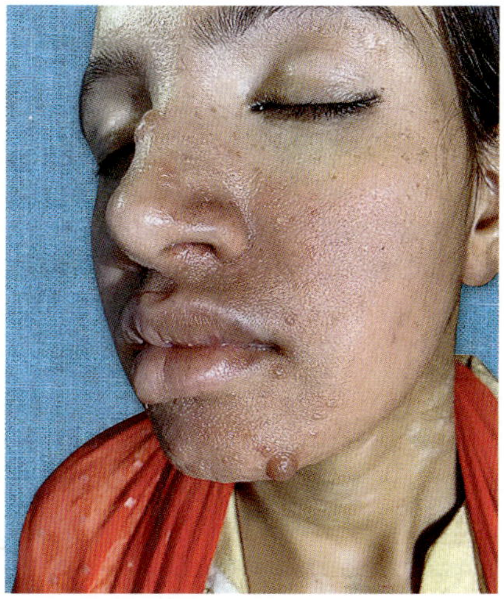

Fig. 56: Infiltrated papules and nodules over face, nose, chin in post-kala-azar dermal leishmaniasis (PKDL).

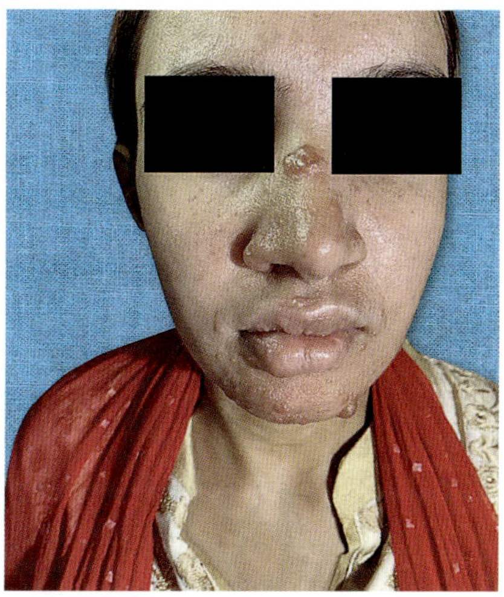

Fig. 57: Same girl, another view.

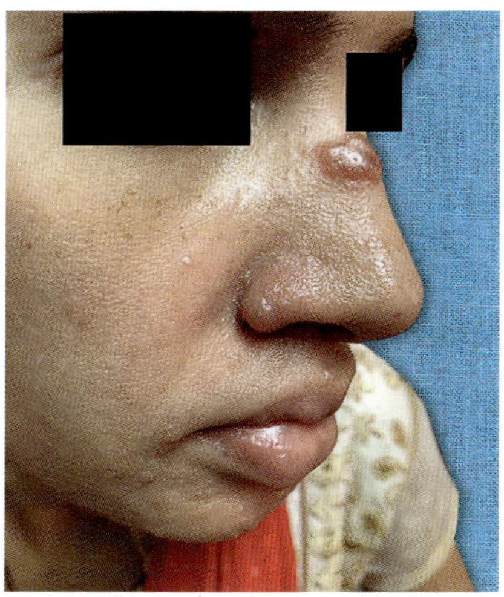

Fig. 58: Close-up view of lesions.

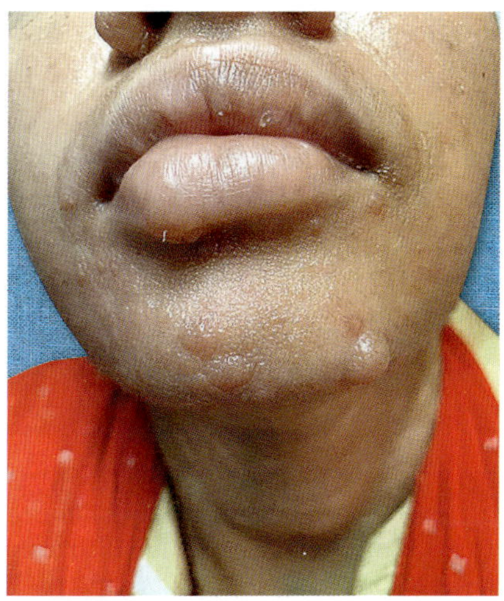

Fig. 59: Nodular lesions of PKDL.

"Success is the sum of all efforts repeated day in and day out." —**Robert Collier**

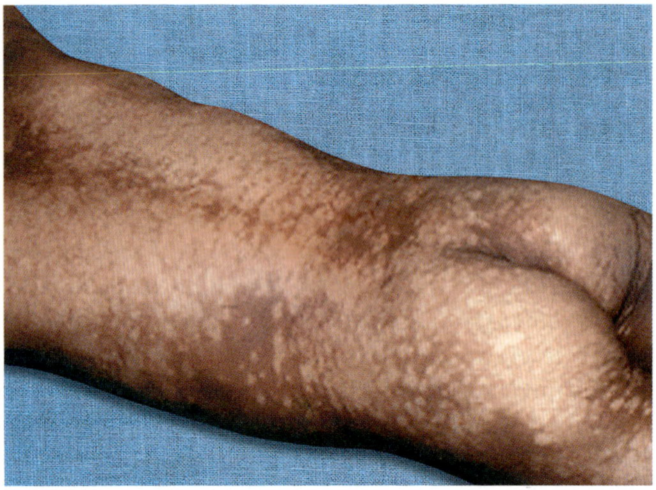

Fig. 60: Post-kala-azar dermal leishmaniasis (PKDL) presenting as hypo-to-mild depigmented macules, widely distributed over trunk and/extremities.

and nodules in an otherwise healthy individual, which start around the mouth and spread to other parts of the body, mostly involving the sun-exposed areas. While polymorphic lesions are prevalent in the South Asian variant, the Sudanese variant has papular or nodular lesions. Atypical variants include erythrodermic, warty, lupoid, and tumor-like forms. PKDL may resemble leprosy, secondary syphilis and sarcoidosis. Multiple lesions can coalesce resulting in gross enlargement of the nose and lips. Occasionally, secondary involvement of nasal mucosa, hard and soft palate, oropharynx, larynx or eyelids and cornea may occur. PKDL patients harbor parasites in their lesions, especially the papulonodules, thus playing a pivotal role in the inter-epidemic transmission of VL.

The pathogenesis of PKDL is largely immunologically mediated. High concentrations of IL-10 in the peripheral blood of VL patients predict the development of PKDL. Diagnosis is mainly clinical. Microscopic examination of smears, PCR and monoclonal antibodies can be used to detect parasites. Serological tests and the leishmanin skin test are of limited value. In Sudan, only severe or chronic cases are treated as self-healing occurs in most patients within 12 months. While, in India, treatment is always needed. Drugs such as sodium stibogluconate, liposomal amphotericin B and newer compounds such as miltefosine are used following which the rash disappears and patients develop immunity which is permanent unless there is associated immunosuppression.

WHAT'S NEW

1. Ozenoxacin, a quinolone antibiotic has been FDA approved for the topical treatment of impetigo secondary to *S. aureus* and *S. pyogenes* in children above 2 months of age.
2. WHO has classified NOMA into 5 stages:
   i. Stage 1 – acute necrotizing ulcerative gingivitis
   ii. Stage 2 – edema
   iii. Satge 3 – gangrene
   iv. Stage 4 – scarring
   v. Stage 5 – sequelae
3. Under dermoscope scabies mite is seen as a dark equilateral triangular structure, referred to as a "jet with contrail". The examination should be focused on external genitalia and finger seams.
4. Efinaconazole topical solution 10% and tavaborole topical solution 5% are FDA approved for the treatment of onychomycosis in children ≥ 6 years; ciclopirox topical solution 8% nail lacquer is approved in children ≥ 12 years.
5. The 2020 International Alliance for the Control of Scabies (IACS) Criteria categorize diagnosis at three levels of diagnostic certainty (confirmed, clinical and suspected scabies) and eight subcategories, and can be adapted to a range of research and public health settings.
6. The off-label use of oral ivermectin in infants and children < 15 kg has been found to be safe and effective. Efficacy is higher when the delay between the two doses is < 10 days.
7. The Ministry of Health and Family Welfare has decided to introduce a three-drug regimen for Paucibacillary (PB) cases of leprosy in place of a two-drug regimen for 6 months and WHO had agreed to supply the revised drug regimen from April 1, 2025.

SUGGESTED READINGS

1. Engelman D, Yoshizumi J, Hay RJ, Osti M, Micali G, Norton S, et. al. The 2020 International Alliance for the Control of Scabies Consensus Criteria for the Diagnosis of Scabies. Br J Dermatol. 2020;183(5):808-20.
2. Torrelo A, Grimalt R, Masramon X, Lopez NA, Zsolt I. Ozenoxacin, a New Effective and Safe Topical Treatment for Impetigo in Children and Adolescents. Dermatology. 2020;236(3): 199-207.
3. Gupta AK, Venkataraman M, Shear NH, Piguet V. Onychomycosis in Children – Review on treatment and management strategies. J Dermatolog Treat. 2022;33(3):1213-24.

CHAPTER

6

Exanthems of Infective Etiology

MEASLES (RUBEOLA) (FIGS. 1 TO 3)

This is one of the most common viral exanthem of childhood. Transmitted by direct contact with droplets from infected persons, rubeola is caused by measles virus [a ribonucleic acid (RNA)-containing paramyxovirus] with an incubation period of 14 days. The prodromal period lasts for 3–4 days and is characterized by fever, chills, malaise, headache, perspiration, prostration, conjunctivitis, photophobia, coryza with mucopurulent discharge, and persistent dry cough. The appearance of the typical morbilliform rash is preceded by Koplik's spots which appear in the buccal mucous membrane opposite the first molar teeth and spread all over the buccal mucosa. The spots are 1–3 mm, white to bluish white elevations resembling grains of salt, sprinkled on a bright erythematous background. Highly diagnostic of measles, the Koplik's spots disappear as the exanthem becomes full blown. The exanthem appears after 3–4 days of onset of illness as an erythematous maculopapular eruption, first seen on the scalp and hairline, the forehead, the area behind the earlobes, and the upper part of the neck. It then spreads downward to involve the face, neck, trunk, and finally the feet by the fourth day. The rash fades in the same order as it appeared. On the second and third day of the rash, the child looks very toxic with high fever, puffy and congested eyes, coryza, and distressing cough. Within the next 24–36 hours, the fever subsides, the conjunctivitis and coryza clear, and cough decreases with the child feeling normal.

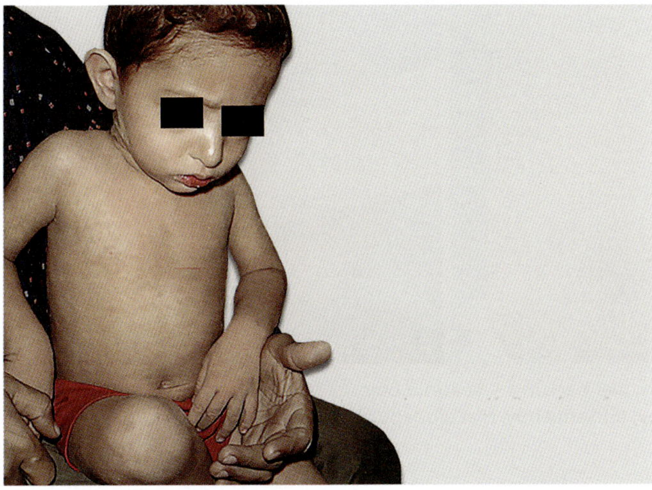

Fig. 1: Generalized maculopapular eruption of measles.

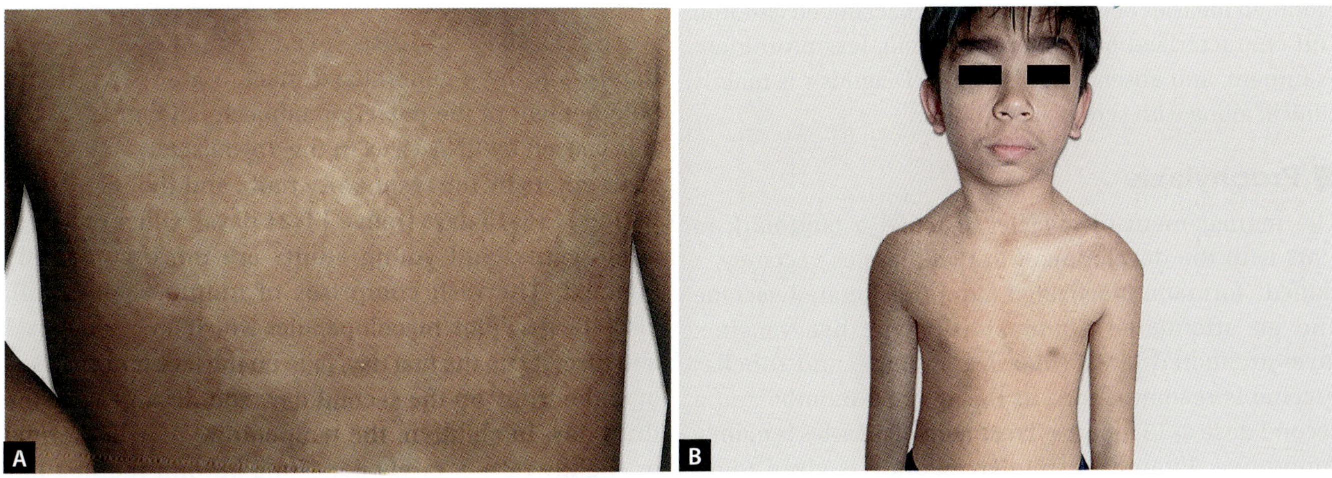

Figs. 2A and B: (A) Measles rash in a 6-year-old boy, note the diffuse maculopapular rash; (B) Same boy with measles rash on trunk and extremities.

"One must be deeply aware of the impermanence of the world." —**Dogen**

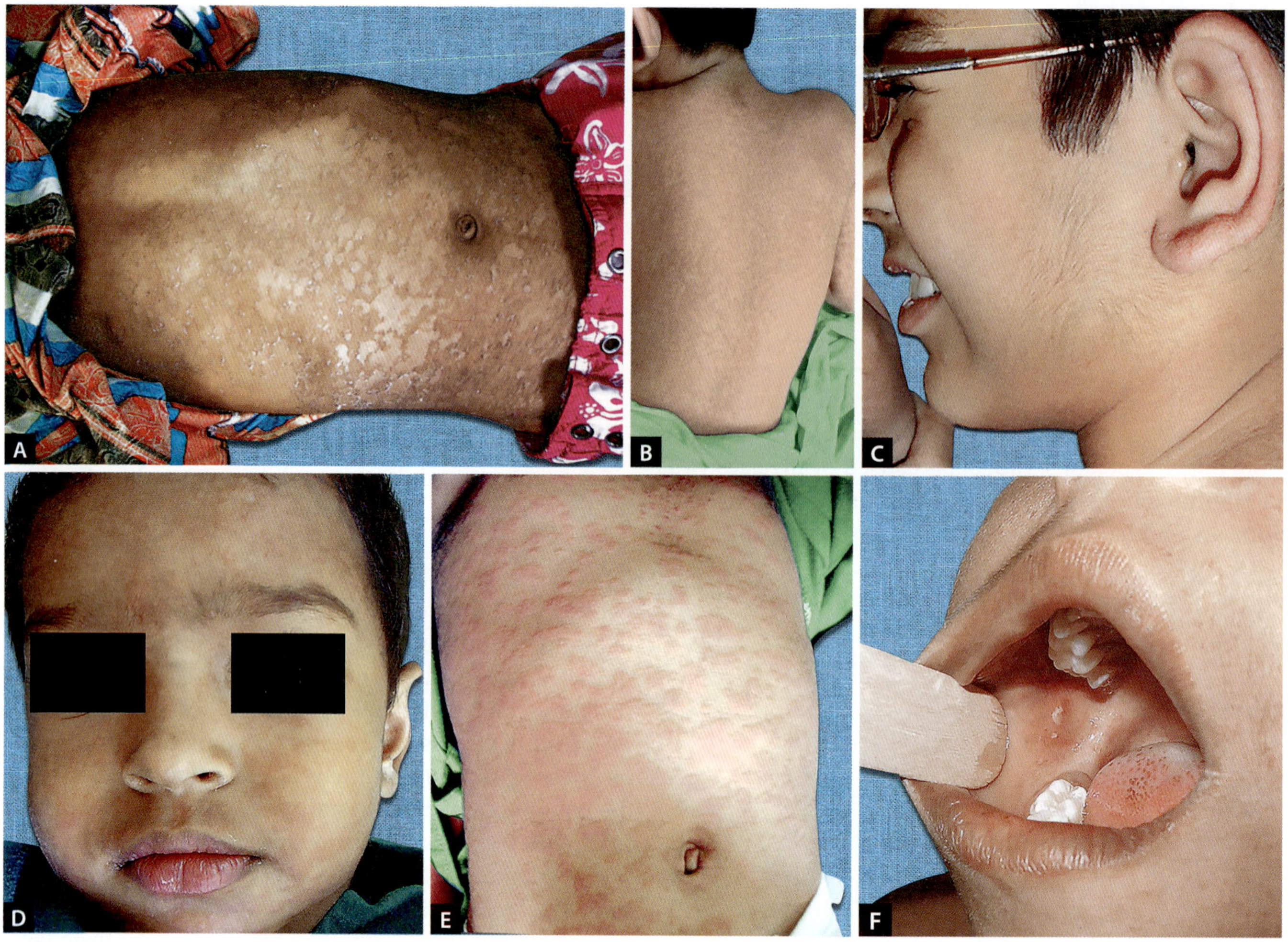

Figs. 3A to F: (A) Subsiding rash of measles with scaling; (B) Measles rash over back in a 4-year-old boy; (C) Measles rash in a 6-year-old boy, note erythema over pinna; (D) Measles rash over face in a 3-year-old boy; (E) Same boy, maculopapular lesions on trunk; (F) Koplik's spots.

Complications include pneumonia, gastroenteritis, myocarditis, laryngotracheobronchitis, and encephalitis. Modified measles occurs in previously vaccinated children and characterized by milder prodrome, less prominent exanthem, and absent Koplik's spots. Diagnosis is mainly clinical along with serological studies.

Prophylaxis

The management of measles reached a landmark in 1963 with the development of two measles vaccines, a "killed" formalin inactivated alum precipitated vaccine and an attenuated Edmonston-B type live vaccine. Live-attenuated MMR (measles, mumps, and rubella) vaccine is recommended at the age of 9 months and a second dose at 15 months. Treatment of measles is mainly supportive. Vitamin A supplementation is given to all children with measles.

GERMAN MEASLES (RUBELLA) (FIGS. 4 AND 5)

It is a common viral disease in children and young adults manifested by a generalized maculopapular rash and enlargement of the posterior suboccipital lymph nodes. It is caused by RNA virus in the *Togaviridae* family. The virus enters by the respiratory route and the incubation period is 16–18 days (range 14–21 days). Older children, adolescents, and young adults are more commonly affected. The rash comprises of innumerable small, discrete, rose pink maculopapules which are generalized and discrete on the first day, fade on the face and coalesce over the trunk on the second day, and disappear by the third day. In children, the temperature may be normal or slightly raised, rarely persisting beyond the first day of exanthem. In adolescents and young adults, however,

"Life is traveling to the edge of knowledge, then a leap is taken." —**DH Lawrence**

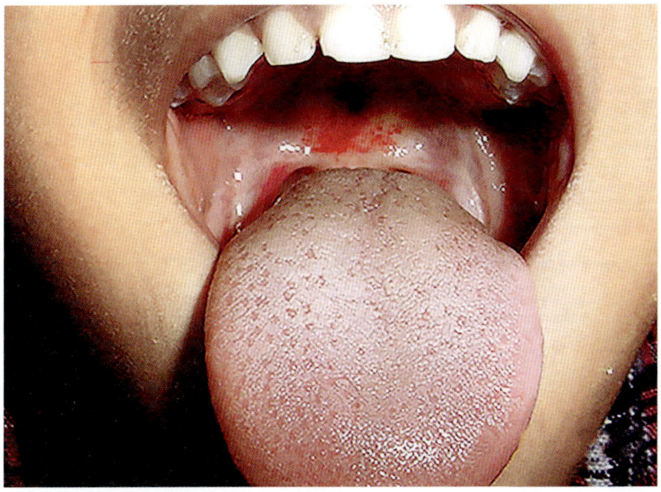

Fig. 4: Palatal hemorrhagic rash in German measles.

there is prodromal phase of headache, malaise, anorexia, conjunctivitis, coryza, sore throat, and cough. Enlargement of posterior auricular and suboccipital lymph nodes precede the appearance of rash by 1–5 days, lasts for 2–7 days and subsides quickly after the rash disappears. Forchheimer spots are the characteristic enanthem seen which presents as erythematous to petechial macules on palate. In older children and adults, arthritis may affect around 30% of females and 5% of males. It characteristically involves the small joints of the hands and feet, occasionally the elbows, shoulders, and spine. A pregnant woman who contracts rubella in the first trimester has a high probability of intrauterine transmission resulting in congenital rubella syndrome. Serologic tests help in confirming the diagnosis.

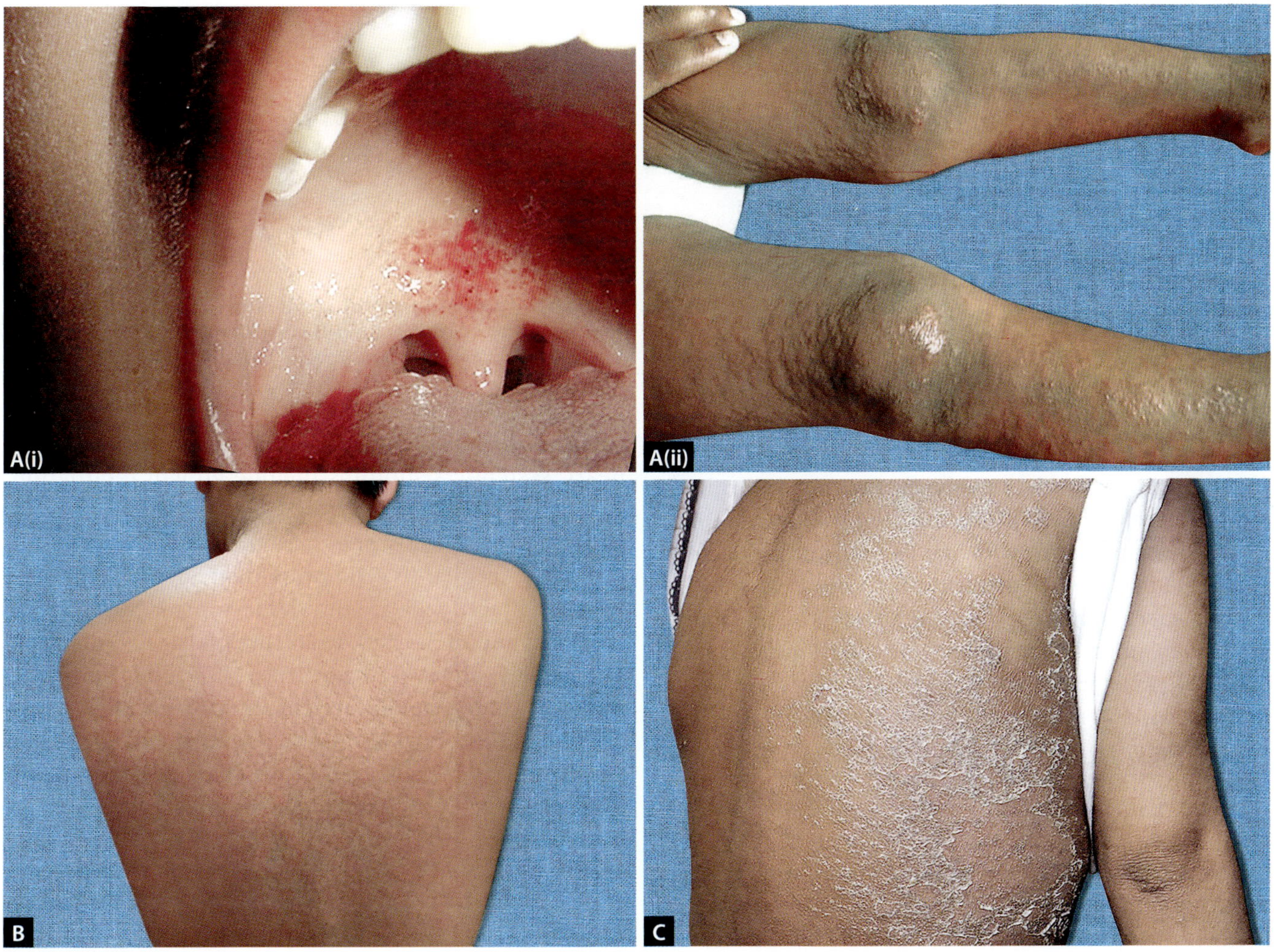

Figs. 5A(i) to C: A(i) Close-up view of palatal rash; A(ii) Rash of German measles in a 16-year-old boy; (B) Rash of German measles over the trunk; (C) Subsiding rash of German measles.

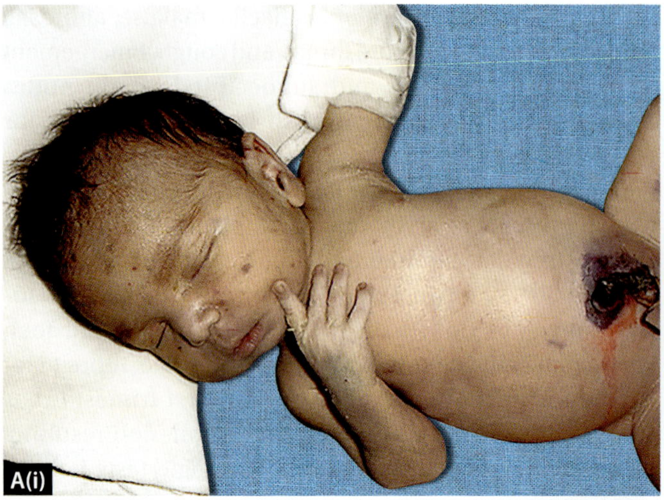

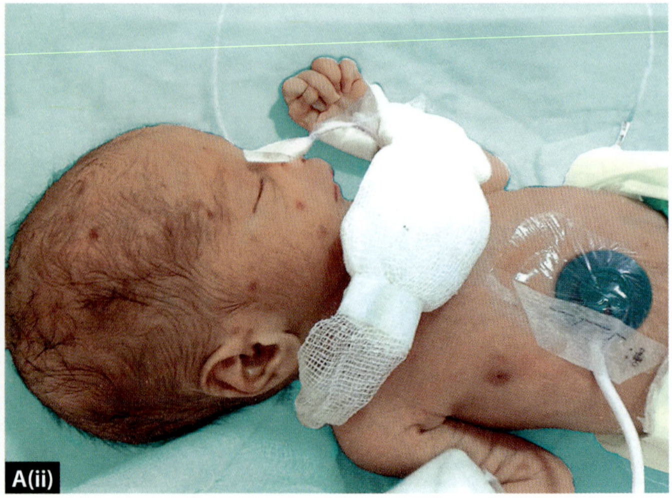

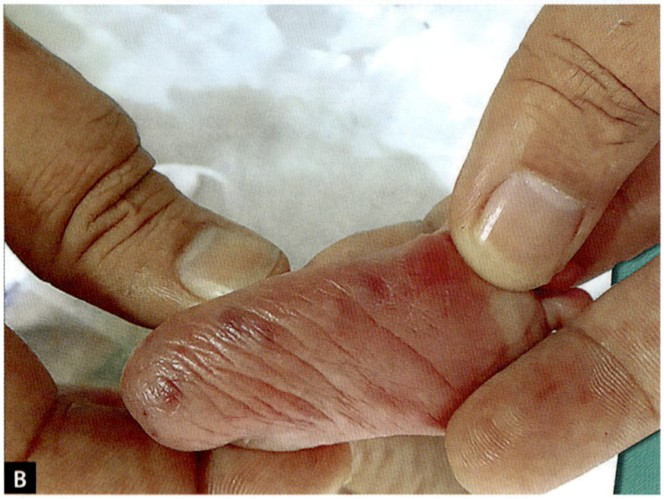

Figs. 6A(i) to B: A(i) Rash of congenital rubella in a newborn; A(ii) Congenital rubella, note blueberry muffin lesions; (B) Same baby, close-up view of blueberry muffin lesions over sole.

Prophylaxis

Current prophylactic recommendations for rubella include vaccination of all children with live-attenuated vaccine in combination with measles and mumps vaccine, at the age of 9 months and a second dose at 15 months. Rubella vaccine, however, should not be administered to pregnant women and pregnancy should be avoided for at least 4 weeks after receiving the vaccine.

CONGENITAL RUBELLA [FIGS. 6A(i) TO B]

Congenital rubella occurs following maternal rubella infection during the first 20 weeks of pregnancy. First trimester infection can lead to congenital rubella syndrome in 90% live-born infants. The earlier in pregnancy the maternal rubella occurs, the greater the risk to the fetus. Affected infants are born at term but have low birth weight. Besides the classic triad of congenital cataract, deafness, and congenital malformations of the heart, systemic symptoms include growth retardation, thrombocytopenic purpura, hyperbilirubinemia, hepatosplenomegaly, pneumonia, osseous defects, and meningoencephalitis. The prominent cutaneous lesions of congenital rubella are thrombocytopenic purpura and blueberry muffin lesions; which are bluish-red infiltrated plaques usually noted at birth. They may be few to numerous and generally appear on the head, neck, trunk, or extremities. They are usually round and vary from a dark blue to purplish red color. The lesions disappear by 3–6 weeks. Other cutaneous manifestations include a generalized maculopapular rash, reticulate erythema over face and extremities, hyperpigmentation of the navel and forehead, eczema, and recurrent urticaria.

The mortality rate is 20–30% within the first year of life. Treatment consists of supportive measures and recognition of potential disabilities.

"Whether you think you can or think you can't, you're right." **—Henry Ford**

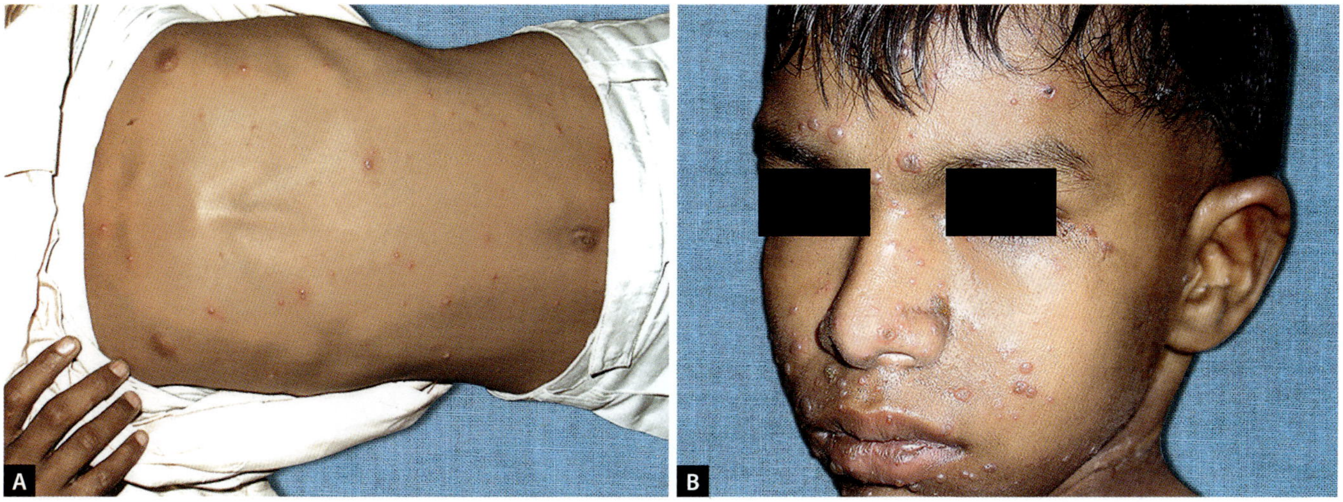

Figs. 7A and B: (A) Polymorphic eruptions of varicella; (B) Varicella lesions, polymorphous.

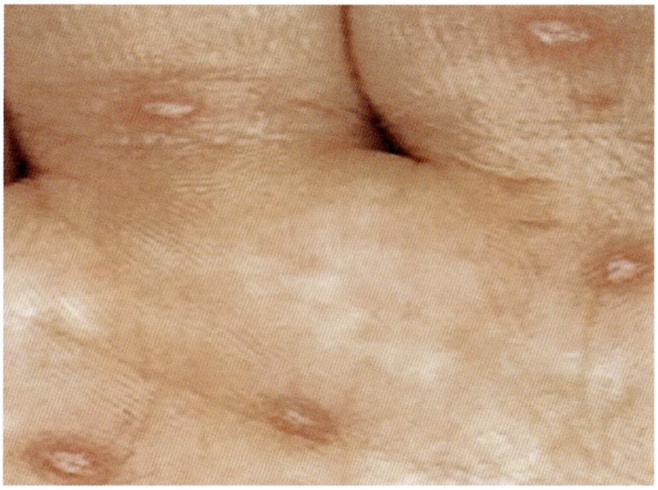

Fig. 8: Chickenpox rash over palm.

Prophylaxis

The live-attenuated rubella vaccine or in combination with measles and mumps is recommended in all children at 9 months and the second dose at 15 months of age.

VARICELLA (CHICKENPOX) (FIGS. 7 TO 9B)

It is a highly contagious disease of childhood and at times adulthood caused by a DNA (deoxyribonucleic acid) virus, the varicella-zoster virus. Transmission is by droplet infection and rarely from skin contact with varicella or herpes zoster patients in immunocompromised individuals. Approximately half of the cases occur before the fifth year of life and 80–90% cases occur before adolescence. The incubation period of the disease is 15–20 days and the disease begins with fever, malaise, and development of an exanthem. The exanthem is characterized by a teardrop vesicle on an erythematous base which develops by 24–48 hours of onset of fever. The eruption usually starts on the trunk and have a centripetal distribution and the involvement of mucous membrane is characteristic. The vesicles are polymorphic in nature, i.e., present in the form of macules, papules, and vesicles, all in different stages of evolution at the same time. The vesicles have an umbilicated appearance and appear in crops at the height of temperature. The diagnosis is quite clear cut from its clinical appearance. However, when only a few vesicles have appeared, one may do a Tzanck smear examination and look for multinucleated giant cells for confirmation of diagnosis. Patients are believed to be contagious from 1–2 days before and for approximately 5 days after the onset of rash. Rare complications include encephalitis, meningoencephalitis, cerebellar ataxia, or Guillain-Barré syndrome.

Breakthrough Varicella (Figs. 9C to F)

Breakthrough chickenpox is an infection with wild type of varicella zoster virus occurring in vaccinated individual 42 days or more after receiving the vaccine. The clinical presentation is milder and atypical. Patients are usually afebrile or with low-grade fever. Cutaneous lesions are chiefly maculopapular with fewer than 50 lesions and usually do not progress to vesiculation and crust formation as seen in unvaccinated varicella. Disease course is shorter and risk of complications is much less. Sometimes, the cases may be misdiagnosed as insect bite reaction. The affected children are less contagious compared to unimmunized children. However, around 25–30% of

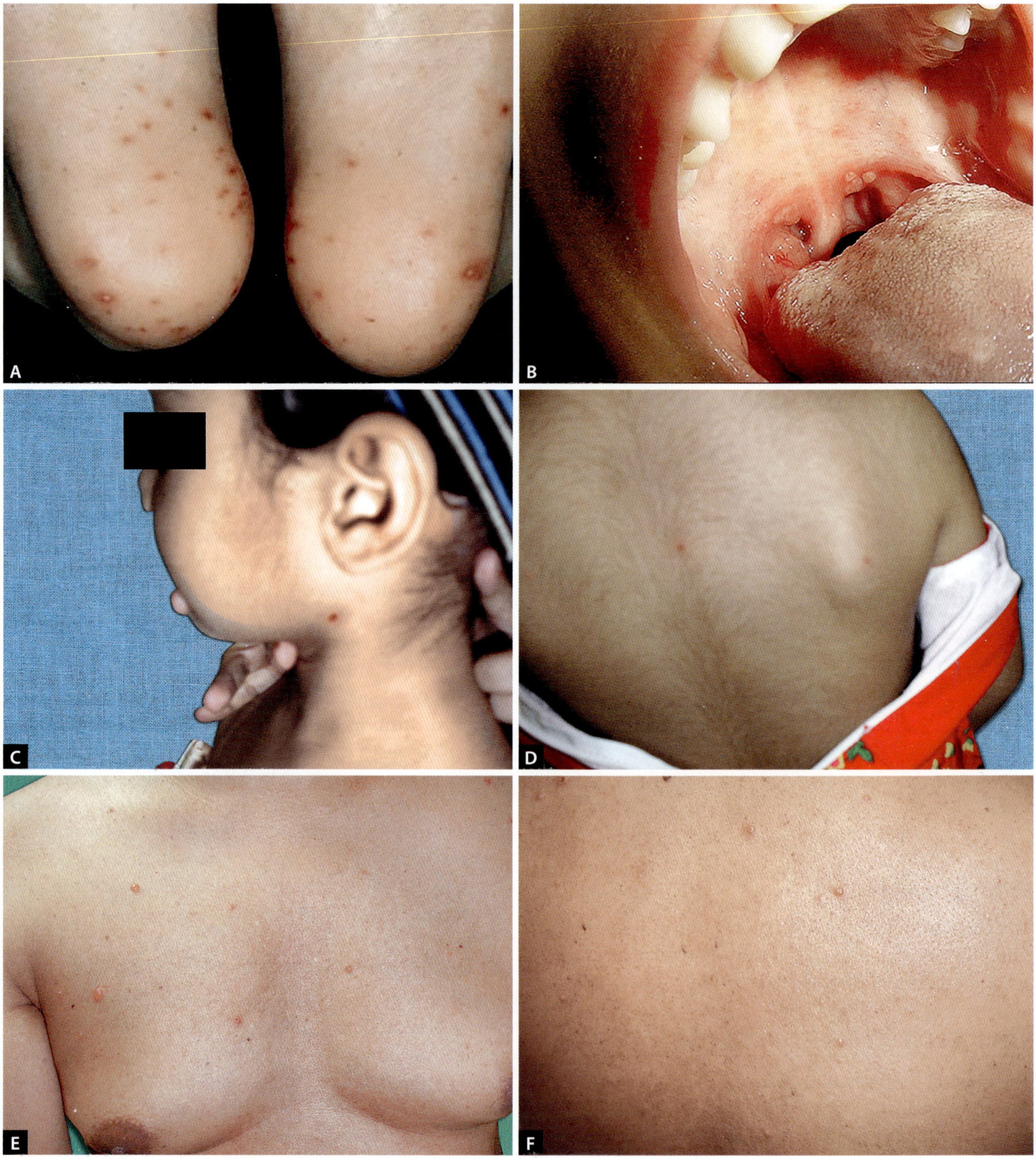

Figs. 9A to F: (A) Varicella lesions over soles; (B) Mucosal erosions in tongue and oral cavity in varicella; (C) Breakthrough varicella; (D) Same girl with breakthrough varicella. Note very few innocuous lesions; (E) Polymorphic lesions of breakthrough varicella over trunk in a 17-year-old child; (F) Same child, close-up view of lesions.

persons with breakthrough varicella may present with features typical of varicella in unvaccinated people and this is usually seen in individuals immunized with single dose of varicella vaccine. Some of the proposed risk factors for vaccine failure are vaccination at younger age, longer time since vaccination (≥5 years), history of asthma or eczema, and autoimmune conditions; though not well supported.

Atypical presentation of breakthrough varicella poses a diagnostic challenge to the clinicians. Laboratory tests are gaining importance for confirming this disease and managing cases and contacts. Detection of viral DNA by polymerase chain reaction (PCR) from skin lesion and varicella immunoglobulin M (IgM) tests during acute or convalescent phase are preferred methods for diagnostic confirmation. Treatment is directed towards symptomatic relief and acyclovir is indicated only in cases of severe disease and in varicella complications. Children with suspected breakthrough varicella should be isolated until 24 hours have elapsed since the appearance of any new lesions. The diagnosis of this entity is of particular importance in schools, day cares, hospitals, or other settings that depend on vaccine-derived immunity to protect against transmission of the infection.

Management

Acyclovir orally at a dose of 20 mg/kg/dose for children 2–12 years of age (up to 500 mg per dose) and 4 g/day for adults for 5–7 days, if started within 24–48 hours, gives good results. This is also useful in immunocompromised children. For immunocompromised patients exposed to varicella, gamma-globulin prophylaxis (1.3 mL/kg) or zoster immune globulin (ZIG) may be used to alter the subsequent course of clinical disease. Only when there is definite evidence of secondary infection, an antibiotic should be used. Regular bathing with soap and water and intake of high protein diet are important. When the vesicles start healing, there may be a sense of itching which may require oral antihistamines. Topical application of soothing agent such as calamine may help relieving the local discomfort. Adequate rest for at least 10–14 days is necessary. Various myths and misconceptions about the disease are to be dealt firmly.

DENGUE FEVER (FIGS. 10 TO 15B)

It is a viral disease, the virus belonging to the family *Flaviviridae* and has four serologically distinct types, viz., DEN-1, DEN-2, DEN-3, and DEN-4. Dengue virus is transmitted by mosquitoes of the species *Aedes*, *Aedes aegypti*, and *A. albopictus*. It is the most common cause of arboviral disease in the world with an estimated annual occurrence of 100 million cases of dengue fever

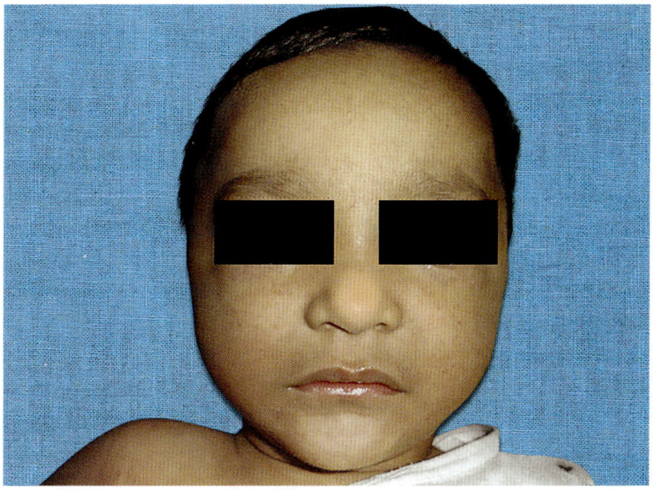

Fig. 10: Flushed cheek and maculopapular rash of dengue.

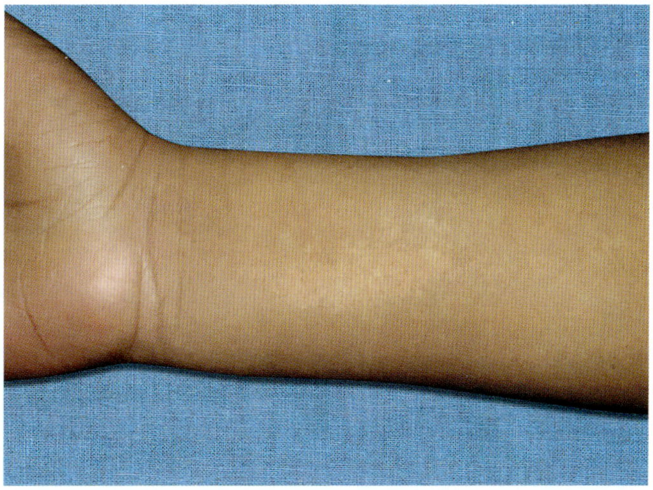

Fig. 11: Maculopapular rash of dengue over forearm and palm.

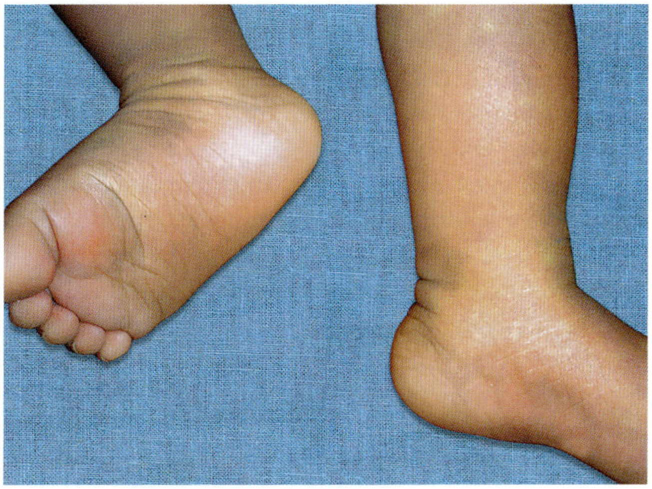

Fig. 12: Dengue rash over legs and soles, note spared island of normal skin.

"If it's a good idea, go ahead and do it, it's much easier to apologize than it is to get permission." —**Grace Hopper**

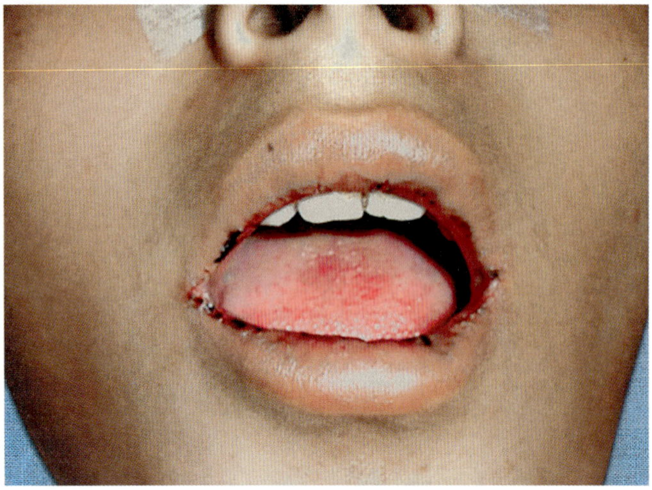

Fig. 13: Hemorrhagic rash of dengue over lips.

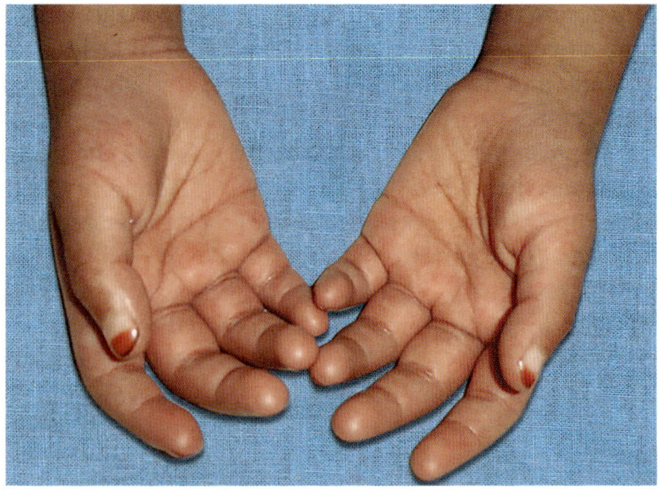

Fig. 14: Erythematous swollen palms in dengue.

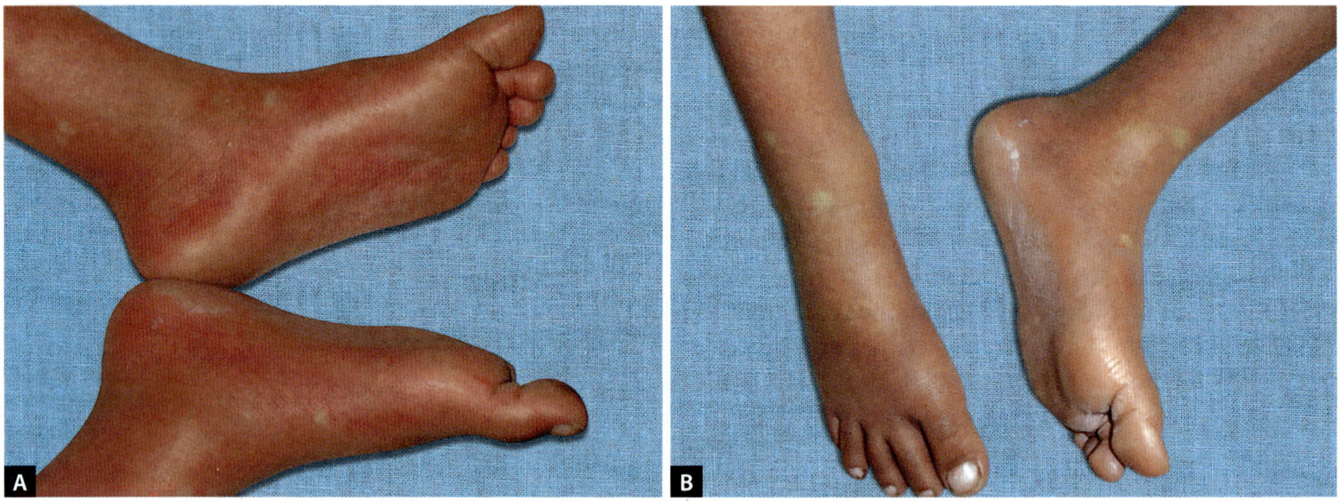

Figs. 15A and B: Erythematous swollen legs and soles in dengue, note island of normal skin.

and 250,000 cases of dengue hemorrhagic fever and a mortality rate of 25,000 per year. The disease has been reported in more than 100 countries with 2.5 billion people living in the area where dengue is epidemic. Most cases of dengue hemorrhagic fever are reported from Asia where it is a leading cause of hospitalization and death in children. Classical dengue fever is characterized by sudden onset of very severe headache, retro-orbital pain, fatigue associated with severe arthralgia and myalgia. The fever usually lasts for 5–7 days after which a rash appears. The rash is usually of maculopapular nature, confluent with sparing of normal islands of circular coin shaped skin (very characteristic). The rash subsides by 3–7 days with scaling and mild pruritus. The patients may have additional hemorrhagic manifestation, e.g., petechiae, purpura, a positive capillary fragility test, etc. Gum bleeding, menorrhagia, epistaxis, and bleeding per anus are occasionally seen. Flagellate purpura can be rarely associated with dengue fever secondary to trauma.

Diagnosis

Laboratory investigations show leukopenia, thrombocytopenia, and mild-to-moderate elevation of hepatic transaminase levels. Dengue NS1 test detects the non-structural protein NS1 of dengue virus. NS1 antigenemia is detectable within 24 hours and up to 9 days following onset of symptoms. Primary infections are characterized by an increase in dengue-specific IgM antibodies 4–5 days after the onset of fever with increase in IgG antibodies after 7–10 days; IgM antibodies are detectable for 3–6 months, while IgG antibodies are detectable throughout life. In secondary infections, the level of IgM antibodies is lower than in primary infections and the antibodies are sometimes absent. However, levels of IgG antibodies rise rapidly in secondary infections, even during the acute phase of the disease.

Management

Treatment is basically symptomatic and supportive. For fever, paracetamol is prescribed. Bed rest and fluid replacement are very important. Patients with platelet count less than 1 lakh/mm^3 require hospitalization and are treated with platelet concentrate and/or fluid replacement when indicated. If there is bleeding or evidence of intravascular coagulation, fresh blood or fresh frozen plasma should be administered. It is very important to go for preventive treatment for travelers in areas where dengue is endemic. Application of insect repellents, protective clothing, and use of insecticides are very important.

GIANOTTI–CROSTI SYNDROME (FIGS. 15C TO G)

It is also known as papular acrodermatitis of childhood. This disease is seen most commonly between the age group of 1 and 6 years. It is a distinctive, self-limiting dermatosis of childhood. The disease is characterized by the abrupt onset of nonpruritic erythematous to lichenoid papules on the face, buttocks, extremities generally lasting about 4–6 weeks, and it is at times associated with mild constitutional symptoms and acute hepatitis.

Etiology

The disease begins abruptly, and the eruption is often preceded by an upper respiratory tract infection, generalized lymphadenopathy, hepatomegaly, and rarely splenomegaly. Evidence of hepatitis manifested by hepatomegaly, elevated serum enzyme levels, virus-like particles in liver and lymph node specimens, and

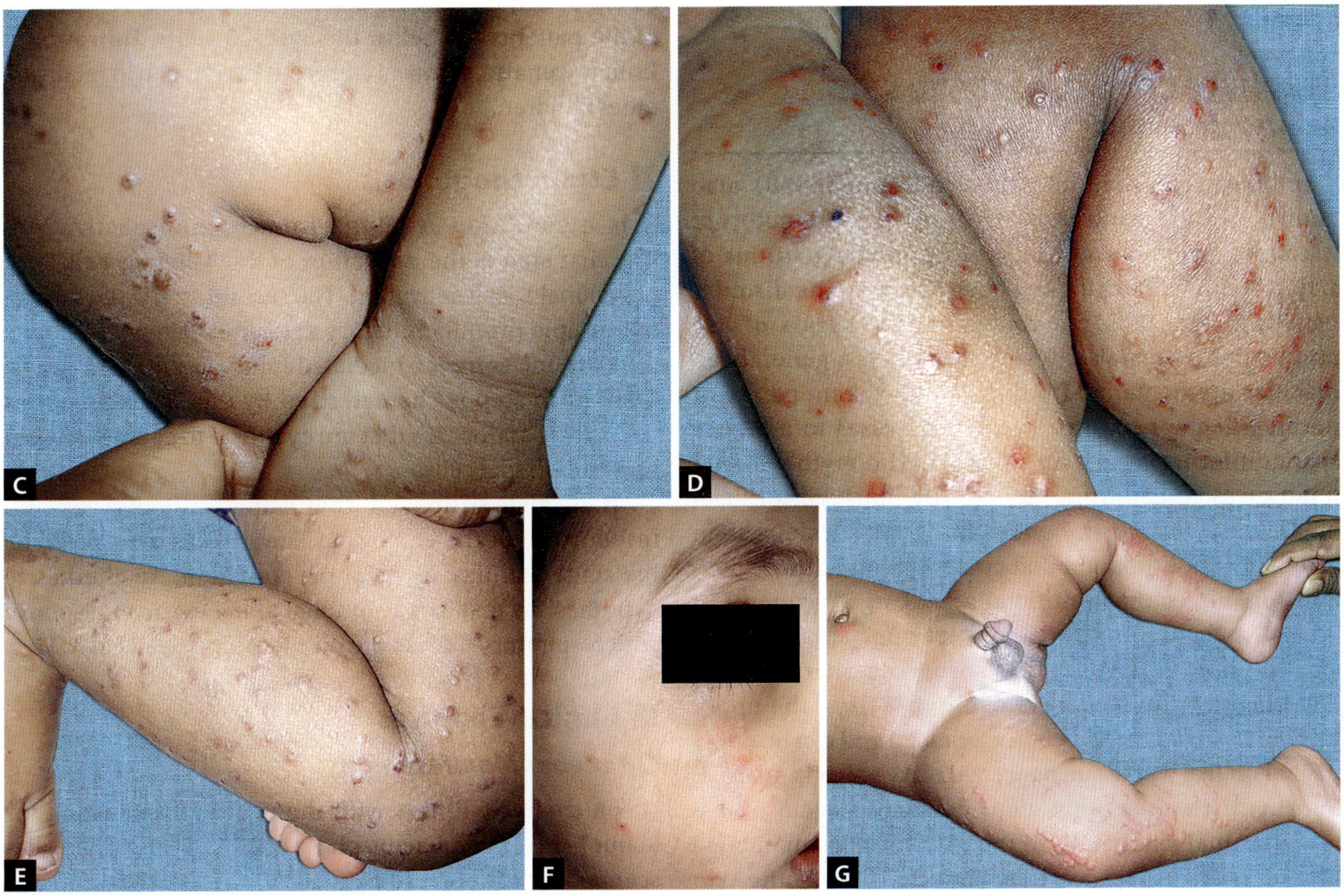

Figs. 15C to G: (C to E) Lichenoid papules of Gianotti–Crosti syndrome (GCS) in a 3-year-old boy; (F) A 4-year-old girl with GCS over the face; (G) Lichenoid papules of GCS over thighs and legs along with Koebner phenomenon.

"If you want to live a happy life, tie it to a goal not to people or objects." **—Albert Einstein**

detection of elevated serum levels of hepatitis B surface antigen suggests viral etiology in some patients. Since the disorder subsequently has also been associated with infection with *Epstein-Barr virus (EBV), parainfluenza virus, coxsackievirus A16, respiratory syncytial virus,* poliovirus vaccine, and *group A β-hemolytic streptococci,* it may actually represent a host response to a variety of infectious agents.

Children between 3 months and 15 years of age are usually affected, although adults have been rarely afflicted by this disorder. The eruption consists of monomorphous, symmetrical, flat-topped 1–10 mm, flesh-colored, pale pink or coppery red papules on the face, buttocks, extremities, palms, soles, and occasionally the back. Nonscaly lesions and noninvolvement of trunk are characteristic.

Treatment

Diagnosis is based on clinical features. Since this syndrome is benign and self-limiting, treatment other than symptomatic measures is unnecessary. Topical corticosteroid creams can be given for severe pruritic lesions.

STAPHYLOCOCCAL SCALDED SKIN SYNDROME (FIGS. 16A TO G)

Staphylococcal scalded skin syndrome (SSSS) also known as Ritter's disease or pemphigus neonatorum is caused by epidermolytic toxin producing strains of staphylococci belonging to phage group 2. The disorder usually affects children younger than 5 years of age and begins as malaise, fever, irritability, a generalized macular erythema, and a fine, stippled, sandpaper, or nutmeg-like appearance which progresses to a tender scarlatiniform phase over 1–2 days. The erythema and tenderness spread from the intertriginous, periorificial areas and trunk to the entire body. The lesions then exfoliate with exudation and crusting around the mouth and sometimes the periorbital area. Large fragments of crusts often become separated leaving radial fissures surrounding that give the disorder its characteristic and diagnostic appearance. Within 2–3 days, the upper layer of the epidermis becomes wrinkled and can be easily peeled off like wet tissue paper. Nikolsky's sign is positive. Shortly, thereafter the patient develops flaccid bullae and eventual exfoliation of the skin (the desquamative phase). If there is no secondary infection, the entire skin heals without scarring within 14 days of the onset of the process.

Prognosis

Staphylococcal scalded skin syndrome has mortality around 4% in children, with most fatalities occurring in newborns.

Treatment

Treatment is aimed at eradication of staphylococci from the focus of infection, thus terminating the production of toxin. Topical antibiotics are ineffective. A penicillinase-resistant antistaphylococcal agent, viz., cloxacillin (12.5–25 mg/kg/day), combination of cloxacillin and clavulanic acid is given for 7–10 days. Parenteral antibiotics are given to those who are severely ill or have extensive skin involvement.

KAWASAKI DISEASE (FIGS. 17A TO T)

It is an acute multisystem vasculitis primarily affecting infants and young children. It is also called as acute febrile mucocutaneous lymph node syndrome. It is a leading cause of acquired heart disease in children. About 80% of the patients are below the age of 5 years. However, in Indian scenario, Kawasaki disease (KD) is seen in relatively older children.

Etiopathogenesis

It is a condition resulting from immune activation. The first step is the activation of the T-helper cells and polyclonal B-cell activation. The second step is the release of multiple proinflammatory cytokines. The third step is the immune complex-mediated injury to the vessel walls. The fourth step is characterized by the development of circulating antibodies that are cytotoxic to cardiac myosin and endothelial cells.

It is also proposed that superantigens may be responsible for the etiology of Kawasaki as manifested by the acute manifestations of the condition. An alternative hypothesis is that a conventional antigen driven response with respiratory tract as the portal of entry leads to KD.

Clinical Features

Cutaneous Manifestations

It is a triphasic illness with the acute phase lasting for about 7–14 days, subacute phase of 25 days, and a convalescent phase of nearly 70 days.

The patient presents with a high fever and appears toxic. About 90% of the patients present with an exanthem

"If you look at what you don't have in life, you'll never have enough." —**Oprah Winfrey**

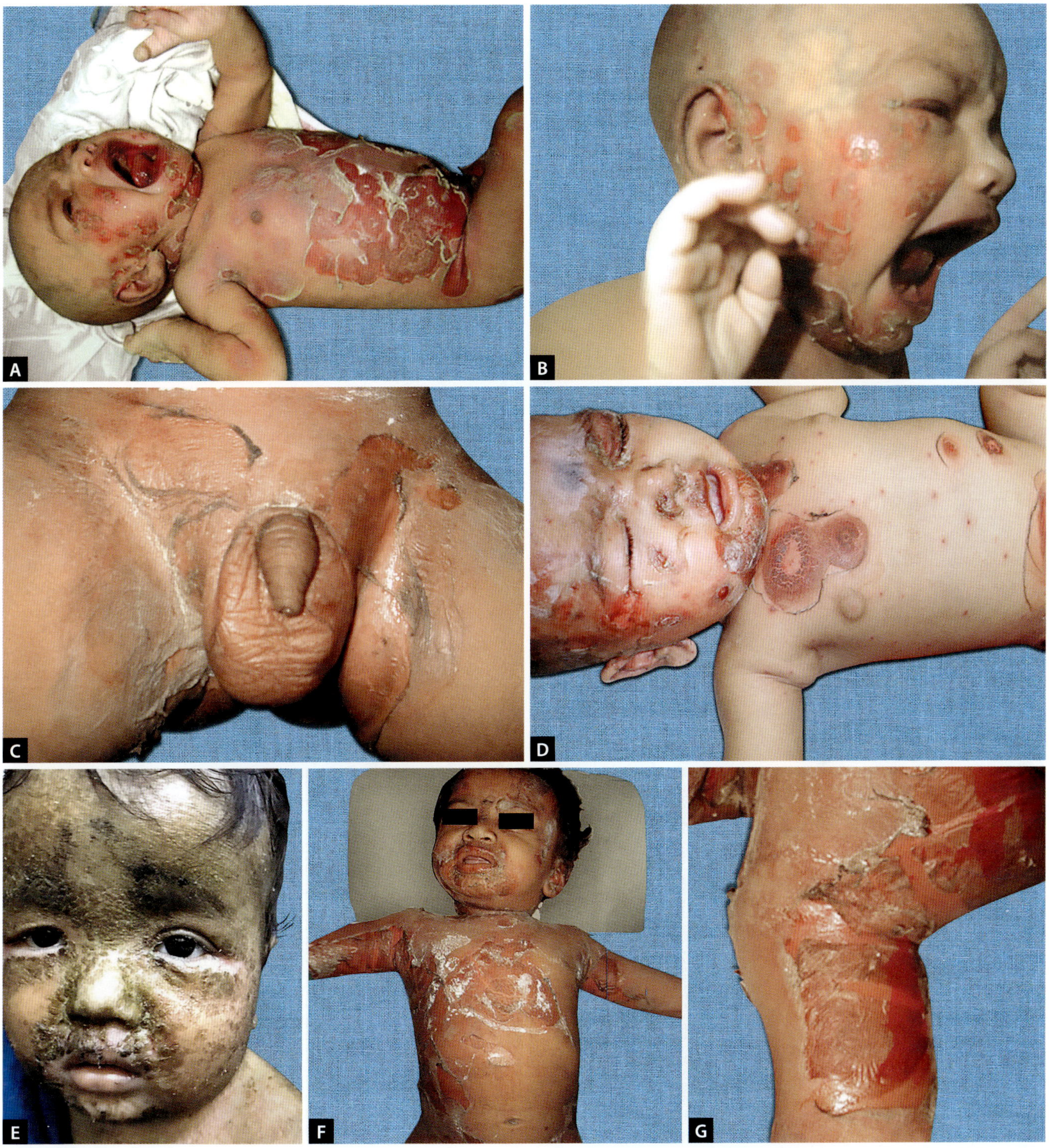

Figs. 16A to G: (A) Rash of staphylococcal scalded skin syndrome (SSSS) over trunk and face; (B) Rash of SSSS over face; (C) SSSS; (D) SSSS in a 5-month-old baby; (E) Same baby, subsiding lesions; (F) SSSS in a 7-month-old baby; (G) Same baby, close-up view of exfoliation seen on axilla and chest.

in the first few days involving the trunk and proximal extremities. The morphology varies from macular, papular, scarlatiniform, morbilliform, urticarial, and targetoid lesions. One of the earliest manifestations is the presence of perineal eruption that starts with an erythema and desquamates in about 48 hours.

"We must accept finite disappointment; we must never lose infinite hope." **—Martin Luther King**

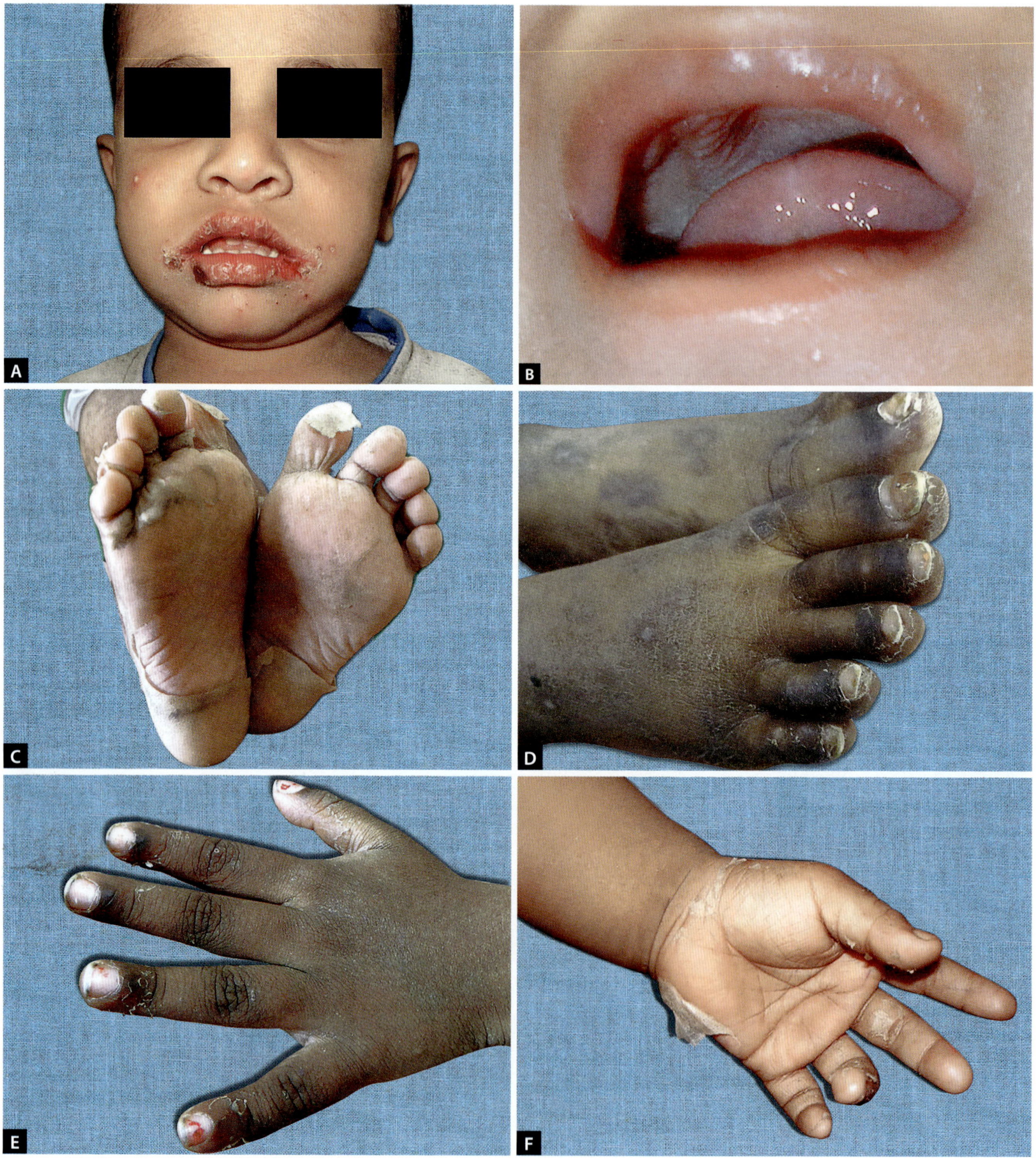

Figs. 17A to F: (A) Kawasaki disease (KD), note cheilitis; (B) KD, erythematous lips, and tongue; (C) KD, plantar exfoliation; (D) KD, lesions over dorsum of feet; (E) KD, note finger-tip exfoliation; (F) Palmar exfoliation.

Edema and erythema of the hands and feet with fusiform swelling of the fingers resolves with desquamation in about 2–3 weeks.

Mucosal involvement occurs in the form of conjunctival congestion which may sometimes also be associated with anterior uveitis. The lips become cherry red,

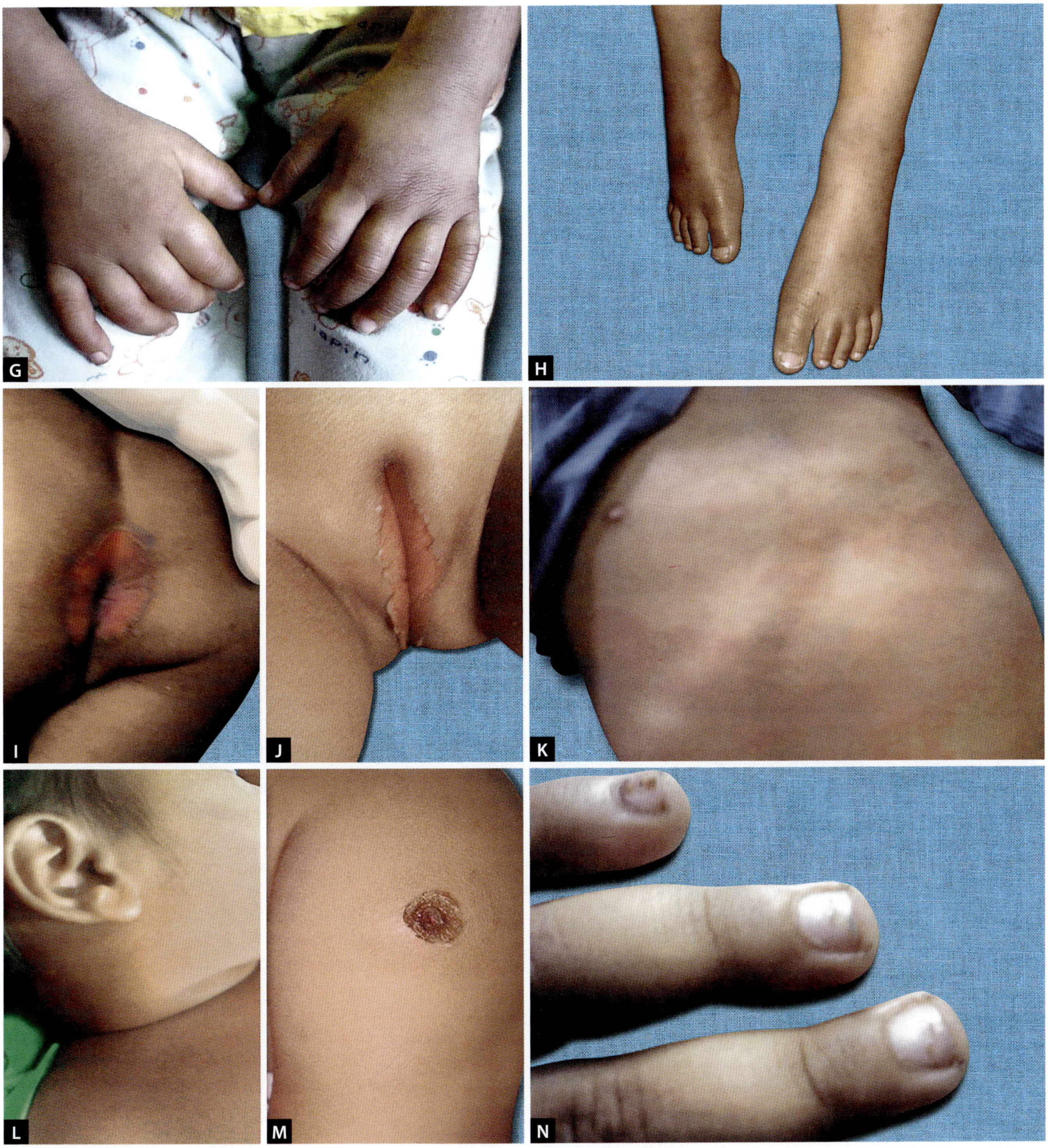

Figs. 17G to N: (G) Edema of hands; (H) Edema of feet; (I) Perianal excoriation; (J) Vulval exfoliation in Kawasaki disease (KD); (K) Polymorphous rash; (L) Unilateral cervical lymphadenopathy; (M) Bacillus Calmette–Guérin (BCG) reactivation; (N) Beau's lines due to KD episode.

fissured, and cracked. The tongue has been described as "strawberry tongue," with the hypertrophied papillae and hyperemia.

Recently diagnosis of KD has been challenging due to the atypical or incomplete presentation. Children present with fever and only desquamation of hand, feet,

"Time you enjoy wasting, was not wasted." —**John Lennon**

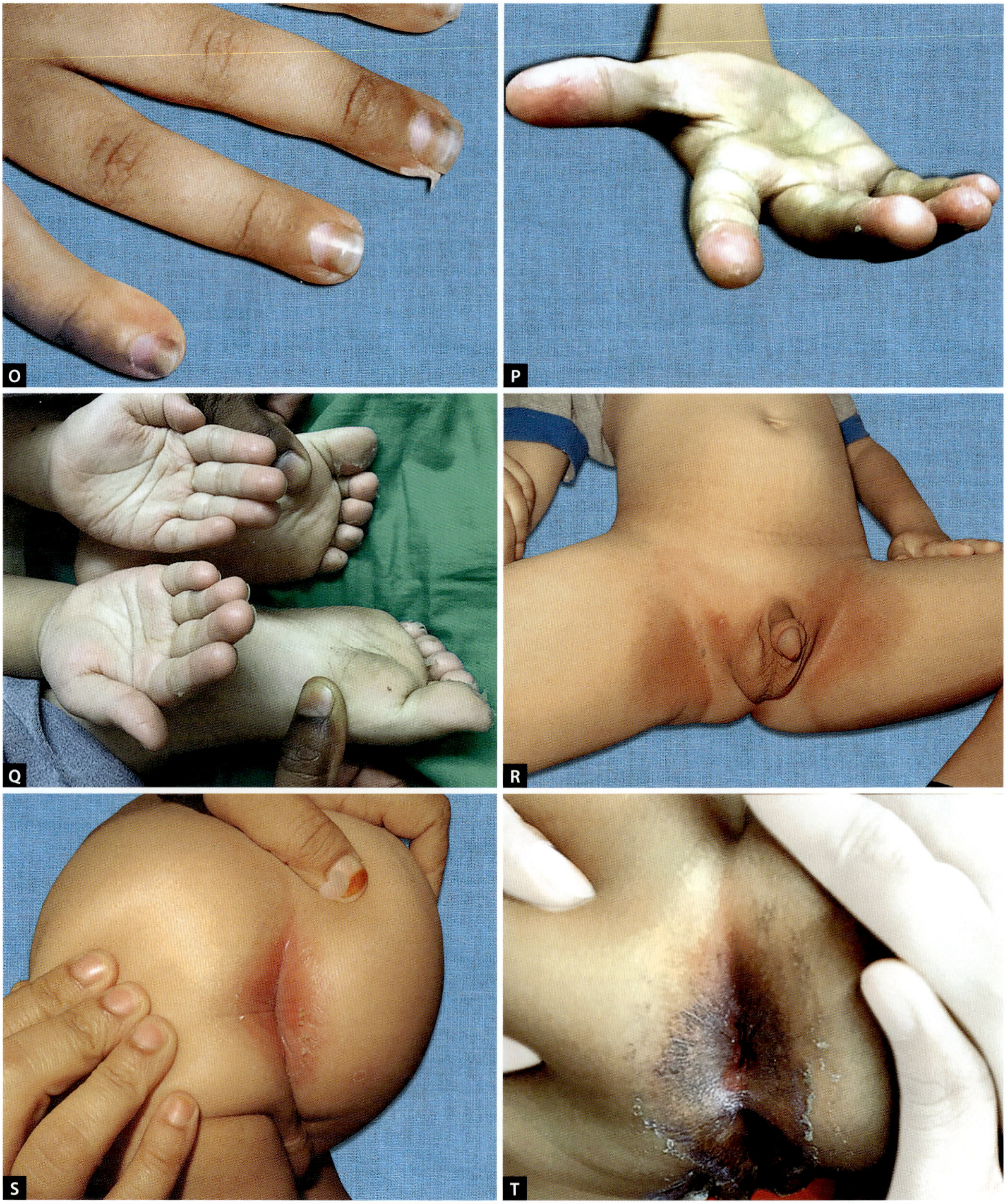

Figs. 17O to T: (O) Orange-brown chromonychia in Kawasaki disease (KD); (P) KD, finger-tip exfoliation; (Q) KD, finger and toe tip exfoliation; (R) KD, lesions over groin; (S) Perianal exfoliation, note marked erythema; (T) Perianal exfoliation.

"Knowledge is like a garden; if it is not cultivated, it cannot be harvested." —**African Proverb**

and perineal area. Any child with persistent fever for >5 days along with periungual desquamation should raise the suspicion of KD.

Systemic Associations

- Cardiovascular abnormalities including pericardial effusion, myocarditis, congestive cardiac failure, and coronary artery ectasia
- Arthralgia and arthritis
- Urethritis with sterile pyuria
- Aseptic meningitis
- Diarrhea and abdominal pain
- Sensorineural hearing loss
- Hepatic dysfunction

Diagnostic Criteria for Kawasaki Syndrome

Fever of 5 days or more with at least four of the following:

1. Bilateral painless bulbar nonexudative conjunctival injection
2. Injected or fissured lips or fissured pharynx or strawberry tongue
3. Erythema of palms and soles or edema of hands and feet or periungual desquamation
4. Polymorphous exanthema
5. Acute nonsuppurative cervical lymphadenopathy (at least 1.5 cm, often unilateral)

Incomplete Kawasaki Disease

Fever for ≥5 days with two or three of the above clinical criteria.

Atypical Kawasaki Disease

Patients who fulfill KD criteria but who have a clinical feature that is not typically seen with KD.

Laboratory Diagnosis

- Transaminitis
- Thrombocytosis
- Sterile pyuria
- Elevation of acute phase reactants
- Electrocardiographic and echocardiographic changes

Differential Diagnosis

- SSSS
- Stevens-Johnson syndrome
- Erythema multiforme
- Scarlet fever
- Toxic shock syndrome
- Viral exanthem

Treatment

The combined use of intravenous immunoglobulin (IVIg) and aspirin has been the basis for treatment. The efficacy of IVIg in prevention of coronary artery complication has been dose-dependent; however, the optimal dose has not yet been established, although reports state administration of IVIg, 2 g/kg over 10–12 hours as a single dose has more benefit.

Approximately 85% of patients treated within the first 10 days of the disease will show resolution. If fever persists after 2–3 doses of IVIg, intravenous methylprednisolone in pulse doses for 3 days may be considered.

Other modalities include plasmapheresis, biologics (infliximab), and cyclophosphamide. Etanercept and rituximab may be useful for resistant KD.

TOXIC SHOCK SYNDROME (FIG. 18)

This severe disorder is an acute febrile illness with multisystem involvement characterized by myalgia, vomiting, diarrhea, pharyngitis, high fever, mucous membrane and conjunctival hyperemia, hypotension, scarlatiniform rash, and in severe cases with shock.

Similar cases were previously described as staphylococcal scarlet fever as early as 1978. Although it is more common in adolescent females and young women, it can also affect males and children. It is mediated by a

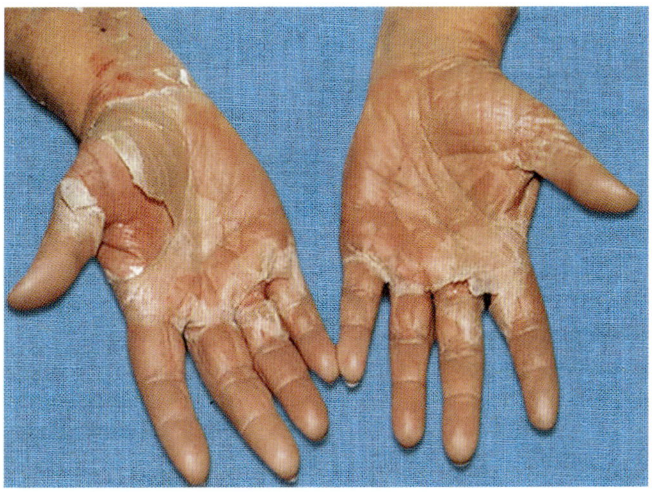

Fig. 18: Maculopapular rash of toxic shock syndrome over palms, along with sheets of exfoliation.

blood-borne toxin produced by *Staphylococcus aureus* at a focal site of infection. These include a phage group 1 *Staphylococcus aureus* toxic shock syndrome toxin 1 (TSS-1) and staphylococcal enterotoxin B in most patients and less commonly other exotoxins such as enterotoxins A, C, D, E, and H. A similar syndrome has been described following infection with toxin producing strains of streptococci. Most cases are related to tampon use during menstruation. However, they can also result from surgical wound infections, infections following sinusitis, nasal packing, ear piercing, deep and superficial abscesses, infected burns, herpes zoster, cellulitis, adenitis, bursitis, empyema, osteomyelitis, septic abortion, etc. The scarlatiniform rash typically desquamates, nails are shed, and telogen effluvium may occur. Flaccid blisters with subepidermal fluid are seen in some infants with toxic shock syndrome.

Treatment

The treatment should be aggressive with early institution of antistaphylococcal antibiotics. In severe cases, fluid replacement is essential. Vasopressors are used to maintain normal blood pressure. Other appropriate measures like respiratory assistance, or dialysis should be provided when necessary.

CHIKUNGUNYA FEVER (FIGS. 19A TO K)

Chikungunya fever is a re-emerging acute viral infection characterized by fever, arthritis, myalgia, conjunctivitis, and mucocutaneous manifestation. It was documented in an outbreak at Tanzania in 1952 and India in 1964. It is usually self-limiting but rarely fatal.

Etiology

It is caused by an arbovirus transmitted by the bite of *Aedes* mosquito. It is also transmitted vertically if mother gets the infection few days prior to delivery or during any phase of pregnancy.

Clinical Features

Chikungunya fever is seen in all age groups from newborn to adults. It affects both sexes equally. There is high-grade fever associated with arthralgia, myalgia, lymphadenopathy, skin eruptions, conjunctivitis, photophobia, meningeal syndrome, and acute encephalopathy. Cutaneous features are seen in 40–50% of cases. Clinically manifests as generalized maculopapular rash, hyperpigmentation, xerosis, desquamation of palms, generalized urticaria lesions, transient nasal erythema, vesiculobullous lesions, vasculitis, erythema multiforme-like lesions, aphthous ulcers, and oral mucosal pigmentation. Skin rash commonly affects extremities, trunk, neck, earlobes, and face.

The cause of hyperpigmentation is not known. It is mainly attributed to postinflammatory hyperpigmentation. Different morphological patterns of hyperpigmentation seen are centrofacial, freckle-like, blotchy, flagellate, palmar pigmentation, or diffuse pigmentation on face, nose, pinna, trunk, and extremities. Neonates affected by vertical transmission can present with only hyperpigmentation. Nasal hyperpigmentation (chik sign) is a very striking clue to diagnose chikungunya in neonates which is not seen in any other viral infections. This pigmentation persists for months even after remission.

Most of the newborns are asymptomatic when maternal infection occurs at the end of gestation and only 12% are symptomatic and most of them develop severe symptoms such as respiratory distress, sepsis, intravascular coagulation, meningoencephalitis, myocarditis, pericarditis, and intracerebral hemorrhage leading to persistent disabilities. Rarely congenital chikungunya can present with dystrophic calcification.

Investigations

Diagnosis of chikungunya rash is mainly clinical. Serological tests include fourfold increase in IgG levels and IgM antibodies specific to chikungunya. Viral culture confirms the diagnosis.

Treatment

The treatment of cutaneous lesions is mainly symptomatic. Bland emollients and calamine lotion can be given. Antihistamines are given for pruritus. Hyperpigmentation persists for few weeks to months. Counseling of parents about the course of the disease is required.

RICKETTSIAL DISEASES (FIGS. 20 TO 24)

Rickettsiae comprise a group of microorganisms that phylogenetically occupy a position between bacteria and viruses. They are obligate intracellular gram-negative coccobacillary forms that multiply within eukaryotic cells. Rickettsiae do not stain well with Gram stain, but they take on a characteristic red color when stained by the Giemsa stain. Rickettsial illnesses, caused by organisms within the

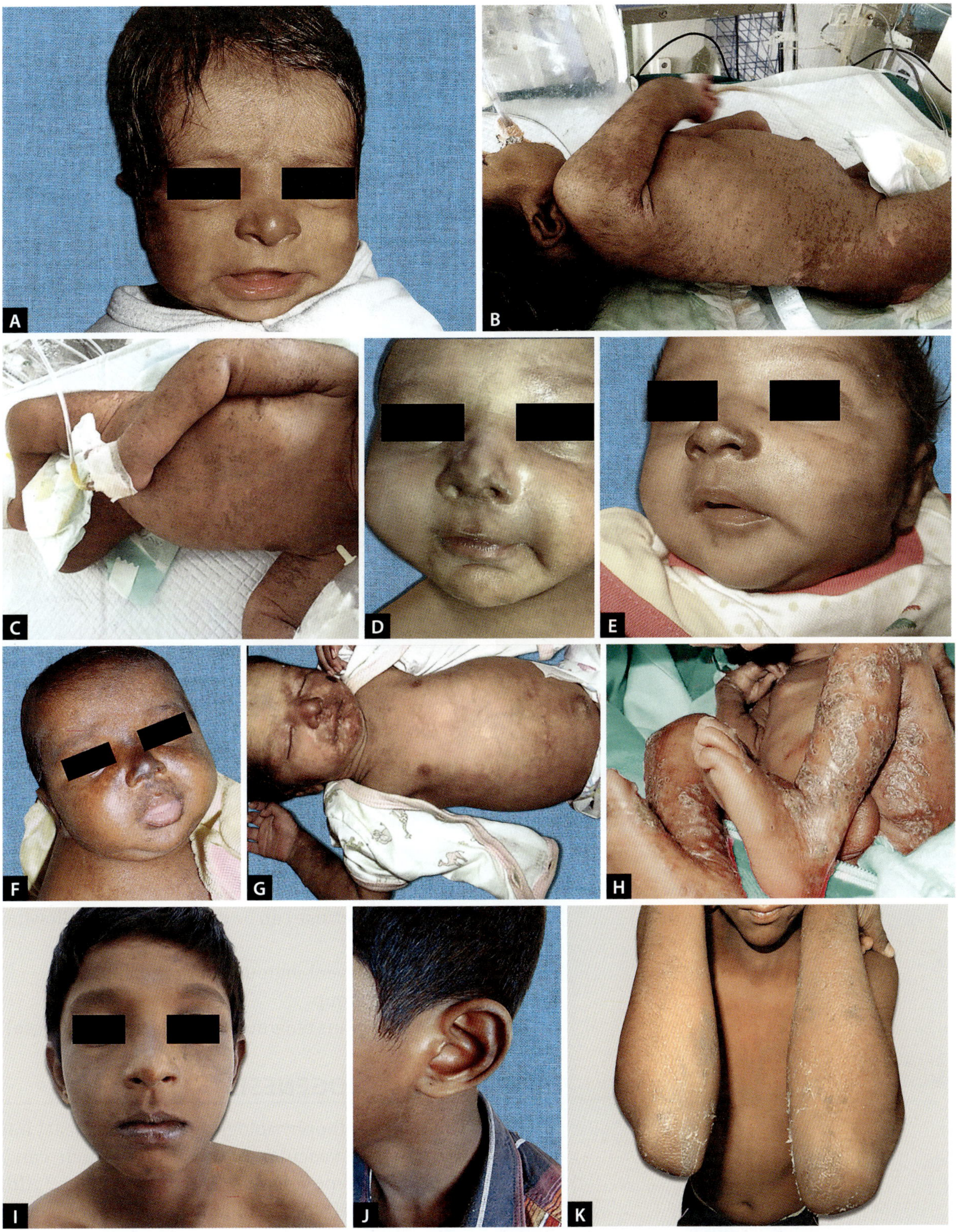

Figs. 19A to K: (A) Classical rash of chikungunya fever; (B) Chikungunya rash in a neonate, note the superficial erosions over trunk and extremities; (C) Same neonate, another view; (D) Rash over face, hyperpigmentation in a butterfly distribution; (E) Facial hyperpigmentation in neonatal chikungunya; (F) Classical chik sign seen in chikungunya along with hyperpigmentation on face and upper chest; (G) Generalized hyperpigmentation; (H) Dystrophic calcification in a case of congenital chikungunya, a very rare event; (I) Childhood chikungunya, note hyperpigmentation; (J) Same child, note hyperpigmentation over pinnae; (K) Subsiding chikungunya rash, note exfoliation.

"And most important, have the courage to follow your heart and intuition." —**Steve Jobs**

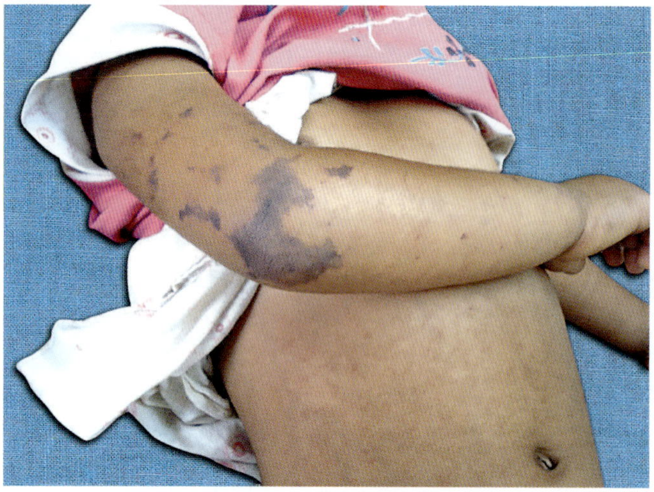

Fig. 20: Purpuric lesions of rickettsial disease.

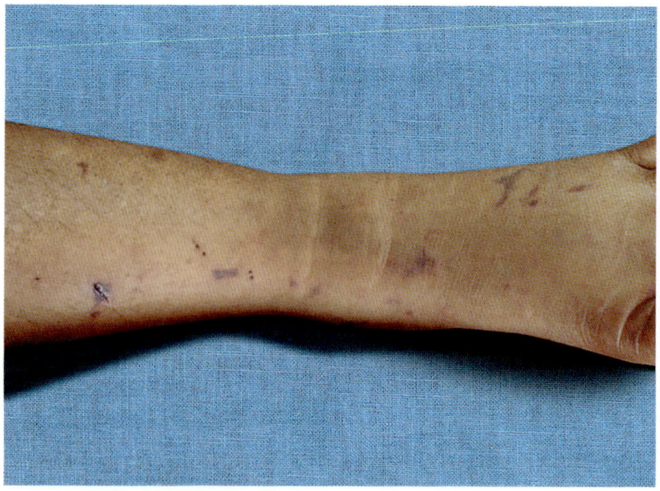

Fig. 21: Classical lesions of rickettsial disease.

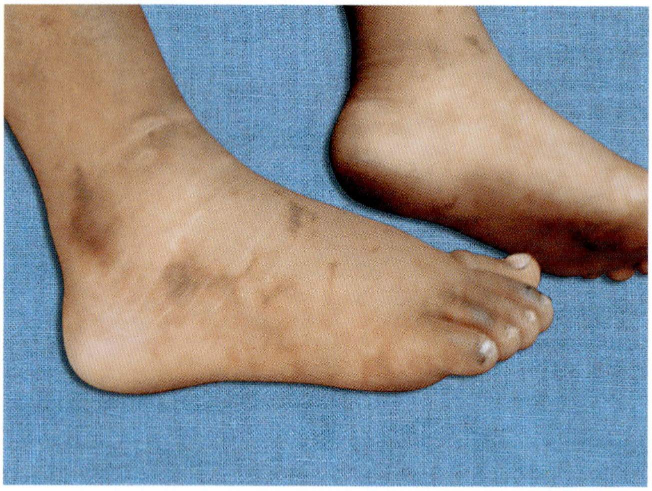

Fig. 22: Same boy, subsiding purpuric rash of rickettsial disease.

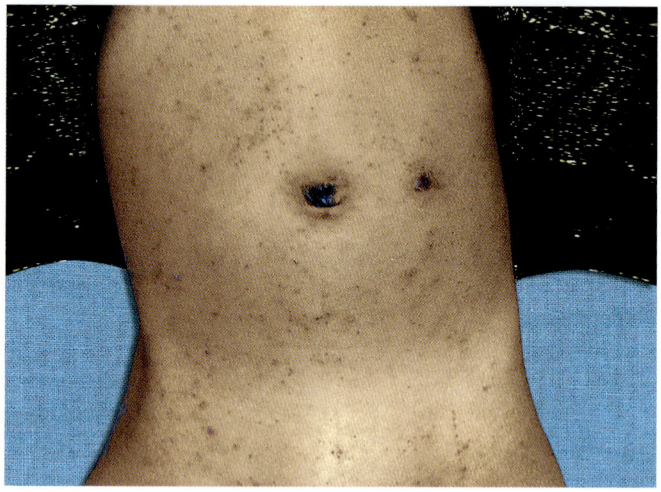

Fig. 23: Rickettsial pox lesions.

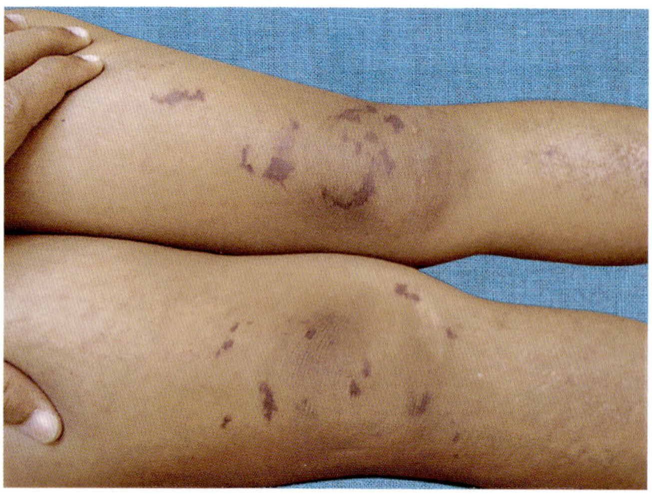

Fig. 24: Rickettsial disease, lesions over knee.

genus of *Rickettsiae* can be divided into the following three biogroups:

1. Spotted fever biogroup (15 rickettsioses)
2. Typhus group
3. Scrub typhus biogroup (Tsutsugamushi disease)

ETIOPATHOGENESIS

The major pathophysiologic effect of rickettsial infection is increased vascular permeability which can result in edema, hypovolemia, and hypotension. Although endothelial cells of the microcirculation of all organs are affected, the critical organs are the lungs and the brain which can cause life-threatening infection. A fatal outcome results if there is pulmonary edema, acute respiratory distress syndrome, and aseptic meningitis.

Clinical Features

Typically begins with a prodrome of fever, headache, nausea, myalgia, vomiting, and abdominal pain. A cutaneous rash develops between the 3rd and 6th day of the disease. Lethargy and confusion may be early features of central nervous involvement. As clinical course progresses, hypotension, acute renal failure, respiratory failure, and coma may develop.

The typical cutaneous feature is the presence of an eschar consisting of a central area of dermal and epidermal necrosis (0.5–2 cm) surrounded by a zone of erythema that appears during the initial 4–10 days. The rash begins at the wrists and ankles in case of spotted fever and axillae in typhus fever. The exanthem involves the entire body with relative sparing of the face. Palms and soles are generally involved with a maculopapular rash. Petechiae and purpura may develop in cases of severe endothelial injury. Cutaneous necrosis can also lead to the necrosis of digits, ear lobes, and tip of nose.

Differential Diagnosis

- Viral exanthem
- Drug rash
- Kawasaki disease
- Measles
- Dengue fever

Laboratory Diagnosis

Serologic testing using specific methods (e.g., immunofluorescence antibody test, indirect immunoperoxidase test, and enzyme immunoassay) is superior to the Weil-Felix reaction.

Treatment

Specific Therapy

Adequate antibiotic therapy initiated early in the first week of illness is highly effective and is associated with the best outcome. Fever usually subsides within 24–72 hours after starting antibiotic therapy. If fever fails to subside with the use of a suitable antibiotic, the diagnosis of rickettsial disease should be reconsidered. Treatment may be terminated 2–3 days after the patient is afebrile and at least 10 days of therapy has been given.

Doxycycline is the drug of choice for all rickettsial infections. It is preferred over other tetracyclines for the treatment of rickettsial infections, and at such low dose and short duration, is rarely associated with staining of teeth in children younger than 8 years.

The first-line drug in cases of scrub typhus is azithromycin.

Supportive Therapy

Thrombocytopenia, hypoalbuminemia, hypotension, and coagulation defects require supportive management. Hyponatremia is best managed with maintenance fluids or even modest fluid restriction.

HAND-FOOT-AND-MOUTH DISEASE (FIGS. 25 TO 35)

Hand-foot-and-mouth disease (HFMD) is a distinctive viral infection caused by *Enterovirus*, member of Picornaviridae. It was first reported in New Zealand in 1957. HFMD is most commonly associated with infections

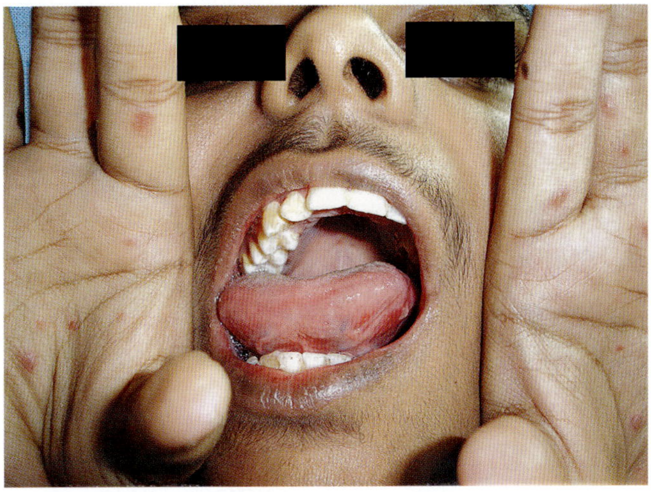

Fig. 25: Hand-foot-and-mouth disease (HFMD) in an adolescent boy.

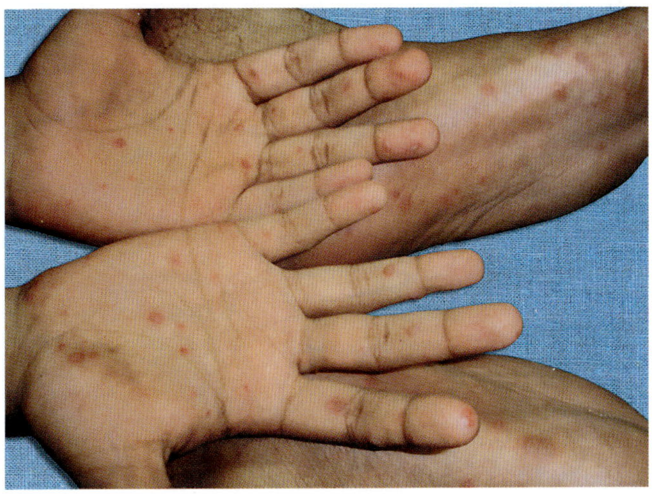

Fig. 26: Same boy with palmoplantar lesions.

"Hardship often prepare ordinary people for an extraordinary destiny." **—CS Lewis**

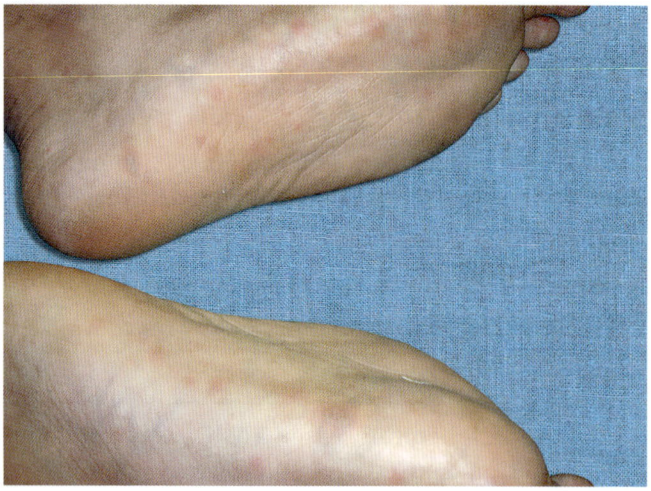

Fig. 27: HFMD, close-up view of plantar lesions.

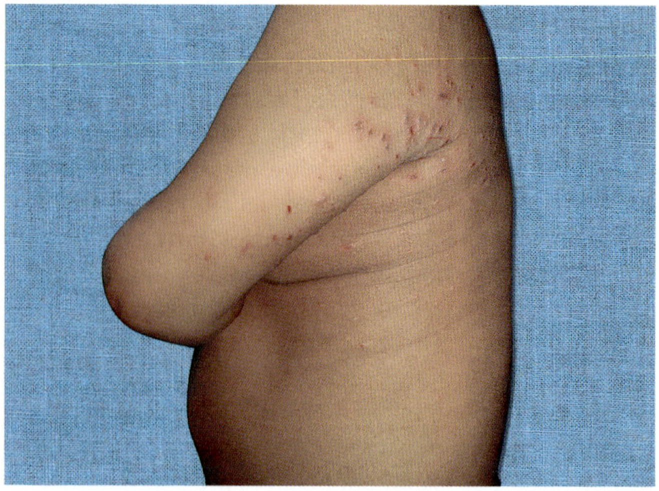

Fig. 28: Grouped vesicles around axillary fold in HFMD.

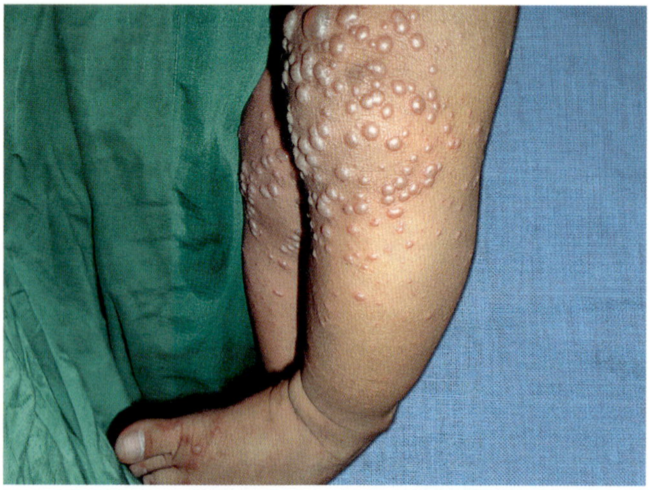

Fig. 29: Clustering of lesions of HFMD around knee.

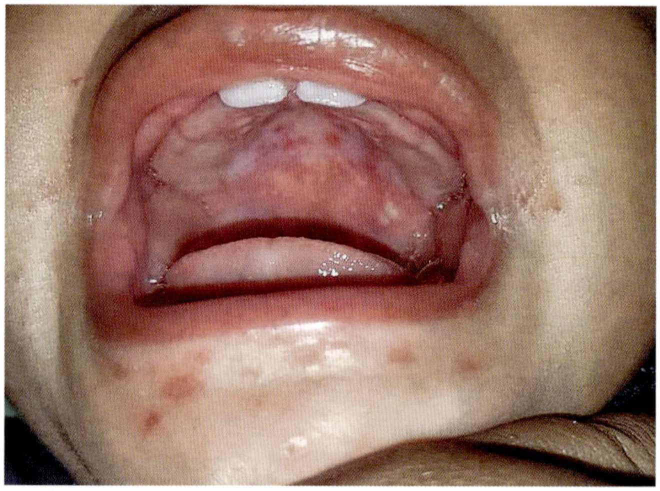

Fig. 30: Oral mucosal lesions in HFMD.

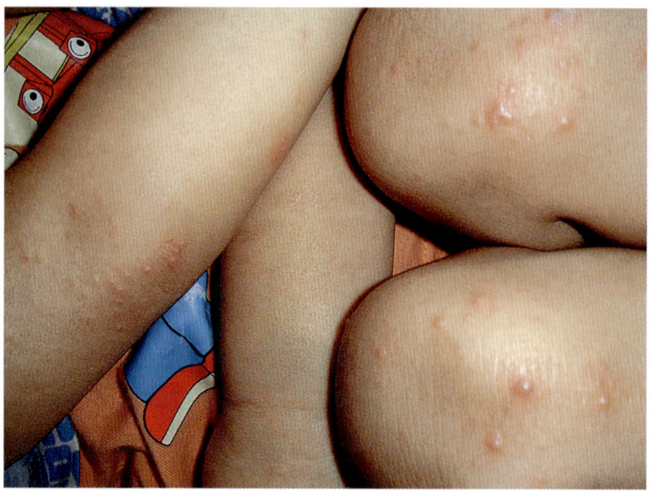

Fig. 31: Lesions over elbow and knee in HFMD.

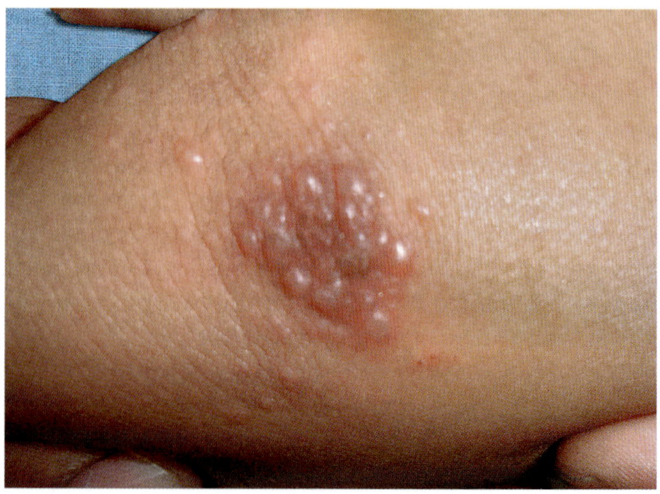

Fig. 32: Grouped vesicles in HFMD.

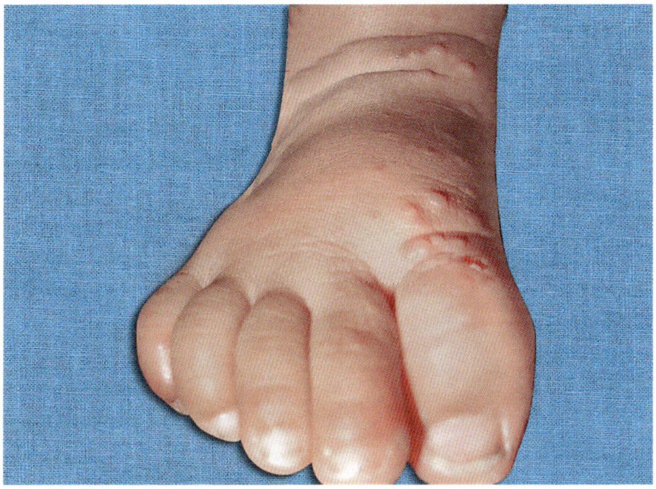

Fig. 33: Lesions over foot in an infant with HFMD.

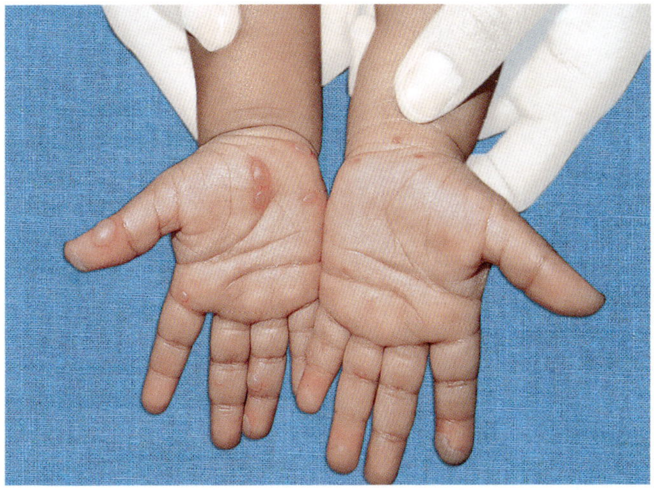

Fig. 34: Large blisters of HFMD over palms.

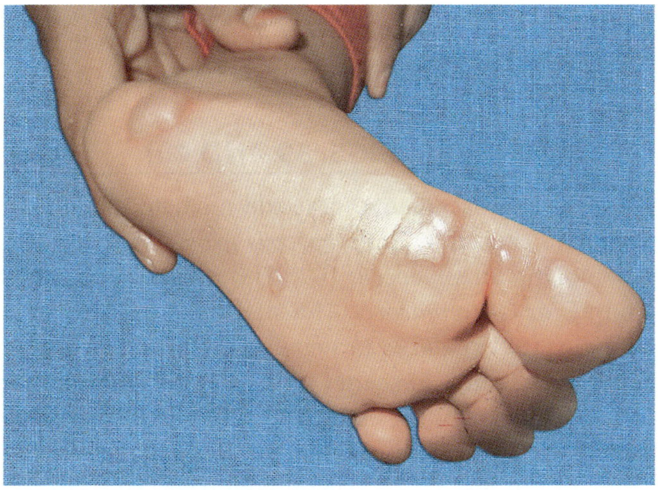

Fig. 35: Large blisters of HFMD on sole.

due to *coxsackie* A16 or *Enterovirus* 71, which are single-stranded, encapsulated RNA viruses. Other etiological agents are *coxsackie* virus A4-A7, A9, A10, B1-B3, and B5. HFMD affects children most commonly between 1 and 10 years of age. It rarely occurs in adults. It is seen in summer and autumn months. It is highly contagious to other family members. The route of transmission is fecal-oral route or through contact with skin lesions or oral secretions. After a short incubation period of 3-6 days, the virus spreads to regional lymph nodes within 24 hours and later disseminate to oral cavity and skin.

Mild fever and constitutional symptoms may precede the skin eruptions. It is characterized by sudden onset of groups of papulovesicles or vesicles on an erythematous base. These vesicles are oval to elliptical and are painful. They occur on specific areas such as hands, feet, perioral region, elbow and knee joints, forearms, legs, and gluteal region. It affects oral mucosa and rarely genitalia. It heals without scarring. Most of the cases improve spontaneously within 7-10 days. Complications are rare and include cardiac dysfunction, fulminant pulmonary edema, myocarditis, meningitis, encephalitis, and acute flaccid paralysis. Atypical forms have become very common in the current scenario and includes bullous, purpuric, desquamation, targetoid lesions, and generalized maculopapular form. Most common nail complications include Beau's lines and onychomadesis which presents after 6-8 weeks post hand-foot-mouth disease.

Differential diagnoses to be considered are varicella, herpes simplex, impetigo, pompholyx, papular urticaria, scabies, and herpangina. Mortality is rare and complications are more seen with *Enterovirus* 71. HFMD is a clinical diagnosis and requires no investigations. Confirmation can be done by culture or by detection of neutralizing antibodies in serum. Management of HFMD is symptomatic. Systemic antibiotics can be given if it is associated with secondary infection. Topical anesthetics can be used for oral mucosa.

UNILATERAL LATEROTHORACIC EXANTHEM (ASYMMETRIC PERIFLEXURAL EXANTHEM) (FIGS. 36 TO 38)

Unilateral laterothoracic exanthem, also called as asymmetric periflexural exanthem of childhood, is a distinct exanthem presenting in a unilateral distribution. It is an underdiagnosed condition. The exact etiology is not known and probably related to viral association

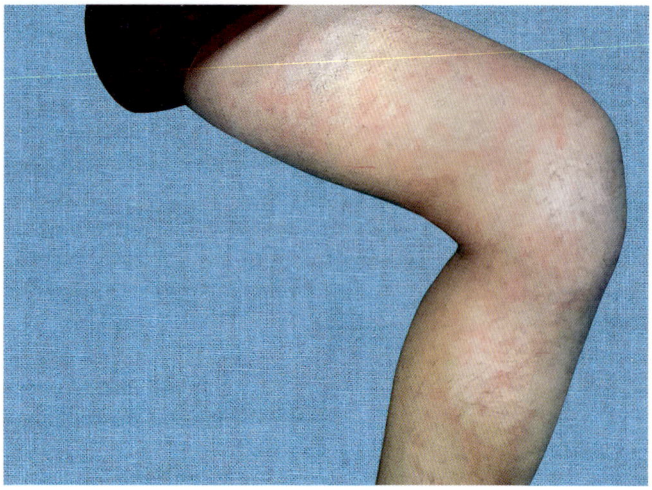

Fig. 36: Asymmetric periflexural exanthem over thigh and leg in an 8-year-old boy.

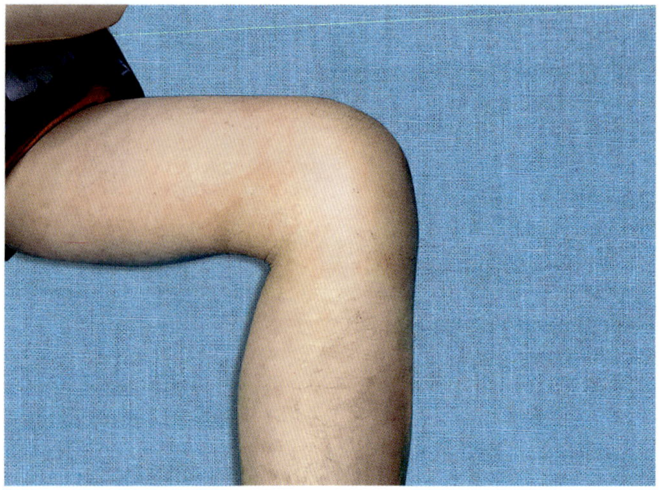

Fig. 37: Same boy, another view.

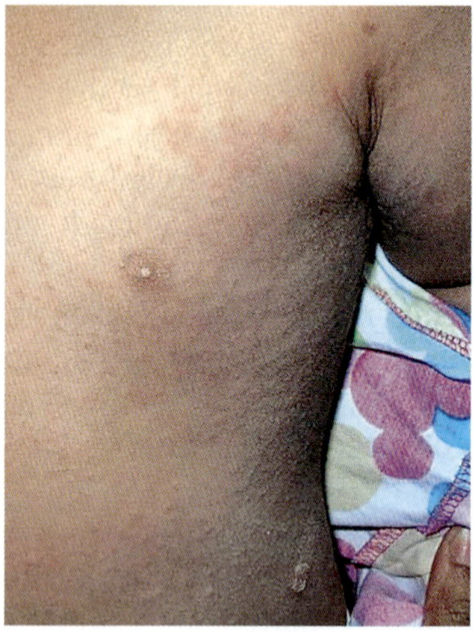

Fig. 38: Asymmetric periflexural exanthem (APE) or unilateral laterothoracic exanthem (ULTE) in an 11-month-old child.

such as adenovirus, parainfluenza virus, and EBV. There is a mild prodrome of low-grade fever, respiratory or gastrointestinal symptoms. The age of onset is between 1 and 5 years of age and usually occurs during winter and spring season. Lesion starts as asymptomatic to pruritic skin colored to erythematous papules on the trunk, in a centrifugal fashion extending toward the axillae or can occur on the extremity. Initially, they are unilateral in distribution and later can become bilateral. Other morphological patterns include eczematous, morbilliform, scarlatiniform, vesicular, and purpuric lesions in an annular or reticulate pattern. Differential diagnoses include contact dermatitis, pityriasis rosea, scarlet fever, miliaria, erythema infectiosum (EI), tinea infections, and papular acrodermatitis of childhood. Lesions resolve by few weeks spontaneously with desquamation leaving behind postinflammatory pigmentation.

SCARLET FEVER (FIGS. 39 AND 40)

Scarlet fever or "scarlatina," is a toxin-mediated childhood exanthem caused by *Streptococcus pyogenes*, a group A β-hemolytic *Streptococcus* (GABHS) and very rarely by group C or G *streptococci*. The streptococcal pyrogenic exotoxins (SPEs) and M protein are important virulence factors. Epidemics of scarlet fever were common in the 18th and 19th centuries after which it had substantially decreased. However, recent studies have shown a resurgence of the disease in several countries. This change might be due to microbial determinants, such as new strains with higher virulence capacities and changes in herd immunity with lack of immunity in young children. Epidemiological changes in the type of SPEs produced over time have been associated with changes in the severity of the disease.

Scarlet fever occurs more commonly in children, especially under 10 years of age. Transmission is by the aerosol route, but may also spread by direct skin contact and rarely can be food-borne. Risk of scarlet fever has been shown to increase along with the degrees of air pollution. It is characterized by the presence of a rash along with a *S. pyogenes* infection, usually pharyngitis, but may also complicate skin and soft tissue or wound infections, as well as varicella in children. The incubation period is short, about 2–3 days, with a sudden onset of fever, headache, malaise, and evidence of tonsillitis and pharyngitis without rhinorrhea or cough. Tonsillopharyngeal erythema and

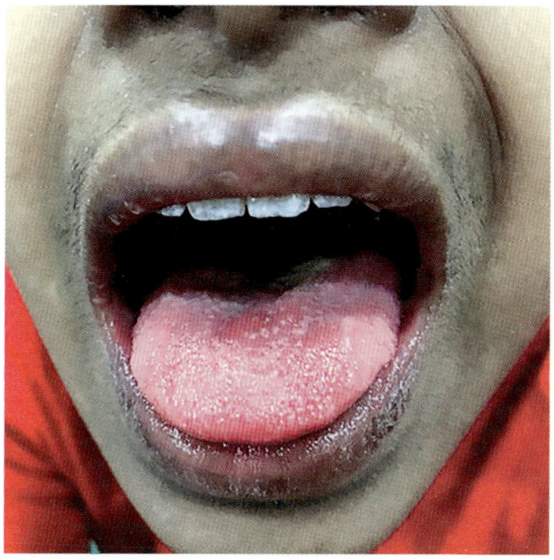

Fig. 39: Strawberry red tongue in scarlet fever.

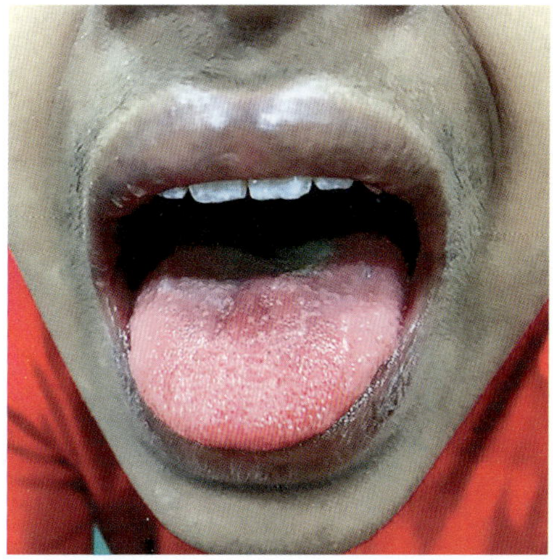

Fig. 40: Same child, close-up view.

exudates and petechial macules on the palate may be seen. Tender anterior cervical adenopathy is commonly present.

The characteristic punctate erythematous rash of scarlet fever appears on the first or second day of illness on the groin, axilla, and trunk and then spreads to the extremities sparing the palms and soles. This exanthem is usually a result of delayed-type skin reactivity to pyrogenic exotoxins (SPEs) produced by the organism. The fine blanchable erythematous macular and papular rash gives the skin a characteristic "sandpaper" feel on a background of erythema. Accentuation of this rash on the flexural creases gives rise to classic linear red streaks of petechiae called Pastia's lines. It may be difficult to identify the exanthem in darkly pigmented skin and may consist of only punctate papules resembling "goose flesh." Facial flushing with circumoral pallor is characteristic. Edematous red papillae on a coated tongue (white strawberry tongue) is seen in the first few days of illness which later becomes red and glistening studded with prominent papillae (red strawberry tongue) following resolution of the white coating. The exanthem usually resolves over 4–5 days followed by thick sheets of desquamation of the palms and soles, which typically begins on the fingertips at the free margin of the fingernails. Complications include toxic and septic forms of scarlet fever with peritonsillar and retropharyngeal abscesses associated with prolonged symptoms or localized pain, acute rheumatic fever (RF), glomerulonephritis, bacteremia, pneumonia, endocarditis, and meningitis. Rarely, hepatitis, gallbladder hydrops or splenomegaly may occur. The differential diagnosis of scarlet fever includes viral exanthems, KD, staphylococcal toxic shock syndrome, and allergic reactions.

Diagnosis is established based on clinical manifestations and confirmed by laboratory examination. The Centor Criteria Score comprising four clinical signs and symptoms can be used to estimate the probability of group A *Streptococcus* (GAS) pharyngitis. Throat swab culture with growth of GAS is the gold standard laboratory examination. Rapid antigen detection tests and antistreptococcal serologies are also used. Scarlet fever and streptococcal pharyngitis usually resolve spontaneously but early initiation of treatment is required to alleviate symptoms and prevent the development of complications. It has been suggested to start antimicrobial therapy within 9 days of onset of pharyngitis in order to prevent RF. Drug of choice for scarlet fever is penicillin V. Amoxicillin has similar efficacy and is often preferred for its longer half-life, especially in children. In case of penicillin allergy, macrolides (erythromycin, azithromycin, and clarithromycin) or clindamycin can be used. First-generation cephalosporins can be used but the possibility of cross-reaction in cases of penicillin allergy should be considered. Intramuscular penicillin G has also been used but is painful. Supportive therapy in the form of analgesics and/or antipyretic agents are usually required. Measures to reduce the spread of the disease is very important. Children should be quarantined for 24 hours after the commencement of appropriate antibiotic treatment.

PAPULAR-PURPURIC GLOVES AND SOCKS SYNDROME (FIGS. 41 AND 42)

Papular-purpuric gloves and socks syndrome (PPGSS) is a rare exanthematous condition that affects mostly young adults and rarely children, predominantly during the

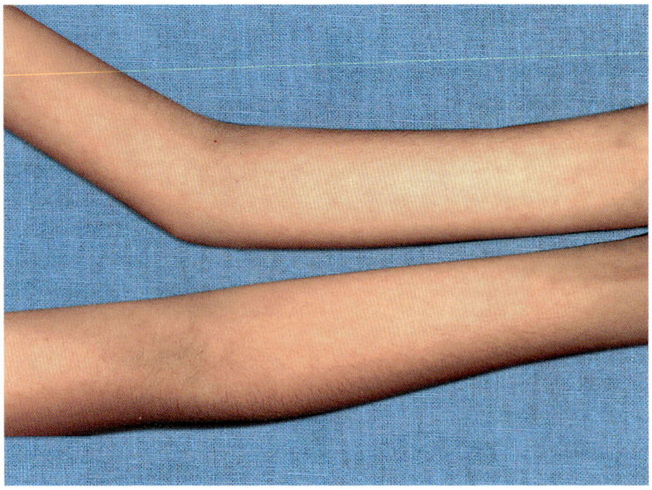

Fig. 41: Papular-purpuric gloves and socks syndrome, lesions over upper limbs.

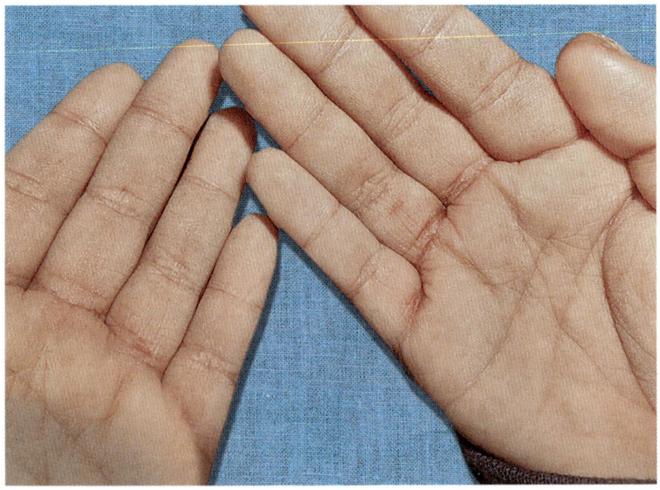

Fig. 42: Papular-purpuric gloves and socks syndrome, lesions over palms.

spring and summer. It is characterized by acute onset of fever with intense erythema, edema, and petechiae on the hands and feet, and oral lesions. Parvovirus B19 is the most common causative organism; however, other viruses, such as *cytomegalovirus (CMV), EBV, measles, rubella, hepatitis B virus, Coxsackievirus B6, human herpesvirus* 6 and 7, bacteria (*Arcanobacterium haemolyticum*), *Mycoplasma pneumoniae*, and drugs such as trimethoprim/sulfamethoxazole have also been implicated as causative agents for PPGSS. Characteristic cutaneous manifestation is acute onset of painful, pruritic erythema, and edema localized symmetrically over the hands and feet with a sharp demarcation at the wrists and ankles, followed by the gradual appearance of erythematous papules, petechiae or purpura and rarely, blisters on the same sites. Less frequently, similar lesions may also occur on the cheeks, elbows, knees, trunk, thighs, and buttocks. Appearance of purpuric rash is accompanied by the development of constitutional symptoms (fever, fatigue, lymphadenopathy, myalgia, arthralgia, diarrhea, and abdominal pain) and oral lesions. Oral erosions, petechiae, and edema involving the lips, buccal mucosa, and palate are often present. Genital mucosa may also be affected with painful edema, erythema, and/or ulcerations of the glans penis and vagina. It is a self-limiting disease with resolution occurring spontaneously in 7–14 days, with slight peeling on palms and soles. Rarely, PPGSS can recur after complete resolution of the lesions. The symptoms are generally mild in children and adolescents, while most severe cases occur in adults. Atypical variants include a unilateral distribution, involvement of the buttocks, genital, and axillary regions, and large hemorrhagic bullae progressing to cutaneous necrosis and skin ulcerations. Patients with PPGSS are considered to be contagious when skin lesions are present as the syndrome develops at the onset of viremia, before the appearance of serum IgM antibodies.

The diagnosis of PPGSS is primarily clinical and may be supported by laboratory and histopathological findings. Nonspecific findings include mild anemia, leukopenia, neutropenia, monocytosis, eosinophilia, thrombocytopenia, unconjugated hyperbilirubinemia, and mild elevation of serum hepatic transaminase levels. The pathogenesis of PPGSS is not clear. The hypothesized mechanism is most likely due to immune complex deposition, supported by histopathological findings of lymphocytic perivascular infiltrates, edema of the papillary dermis, and extravasation of red blood cells. These findings are not specific for vasculitis, though focal vasculitic changes have been reported. Direct immunofluorescence shows deposition of IgM and C3 at the dermoepidermal junction in a granular pattern and in the walls of the papillary dermal vessels, suggesting a vascular reaction to antigenic challenge. PVB19 viral particles have been isolated in the endothelial cells of the dermal vessel walls and in the basal cells of the epidermis. Serum anti-Parvovirus B19 IgM antibodies testing helps in diagnosing acute infection in immunocompetent patients. An early negative serology result does not rule out parvovirus B19 infection. Parvovirus B19 DNA can be detected by PCR in serum during the early stages of disease. This is more helpful in patients with transient aplastic crisis or in immunocompromised patients where the antibody response is deficient.

The symptomatic variety of PPGSS should be differentiated from lymphoproliferative disorders, thrombocytopenic syndromes, KD, leukocytoclastic or hypersensitivity vasculitis (cryoglobulinemic vasculitis and Henoch-Schönlein purpura) and still's disease, Gianotti-Crosti syndrome, hand foot mouth disease, erythema multiforme and meningococcal sepsis. In most cases of PPGSS, only symptomatic treatment with antipyretics and nonsteroidal anti-inflammatory drugs is sufficient as it resolves spontaneously. Immuno-suppressive therapy is avoided as it may promote the persistence of the virus.

ERYTHEMA INFECTIOSUM (FIGS. 43 TO 45)

Erythema infectiosum or "fifth disease" is a common viral exanthem caused by parvovirus B19 and typically occurs in outbreaks among children 5–15 years old during spring and early summer months. It is transmitted via droplets from respiratory secretions and can also spread via blood exposure. Viremia usually occurs within 5–10 days, and the patient remains contagious for approximately 5 days until the production of IgM anti-B19 antibody. Symptoms range from nonspecific flu-like symptoms to the classic symptoms of facial rash and arthralgia. Once patients have symptoms of arthralgia and exanthem, they are no longer contagious. In the fetus, it affects red blood cell production causing hydrops fetalis.

Prodromal symptoms include fever, chills, runny nose, nausea, and headache. The illness occurs in three phases. First phase is marked by the appearance of characteristic fiery red facial erythema sparing the nasal bridge and perioral area, called as the slapped-cheek appearance. It occurs 2–3 days after the prodrome and is related to the formation and deposition of immune complexes. In the second phase, lace-like or reticulated eruption occurs on the trunk and extremities after several days of the facial rash. It is evanescent and may be pruritic and spares the palms and soles. This rash usually fades away in 2–3 weeks. The rash may be very "fleeting" (<24 hours), but may intermittently recur in response to sunlight exposure, heat, emotional stress, or strenuous exercise. This intermittent waxing and waning marks the third stage of the disease. Older infected children may also have lymphadenopathy and an atypical rash. Other viral exanthems such as measles, rubella, roseola, and scarlet fever should be differentiated from EI. Joint symptoms,

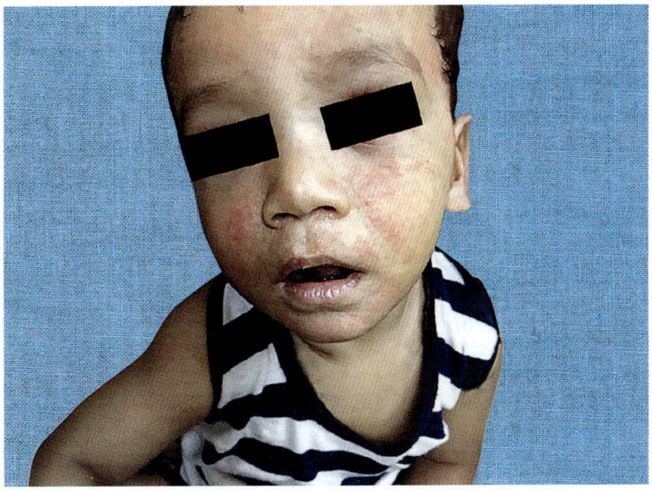

Fig. 44: Same child, another view.

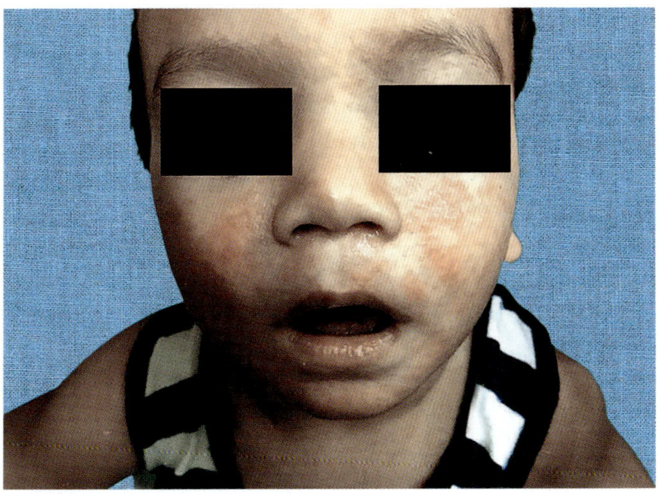

Fig. 43: Erythema infectiosum, note "slapped cheek" appearance.

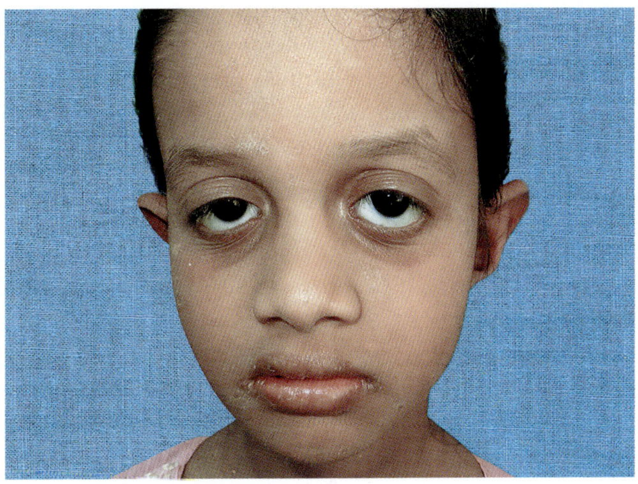

Fig. 45: Another girl with erythema infectiosum.

"Life doesn't get easier or more forgiving; we get stronger and more resilient." —**Steve Maraboli**

thought to be immune-mediated, are more common in adult females and occur only in 8–10% of children with EI. There is symmetric involvement of joints of hands, wrist, knees, and feet. Signs of physical destruction of the joints from the virus are not present and the symptoms are transient and self-limited, resolving after about 3 weeks of onset. Chronic arthritis may occasionally be seen in children. Manifestations of rash and joint symptoms are absent in immunocompromised individuals as they would not have an adequate immune response to this infection for these symptoms to develop. They may instead develop chronic parvovirus B19 infection which can lead to neutropenia, thrombocytopenia, or complete bone marrow suppression.

Symptoms of EI are usually mild and self-limiting in immunocompetent hosts. So, laboratory diagnosis is usually not warranted in the presence of typical clinical manifestations. Serological testing for specific parvovirus B19 IgM antibody can confirm acute infection in immunocompromised patients and in those with aplastic crisis. In pregnant women exposed to B19, serologic testing for IgM and IgG antibodies is recommended, and if acute infection is documented, serial fetal ultrasonography is indicated. Prenatal presence of protective Ig G antibodies against B19 in the mother prevents vertical transmission of B19 infection. Treatment consists of symptom control [e.g., use of acetaminophen and/or nonsteroidal anti-inflammatory drugs (NSAIDs) for fever, headache, arthralgia] and supportive management.

NOVEL CORONA VIRUS (COVID-19) INFECTION

Severe acute respiratory syndrome coronavirus 2 (SARS-CoV-2) is a new strain of coronavirus.

The disease caused by the novel coronavirus was first identified in Wuhan, the largest metropolitan area in China's Hubei province. It has been named coronavirus disease 2019 (COVID-19): "CO" stands for corona, "VI" for virus, and "D" for disease. Formerly, this disease was referred to as "2019 novel coronavirus" or "2019-nCoV". The COVID-19 virus is a new virus linked to the same family of viruses as "Severe Acute Respiratory Syndrome (SARS)" and some types of common cold. COVID-19 is an illness that may lead to serious respiratory disease and may be fatal. The first human case occurred in Wuhan, China in December 2019, and the infection rapidly spread throughout the world. COVID-19 is a RNA virus which belongs to human beta-coronavirus group. Some mutations emerging in the SARS-CoV-2 genome are speculated to modulate viral transmission, replication efficiency and virulence in different parts of the world.

Other coronaviruses cause the common cold, pharyngitis, laryngitis, and "flu-like symptoms". On 11th March 2020, the World Health Organization declared the COVID-19 outbreak as a pandemic, as it had spread rapidly worldwide. COVID-19 affects people of all ages. Older persons, those with underlying chronic medical conditions, and those who are immunosuppressed have a higher risk of developing severe, life-threatening illness. However, young and otherwise healthy people can also be affected significantly with increased mortality. The most common underlying chronic medical conditions that are reported to result in more severe disease include: diabetes, cardiovascular disease including hypertension, and obstructive pulmonary disease. The incubation period is 2–10 days in most individuals. Patients are infectious for a couple of days before becoming symptomatic, during active phase and after recovery. Infected people without symptoms are also infectious. Although the rate of spread of infection is about 55% of those with symptoms, worldwide, this group is thought to contribute to the spread of the virus ten-fold. In countries where there is evidence of community spread, physical distancing and face masks are required to prevent an exponential increase in cases.

How does COVID-19 Spread?

The SARS-CoV-2 virus is found in droplets spread by an infected individual while he/she is coughing, sneezing, talking, or touching items. The droplets may land on surfaces such as door handles, computer keyboards, and table-tops. The virus remains infectious for several days on smooth surfaces but shorter periods on paper, wood, or cloth. An uninfected individual who has touched an invisible droplet may then touch his/her face, transmitting the virus through the mucous membranes of their mouth, nose, and eyes, resulting in infection.

What are the Symptoms of COVID-19?

The severity of COVID-19 is variable. Some individuals infected with SARS-CoV-2 do not develop any symptoms. The most common symptoms of COVID-19 are fever, cough, shortness of breath and tiredness.

Other common symptoms include:

- Body aches and pains
- Runny nose
- Loss of smell and taste

"Courage is not the absence of fear, but rather the judgement that something else is more important than fear." —**Ambrose Redmoon**

- Sore throat
- Abdominal pain
- Diarrhea

Skin Rash of COVID-19 Infection

More and more data on cutaneous presentations of COVID-19 are coming up. Skin manifestations have been uncommonly described in patients with COVID-19. They are reported to be similar to other viral infections: an erythematous exanthema, acute urticaria, chickenpox-like vesicles, pseudo-chilblain lesions (referred to as COVID toes), retiform purpura or necrosis.

In Italy, cutaneous manifestations were seen in 20% of patients with most having nonspecific viral rash. Often, it develops in already hospitalized patients and can possibly be misdiagnosed as drug reaction. In China, ischemic lesions suggesting coagulopathy, and urticarial rash were seen. Dengue-like rash was observed in a few patients with COVID-19 infection in Singapore and Bangkok. In France, various skin rash observed were pseudo-frostbite, persistent painful redness of different parts of skin. Foot sore is another type of skin rash seen in some patients and termed as 'COVID toes'.

Diagnosis

COVID-19 is diagnosed using respiratory swabs. These real-time reverse transcription-polymerase chain reaction (rRT-PCR) tests detect the SARS-CoV-2 virus. Tests for other respiratory infections such as influenza and respiratory syncytial virus (RSV) may be done at the same time.

- A positive result means the patient has active COVID-19 (or one of the other infections tested).
- A negative swab does not always rule out infection.
- The test may be repeated if symptoms progress or for public health purposes.

The diagnosis of COVID-19 may also be made clinically where the patient has been in contact with a COVID-19 patient, where community infection is widespread, or the patient has recently traveled from a country with community infection.

Treatment and Prevention

Isolation of the patient is extremely important. Azithromycin and hydroxychloroquine have shown variable success. In in vitro study, ivermectin has been found to be effective. Various antivirals tried in cases of COVID-19 with variable success are lopinavir, ritonavir, favipiravir, and remdesivir. For severe infection, tocilizumab was found to be quite effective in some patients.

Quarantine of all contacts for at least 14 days is very important.

For prevention of the disease spread, use of mask among all patients having cough and cold, their contacts, social distancing, etc. are to be strictly practiced. Doctors and all healthcare workers must use personal protective equipment and mask.

ROSEOLA INFANTUM (FIGS. 46 AND 47)

Roseola infantum is a common disease of childhood caused primarily by human herpesvirus 6 (HHV-6) and less frequently by human herpesvirus 7 (HHV-7). It is also known as sixth disease or exanthema subitem which occurs in children of age 6-12 months, usually before

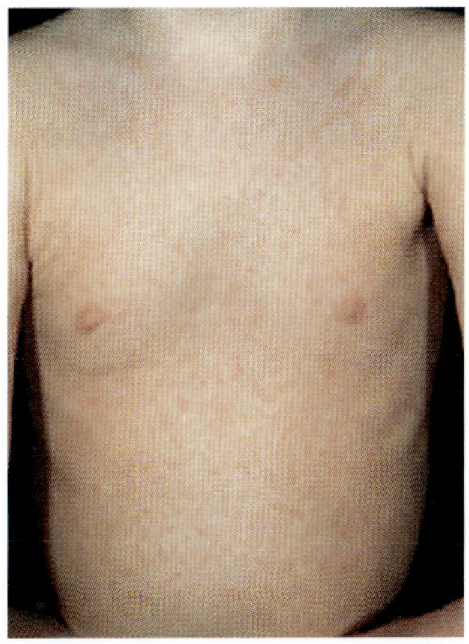

Fig. 46: Roseola infantum in a 6-year-old boy.

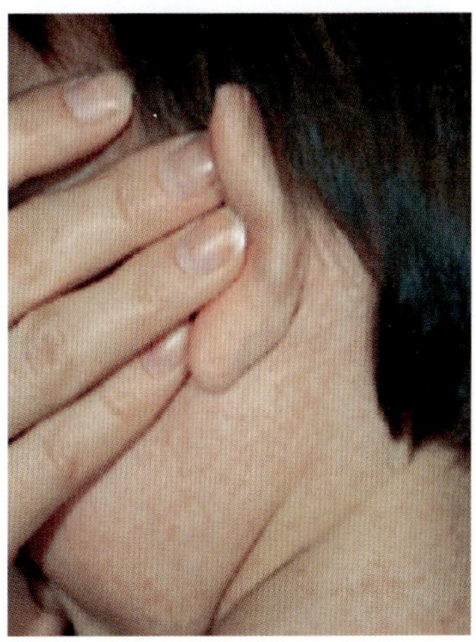

Fig. 47: Same boy, retroauricular region.

"Happiness is not by chance but by choice." —**Jim Rohn**

2 years. It presents as acute onset of high-grade fever up to 40 C for 3–5 days. Fever subsides rapidly with occurrence of nonpruritic, pink papular rash (2–5 mm) that begins on the trunk and spreads to the neck, extremities and face. As the virus can cross the blood brain barrier, children can have acute febrile seizure during the febrile phase. Uvulo-palatoglossal spots also known as Nagayama spots, are erythematous papules found on the soft palate and uvula. It is a clinically diagnosed, self-limited illness that is usually treated symptomatically. Other symptoms like malaise, irritability, conjunctivitis, lymphadenopathy, orbital edema, inflammation of the tympanic membranes, anorexia, a bulging fontanelle, diarrhea, cough and other upper respiratory tract symptoms are also seen.

Management

The disease is usually self-limiting and no specific treatment is required. Supportive therapy like rest, fluid management and antipyretics for fever can be given. Adequate hand washing is advised to prevent the spread of disease. Currently no vaccine or antiviral therapy is available for the acute phase of the disease.

SUGGESTED READINGS

1. Adem PV. Emerging and re-emerging rickettsial infections. Semin Diagn Pathol. 2019;36(3):146-51.
2. Alexender Otto M. Skin Manifestations are emerging in the corona virus pandemic. Dermatology News; April 3, 2020.
3. Esposito S, Principi N. Hand, foot and mouth disease: current knowledge on clinical manifestations, epidemiology, aetiology and prevention. Eur J Clin Microbiol Infect Dis. 2018;37(3):391-8.
4. Keighley CL, Saunderson RB, Kok J, Dwyer DE. Viral exanthems. Curr Opin Infect Dis. 2015;28(2):139-50.
5. Son MBF, Newburger JW. Kawasaki disease. Pediatr Rev. 2018;39(2):78-90.
6. Vasani R, Kanhere S, Chaudhari K, Phadke V, Mukherjee P, Gupta S, et al. Congenital chikungunya: a cause of neonatal hyperpigmentation. Pediatr Dermatol. 2016;33:209-12.
7. www.thelancet.com/child-adolescent. Published online April 8, 2020. [online] Available from https://doi.org/10.1016/S2352-4642(20)30105-XApril 08.

CHAPTER

7

Eczema and Dermatitis

NAPKIN DERMATITIS (FIGS. 1 TO 2B)

The term "napkin dermatitis" refers to an inflammatory eruption of the napkin area. Hydration of skin, friction between skin and the fabric of the napkin, urine and its degradation products, proteolytic and lipolytic enzymes, and microorganisms such as *Candida albicans* and *Staphylococcus aureus* are supposed to play an etiologic role. Onset is from 3rd to 12th week and the peak prevalence is seen between the 7th and 12th month. Both sexes and all races appear to be equally affected. It manifests as confluent erythema on the convex surfaces in closest contact with the napkin, i.e., buttocks, genitalia, lower abdomen and pubic area, and upper thighs sparing the inguinal folds. Where the reaction is acute, peeling of skin in sheets may occur. Postinflammatory hypopigmentation may be a striking feature. In both sexes, involvement of the genitalia may lead to dysuria.

Jacquet's Dermatitis (Fig. 2C)

Jacquet's dermatitis is a severe erosive form of irritant contact napkin dermatitis. This clinical entity was first recognized by Jacquet in 1905. It tends to affect more in older children wearing napkin or with infrequent diaper change. The frequency of its occurrence recently has decreased due to the use of good modern diapers. Persistent occlusion, maceration, friction, and prolonged contact with urine and feces contribute to the development of Jacquet's dermatitis. It persists for a long time if the child has incontinence. They are also called as "ammoniacal ulcers." It clinically presents as papuloerosive and nodular lesions, superficial erosions or punched out ulcers with raised erythematous border. Mucosae are spared. The most common sites affected are penis, labia, and concave surface of perianal region. Jacquet's dermatitis is difficult to differentiate from perianal pseudoverrucous papules and nodules (PPPN), and granuloma gluteale infantum.

Management

Napkin dermatitis is self-limiting in most of the cases as the children outgrow this problem after successful potty training. The mother or the caregiver should be advised regarding increasing the frequency of napkin changes and proper cleansing of the skin, either with

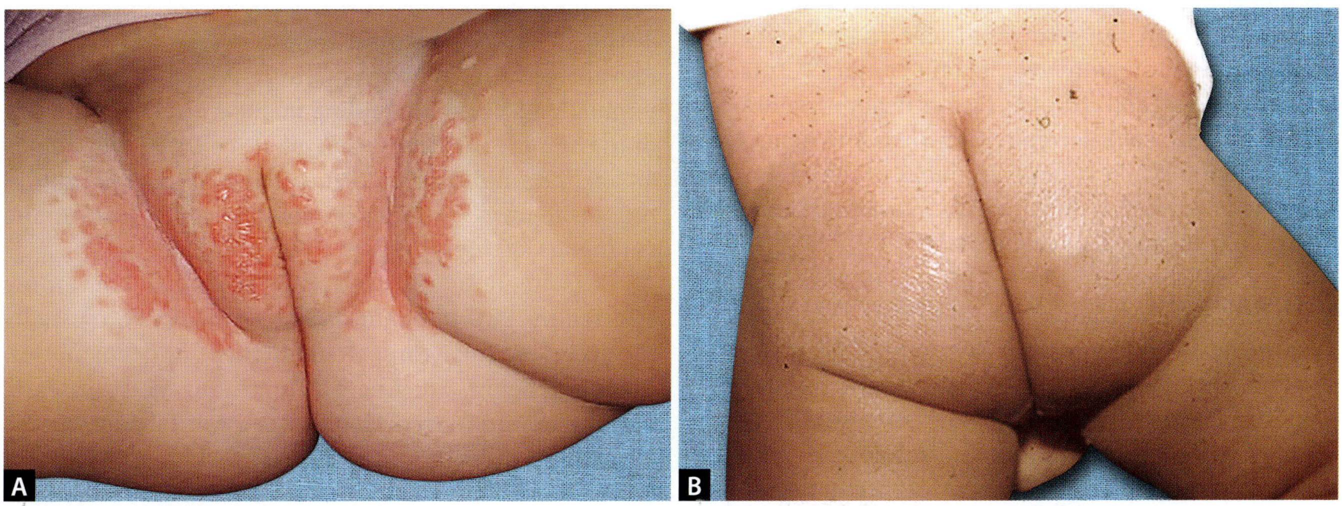

Figs. 1A and B: (A) Napkin dermatitis, note involvement of convex surfaces; (B) Erythema and chapping over buttock in napkin dermatitis.

"I have noticed that even those who assert that everything is predestined and that we can change nothing about it still look both ways before they cross the street." —**Stephen Hawking**

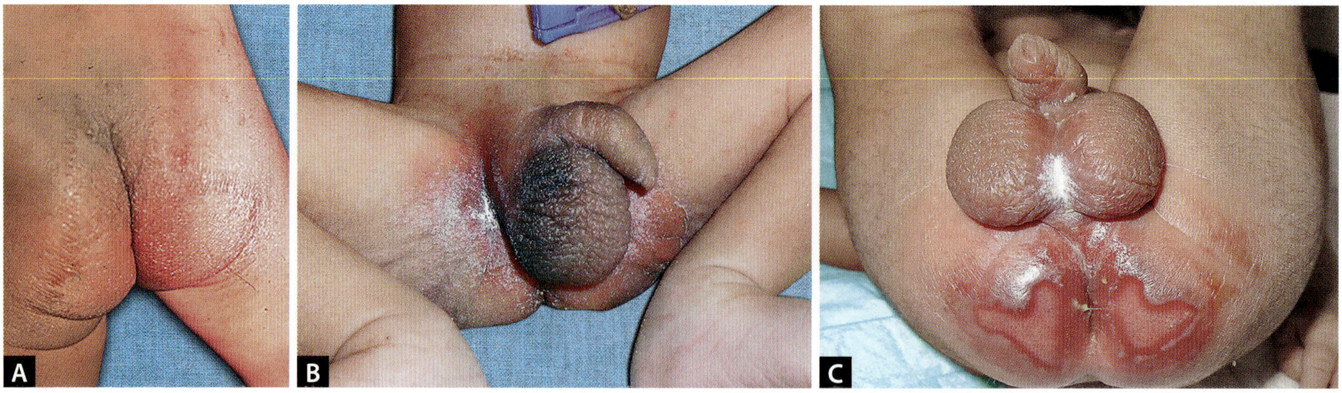

Figs. 2A to C: (A) Same child, close-up view; (B) Candidal diaper dermatitis; (C) Jacquet's dermatitis.

a baby soap or a nonsoap nondetergent cleanser. The skin should be cleaned with lukewarm water without rubbing. The nondisposable nappies should be cleaned with a mild detergent and antiseptics should be preferably avoided. Various barrier creams containing zinc oxide, titanium dioxide, and white petrolatum jelly are useful. Antibacterials and antifungals are to be used only in cases of secondary infections. Application of baby powder is better avoided as the starch content of it can enhance growth of *C. albicans*. Mild topical corticosteroid can be used for 5–7 days if rash is not improving with the above measures.

IRRITANT CONTACT DERMATITIS [FIGS. 3A(i) TO (iv)]

It develops as a result of direct irritant potential of various substances in contact with the skin of infants and newborns. The dermatitis develops as a result of nonimmunologic mechanisms. Mild irritants, when kept in contact with skin in sufficient concentration and over a significant period, can produce chronic irritant dermatitis. This is known as cumulative irritant contact dermatitis. Various physical and chemical factors include friction, low humidity, heat, cold, solvents, and soaps and detergents. Babies with atopic diathesis are more prone to develop this type of dermatitis. It manifests as localized patches of dry, slightly inflamed, or chapped skin.

Treatment

Treatment of acute irritant dermatitis comprises of cleaning the area with water and mild soap or neutralizing solution. Frequent wet compresses with application of a bland emollient or mild corticosteroid is helpful. All incriminating physical and chemical factors are to be removed. Barrier creams may be useful.

ALLERGIC CONTACT DERMATITIS [FIGS. 3A(v) AND (vi)]

Contact dermatitis can be defined as an inflammatory process affecting the surface of the skin that is induced by contact with chemical, physical, and/or biotic agents in the environment, and which lesions the skin, mucosae, and semi-mucosae by means of allergic and irritant pathogenetic mechanisms.

The skin of a child is thinner with a thin stratum corneum and incompletely formed layers of the epidermis. Adult morphology is not reached until puberty. As a result, substances have a greater chance of being absorbed through the skin of newborns and infants. The ratio between the skin surface area and body is also higher which increases absorption.

Allergic contact dermatitis (ACD) can start as early as 6 months and generally develops around 2–3 years when the immune system starts developing in contrast to irritant contact dermatitis which can happen at any time after birth.

Typical clinical features include eczematous lesions at the site of contact and sometimes at a distant site. Prevalence varies between 14.5 and 70% depending on the population selected, sampling method used, and the size of the sample. ACD develops in susceptible individuals as an immunological process. There is a sensitization process followed by an elicitation phase that leads to the cutaneous features.

Legs, feet, hands, and face are most commonly affected by ACD in children. Suspect agents are usually footwear, metals, topical medicines, and cosmetics. Cosmetic agents may be an important cause in early infancy as mothers may often use herbal ingredients whose allergenic potential is unknown. Certain preservatives such as parabens, Kathon G and Euxyl 400, can cause sensitization if kept for long periods of time and

"If you are unable to find the truth right where you are, where else do you expect to find it?" —**Dogen**

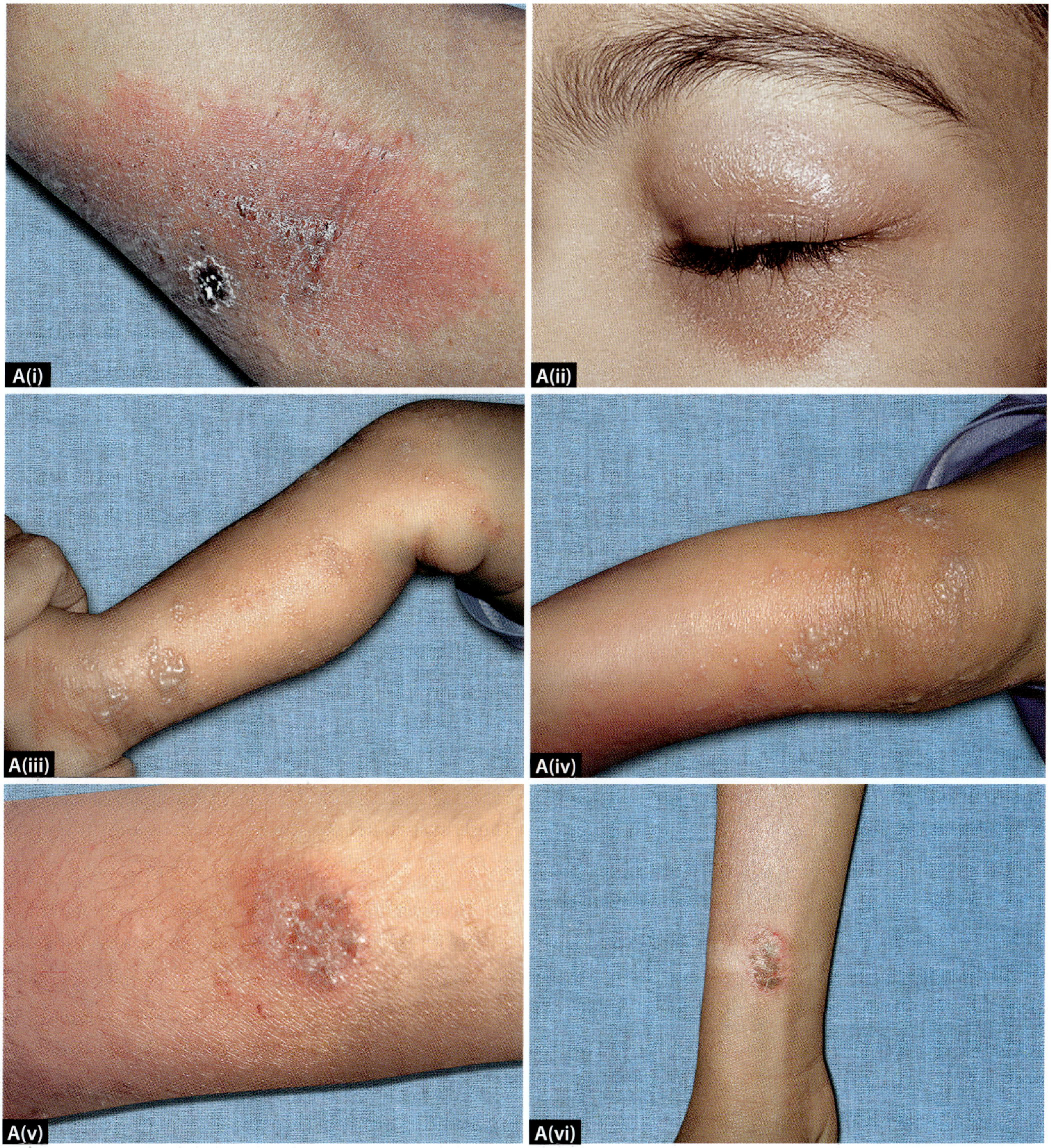

Figs. 3A(i) to (vi): A(i) Irritant dermatitis; A(ii) Irritant dermatitis of eyelid; A(iii) Acute irritant dermatitis in a 3-year-old girl; A(iv) Irritant dermatitis, close-up view; A(v) Allergic contact dermatitis (ACD) to wrist watch band; A(vi) ACD to wrist watch band in another adolescent boy.

not washed off. Propolis and tea tree oil can also cause ACD. Another important role is played by antibiotics, topical cortisones, antiseptics, and disinfectants such as mercurochrome, thiomersal, neomycin to name a few. Metal contact increases sharply in childhood and adolescence. In this period, nickel, chrome, and cobalt become important sensitizers. Another important source of nickel exposure is the use of cleansing agents

"Muddy water is best cleared by leaving it alone." —**Alan Watts**

and cosmetics by children while trying to emulate their mothers. Common items are mascara, eyeliners, eye pencils, eye shadows, etc. Girls can also become sensitized by using perfumed products which contain essential oils and perfumed preservatives such as benzyl alcohol. The corresponding hapten positives are "fragrance mix" and balsam of Peru.

Leather shoes can cause sensitization as they may contain traces of potassium dichromate that is used for tanning leather. Even wearing rubber shoes may lead to sensitization due to the presence of vulcanization accelerators, rubber antioxidants (the thiurams and p-phenylenediamine), and resin glues. Braces and other orthodontic appliances used during childhood may cause sensitization due to presence of steel, chrome-cobalt, and nickel-titanium. These can lead to perioral dermatitis and cheilitis. Adolescents may experience ACD involving the scalp, face, and eyelids due to exposure to hair dyes containing p-phenylenediamine.

Clothing-related ACD has been reported from dyes and fixing resins, glues, and metal accessories. ACD to clothing may occur at sites which are not touched by the cloth, e.g., the hands.

Presence of pre-existing skin disease such as atopic dermatitis (AD) increases the susceptibility to all forms of contact dermatitis. During periods of quiescence, sensitization increases. Also, many a times the medicines used to treat AD, e.g., antibiotics, can cause sensitization. Topical antivirals, antifungals, and antihistamines can cause ACD. The lesions of AD and ACD can overlap and coexist and eczematous lesions are often worsened by medications. In cases of AD, patch tests may be carried out in suspect cases when lesions are present at atypical sites not suggestive of AD, but present at the site of suspected contact with an allergen. Diagnosis of ACD is made by carrying out patch tests or epicutaneous tests. But only 15–25% of patch tests turn out to be positive since the tests are not standardized for children.

Treatment of pediatric ACD requires topical or systemic steroids depending on the severity of the disease. At the same time, avoidance of exposure to the allergen is important along with avoiding substances that may show cross reactivity.

LIP LICKER'S DERMATITIS (FIGS. 3B TO G)

It is mostly seen in preschool children and children of early school going age. The lips and adjacent skin frequently become dry and, as a result of a licking habit, inflamed, irritated, and scaly. The vermillion border of the lip is spared. In addition, saliva frequently becomes trapped between the thumb and mouth of thumbsuckers, and a similar reaction is commonly seen in toddlers. These are more commonly seen in atopic children.

Treatment

Counseling of the children regarding avoidance of lip licking or thumb sucking is important. Bland emollients are the mainstay of management.

CRADLE CAP (FIGS. 4A TO C)

This term is used when there is adherent scaling of the scalp seen in newborns mostly between 3rd week and 3 months of life. This occurs as a part of infantile seborrheic dermatitis secondary to maternal circulating hormones resulting in overactivity of sebaceous glands. Greasy scaling is seen on vertex, frontal region, forehead, eyebrows, ears, and neck.

Treatment

Cradle cap is a self-limiting condition. Oiling the scalp to loosen the scales and shampooing should be considered. For persistent and extensive lesions, mild topical steroid such as hydrocortisone cream or ketoconazole shampoo can be useful. Counseling of parents is important.

INFANTILE SEBORRHEIC DERMATITIS (FIGS. 4D TO 7)

The term infantile seborrheic dermatitis is used to describe an eruption having a predilection for the scalp and the proximal flexures and a favorable prognosis compared to AD. However, the term is used by clinicians to describe a clinical presentation that may reflect a variety of different skin disorders and may, therefore, have a number of different causes.

There is considerable debate about the relationship between seborrheic dermatitis and AD. Some authors propose that infantile seborrheic dermatitis is merely a characteristic pattern of AD and not a separate entity on the basis of the observation that apparently typical infantile seborrheic dermatitis not infrequently transforms into equally typical AD. No specific etiologic agent has been identified, although nutritional factors and the fungus *Malassezia furfur* are thought to play a role. The eruption first appears between the 2nd week and the 6th month of life but most commonly between 3 and 8 weeks. It usually starts on the napkin area but may also appear first on the

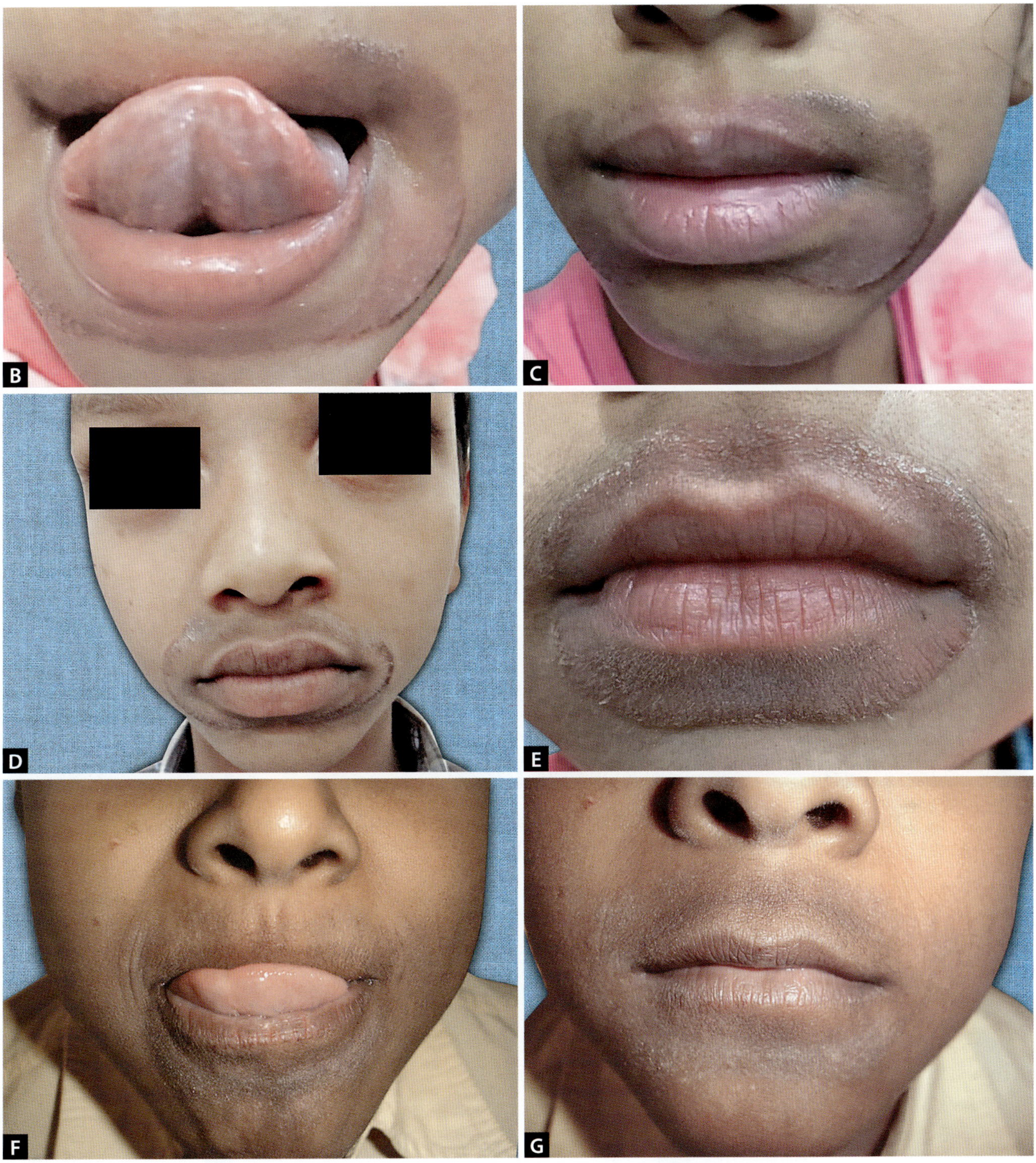

Figs. 3B to G: (B to F) Lip licker's dermatitis; (G) Lip licker's dermatitis, close-up view.

face, scalp, or trunk. It spreads rapidly to involve the scalp, particularly the vertex and frontal areas, face, neck, napkin area, and axillae. On the face, the forehead, eyebrows, eyelids, and nasolabial folds are most commonly affected.

The rash comprises of well-defined areas of erythema and scaling with fine vesicles. The scales are adherent, yellow-brown in color, large and greasy in the scalp but smaller, whiter and drier in other areas. Rarely infants present with pruritus which is in contrast to AD.

"To accept some idea of truth without experiencing it is like a painting of a cake on paper which you cannot eat." —**Suzuki Roshi**

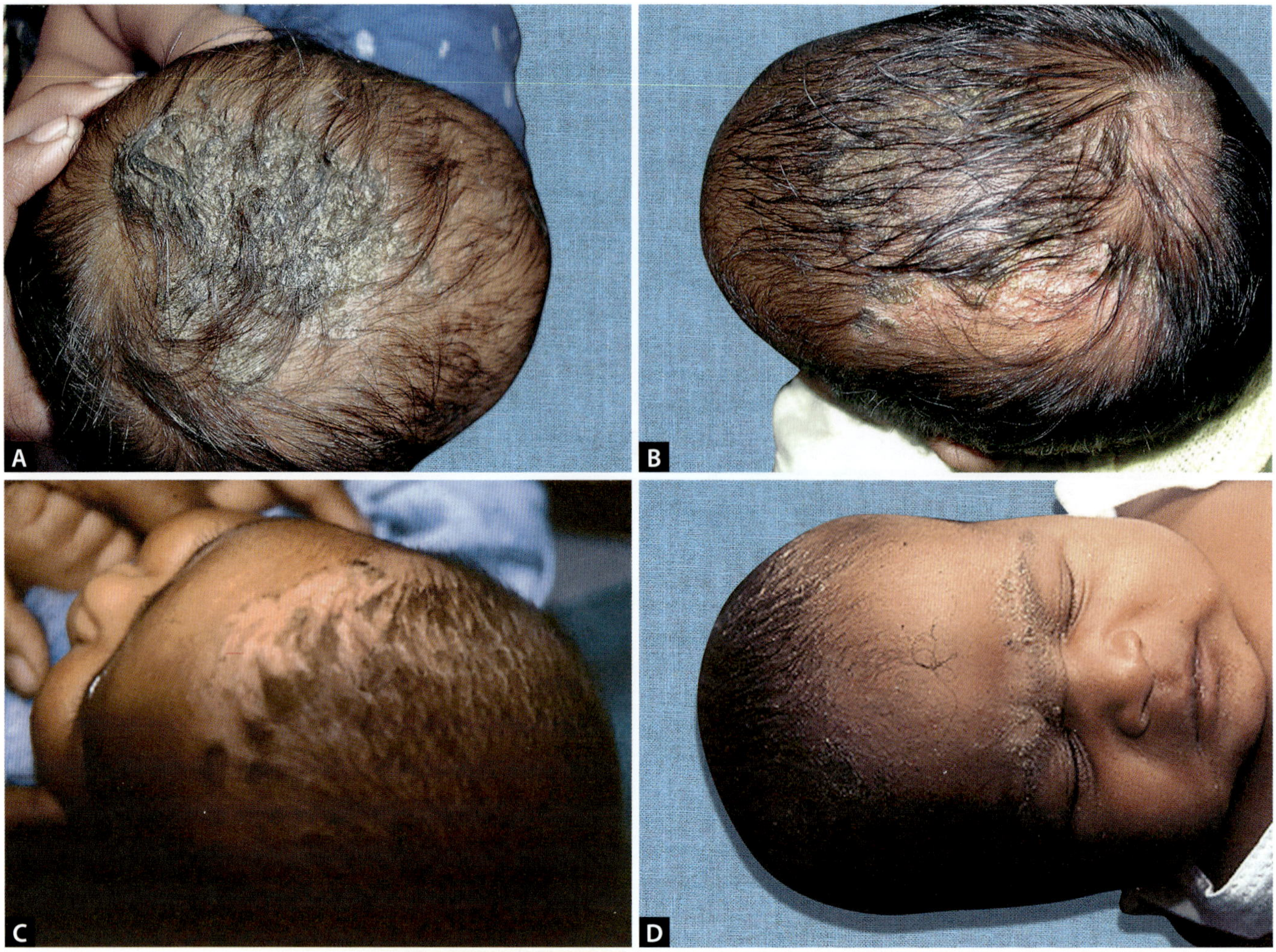

Figs. 4A to D: (A) Cradle cap (localized); (B) Cradle cap involving entire scalp; (C) Cradle cap (subsiding); (D) Involvement of face, eyebrows and eyelids in infantile seborrheic dermatitis.

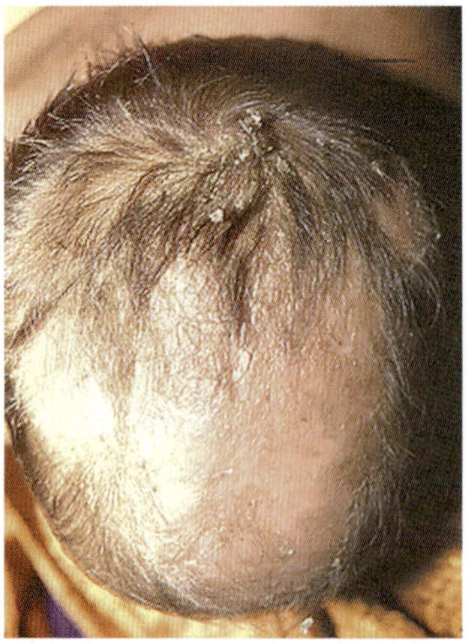

Fig. 5: Diffuse scaling and crust formation over the scalp in infantile seborrheic dermatitis.

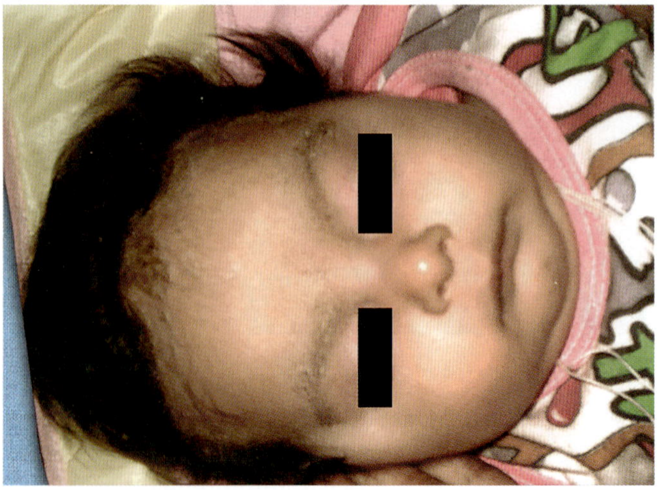

Fig. 6: Scales and crust of infantile seborrheic dermatitis.

"We are drowning in information but starved for knowledge." —**John Naisbitt**

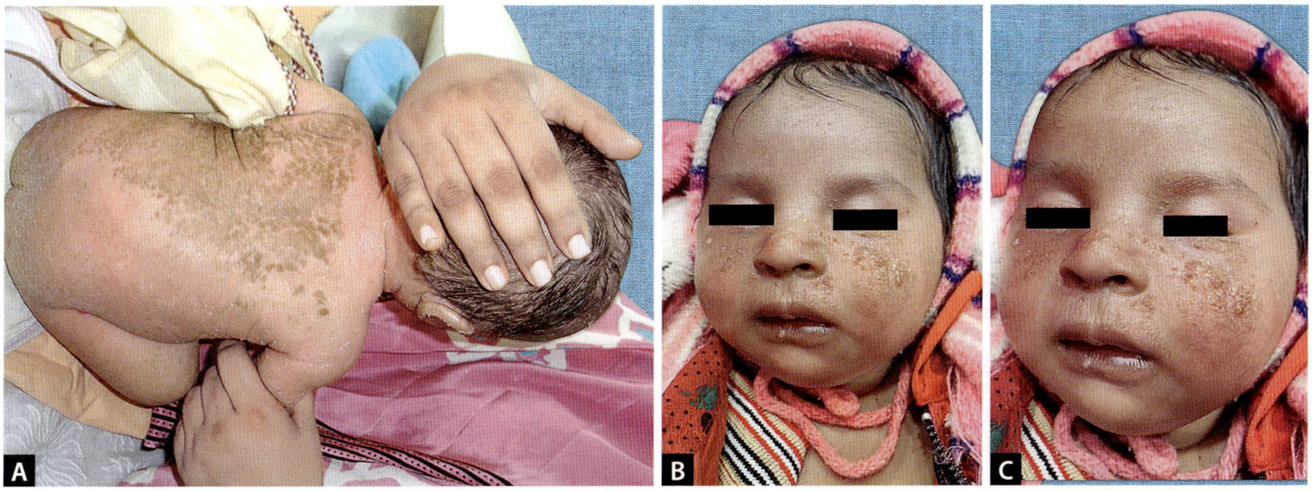

Figs. 7A to C: (A) Infantile seborrheic dermatitis (ISD); (B) ISD in a 3-month-old baby; (C) Same baby, close-up view.

Differential Diagnosis

There is considerable diagnostic overlap with cradle cap, intertrigo, disseminated primary irritant napkin dermatitis, AD, infantile psoriasis, multiple carboxylase deficiency, and primary immunodeficiencies. Differentiation from AD is desirable because of the more favorable prognosis of infantile seborrheic dermatitis.

Axillae are not commonly affected in AD, whereas flexors of forearms and shins which are affected in AD, are not involved in infantile seborrheic dermatitis.

Treatment

Prognosis of infantile seborrheic dermatitis is good. Cleansing and antiseborrheic shampoos over the scalp are more or less same as in cases of cradle cap. In milder cases, a mild topical steroid should be applied over forehead, retroauricular folds, eyebrows, earlobes, groin, etc., once per day for 2–3 weeks. Topical antifungals are helpful for areas other than the scalp. Application of body oil and soap should be as in cases of normal babies. For severe cases, where pruritus is often present, either promethazine (in early infancy) or cetirizine (in infants above 6 months of age) may be given. However, application of topical corticosteroid cream or lotion over extensive area of the body is not recommended. Oral antistaphylococcal antibiotics may be given in cases where secondary infection is suspected.

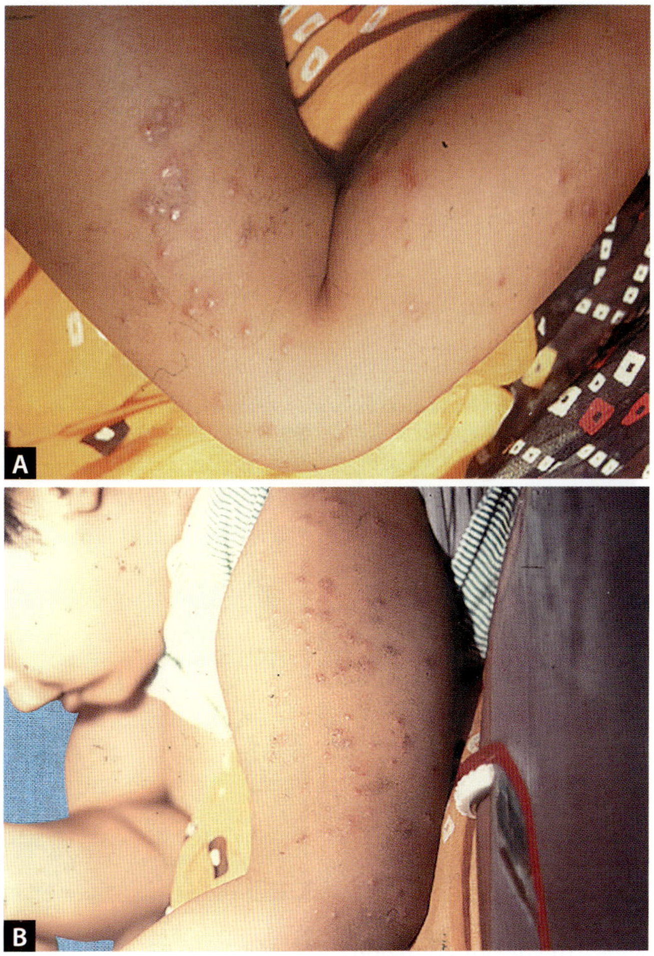

Figs. 8A and B: (A) Papular urticaria over thigh and leg (common sites); (B) Same child close-up view.

PAPULAR URTICARIA (FIGS. 8 AND 9)

Injection of foreign protein by biting insects into skin of the most sensitive subjects may cause an immediate immunoglobulin E (IgE)-mediated reaction which starts as an extremely itchy urticarial weal at the site of the bite. This is succeeded by a firm pruritic papule, which persists for several days. The weal and papule may show a central

"It really boils down to this: that all life is interrelated. We are all caught in an inescapable network of mutuality, tied in a single garment of destiny. Whatever affects one directly, affects all indirectly." —**Martin Luther King, Jr.**

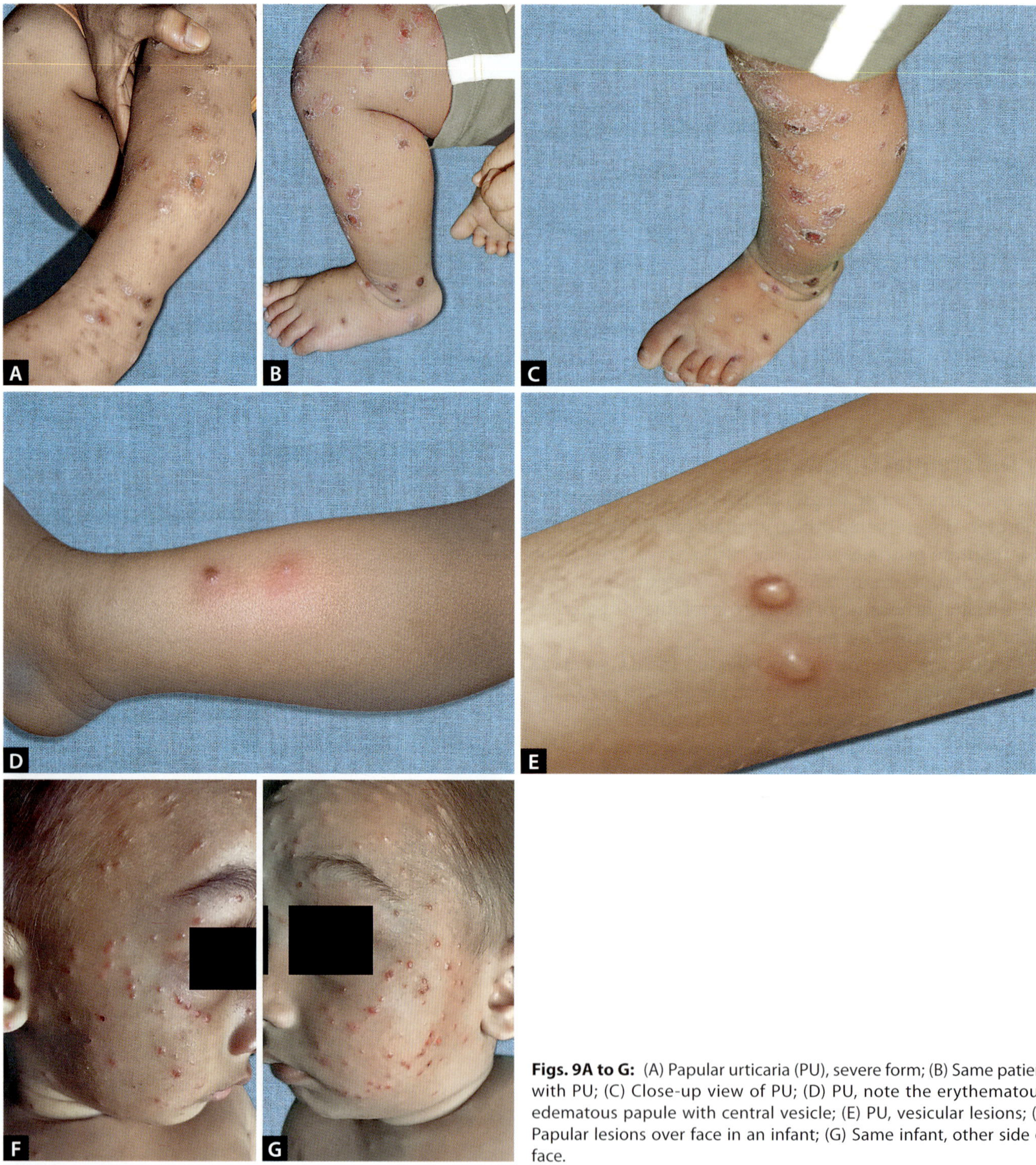

Figs. 9A to G: (A) Papular urticaria (PU), severe form; (B) Same patient with PU; (C) Close-up view of PU; (D) PU, note the erythematous, edematous papule with central vesicle; (E) PU, vesicular lesions; (F) Papular lesions over face in an infant; (G) Same infant, other side of face.

hemorrhagic punctum and the papule may be surmounted by a tiny vesicle. Lesions are grouped in clusters and develop in crops at irregular intervals. Bullous reactions are common on the lower legs. Irritation is an almost constant symptom and rubbing and scratching may increase the inflammatory changes and induce eczematization.

Complication

Secondary infection is a common complication and may manifest as impetigo, folliculitis, cellulitis, and lymphangitis.

"To follow the path, look to the master, follow the master, walk with the master, see through the master, become the master." —**Zen Proverb**

Treatment

Full-sleeve clothes give protection from insect bite and help to prevent development of new papules to an extent. Use of mosquito repellents, mosquito nets, spraying of beddings, and their exposure to sunlight are advocated. For skin lesions, topical application of a mild steroid, e.g., hydrocortisone for infants and young children, and fluticasone or mometasone for older children can be given for initial 3–5 days to accelerate resolution of papular urticaria lesions. Topical antibiotics can be given for secondary infections. The author prefers to give calamine lotion for application over legs to prevent direct contact of smaller insects such as ants on the child's skin. Antihistamines such as cetirizine can be given for pruritus.

NODULAR PRURIGO (FIGS. 10A TO D)

This is characterized by chronic intensely itchy nodules which can occur at any age between 20 and 60 years. In children, it is more common in atopics. The individual lesion is a hard nodule of 1–3 cm in diameter, with a raised warty surface. The lesions are usually pigmented, grouped, numerous and symmetrical, initially on the distal parts of the limbs and are more prominent on the extensor surfaces. The trunk, face, and even the palms can be affected. Crusts and scales may cover recently excoriated lesions. The patient is troubled by crises of pruritus of intense severity. The nodules may remain pruritic indefinitely although some may regress spontaneously to leave scars. The disease runs very protracted course.

Treatment

Symptomatic relief of pruritus is very important and sedating antihistamines at night is required for long-term control of the disease. Topical corticosteroids are better applied on early erythematous lesions to control inflammation for 2–3 weeks. Intralesional triamcinolone acetonide helps to reduce nodularity of chronic lesions.

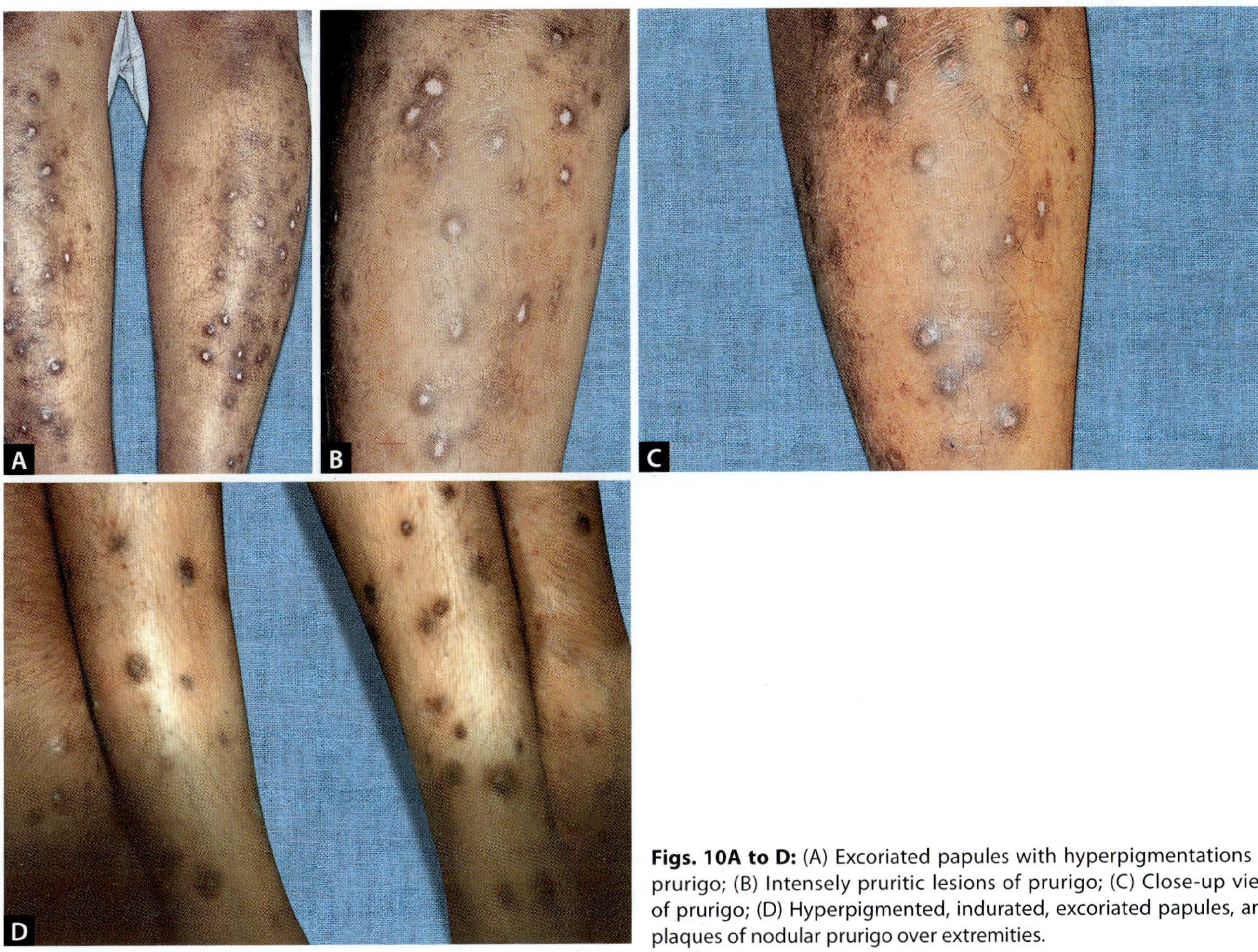

Figs. 10A to D: (A) Excoriated papules with hyperpigmentations in prurigo; (B) Intensely pruritic lesions of prurigo; (C) Close-up view of prurigo; (D) Hyperpigmented, indurated, excoriated papules, and plaques of nodular prurigo over extremities.

It may be combined with cryosurgery. Topical capsaicin, ultraviolet (UV) radiation, and rarely oral thalidomide are the other treatment modalities. Associated xerosis is controlled by application of emollients.

ATOPIC DERMATITIS (FIGS. 11 TO 35N)

Atopic dermatitis is a chronic, inflammatory skin condition characterized by itchy papular (vesicles in infants) rash typically in a flexural distribution, which become excoriated and lichenified with time. There is often associated personal or family history of "atopy."

Clinical Features

This itchy chronic and fluctuating condition usually starts between 2 and 6 months and has a slight male predilection.

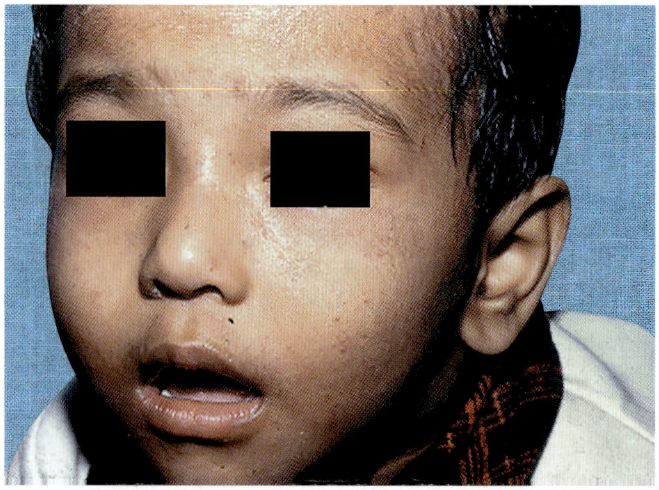

Fig. 11: Xerosis over the face in atopic dermatitis.

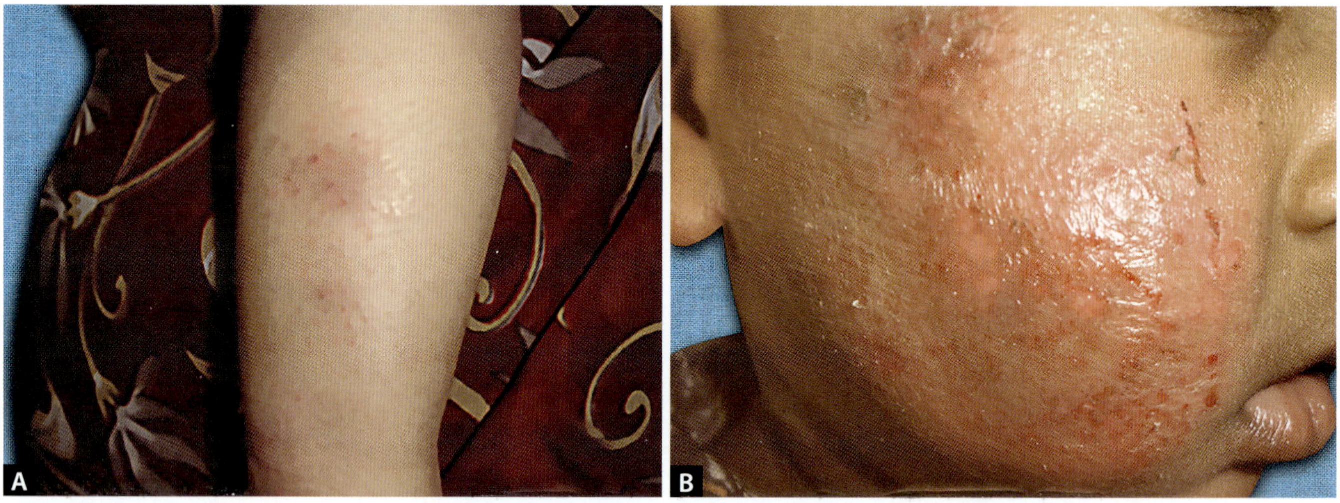

Figs. 12A and B: (A) Nummular eczema over leg; (B) Acute eczema in atopic dermatitis.

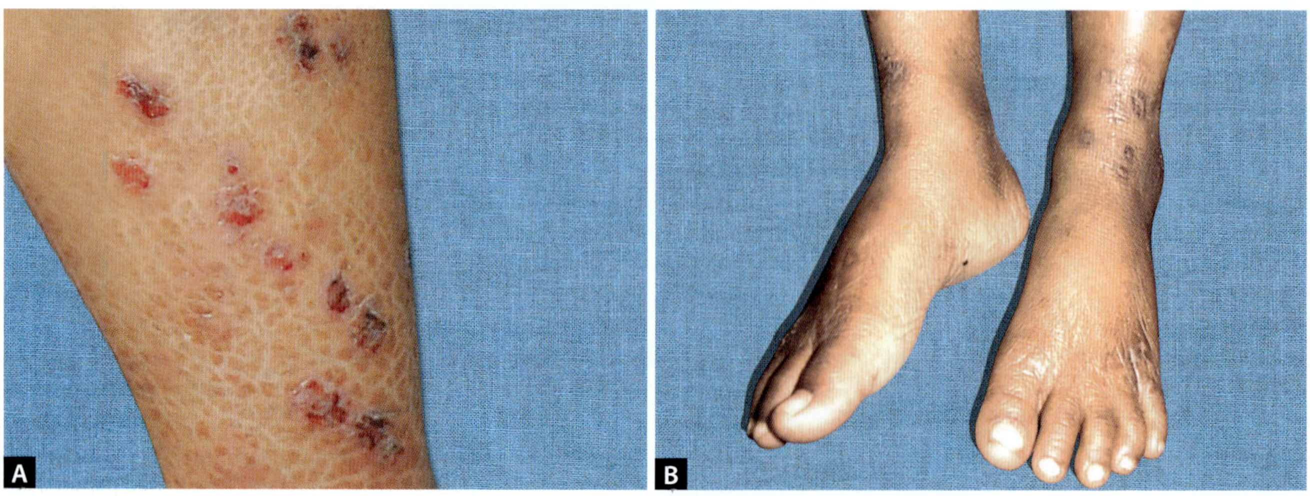

Figs. 13A and B: (A) Subacute eczema; (B) Subacute eczema over both the legs.

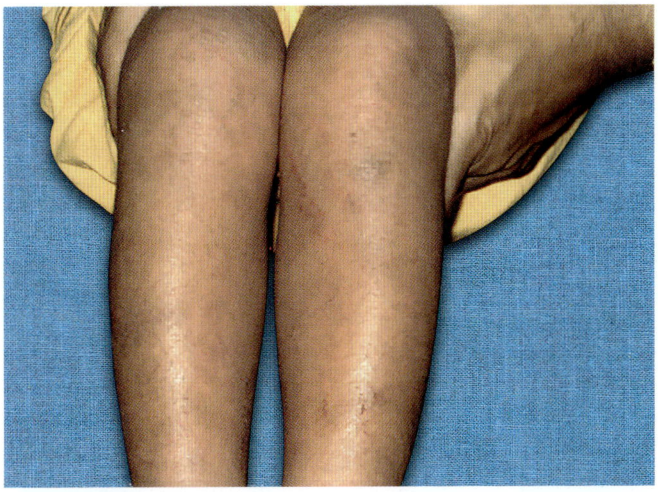

Fig. 14: Severe xerosis in a case of atopic dermatitis.

The symptoms are as follows:
- Itching
- Macular erythema and papules/papulovesicles
- Eczematous areas with crusting
- Lichenification and excoriation
- Xerosis
- Secondary infection

Infantile Phase (Figs. 31A and B)

Infantile phase manifests from 3 months to 2 years of age. Most frequently starts on face and there is relative sparing of napkin area. When the child begins to crawl, the exposed surfaces become involved with erythema, and intensely itchy papules (discrete/confluent) which may become exudative and crusted as a result of rubbing. The disease runs a chronic course varying with teething, respiratory infections, emotional upsets, and climatic changes.

Childhood Phase (Figs. 32A to C)

It starts from 2 to 12 years, and the areas commonly involved are elbow and knee flexures, sides of the neck, wrists and ankles. Sides of neck may show striking reticulate pigmentation called as "atopic dirty neck" **(Fig. 29)**. The erythematous and edematous papules tend to lichenify. However, in some patients, even after prolonged rubbing, lichenification does not occur and is difficult to treat.

Adult Phase (Figs. 33A to C)

The clinical features are similar to that in childhood with lichenification of the flexures and hands. Childhood AD may progress to adult phase or it may occur for the first time in adults.

INFECTED LESIONS OF ATOPIC DERMATITIS (FIGS. 34A AND B)

It is commonly seen over body folds where *S. aureus* colonization is high. Toxins produced by *S. aureus* act as superantigens and induce inflammatory cascade. There is disease flare with impetiginization of pre-existing lesions. It manifests as pustules, erosions, and honey-colored crusts.

ATOPIC HAND ECZEMA

Patchy vesicular and lichenified hand eczema with coarsening and pitting of nails is also seen in AD children. Fingertip eczema is more common in children and presents as diffuse erythema with scaling on the volar aspect of the fingertips.

Associated Disorders

- Asthma and allergic rhinitis occur in 30–50% of cases of AD and their onset is later than that of eczema.
- Xerosis is a common problem in AD patients.
- Sometimes, infantile seborrheic dermatitis may turn to typical AD.
- There is greater risk of developing contact dermatitis than nonatopics.
- Moist or fissured eczema around the mouth is common in children with AD.
- Drug reactions of the anaphylactic type are more common in atopic persons.
- Food allergy is frequent in patients of AD.
- Statistically significant association has been found between alopecia areata and atopy.
- Urticaria with allergic basis is more common in atopics.

PITYRIASIS ALBA (FIGS. 15A TO E)

This is a type of nonspecific dermatitis of unknown origin which characteristically produces erythematous scaly patches which subside to leave areas of hypopigmentation. Peak age of onset is between 3 and 16 years with equal prevalence in both sexes. The individual lesion is a rounded, oval, or irregular plaque which is red, pink, or skin colored and has fine lamellar or branny scaling. Initially, erythema is conspicuous but by the time the physician sees the patient, there is fine scaling and hypopigmentation which prompts the patient to seek advice. There are usually

"The resistance to the unpleasant situation is the root of suffering." —**Ram Dass**

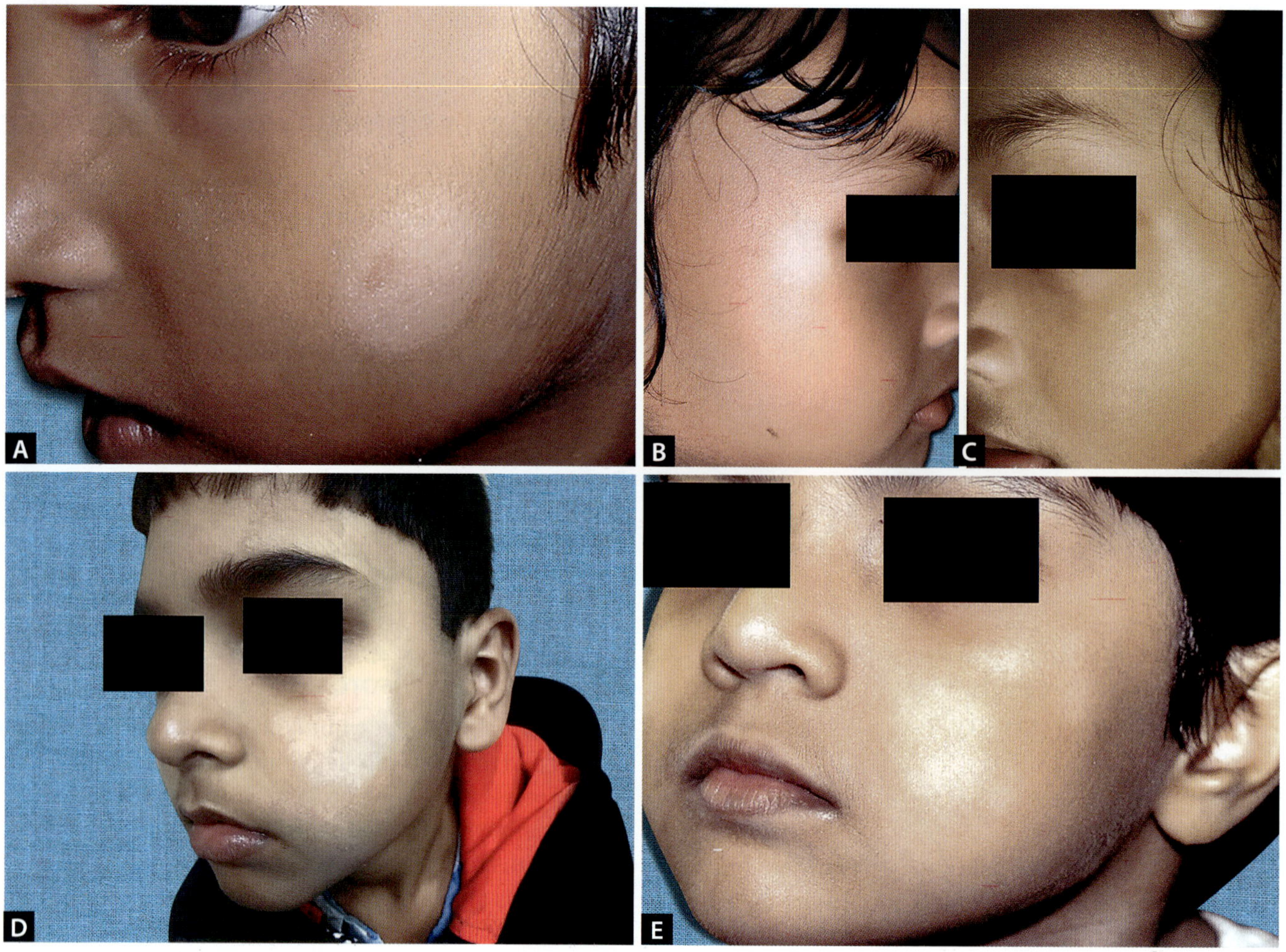

Figs. 15A to E: (A) Hypopigmented and scaly patch of pityriasis alba over the cheek; (B) Pityriasis alba over the face; (C) Same patient, different view; (D) Pityriasis alba, large hypopigmented scaly macule; (E) Pityriasis alba, multiple hypopigmented macules.

several patches which range from 0.5 to 2 cm in diameter. In children, the lesions are often confined to the face, and are most common around the mouth, chin, and cheeks. The course is variable. Most cases persist for some months and some may still show leukoderma for a year or more after scaling subsides. Recurrent crops of new lesions may develop at intervals. The average duration of the facial lesions in children is a year or more. The conspicuous leukoderma may lead to a misdiagnosis of vitiligo. In older children and adults, the lesions on the trunk, during the early erythematous phase may be mistaken for psoriasis, but the distribution, the sparing of scalp, elbows and knees, and the lack of psoriatic scale should exclude the diagnosis.

KERATOSIS PILARIS (FIGS. 16A AND B)

It is a common autosomal dominant disorder comprising keratinous plugs in the follicular orifices with varying degrees of perifollicular erythema. In its isolated form, it appears in childhood and reaches its peak in adolescence. Small gray-white plugs of keratin obstruct the follicular openings entrapping the body hair. The sites of predilection are the cheeks, extensor surface of upper arms, thighs, and buttocks. Uneven involvement of a given area is usual with some follicles completely spared, while adjacent ones are grossly plugged. Perifollicular erythema is often present. When redness is marked, the term keratosis rubra pilaris is used. Often the lesions improve during summer.

DENNIE–MORGAN FOLDS (FIGS. 17A TO C)

Dennie–Morgan infraorbital fold has been included in most descriptions of atopic eczema. This sign is thought to be present when there is a definite double fold or if one or more creases, outlining skin folds starting at the inner canthus extend laterally at least beyond an imaginary perpendicular line through the pupil. The percentage of

"For things to reveal themselves to us, we need to be ready to abandon our views about them." **—Thích Nhat Hanh**

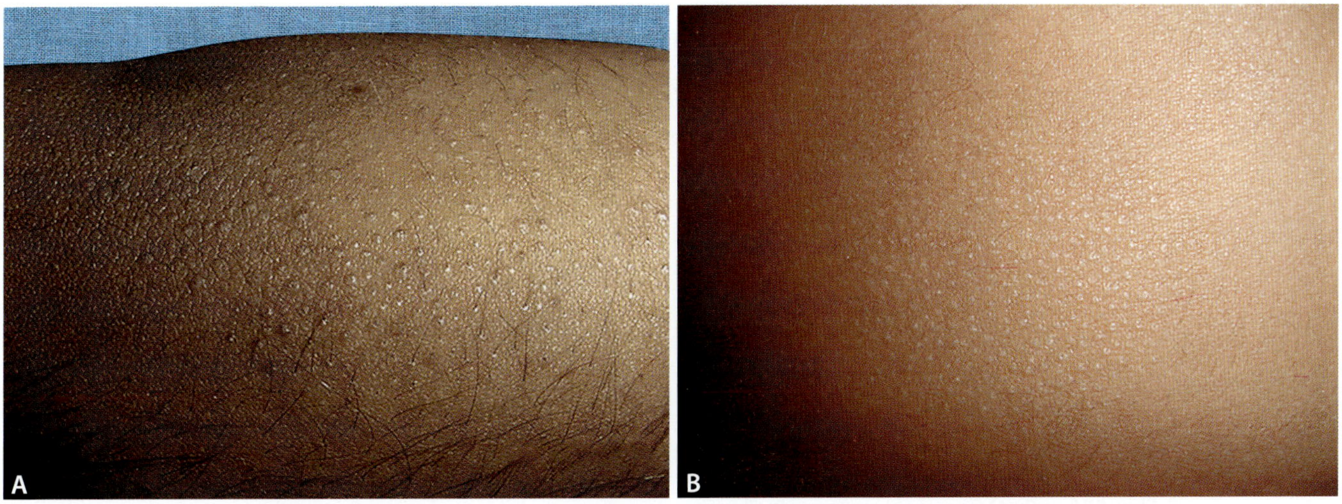

Figs. 16A and B: (A) Follicular keratotic papules of keratosis pilaris; (B) Keratosis pilaris.

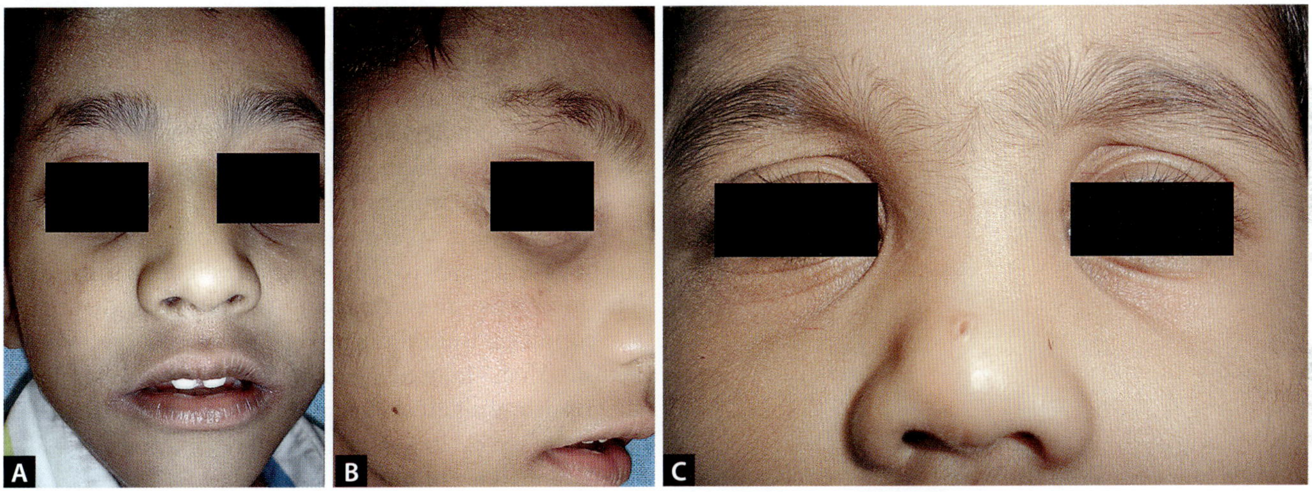

Figs. 17A to C: (A) Dennie–Morgan infraorbital folds; (B) Close-up view of Dennie–Morgan infraorbital folds; (C) Dennie–Morgan infraorbital folds in a child with atopic dermatitis.

atopic eczema patients exhibiting infraorbital folds was found to be 50–60% in most studies.

GEOGRAPHIC TONGUE (BENIGN MIGRATORY GLOSSITIS) (FIGS. 18A TO C)

Geographic tongue may be asymptomatic or may cause a sore tongue. Patients of any age may be affected. Some studies have shown that patients with a personal or family history of atopy, and high serum IgE levels are more likely to present with geographic tongue. Clinically, it is characterized by map-like red areas with increased thickness of intervening filiform papillae. Alternatively, there are rounded, sometimes scalloped, reddish areas with a white margin. Patterns may change from day-to-day and even within a few hours. Rarely labial or palatal mucosa may be affected. There are no associated complications and the only differential diagnoses are psoriasis and larva migrans. Clinical examination usually suffices to differentiate the condition from lichen planus, candidiasis, or deficiency glossitis.

JUVENILE PLANTAR DERMATOSIS (FIGS. 19 AND 20)

This condition is characterized by dry, fissured dermatitis of the plantar surface of the forefoot. It occurs almost exclusively in children aged 3–14 years. Atopy is thought to have an association with this condition. Many children

"Tough times don't last. Tough people do." —**Robert H Schuller**

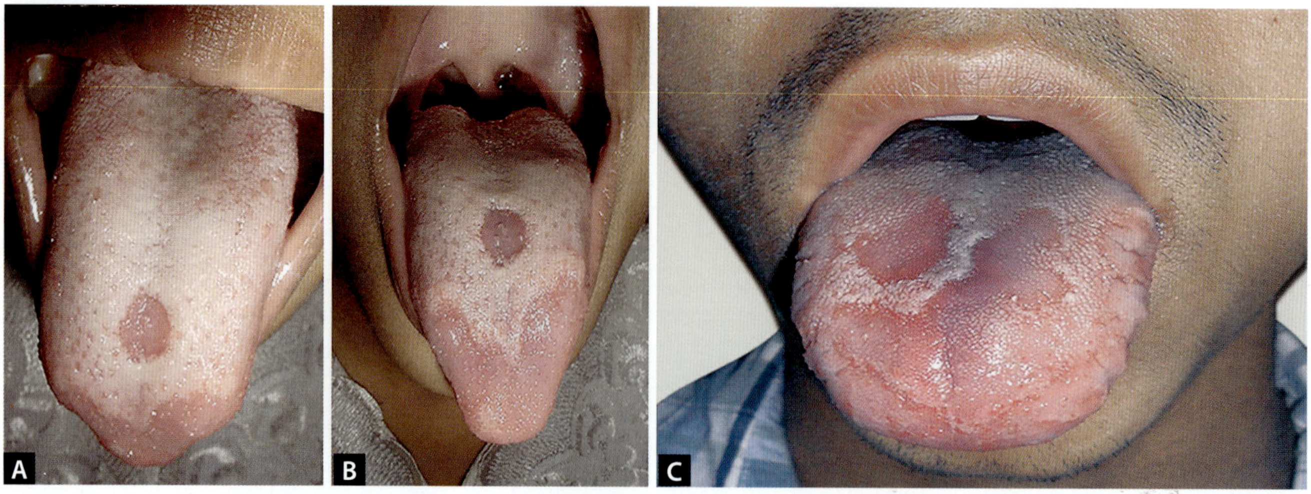

Figs. 18A to C: (A) Geographic tongue; (B) Close-up view of a geographic tongue; (C) Geographic tongue.

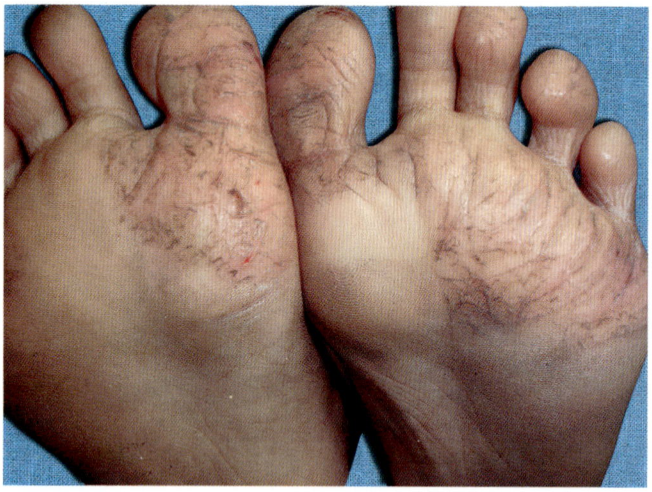

Fig. 19: Bilateral symmetrical lesions of juvenile plantar dermatosis.

with this condition have an increased personal or family history of atopy. Exacerbation can occur due to hyperhidrosis, occlusive footwear, and plastic shoes. There is a slight preponderance of male children. The presenting features are redness and pain on the plantar surface of the forefoot, which assumes a glazed and cracked appearance. The condition is most severe on the ball of the foot and toe pads and tends to spare the nonweight bearing instep. The toe clefts are normal and this helps to distinguish the condition from tinea pedis. The lesions are strikingly symmetrical. Juvenile plantar dermatosis is a clinical diagnosis although skin scrapings to exclude fungus and patch tests to exclude footwear allergy may be advisable if the diagnosis is doubtful.

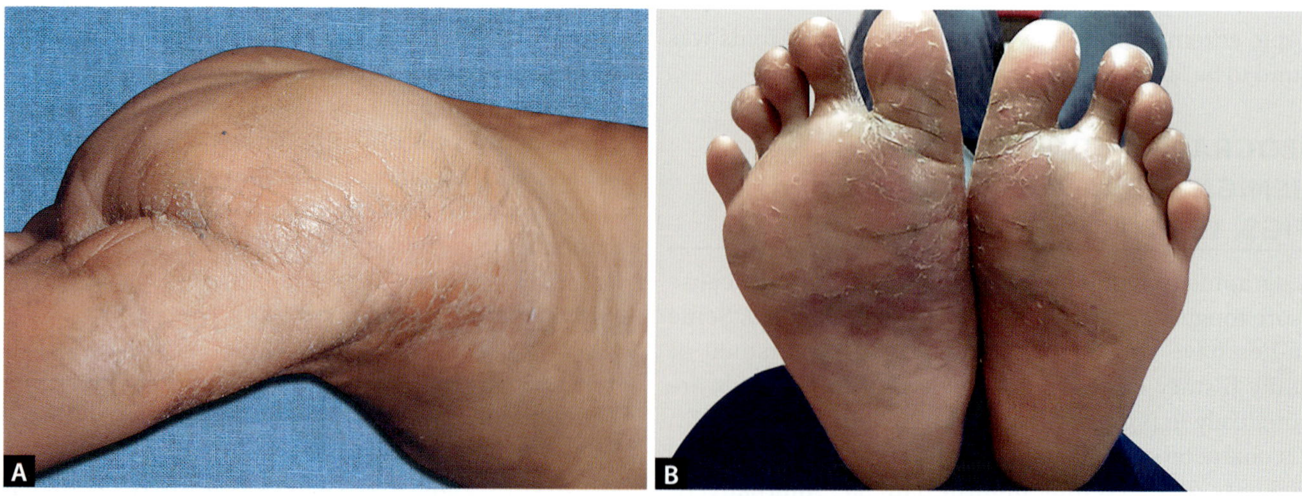

Figs. 20A and B: (A) Classical lesion of juvenile plantar dermatitis (JPD) in a young boy; (B) Another view of JPD.

POMPHOLYX (FIGS. 21A TO D)

Pompholyx is a form of eczema of the palms and soles, in which edema fluid accumulates to form visible vesicle or bullae. Onset before 10 years is unusual. It is characterized by the sudden onset of crops of clear vesicles, which appear deeply seated and sago-like. There is no erythema, but a sensation of heat and prickling of the palms may precede the attacks. Vesicles may become confluent and present as large bullae, especially on the feet. Itching may be severe, preceding the eruption of vesicles. The lesion subsides spontaneously, and resolution with desquamation occurs in 2–3 weeks in most cases, but recurrent attacks may cause a wave-like continuation of symptoms with lesions occurring symmetrically on the palms and soles. It may be confused with contact dermatitis where the lesions are usually unilateral and asymmetrical. Dermatophytosis which presents as localized and asymmetrical area of scaling and vesiculation of the palm or sole can be confirmed by scrapings for fungus.

SEVERE ATOPIC DERMATITIS (FIGS. 35A TO G)

In the west, a good number of children suffer from severe AD. In India, however, the severity of the disease is much less in majority of the children suffering from AD. The various probable reasons put forth are a different kind of season and environment in our country, practice of prolonged breastfeeding, different dietary habits of mothers during pregnancy and lactation, different dietary habits of the children, and genetic makeup of our population. Recently, there has been a paradigm shift over the last one and a half decade in Indian subcontinent and we are seeing more than 15% of total cases of AD to be moderately severe or severe AD.

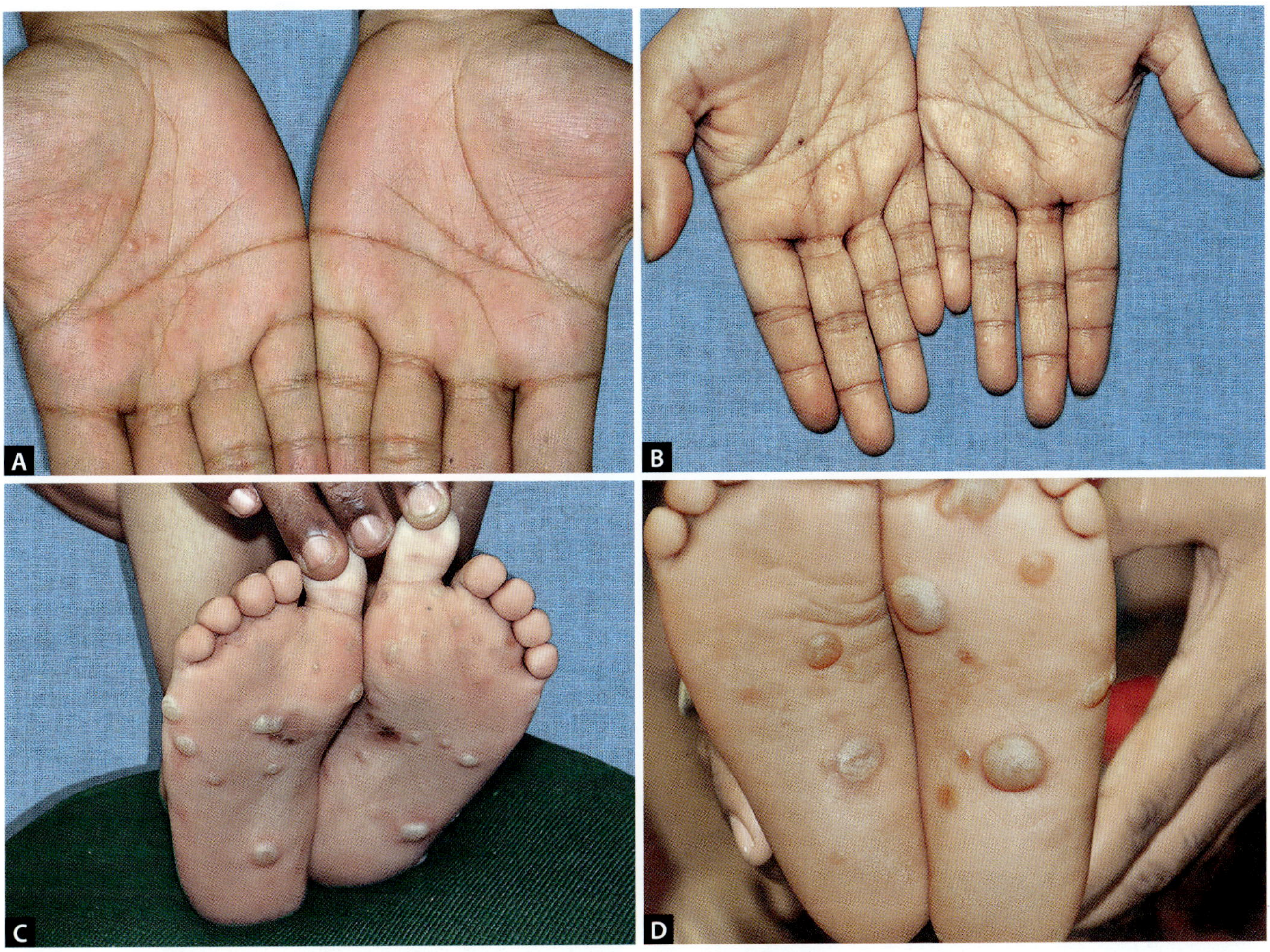

Figs. 21A to D: (A) Pompholyx lesions over palms; (B) Pompholyx over palms and fingers; (C) Large vesicles of pompholyx; (D) Same patient, close-up view.

"It does not matter how slowly you go as long as you do not stop." —**Confucius**

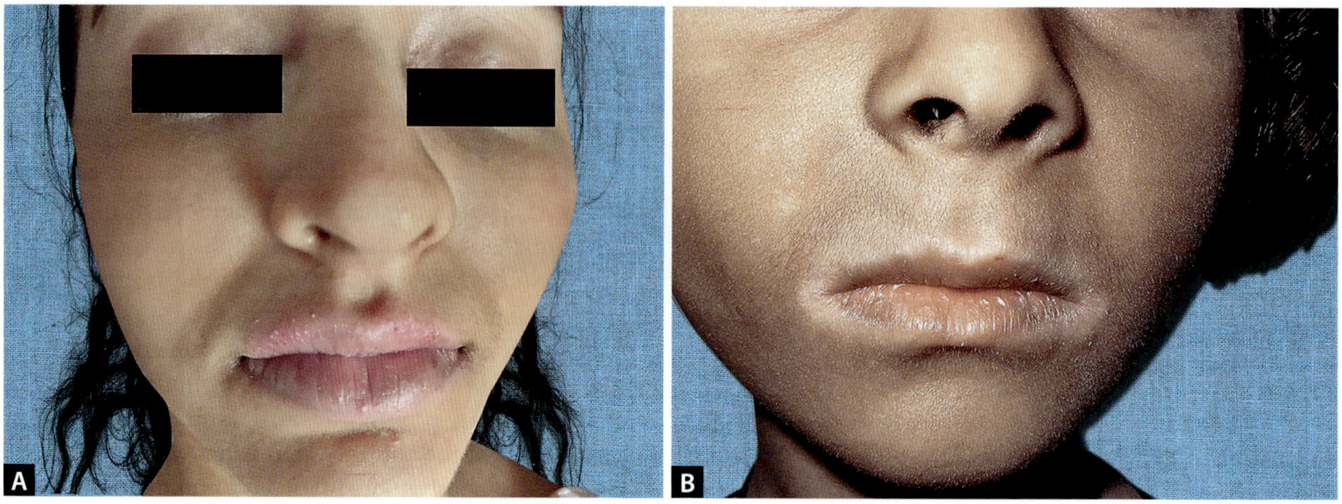

Figs. 22A and B: (A) Atopic cheilitis; (B) Atopic cheilitis, note perioral hypopigmentation.

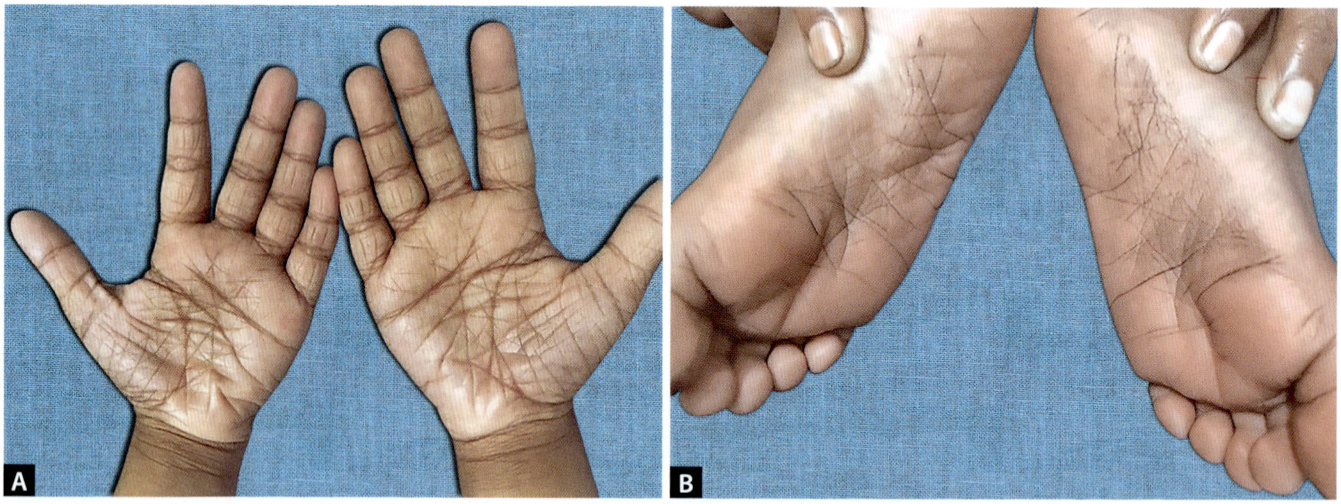

Figs. 23A and B: (A) Hyperlinear palms in atopics; palmar hyperlinearity; (B) Plantar hyperlinearity.

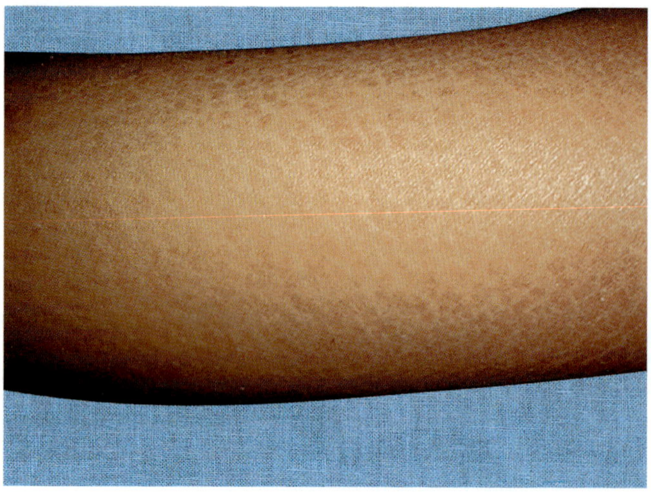

Fig. 24: Fine fixed scales of ichthyosis vulgaris.

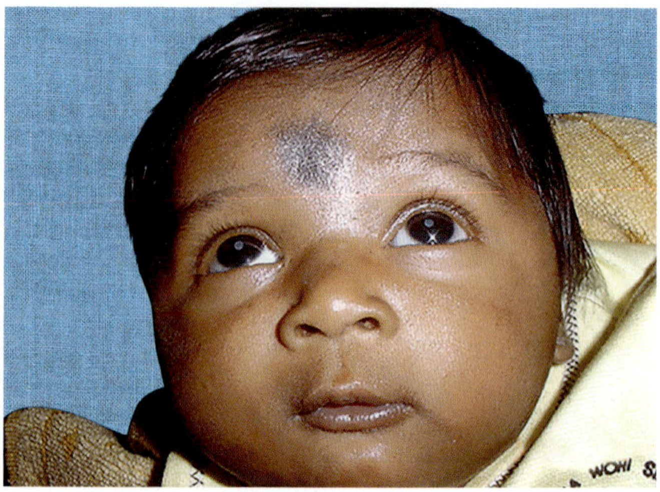

Fig. 25: Atopic cataract.

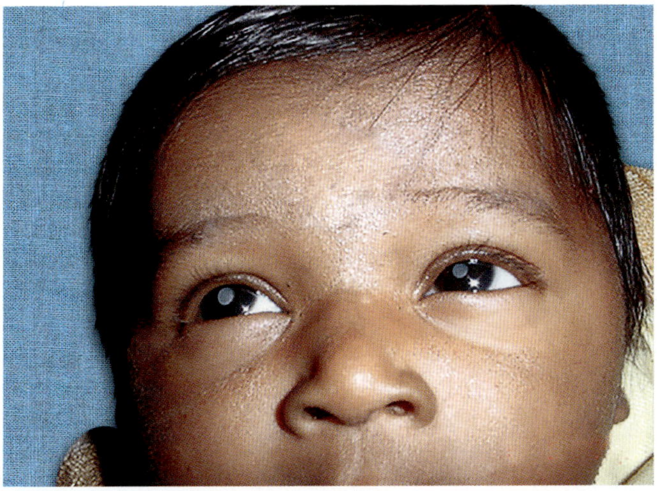

Fig. 26: Close-up view of atopic cataract.

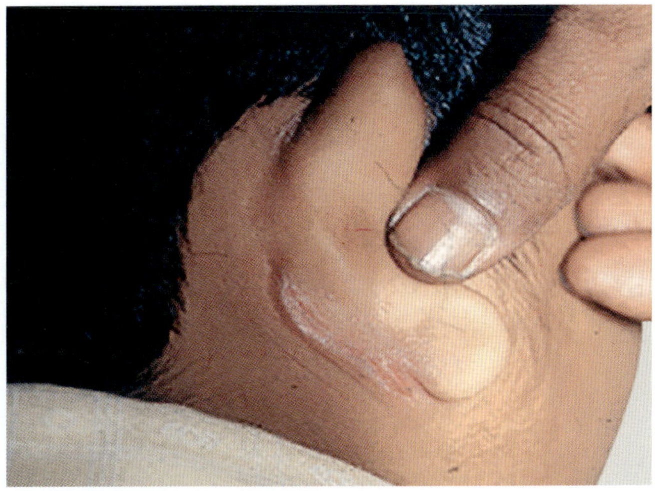

Fig. 27: Infra-auricular fissuring in atopic dermatitis.

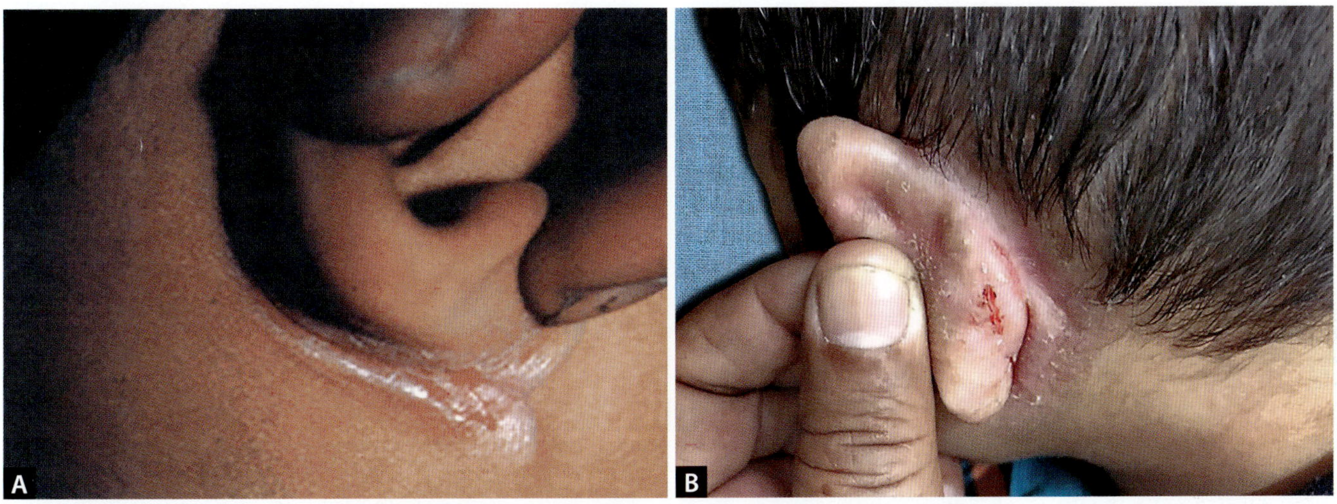

Figs. 28A and B: (A) Same boy having infra-auricular fissuring at a later date; (B) Infra- and retroauricular fissuring and eczema.

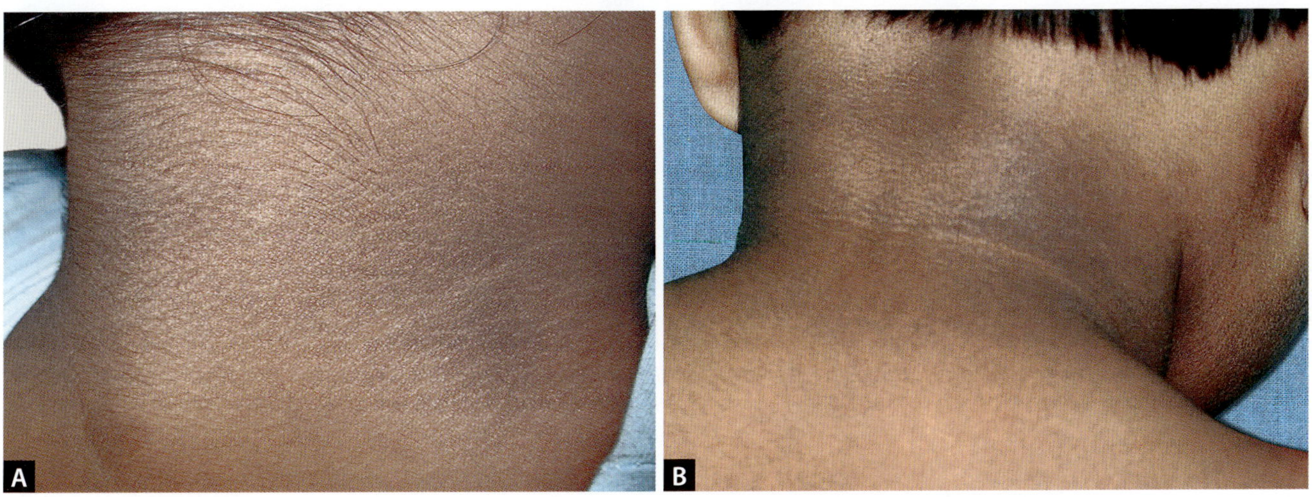

Figs. 29A and B: (A) "Dirty neck" of atopic child; (B) Atopic "dirty neck" along the sides of neck.

"Everything you've ever wanted is on the other side of fear." —**George Addair**

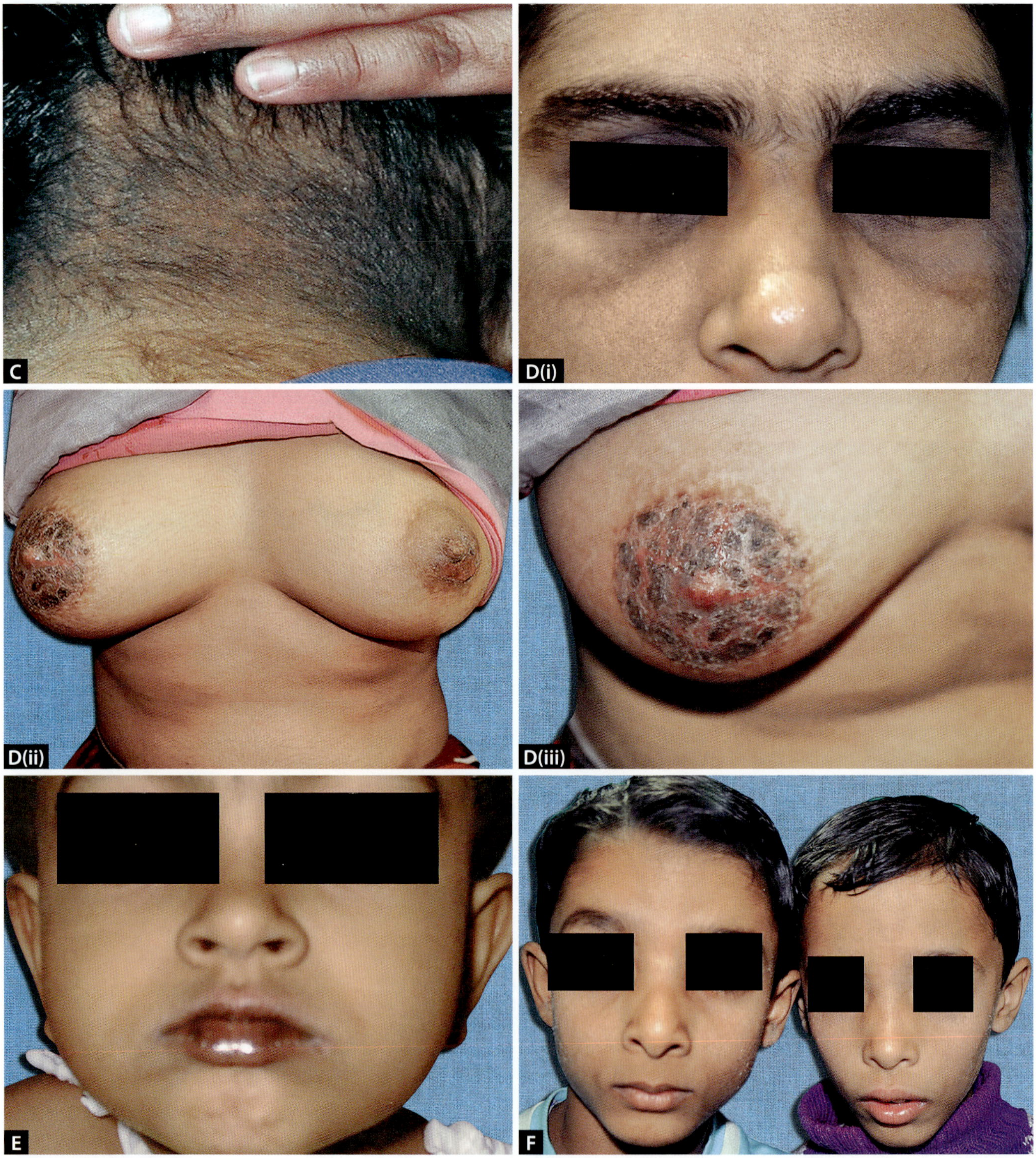

Figs. 29C to F: (C) Hyperpigmentation of neck in atopic dermatitis; D(i) Periorbital melanosis in atopic patient; D(ii) Nipple eczema of atopic dermatitis; D(iii) Close-up view of nipple eczema; (E) Atopic cheilitis; (F) Atopic dermatitis seen in twins, note the eczematous lesions on face.

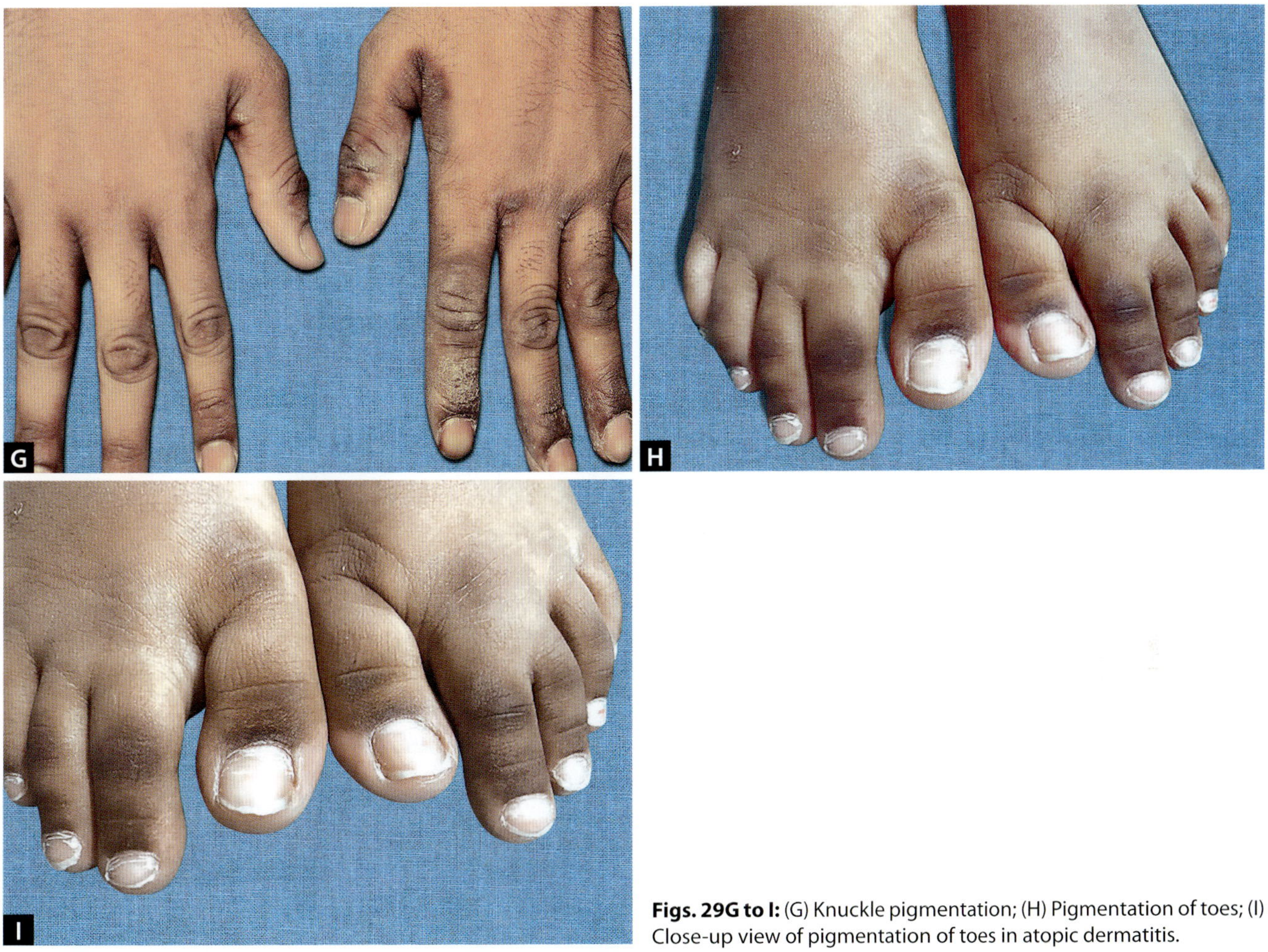

Figs. 29G to I: (G) Knuckle pigmentation; (H) Pigmentation of toes; (I) Close-up view of pigmentation of toes in atopic dermatitis.

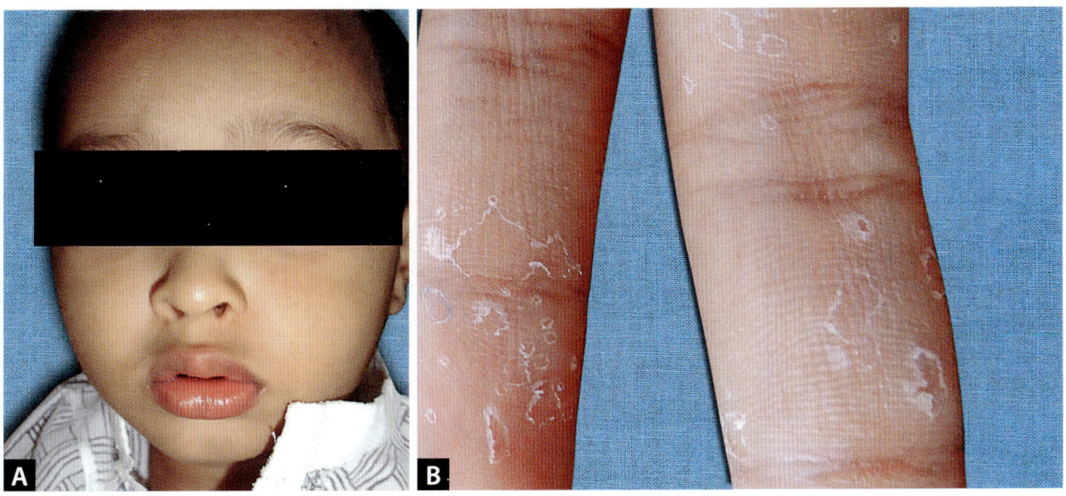

Figs. 30A and B: (A) Atopic cheilitis; (B) Keratolysis exfoliativa (KE).

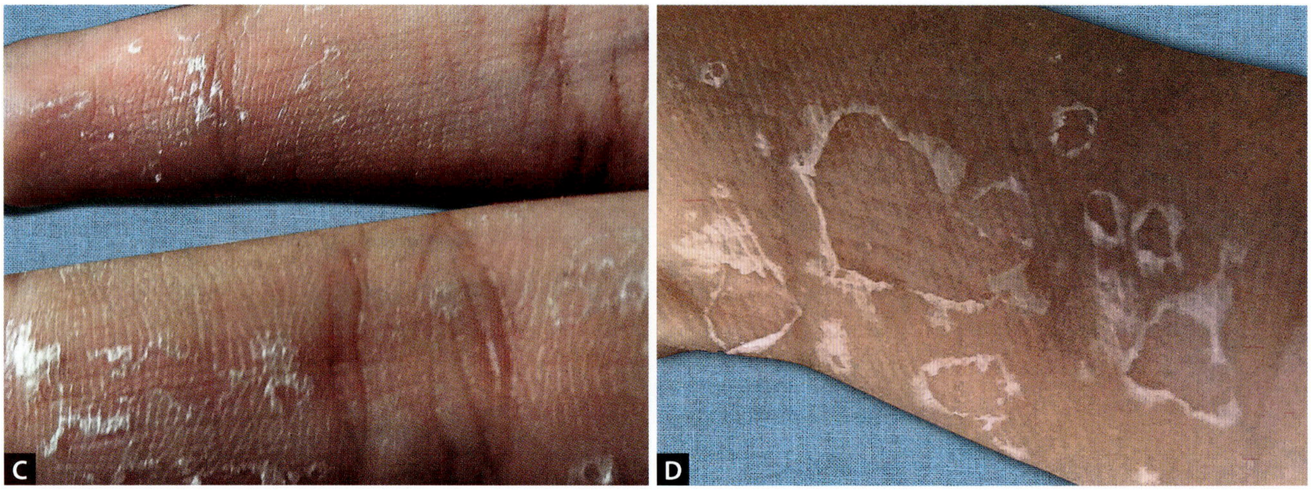

Figs. 30C and D: (C) Keratolysis exfoliativa (KE) over fingers; (D) KE, close-up view.

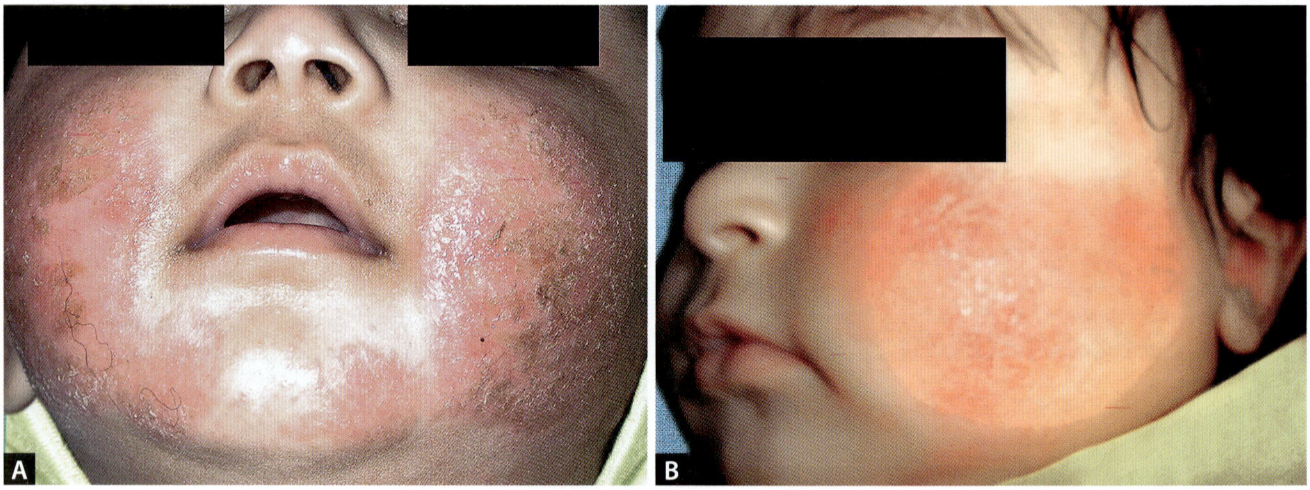

Figs. 31A and B: (A) Acute lesions of atopic dermatitis (AD) over face; (B) Classical lesions of AD over face.

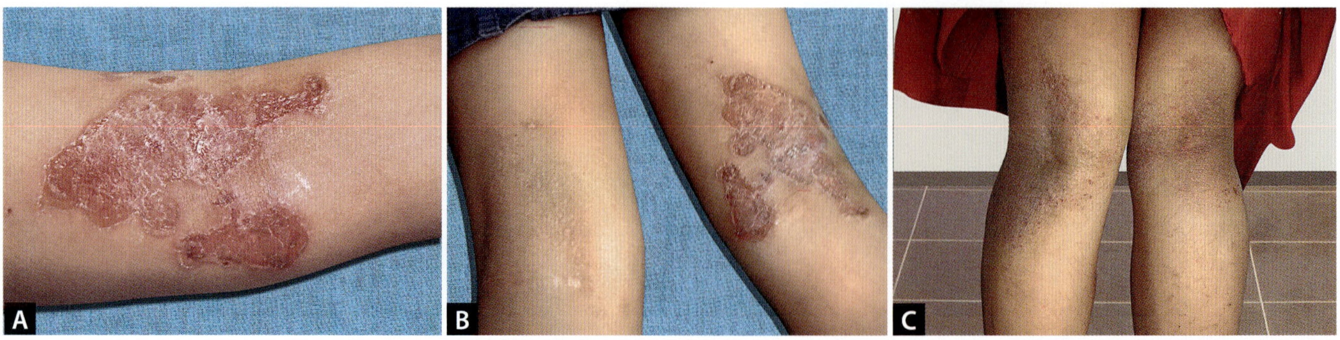

Figs. 32A to C: (A) Subacute eczema of atopic dermatitis (AD); (B) Subacute eczema of AD over popliteal fossae; (C) Flexural eczema of childhood AD.

"No man's knowledge here can go beyond his experience." —**John Locke**

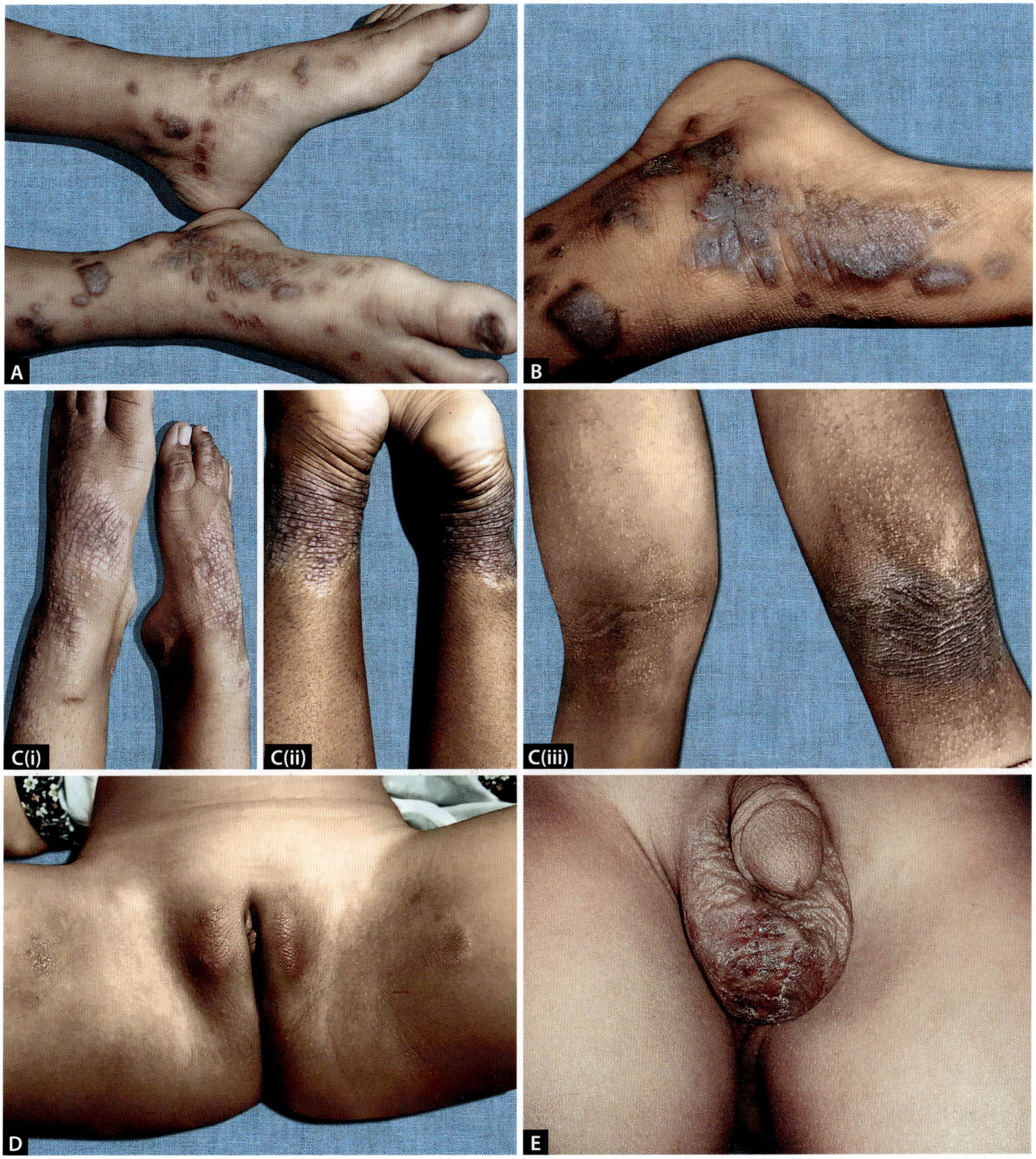

Figs. 33A to E: (A) Chronic lichenified eczema of atopic dermatitis (AD); (B) Close-up view; C(i) Lichenified eczema; C(ii) Same patient, another view; C(iii) Lichenified eczema with postinflammatory hyperpigmentation; (D) AD vulva; (E) AD scrotum.

"We must embrace pain and burn it as fuel for our journey." —**Kenji Miyazawa**

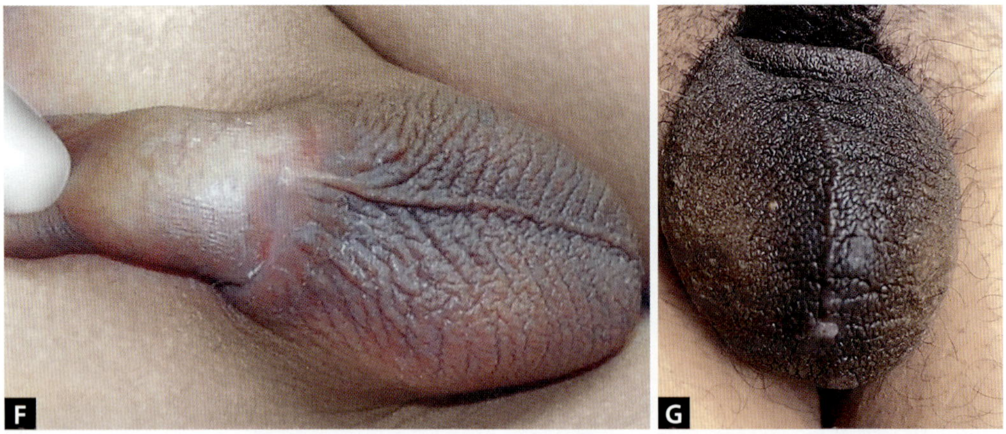

Figs. 33F and G: (F) Atopic dermatitis (AD) penoscrotal junction; (G) AD scrotum with postinflammatory hyperpigmentation.

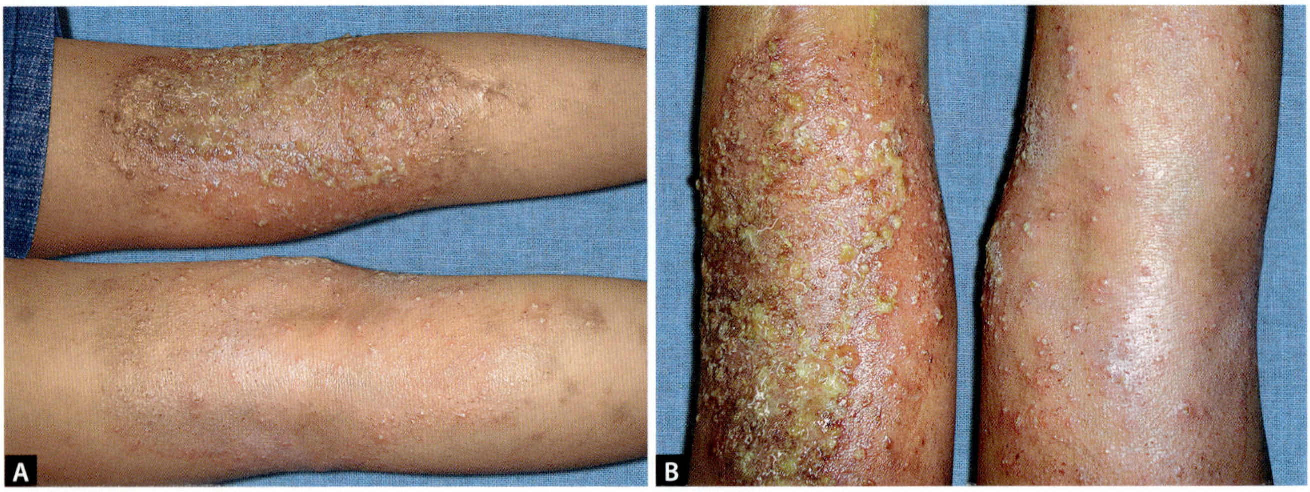

Figs. 34A and B: (A) Secondary infection in flexural eczema; (B) Gross secondary infection of eczema in atopic dermatitis (AD).

POSTERIOR THIGH DERMATITIS (FIGS. 35H AND I)

This is an atypical pattern of AD seen more commonly in school-going children. Toilet seat and car leather cover causing allergic sensitization can produce dermatitis over back of the thighs. It manifests due to contact allergy with nickel, cobalt, and chromium.

REGIONAL DERMATITIS

Regional dermatitis in atopic dermatitis includes the following entities:

1. Head and neck dermatitis: Predominantly head and neck areas are involved. "Portrait dermatitis" is a variant where lesions are mostly confined to seborrheic areas resembling bust sculpture. This variants is most commonly seen in adolescents probably owing to *Malassezia*.
2. Hand eczema: Three patterns of hand eczema are described in atopic dermatitis, they are
   i. Dyshidrosiform: Acute relapsing type typically involving palms and soles presenting as itchy vesiculobullous lesions
   ii. Hyperkeratotic: Chronic type mostly present over dorsum of hands, resembling irritant contact dermatitis
   iii. Dry pulpitis: Chronic erythematous desquamative type involving the distal phalynx
3. Eyelid eczema: Lesions usually presents bilaterally and mostly involving the lower eyelids, where as unilateral and upper eyelid involvement favors contact dermatitis.
4. Vulval eczema
5. Nipple eczema

"A problem is a chance for you to do your best." —**Duke Ellington**

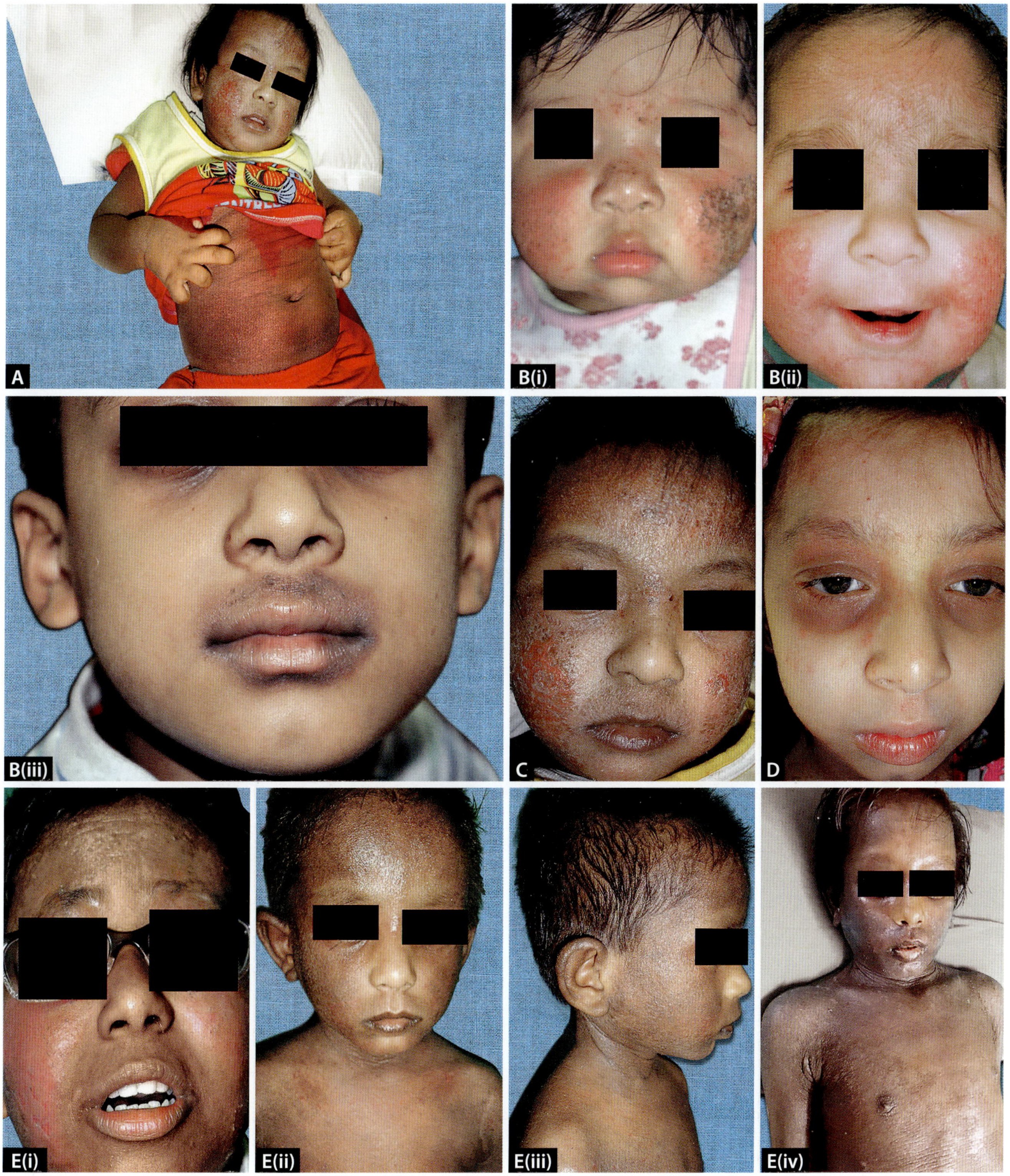

Figs. 35A to E(iv): (A) Severe atopic dermatitis (AD) in an infant, whole body; B(i and ii) Eczema over face; B(iii) Perioral lichenification in AD; (C) Severe AD, note facial lesions; (D) Severe AD, note periorbital lesions; E(i) Severe AD with excruciating pruritus; E(ii) Severe AD with diffuse postinflammatory hyperpigmentation; E(iii) Same child, note the lesions on the side of face; E(iv) Severe atopic dermatitis.

"Hard times don't create heroes. It is during the hard times when the 'hero' within us is revealed." —**Bob Riley**

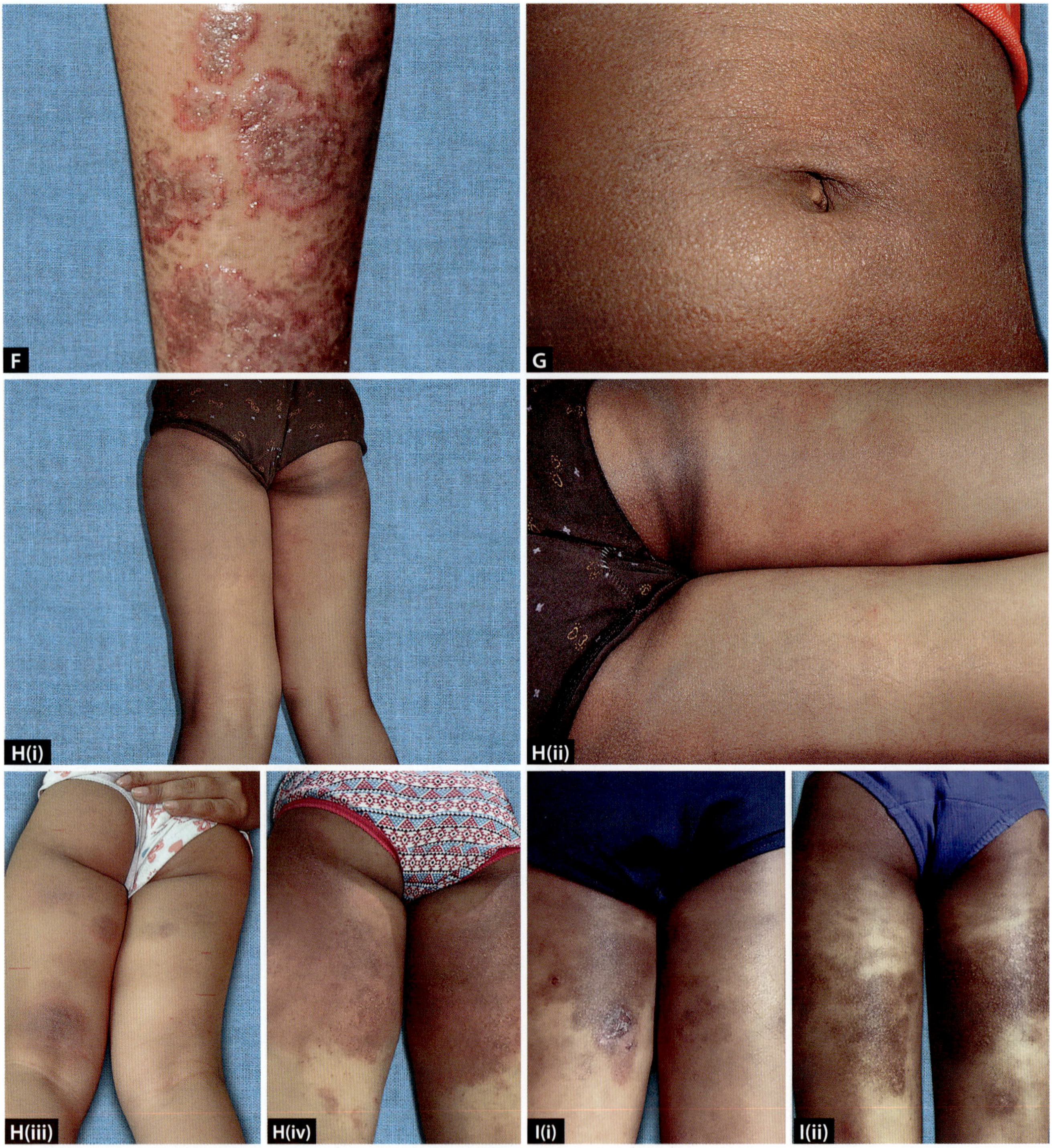

Figs. 35F to I(ii): (F) Severe atopic dermatitis (AD), note acute oozy lesions; (G) Severe and extensive AD; H(i) Posterior thigh dermatitis; H(ii) Close-up view; H(iii) Posterior thigh dermatitis in a 4-year-old girl; H(iv) Posterior thigh dermatitis, another patient; I(i) Posterior thigh dermatitis, note erythema; I(ii) Posterior thigh dermatitis (close-up) view.

Treatment of Atopic Dermatitis (Figs. 35J to N)

Management of AD has several facets. The treatment is basically aimed at effective control of the disease and improved quality of life (QOL) to the children with AD. Counseling parents goes a long way in the control of the disease.

"It's not about perfect. It's about effort." —**Jillian Michaels**

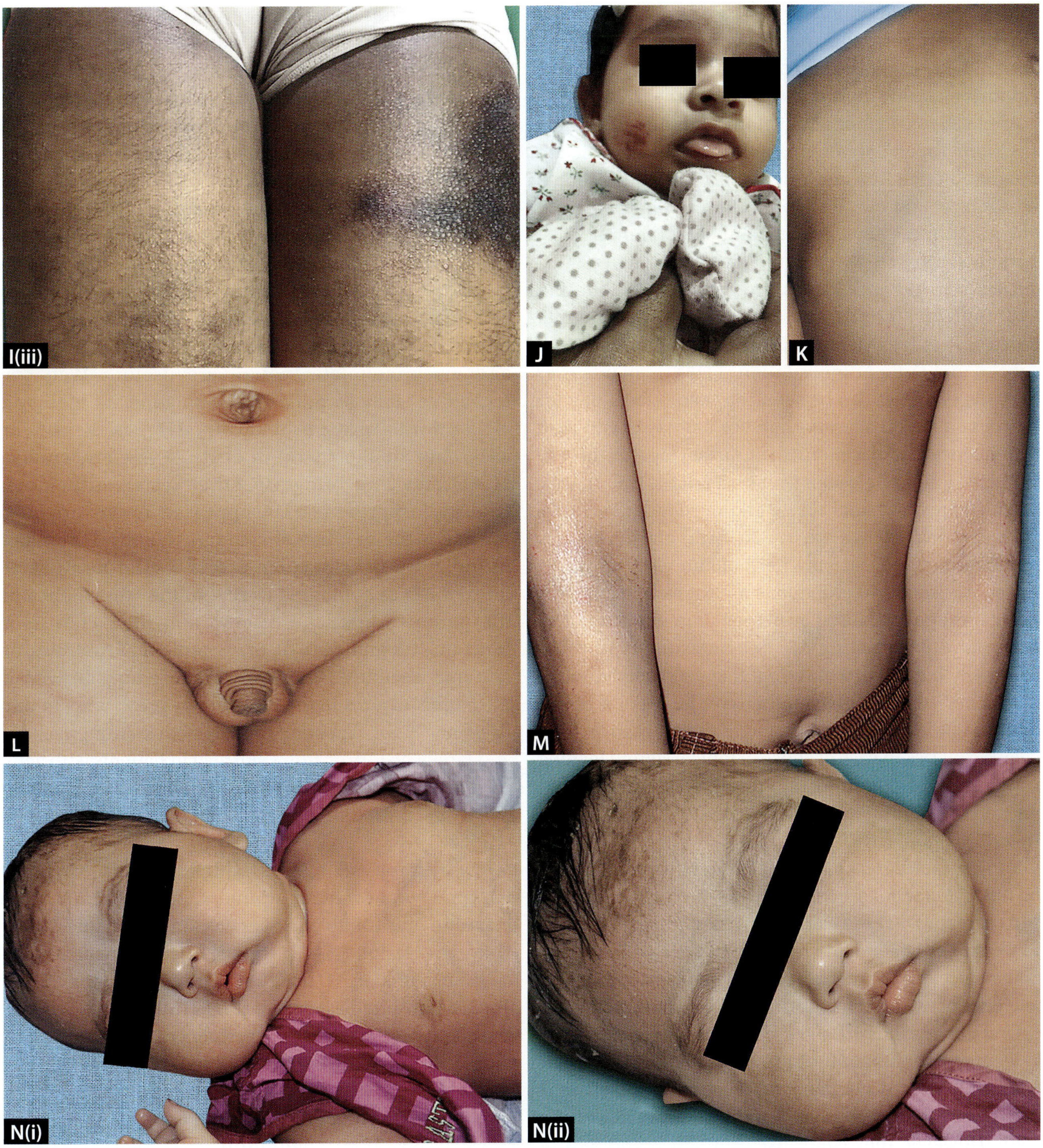

Figs. 35I(iii) to N(ii): I(iii) Posterior thigh dermatitis with postinflammatory hyperpigmentation; (J) Mittens to prevent scratching in a child; (K) Multiple erythematous papules seen on chest after wearing charms and amulets in atopic dermatitis (AD); (L) AD, note the eczematous lesions on lower abdomen and thighs after wearing charms; (M) Exacerbation of flexural eczema after wearing sacred thread; N(i) A 5-month-old infant with cushingoid features secondary to topical steroid abuse; N(ii) Same baby, close-up view.

Cleansing of the skin is very important and in this regard regular bathing has no alternative. Either a moisturizing soap (syndet soap) or a synthetic nonsoap nondetergent cleanser should be used. There is no role of antiseptic bathing and it should be avoided. Maintaining proper temperature and humidity, not touching plants, avoiding pets, avoiding dusty atmosphere and contact with wool, wearing full sleeve clothing, and avoiding constant touching of the skin by metals, e.g., rings, bangle, or amulet make life more comfortable for the children.

Application of emollients within 3 minutes of bathing is helpful. Topical steroids should be applied over the eczematous patches and emollient all over the body. The strength and mode of application of topical steroid depend upon the severity, site, and age of the patients. In infants, as well as over the sites such as eyelids, face, axillae, and groins a less potent steroid is chosen. Mild topical steroids include 1% hydrocortisone. Fluticasone is a moderately potent steroid approved by US Food and Drug Administration (FDA) in infants over 3 months of age. It can be safely applied once a day for 2–3 weeks, then on alternate days for 2–3 weeks and then the frequency of application can be further tapered. In case of infected lesions or lesions over finger or toe web spaces, anterior nares, perianal areas, and retroauricular folds, where *S. aureus* counts are usually high, oral antibiotics are recommended. Eczema herpeticum also known as Kaposi's varicelliform eruption is an extensive cutaneous vesicular eruption, caused by herpes simplex virus (HSV) arising in a pre-existing AD. Mometasone is another moderately potent topical steroid that can be used safely in children. But their use should never be over extensive body area or for prolonged period of time. Because there is significant risk in case of abuse of topical steroid leading to alteration of hypothalamic-pituitary-adrenal (HPA) axis and development of iatrogenic Cushing's disease **[Figs. 35N(i) and (ii)]**.

Topical tacrolimus in two different strengths (0.03%) and (0.1%) ointment or pimecrolimus 1% cream have been used to treat AD. These calcineurin inhibitors are used in the treatment of acute or chronic phase as well as in the maintenance of AD. They can be used in proactive management once or twice per week on areas of repeated outbreaks.

Oral medications are given when lesions are extensive. H_1-receptor antihistamines are basically used for their sedative effects. Cetirizine or levocetirizine given 1 hour before bedtime from 3 months onward can be useful. However, they can cause drowsiness and lack of concentration in the next morning. They can be used for 10–14 days as prolonged use can cause tachyphylaxis. Hydroxyzine, and cyproheptadine can be used as a long-term antihistamine in children above 1 year of age. The first author has been using it for this purpose in infants above 6 months of age safely for the last two decades. In school-going children nonsedating second generation antihistamines have been used over a prolonged period (6 months to 1 year) by the authors, particularly fexofenadine.

Oral antistaphylococcal antibiotics such as cloxacillin, amoxicillin, and cloxacillin combination or erythromycin are used when there is exudation and pustule formation. In patients with recurrent flares of AD associated with infection, long-term antibiotic treatment, and measures to reduce staphylococcal colonization of nose and perineum should be taken by using mupirocin cream.

In severe cases of AD, apart from basic skin care and emollients, systemic immunosuppressants are recommended. Cyclosporine, methotrexate, azathioprine, and mycophenolate mofetil are useful. "Wet wrap technique" may be indicated as an adjuvant therapy in children with severe or refractory AD. Oral steroids are used only for short term in acute, severe exacerbation of AD and as a bridge to other systemic therapies. Oral cyclosporine is FDA approved for treatment of AD and is the first line of systemic therapy. Fortunately in India, we usually come across a mild-to-moderate form of AD as compared to that in the West. Educating the parents about the disease and their counseling form an integral part of management. Probiotics are currently used in AD, not only in preventing or delaying the atopic features in the offspring by prescribing in third trimester in an expecting mother with a strong personal and family history of atopy, but also in patients with active AD to prevent gut-related allergen absorption. The most widely used probiotic in AD is *Lactobacillus rhamnosus* GG (LGG).

Newer topical agents which include extract of bacteria *Rhodobacter sphaeroides*, UR-1505, with immune modulator properties and thiol derivative N-acetylcysteine (NAC), topical oligodeoxynucleotides have been tried in AD but there is no convincing evidence. Topical phosphodiesterase-4 (PDE4) inhibitor, crisaborole is recently approved for the treatment of mild-to-moderate atopic dermatitis in children aged ≥2 years. Oral and topical Janus kinase (JAK) inhibitors represent a potential new treatment strategy for AD. Interferon gamma (IFN-γ), intravenous immunoglobulin, and allergen-specific immunotherapy, alitretinoin have been tried in AD but there is lack of data on its usage in children and hence not recommended. Biologics that have shown promising results and still in trial are dupilumab, nemolizumab, tralokinumab, and lebrikizumab. Dupilumab has shown promising results in the treatment of AD. Dupilumab has also shown to improve moderate-to-severe asthma

"Remember to look up at the stars and not down at your feet. Try to make sense of what you see and wonder about what makes the universe exist. Be curious. And however difficult life may seem, there is always something you can do and succeed at." —**Stephen Hawking**

(phase II studies). Recommended dose in children aged ≥12 years weighing <60 kg is initial dose of 400 mg, followed by a maintenance dose of 200 mg subcutaneous every other week.

ATOPIC DERMATITIS-LIKE ECZEMAS

Some of the conditions which mimic AD and need to be identified are as follows.

Scabies with Eczematization [Figs. 350(i) to (iv)]

Scabies is a highly contagious disorder caused by *Sarcoptes scabiei*, an itch mite. Infestation begins when a fertilized female mite attaches to a new host. She burrows deep into the stratum corneum and lives inside a burrow while laying eggs. These parasites favor a thin stratum corneum and low density of pilosebaceous units, thus explaining the distribution of lesions in children and young infants. Primary lesions consist of pruritic papules, vesicles, pustules, and linear burrows. But most patients will present with a mixture of lesions along with excoriations, eczematization, crusting, and secondary infection. The symptoms in scabies are due to hypersensitivity reaction to the mites, eggs, and scybala (feces). This sensitization leads to the itching and can persist up to 6 weeks.

Diagnosis depends on the characteristic symptoms, distribution of lesions, identification of the burrow when present, and presence of the disease among family members and contact. Definitive diagnosis is based on the demonstration of adult mite, ova, larva, or fecal matter.

Diagnosis in children is sometimes difficult as the disease has an atypical distribution with involvement of the head, neck, palms, and soles.

The primary lesions are also often not demonstrable due to excoriations, crusting, eczematization, and secondary infection. In children, disseminated secondary eczema can often be seen in scabies infestation. This occurs due to an immune response to some component of the infectious agent or due to overzealous hygiene practice leading to excessive skin dryness and subsequent xerosis and eczematization.

The eczema is often acute generalized and symmetrical. Sites commonly affected are the forearms, legs, thighs, and trunks. Vesiculation, blistering, and crusted plaques are often seen. Erythematous rash of the body and pompholyx of the palms and soles can also be seen.

Management of eczematous scabies is by initial treatment of the eczema followed by antiscabietic therapy. Wet wraps and dressing are recommended for oozing eczematous plaques.

Use of any antiseptic soap containing elestab or triclosan topical and systemic steroids, antibiotics for impetiginization, and sedating antihistamines at night are recommended. Once the eczema has subsided, appropriate antiscabietic therapy may be started.

Topical medications for scabies include 5% permethrin cream, 1% gamma-benzene hexachloride, 10% crotamiton, 6–10% precipitate of sulfur (especially in infants less than 2 months), and suspension of benzyl benzoate (12.5-25%). However, the authors prefer to use only 5% permethrin cream.

Oral ivermectin (200 μg/kg body weight) two doses 2 weeks apart have excellent cure rates.

Complications of eczematous scabies include persistent pruritus and possible glomerulonephritis when there is secondary impetiginization with nephritogenic *Streptococcus*.

Wiskott–Aldrich Syndrome

It is dealt with in more detail in Chapter 23: Primary Immunodeficiency Disorders and Skin. It is an X-linked recessive syndrome characterized by triad of chronic eczematous dermatitis resembling AD, recurrent infections, and thrombocytopenia with small platelets. There is increased susceptibility to bacterial (pyoderma or otitis media) as well as viral and fungal infections. Thrombocytopenia manifests as petechiae, epistaxis, bloody diarrhea, and/or hematemesis. There are elevated levels of IgA and IgE with normal levels of IgM and IgG. Death ensues from infection, bleeding, or lymphoma.

Hyperimmunoglobulin E Syndrome

It is dealt with in more detail in Chapter 23: Primary Immunodeficiency Disorders and Skin. It is a primary immunodeficiency syndrome. Autosomal-dominant form is more common, and is also called Job syndrome. It is characterized by triad of eczema, recurrent skin and lung infections, and high-serum IgE. The disease begins within the first month of life. Initial lesions are folliculocentric papulopustular eruption involving the face, scalp, neck, axillae, and diaper area. Cutaneous staphylococcal infections are common. The child later develops

"You are so much more than what you are going through." —**John Tew**

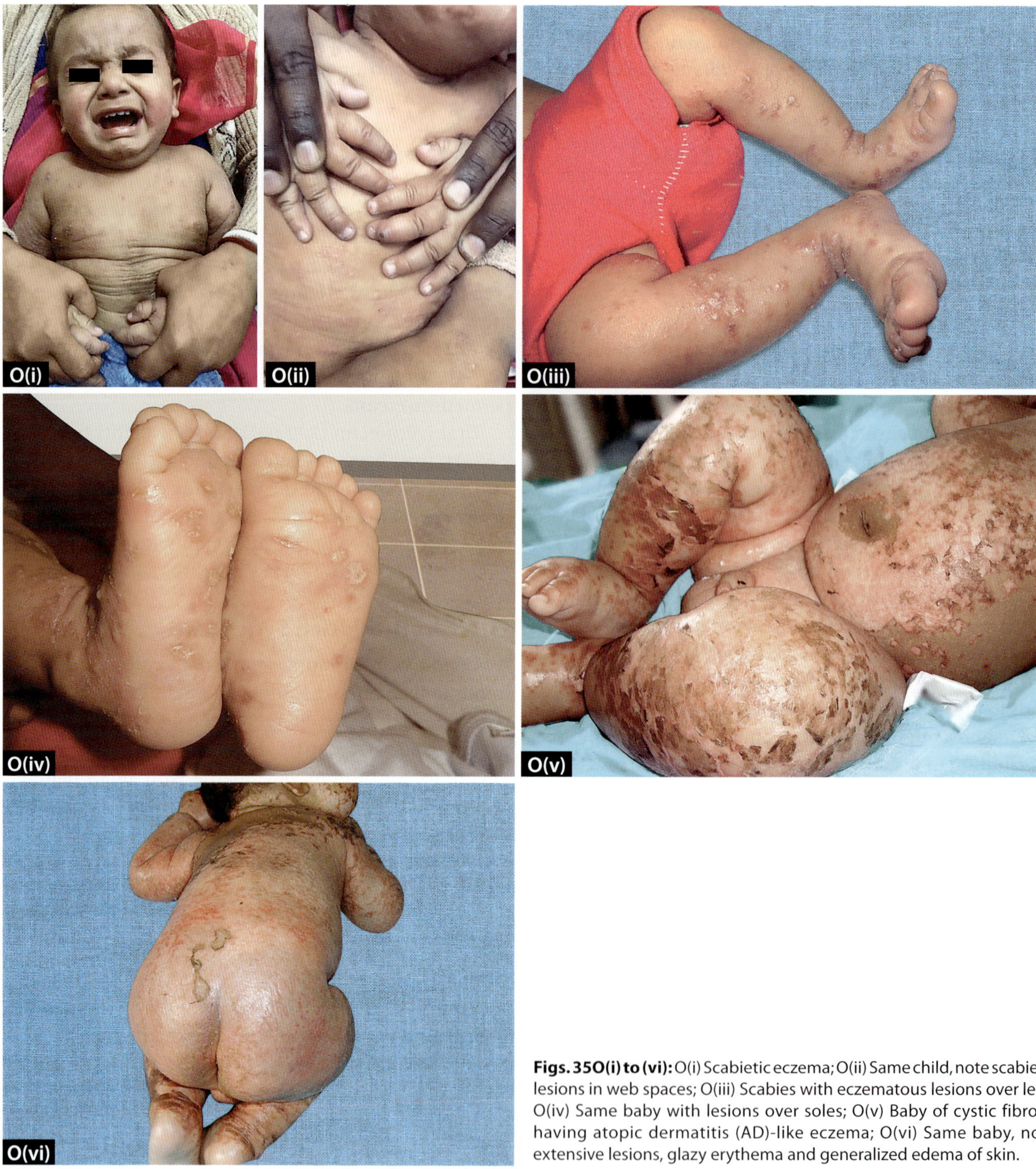

Figs. 35O(i) to (vi): O(i) Scabietic eczema; O(ii) Same child, note scabietic lesions in web spaces; O(iii) Scabies with eczematous lesions over legs; O(iv) Same baby with lesions over soles; O(v) Baby of cystic fibrosis having atopic dermatitis (AD)-like eczema; O(vi) Same baby, note extensive lesions, glazy erythema and generalized edema of skin.

skeletal and dental abnormalities. Eczematous rash of hyperimmunoglobulin E syndrome (HIES) shares many clinical features with AD but they do not have allergic rhinitis, asthma, or other cutaneous signs of atopy unlike individuals with AD.

Severe Combined Immunodeficiency

This is a disorder with deficient cell-mediated and humoral immunity. It presents with failure to thrive in early infancy, diarrhea, and recurrent infections. Initial cutaneous eruptions may be seborrheic-like dermatitis or morbilliform eruptions. Severe eczematous dermatitis and erythroderma may develop with alopecia. Persistent mucocutaneous candidiasis is often present.

Phenylketonuria

This is an autosomal recessive disorder of amino acid metabolism characterized by mental retardation, diffuse hypopigmentation, seizures, dermatitis, and photosensitivity. Early infantile eczema, indistinguishable from AD, may be one of the first signs of phenylketonuria (PKU). Edematous scleroderma of the extremities sparing the hands and feet is also characteristic.

Cystic Fibrosis [Figs. 35O(v) and (vi)]

It is an autosomal recessive disorder due to homozygous or compound heterozygous mutation in the cystic fibrosis transmembrane conductance regulator gene leading to the production of a defective epithelial chloride channel. The classical triad of cystic fibrosis includes chronic obstructive pulmonary disease, exocrine pancreatic insufficiency, and elevation of sodium and chloride concentration in sweat. Cutaneous features in cystic fibrosis present with AD or acrodermatitis enteropathica-like lesions. The characteristic presentation is periorificial and truncal dermatitis. Dermatitis presenting as an initial manifestation of cystic fibrosis is rare and typically presents with erythematous scaly papules to plaques on the perineum and later progresses to involve the perioral region, trunk, and extremities. Occasionally, other features include alopecia, failure to thrive, diarrhea, irritability, hepatomegaly, and pitting edema of the extremities. The exact cause of cutaneous features is not known, but thought to be due to deficiency of zinc, protein, and essential fatty acids. Differential diagnoses include acrodermatitis enteropathica, biotin deficiency, immunodeficiency disorder, and aminoaciduria disorders. Any child with dermatitis along with signs of malnutrition, differential diagnosis of cystic fibrosis should be considered.

Other eczematous dermatoses which have been discussed separately are biotinidase deficiency, infantile seborrheic dermatitis and infectious eczematoid dermatitis, etc.

INFECTIOUS ECZEMATOID DERMATITIS (FIGS. 36 AND 37)

It develops following secondary eczematization from a primary pyogenic infection. The purulent material discharged causes eczematization of the normal looking skin around. Eczematous lesions on the skin over the pinnae in case of otitis externa and eczematization around pyoderma lesions are classical examples.

Treatment

Oral antistaphylococcal antibiotics, e.g., cloxacillin, combination of amoxicillin, and clavulanic acid or erythromycin for 7–10 days, form the mainstay of treatment. It is to be supplemented with application of a moderately potent steroid, e.g., fluticasone and mometasone, for 7–14 days. After oral antibiotic is stopped, one may use a combination of fluticasone and mupirocin for 7 days followed by fluticasone/mometasone only for another 7 days. Associated pruritus is treated with oral

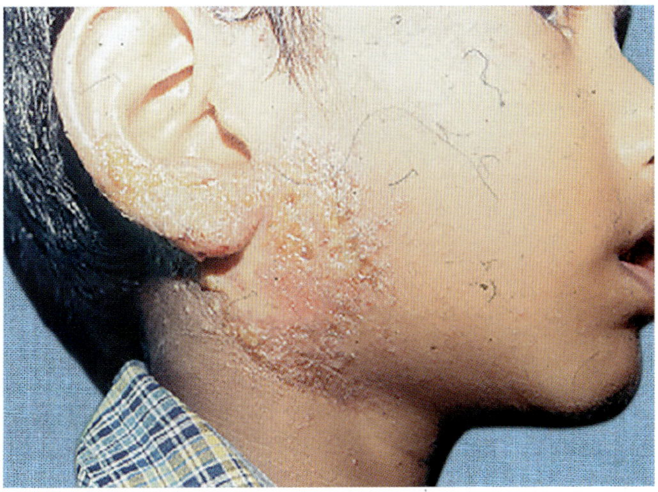

Fig. 36: Infectious eczematoid dermatitis.

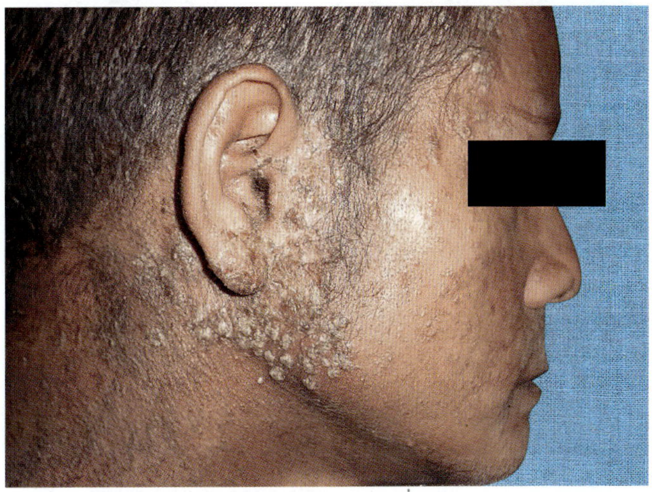

Fig. 37: Infectious eczematoid dermatitis, in the preauricular and retroauricular regions.

"Difficult roads always lead to beautiful destinations." —**Zig Ziglar**

antihistamines. Cleansing of the local skin with lukewarm water and soap is to be done. Cleansing of the skin with antiseptics is avoided. In resistant cases (which is very rare), pus is to be sent for culture and sensitivity testing and antibiotic is to be chosen accordingly.

MILIARIAL ECZEMA (FIGS. 38 TO 40)

This entity has not been described in the standard text and literature published from the west. This is mostly seen in tropical climate like in India. During summer months due to increased sweating, infants and children often develop extensive miliaria. This is more common in hospitalized babies who mostly remain in bed. The miliaria on getting ruptured, undergo eczematization. The lesions are usually distributed over trunk. However, face and extremities may also be affected. With the involvement of face, it may closely simulate AD.

Treatment

The eczematized areas are to be treated with mild topical corticosteroids. However, rest of the treatment of miliaria remains the same.

ALLERGIC CONTACT DERMATITIS (FIGS. 41 TO 44)

This discussion is in addition to earlier discussion on ACD in this chapter.

The occurrence of ACD increases with age; prevalence rates of 13.3–24.5% have been reported, but the highest sensitization rate has been found in children aged 0–3 years. Unlike irritant contact dermatitis (ICD), ACD develops in predisposed subjects and involves an immunological mechanism that requires an initial sensitization phase followed by the elicitation phase that

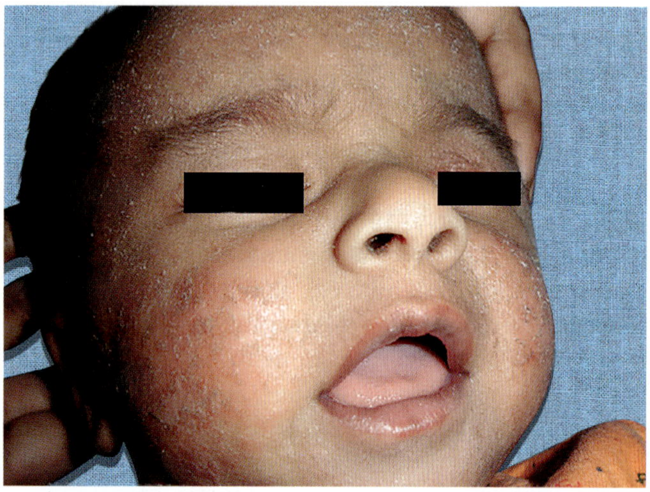

Fig. 38: Miliarial eczema over face in an 3-month-old baby.

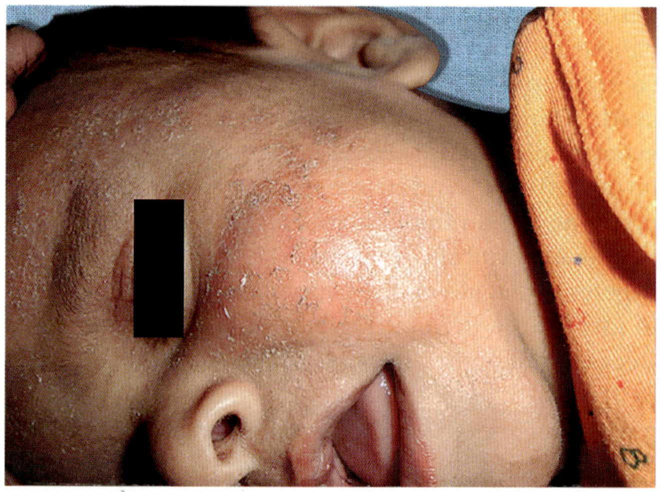

Fig. 39: Same baby, note erythema and scaling.

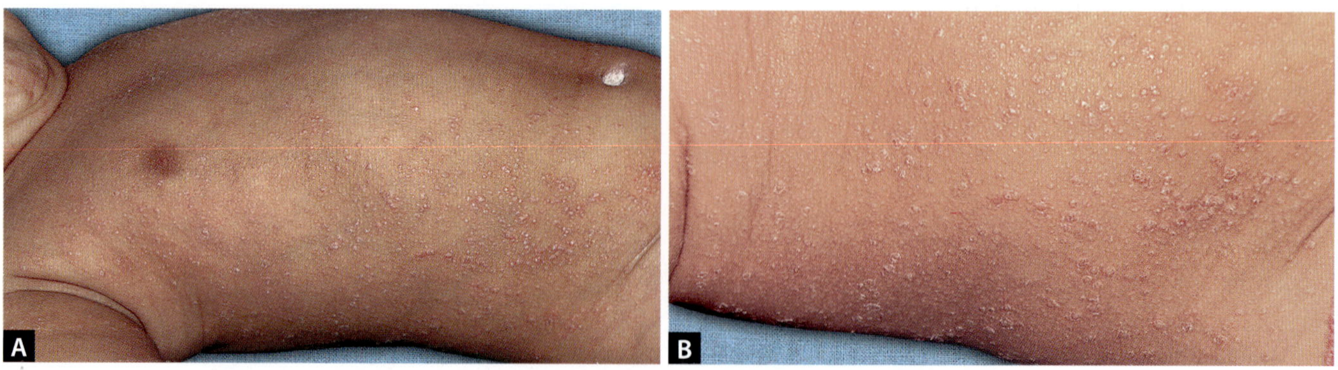

Figs. 40A and B: (A) Miliarial eczema; (B) Same boy, note trunk lesions.

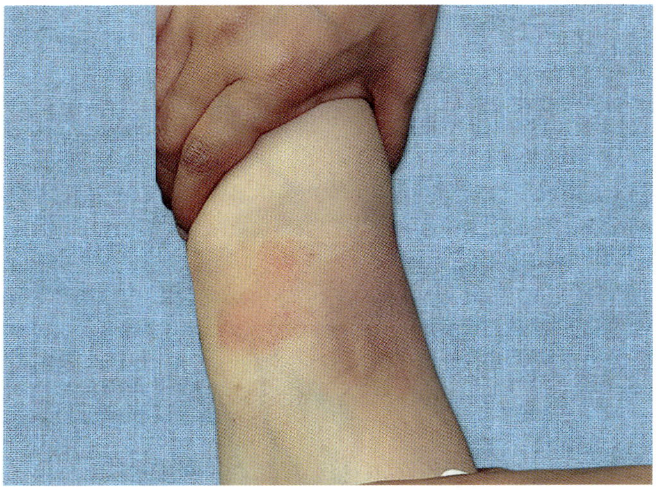

Fig. 41: Contact dermatitis to amulets.

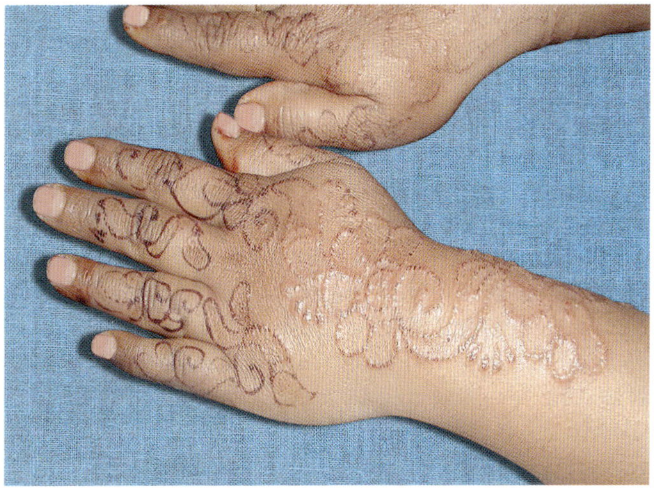

Fig. 42: Contact dermatitis to decorative tattoo.

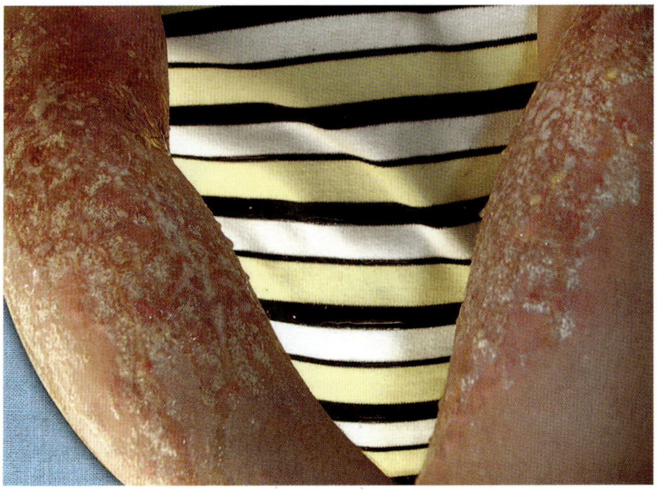

Fig. 43: Contact dermatitis to henna tattoo.

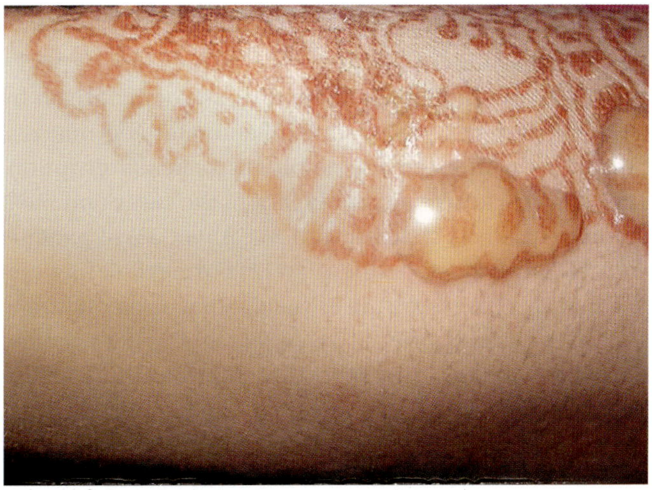

Fig. 44: Acute irritant dermatitis to henna tattoo.

causes the skin lesions. The sensitization phase begins when the hapten penetrates the skin, where it is first biochemically transformed by epidermal enzymatic processes and then conjugated with a carrier protein to become immunogenic. The antigen is thus captured by antigen-presenting cells (APCs), particularly Langerhans cells, processed, bound to class II major histocompatibility complex (MHC) molecules, and expressed on the cell surface. At this point, under the influx of the numerous cytokines produced by keratinocytes and APCs, the Langerhans cells migrate toward the locoregional lymph nodes where specific effector and memory T-lymphocytes are selected and clonally proliferated before leaving the lymph node, entering the bloodstream, and reaching the skin. The legs and feet, hands, and face are the sites most frequently affected by pediatric ACD, which is mainly caused by metals, footwear, topical medications, and cosmetics. Cosmetics are the main cause of ACD in early infancy because mothers are using herbal or other products containing active ingredients. Irritant forms are more frequent than allergic forms, and are due to the application of topical agents that are too aggressive. Even so-called "natural" products such as propolis or tea tree oil can cause ACD. Contact with metals increases exponentially during school age and adolescence. Those responsible for the highest incidence of ACD during childhood are nickel, chromium, and cobalt, which can also induce cosensitization to other metals. Nickel sulfate is contained in multiple products including artificial jewellery buttons of clothes, watch, and even in chocolates.

"Don't wish it were easier. Wish you were better." —**Jim Rohn**

Girls are also frequently sensitized to the perfumes contained in numerous products (often including those that are claimed to be "fragrance-free") in the form of essential oils or perfumed preservatives such as benzyl alcohol. As chrome (potassium dichromate) is one of the ingredients used in the tanning of leather, wearing leather shoes is the main cause of sensitization, particularly in the summer when shoes may be worn without socks. In adolescence, the substances used in hair dyes (such as p-phenylenediamine) can cause ACD of the scalp, face, and eyelids. Once the hapten to which a child has been sensitized has been identified, it is possible to treat the ongoing lesions, but it is also essential to avoid any future contact with the causative substance. This is easy in some cases, but may be difficult in the case of ubiquitous haptens (e.g., nickel), or impossible if the hapten is unknown.

ECZEMA HERPETICUM (FIGS. 45 TO 47)

Eczema herpeticum (EH), also known as Kaposi's varicelliform eruption, is a rare disease characterized by HSV infection of a pre-existing inflammatory dermatosis, presenting with extensive cutaneous vesicular eruption. HSV-1 is the causative agent in 90% of the cases and most commonly affects children with AD. About 3% of patients with AD are estimated to develop EH during their lifetime. It can also occur concomitantly with other skin conditions such as psoriasis, Darier's disease, eczema, irritant contact dermatitis, burns, and seborrheic dermatitis. Primary infection as well as reactivation of the latent virus can lead to EH. It is independent of season and time of the year. Risk factors for development of EH in AD patients include early-onset and persistent severe AD, head and neck AD, extrinsic AD, and administration of immunosuppressive agents. Early-onset AD is also a risk factor for recurrent EH. Pathophysiological risk factors for the development of EH include cathelicidin deficiency, filaggrin mutations, reduced interferon responses, and higher type 2 inflammation.

Clinically, it presents with abrupt onset of fever, malaise, and widespread eruption of monomorphous, small, dome-shaped, grouped papulovesicles on an erythematous base that rupture leaving behind punched-out ulcers. Lymphadenopathy may occur. Most commonly affected areas are the face, neck, and upper trunk. Usually, lesions completely dry and heal after 2–6 weeks. Atypical manifestations such as absence of vesicles or presence

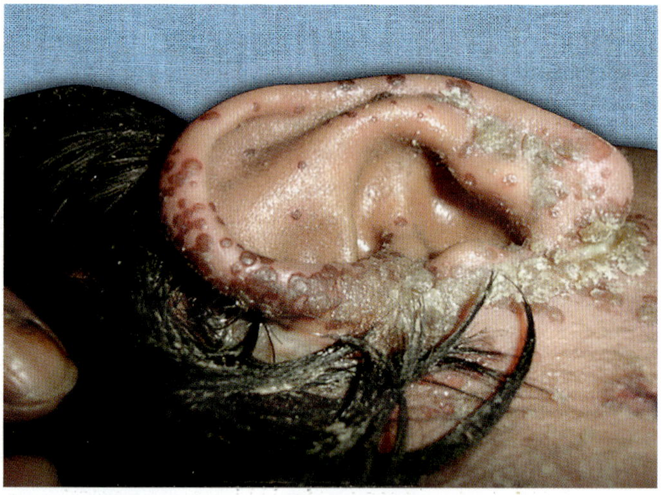

Fig. 46: Same boy, see grouped vesicular lesions on background eczema and erythema.

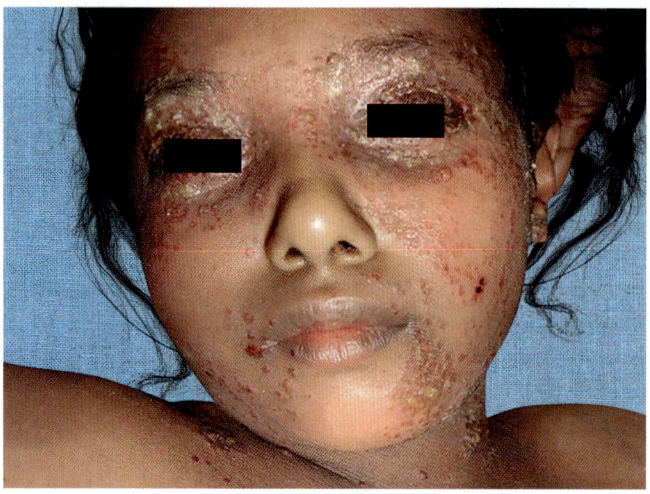

Fig. 45: Eczema herpeticum in an 11-year-old boy.

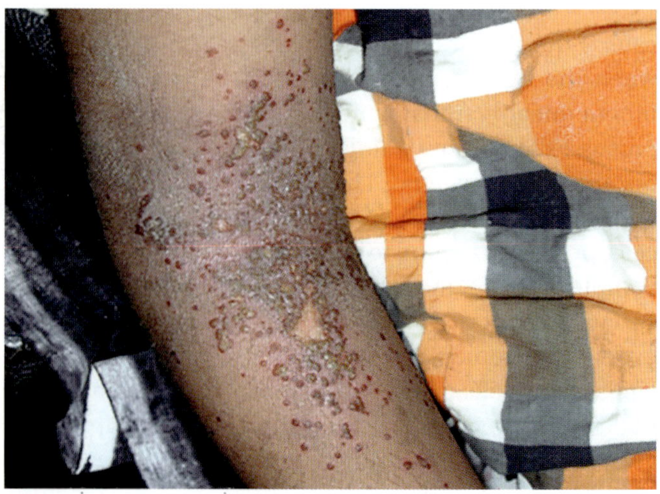

Fig. 47: Same boy, close-up view of cubital fossae with eczema herpeticum.

of only small papules have been described. EH can recur and patients might present with localized HSV infection in previously involved areas. The differential diagnoses include impetigo, scabies, eczema vaccinatum, contact dermatitis, and primary varicella infection.

Early diagnosis and prompt treatment of EH is required to prevent functional complications such as HSV keratoconjunctivitis or keratitis which may lead to blindness, HSV gingivostomatitis causing decreased oral intake leading to dehydration and life-threatening complications such as widespread viremia causing meningitis or encephalitis. Secondary *S. aureus* infection is common and can lead to septicemia causing multiorgan failure and death. In immunocompromised patients, EH can cause severe hepatitis that may progress to fulminant or acute liver failure.

The standard method for diagnosis of HSV infection is virus culture. Tzanck test showing multinucleated giant cells can provide rapid diagnosis and direct fluorescence antigen testing can also be done. Mainstay of treatment is prompt administration of systemic antiviral therapy. Hospitalization and administration of intravenous (IV) acyclovir is recommended in cases of severe disease and immunocompromised patients. IV acyclovir to be given at 25 mg/kg/day in four divided doses for 5–7 days, then orally same dose for at least 4–6 weeks as the chances of relapse is very high. Prophylactic antibiotic therapy to prevent superadded bacterial infection, measures for pain control, hydration with attention to electrolyte balance, and ophthalmological examination in cases of facial involvement is also required. Meticulous skin care with application of bland emollients is important. Use of topical steroids for underlying dermatitis in the setting of EH is controversial.

ECZEMA COXSACKIUM (FIGS. 48 TO 53)

Eczema coxsackium represents an atypical form of hand-foot-and-mouth disease (HFMD) caused by *Coxsackievirus* (CV) A6 and A16, characterized by uniform, clustered, 2–4-mm vesiculobullous and erosive lesions in areas affected by AD, similar to EH. Vesicles may evolve into hemorrhagic crusts or confluent hemorrhagic bullae. It can also occur in association with Darier's disease and epidermolytic ichthyosis. There is also a tendency for localization to sites of skin injury or inflammation, such as sunburns, irritant/diaper dermatitis, healing lacerations, and tinea pedis. Compared to CVA16 virus, disseminated lesions, including perioral and buttock lesions, are more often associated with CVA6. Rarely, CVA9 has also been reported as the causative agent. Eczema coxsackium most commonly occurs among preschoolers in the summer through late fall. Lesions are usually painless and children remain reasonably well, unlike with EH. Brief history of fever or diarrhea may be present during the week before the appearance of the exanthem. Rarely, serious complications including aseptic meningitis may occur. Onychomadesis, Beau's lines, and desquamation of the palms and soles develop 1–3 weeks after resolution of the rash, which may persist for 2–3 weeks.

Eczema coxsackium has to be differentiated from EH (itchy, painful, sometimes blood-stained blisters in an unwell child), varicella, contact dermatitis, and blistering drug reactions. Diagnosis is based on clinical features and

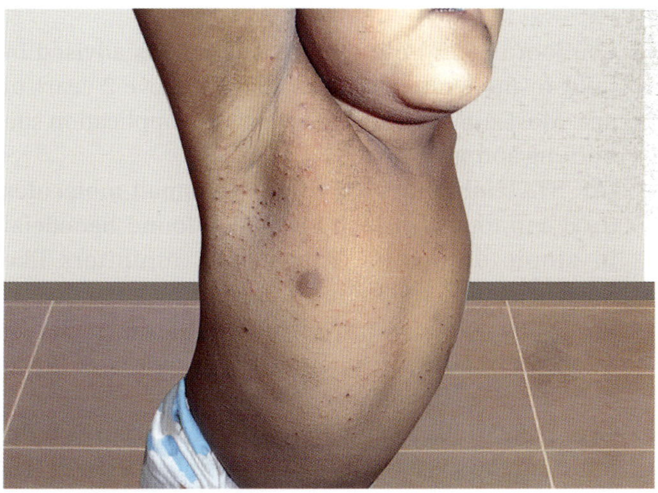

Fig. 48: Eczema coxsackium, note collapsed vesicles (some hemorrhagic) with background eczema over right axilla.

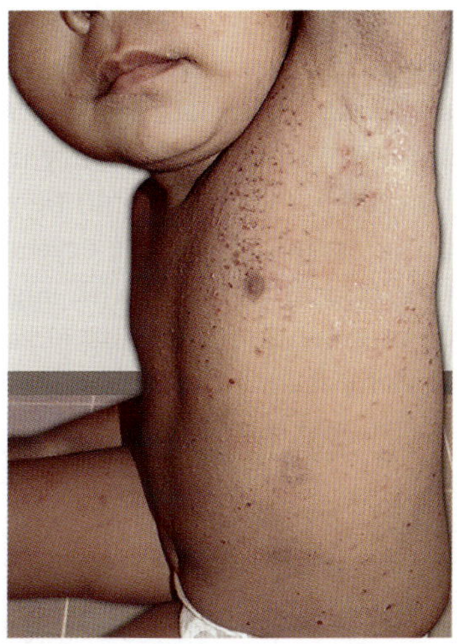

Fig. 49: Same boy, similar lesions over left axilla.

"Experience is a name everyone gives to their mistakes." —**Oscar Wilde**

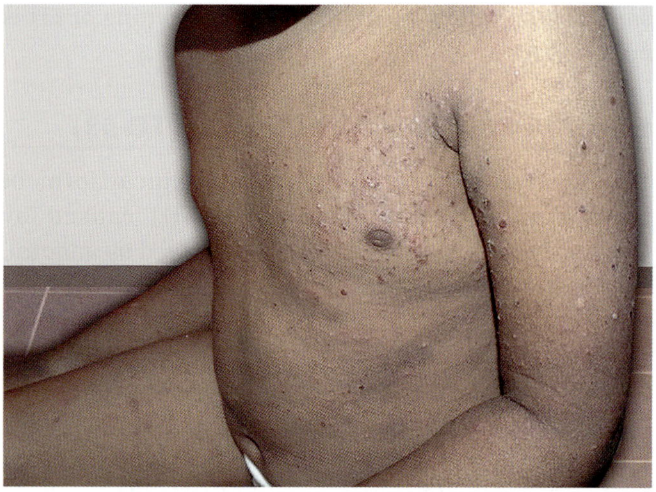

Fig. 50: Note clustered grouped collapsed vesicles over eczematous background.

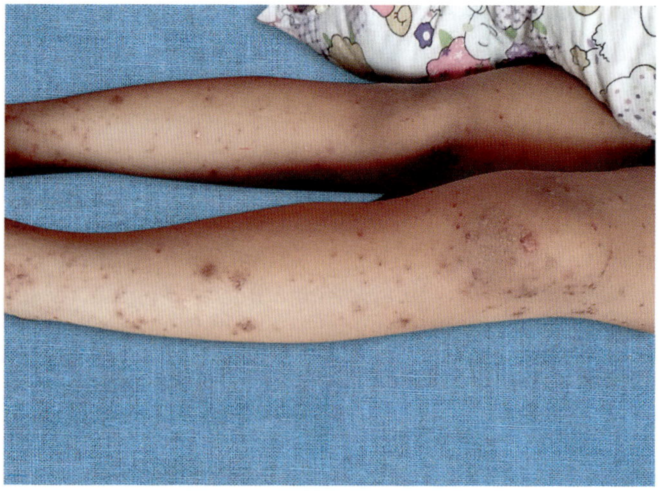

Fig. 51: Eczema coxsackium in a 5-year-old girl.

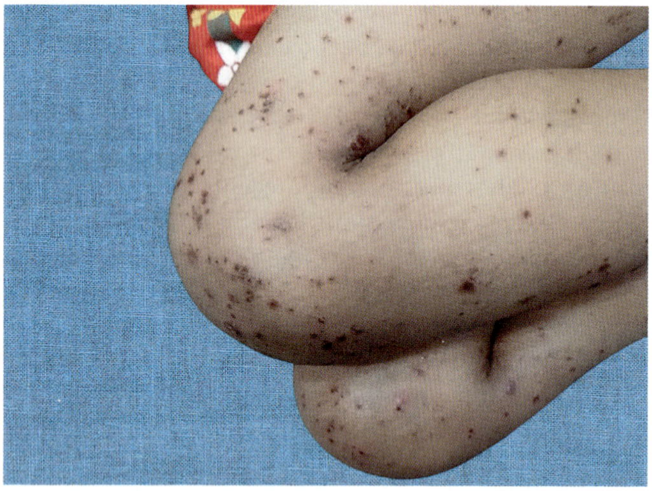

Fig. 52: Eczema coxsackium in a 7-year-old girl. Note collapsed vesicles of hand-foot-and-mouth disease (HFMD).

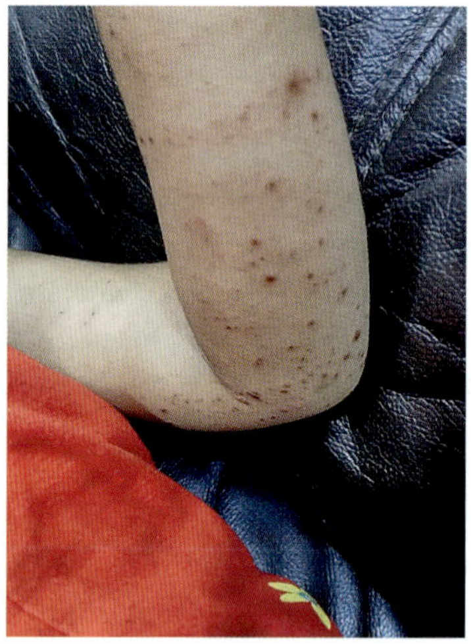

Fig. 53: Same girl, another view.

reverse transcription polymerase chain reaction (RT-PCR) assay from vesicular fluid, throat swabs, or stool samples, which will help in avoiding unnecessary treatment with antibiotics or acyclovir. Parents should be reassured that it is a self-limiting eruption, but the erythema may take weeks to subside. Supportive care with aggressive use of moisturizer for managing underlying eczema and low-potency topical steroids for managing itch are helpful. Wet wrap therapy has shown to be beneficial.

WHAT'S NEW

- Newer molecules which were recently approved for the topical use in atopic dermatitis are crisaborole (PDE4 inhibitor) and JAK STAT inhibitors.
- Crisaborole (2%) ointment twice daily is advised in mild-to-moderate atopic dermatitis above 2 years of age. Most common adverse effects are application site burning and stinging.
- JAK STAT inhibitors are the newer small molecules (oral and topical) which have been found beneficial in atopic dermatitis. Topical JAK inhibitors like Tofacitinib (2% ointment), Ruxolitinib (1.5% cream) have shown good improvement in mild-to-moderate atopic dermatitis. Delgocitinib 0.5% ointment is the only approved topical JAK STAT inhibitor.
- Oral Tofacitinib 5 mg twice daily was approved for other conditions, but when tried as off label use, it has shown favorable results in moderate-to-severe atopic dermatitis where long-term steroids cannot be given.

"All a writer needs is talent and ink." —**JK Rowling**

- Brepocitinib is tried for both oral and topical therapy in atopics. Baricitinib, Upadacitinib, Abrocitinib and Gusacitinib are the other JAK STAT inhibitors under trials for atopic dermatitis.
- Abrocitinib, both 100 mg and 200 mg tablets has shown very good control of moderate-to-severe AD in various global trials and expected to launched in Indian market soon for children above 12 years of age.

SUGGESTED READINGS

1. Dhar S, Parikh D, Rammoorthy R, Srinivas S, Sarkar R, Inamadar A, et al. Treatment guidelines for atopic dermatitis by ISPD Task force 2016. IndianJ Paediatr Dermatol. 2017;18:174-82.
2. Dhar S, Parikh D, Rammoorthy R, Srinivas S, Sarkar R,Inamadar A, et al. Maternal dietary antigen avoidance during pregnancy or lactation. Indian J Paediatr Dermatol. 2017;18:181-2.
3. Paller AS, Mancini AJ. Eczematous eruptions in childhood. In: Paller AS, Mancini AJ (Eds). Hurwitz Clinical Pediatric Dermatology, 5th edition. Edinburgh: Elsevier; 2016. pp. 38-72.
4. Dhar S, Srinivas SM. Food allergy in atopic dermatitis. Indian J Dermatol. 2016;61:645-68.
5. Dhar S, Srinivas SM, Bajaj AK. Allergic contact dermatitis in atopic dermatitis. Indian J Paediatr Dermatol. 2018;19:304-7.
6. McDowell L, Olin B. Crisaborole: A Novel Nonsteroidal Topical Treatment for Atopic Dermatitis. J Pharm Technol. 2019;35(4):172-8.
7. Chovatiya R, Paller AS. JAK inhibitors in the treatment of atopic dermatitis. J Allergy Clin Immunol. 2021;148(4):927-40.

"Life is a journey, not a destination." — **Ralph Emerson**

CHAPTER

8

Papulosquamous Disorders

CHILDHOOD PSORIASIS (FIGS. 1 TO 9A)

Psoriasis is quite common in children affecting 0.5–2% of pediatric population. Besides the common forms, several forms are peculiar to children. Interdigital tinea is uncommon in children and a toe-cleft intertrigo may be psoriatic. Other flexural forms also occur. The disease may mimic chronic blepharitis or perleche, usually unilaterally with a small plaque of psoriasis on one eyelid extending to the lid margin or on the cheek at the angle of the mouth. Psoriasis on the face is more common in children. Other common sites are the scalp and extensor of the limbs. The disease at first appears on the scalp where it may present as pityriasis amiantacea. An indolent pustular acrodermatitis, sometimes of only one digit, eventually proves to be psoriatic. More extensive chronic lesions of the hands and feet may occur with persistent dryness, hyperkeratosis, and fissuring. Chronic plaque psoriasis is the most common type seen in childhood psoriasis followed by guttate psoriasis. It presents as sudden appearance of showers of 2–3 mm scaly papules, mostly on the trunk. Pitting of the finger nails may be the only manifestation for months or even years. Follicular psoriasis occurs on the extensor prominences of elbows and knees, seen only in children. Napkin psoriasis and inverse psoriasis are the most common presentations in infants. Peculiarities of childhood psoriasis include pruritic, thinner, less erythematous, and less scaly plaques and association with comorbid conditions. Geographic tongue can precede the development of psoriasis in children.

Various types of psoriasis seen in childhood are described here.

Guttate Psoriasis (Figs. 9B and C)

It is also known as eruptive psoriasis and is derived from the Latin word *"gutt"* meaning a drop. This type of psoriasis is generally seen in children and adolescents. It is characterized by an eruption of small salmon pink-colored scaly plaques and papules ranging in size from 0.5 to 1.5 cm. Human leukocyte antigen (HLA)-Cw6 has been associated with guttate psoriasis and has a major role in determining the early and younger onset, positive family history, and extensive disease. Association of guttate

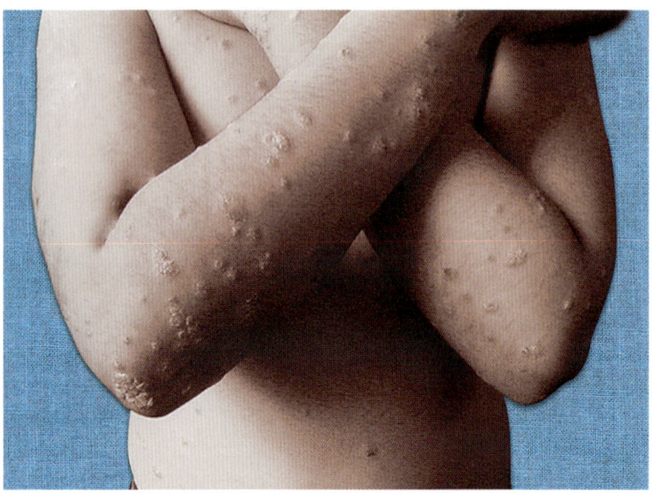

Fig. 1: Psoriasis vulgaris in a child.

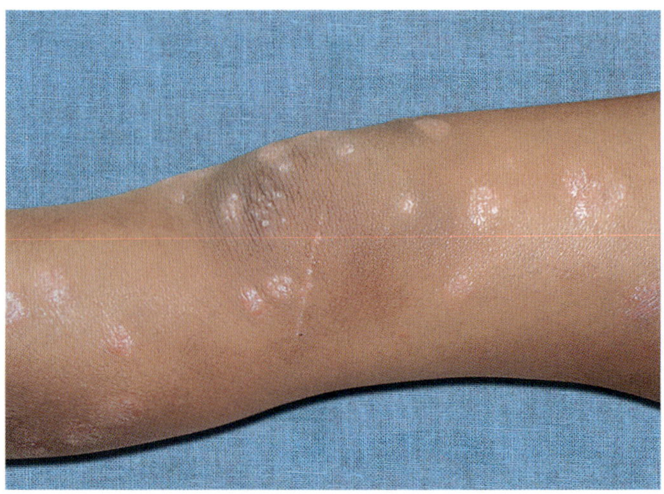

Fig. 2: Close-up view of lesions of psoriasis vulgaris, note Koebner phenomenon.

"The moment you doubt whether you can fly, you cease for ever to be able to do it." **—JM Barrie**

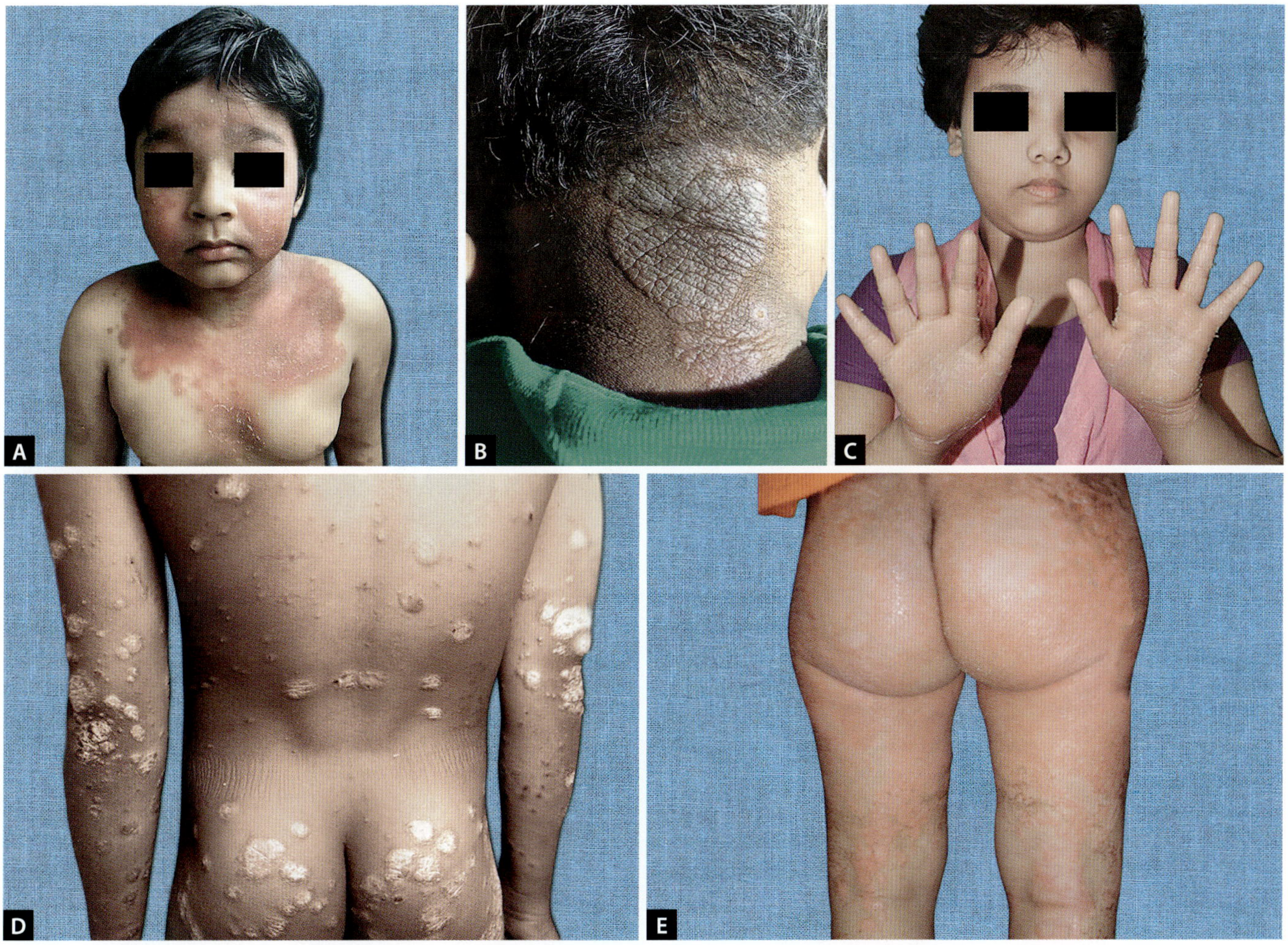

Figs. 3A to E: (A) Psoriasis over face and chest; (B) Psoriasis over nape of neck; (C) Palmar psoriasis; (D) Psoriasis vulgaris; (E) Psoriasis vulgaris in acute flare-up.

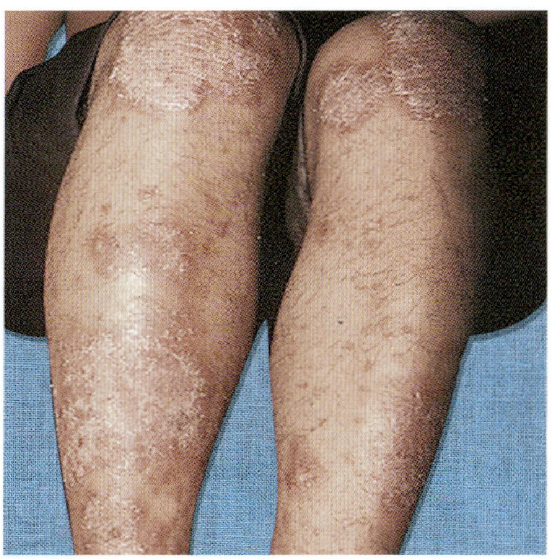

Fig. 4: Involvement of knee and shin in a 15-year-old boy with psoriasis.

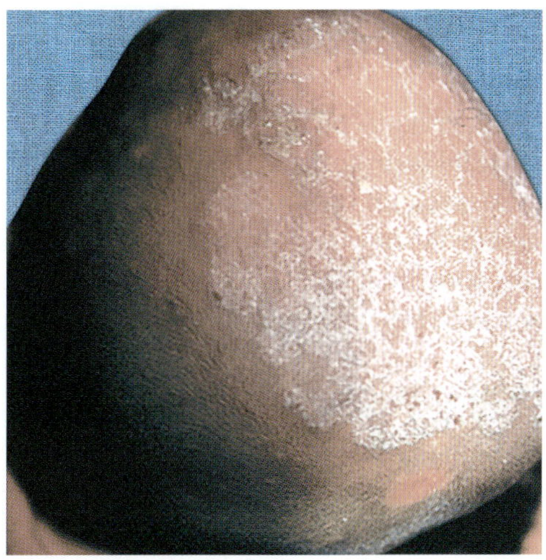

Fig. 5: Psoriasis over the scalp in a 2-year-old boy. The lesions spread following shaving of scalp done as a part of sacred ritual.

"Be so good they can't ignore you." —**Steve Martin**

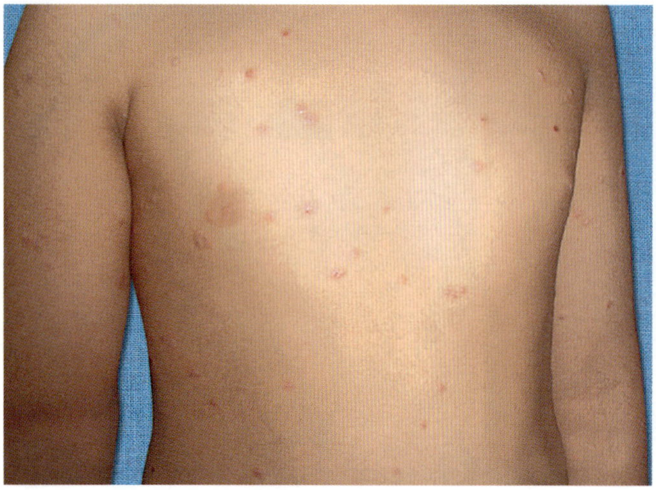

Fig. 6: Pinpoint to few millimeters sized scaly papules of guttate psoriasis.

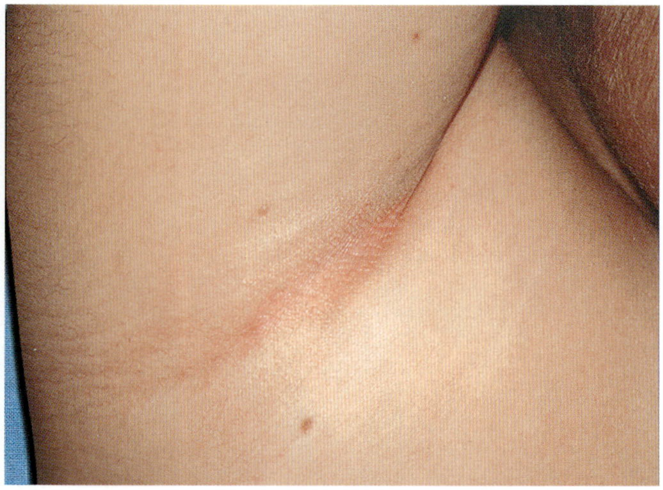

Fig. 7: Mild erythema and scaling in flexural psoriasis.

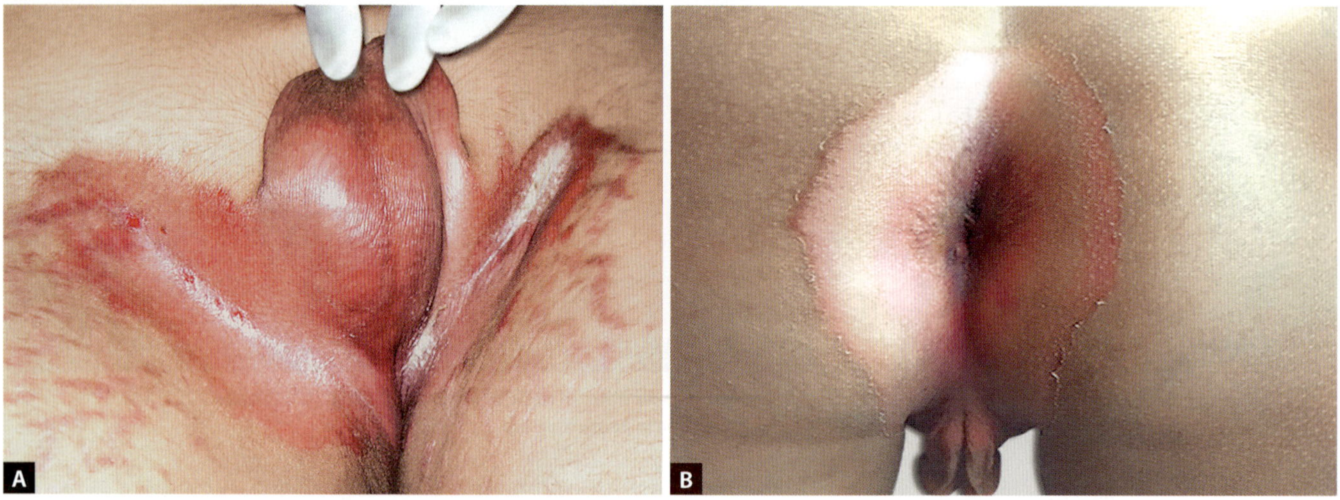

Figs. 8A and B: (A) Flexural psoriasis over inguinal region; (B) Flexural psoriasis.

psoriasis with group A β-hemolytic streptococci has been controversial till date. Laboratory parameters may show a raised antistreptolysin O (ASO) titer, increased anti-DNase B, or streptozyme activity. However, in spite of a definite association with infection, usage of antibiotics has not been shown to be beneficial or alter the course of the disease.

Diaper Psoriasis (Fig. 9D)

This condition, also known as napkin psoriasis, usually presents between the age of 3 and 6 months. True psoriasis does occur in infancy, generally appears in the napkin area as an isomorphic response in a genetically predisposed child with primary irritant napkin dermatitis. It first appears in the diaper area as a bright red, well-demarcated, glazed, rash that may be followed by widespread dissemination of small psoriasis-like lesions. This clinical variant can be differentiated from irritant diaper dermatitis by its unique presentation and poor response to conventional treatment for diaper dermatitis. Unlike other psoriasis, it is generally treatment responsive and disappears by the age of 1 year.

Scalp Psoriasis (Figs. 9E to G)

It presents with discrete, well-defined areas of scaly plaques on an erythematous base. The lesions may extend onto the periphery of the face forming the corona psoriatica, retroauricular area, and upper neck. The scales sometimes have an asbestos-like appearance and can

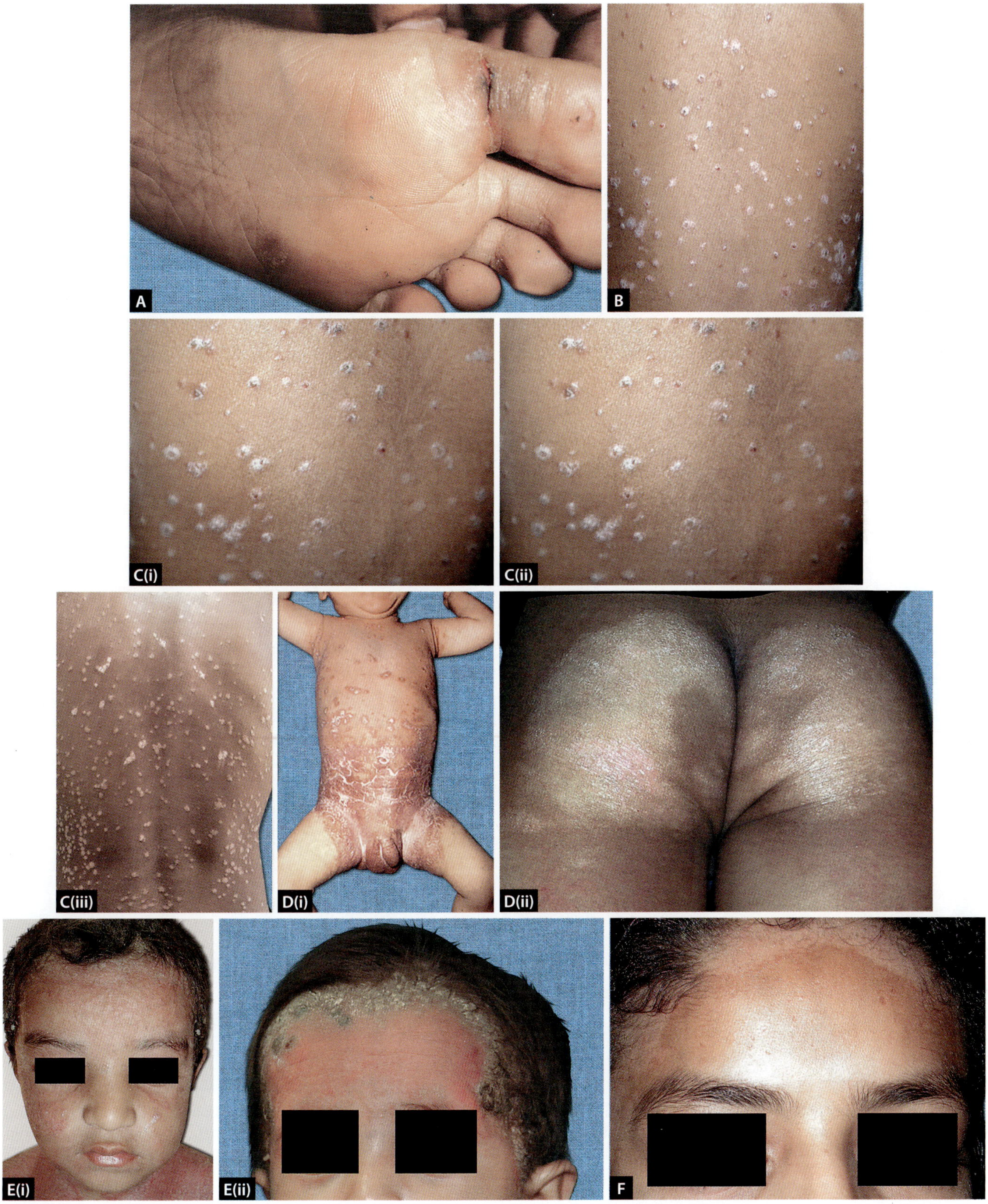

Figs. 9A to F: (A) Plantar psoriasis; (B) Guttate psoriasis; C(i) Same child, close-up view; C(ii) Guttate psoriasis in a 7-year-old boy; C(iii) Guttate psoriasis; D(i and ii) Napkin psoriasis; E(i) Severe psoriasis of scalp and face; E(ii) Scalp psoriasis with corona psoriatica; (F) Corona psoriatica.

"I'm not telling you it is going to be easy, I'm telling you it's going to be worth it." —**Art Williams**

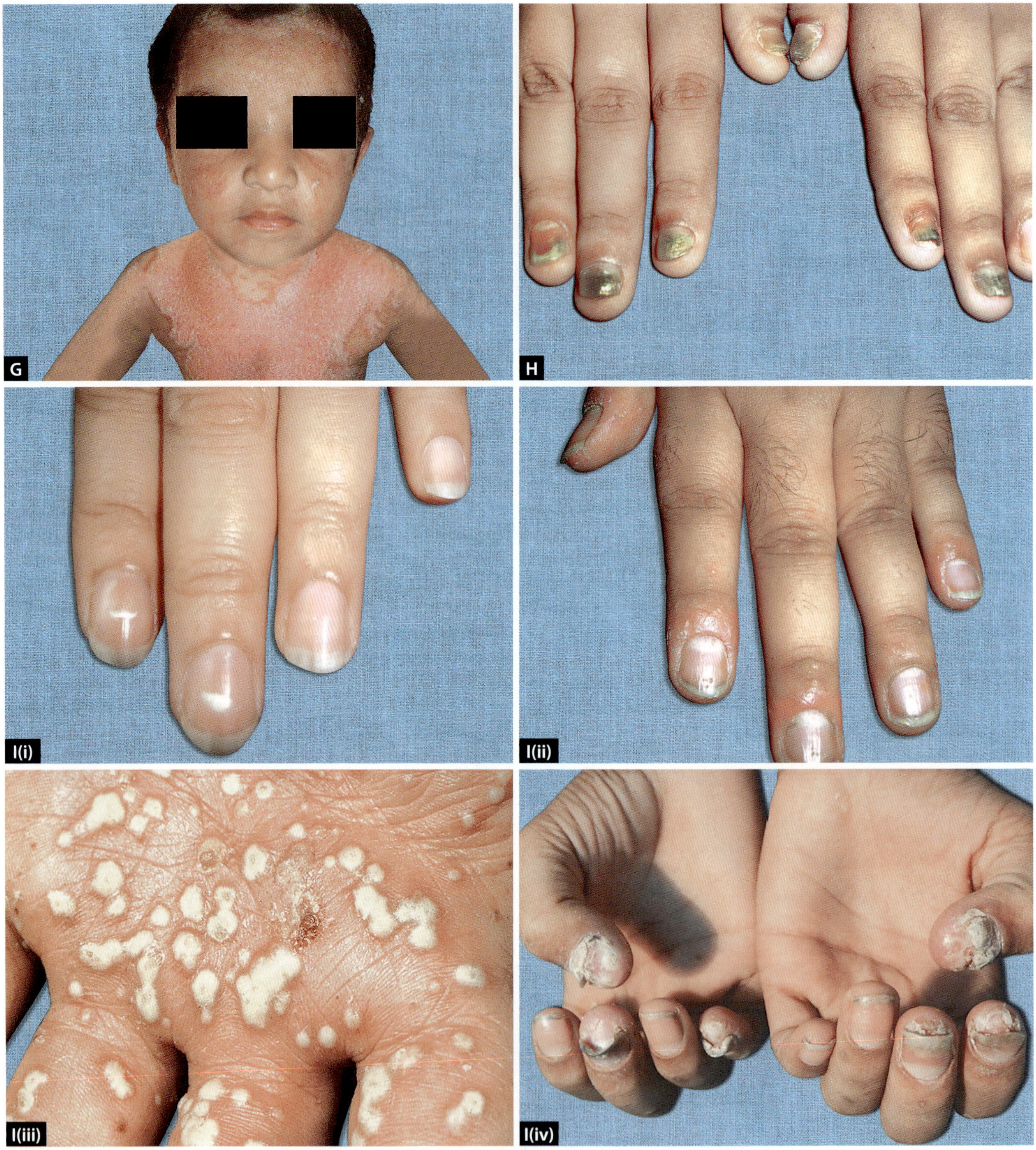

Figs. 9G to I(iv): (G) Extensive psoriasis in a 5-year-old boy; (H) Nail involvement in psoriasis, note onycholysis; I(i) Nail psoriasis presenting as leukonychia; I(ii) Acrodermatitis continua; I(iii) Acrodermatitis continua, note pustular lesions; I(iv) Acrodermatitis continua, note fingertip involvement and destruction of nails.

be attached for some distance to the scalp hair, the so called pityriasis amiantacea. This condition is not easily distinguished from seborrheic dermatitis and at times both may coexist giving rise to sebopsoriasis.

"For my part, I travel not to go anywhere, but to go. I travel for travel's sake. The great affair is to move." —**Robert Louis Stevenson**

Nail Psoriasis (Figs. 9H and I)

Nail psoriasis occurs in 7–40% of children with psoriasis, with a similar pattern of clinical presentation to that of adults and the severity increases with increase in age, duration of the disease, palmoplantar psoriasis and arthropathy. In 0.6–2.3% of the patients, nail changes appears to be the only sign of the disease, preceding other skin and articular involvement. Coarse nail pits involving the fingers and toes is the most common finding. Other alterations include onychodystrophy, leukonychia, red lunula, and crumbling of the nail plate. Oil spots and salmon patches are yellow red discolorations beneath the nail plate. Splinter hemorrhages may result from capillary bleed. Subungual hyperkeratosis may be noted on the distal end of the nail plate. Anonychia or total loss of nail may be seen in advanced disease. Nail psoriasis may affect individual nails of toes and fingers or may involve all the nails of fingers and toes giving rise to twenty-nail dystrophy.

Erythrodermic Psoriasis (Figs. 9J to M)

It represents the generalized form of the disease that affects the entire body. Erythema is the most constant feature with superficial scaling of >90% of the body surface area. Erythroderma may be precipitated by the use of certain drugs, topical application of irritant medications, infections, pustular psoriasis, or withdrawal of systemic steroids. The skin barrier is impaired and hereby the protective functions of the skin are altered giving rise to a state of skin failure. The patient shows signs of impaired thermal regulation, fluid electrolyte imbalance, hypoproteinemia due to excessive loss of proteins in the form of scales, high output cardiac failure, aspiration pneumonitis, and increased

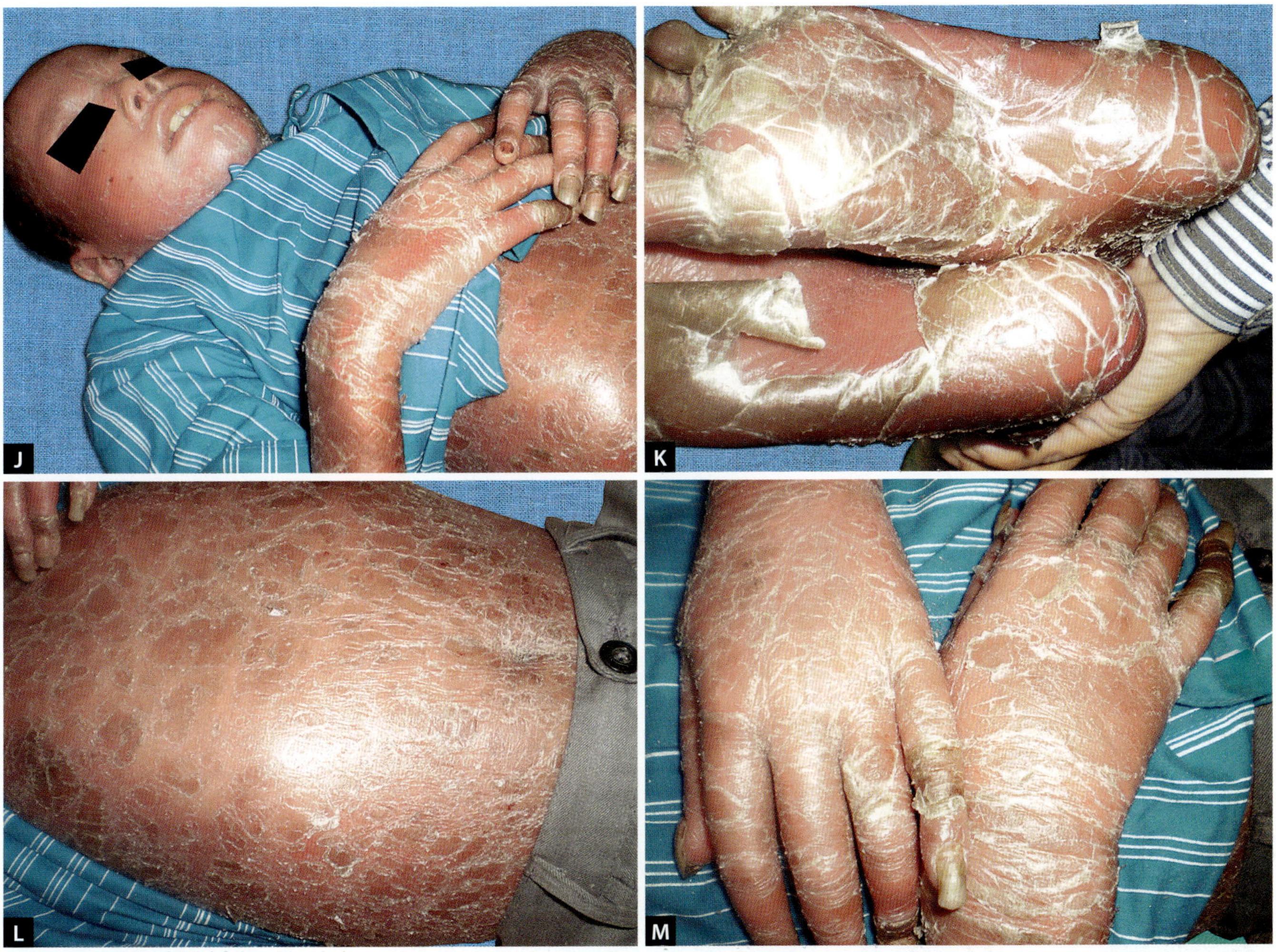

Figs. 9J to M: (J) Psoriatic erythroderma; (K) Thick scales of psoriasis over soles; (L) Close-up view of erythroderma; (M) Erythroderma involving hands.

"The only impossible journey is the one you never begin." —**Tony Robbins**

susceptibility to infections. As a compensatory mechanism for heat loss, there is a rise in basal metabolic rate (BMR) giving rise to a catabolic state. Peripheral edema results due to hypoproteinemia, inflammation, and associated cardiac failure. Generalized or localized lymphadenopathy may occur, known as dermatopathic lymphadenopathy, as a result of the immunological response.

Drug-induced Psoriasis

The etiology of psoriasis is multifactorial and the importance of medications causing either eruption or aggravation of psoriasis must be acknowledged.

Drugs responsible for the induction of psoriasis are as follows:

- Acetazolamide
- Aminoglutethimide
- Amiodarone
- Amoxicillin
- Ampicillin
- Aspirin
- Atenolol
- Chloroquine
- Cimetidine
- Corticosteroids
- Cyclosporine
- Diclofenac
- Diltiazem
- Hydroxychloroquine
- Indomethacin
- Lithium
- Methicillin
- Penicillins
- Potassium iodide
- Propranolol
- Terbinafine

The drugs may cause *de novo* psoriasis or may be responsible for exacerbation of psoriasis. It is clinically indistinguishable from psoriasis vulgaris. Drug-induced psoriasis can manifest as plaque, pustular, or erythrodermic type.

Infantile and Juvenile Pustular Psoriasis (Figs. 10 to 12F)

The term pustular psoriasis refers to those forms of psoriasis in which macroscopic pustules appear. There are two main forms, localized and generalized. In the localized forms, the disease is confined to the hands and feet and tends to be

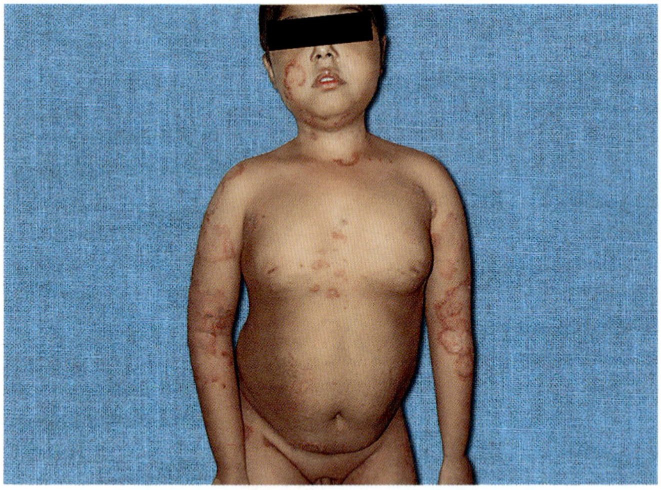

Fig. 10: Annular erythematous plaques with pustules at the periphery.

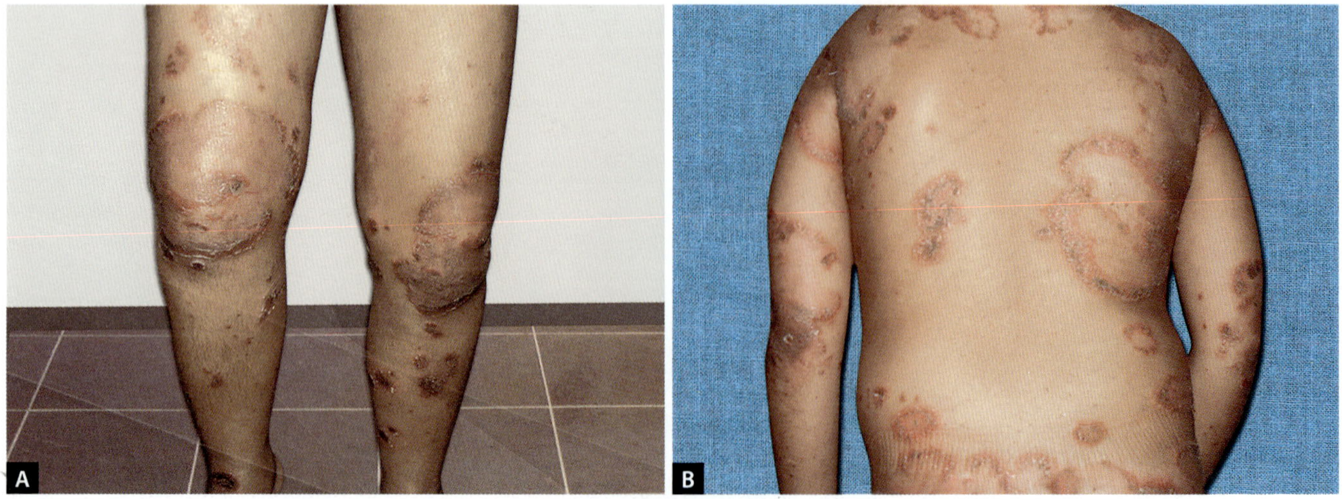

Figs. 11A and B: (A) Generalized pustular psoriasis over thighs and legs; (B) Same child, close-up view of back lesions.

"I have found out that there ain't no surer way to find out whether you like people or hate them than to travel with them." —**Mark Twain**

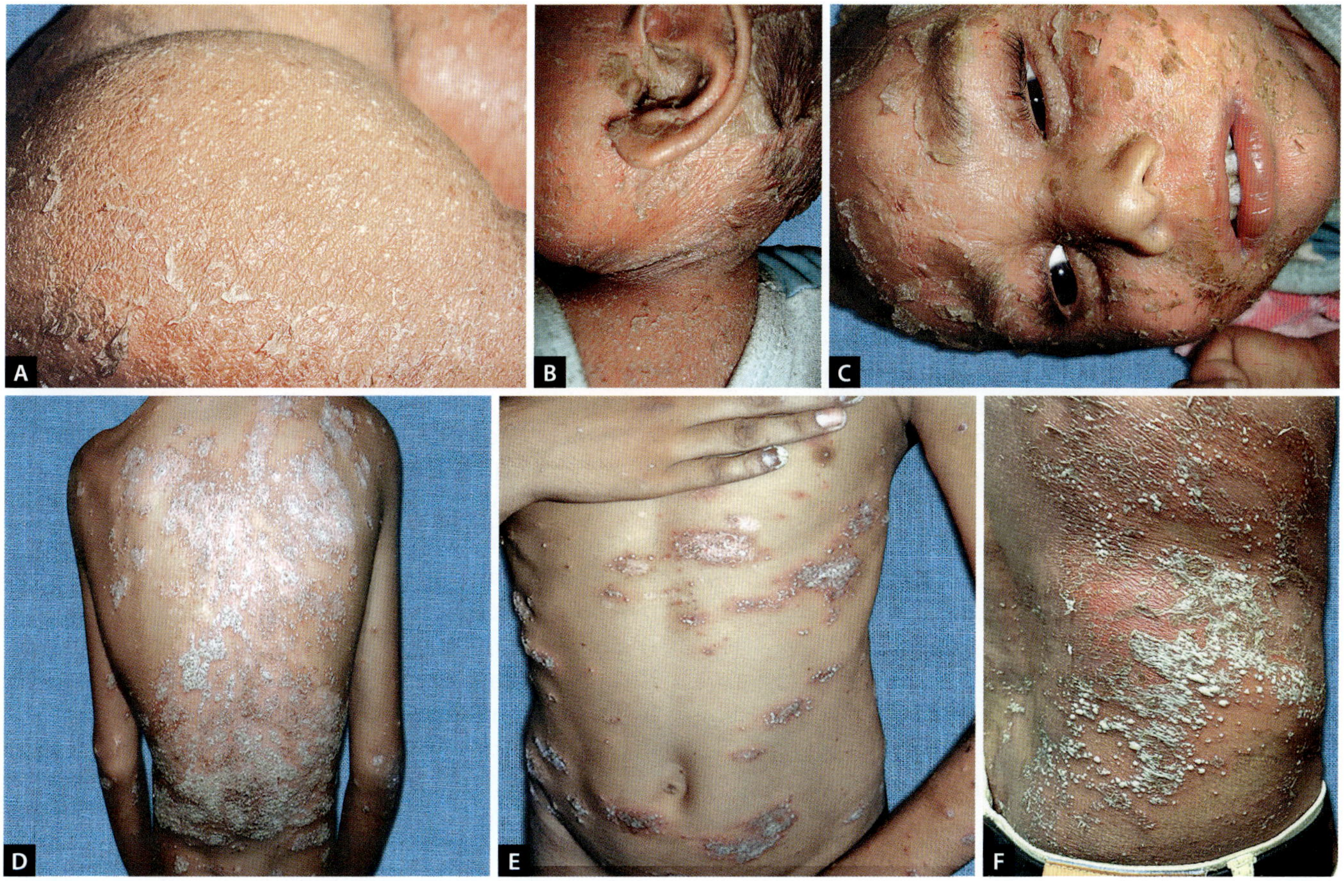

Figs. 12A to F: Close-up view of pustular psoriasis lesions. (A) Generalized pustular psoriasis in a 5-year-old boy; (B) Same child, erythrodermic lesions over nape of neck and upper back; (C) Same child, face lesions; (D) Psoriasis with pustules over back; (E) Same boy, lesions over chest and abdomen; (F) Severe generalized pustular psoriasis.

chronic. In the generalized form, the whole body may be involved and the course is subacute, acute or fulminating, and life-threatening. All forms of pustular psoriasis are rare in childhood. Infantile cases are often benign. Systemic symptoms are often absent and spontaneous remissions occur. The age of onset in majority of the children is 2–10 years. The disease may be Zumbusch pattern, but annular and circinate forms can also be seen. In Zumbusch pattern of psoriasis, lesions start abruptly in a background of erythema along with systemic symptom of toxicity and later becomes generalized. Attacks often settle within a few days but repeated waves of inflammation may follow. In older children, the disease resembles that in adults.

Treatment modalities of psoriasis are divided into two categories: (1) Topical and (2) Systemic.

Topical Treatment

Various topical modalities are topical emollient, corticosteroids, coal tar, dithranol, calcipotriol, tazarotene, etc. Topical coal tar in combination with salicylic acid forms the age old treatment modality for psoriasis. It is an effective modality for lesions over body, palms, and soles. It is kept over these areas for 8–10 hours and then washed off, once daily for 3–6 months. It is also used as shampoo for scalp lesions for about 6 months. It is, however, cosmetically not acceptable as it is messy, has an unpleasant smell, and causes discoloration of skin and scalp.

Anthralin is an effective antipsoriatic substance mostly used for resistant plaque psoriasis, hyperkeratotic psoriasis, plantar psoriasis, etc. It is not recommended over intertriginous areas, face, head, neck, and genitalia. It also stains skin, clothing, and bed linens irreversibly. Short-contact dithranol therapy (SCDT) is an effective but less irritant modality. The ointment is to be kept for 20–30 minutes, and then washed off once every day. The regimen is continued for few months till the clearance of psoriasis lesions.

Topical corticosteroids are often prescribed for psoriatic lesions over trunk, extremities, scalp, flexures, palms, and soles. Clobetasone, fluticasone, hydrocortisone, mometasone, etc., are usually chosen for their less atrophogenic potential. Topical calcipotriol (vitamin D_3 analog), calcitriol, and tazarotene can also be used for psoriasis in children, but their efficacy has not yet been proved beyond doubt.

Systemic Therapy

Phototherapy (PUVA) is given along with trimethylpsoralen or 8-methoxypsoralen. It is, however, not recommended below 8 years (according to some 12 years) of age because of the chance of development of premature cataract (in mice, not documented in human beings). After intake of psoralens, serum level peaks at 2 hours when ultraviolet-A exposure is given either from ultraviolet chamber or by exposure to sunlight. It is given at a dose of 0.6 mg/kg of body weight preferably with breakfast. After 2 hours, the affected parts are exposed to sunlight for 10–15 minutes initially. The duration of exposure is gradually escalated weekly. The regimen is repeated twice a week (not consecutive days) till the clearance of lesions. Nausea, vomiting, and phototoxic reactions are some of the early adverse effects, although not very common. Long-term side effects can cause hepatotoxicity. Hence, pretreatment liver function test is to be carried out in every patient. Narrow band UVB (NBUVB) remains the safest method in children in management of generalized psoriasis due to its relatively less side-effect profile and nonrequirement for post-treatment sun and eye protection. It is started at 70–75% of the minimal erythema dose and increased by about 10–20% with each treatment.

Methotrexate (MTx) may be given in extensive and severe psoriasis at a dose of 0.2–0.4 mg/kg divided into three doses given at 12 hours interval once every week. The author has good experience of treating psoriasis in children with MTx. The drug is usually tolerated well in children. Before starting MTx, complete blood count (CBC), liver function test (LFT), renal function test (RFT), and a baseline chest X-ray are to be carried out. In cases of accidental ingestion of MTx in large amounts, leucovorin (folinic acid) rescue is done at a dose of 20–200 mg 6th hourly depending upon serum MTx levels. Reduction of doses of MTx is needed with concomitant use of nonsteroidal anti-inflammatory drugs (NSAIDs), ampicillin, cephalosporins, and allopurinol. Maintenance with narrow band ultraviolet B (UVB) therapy has been useful.

Oral retinoids (Acitretin: 0.5–1 mg/kg/day) and cyclosporine (3–6 mg/kg/day) have shown good results in pediatric psoriasis. Acitretin is the treatment of choice in pustular psoriasis. Systemic steroids have very limited role in the treatment of childhood psoriasis. Both psoriatic arthritis and nail involvement in psoriasis are fairly uncommon and do not pose much problem in pediatric age group.

Extracutaneous Involvement in Psoriasis (Figs. 12G to J)

Psoriasis is predominantly a cutaneous condition but mucosal involvement may be seen in generalized pustular psoriasis (GPP). Psoriatic arthropathy affects the spine and the interphalangeal joints giving rise to arthralgia and deformities in advanced stages. Patients with psoriasis are at an increased risk of metabolic syndrome characterized by hypertension, dyslipidemia, diabetes mellitus, and obesity. There is increased incidence of anterior uveitis with psoriasis and psoriatic arthritis. This condition is also emotionally disabling as it is associated with significant psychosocial comorbidities arising from the appearance, social rejection, guilt, isolation, and embarrassment. Risk of myocardial infarction is elevated. Lymph node involvement in cases of erythrodermic psoriasis in the form of dermatopathic lymphadenopathy can occur. Pediatric psoriasis has also been associated with rheumatoid arthritis and Crohn's disease.

LICHEN PLANUS (FIGS. 13 TO 16J)

Lichen planus (LP) is characterized by shiny, flat papules, which individually vary in size from pinpoint to a centimeter or more and may be closely aggregated or widely dispersed. On the surface, there may be white lines known as Wickham's striae. The overall color is violaceous. In most cases, the papules flatten after a few months but are often replaced by an area of pigmentation that retains the shape of the papules and persists for months or years. New papules may form while others are clearing. LP can affect any part of the body but certain sites are more commonly affected, e.g., front of the wrists, lumbar region, and around the ankles. Vesicles and bullae in LP may occasionally occur and create diagnostic confusion. Itching is fairly common in LP. Burning and stinging are least common complaints. Oral and nail LP is less commonly seen in children.

Association

Lichen planus may be associated with vitiligo and alopecia areata or there may be a family history of these diseases or family history of autoimmune disorders such as diabetes mellitus, hypertension, thyroid disease, and ulcerative colitis.

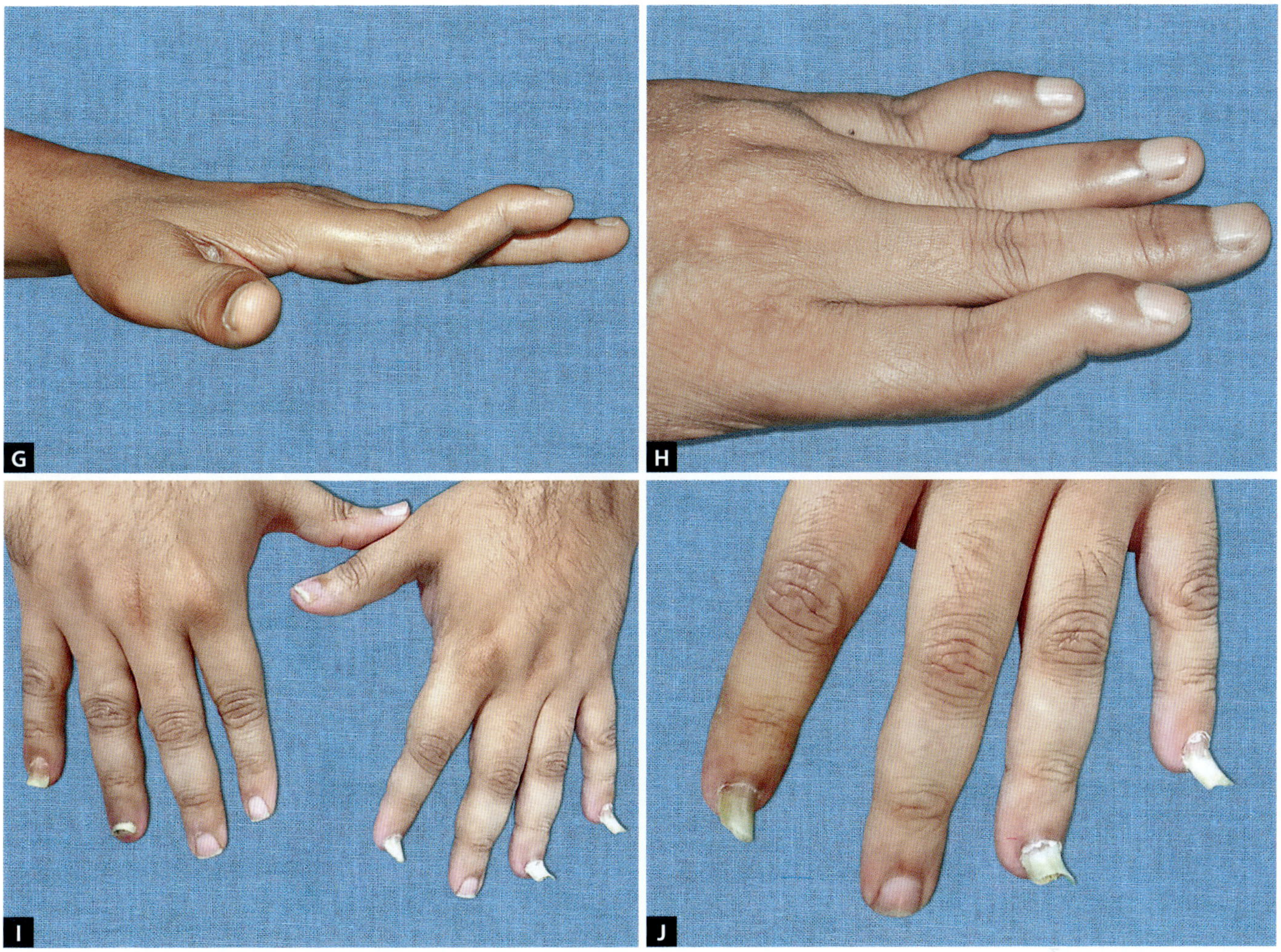

Figs. 12G to J: (G) Psoriatic arthritis, note deformity of finger; (H) Close-up view of swan neck deformity; (I) Psoriatic arthritis with nail dystrophy; (J) Same patient, close-up view.

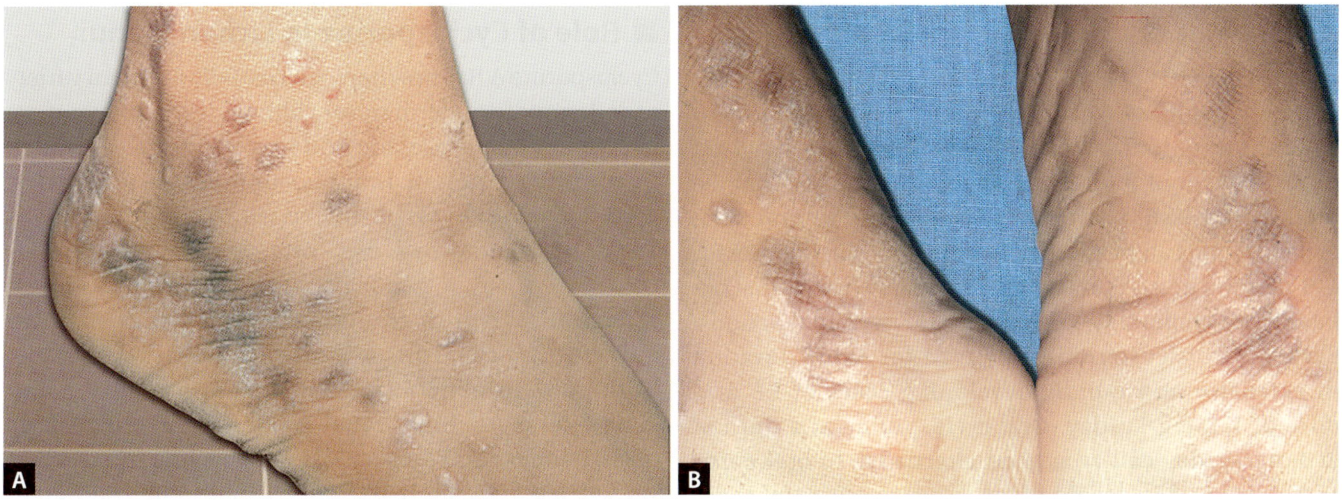

Figs. 13A and B: (A) Flat-topped violaceous papules and plaques of LP over foot; (B) Close-up view of flat-topped papules of LP.

"Everything I was I carry with me, everything I will be lies waiting on the road ahead." —**Ma Jian**

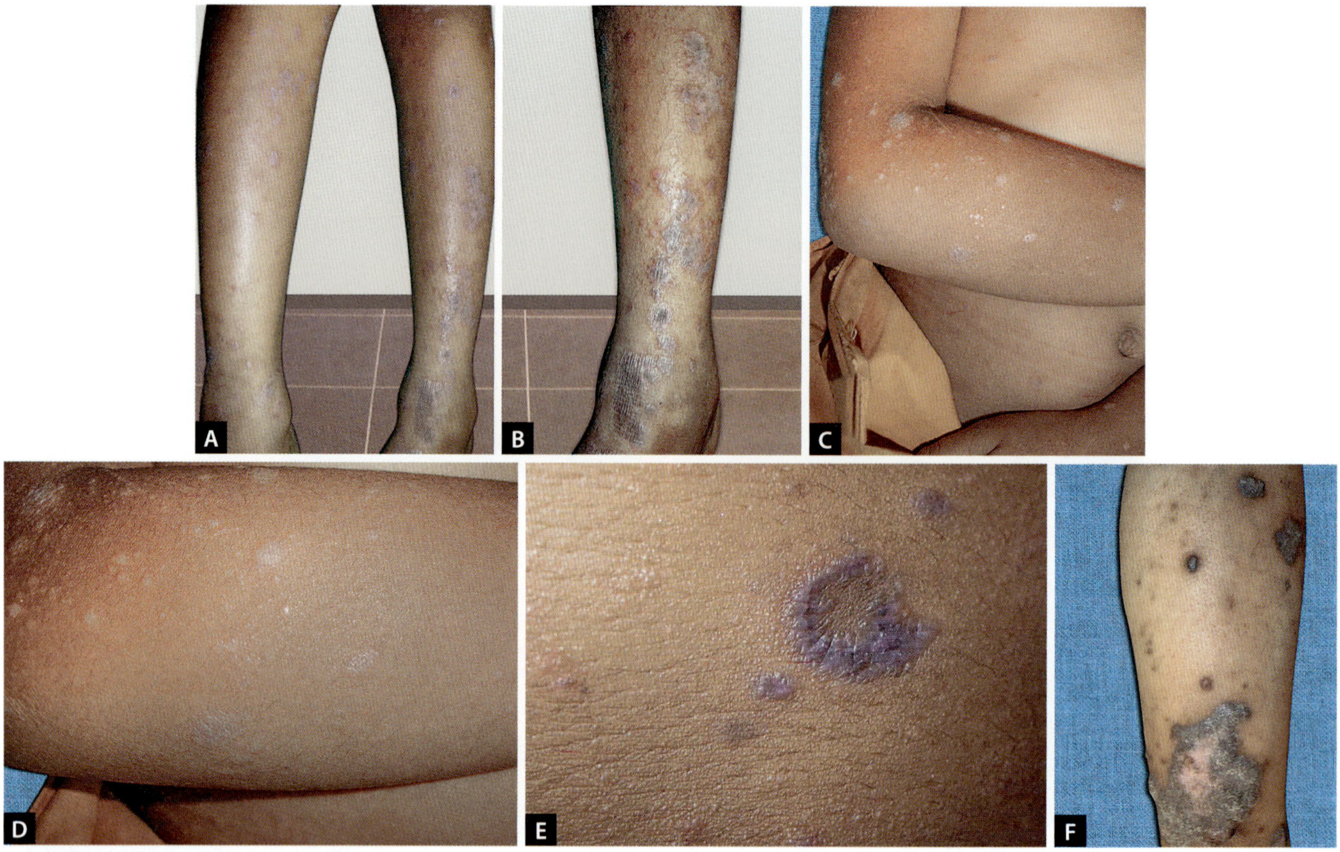

Figs. 14A to F: Classical lesions of lichen planus (LP), note bilateral symmetrical distribution. (A) Eruptive LP over legs; (B) Close-up view; (C) Classical violaceous papules of LP; (D) Close-up view of LP lesions; (E) Flat-topped violaceous papules of LP; (F) Hypertrophic lesions of LP over legs.

Natural History

In majority of the cases of LP, the lesions tend to resolve spontaneously over a period of 9–12 months. Lichen planopilaris and hypertrophic LP tend to persist for years together. Fortunately, such cases are rare in children.

Treatment

For majority of cases of childhood LP, moderately potent topical steroids are quite useful. They may be used for 3 weeks to 3 months. Mild topical steroids may be required for lesions over the face, flexures, or genitalia. Oral dapsone can be given at a dose of 1–2 mg/kg/day for 1–3 months in cases of extensive LP; however, it has not been used commonly in children due to drug reactions. Systemic corticosteroids are given for short duration in extensive and rapidly developing cases of LP at a dose of 1–2 mg/kg/day. Oral cyclosporine at a dose of 2–3 mg/kg/day can be a good alternative to oral corticosteroids and is devoid of any adverse effects of long-term use of corticosteroid, viz., growth retardation and suppression of hypothalamic-pituitary-adrenal (HPA) axis, etc. However, it is costly and may cause hypertrichosis in older children and adolescents. The hypertrichosis induced by cyclosporine is usually reversible.

Role of Cyclosporine in Lichen Planus

Cyclosporine A has now been successfully used in a variety of inflammatory dermatoses, although the mechanism of action remains obscure and may not be solely related to the drug's potent immunosuppressive properties. LP is a disease that is characterized by a predominantly T-cell inflammatory infiltrate. Cyclosporine A is postulated to act via its selective inhibition of T-lymphocyte proliferation or by some other as yet unknown mechanism. It has been used as a first line of therapy in generalized LP in children. The major side effects include renal dysfunction, electrolyte disturbances, and hypertension. The mucocutaneous side effects include hypertrichosis and gingival hyperplasia. It is given at dose of 3 mg/kg/day for 4–6 weeks

"Once you have traveled, the voyage never ends, but is played out over and over again in the quietest chambers. The mind can never break off from the journey."
—Pat Conroy

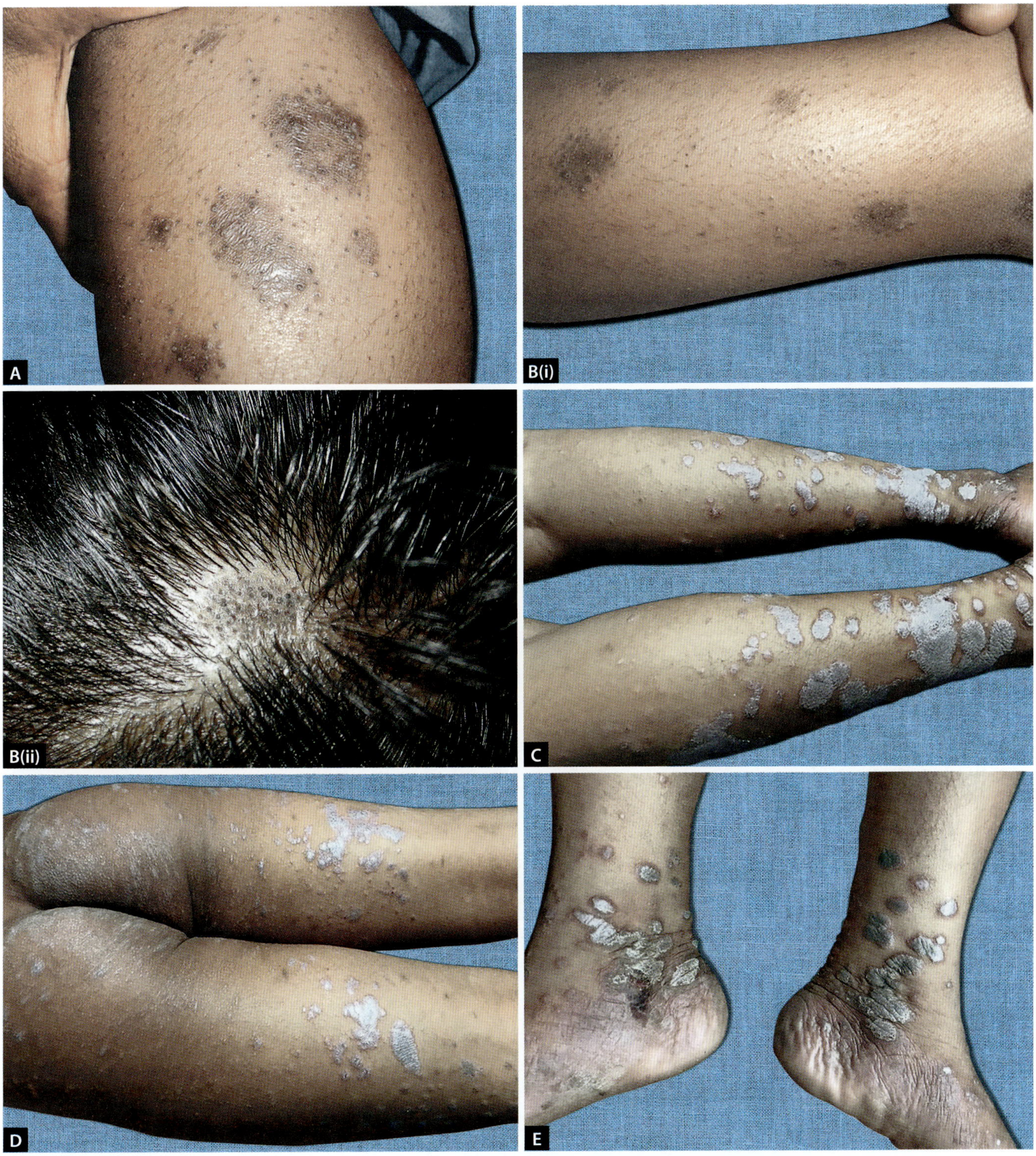

Figs. 15A to E: (A) Lichen planus (LP) lesions, note follicular lesions; B(i) Follicular lesions of LP; B(ii) Follicular LP over scalp; (C) Classical lesions in acute eruptive LP; (D) Same child, lesions over buttock and back of thighs; (E) Same child, lesions around ankle.

followed by maintenance with narrow band UVB therapy. One advantage of starting cyclosporine is early resolution of postinflammatory hyperpigmentation.

Role of Oral Retinoids in Lichen Planus

Systemic retinoids are able to affect pathways involved in cellular differentiation, apoptosis, inflammation, and sebaceous glandular activity. In children, the use of systemic retinoids for LP depends more on the severity of disease rather than the age and weight of the patient. Most patients are seen to respond in about 4 weeks.

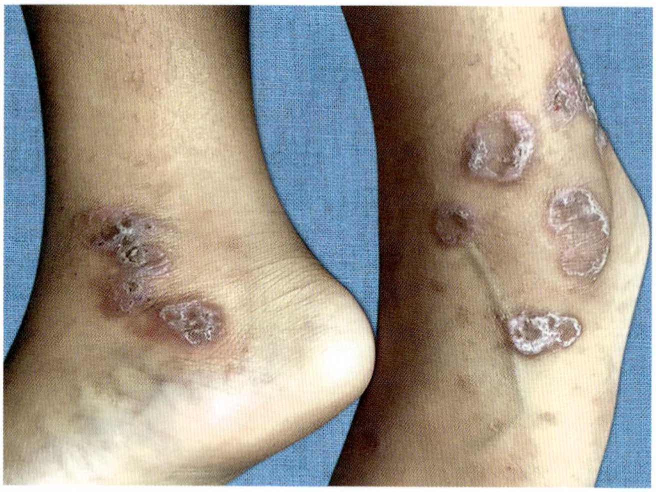

Fig. 15F: Hypertrophic LP, uncommon in pediatric age group.

Retinoids may be combined with systemic steroids in case of extensive disease, hypertrophic lesions, or oral erosive LP. Few reports have also mentioned the absolute necessity to combine retinoids with oral steroids for the control of severe disease. It is given at a dose of 0.5–1 mg/kg/day. The most common side effects include retinoid dermatitis, telogen effluvium, onycholysis, keratoconjunctivitis, cheilitis, and epistaxis. Effects on other system include deranged lipid profile, diffuse skeletal hyperostosis, and premature closing of epiphysis in the bone, transaminitis, pseudotumor cerebri, and depression.

LICHEN NITIDUS (FIGS. 17 AND 18)

This condition is clinically characterized by minute papules pinpoint to pinhead-sized and have a flat or dome-shaped shiny surface. They usually remain discrete, although they may be closely grouped. Sites of predilection are the forearms, penis, abdomen, chest,

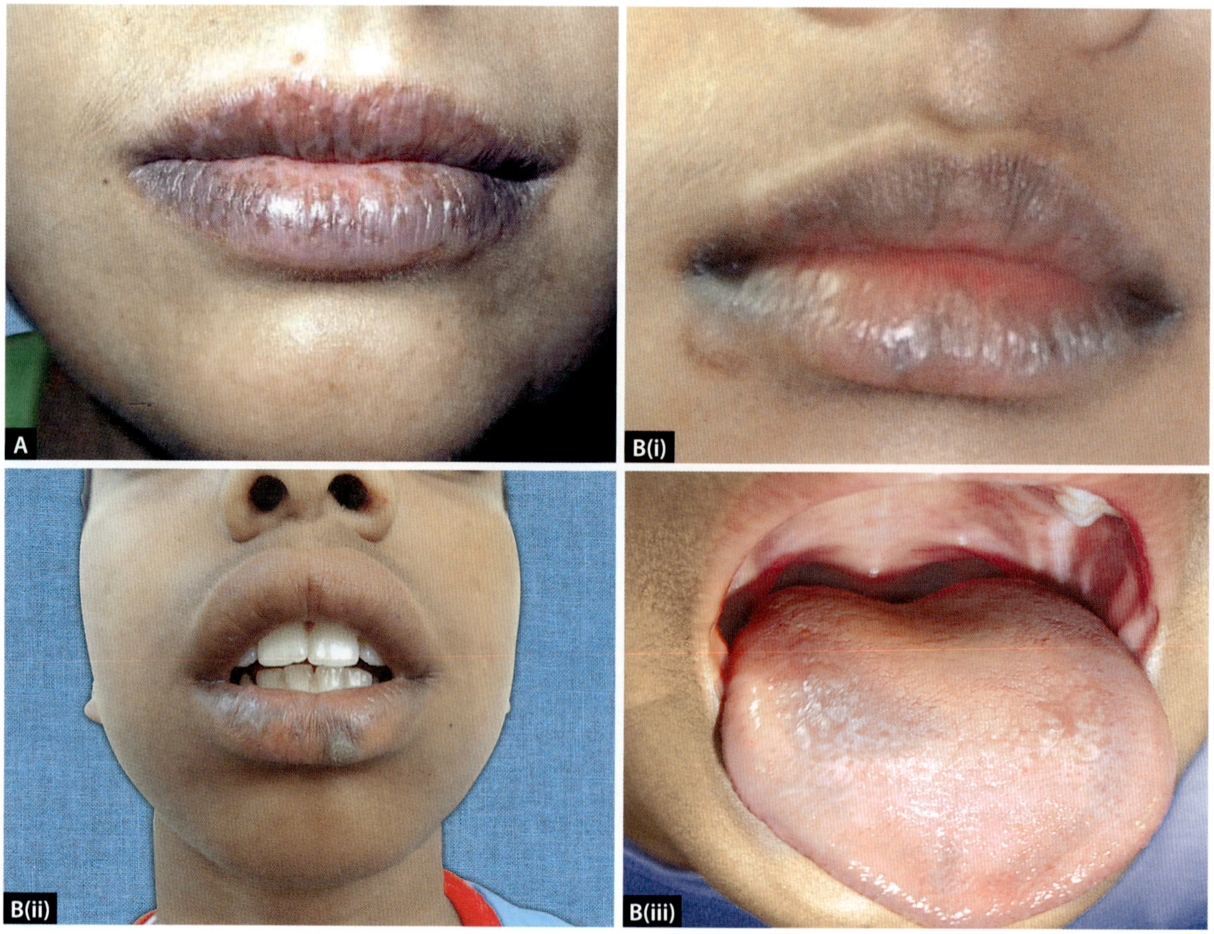

Figs. 16A to B(iii): Lichen planus (LP) over lips. (A) LP over lips; B(i to iii) LP affecting the lips and tongue.

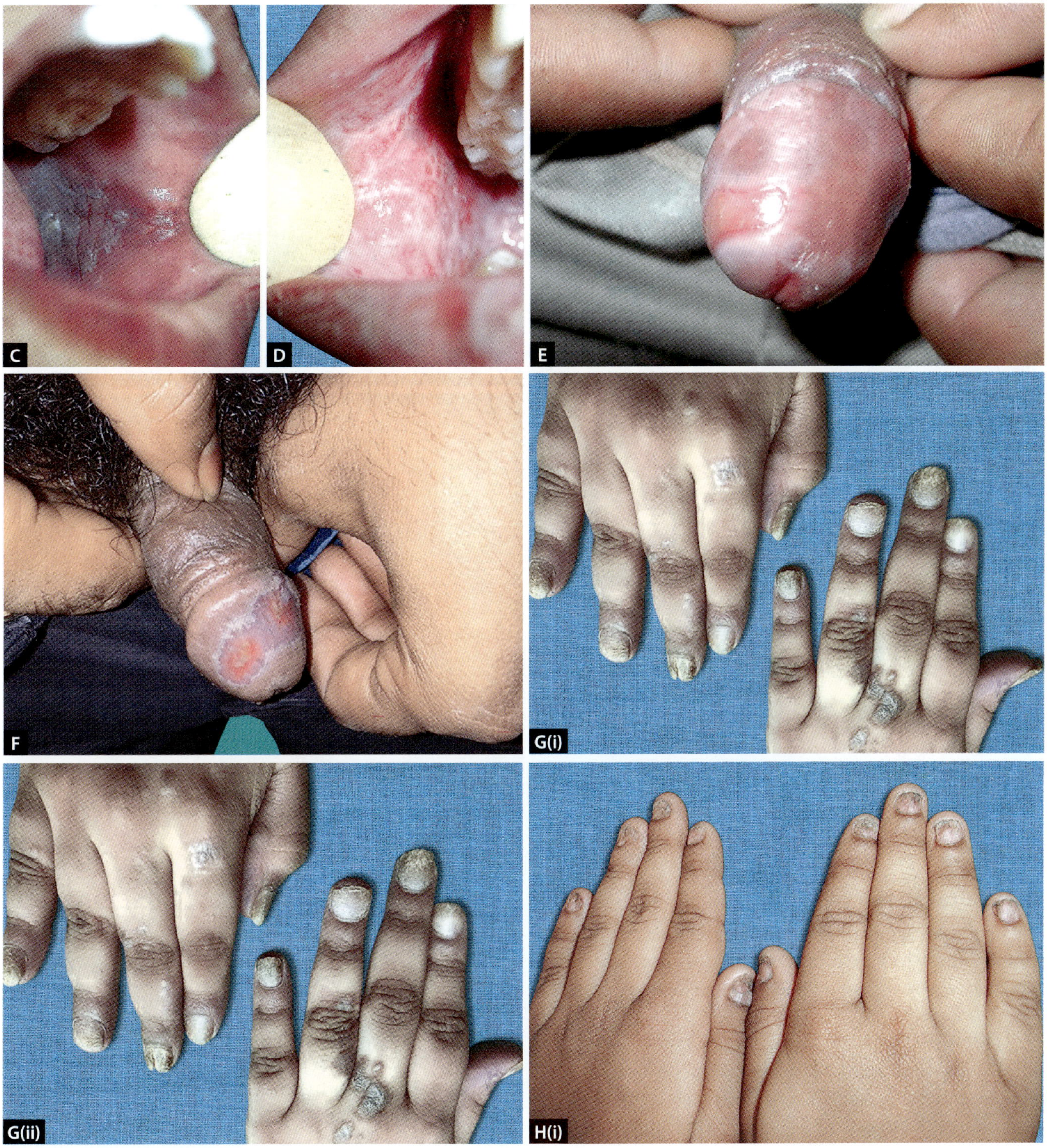

Figs. 16C to H(i): (C) Lichen planus (LP) of oral mucosa, note violaceous color; (D) Classical white lacy pattern of oral LP; (E) LP of glans and prepuce in a 17-year-old boy; (F) LP over glans penis; G(i) LP lesions with nail dystrophy; G(ii) Same patient, close-up view; H(i) Nail involvement in LP.

and buttocks. Generalized lichen nitidus is not uncommon in children. Coexistence with LP is quite common. Lichen nitidus must be distinguished from lesions of lichen scrofulosorum where there are grouped follicular papules in small patches on the trunk, and from keratosis pilaris where there are horny follicular papules mainly on the extensor surface of the limbs.

"Mankind's greatest achievements have come about by talking and its greatest failures by not talking. It doesn't have to be like this. Our greatest hopes could become reality in the future. With the technology at our disposal, the possibilities are unbounded. All we need to do is make sure we keep talking." —**Stephen Hawking**

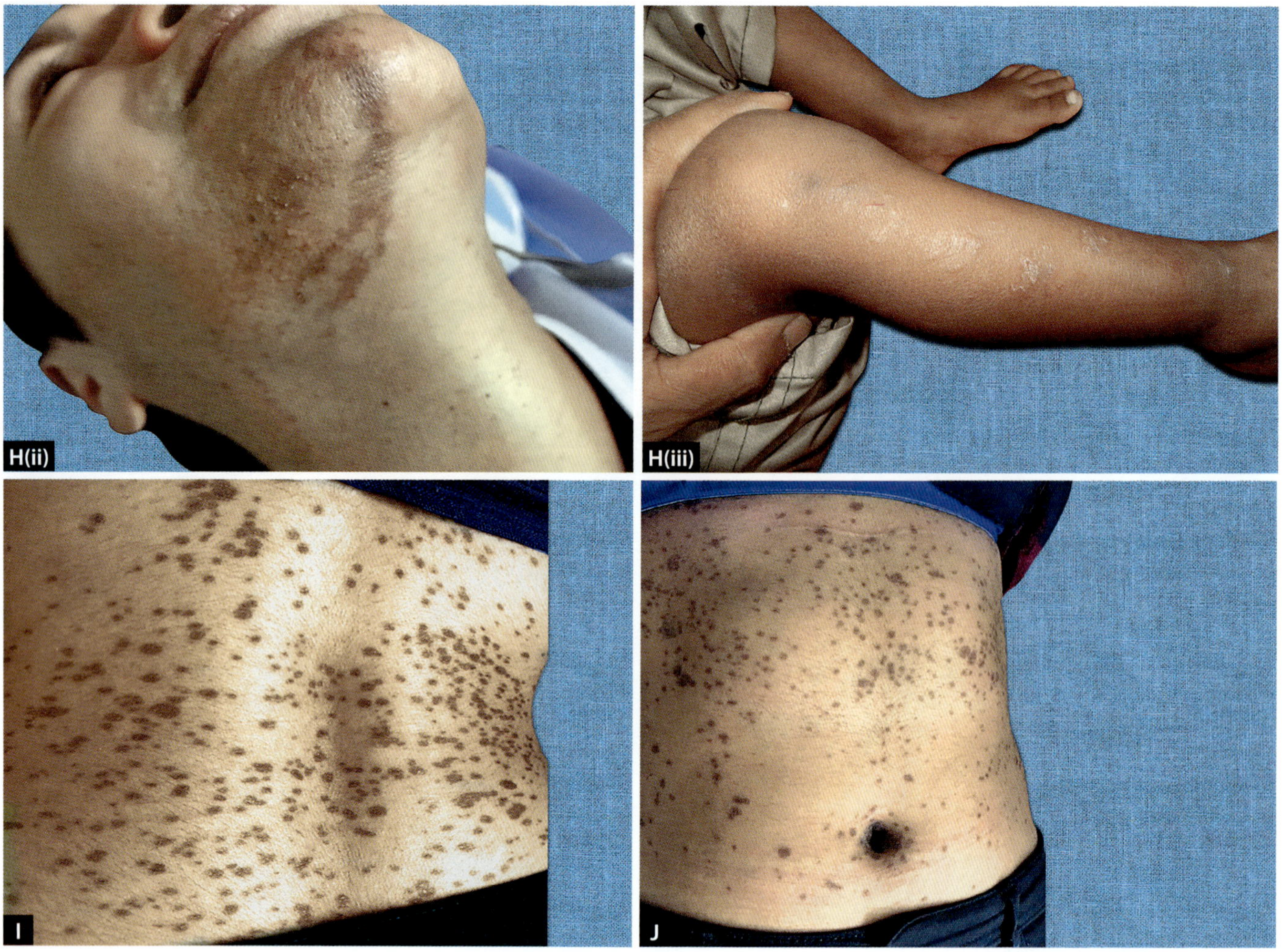

Figs. 16H(ii) to J: H(ii) Linear LP in an 18-year-old girl; H(iii) LP linearis in a 4-year-old boy; (I) Eruptive LP with postinflammatory hyperpigmentation; (J) Another view of postinflammatory hyperpigmentation (PIH) in eruptive LP.

Natural History

The condition is mostly self-limiting and tends to subside spontaneously by 6 months to 1 year. However sometimes lesions may remain unresolved for years together.

Treatment

Emollients and mild to moderately potent topical corticosteroids are useful in most of the cases. Itching is an exception rather than the rule (c.f. LP). Oral antihistamines are not required in majority of the cases. Recent treatment modalities that have shown good results for generalized lichen nitidus include narrow band UVB therapy, cyclosporine, and oral retinoids.

LICHEN PLANUS ACTINICUS (FIGS. 19A TO D)

Actinic lichen planus (ALP) is a rare photosensitive variant of LP affecting primarily the sun-exposed areas of the face, hands, and forearm of children and young adults. It typically occurs during spring and summer in dark skin-type (mainly phototype IV) in the tropics and subtropics. It has been reported with a variety of different names such as LP subtropicus, LP tropicus, summer time actinic lichenoid eruption, lichenoid melanodermatitis, and LP actinicus. Children aged 10–19 years constitute 83% cases of pediatric actinic LP, while 17% of the cases occur in those aged <10 years. There are four morphologic patterns

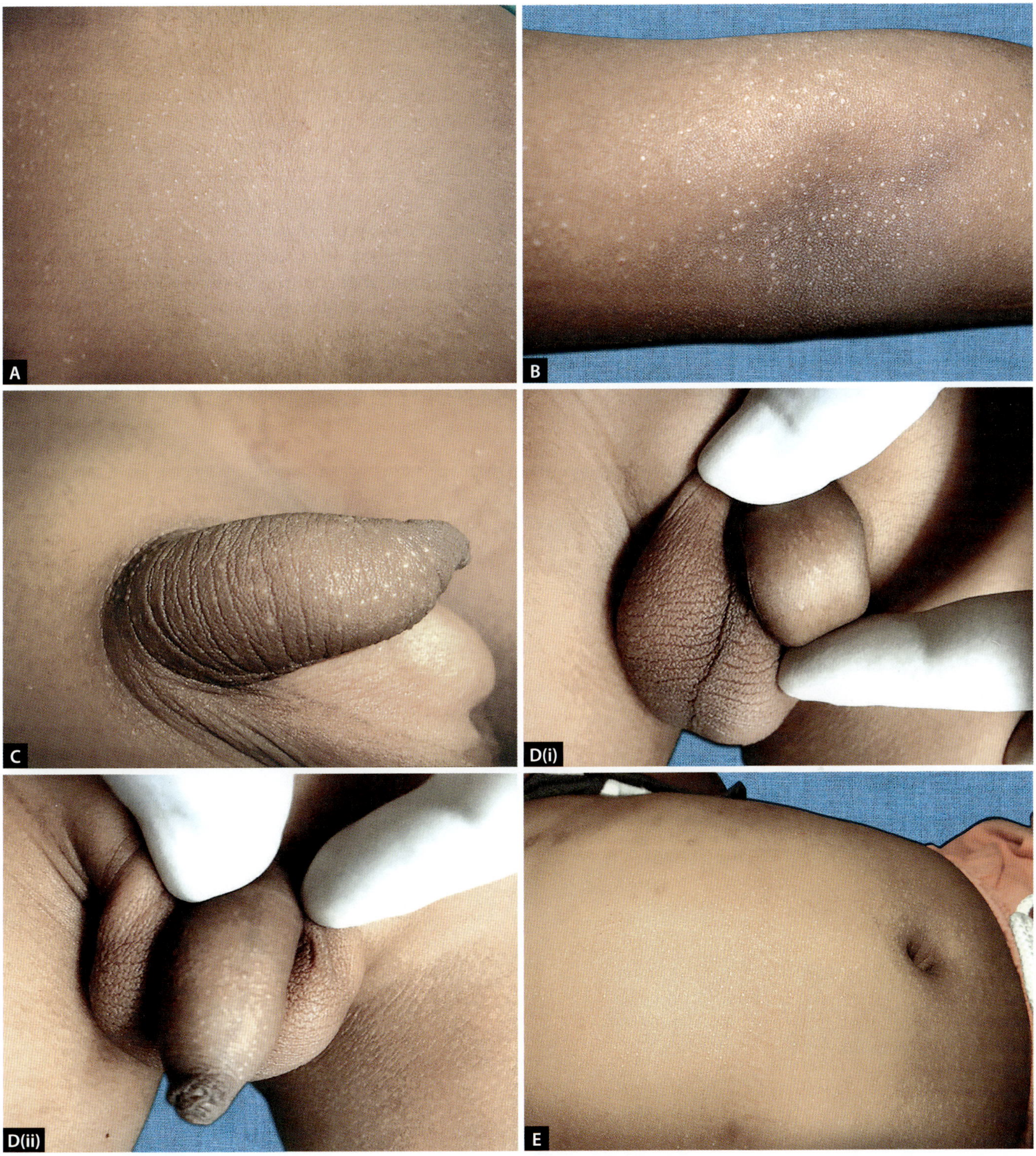

Figs. 17A to E: (A) Lichen nitidus over back, note Koebner phenomenon; (B) Lichen nitidus over elbow; (C) Lichen nitidus lesions over penile skin; D(i) Lichen nitidus lesions over penile skin, a very common site in boys; D(ii) Same child, another view; (E) Generalized lichen nitidus in a 3-year-old boy.

"It is not the destination where you end up but the mishaps and memories you create along the way." —**Penelope Riley**

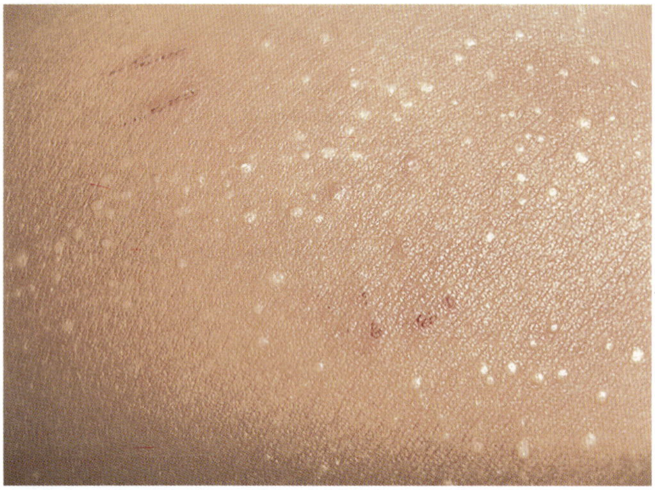

Fig. 18: Close-up view of lichen nitidus lesions.

of ALP, namely annular, dyschromic, classic plaque-type, and pigmented forms.

Annular type, which is the most common form, consists of erythematous to brownish annular atrophic plaques mostly over the face, surrounded by a hypopigmented halo. Mucosal involvement, pruritus, and koebnerization are usually absent in this variant, unlike in classical form. Dermoscopy shows diffuse peppering pigment pattern arising on a brown background in the early phase, fading in color without other identifiable features (absence of Wickham striae pattern and vascular patterns). Hyperpigmented follicular openings and recently, rosettes have also been seen. Although pathogenesis has not been well-established, sunlight appears to be the major triggering factor in genetically predisposed people.

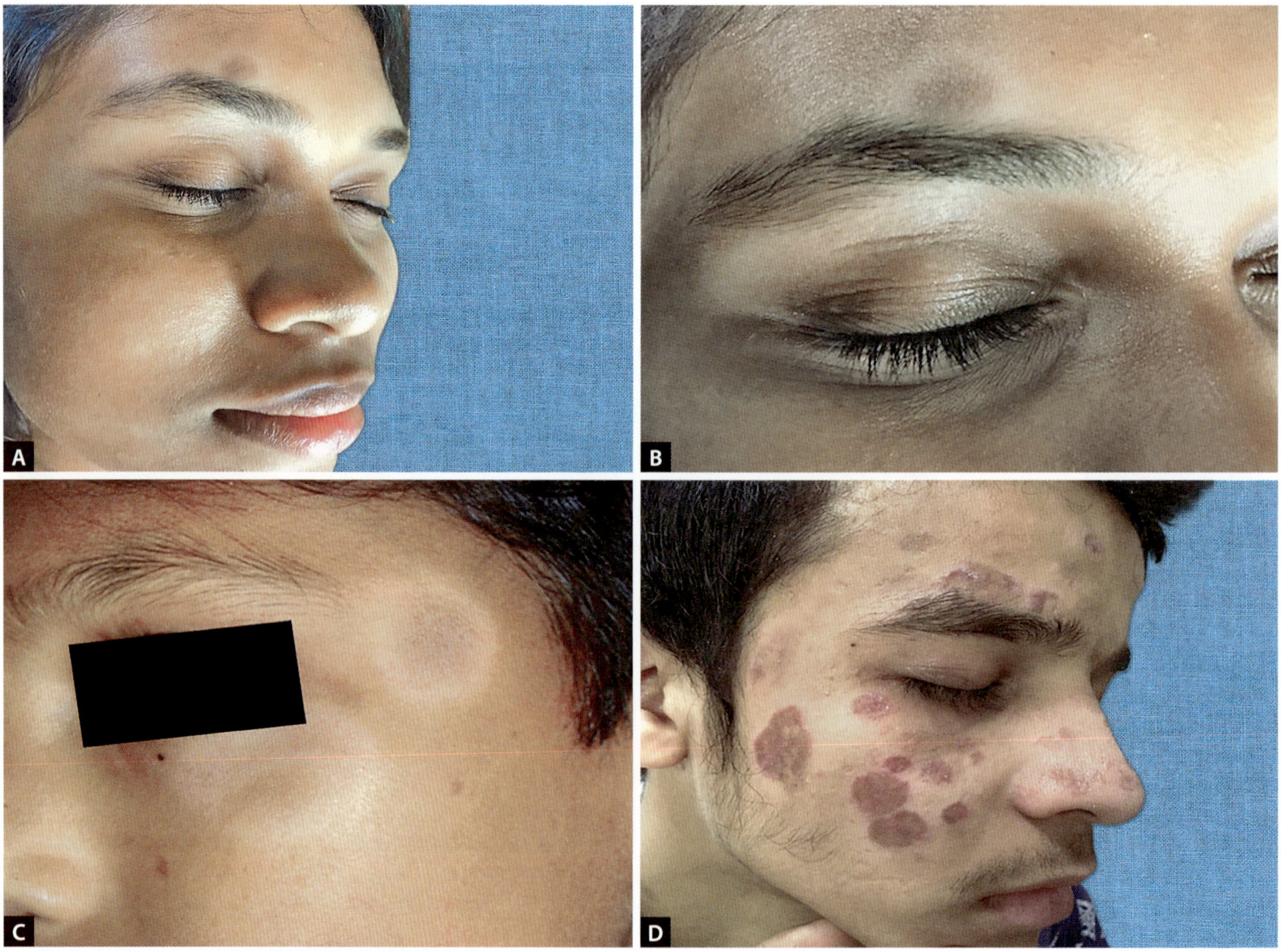

Figs. 19A to D: (A) Lichen planus (LP) actinicus; (B) Same patient, close-up view; (C) LP actinicus, classical lesion; (D) Extensive LP actinicus on face.

"If you have the guts to keep making mistakes, your wisdom and intelligence leap forward with huge momentum." —**Holly Near**

The differential diagnosis of actinic LP includes other photodermatosis, like polymorphous light eruption, DNA repair-defective disorders, nutritional and metabolic aberrations, dermatoses exacerbated by UV radiation, and photosensitization by exogenous or endogenous chemicals, discoid lupus erythematosus, LP pigmentosus, granuloma annulare, sarcoidosis, and postinflammatory hyperpigmentation. Presence of characteristic lesions on the sun-exposed areas and histopathology confirms the diagnosis. The histopathological findings resemble that of the classic LP (hyperkeratosis with focal parakeratosis, hypergranulosis, a marked lymphocytic band infiltrate, Civatte bodies, and pigmentary incontinence). Atypical histopathological patterns (dermatitis-like, lichenoid tissue reaction, lupus erythematosus like and polymorphic light eruption like) have also been reported. Pigmented ALP presents a variable degree of solar elastosis with thinning of the epidermis at the center of the lesion and striking pigment incontinence in the upper dermis and melanophages. Spontaneous remission can occur in the winter season, but they can relapse during the subsequent summer. Sun avoidance and corticosteroids are the mainstay of treatment. Photoprotection with broad-spectrum sunscreens is necessary. Other treatment options include oral hydroxychloroquine, dapsone, glucocorticoids, cyclosporine, and retinoic acid derivatives.

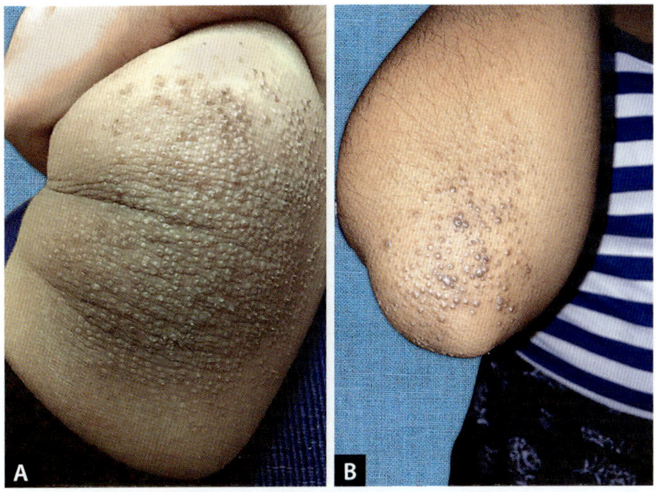

Figs. 20A and B: (A) Lichen spinulosus; (B) Close-up view of lichen spinulosus.

LICHEN SPINULOSUS (FIGS. 20A AND B)

Lichen spinulosus (LS) is a rare idiopathic follicular keratotic disorder occurring mostly in children and adolescents characterized by an acute onset of crops of asymptomatic, skin-colored, or hypopigmented minute (1–3 mm) follicular papules with projecting keratinous spines without erythema that appear as nutmeg grater or goosebumps-like. The horny spine of LS can be removed, leaving behind a tiny funnel-like orifice. These grouped round to oval plaques measuring 2–6 cm are distributed symmetrically on the neck, buttocks, abdomen, and extensor aspects of the arms. Generalized eruption has been rarely reported, mostly in adults in association with systemic disease (HIV and Crohn's disease). LS is slightly more common in boys than girls with no racial predilection or seasonal variations.

Though the exact cause of LS is unknown, it appears to be an abnormal reaction pattern of follicles to various triggers such as atopic diathesis, infections, id reaction to fungal infection, trauma and drug-related reactions, including reactions to thallium, gold, diphtheria toxin, and arsphenamine and malnutrition, specifically vitamin A deficiency. Genetic predisposition has been proposed to play a role. LS-like lesions on the face have been reported with folliculodystrophy of immunosuppression (trichodysplasia spinulosa), demodicosis, follicular mucinosis, and multiple myeloma. There are few reports of coexistence of LS with lichen nitidus and palmoplantar keratoderma. Histopathologically, it shows a dilated follicle protruding above the epidermal surface with a central, infundibular, keratotic plug. Follicular hyperkeratosis, parakeratosis, acanthosis, dermal perifollicular, and perivascular lymphocytic infiltrate may be present. LS has to be differentiated from keratosis pilaris, follicular mucinosis, lichen nitidus, Darier's disease, phrynoderma, pityriasis rubra pilaris, and multiple minute digitate hyperkeratosis (MMDH). LS does not usually spontaneously remit and persists for weeks to months though rarely persists indefinitely, if left untreated. Treatment is usually considered because of cosmetic reasons. It mainly consists of emollients, keratolytics, and mid potency topical corticosteroid. Variable response has been shown to topical lactic acid, salicylic acid, urea gels or ointments, topical tretinoin, topical adapalene, and topical calcipotriene. Treating underlying conditions and correcting vitamin deficiencies have shown to offer some improvement.

"The end of all our exploring will be to arrive where we started." —**TS Eliot**

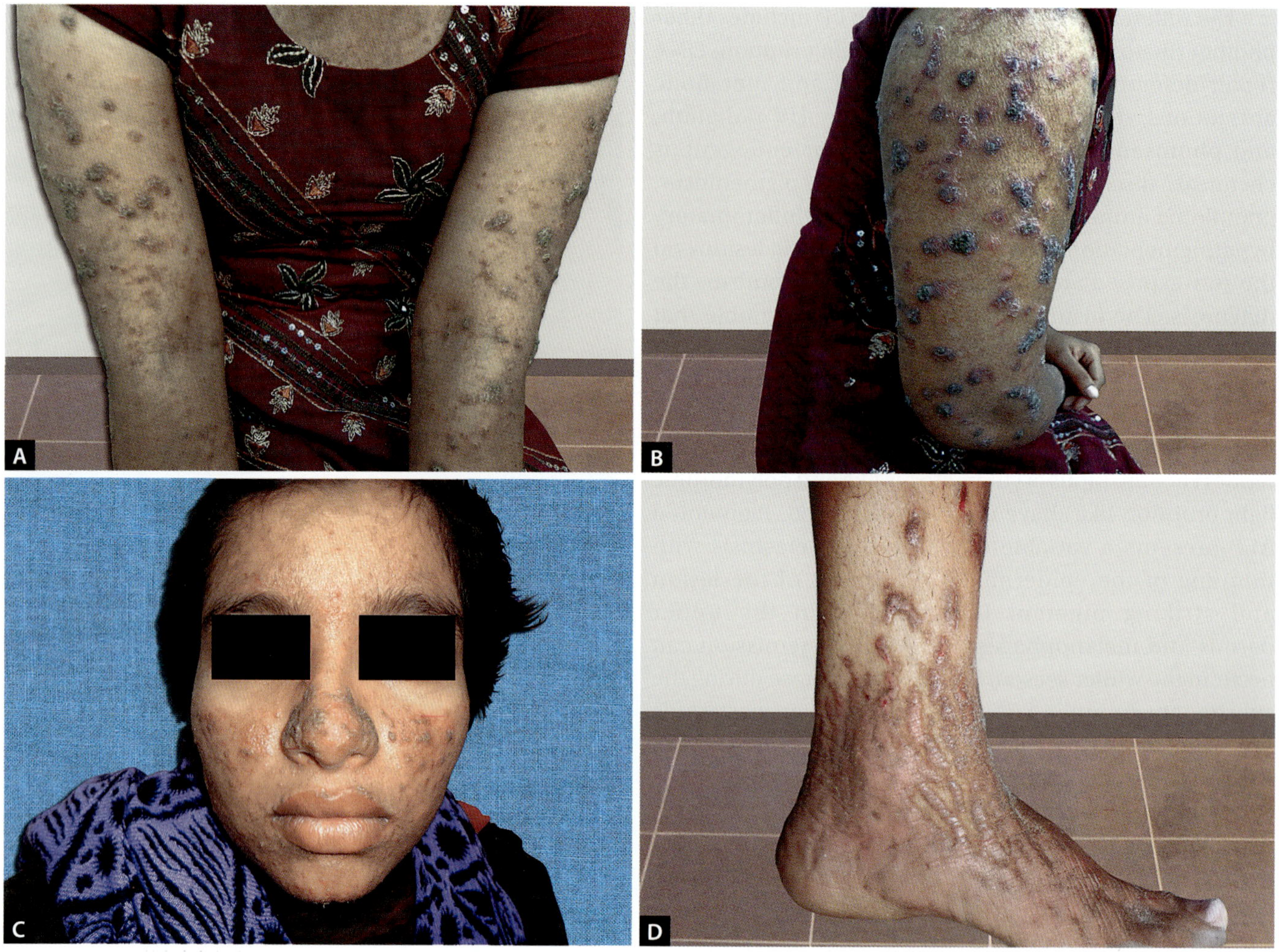

Figs. 21A to D: (A) Nekam's disease in a 17-year-old girl; (B) Close-up view of lichenoid lesions; (C) Same girl, facial lesions, note crusting and few comedonal lesions; (D) Linear lichenoid plaques around ankle.

NEKAM'S DISEASE (FIGS. 21A TO D)

Nekam's disease also called as keratosis lichenoides chronica is a rare mucocutaneous disorder seen in children. It is characterized by violaceous, keratotic papules, plaques, and nodules in a linear or a reticulate pattern distributed symmetrically on the trunk and extremities. Histopathological features include vacuolar degeneration of keratinocytes at dermoepidermal junction, necrotic keratinocytes with lymphohistiocytic infiltrate in dermis. Other clinical features associated are seborrheic dermatitis or rosacea-like rash, recurrent aphthous-like ulcers, palmoplantar keratoderma, and ungual dystrophy. It should be differentiated from Darier's disease, LP-psoriasis overlap, lichen planopilaris, and lupus erythematosus. Systemic treatment with oral steroids, MTx, retinoids, dapsone, antimalarials, photochemotherapy (PUVA) therapy, and efalizumab may be helpful.

PITYRIASIS RUBRA PILARIS (FIGS. 22A AND B)

Pityriasis rubra pilaris (PRP) is a rare papulosquamous disorder which is characterized by keratotic follicular papules, plaques with branny scaling, reddish orange erythema and palmoplantar keratoderma. Etiology is usually multifactorial—can be genetic (CARD 14 mutation), associated with HIV, infections (especially juvenile variant), autoimmune disorders and malignancy associated.

They are broadly classified into 6 types—classic adult (most common), atypical adult, classic juvenile, circumscribed juvenile, atypical juvenile and HIV associated.

"Think before you speak, read before you think". —**Lebowitz**

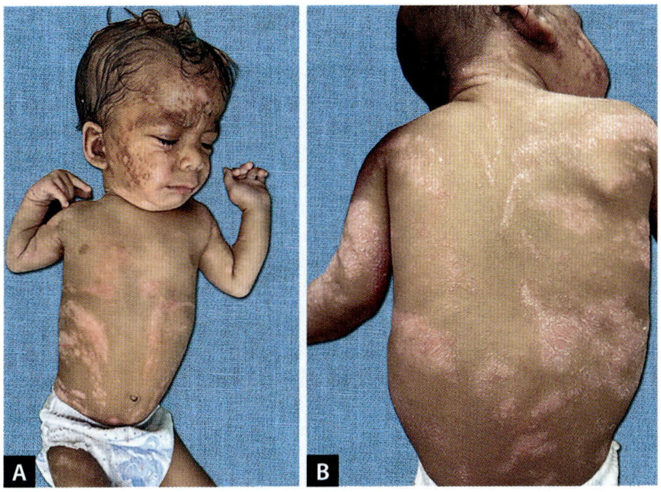

Figs. 22A and B: (A) CARD14 associated papulosquamous eruption (CAPE) in a 1-year-old boy; (B) Same patient, back.

Classic juvenile variant resembles the classic PRP which presents as erythroderma with islands of sparing, waxy palmoplantar keratoderma and follicular hyperkeratosis. It usually resolves within 1–2 years. Circumscribed juvenile variant is the most common variant among children which is seen mostly in prepubertal age group characterized by well-defined erythematous scaly plaques on elbows and knees resembling psoriasis. Atypical juvenile is usually familial and presents as follicular hyperkeratosis, scleroderma like changes of hands and feet. This variant has a chronic relapsing course which improves on treatment and recurs after stoppage of therapy.

Treatment

Topical therapy includes topical emollients, mild keratolytics (3% salicylic acid, 20% urea), retinoids (tazarotene), vitamin D analogues and calcineurin inhibitors are beneficial. However, first line therapy in cases of PRP is oral retinoids. Oral isotretinoin (1–2 mg/kg/day) or etretinate (0.4 mg/kg/day) is recommended in generalized variants in children. Oral vitamin A (50,000 IU) has also shown beneficial results in some patients. Narrow band UVB along with acitretin is found to be very effective in hyperkeratotic lesions.

PITYRIASIS LICHENOIDES

Pityriasis lichenoides is a rare papulosquamous disorder which occurs in two forms acute and chronic. Acute form is known as pityriasis lichenoides et varioliformis acuta (PLEVA) and chronic as pityriasis lichenoides chronica (PLC). This spectrum of disease occurs in both adults and children, with infection being the commonest trigger in children.

PLEVA usually occurs as crops of small erythematous papules and plaques with fine scales which later becomes vesicular, hemorrhagic and crusting. PLC usually appears as erythematous papules with centrally adherent scales. Both heal leaving behind postinflammatory pigmentation with hypopigmentation being the most common. Patients are usually asymptomatic with lesions distributed often over trunk and extremities. Children are more prone to have facial involvement and postinflammatory hypopigmentation. Mucosal involvement is rare. Systemic features like fever and lymphadenopathy is only seen with severe, rare variant of PLEVA, febrile ulceronecrotic Mucha–Habermann disease.

Treatment

Topical therapy with corticosteroids is not useful as monotherapy. Systemic therapy with oral antibiotics is often the first line therapy. Oral erythromycin (30–50 mg/kg/day) is the most effective therapy. Treatment should be continued for atleast 2–3 months and slow tapering should be done to prevent recurrences. Oral azithromycin ahs also been tried with more compliance compared to erythromycin. Narrow band UVB (NB-UVB) phototherapy with similar doses to psoriasis and atopic dermatitis was found to be more effective in PLC than in PLEVA. Other systemic treatment like methotrexate, oral doxycycline and clarithromycin were also effective in children.

WHAT'S NEW?

- Biologics in cases of pediatric psoriasis is the current area of research. TNF alpha inhibitors (etanercept, infliximab and adalimumab) and IL-17 inhibitors (secukinumab, ixekizumab) are approved in pediatric patients. Ustekinumab (IL-12/23 inhibitors) are also tried in childhood psoriasis.
- Secukinumab is also been found to be effective pediatric pustular psoriasis. Role of IL-36 inhibitors is established in adults pustular psoriasis.
- CARD-14 associated papulosquamous eruption (CAPE) is a new entity which is characterized by overlap of psoriasis and PRP like lesions. All these patients have CARD 14 mutation. Genetic testing should be done in suspected cases and their close family. Treatment options are the same as for psoriasis and PRP.
- In juvenile PRP, various biologics like secukinumab, risankizumab and ustekinumab have been tried with beneficial results.

SUGGESTED READINGS

1. Eichenfield LF, Paller AS, Tom WL, Sugarman J, Hebert AA, Friedlander SF, et al. Pediatric psoriasis: evolving perspectives. Pediatr Dermatol. 2018;35(2):170-81.
2. Gautam M, Tahiliani H, Nadkarni N, Patil S, Godse K. Acitretin in pediatric dermatoses. Indian J Paediatric Dermatol. 2016;17:87-94.
3. Kumar A, Mendiratta V, Agarwal S, Chander R, Sanke S. Childhood lichen planus: a series of 42 patients. Indian J Paediatr Dermatol. 2018;19:116-9.
4. Tziotzios C, Brier T, Lee JYW, Saito R, Hsu CK, Bhargava K, et al. Lichen planus and lichenoid dermatoses: conventional and emerging therapeutic strategies. J Am Acad Dermatol. 2018;79(5):807-18.
5. Frare CP, Blumstein AJ, Paller AS, Pieretti L, Choate KA, Bowcock AM, et al. CARD14-associated papulosquamous eruption (CAPE) in pediatric patients: Three additional cases and review of the literature. Pediatr Dermatol. 2021;38(5):1237-42.
6. Katakam BK, Munisamy M, Rao TN, Chiramel MJ, Panda M, Gupta S, et al. Recommendations for Management of Childhood Psoriasis. Indian Dermatol Online J. 2021;12(Suppl 1):S71-S85.
7. Guenther J, Novack D, Kamath S, Worswick S. Treatment Options for Juvenile Pityriasis Rubra Pilaris. Paediatr Drugs. 2023;25(2):151-64.
8. Albela H, Lee WQ, Nordin SN, Gopinathan LP, A Ramli MN, Leong KF. Juvenile Pityriasis Rubra Pilaris in a 4-year-old Child Treated Successfully with Secukinumab. Indian J Dermatol. 2022;67(5):601-3.

"Life is short and it is here to be lived". —**Unknown**

CHAPTER 9

Vesiculobullous Diseases

CHRONIC BULLOUS DERMATOSIS OF CHILDHOOD [FIGS. 1 TO 4H(ii)]

Linear IgA bullous dermatosis has a bimodal age of onset; in adults referred to as linear IgA disease, and the childhood variant was formerly known as chronic bullous dermatosis of childhood (CBDC). CBDC is a chronic, acquired, autoimmune, subepidermal disease of children with cutaneous and mucosal involvement, characterized by immunoglobulin A (IgA) basement membrane antibodies. The mean age of onset is under 5 years; it is usually acute and the initial attacks are more severe than subsequent recurrences. It may be idiopathic or due to different triggering factors, including drugs. Symptoms vary from absent or mild pruritus to severe burning. The face and perineum are involved, particularly in younger children. The perioral area, eyelids, ears, and scalp may be affected. The involvement of the perineum and vulva has been mistaken for sexual abuse in some patients. The eruption may spread to the trunk, thighs, arms, hands, and feet. The lesions comprise urticated papules and plaques, annular, polycyclic lesions often with blistering around the edge, the "string of pearls" or "cluster of jewels" sign. The blisters may occasionally turn hemorrhagic. Mucosal involvement is common. Oral mucosa may be involved with ulcers and erosions, and hoarseness may indicate pharyngeal involvement. The nose may bleed. The eyes may be sore and gritty with conjunctival involvement. Immunofluorescence shows deposition of IgA in the dermoepidermal junction.

Natural History

Spontaneous remission occurs in the majority after an average of 3–6 years. Usually, the disease does not extend beyond puberty.

Treatment

Dapsone is the drug of choice since sulfapyridine is not available in our country. It is given in a dose of 1–2 mg/kg/day in two divided doses. The drug may be discontinued when the old lesions heal and the new lesions have stopped coming. However, several such courses may be

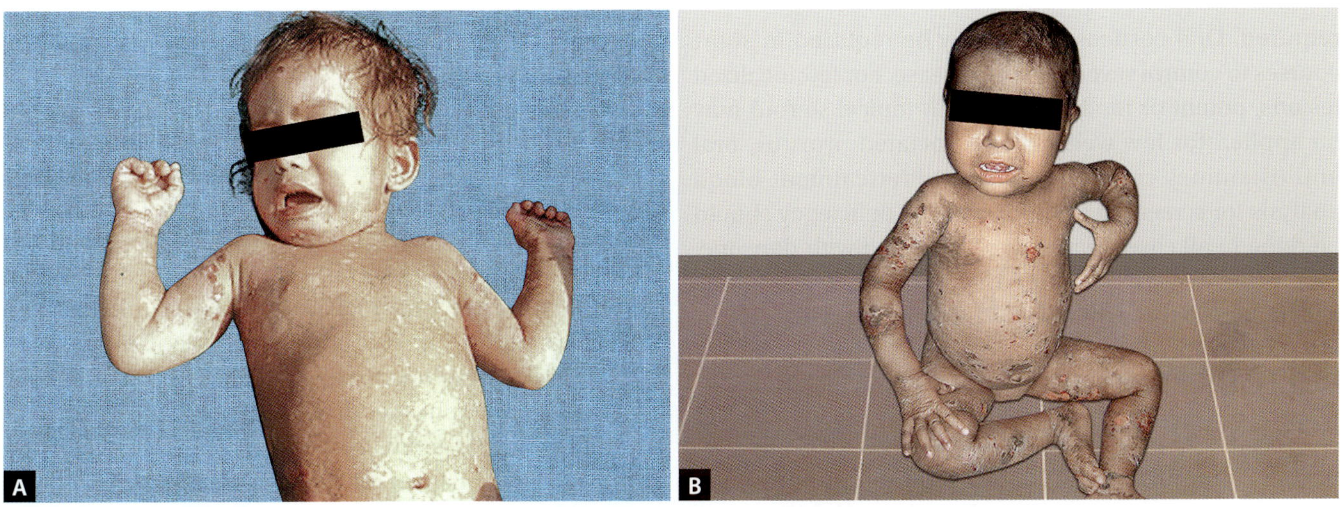

Figs. 1A and B: (A) Vesicles and tense bullae of chronic bullous dermatosis of childhood (CBDC) over trunk; (B) CBDC over trunk, mostly ruptured bullae.

"Change your thoughts and you change your world." **–Norman Vincent Peale**

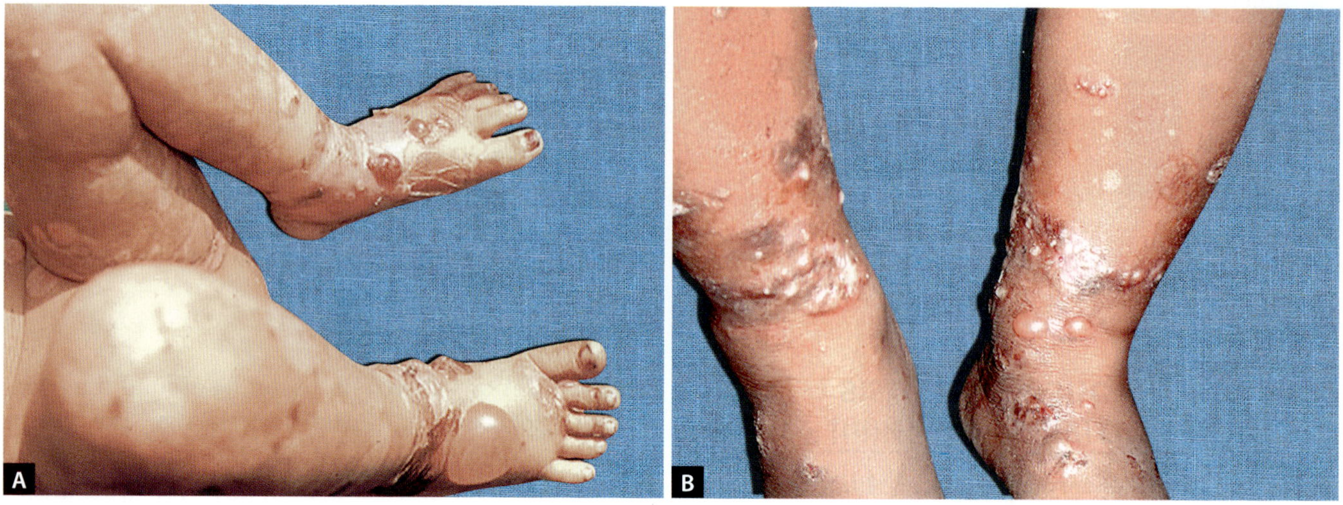

Figs. 2A and B: (A) Involvement of legs and feet in chronic bullous dermatosis of childhood (CBDC), note hemorrhagic bullae; (B) Distribution of bullae in CBDC over legs.

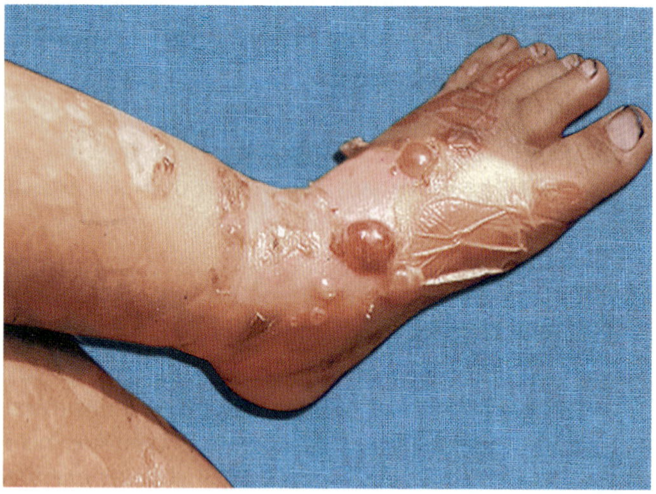

Fig. 3: Same child with hemorrhagic bullae (close-up view).

required. Oral corticosteroids may be required in short courses to control severity of the disease. For few localized lesions, potent or moderately potent topical steroid may be applied for few weeks. For associated pruritus, oral antihistamines can be prescribed. Pretreatment blood analysis for screening of G6PD enzyme deficiency should be done in all cases planned to be treated with dapsone. In refractory cases, systemic corticosteroids, cyclosporine, colchicine, erythromycin, and IVIg, may be used.

BULLOUS PEMPHIGOID IN PEDIATRIC AGE GROUP (FIGS. 4I TO L)

Bullous pemphigoid (BP) is an acquired autoimmune disorder presenting with subepidermal blistering, eosinophilia, and severe pruritus. It mostly affects the elderly, rare in pediatric age group but cases have been increasingly reported. Most cases are seen in infants and adolescent age group. Palmoplantar involvement is characteristic of infantile BP. Mucous membrane involvement is seen more commonly in children than adults. Diagnosis requires identification of subepidermal blisters under hematoxylin and eosin (H&E) and positive direct immunofluorescence (DIF). Childhood BP has a short and benign course. Topical steroids and oral erythromycin are preferred. Treatment for severe BP includes prednisone and dapsone, but prednisolone (1–2 mg/kg/day) is preferred in children. Childhood BP can be associated with increased levels of IgE and atopic eczema, in such situation IVIg has been tried.

CICATRICIAL PEMPHIGOID (FIGS. 5A TO D)

It affects mucosal surfaces, and a localized form (chronic pemphigoid of Brunsting–Perry) is seen which is usually limited to the head and neck. In this disorder, recurrent bullae are seen in the oral mucosa and conjunctiva and other mucous membranes such as nasopharynx, esophagus, larynx, genitalia, and anal canal. Until many years after onset of the condition, the ocular form may not occur and oral involvement often takes the form of a desquamative gingivitis (DG). Entropion, trichiasis, symblepharon, dryness of the cornea, corneal ulceration, and, at times, eventual blindness can develop. Esophageal lesions can result in stricture formation and laryngeal lesions when present, may be life-threatening.

"There is no royal road to anything. One thing at a time, all things in succession. That which grows fast, withers as rapidly. That which grows slowly, endures."

–Josiah Gilbert Holland

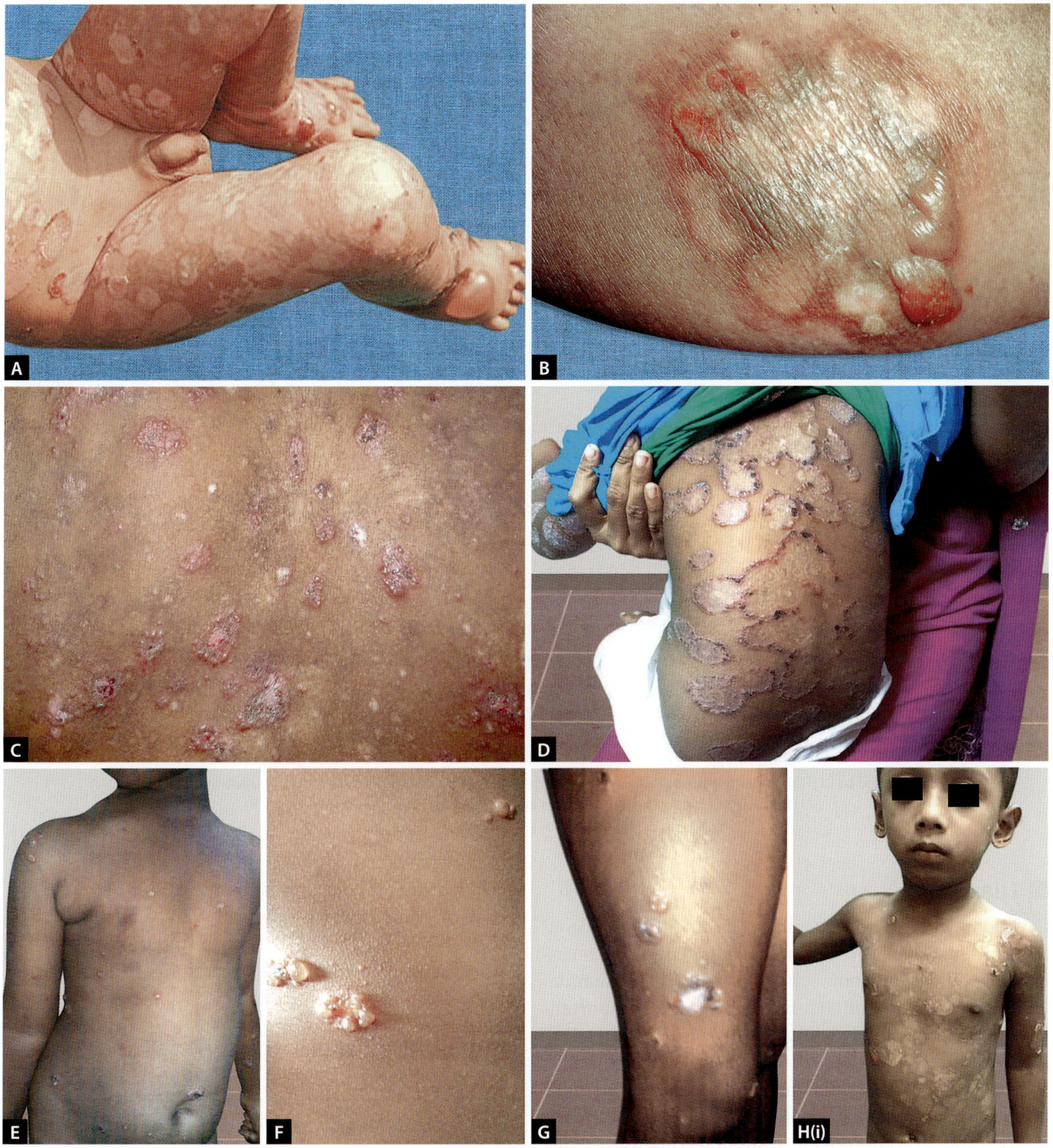

Figs. 4A to H(i): (A) Bullae with erosions on extremities; (B) Close-up view of chronic bullous dermatosis of childhood (CBDC) lesions, "cluster of jewels" appearance; (C) Lesions of CBDC over back; (D) CBDC, note "string of pearls" arrangement of vesicles; (E) CBDC in a 4-year-old boy; (F) "Cluster of jewels" sign in CBDC; (G) Around healed vesicles, new vesicles in a ring-like fashion makes "cluster of jewels" appearance; H(i) Healed vesicles with postinflammatory hypopigmentation.

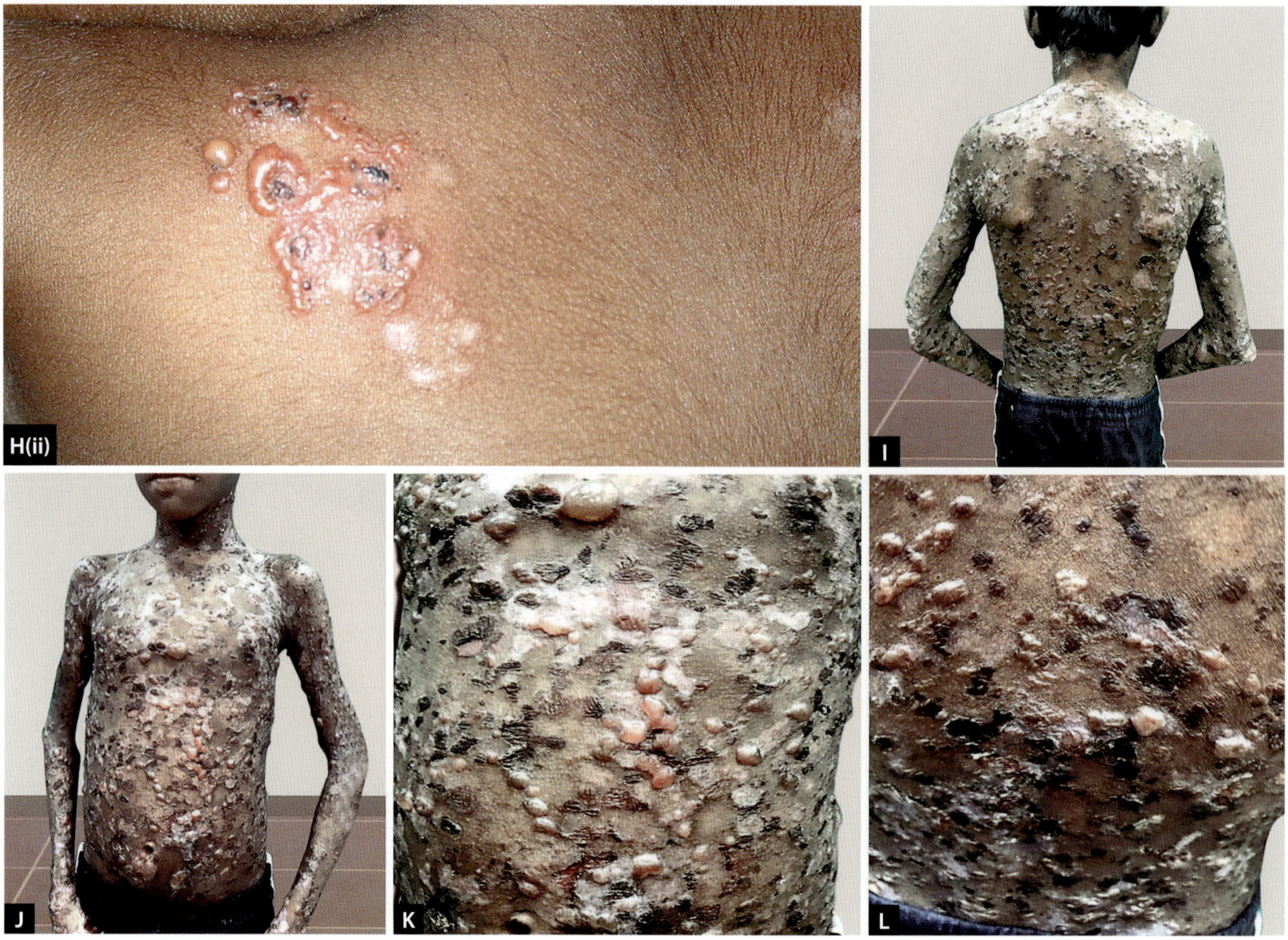

Figs. 4H(ii) to L: H(ii) Linear immunoglobulin A (IgA) disease; (I) Extensive bullous lesions in bullous pemphigoid; (J) Same boy, front view; (K) Close-up view of trunk; (L) Close-up view of back.

Diagnosis

In childhood, the clinical features of cicatricial pemphigoid are indistinguishable from those in adults. Biopsy specimens of cutaneous lesions show subepidermal blister formation, usually without papillary microabscesses [important diagnostic feature of dermatitis herpetiformis (DH)]. DIF reveals deposition of C3 and IgG at the BMZ. Indirect testing of serum for circulating IgG anti-BMZ antibodies is positive in approximately 70% of patients. Antibody titers do not correlate with clinical disease activity.

Treatment

The response to treatment of this disease in childhood is variable. The eruption may be suppressed by systemic corticosteroids. A combination of dapsone or chlorambucil with corticosteroids may be helpful. In some patients, cyclosporine and cyclophosphamide (alone or with low doses of corticosteroids) appear to have been effective. For few lesions, topical corticosteroids may be given. If there is associated itching, oral antihistamines may be prescribed.

DERMATITIS HERPETIFORMIS (FIGS. 5E TO H)

Dermatitis herpetiformis is a rare, intensely pruritic, relapsing, chronic, papulovesicular disease. It can present in childhood and old age. Males are more commonly affected than females. The onset may be acute or gradual and pruritus is usually the first and predominant symptom. Early lesions on the skin are erythematous papules, urticarial weals, or groups of small vesicles often excoriated so rapidly that it may be impossible to find an

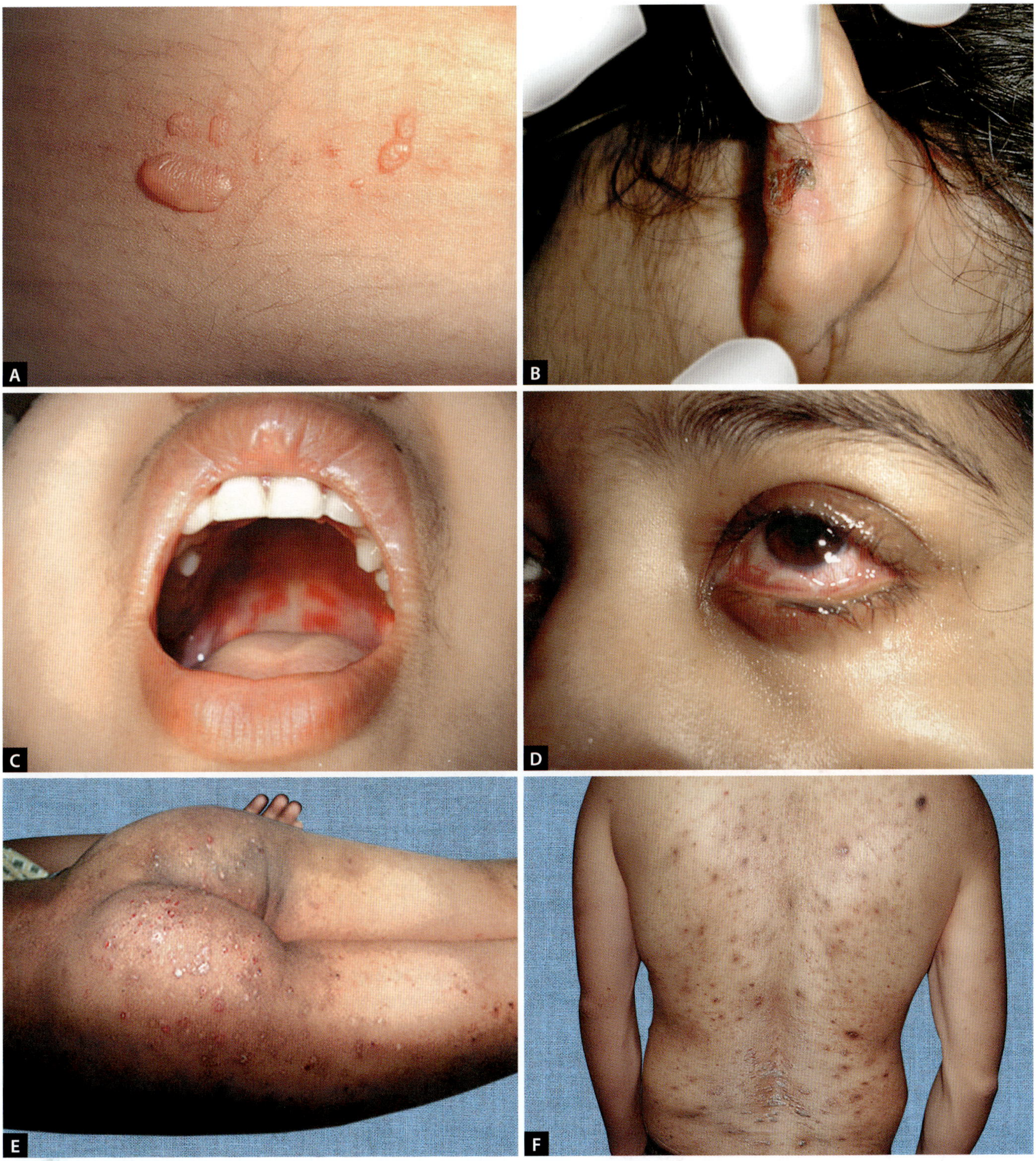

Figs. 5A to F: (A) Subepidermal bullae in a case of cicatricial pemphigoid; (B) Subepidermal bullae over pinna with scarring in cicatricial pemphigoid; (C) Same girl, note palatal ulcer; (D) Conjunctival scarring in the same girl; (E) Excoriated papulovesicles of dermatitis herpetiformis (DH) over buttocks and thighs; (F) Dermatitis herpetiformis in an 18-year-old boy.

intact vesicle. The vesicles are usually grouped together on plaques of erythema and rarely blisters, 1–2 cm in diameter, develop. The sites of predilection are the extensor aspects of the limbs, especially the knees, just below the point of the elbows, buttocks, and the natal cleft. The axillary folds, shoulders, trunk, face, and scalp

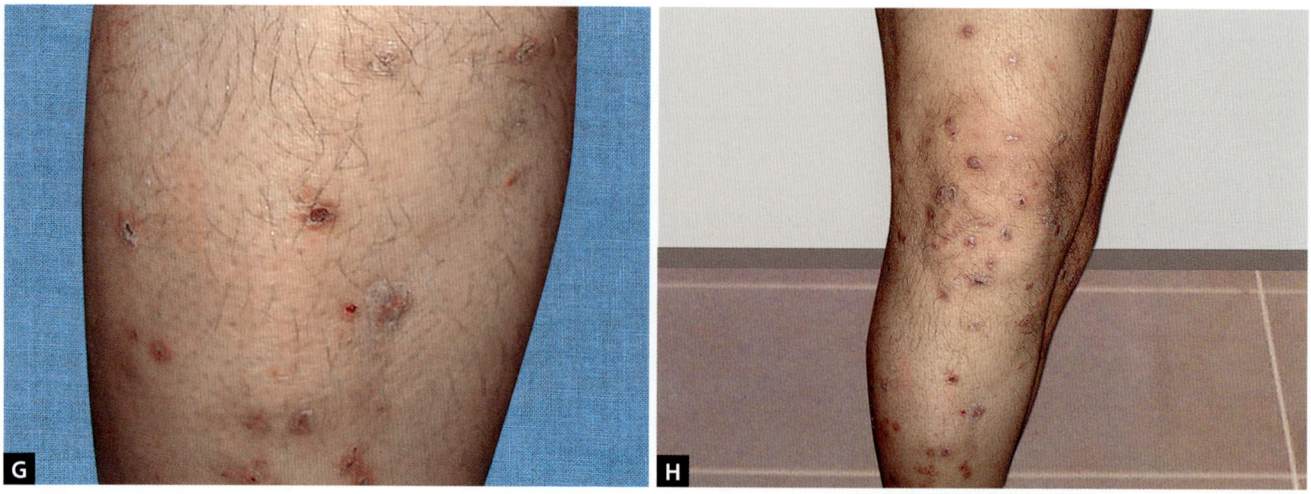

Figs. 5G and H: (G) Close-up view of DH lesions; (H) DH lesions over thighs and legs.

can be frequently involved. Oral lesions are common but asymptomatic. Active disease may be associated with a feeling of malaise. In addition, constitutional symptoms due to gluten sensitive enteropathy may be present. Differential diagnoses include papular urticaria, atopic dermatitis, scabies, and pityriasis lichenoides et varioliformis acuta.

Treatment

The drug of choice for DH is dapsone. The dosage and duration of treatment is more or less same as in cases of CBDC. The initial dose is 2 mg/kg/day, with an increase or decrease in dosage depending on the clinical response and the side effects associated with therapy. Once a favorable response is achieved, the dose is decreased gradually to a minimum level of 25–50 mg/day. Various adverse effects observed are nausea, vomiting, headache, giddiness, fever, lymphadenopathy, exfoliative dermatitis, or hemolysis, particularly in G6PD enzyme deficient cases. The condition is extremely pruritic. Oral antihistamines form an integral part of management of cases with DH. Gluten-free diet in children has shown resolution of skin lesions as well as gastrointestinal symptoms and this has to be maintained for few years.

EPIDERMOLYSIS BULLOSA (FIGS. 6 TO 16)

In between the cells of the epidermis there is desmosome-tonofilament complex which keep the cells knit together. The epidermis is attached to the dermis by anchoring fibrils and anchoring filaments. Epidermolysis bullosa (EB) is a group of inherited disorders in which there is defective formation of keratin, anchoring fibrils and filaments. As a result, on slightest trauma, there is separation either in the epidermis or dermoepidermal junction with formation of blisters. Therefore, these diseases are called "mechanobullous disorders." On the basis of clinical, histopathological, and electron microscopic findings, four groups of EB are recognized: Simplex, junctional, dystrophic, and mixed variant **(Table 1)**. Subtypes of EB are classified based on phenotypic features, distribution (localized/generalized), severity, and some additional features such as exuberant granulation tissue, mottled pigmentation, and pseudosyndactyly. Because of great differences in prognosis, identification of type of EB is often very important. The hallmarks of the disease are mechanical fragile skin, easily inducible

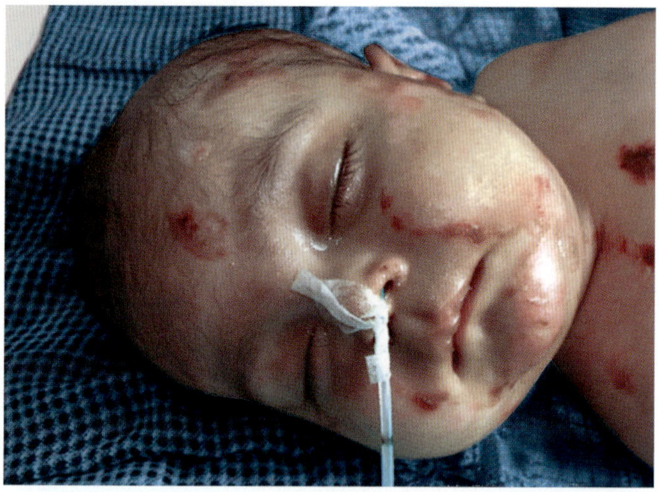

Fig. 6: Erosion and crusting of epidermolysis bullosa in a newborn.

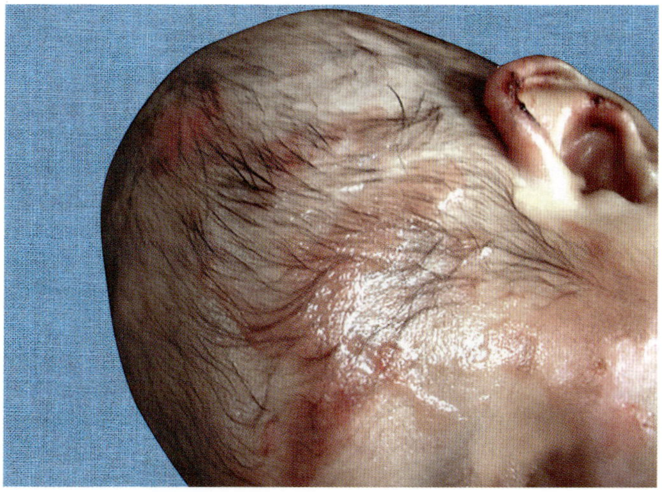

Fig. 7: Bullae and erosion of epidermolysis bullosa.

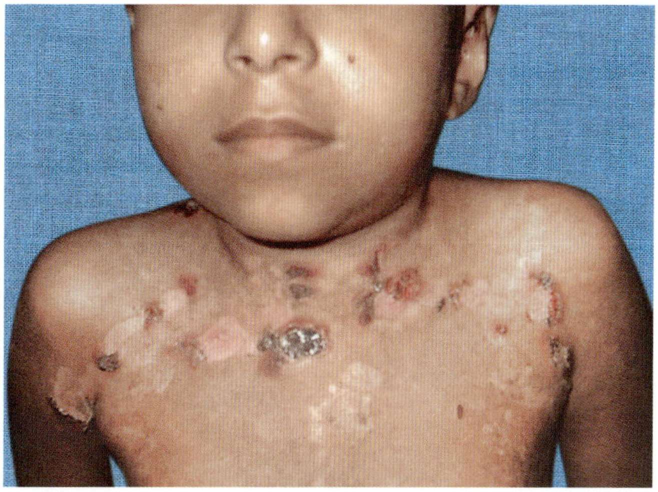

Fig. 8: Epidermolysis bullosa in an 8-year-old girl, note erosion, crusting and hypopigmentation.

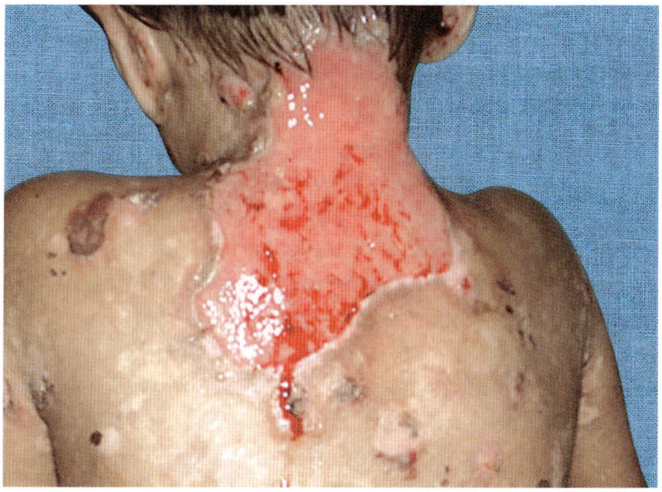

Fig. 9: Large area of erosion over back.

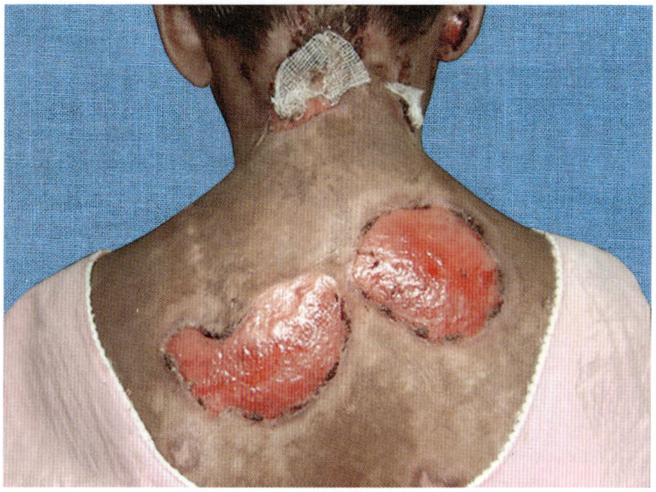

Fig. 10: Reappearance of erosions after skin grafting.

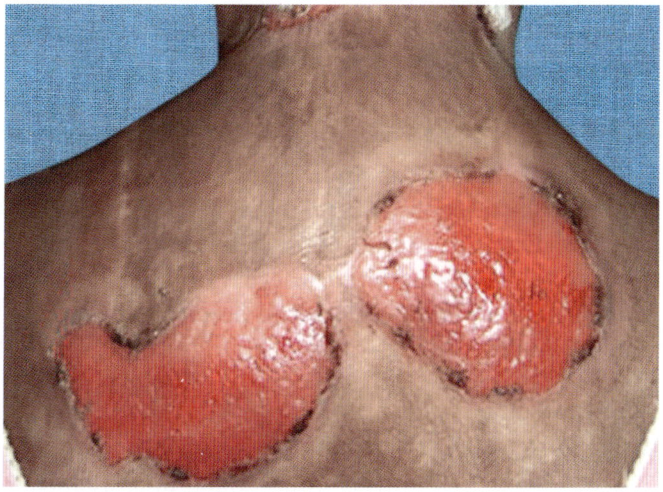

Fig. 11: Same girl, close-up view.

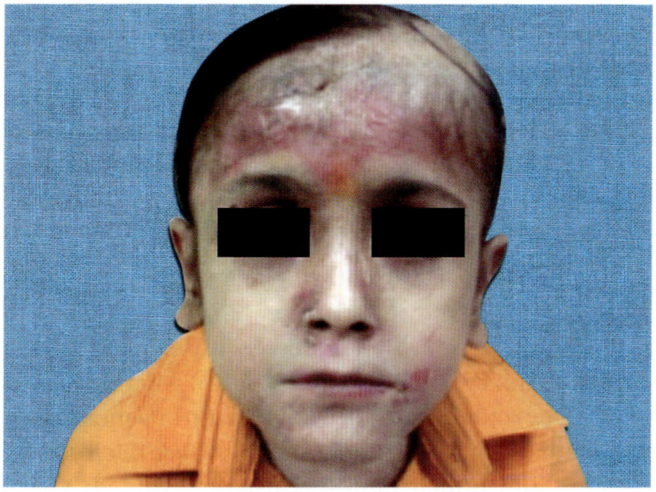

Fig. 12: A 15-year-old boy with AR dystrophic epidermolysis bullosa since birth.

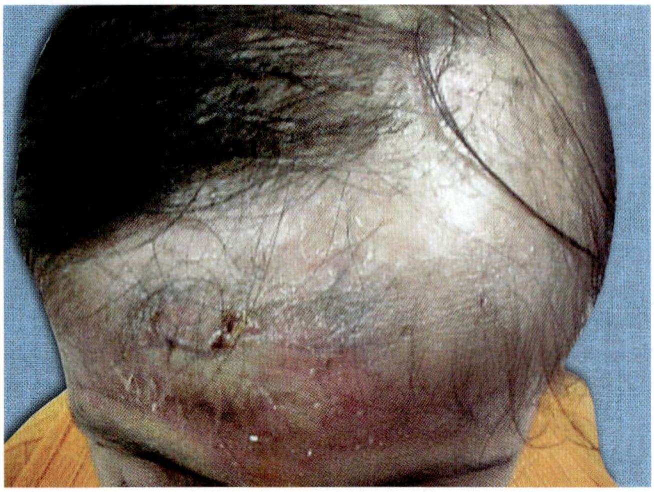

Fig. 13: Same boy, close-up view of scarring alopecia.

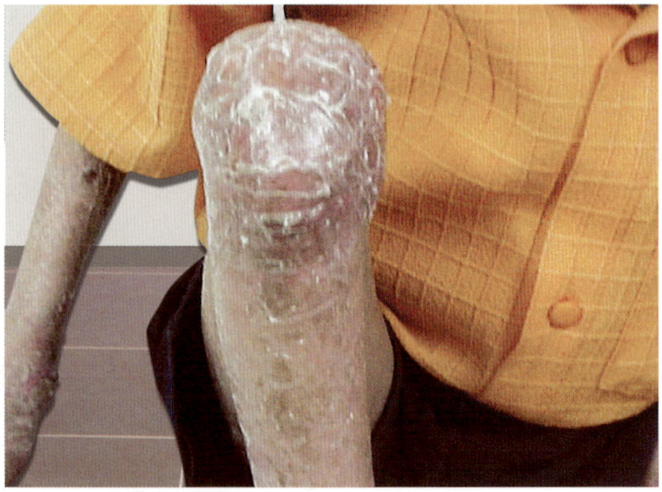

Fig. 14: Scarring and psoriasiform scaling over knee.

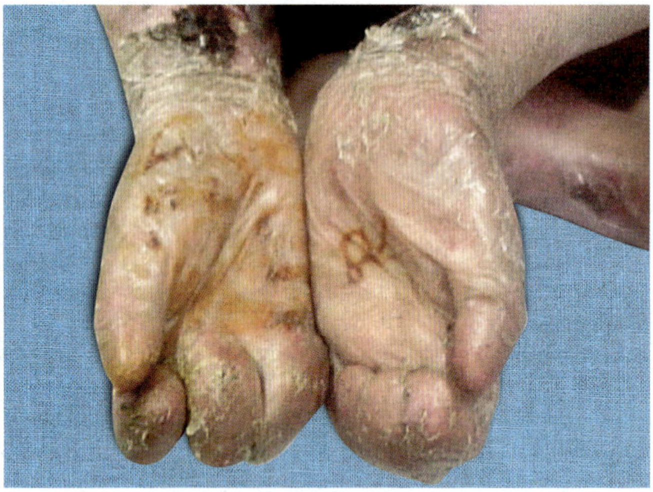

Fig. 15: Mitten-like deformity of hands.

blisters, and erosions from birth or early infancy. Inherited EB encompasses over 30 phenotypically or genetically distinct entities. The clinical features of the major forms of EB have been highlighted in **Tables 2 to 4**. In Kindler syndrome, blisters are generalized, usually subsides in late childhood giving rise to poikilodermatous appearance.

Investigations

Although EB is a clinical diagnosis, skin biopsy for histopathology and antigen mapping is necessary to determine the type of EB and predict the prognosis. Biopsy is usually taken from unaffected skin. Microblister is induced by rubbing the skin with fingertip or pencil eraser. Skin should be stroked 30–40 times to induce microblister. Incision and punch biopsy is usually avoided. Shave biopsy would be ideal in EB.

Management

Treatment depends on the severity of EB. In mild variants, parents are educated about the wound care and how to avoid trauma. Pain and progression of large blisters may be controlled by gently popping the blister or cutting a square skin window. Nonadhesive dressings/vaseline impregnated gauzes are useful. Prevention of trauma and treatment of infection with topical and/or oral antibiotics are important. Bland emollients or liquid paraffin can be used all over the body for lubrication.

In severely affected children, a multidisciplinary approach is necessary. The dermatologist, pediatric internist, ophthalmologist, gastroenterologist, otolaryngologist, pediatric surgeon, dentist, and a physical therapist may be involved in the care of such infants and children.

Oral zinc, multivitamins, and minerals, particularly iron supplementation, may facilitate wound healing. Good nutrition is mandatory for maintenance of good health and early healing of erosions/ulcers.

Future Therapies of Epidermolysis Bullosa

Epidermolysis bullosa requires a multidisciplinary approach for the holistic care of the affected individual. Keeping in mind this necessity, the concept of all in one clinic has been started wherein in a single clinic, specialists from various branches are available to deal with the multisystem disorder.

Wound Care

Wound infection is the most common complication in these patients. The most common offending organisms include *Staphylococcus aureus*, *Staphylococcus*

"I would rather die of passion than of boredom." **–Vincent van Gogh**

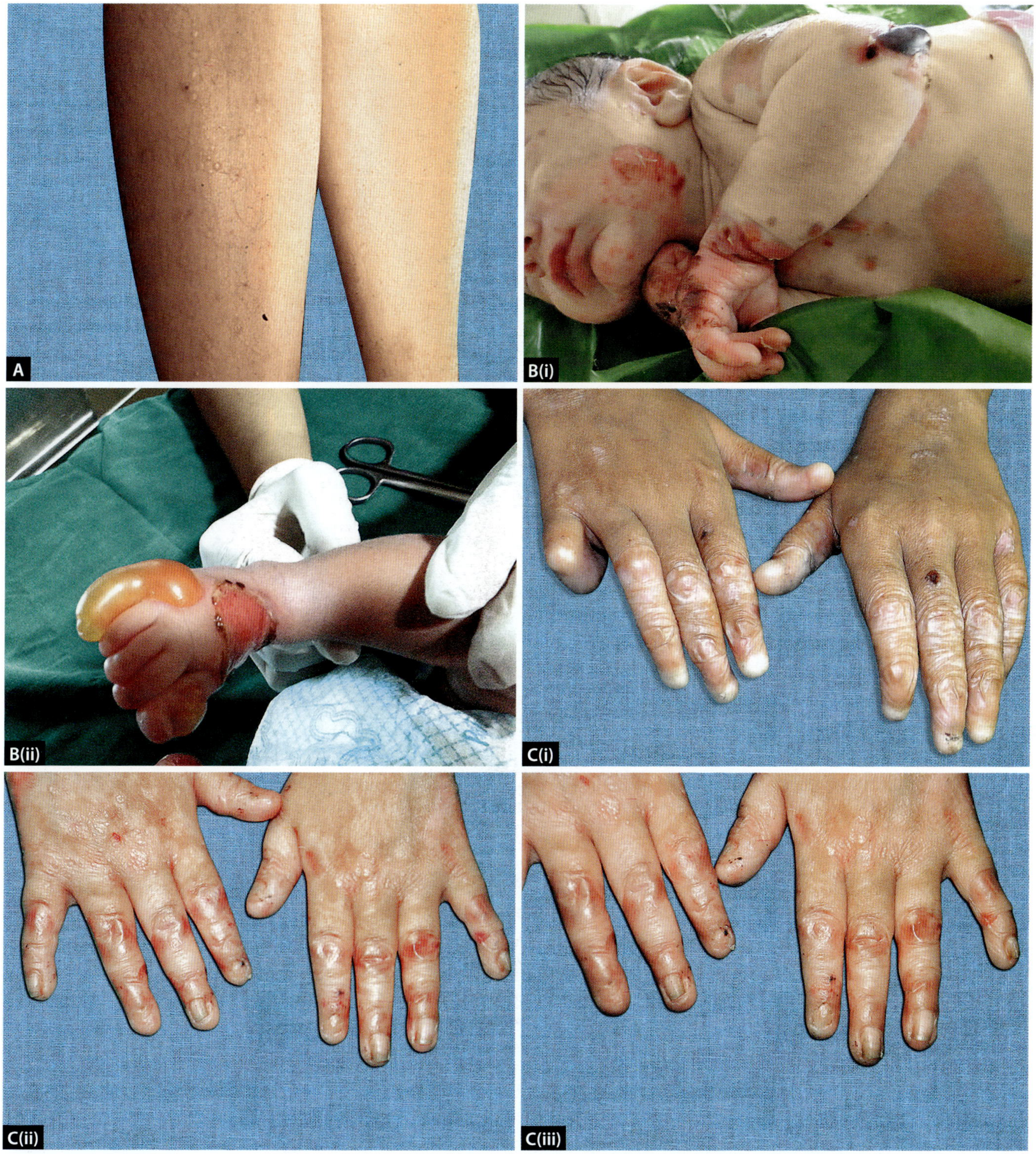

Figs. 16A to C(iii): (A) Multiple skin-colored scar-like spontaneously appearing lesions over the leg (albopapuloid lesions) in dominant dystrophic EB; B(i) Epidermolysis bullosa (EB) in a newborn. Note hemorrhagic bulla; B(ii) EB simplex; C(i) Dystrophic EB, note anonychia; C(ii) EB dystrophica, note milia; C(iii) Same patient, close-up view.

epidermidis, and *Pseudomonas aeruginosa*. The dressings include nonadherent dressings such as mepitel dressings, silicone mesh, lipid colloid contact layer, vaseline gauze impregnated dressings, and burns mesh. Foam dressings are being used to separate the toes in order to avoid formation of adhesions. Silver and honey impregnated

"A person who never made a mistake never tried anything new." **–Albert Einstein**

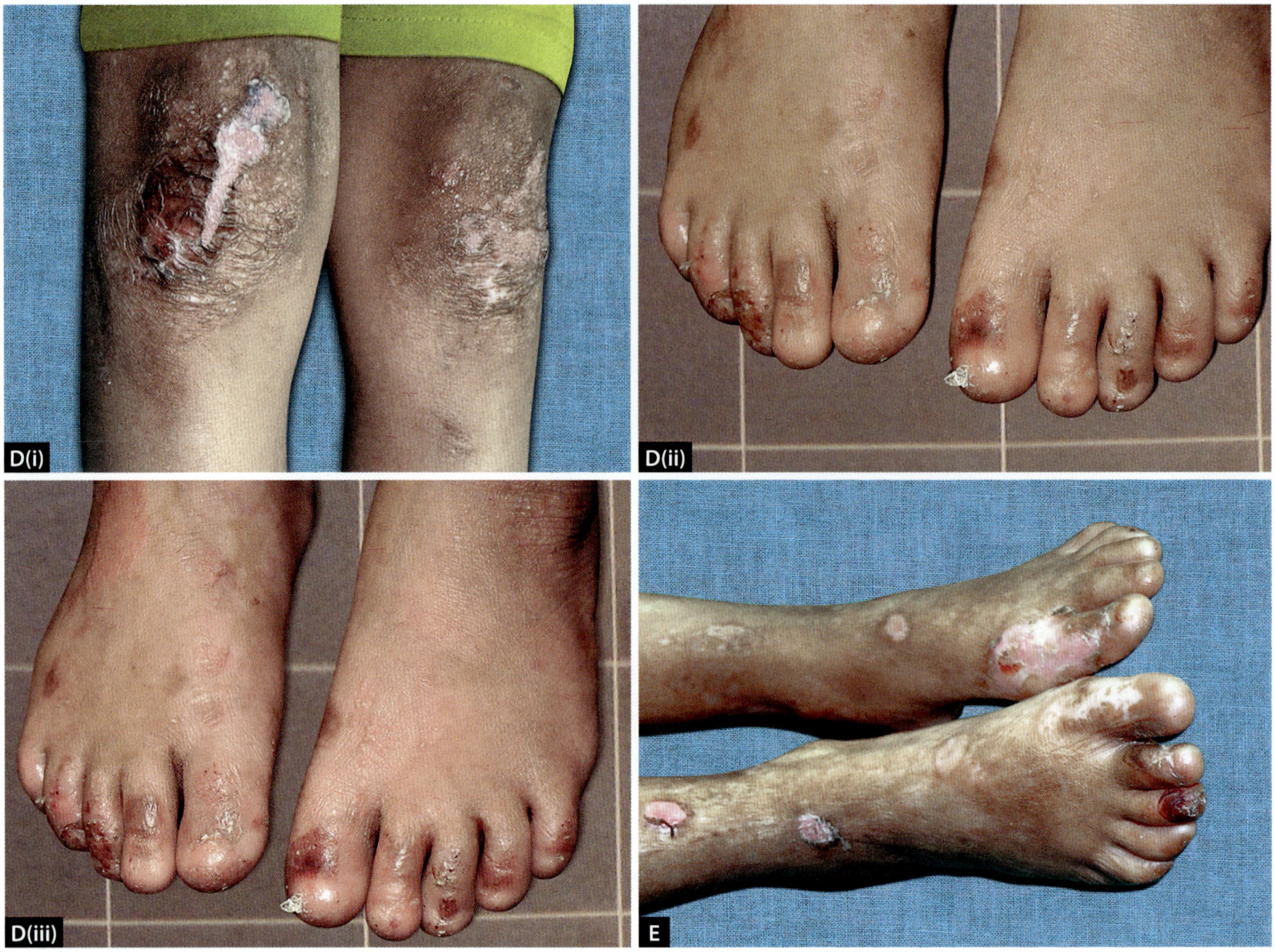

Figs. 16D(i) to E: D(i) Dystrophic EB, note cigarette paper-like scars over knees; D(ii and iii) Scarring along with anonychia in dystrophic EB; (E) Dystrophic epidermolysis bullosa.

Table 1: Recent classification of epidermolysis bullosa.

Type	*Major types*	*Subtypes*	*Target proteins*
Epidermolysis bullosa simplex (EBS)	Suprabasal	Acral peeling skin syndrome	Transglutaminase 5
		EBS superficialis (EBSS)	Unknown
		Acantholytic EBS (EBS-acanth)	Desmoplakin and plakoglobin
		Skin fragility syndromes	Desmoplakin, plakoglobin, and plakophilin
	Basal	EBS, localized (EBS-loc)	K5 and K14
		EBS, generalized severe (EBS-gen sev)	K5 and K14
		EBS, generalized intermediate (EBS-gen intermed)	K5 and K14
		EBS with mottled pigmentation (EBS-MP)	K5
		EBS, migratory circinate (EBS-migr)	K5
		EBS, autosomal recessive K14 (EBS-AR K14)	K14
		EBS with muscular dystrophy (EBS-MD)	Plectin
		EBS with pyloric atresia (EBS-PA)	Plectin, α6β4 integrin
		EBS-Ogna (EBS-og)	Plectin
		EBS, autosomal recessive-BP230 deficiency	Bullous pemphigoid antigen-1
		EBS, autosomal recessive-exophilin 5 deficiency	Exophilin 5

Continued

"What's money? A man is a success if he gets up in the morning and goes to bed at night and in between does what he wants to do." **–Bob Dylan**

Continued

Type	Major types	Subtypes	Target proteins
Junctional epidermolysis bullosa (JEB)	JEB, generalized	JEB, severe generalized	Laminin-332
		JEB, generalized intermediate	Laminin-332
		JEB, with pyloric atresia	Collagen XVII
		JEB, late onset	Collagen XVII
		JEB, with respiratory and renal involvement	Integrin α3 subunit
	JEB, localized	JEB, localized (JEB-loc)	Collagen XVII, α6β4 integrin, Laminin 332
		JEB, inversa	Laminin 332
		JEB-loc syndrome	Laminin -332 Isoform α3 chain
Dystrophic epidermolysis bullosa (DEB)	Dominant dystrophic epidermolysis bullosa (DDEB)	DDEB, generalized (DDEB-gen)	Collagen VIIda
		DDEB, acral (DDEB-ac)	Collagen VII
		DDEB, pretibial (DDEB-pt)	Collagen VII
		DDEB, pruriginosa (DDEB-pr)	Collagen VII
		DDEB, nails only (DDEB-na)	Collagen VII
		DDEB, bullous dermolysis of newborn (DDEB-BDN)	Collagen VII
	Recessive dystrophic epidermolysis bullosa (RDEB)	RDEB, generalized severe	Collagen VII
		RDEB, generalized intermediate	Collagen VII
		RDEB, inversa	Collagen VII
		RDEB, localized	Collagen VII
		RDEB, pretibial	Collagen VII
		RDEB, pruriginosa	Collagen VII
		RDEB, centripetalis	Collagen VII
		RDEB, bullous dermolysis of newborn	Collagen VII
Kindler syndrome			Kindlin-1 (Fermitin family homolog 1)

Source: Adapted from Fine JD, Bruckner-Tuderman L, Eady RAJ, Bauer EA, Bauer JW, Has C, et al. Inherited epidermolysis bullosa: updated recommendations on diagnosis and classification. J Am Acad Dermatol. 2014;70(6):1103-26.

Table 2: Clinical features of major types of epidermolysis bullosa simplex (EBS).

Clinical features	EBS, localized	EBS, generalized	EBS, other generalized
Mode of transmission	Autosomal dominant	Autosomal dominant/sporadic	Autosomal dominant/sporadic
Onset	Birth to early adulthood	Birth/within first week	Birth/infancy
Skin distribution	Hands and feet	Generalized	Generalized, infancy on occiput, back, and legs
Skin features	Nonscarring bullae, worse during summer, increases with trauma	Grouped herpetiform blisters on trunk, proximal limbs, tendency of blistering decreases with age—milia, scarring present	Nonscarring bullae, tense, serous, blister worse in summer, improvement with puberty—milia, scarring present
Other features	Dystrophic nails, palmoplantar keratoderma (PPK)	Nail shedding, flexion deformities of digits	Associated with congenital absence of skin, focal PPK
Extracutaneous features	Intraoral, palatal erosions	Intraoral blistering, hoarse cry due to laryngeal involvement, constipation, gastroesophageal reflex	Soft tissue abnormalities are variable
Improvement with age	Persistent, learn to modify lifestyle	Reduces, can be troublesome	Improves

"I have been impressed with the urgency of doing. Knowing is not enough; we must apply. Being willing is not enough; we must do." **–Leonardo da Vinci**

Table 3: Clinical features of major subtypes of junctional epidermolysis bullosa (JEB).

Clinical features	*JEB, generalized severe*	*JEB, generalized Intermediate*	*JEB, localized*
Mode of transmission	AR	AR	AR
Onset	Birth	Birth	Birth
Skin distribution	Generalized	Generalized	Localized
Skin features	Blisters, milia, atrophic scarring, granulation tissue	Blisters, milia, scarring, granulation tissue absent or rarely present	Blisters, milia, no scarring, no granulation tissue
Other features	Scalp erosions, PPK absent	Diffuse nonscarring to scarring alopecia, focal PPK, EB nevi	Nail dystrophy
Extracutaneous features	Anemia, growth retardation, soft tissue abnormalities, enamel hypoplasia, caries, gastrointestinal tract involvement, genitourinary tract, ocular abnormalities, pseudosyndactyly, and delayed puberty	Anemia, growth retardation, soft tissue abnormalities, enamel hypoplasia, caries, gastrointestinal tract, and ocular not involved	Soft tissue abnormalities and excessive caries
Death	Common	Uncommon	None

(AR: autosomal recessive; PPK: palmoplantar keratoderma)

Table 4: Clinical features of major subtypes of DEB.

Clinical features	*DDEB, generalized*	*RDEB, severe generalized*	*RDEB, generalized intermediate*
Mode of transmission	AD	AR	AR
Onset	Birth	Birth	Birth
Skin distribution	Generalized, trunk, limbs, bony prominences	Generalized, frictional areas	Generalized
Skin findings			
Blisters	Follow sharp knocks rather than mild friction	Mildest trauma produces blister, erosions, and crusting	Milder, localized
Milia	Present	Constant feature	Present, not significant
Atrophic scarring	Present	Present	Present
Granulation tissue	Absent	Rare	Absent
Nail involvement	Dystrophy, scarring of nail bed, flexion contractures of fingers	Dystrophic	Dystrophic
Scalp abnormalities	Telogen effluvium	Scarring alopecia, decreased body hair	Scarring alopecia, less pronounced
Palms and soles (Keratoderma)	Absent	None	None
Other features	Albopapuloid lesions, congenital absence of skin	Pruritus present, flexion contractures at axillae, knees, elbows by adulthood, delayed puberty, dilated cardiomyopathy, decreased bone mineralization, bone pain, fracture of calcanei, vertebral bodies	None
Extracutaneous involvement			
Anemia	25%	Present	Less common
Growth retardation	Rare	Present, thin, and short stature	Less common
Oral cavity			
Soft tissue abnormalities	Mild	Ankyloglossia, microstomia, gums fragile, and tongue atrophic	Oral blisters
Enamel hypoplasia	Absent	Absent	Absent
Caries	Normal frequency	Excessive	Normal frequency
Gastrointestinal tract	Dysphagia, microstomia, constipation, and anal fissures	Constipation, dysphagia, fibrosis, stricture, and poor nutrition	Dysphagia and anal fissures

Continued

Continued

Clinical features	*DDEB, generalized*	*RDEB, severe generalized*	*RDEB, generalized intermediate*
Genitourinary tract	Rare	Urethral stenosis, urinary retention, postinfectious glomerulonephritis, hydronephrosis, renal amyloid, IgA nephropathy, and renal failure	Rare
Ocular findings	Absent	Symblepharon, limbal broadening, ectropion, pannus, and corneal opacities	Present, less common
Pseudosyndactyly	Rare	Present, mitten-like appearance of hands, feet in 90–100%	Rare
Respiratory tract	Absent		Absent
Malignancy			
SCC	Present in older patients	Multiple SCC by 35 years (67.8%), 90.1% by 55 years	SCC less common
Death	None	Death by third to forth decade	Death less common

(AD: autosomal dominant; AR: autosomal recessive; DDEB: dominant dystrophic epidermolysis bullosa; DEB: dystrophic epidermolysis bullosa; RDEB: recessive dystrophic epidermolysis bullosa; SCC: squamous cell carcinoma)

dressings are available which are said to have antibacterial activity thereby preventing secondary infections. Collagen-based dressings modify the cell kinetics and provide faster wound healing. Artificial skin substitutes are available in the form of dermal allograft and apligraft. Synthetically prepared skin products such as bioengineered skin products and biological dressings in the form of amniotic membranes are being increasingly used.

Gene Therapy

It implies the use of keratinocyte cultures from normal skin of affected patient. These cells are then propagated and transduced with a DNA-containing vector in culture and the corrected keratinocytes are allowed to grow in sheets, which are then grafted back to the affected site. However, the major limitation of this concept is the concern of carcinogenesis.

Protein Replacement Therapy

This concept makes use of recombinant proteins which are topically applied or injected or administered systemically. The goal is to replace the defective protein or replenish a missing protein. This concept has been successfully used in mice with recessive dystrophic epidermolysis bullosa (RDEB); however, the efficacy in human models is yet to be studied.

Cell-based Techniques

The latest attempts in molecular strategies revolve around the use of fibroblasts and stem cell therapy. Fibroblasts are artificially cultured and injected to the skin of the affected patients which results in increased collagen VII in cases of RDEB.

Bone Marrow Stem Cell Transfer

The rationale is the existing ability of bone marrow cells to differentiate into skin cells given the right microenvironment. It is hypothesized that in RDEB chronic skin injury generates a microenvironment that promotes the homing of bone marrow derived stem cells which can differentiate into skin cells, produce type VII collagen and restore the defective anchoring fibrils. Bone marrow transplant results in long-term survival and reversion of phenotype with normalization of basement membrane and formation of anchoring fibrils.

EPIDERMOLYSIS BULLOSA PRURIGINOSA (FIGS. 17 TO 19)

Epidermolysis bullosa pruriginosa (EBP) is an unusual clinical variant of dystrophic EB caused by mutation in *COL7A1* gene, which is responsible for encoding type VII collagen, a major structural component of anchoring fibrils at the dermoepidermal junction. It is inherited either as autosomal dominant or less commonly as autosomal recessive form. It presents either at birth, or during infancy, or childhood with mild acral blistering and erosions. In teenage years and in adults, it typically presents as severely pruritic, hypertrophic, and lichenified plaques or nodules, especially on the shins of tibia and

"When I stand before God at the end of my life, I would hope that I would not have a single bit of talent left and could say, I used everything you gave me."

–Erma Bombeck

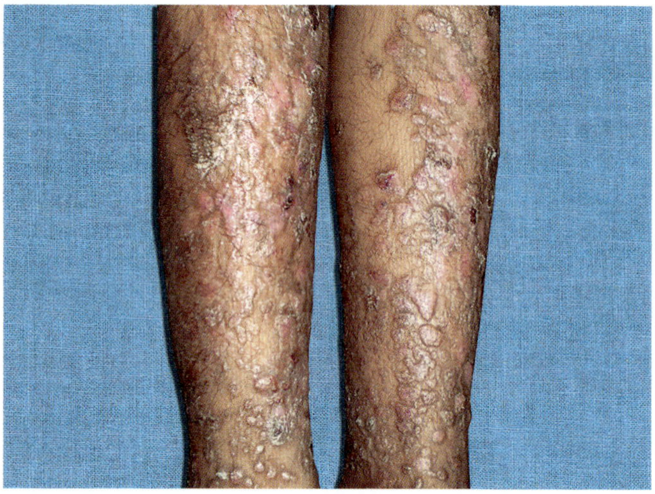

Fig. 17: Epidermolysis bullosa pruriginosa.

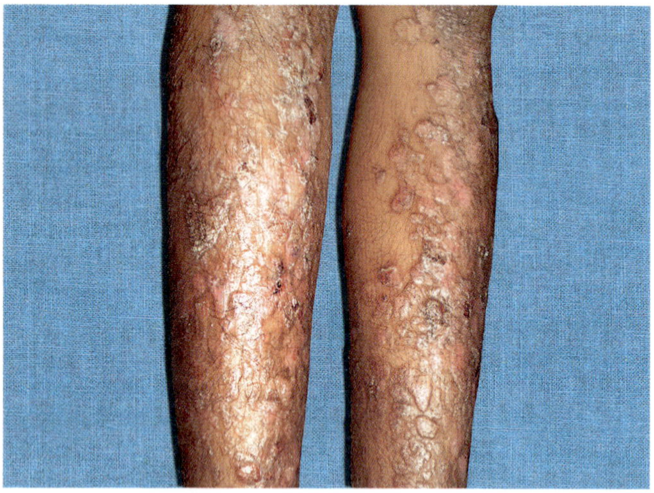

Fig. 18: Same patient, close-up view.

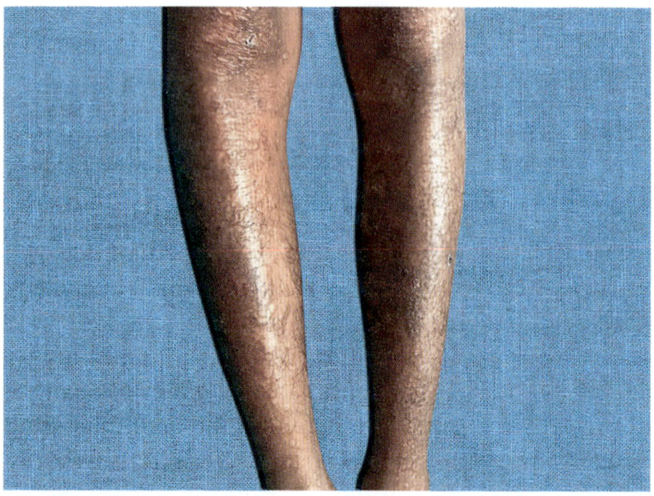

Fig. 19: Same patient, note excellent clearance after 6 months with oral acitretin treatment.

forearms with marked scarring. There is relative sparing of the face and flexures. The main characteristics of EBP include extremely pruritic linear lichenified or nodular prurigo-like lesions predominantly over legs, occasional trauma-induced blistering, excoriations, milia, nail dystrophy, and in some cases, albopapuloid lesions on the trunk. Pruritus may present either before or with the cutaneous manifestations. Flagellate scarring has also been reported. The exact cause of pruritus is unknown, but has been attributed to bradykinin interacting with other mediators. The exposure of type VII collagen might trigger the activation of the kinin cascade, thereby resulting in severe pruritus. Also, raised IgE levels reacting to environmental allergens could contribute to the severe itching sensation and scratching response.

Histopathology shows hyperkeratosis, mild acanthosis, disruption of the dermoepidermal junction with frank subepidermal blister formation in some areas, fibrosis, vascular proliferation, milia, and a lymphohistiocytic infiltrate. Ultrastructurally, there are alterations in the number and structure of anchoring fibrils in the lesional and perilesional skin consistent with a diagnosis of dystrophic EP. EBP has to be differentiated from lichen planus hypertrophicus, lichen simplex chronicus, cutaneous amyloidosis, Nekam's disease and dermatitis artefacta. Absence of intact blisters in most cases, prominent scars, and the marked lichenification with severe pruritus show overlap with these conditions. Presence of subepidermal cleft on histopathology rules out these conditions.

Diagnosis is based on characteristic clinical features, history of trauma-induced blistering, family history of similar cutaneous manifestations inherited in a dominant or recessive fashion, and a consistent histologic picture. Mutation analysis can be used to confirm the diagnosis.

There is no definite treatment to date and EBP is known to be resistant to various treatment modalities. Genetic counseling and gene therapy are the most promising approaches. Prenatal diagnosis can be done using fetal skin biopsy samples taken at 15–18 weeks of gestation. Rapid diagnosis may be possible by using LH 7:2 monoclonal antibody staining of skin samples obtained from 18 weeks fetus at risk. Symptomatic treatment is mainly aimed at controlling pruritus and halting the progression of cutaneous lesions and includes use of topical (corticosteroids and calcineurin inhibitors), intralesional (steroids) as well as systemic (antihistamines, cyclosporine, thalidomide, retinoids, naltrexone) drugs. Recently, dupilumab has also been used. Cryotherapy, topical ketamine 0.5%, amitriptyline 2% (KA) gel, and surgical modalities (dermabrasion, excision, and grafting) have also been tried.

PEMPHIGUS VULGARIS AND PEMPHIGUS FOLIACEUS (FIGS. 20 TO 25)

In pemphigus vulgaris (PV), erosions inside the mouth or tongue or blisters over the scalp precede widespread cutaneous lesions in >50% of children. Vesicles and bullae develop gradually over face, scalp, trunk, and extremities. The bullae may subsequently rupture to form large areas of erosions. Blisters heal insidiously without scarring. However, often they have a tendency to get secondarily infected. Pruritus, pain and burning of the skin and mucous membranes may be severe. On tangential pressure on

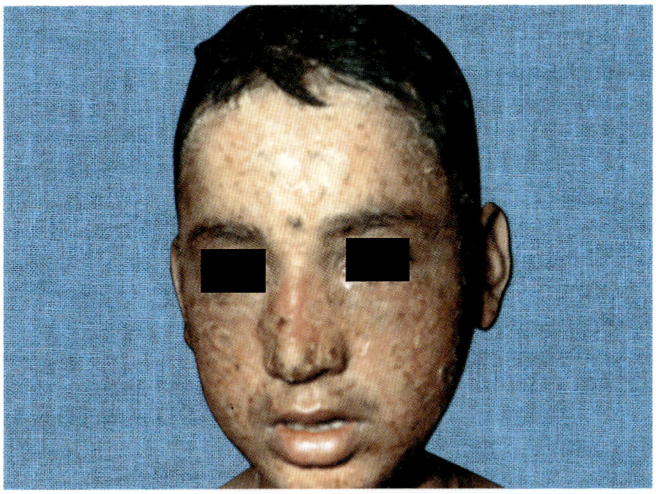

Fig. 22: Close-up view of face in another boy with pemphigus foliaceus.

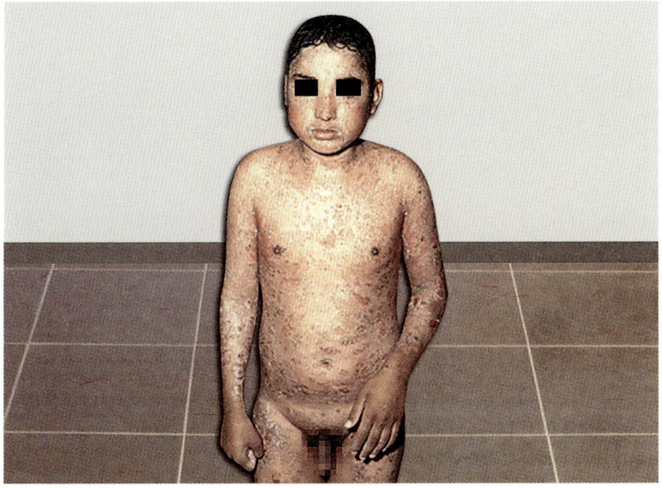

Fig. 20: Dried-up vesicles, crust and scab of pemphigus foliaceus, distributed over seborrheic areas.

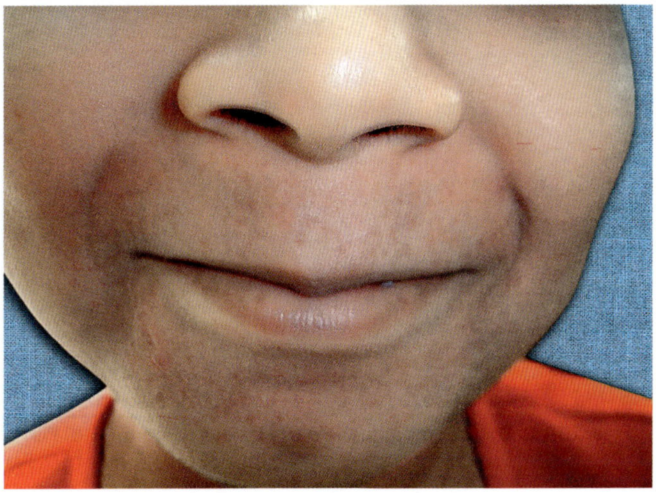

Fig. 23: A 6-year-old boy with pemphigus vulgaris, note facial erythema but no bulla/erosion.

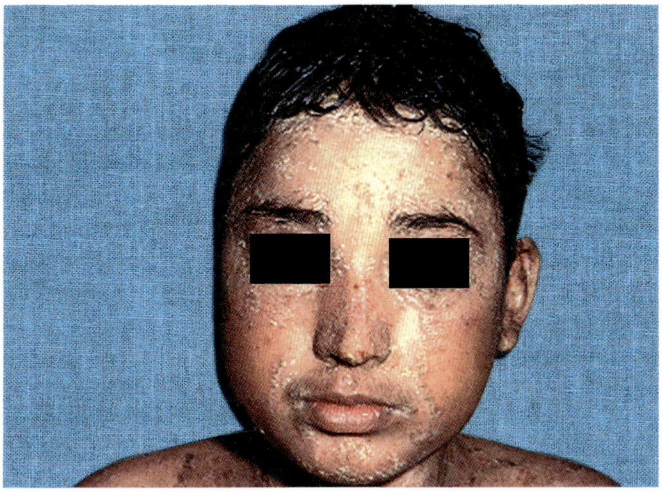

Fig. 21: Face of the same boy.

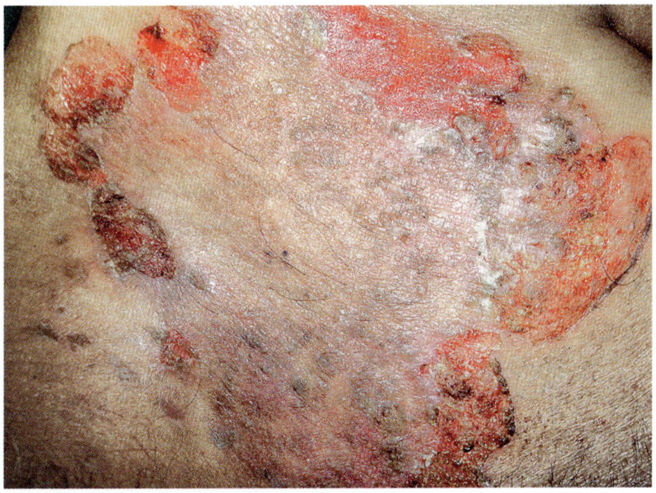

Fig. 24: Infected erosions.

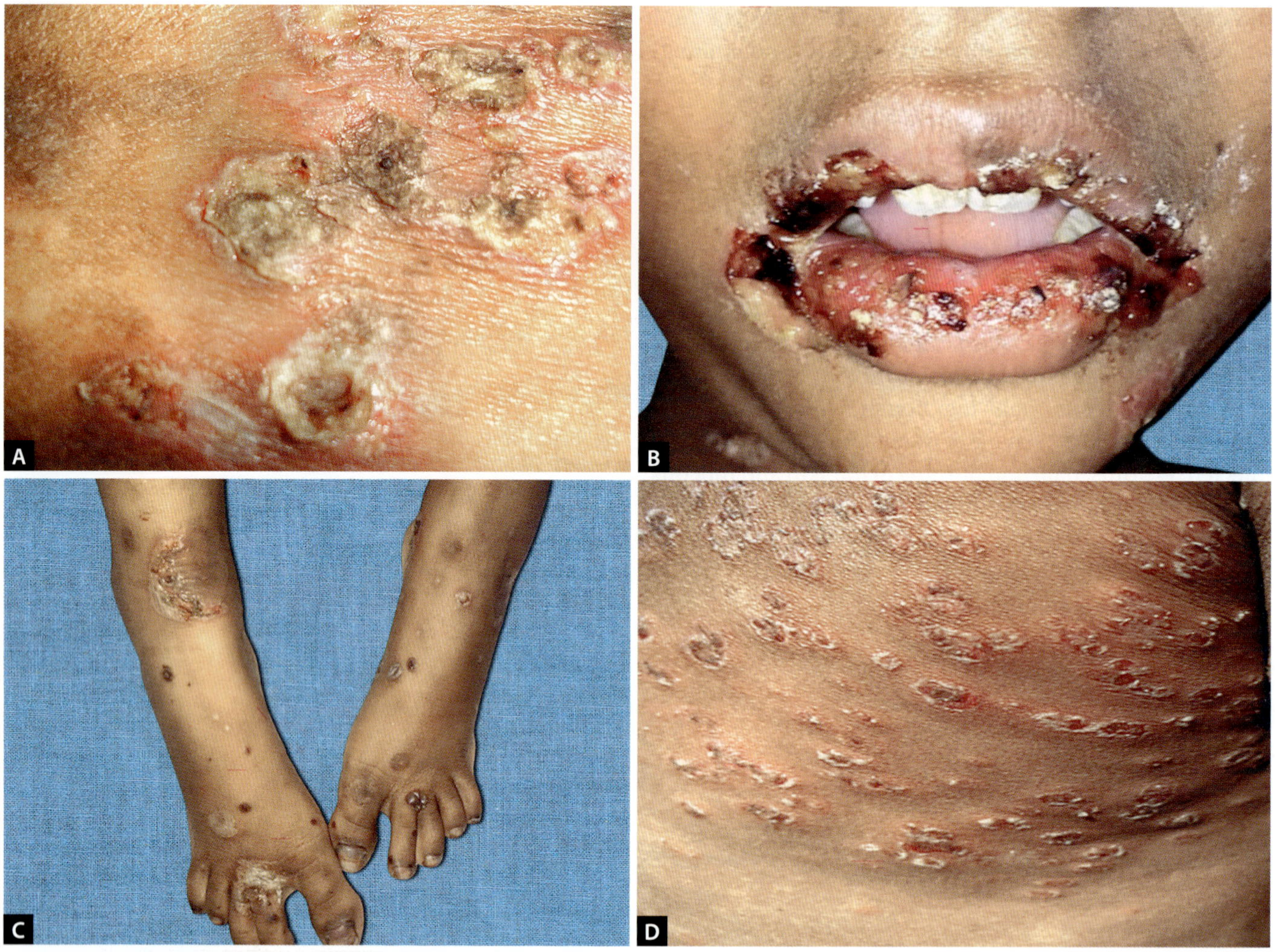

Figs. 25A to D: (A) Pemphigus vulgaris; lesions over trunk; (B) Pemphigus vulgaris in a 14-year-old boy; (C) Same boy with lesions over legs, note nail involvement; (D) Pemphigus foliaceus, close-up view.

the skin surrounding the blisters, the normal looking skin peels off like the peel of a boiled potato. This is known as Nikolsky's sign. The bullae are formed suprabasally as a result of acantholysis. There is deposition of IgG, IgM, and C3 in the intercellular spaces. Pemphigus foliaceus (PF), although rare in children, is a superficial and milder form of pemphigus in seborrheic distribution characterized by small flaccid bullae that rupture easily to form superficial shallow erosions. Oral lesions are rarely seen in PF.

Drug-induced Pemphigus

The incidence of drug-induced pemphigus reported in children is very rare. Drugs causing pemphigus can be divided into sulfhydryl containing or the thiol group and the non-thiol group. Drugs belonging to the thiol group such as penicillamine and captopril have a sulfhydryl group that is postulated to interact with the sulfhydryl groups in desmoglein 1 and 3, thus modifying the antigenicity of desmogleins. The non-thiol group drugs include ceftazidime, penicillin, rifampicin, and progesterone. Drug-induced pemphigus requires several months of exposure before the onset. It generally presents as nonspecific morbilliform, annular, or urticarial eruption which further progresses to form vesiculobullous lesions. Drug-induced pemphigus more often clinically resembles PF than PV. Oral lesions are rare. Treatment includes withdrawal of offending drug and initiation of oral steroids along with supportive measures.

Diagnosis

The clinical diagnosis is supported by histopathological examination of the skin biopsy specimen and confirmed by DIF testing. Circulating immune complexes may be picked up by indirect immunofluorescence testing (IIF). In both

"When I hear somebody sigh, 'Life is hard,' I am always tempted to ask, 'Compared to what?" **–Sydney Harris**

diseases, there is separation and destruction of epidermal cells called acantholysis. While in PF, the acantholysis is at granular cell layer with formation of subcorneal blisters, in PV, the separation is at suprabasal level with formation of suprabasal intraepidermal bullae. In both the conditions, there is deposition of IgG, IgM, and C3 in the intercellular spaces.

Treatment

Before the advent of corticosteroids, most of the patients with PV used to die of septicemia and related complications. Corticosteroids are given in high dosage (2–5 mg/kg/day) Subsequently, immunosuppressive, e.g., azathioprine or cyclophosphamide, may be added while tapering off the steroids once the severity of PV is brought under control. Pulse therapy of steroid using either methylprednisolone or dexamethasone along with cyclophosphamide has also been used successfully in the treatment of PV in children.

Pemphigus foliaceus usually follow a less severe course as compared to PV. It may be treated successfully with dapsone 1–2 mg/kg/day. If dapsone fails, oral corticosteroids may be used, but at a much lower dosage (1–2 mg/kg/day) for shorter duration than PV. Immunosuppressives are usually not required. For localized lesions, moderately potent or potent topical corticosteroids may prove useful. For both PV and PF, oral antistaphylococcal antibiotics may be required from time to time, since the skin erosions may get secondarily infected mostly by *S. aureus*.

SUBCORNEAL PUSTULAR DERMATOSES (FIGS. 26 TO 29)

It is a rare, chronic, vesicopustular disease characterized by exacerbation and remission and chiefly affects middle-aged women.

However, occasionally, it can affect adolescent boys and girls also. Pathogenesis is poorly understood. Cytokines such as interleukin 8 (IL-8), tumor necrosis factor-alpha (TNF-α) liberated from keratinocytes and monocytes may have some role in neutrophilic activation. Some cases are reported to be associated with monoclonal gammopathy.

Clinically, the disease is characterized by crops of small, flaccid, superficial pustules on an erythematous or normal base and arranged in a serpiginous or annular pattern. Lesions are chiefly distributed over axilla, groin, abdomen, inframammary region, and flexor aspect of limbs. Palms, soles, face, and mucous membranes are usually spared. Within a few days, lesions resolve with thin, dry, superficial crust. Healed lesions may leave some residual hyperpigmentation without atrophy or scarring. Patient may complain of mild pruritus but systemic symptoms are characteristically absent.

Histopathology reveals subcorneal pustules filled with polymorphonuclear leukocytes. Though acantholytic cells are usually absent, some of the older lesions show acantholytic cells near the base. Spongiform pustules may be noted in the upper epidermis. Though negative immunofluorescence is the usual feature, some cases are found to be associated with intercellular IgA staining in the upper epidermis. Pustules are sterile on bacterial culture.

Differentiation between subcorneal pustular dermatoses (SCPD) and impetigo can be made by

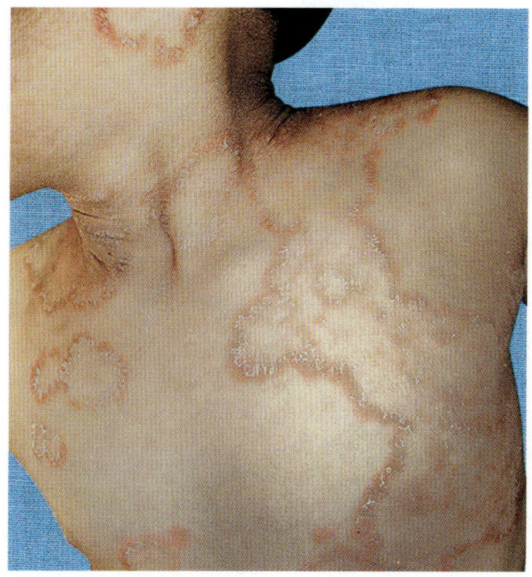

Fig. 26: Subcorneal pustular dermatoses in a 7-year-old boy.

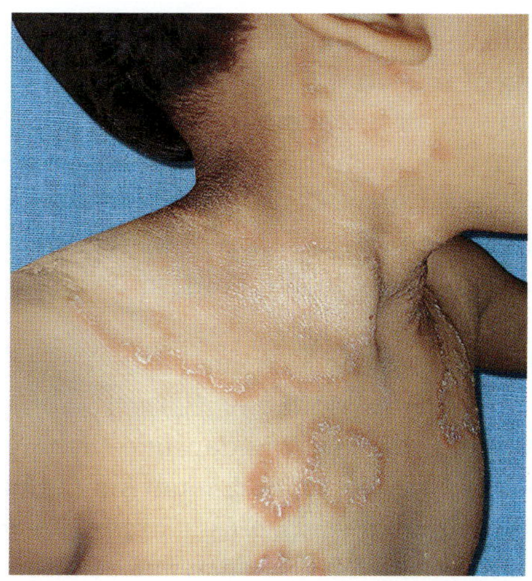

Fig. 27: Annular scaly lesions of subcorneal pustular dermatoses.

"Everything has beauty, but not everyone can see." **–Confucius**

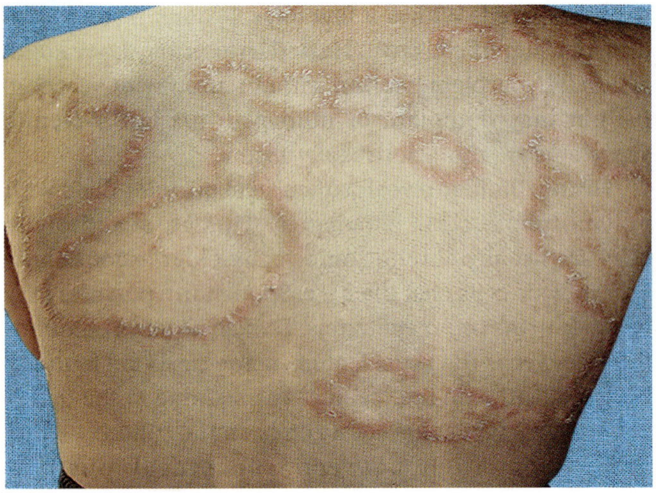

Fig. 28: Same boy, lesions over back.

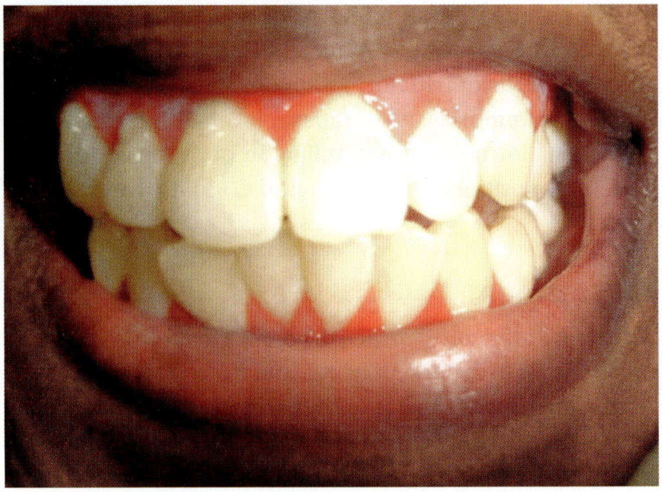

Fig. 30: Desquamative gingivitis in an 18-year-old girl (was diagnosed as bullous pemphigoid after gum biopsy).

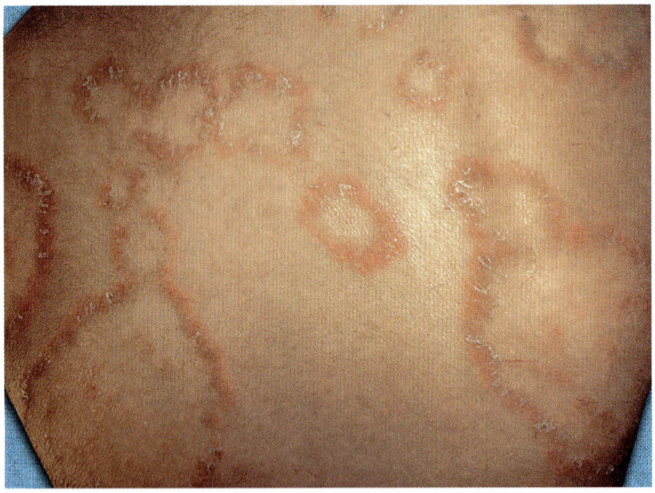

Fig. 29: Close-up view of subcorneal pustular dermatoses lesions.

negative culture of the former and excellent response to antibiotics of the latter. Findings favoring diagnosis of subcorneal type of IgA pemphigus and PF are abundant acantholytic cells in histopathology and positive immunofluorescence. Generalized pustular psoriasis can be diagnosed by presence of systemic symptoms, spongiform pustules in the epidermis, and failure to respond to sulfones.

Localized cases may be treated with topical steroids. Drug of choice is dapsone (50–200 mg). Sulfapyridine is also very effective. During dapsone therapy, regular monitoring of complete blood count should be kept in mind. Other modalities such as acitretin, narrow band UVB therapy, colchicine, biologics, and azithromycin can be tried.

DESQUAMATIVE GINGIVITIS (FIG. 30)

Desquamative gingivitis is a descriptive term for nonspecific gingival manifestation associated with different diseases. Different types of mucocutaneous disorders represent gingival manifestations as either desquamative lesions or in the form of gingival ulceration. Some diseases which present with DG are: Lichen planus, pemphigoid, pemphigus, erythema multiforme as well as allergic stomatitis and psoriasis vulgaris.

The classical features in making a clinical diagnosis of DG: Erythema of gingiva not caused by dental plaque, desquamation of gingiva, other intraoral and sometimes extraoral lesions, and mouth soreness due to spicy food items.

INSECT BITE REACTION (PAEDERUS DERMATITIS) (FIGS. 31 TO 34)

Paederus dermatitis or "blister beetle dermatitis" is a peculiar irritant contact dermatitis characterized by erythematous and bullous lesions of sudden onset predominantly on exposed areas of the body. A very unique feature of blister beetle dermatitis is "kissing lesions" over two adjacent areas of any flexural fold. The lesions are erythematous or edematous which may be linear, giving a whiplash appearance. Usually, there is severe burning or stinging sensation and children refer to it as "feeling of acid/alkali burn" typically. A venomous insect can produce a hemorrhagic large blister on the site of sting or contact. The condition is treated with use of oral antihistamines, topical corticosteroids, and in severe cases, a short course (3–5 days) of oral corticosteroid can be tried. Oral antibiotics have no role.

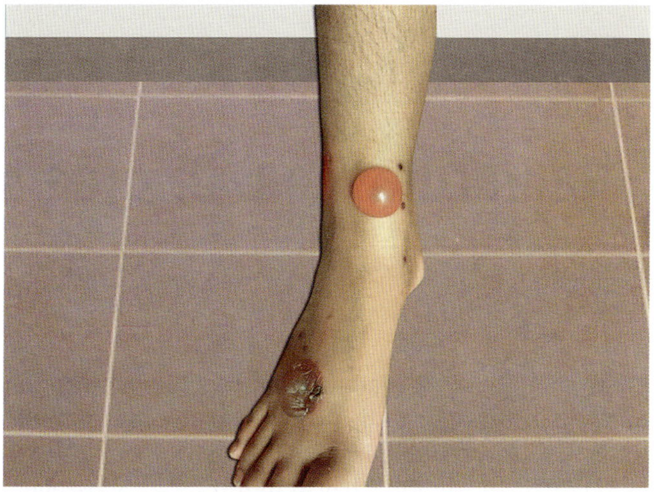

Fig. 31: Insect bite blister.

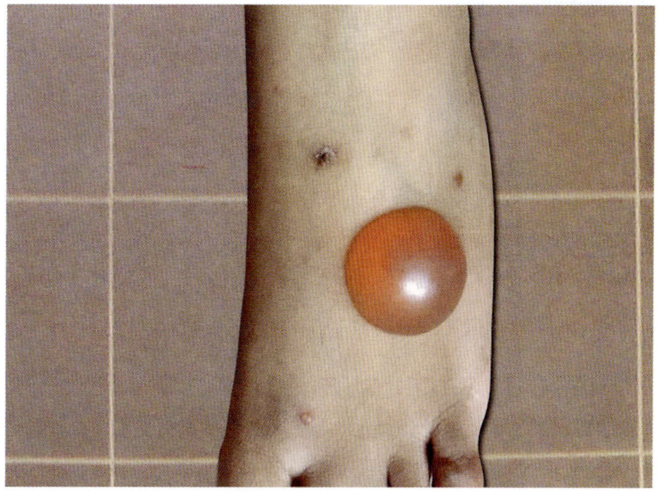

Fig. 32: Close-up view.

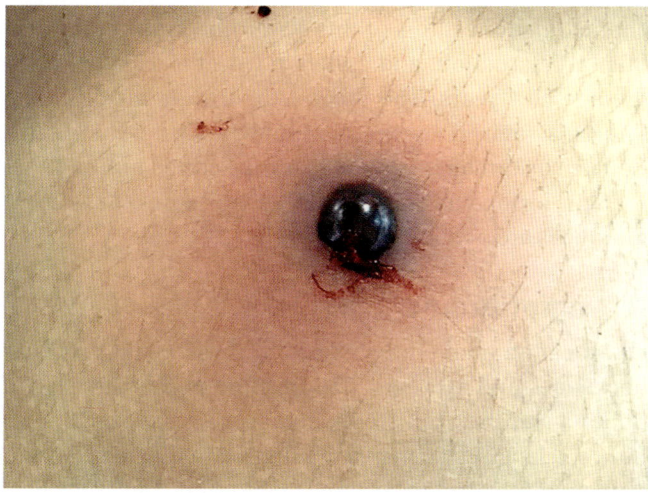

Fig. 33: Hemorrhagic blister from bite of a venomous insect.

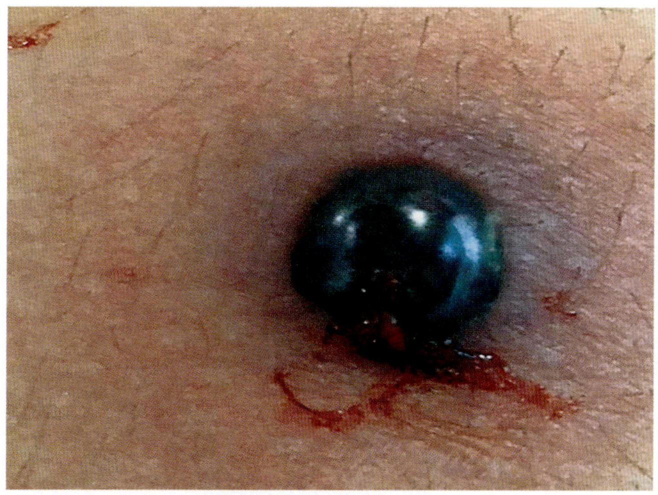

Fig. 34: Close-up view.

WHAT'S NEW?

- In a recent study conducted in Northern part of India, Pemphigus vulgaris was found to be the most common autoimmune bullous disorder in children.
- Rituximab, an anti-CD20 monoclonal antibody which is the first line treatment modality in adults, in combination with corticosteroids has shown better results compared to other modalities.

SUGGESTED READINGS

1. Bruckner Tuderman L. Newer treatment modalities in epidermolysis bullosa. Indian Dermatol Online J. 2019;10(3): 24450.
2. Has C, Bauer JW, Bodemer C, MC Bolling, L Bruckner-Tuderman, A Diem et al. Consensus re-classification of inherited epidermolysis bullosa and other disorders with skin fragility Br J Dermatol. 2020 Oct;183(4):614-27.
3. Peterman CM, Vadeboncoeur S, Schmidt BA, Gellis SE. Pediatric pemphigus herpetiformis: case report and review of the literature. Pediatr Dermatol. 2017;34(3):3426.
4. Mahajan R, Handa S, Kumar S, Chatterji D, Saikia UN, De D. Pediatric autoimmune blistering disorders - a five-year demographic profile and therapy experience. Int J Dermatol. 2022;61(12):1511-8.
5. Goyal T, Varshney A, Bakshi SK. Incidence of Vesicobullous and Erosive Disorders of Neonates: Where and How Much to Worry? Indian J Pediatr. 2021;88(6):574-8.
6. Karmakar S, Basu K, Sengupta M, Chatterjee G, Sarkar S, Bandopadhyay M. Genetic and acquired blistering disorders of pediatric age group: An experience from Eastern India. Indian J Pathol Microbiol. 2021;64(3):509-17.

"When I was 5 years old, my mother always told me that happiness was the key to life. When I went to school, they asked me what I wanted to be when I grew up. I wrote down "happy". They told me I didn't understand the assignment, and I told them they didn't understand life." **–John Lennon**

CHAPTER 10

Neurocutaneous Disorders

TUBEROUS SCLEROSIS COMPLEX (BOURNEVILLE DISEASE, EPILOIA) (FIGS. 1 TO 6)

This represents a genetic disorder of hamartoma formation in many organs such as the skin, brain, eye, kidney, and heart. It is an autosomal dominant disorder and initial linkage studies showed that about half the tuberous sclerosis complex (TSC) families were linked to 9q34 (*TSC1*) and the other half to 16p13 (*TSC2*). Subsequent mutational analysis has shown *TSC1* mutations in 10–20% of affected individuals and *TSC2* mutations in 80–90%. The characteristic features of this syndrome are skin lesions, mental retardation, and epilepsy. Onset is usually before the age of 5 years. The diagnostic criteria for tuberous sclerosis revised by the National Institutes of Health Consensus Conference in 1998 are described in **Box 1**.

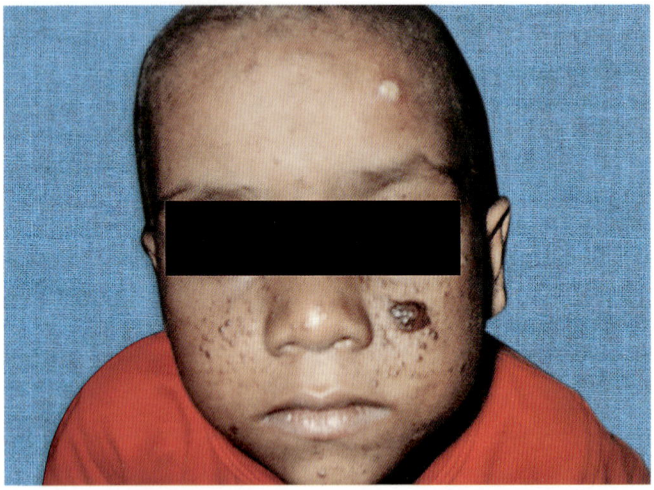

Fig. 1: Adenoma sebaceum over the face.

Skin lesions are seen in 60–70% of cases. Lesions of four types are pathognomonic.

Angiofibroma

Often called adenoma sebaceum, these usually appear between 3 and 10 years, and become more extensive at puberty and then remain unchanged. Firm, discrete, red-brown, telangiectatic papules, 1–10 mm in diameter, extend from the nasolabial folds to the cheeks and chin. They may be numerous and conspicuous. They may be overlooked, when confined to a small area on each side of the nose or chin.

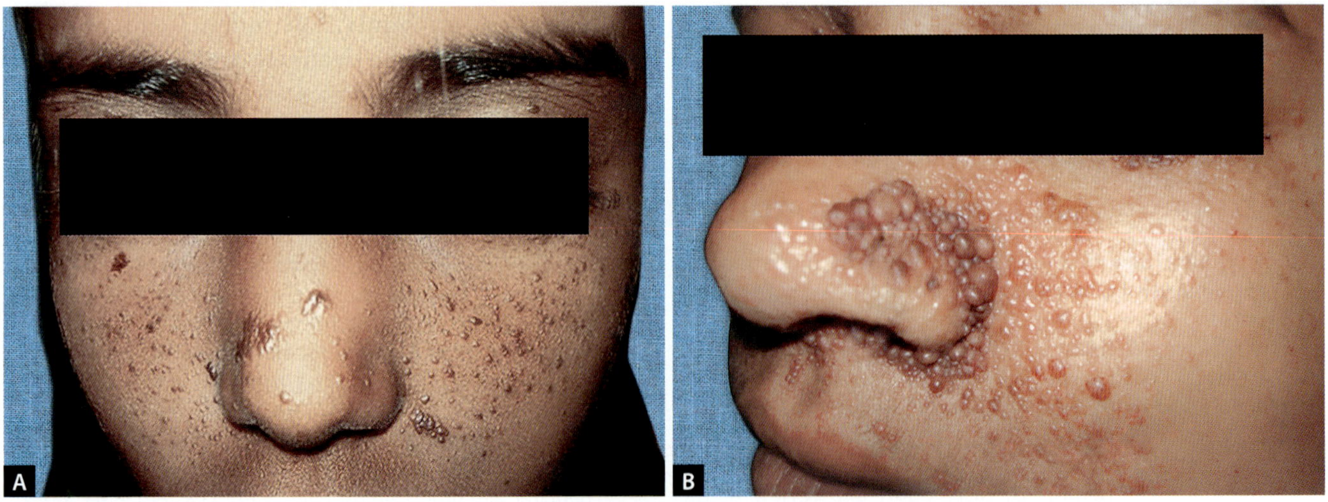

Figs. 2A and B: (A) A full blown case of epiloia with angiofibroma over face; (B) Classical angiofibroma (adenoma sebaceum).

"Every great dream begins with a dreamer. Always remember, you have within you the strength, the patience, and the passion to reach for the stars to change the world." —**Harriet Tubman**

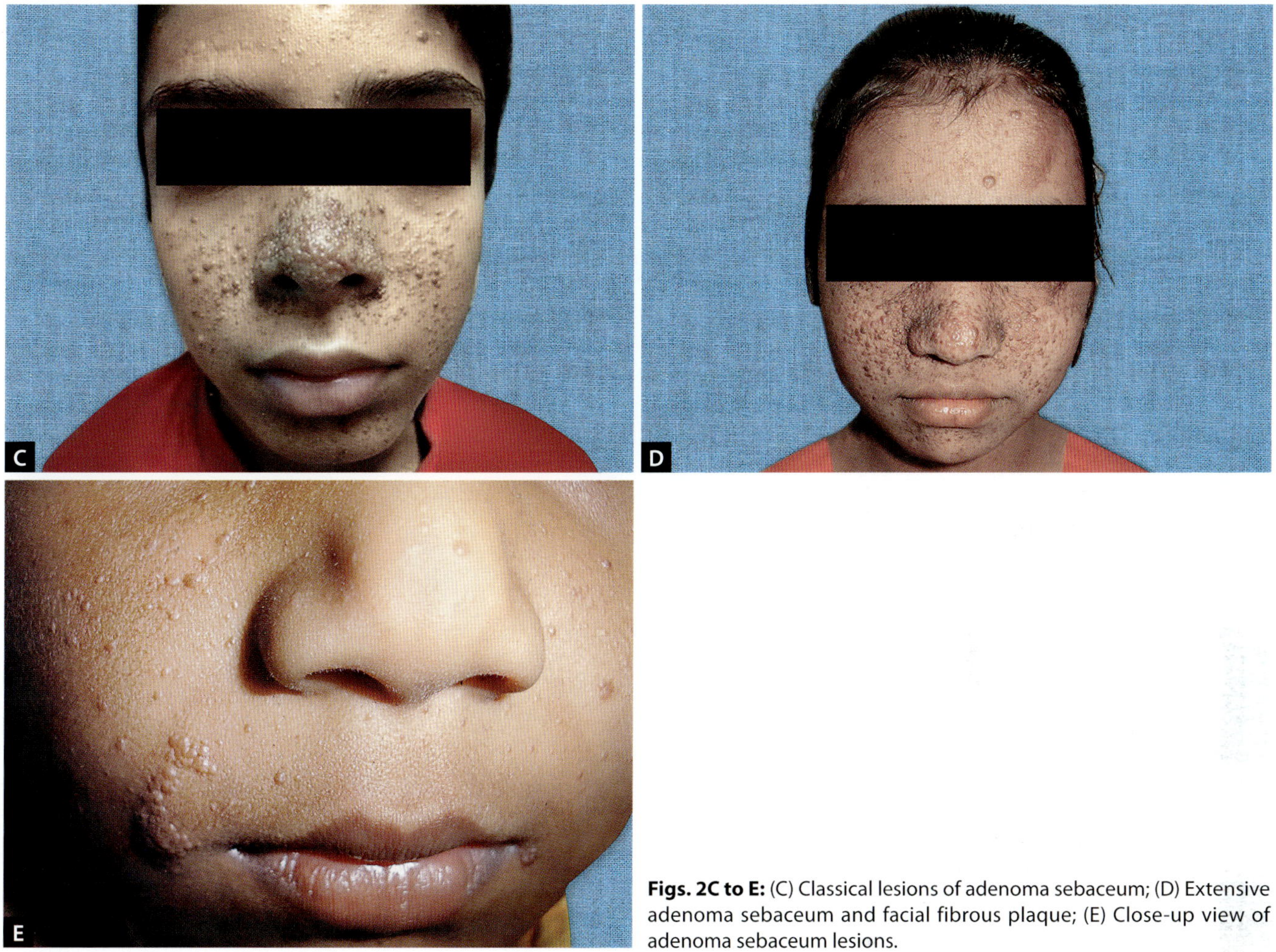

Figs. 2C to E: (C) Classical lesions of adenoma sebaceum; (D) Extensive adenoma sebaceum and facial fibrous plaque; (E) Close-up view of adenoma sebaceum lesions.

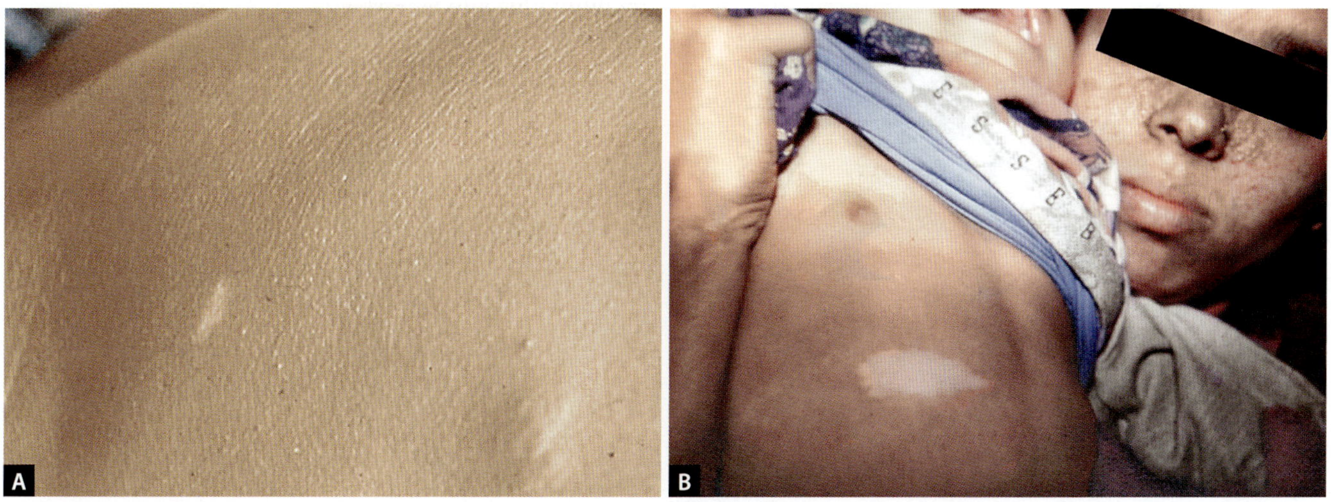

Figs. 3A and B: (A) Shagreen patch and ash leaf macule over back; (B) Adenoma sebaceum in mother and ash leaf macule in child.

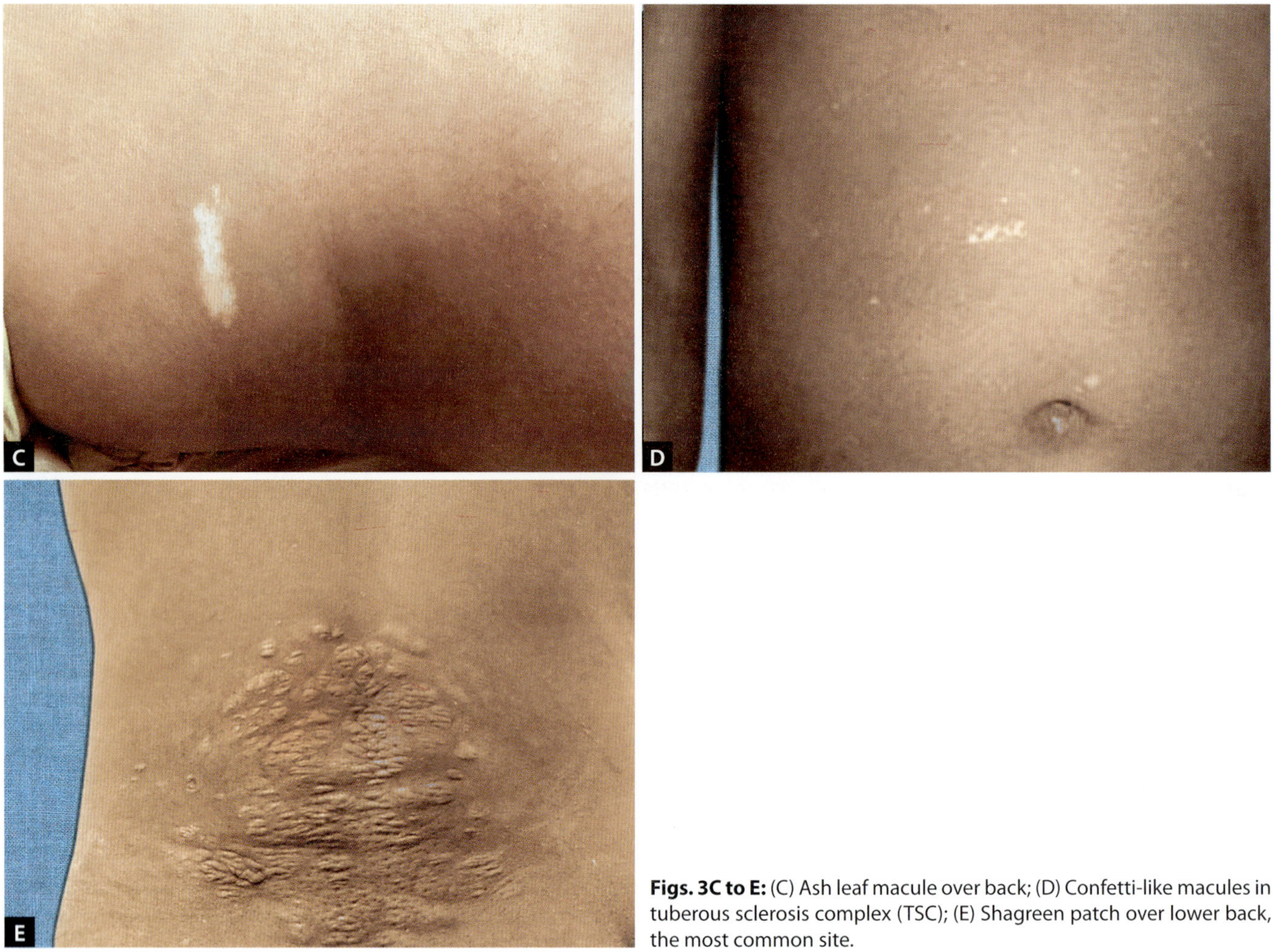

Figs. 3C to E: (C) Ash leaf macule over back; (D) Confetti-like macules in tuberous sclerosis complex (TSC); (E) Shagreen patch over lower back, the most common site.

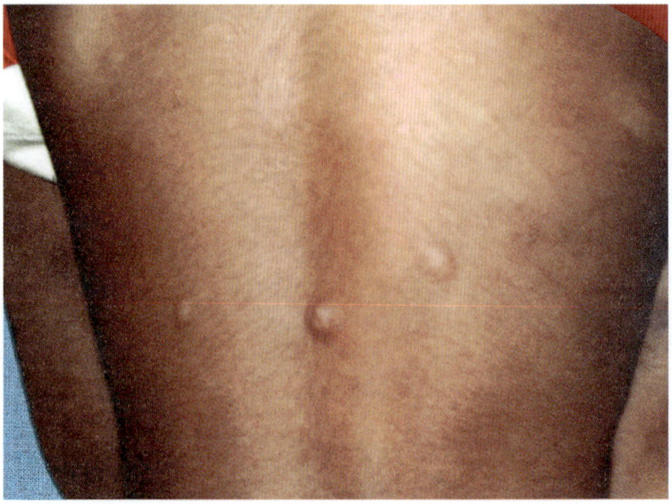

Fig. 4: Collagenoma or Shagreen patches over back.

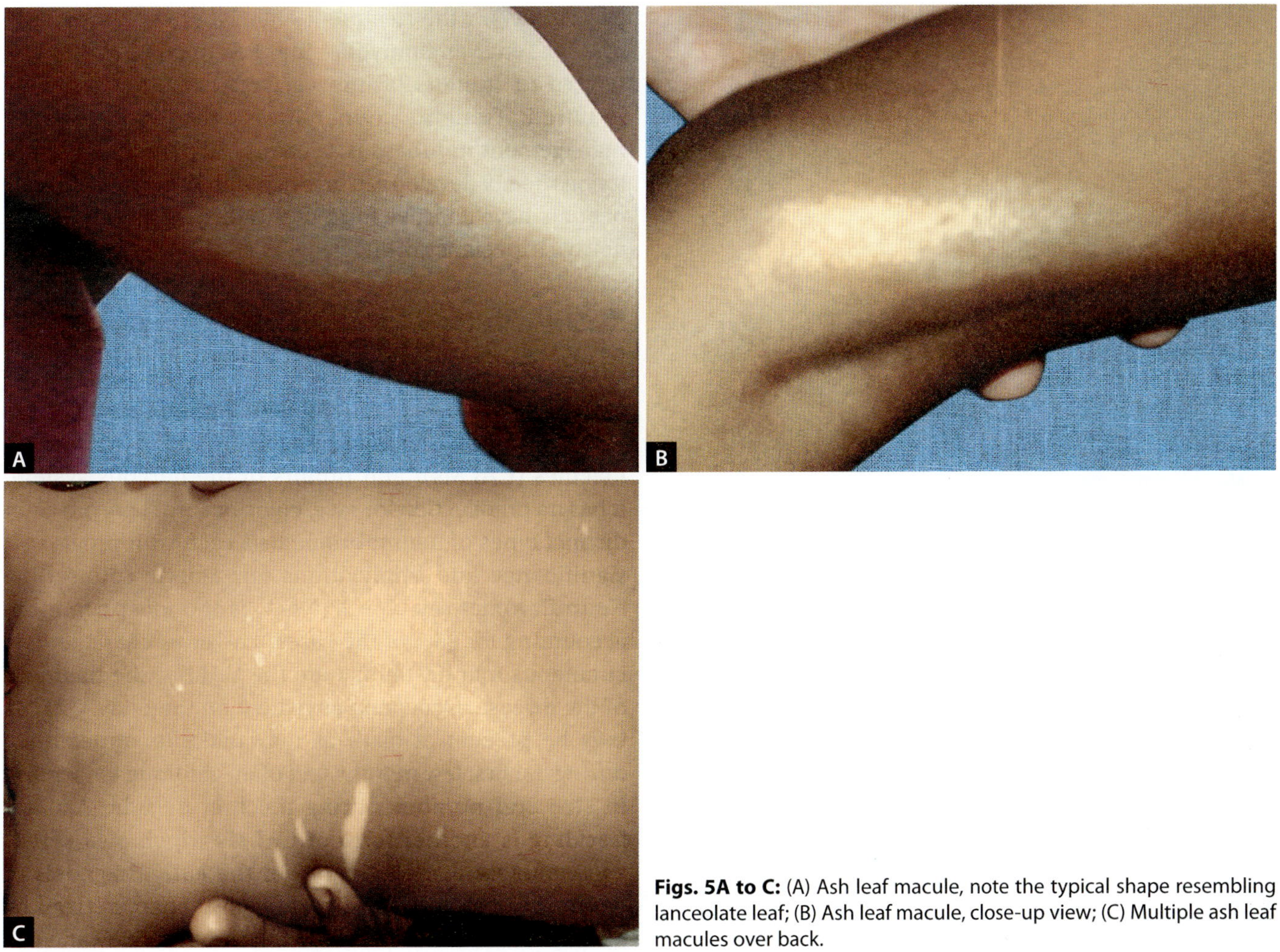

Figs. 5A to C: (A) Ash leaf macule, note the typical shape resembling lanceolate leaf; (B) Ash leaf macule, close-up view; (C) Multiple ash leaf macules over back.

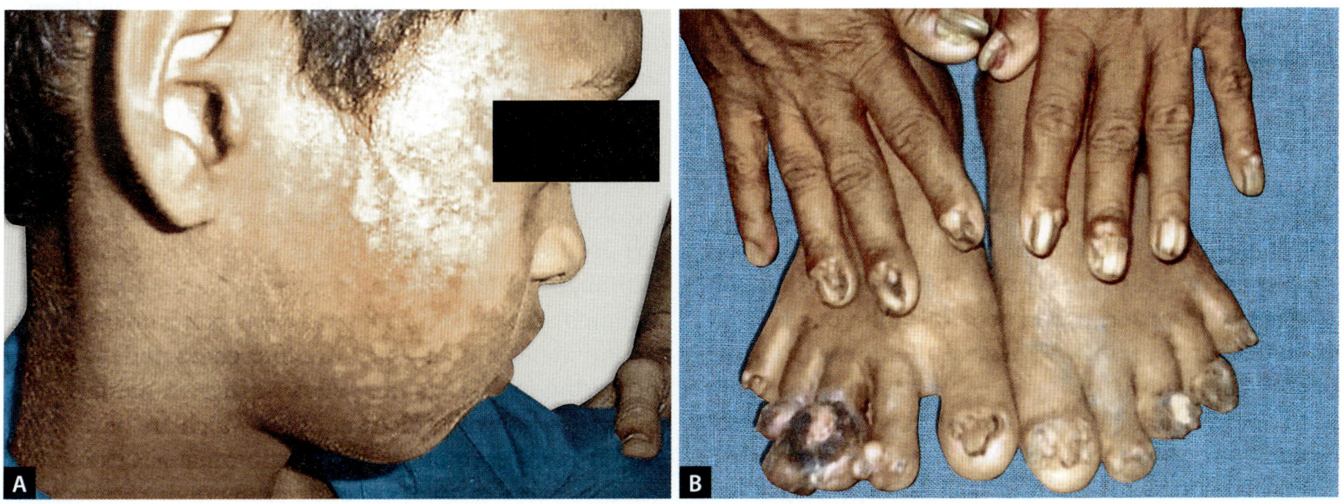

Figs. 6A and B: (A) Hypopigmented macules of tuberous sclerosis; (B) Periungual fibroma or Koenen's tumor.

"Faith gives us strength and reassurance and leaves us bathed in the wisdom that we are never alone." —**Debbie Ford**

Box 1 Diagnostic criteria of tuberous sclerosis.

Major features:
- Hypopigmented macules (≥5 mm across) (≥3)
- Angiofibroma (>3) or fibrous cephalic plaque
- Shagreen patch (connective tissue nevus)
- Ungual fibroma
- Cortical dysplasia
- Subependymal nodules
- Subependymal giant-cell astrocytoma
- Cardiac rhabdomyoma
- Multiple retinal hamartomas
- Angiomyolipomas (≥2)
- Lymphangioleiomyomatosis

Minor features:
- Confetti skin lesions
- Intraoral fibromas
- Dental enamel pits (more than 3 is suggestive)
- Multiple renal cysts
- Nonrenal hamartomas
- Retinal achromic patch

Definite diagnosis: 2 major OR 1 major + ≥2 minor features OR presence of a *tuberous sclerosis complex 1 (TSC1/TSC2 mutation of confirmed pathogenicity)*

Possible diagnosis: Either 1 major feature OR ≥2 minor features

Periungual Fibromas

These appear at or after puberty as smooth, firm flesh-colored excrescences emerging from the nail-folds. They are usually 5–10 mm in length, but may be very large.

Shagreen Patch

This presents as an irregularly thickened, slightly elevated, soft, skin colored, plaque usually over the lumbo-sacral region.

Ash Leaf Macules

These white macules, 1–3 cm in length, most easily detectable by examination under Wood's light, are frequently present on the trunk or limbs. This valuable sign may be found at birth or in early infancy, some years before the other signs of the disease develop and may suggest the diagnosis in infants with convulsions.

Seizure disorders associated with tuberous sclerosis often respond to anticonvulsant therapy. Death may result from status epilepticus, pulmonary or renal insufficiency, cardiac failure, etc. Adenoma sebaceum is a cosmetic problem and may be removed by electrosurgery, cryosurgery, dermabrasion, or laser therapy. Application of low-dose topical rapamycin (0.003–0.015%) over facial angiofibromas has shown good results. Currently Food and Drug Administration (FDA) has approved topical everolimus for the treatment of facial angiofibroma and oral for renal angiomyolipoma. For relief of symptoms related to tumors of internal organs, surgery may be required. Genetic counseling is the main stay of management in tuberous sclerosis. All patients with skin lesions do not develop seizures or mental retardation. Many patients have abortive form of this disease and may have normal expectancy of life.

NEUROFIBROMATOSIS AND CAFÉ-AU-LAIT MACULES (FIGS. 7 TO 8C)

Neurofibromatosis is an autosomal dominant disorder characterized by cutaneous pigmentation [café-au-lait macules (CALMs)] and tumors of the nervous system. It has no predilection for race, color, or sex. There are eight distinct types of neurofibromatosis each with prognostic significance and implications for genetic counseling. Neurofibromatosis type 1 (NF-1) is the most common, accounting for 85% of the cases. The most characteristic cutaneous manifestations are the CALMs, the hallmark of the disease. Occurring anywhere on the body, CALMs may be present at birth or may make its appearance during the first few months and often continue to increase in size and number during the first decade. Axillary freckling is another form of CALMs which also serves as a valuable diagnostic tool in the early diagnosis of neurofibromatosis. The disease is also characterized by dermal and subcutaneous neurofibromas of Schwann cell origin derived from peripheral nerve sheaths.

These cutaneous tumors usually appear in the late childhood or adolescence. They vary in number from a few to hundreds with a progressive increase in the size and number with increasing age. They may appear as superficial tumors 1–2 mm to several centimeters in diameter or as discrete beaded, nodules, elongated masses along the course of the nerves. Plexiform neurofibromas involve deeply located large nerves, may reach enormous proportions, and have a bag of worm consistency. Although, most of these tumors are benign, some may undergo malignant transformation, which is however, rare before the age of 40 years. Another characteristic lesion occurring in NF-1 is the yellowish-brown hamartomas on the iris known as Lisch nodules, which are best visible on slit-lamp examination. Neurofibromatosis eventually leads to some form of systemic problem or compromise before the age of 20 years. The severity and progression is however variable and the cutaneous involvement is not indicative of the extent of the disease in other organs.

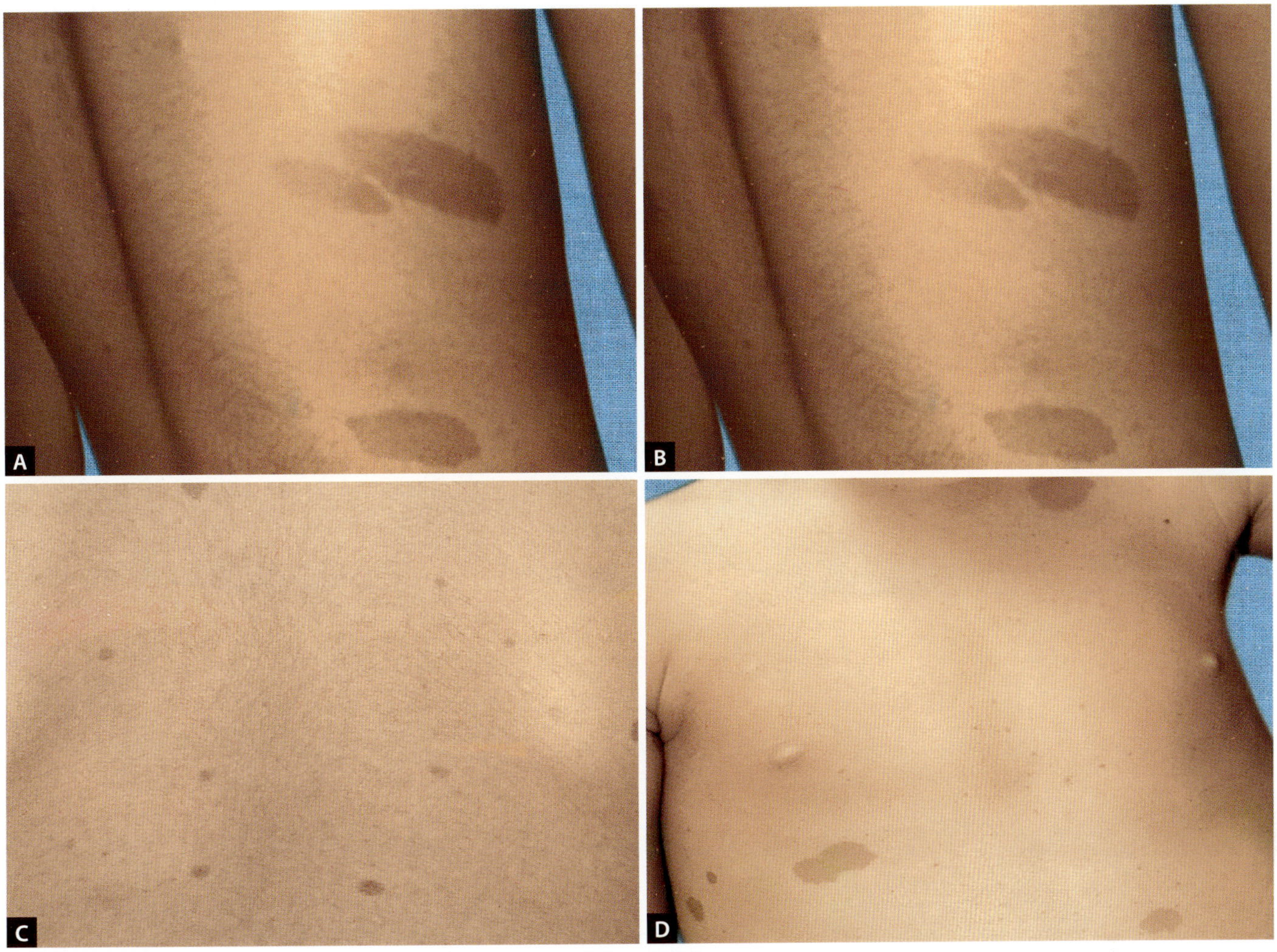

Figs. 7A to D: (A) Café-au-lait macules of neurofibromatosis, note regular border of macules; (B) Large café-au-lait macules suggestive of neurofibromatosis (NF); (C) Multiple small café-au-lait macules; (D) Café-au-lait macules, small sized and few in number.

Various systemic associations with NF-1 reported are rickets, pheochromocytoma and juvenile myelomonocytic leukemia. Neurologic manifestations occur in 40% of the patients. Acoustic neuromas and optic gliomas are the most common lesions of the cranial nerves. Mental retardation, seizures, and tumors are the neurologic manifestations of neurofibromatosis. Skeletal defects include scoliosis, kyphosis, pseudoarthrosis of forearm or leg bones and sphenoid dysplasia. The diagnostic criteria for NF-1 are described in **Box 2**.

Legius Syndrome

It is an NF-1-like syndrome characterized by multiple CALMs with or without axillary or inguinal freckling. Other NF-1 specific features such as Lisch nodules, optic gliomas, neurofibromas, associated bony changes and malignant peripheral nerve sheath tumors are absent in this condition.

Plexiform Neurofibroma (Figs. 8D to F)

Plexiform neurofibromas are essentially pathognomonic for NF-1. Plexiform neurofibromas occur in up to 30% of cases of NF-1, most frequently in the craniomaxillofacial region. These almost always develop during childhood. Neurofibromas arise from multiple nerves as bulging and deforming masses involving connective tissue and skin folds. The clinical description of lesions is called as "bags of worms." Large tumors are attached to major nerve trunks in neck or extremities. Histopathology shows hypocellularity with myxoid background, containing Schwann cells, fibroblasts, and mast cells. These stain positive with S100.

"Knowledge is life with wings." —**William Blake**

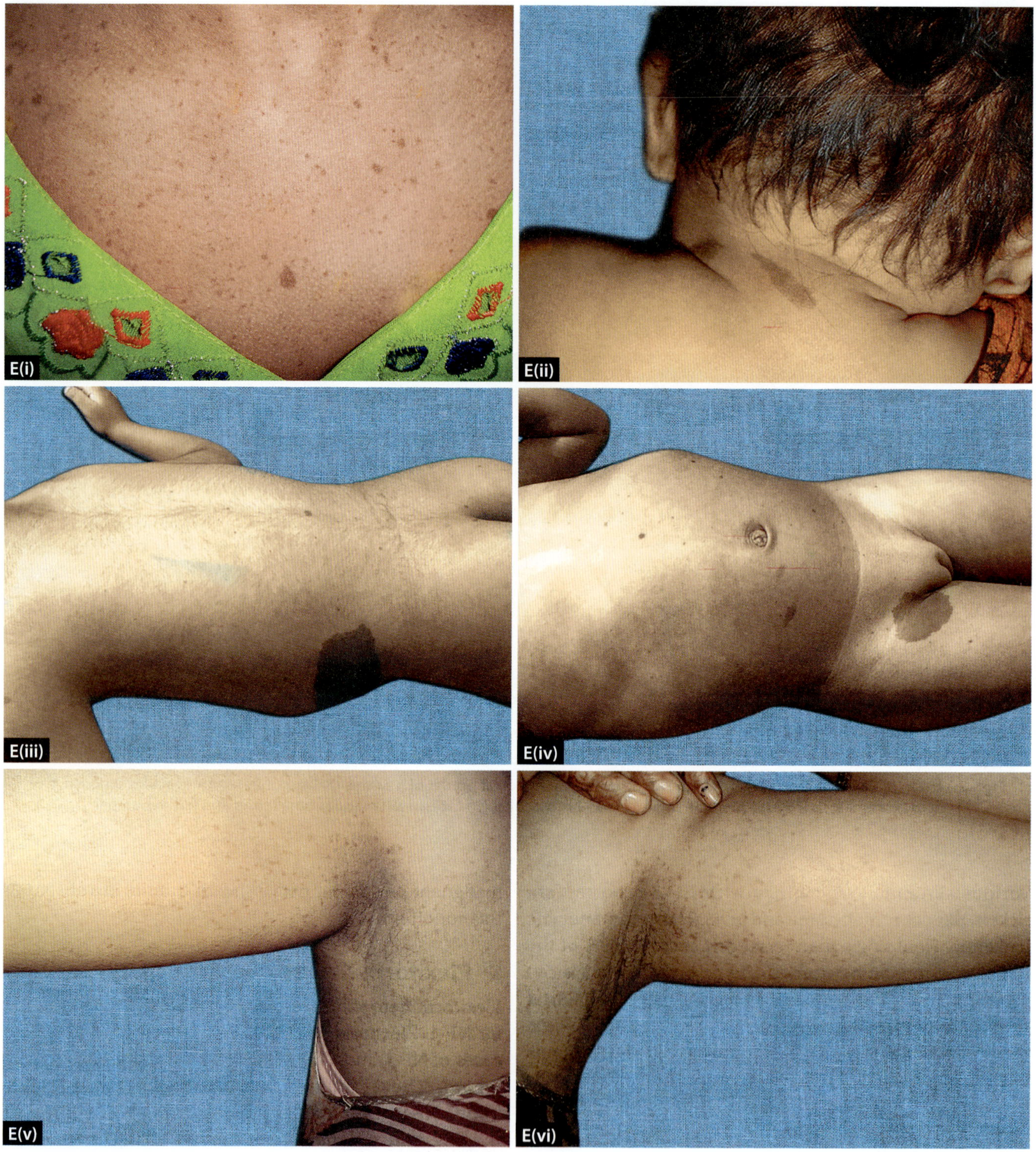

Figs. 7E(i) to (vi): E(i) Café-au-lait macule, multiple but very small sized; E(ii) Café-au-lait macule in a newborn; E(iii) Café-au-lait macule, both large and small macules; E(iv) Same child, front view; E(v) Axillary freckling, an important feature of neurofibromatosis type 1 (NF-1); E(vi) Same patient, another view.

These neurofibromas tend to transform to malignant peripheral nerve sheath tumors (MPNSTs) in some cases. Malignant progression is generally considered the main cause of mortality. Therapy for plexiform neurofibromas is usually surgical, aiming at resecting deforming masses and cancerous tissue when malignant transformation

"If you have knowledge, let others light their candles in it." **—Margaret Fuller**

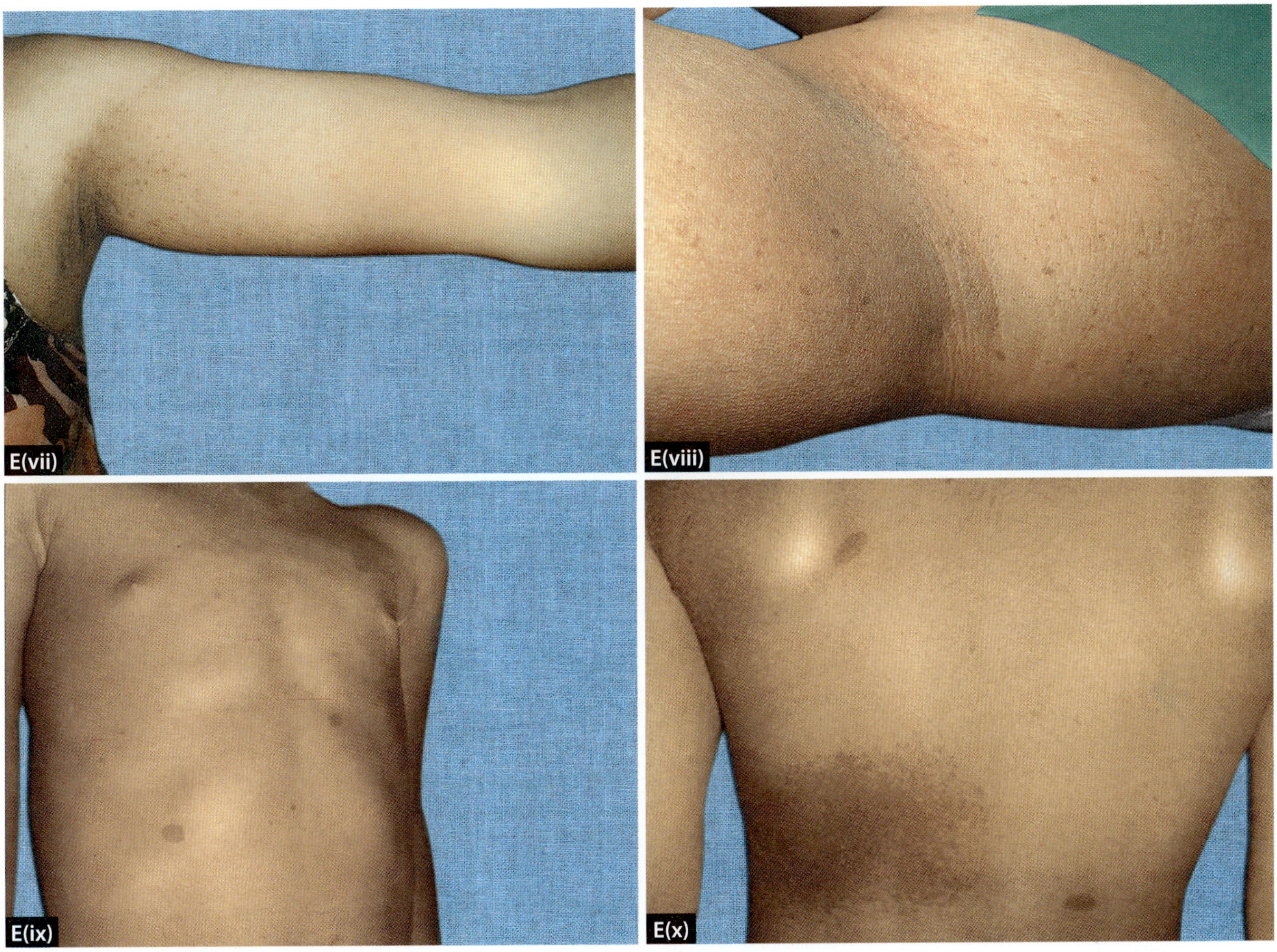

Figs. 7E(vii) to (x): E(vii) Same patient, close-up view; E(viii) Axillary freckling; E(ix) Café-au-lait macule of neurofibromatosis; E(x) Same patient, back view.

occurs. However, these masses tend to recur in 20% of cases despite an appropriate approach. In unresectable cases, administration of interferon-α may show good result.

Management

Since many patients have minor or incomplete forms, reassurance for the parents and children affected with mild form is helpful. Treatment of the cutaneous tumors comprises of surgical excision. Dermabrasion is targeted toward removal of the tumors which are either disfiguring or interfere with the function or are subject to irritation. Genetic counseling is important.

McCUNE–ALBRIGHT SYNDROME (FIGS. 9A TO C)

McCune-Albright syndrome consists of cafe-au-lait macules, polyostotic fibrous dysplasia, endocrine dysfunction, sexual precocity, and precocious somatic development, especially in girls. In this disorder, the pigmented lesions are few, light-to-dark brown, usually large and unilateral, frequently have a jagged irregular border (resembling the coast of Maine), and generally stop abruptly at the midline. This is in contrast to the smooth outline (resembling the coast of California) and light brown color of the spots seen in von Recklinghausen disease (NF-1).

INCONTINENTIA PIGMENTI (FIGS. 10 AND 11)

Incontinentia pigmenti (IP) is a complex hereditary syndrome in which vesicular, verrucous, and pigmented cutaneous lesions are associated with developmental defects of the eye, skeletal system, and central nervous system. This syndrome is due to an X-linked dominant trait that is lethal

"Turn your wounds into wisdom." —**Oprah Winfrey**

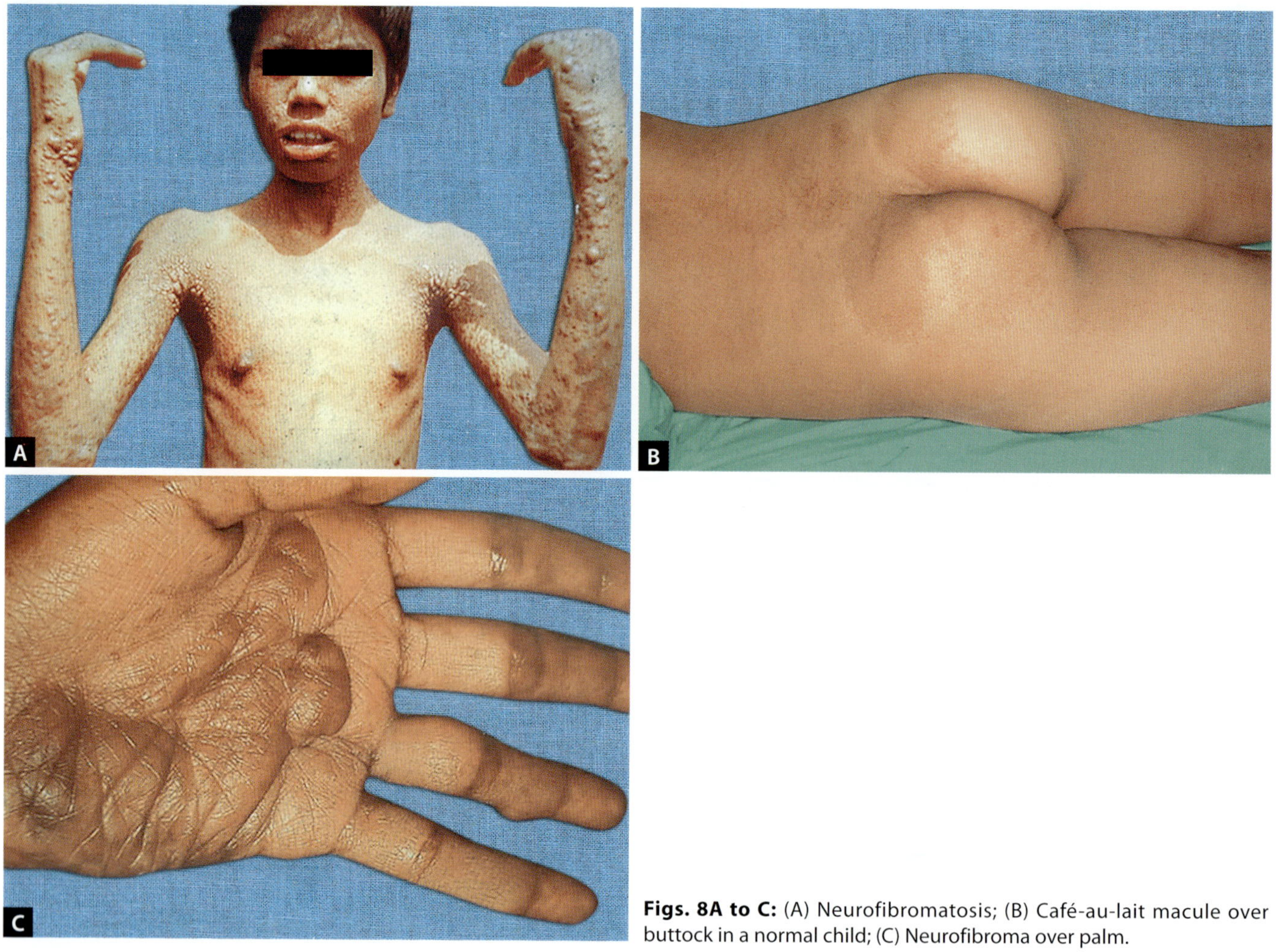

Figs. 8A to C: (A) Neurofibromatosis; (B) Café-au-lait macule over buttock in a normal child; (C) Neurofibroma over palm.

Box 2 Diagnostic criteria for NF1 (National Institutes of Health Consensus Development Conference, 1988).

Presence of two or more of the following criteria is needed for diagnosis:
1. Six or more café-au-lait macules (CALMs), >5 mm in greatest diameter at prepubertal age and >15 mm in greatest diameter in adults
2. Two or more neurofibromas of any type or one plexiform neurofibroma
3. Axillary or inguinal freckling
4. Optic glioma
5. Two or more Lisch nodules
6. A distinctive osseous lesion, e.g., sphenoid dysplasia/thinning of cortex of long bones with or without pseudoarthrosis
7. First-degree relative (parent, sibling, and offspring) with NF-1 by the above criteria

in males. The skin changes are often present at birth, or develop before the end of the first week and rarely appear after the first 2 months. Four clinical stages are recognized: vesicular, hyperkeratotic, hyperpigmentation and hypopigmentation, but their sequence is irregular, their duration variable, and they may overlap. Clear tense vesicles, often in linear groups, develop in the limbs in recurrent crops. The crops continue for a few days or for a month or two. They are accompanied or followed by smooth, red nodules or plaques, often irregularly linear, on the limbs and trunk. The plaques may be extensive and may precede the vesicles. Linear warty lesions may appear on the back of hands and feet, particularly on the fingers and toes. The pigmentation which may be the only abnormality, may present from birth or may appear as the inflammatory lesions, which are subsiding although not necessarily in the same sites, and the inflammatory lesions can develop in areas already pigmented.

The pigmentation ranging in color from blue-gray or slate to brown is characteristic of the syndrome and the bizarre-splashed or Chinese figure distribution is characteristic. The pigmentation persists for many years slowly fading until it is imperceptible by the second or third decade.

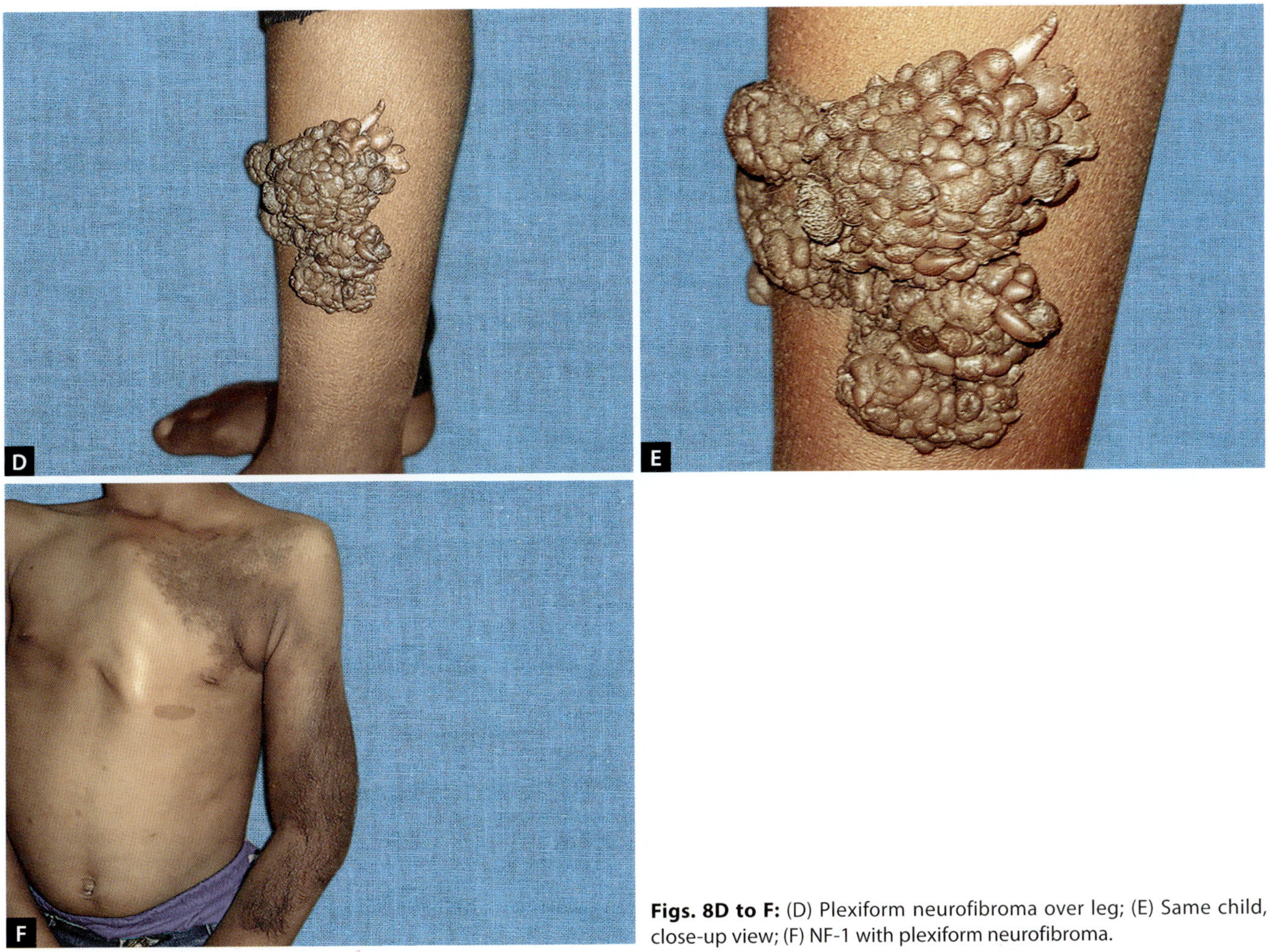

Figs. 8D to F: (D) Plexiform neurofibroma over leg; (E) Same child, close-up view; (F) NF-1 with plexiform neurofibroma.

Systemic Association

Other associated defects found in this condition are dental defects, ocular defects, central nervous system disorders, and skeletal system abnormalities.

Treatment

There is no specific treatment. Genetic counseling for carrier females is advisable. Associated systemic defects are to be addressed. Normal developmental milestones and absence of seizure early in life offer a better prognosis.

HYPOMELANOSIS OF ITO (FIGS. 12A TO C)

This is manifested by whorled appearance of depigmented areas of varying extent, unilateral or bilateral. The appearance resembles the late stage of IP, but this is a separate disease without the preceding inflammatory stages and without the sex-linked inheritance of IP. There may be associated disorders in the musculoskeletal system, teeth, eyes, and central nervous system.

Appearance of hypopigmented lesions in absence of previous inflammatory dermatosis should alert a pediatrician/dermatologist about hypomelanosis of Ito. Now this entity comes under pigmentary mosaicism.

Treatment

All patients with multiple and bilateral hypopigmented lesions should be evaluated for musculoskeletal, developmental, ocular, dental, and other anomalies. Neurologic assessment and an electroencephalogram (EEG) are also mandatory.

"Physical fitness is the first requisite of happiness." —**Joseph Pilates**

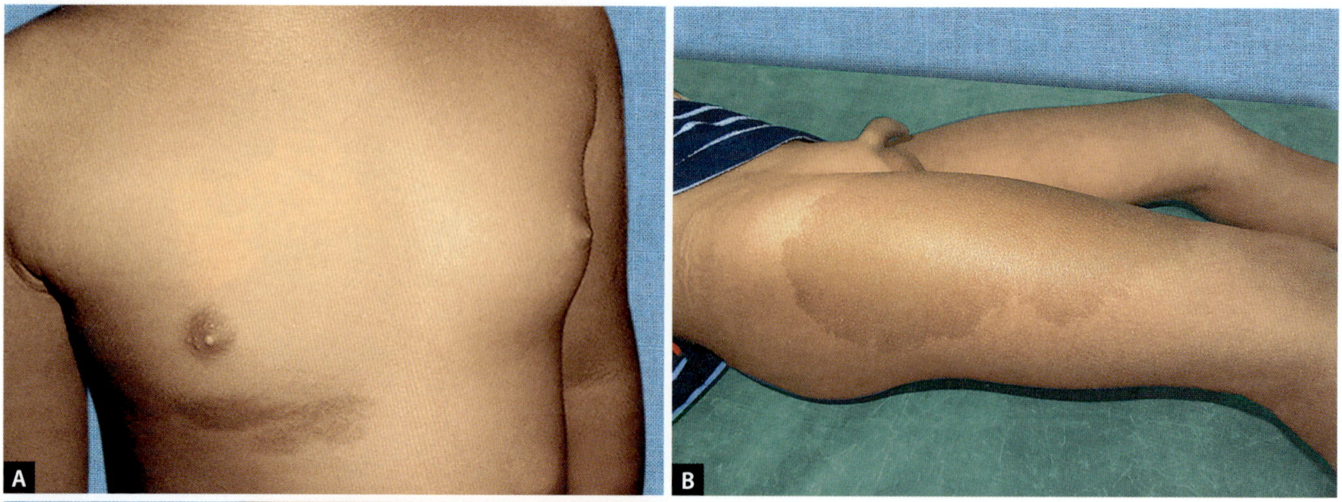

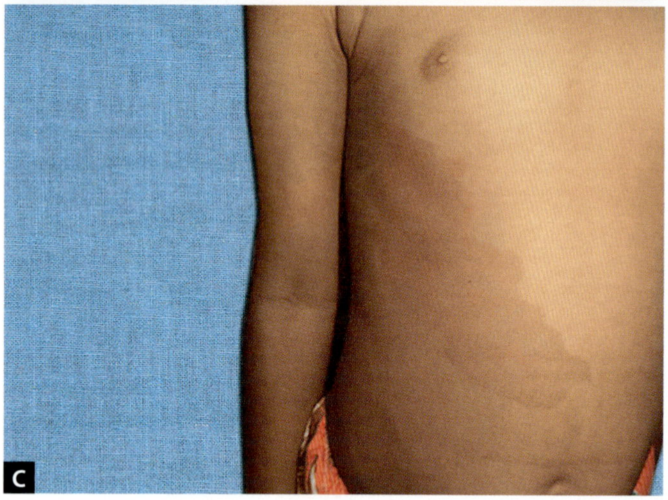

Figs. 9A to C: (A) Café-au-lait macule of McCune–Albright syndrome, note irregular border and midline restriction of the macule; (B) McCune–Albright syndrome, giant café-au-lait macule (CALM); (C) Giant café-au-lait macule (CALM) in a 7-year-old girl with McCune–Albright syndrome.

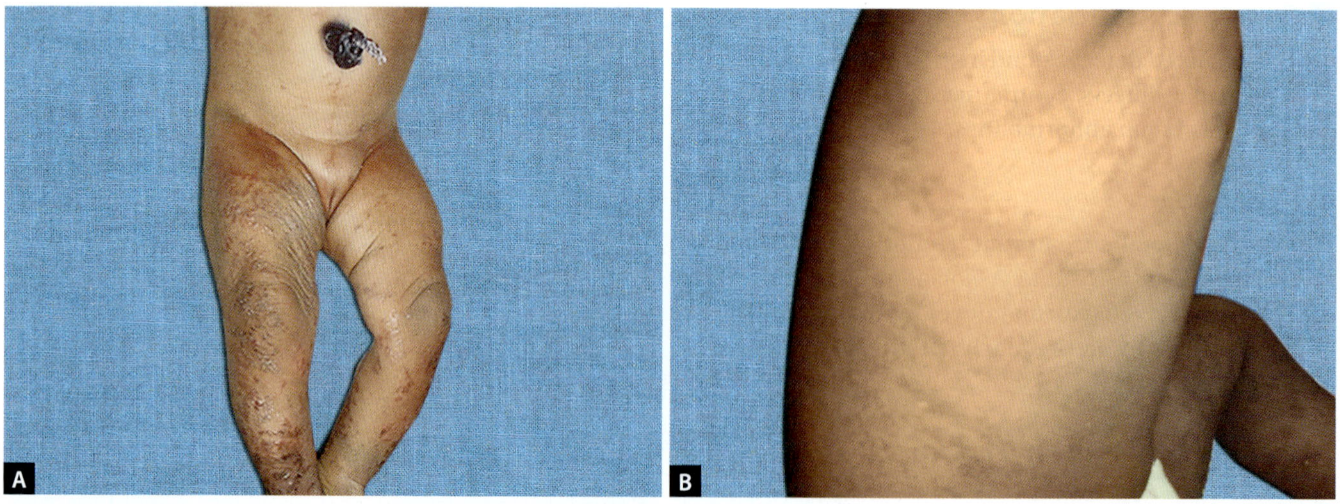

Figs. 10A and B: (A) Papules, vesicles, and crusting along the Blaschko's lines over leg, thigh, and trunk in a female child with incontinentia pigmenti; (B) Incontinentia pigmenti over trunk (hyperpigmentation stage).

"The human body has been designed to resist an infinite number of changes and attacks brought about by its environment. The secret of good health lies in successful adjustment to changing stresses on the body." —**Harry J Johnson**

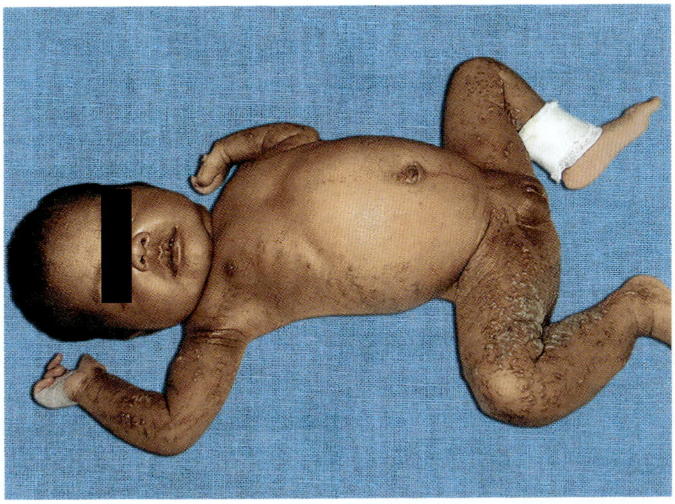

Fig. 10C: Papulovesicular and verrucous stage of incontinentia pigmenti.

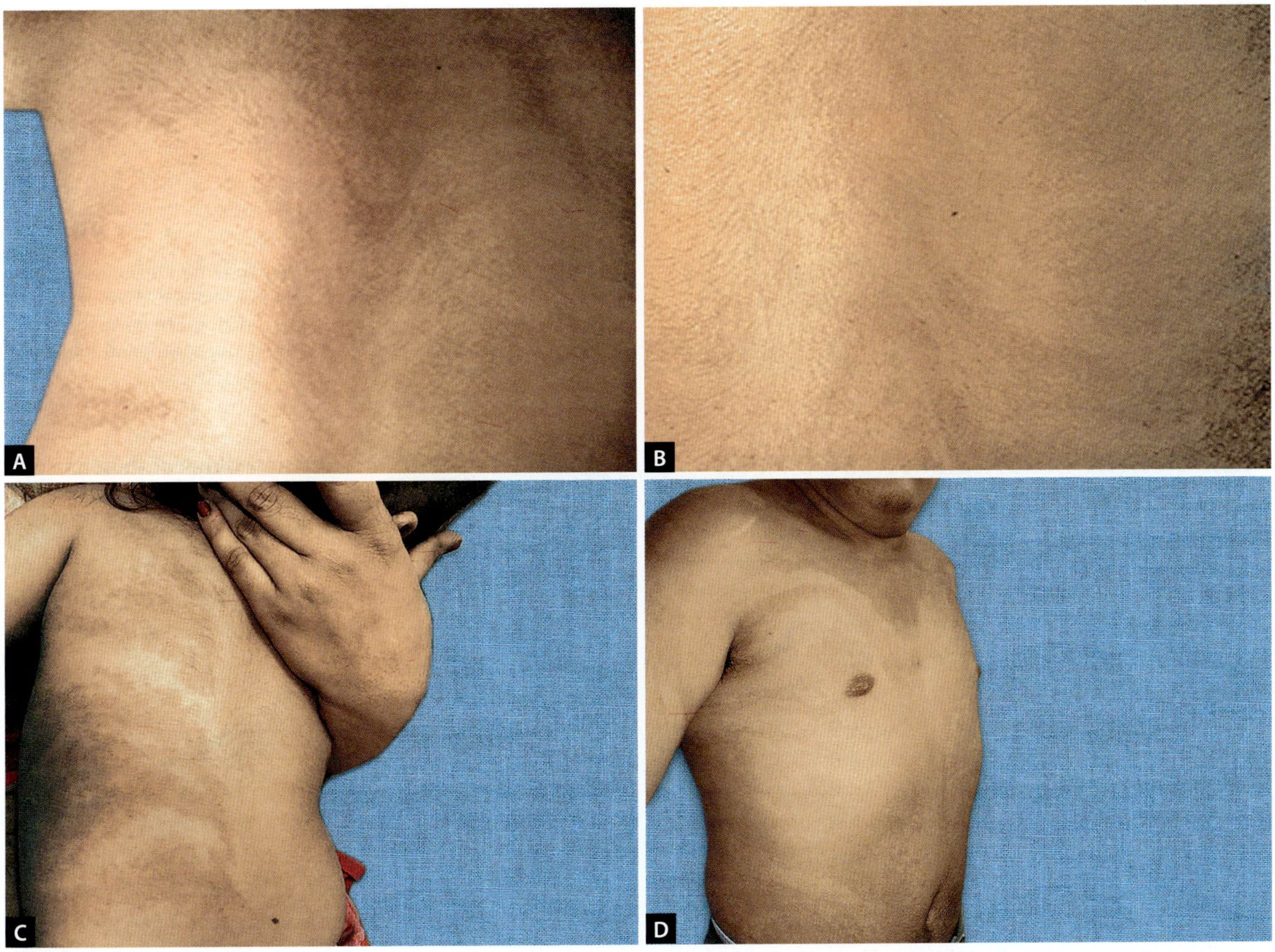

Figs. 11A to D: (A) Wavy bilateral symmetrical pigmented streaks of patches of incontinentia pigmenti (IP) over back; (B) Close-up view of back of the same child; (C) Whorled streaks of hyperpigmented macules over back in a child with IP; (D) Whorled streaks of hyperpigmented macules over front of the trunk in an adolescent boy with IP.

"To keep the body in good health is a duty...otherwise we shall not be able to keep the mind strong and clear." **—Buddha**

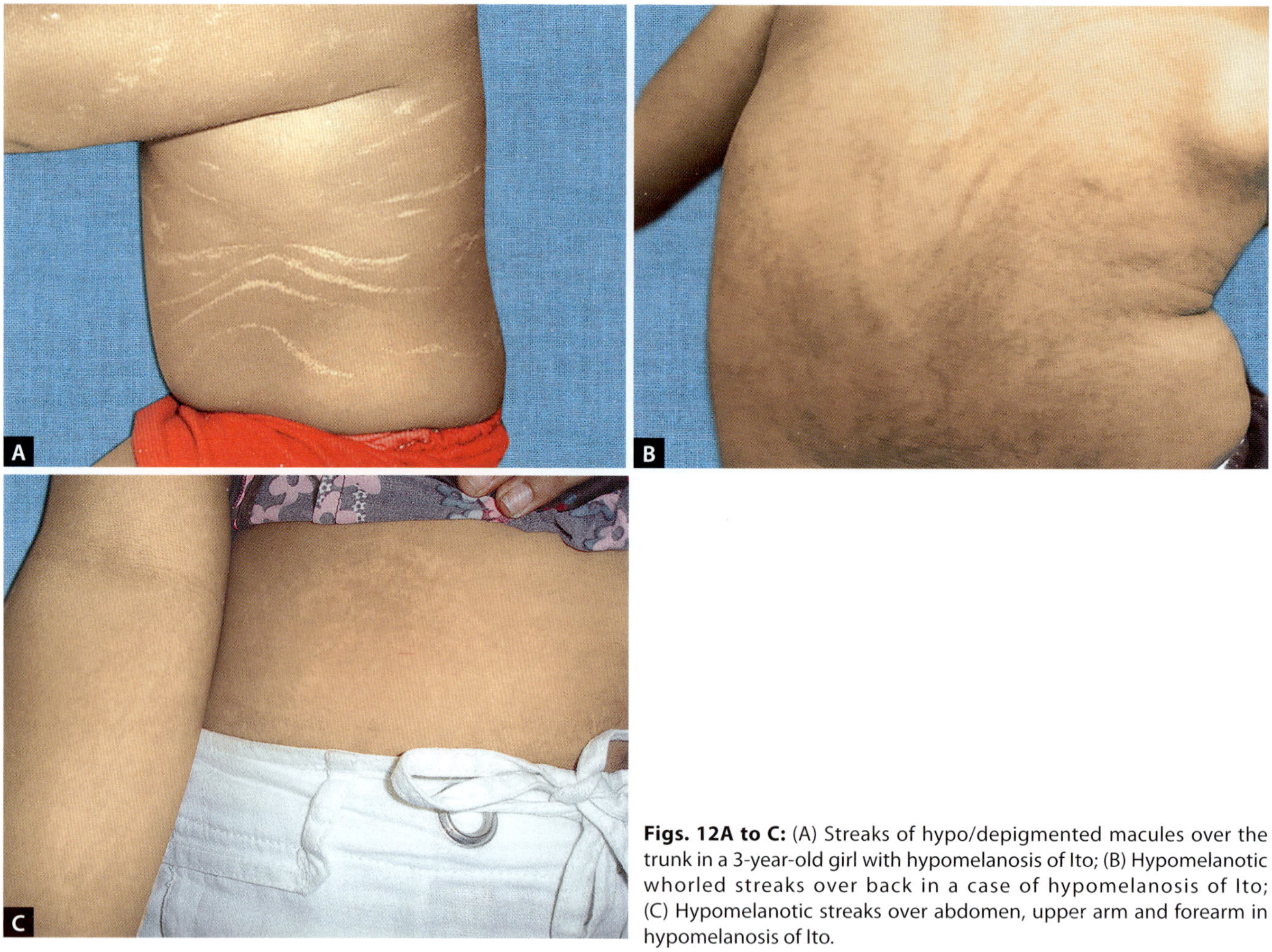

Figs. 12A to C: (A) Streaks of hypo/depigmented macules over the trunk in a 3-year-old girl with hypomelanosis of Ito; (B) Hypomelanotic whorled streaks over back in a case of hypomelanosis of Ito; (C) Hypomelanotic streaks over abdomen, upper arm and forearm in hypomelanosis of Ito.

PIGMENTARY MOSAICISM ASSOCIATED WITH EXTRACUTANEOUS INVOLVEMENT (FIGS. 13A TO C)

Pigmentary mosaicism is a term used for all pigment anomalies caused by chromosomal mosaicism. It is characterized by hypo- or hyperpigmented lesions along the lines of Blaschko, phylloid, checker-board pattern, patchy pigmentation without midline separation, lateralization, and sash pattern. It is an umbrella term that includes conditions like hypomelanoses of Ito, linear and whorled nevoid hypermelanosis, phylloid hypo- and hypermelanosis, and pigmentary mosaicism of hypopigmented and hyperpigmented type. This group of disorders may be associated with or without systemic abnormalities. Pigmentary mosaicism has been associated with extracutaneous features in 50% cases. Most common association is neurological deficits such as epilepsy, learning difficulties, spasticity, hypotonia, and microcephaly, and musculoskeletal features facial dysmorphism, asymmetry of limbs, short stature, syndactyly, and kyphoscoliosis. Pigmentary mosaicism should be differentiated from IP, nevus depigmentosus, and Goltz syndrome.

FAUN TAIL NEVUS (FIGS. 14A TO E)

Spina bifida occulta usually involves lumbar spine (diastematomyelia) and may occur in as many as 20% of all individuals; only a small percentage will have significant associated neurological defect. In about 50% of cases, there is a dermal dimple or sinus, a lipoma, soft silky hairs (called faun tail), a pigmented macule, a skin tag, a dermoid cyst, an infantile hemangioma, or a port-wine stain.

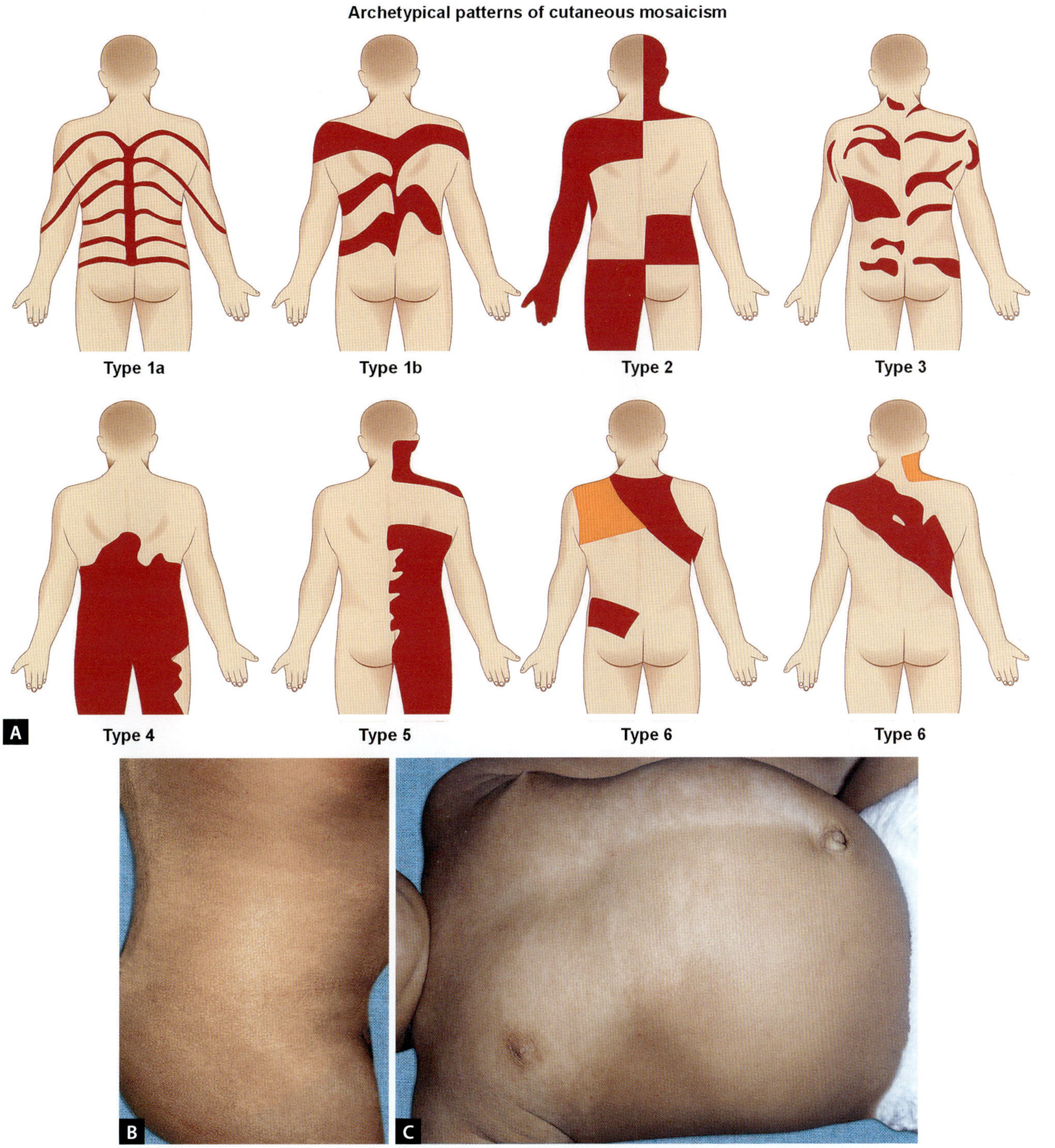

Figs. 13A to C: (A) Archetypal patterns of pigmentary mosaicism; (B and C) Pigmentary mosaicism.

Treatment

Underlying neurological defect is to be treated by a pediatric neurologist. For cosmetic purpose, hair can be removed by epilating creams, or may be shaved off time-to-time. Laser epilation will give long-term cosmetic benefit.

"Nothing is impossible, the word itself says "I'm possible"!" —**Audrey Hepburn**

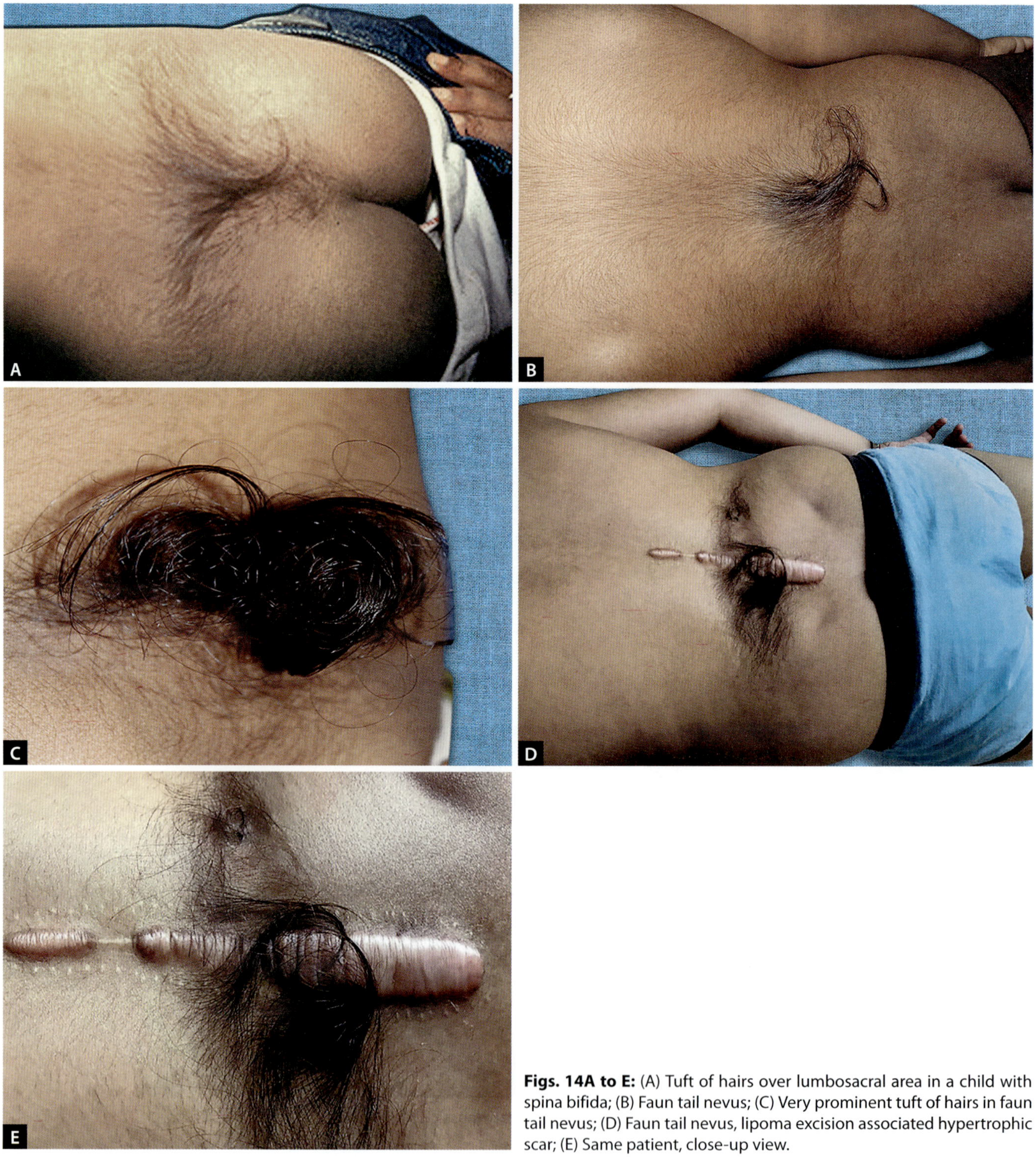

Figs. 14A to E: (A) Tuft of hairs over lumbosacral area in a child with spina bifida; (B) Faun tail nevus; (C) Very prominent tuft of hairs in faun tail nevus; (D) Faun tail nevus, lipoma excision associated hypertrophic scar; (E) Same patient, close-up view.

MENINGOMYELOCELE (FIGS. 15 AND 16)

Meningomyelocele is a common form of spinal dysraphism. It is the most common neurological congenital anomaly affecting approximately 300,000 newborns yearly worldwide. They affect 1 in 1,000 established pregnancies. Meningomyeloceles are open neural tube

"I've learned that people will forget what you said, people will forget what you did, but people will never forget how you made them feel." **—Maya Angelou**

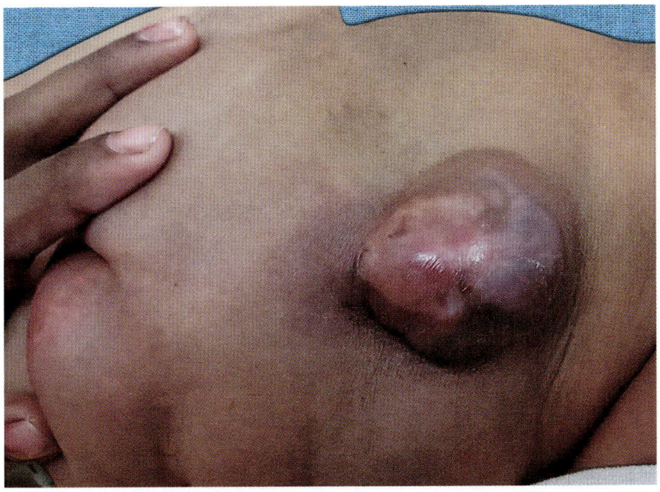

Fig. 15: Meningomyelocele in a newborn.

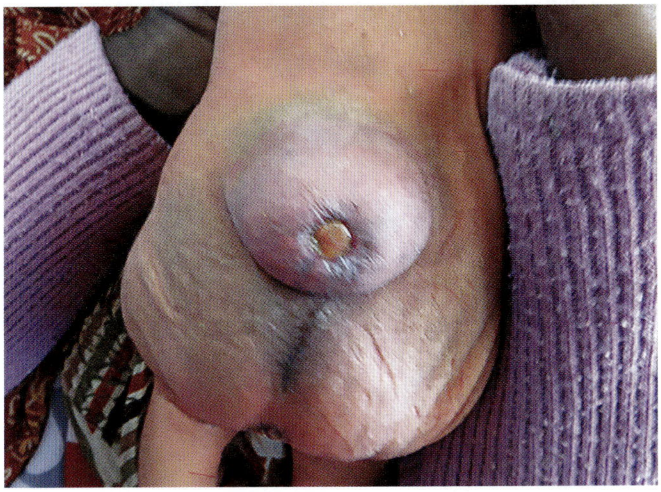

Fig. 16: Meningomyelocele in a newborn, note classical site and morphology.

defects resulting from incomplete closure of vertebral column during embryogenesis resulting in the exposure of the meninges or spinal cord. The progression of spinal neurulation along the body axis is delayed or halted. The inheritance of meningomyelocele is mutifactorial. Maternal folic acid deficiency is strongly associated with neural tube defects.

Clinically, meningomyelocele presents with swelling over the back noticed from birth. Initially, presents as cerebrospinal fluid (CSF) leak since the skin is poorly developed. Sites involving meningomyelocele are thoracolumbar, lumbosacral, lumbar, sacral, and cervical. Cutaneous lesions associated with spinal dysraphism include hypertrichosis, dimples, acrochordons, lipomas, hemangioma, aplasia cutis, dermoid cyst, telangiectasia, capillary malformation, hyperpigmentation, melanocytic nevi, small sacral dimples, and teratomas. Meningomyelocele is associated with various neurological and skeletal defects. Management of meningomyelocele is multidisciplinary. Surgery with treatment of complication is the main stay of management. Parents must be counseled about the prognosis.

STURGE-WEBBER SYNDROME

Sturge-Webber syndrome is a common neurocutaneous disorder caused by the mutation in GNAQ gene or GNA11 gene which effects the skin, brain, eye, spine and nerves. It affects the blood vessels especially those vessels in the skin, eye and the brain tissue. Capillary malformations are the most common cutaneous changes, which usually appears over the sensory distribution of trigeminal nerve. Bony or soft tissue overgrowth are also noted especially of upper lip and maxilla. Risk factors for CNS involvement are extensive bilateral involvement, median port wine-wine birthmark, >50% of contiguous hemi forehead involvement.

Neurological features include seizures due to cerebral vascular malformations, migraine-like headaches, stroke/transient or permanent hemiparesis, leptomeningeal angiomatosis (usually ipsilateral to portwine stain), cognitive impairment, emotional, attention and behavioral problems.

Ocular features include glaucoma (ipsilateral), choroidal hemorrhage, ocular melanocytosis, iris heterochromia and mammillations, cilioretinal occlusion.

ROACH SCALE CLASSIFICATION

- *Type 1 (Classic SWS)*: Facial + leptomeningeal malformations; may have glaucoma.
- *Type 2*: Facial capillary malformation alone; may have glaucoma.
- *Type 3*: Isolated leptomeningeal angiomatosis; usually no glaucoma.

Management

Antiepileptic medications are the mainstay of treatment. However, newer targeted therapies like sirolimus, rapamycin have been found to be effective in vascular malformations. Rapamycin along with low dose aspirin is

"To teach is to learn twice". —**Joseph Joubert**

found to be effective in reducing the chances of seizures. Other treatment modalities include lasers like pulsed dye laser (PDL), intense pulse light layers (IPL) or ablative methods like fractional CO_2 lasers and erbium YAG lasers. Choroidal hemorrhages causing vision loss can be treated by external beam radiotherapy, proton beam radiotherapy. Photodynamic therapy with verteporfin was also found effective.

SUGGESTED READINGS

1. Barros FS, Marussi VHR, Amaral LLF, da Rocha AJ, Campos CMS, Freitas LF, et al. The rare neurocutaneous disorders: update on clinical, molecular, and neuroimaging features. Top Magn Reson Imaging. 2018;27(6):433-62.
2. Becker B, Strowd RE 3rd. Phakomatoses. Dermatol Clin. 2019;37(4):583-606.
3. Belzile E, McCuaig C, Le Meur JB, Coulombe J, Hatami A, Powell J, et al. Patterned cutaneous hypopigmentation phenotype characterization: a retrospective study in 106 children. Pediatr Dermatol. 2019;36(6):869-75.
4. Curatolo P, Specchio N, Aronica E. Advances in the genetics and neuropathology of tuberous sclerosis complex: edging closer to targeted therapy. Lancet Neurol. 2022;21(9):843-56.
5. Kromann AB, Ousager LB, Ali IKM, Aydemir N, Bygum A. Pigmentary mosaicism: a review of original literature and recommendations for future handling. Orphanet J Rare Dis. 2018;13(1):39.
6. Sewell MJ, Chiu YE, Drolet BA. Neural tube dysraphism: review of cutaneous markers and imaging. Pediatr Dermatol. 2015;32(2):161-70.
7. Sánchez-Espino LF, Ivars M, Antoñanzas J, Baselga E. Sturge-Weber syndrome: A review of pathophysiology, genetics, clinical features, and current management approache. Appl Clin Genet. 2023;16:63-81.
8. Tamura R. Current Understanding of Neurofibromatosis Type 1, 2, and Schwannomatosis. Int J Mol Sci. 2021;22(11):5850.

CHAPTER

11

Pigmentary Disorders

VITILIGO [FIGS. 1 TO 4D(x)]

Vitiligo results from autoimmune destruction of the melanocytes, the exact etiology of which is still elusive. Depending on the distribution of lesions, it can be of several types: Focal, segmental, vulgaris, universal, lip-tip (involvement of lips and tip of the fingers and toes), etc. The disease is often associated with other autoimmune cutaneous and systemic disorders, e.g., alopecia areata, lichen planus, psoriasis, Addison's disease, autoimmune thyroiditis, autoimmune hepatitis, pernicious anemia, and diabetes mellitus. Positive family history in childhood vitiligo is seen in 11–46% in various studies. Childhood vitiligo differs from adult vitiligo as they have distinct epidemiological and clinical features and is strongly associated with family history and other autoimmune disorders. Various studies have shown that the most common clinical type of vitiligo in children is vitiligo vulgaris followed by focal and segmental vitiligo. Universal vitiligo is rare in children.

Repigmentation of the perifollicular and at the border of patches, is fairly good with topical steroid(s).

Prognosis

Presence of leukotrichia over vitiligo patches is a bad prognostic sign as far as the repigmentation is concerned. Scalp leukotrichia is a common finding in children with family history of vitiligo and other autoimmune disorders.

Differential Diagnosis

Presence of leukotrichia helps to differentiate vitiligo from other hypo/depigmentary disorders, e.g., leprosy, nevus depigmentosus, post-kala-azar dermal leishmaniasis (PKDL), and postinflammatory hypopigmentation.

Treatment

Treatment is broadly classified into medical therapy and surgical therapy. Medical therapy includes topical corticosteroids; mild for face and flexures, e.g., clobetasone, desonide, hydrocortisone, moderately potent steroid, e.g., fluticasone, mometasone or potent steroid, e.g., clobetasol and betamethasone dipropionate, are to be applied once/day for 2–3 months depending upon the response. Topical calcineurin inhibitors tacrolimus and pimecrolimus have shown good results with twice daily application.

The other popular medical therapy for vitiligo is photochemotherapy (PUVA), where psoralen is combined with ultraviolet A (UVA), also known as PUVA therapy. Psoralens used are either trimethylpsoralen (TMP), 8-methoxypsoralen, or 5-methoxypsoralen. Since 8-methoxypsoralen can cause marked phototoxicity, the preferred psoralen is TMP. It is given in a dose of 0.6 mg/kg/day with milk or light breakfast. Two hours after the intake of medicine, exposure to sunlight is given 10–15 minutes initially followed by increments of 5 minutes every week to a maximum of 30 minutes. It is given 2–3 days a week. PUVA therapy is recommended only above 8 years (according to some experts 12 years) of age. PUVA therapy is now rarely used in children due to its toxicity. Narrow-band ultraviolet B (NBUVB) therapy has become the treatment of choice in childhood vitiligo. The peak emission of NBUVB is 311 nm and this peak in vitiligo stimulates the dormant skin melanocytes and also modulates the cutaneous immune system. However, the exact mechanism of repigmentation is not known. It can be given twice/thrice weekly. The starting dose is 200 mJ/cm^2 and up to a maximum dose of 3,000 mJ/cm^2 can be given for the entire body. Around 18–36 exposures are necessary to assess the treatment response. There are reports of low serum levels of vitamin D and its expression of receptor. The cumulative dose of vitamin D could improve vitamin D levels and influence the rate of pigmentation. Excimer laser has also shown good improvement in childhood vitiligo.

Other treatment modalities for extensive and unstable vitiligo include immunosuppressants such as short

"Life is a daring adventure or nothing at all." —**Helen Keller**

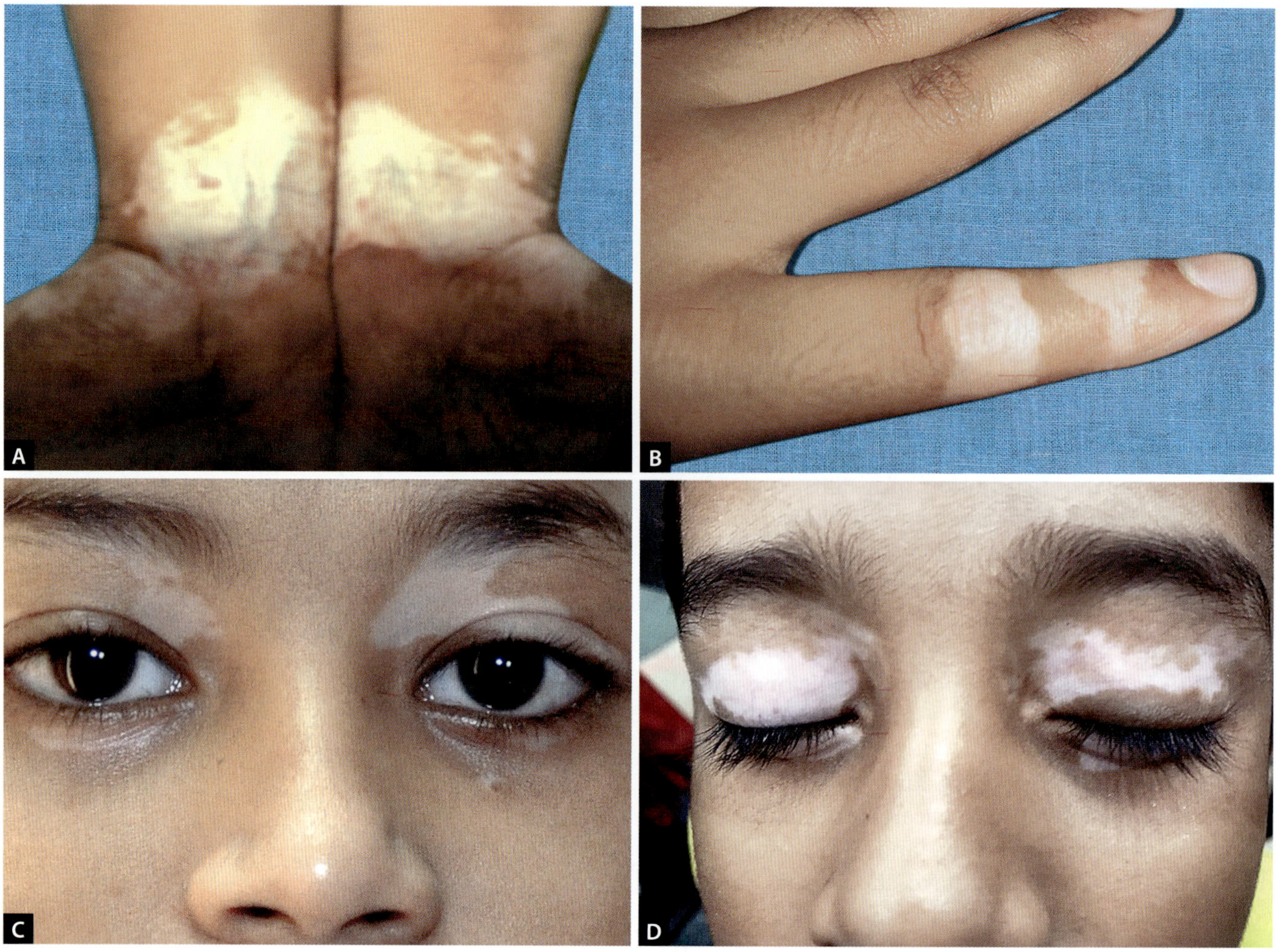

Figs. 1A to D: (A) Depigmented patches of vitiligo in a mirror-image distribution over the wrists; (B) Focal vitiligo; (C) Vitiligo of eyelids—a very common site in children where the disease often starts; (D) Another child with eyelid vitiligo.

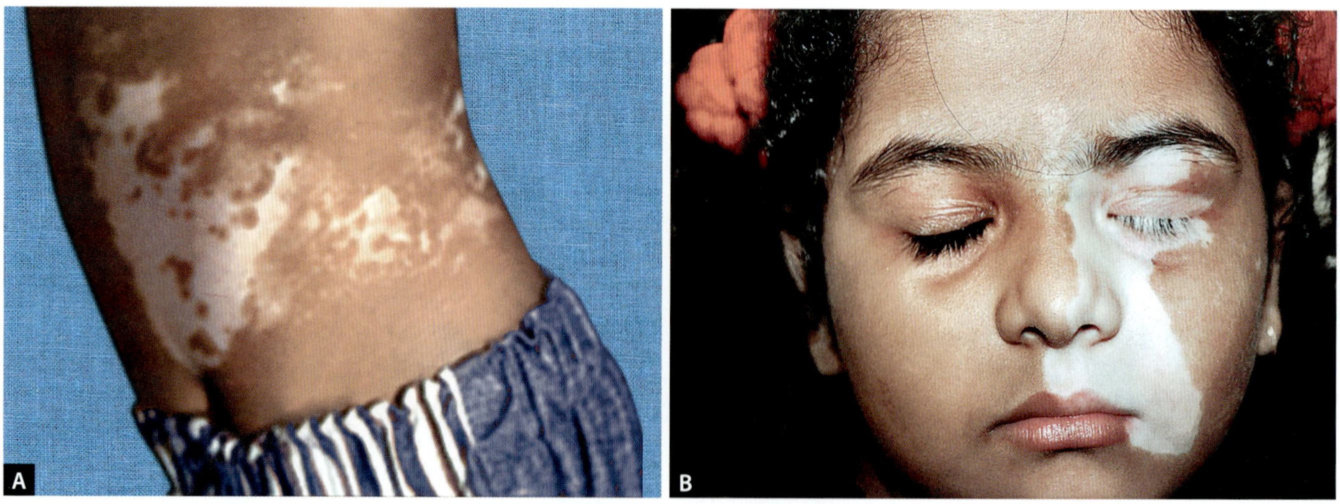

Figs. 2A and B: (A) Perifollicular repigmentation in vitiligo patch; (B) Segmental vitiligo, note leukotrichia of eyelashes.

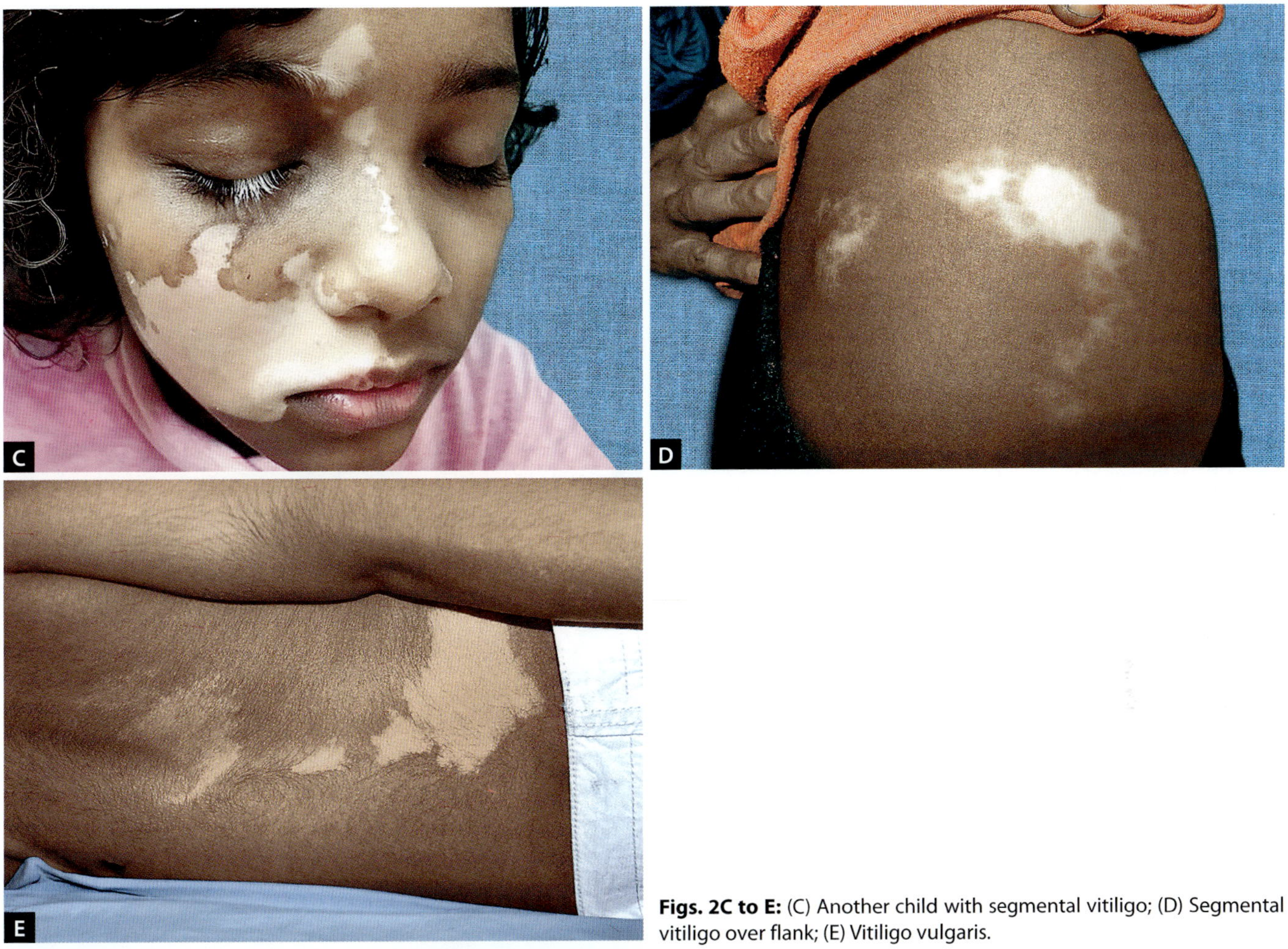

Figs. 2C to E: (C) Another child with segmental vitiligo; (D) Segmental vitiligo over flank; (E) Vitiligo vulgaris.

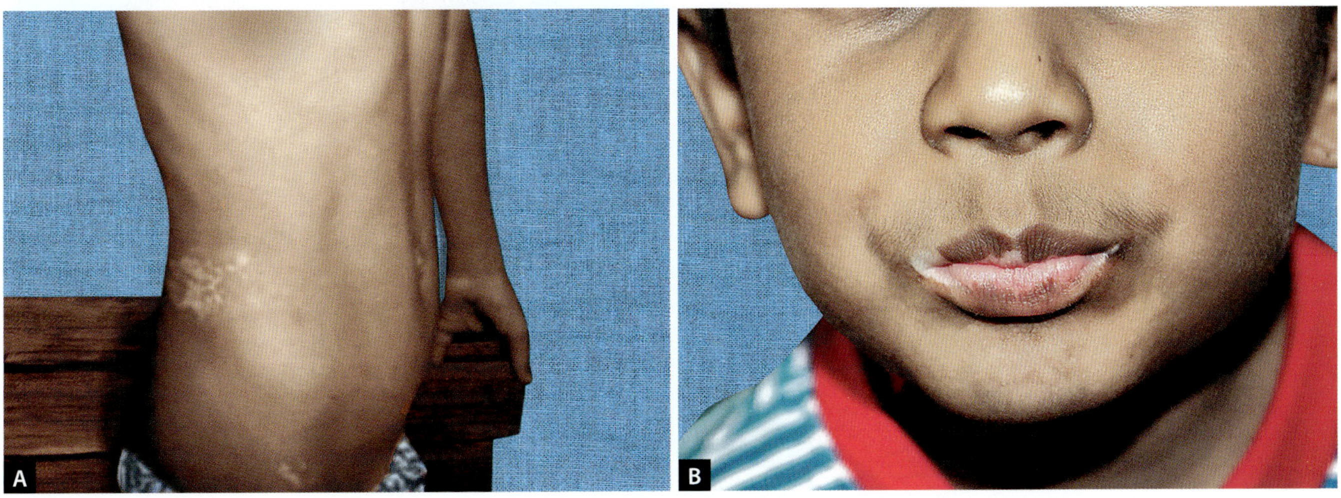

Figs. 3A and B: (A) Repigmenting vitiligo with topical corticosteroid; (B) Lip vitiligo.

course of oral steroids, cyclosporine, azathioprine, and methotrexate.

Once the spread of vitiligo is brought under control or the stability of vitiligo is achieved, various surgical procedures which can be undertaken are micropigmentation or tattooing, punch grafting, dermabrasion, split thickness skin grafting, melanocyte transfer, etc. One must remember that there is no dietary restriction required

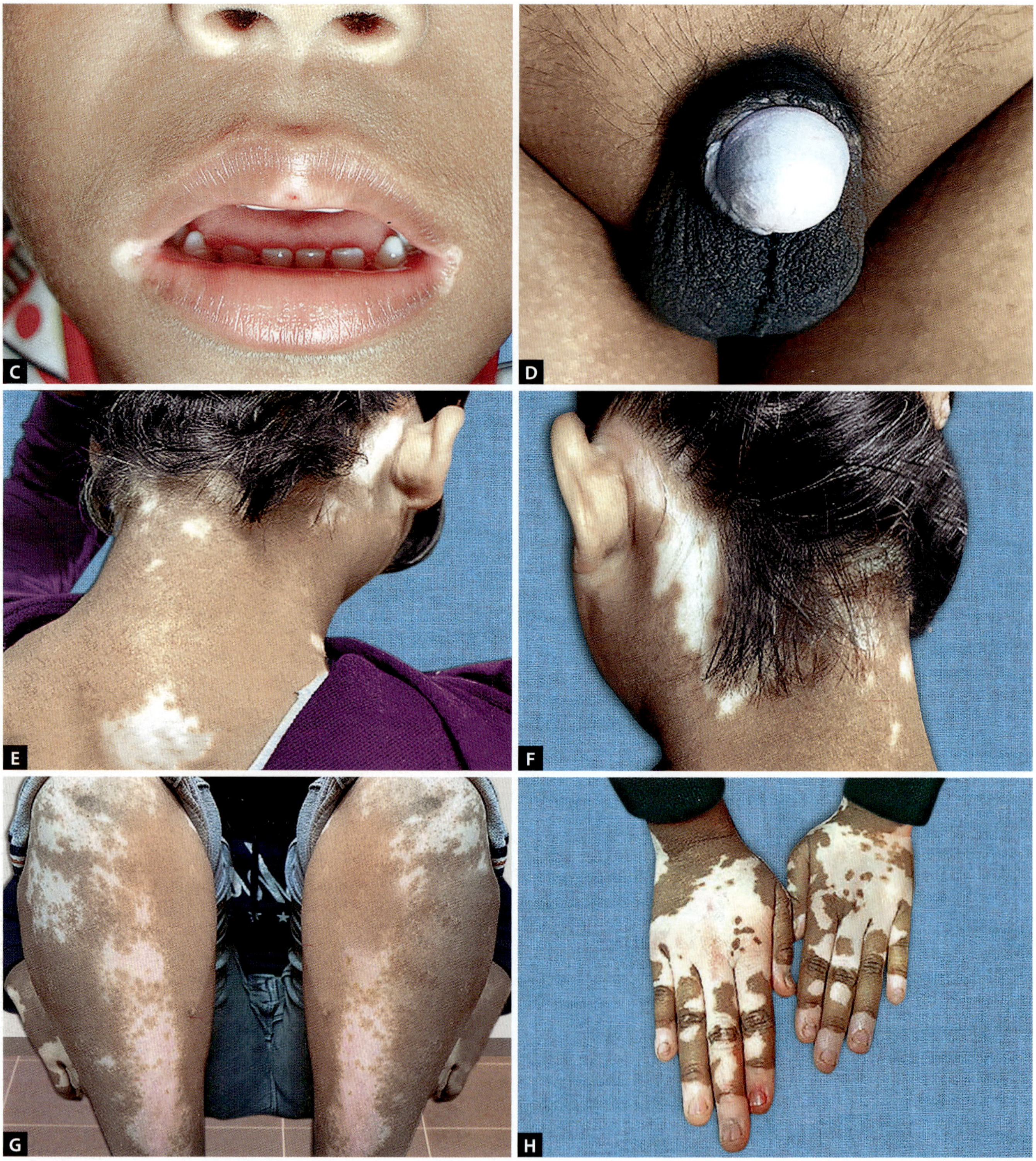

Figs. 3C to H: (C) Another child with lip vitiligo; (D) Vitiligo of glans penis; (E) Vitiligo over retroauricular area, nape of the neck in an 11-year-old girl; (F) Same girl, close-up view; (G) Lesions over knee, shin in the same girl; (H) Involvement of dorsum of hands and fingers, difficult sites for treatment.

"Each life is made up of mistakes and learning, waiting and growing, practicing patience and being persistent." —**Billy Graham**

in such patients. There is no scientific documentation in favor of avoidance of sour food/drink, vitamin C or fruit juice, etc. Reassurance explaining, and counseling of children and/or parents are required in the management of vitiligo.

Factors to be considered before selecting a patient for vitiligo surgery are stability, age, size, morphological type, and anatomical site. Grafting has shown at least 75% repigmentation in 30–90% patients and is most useful for focal and segmental lesions. Vitiligo in children is unstable with frequent relapses; hence, vitiligo surgery in children is not a favorable treatment modality. There are two types of vitiligo surgery: Tissue grafts and cellular grafts. Noncultured cellular transplants have been conducted in children with good and long-lasting results. Minipunch grafting is the simplest grafting procedure but has a risk of cobblestoning and mismatch. This method is used for fingertips, toes, areola, and palms and soles. Split thickness grafting gives good repigmentation and large areas can be treated in a single session. In noncultured epidermal suspension (keratinocytes and melanocytes), large areas can be treated by harvesting grafts one-fourth to one-tenth smaller size than the treated area and there is uniform pigmentation. Studies have shown that this method has been used in children between 4 and 16 years with excellent repigmentation by 16 weeks.

WOOD'S LAMP [FIGS. 4D(xi) AND (xii)]

Wood's lamp was invented in 1903 by a Baltimore physicist Robert W Wood. It is a small, inexpensive, safe, and handy device used for diagnosis of infective and pigmentary disorders. Wood's lamp emits Wood's light of low intensity, long wave ultraviolet light (320–400 nm), also called as

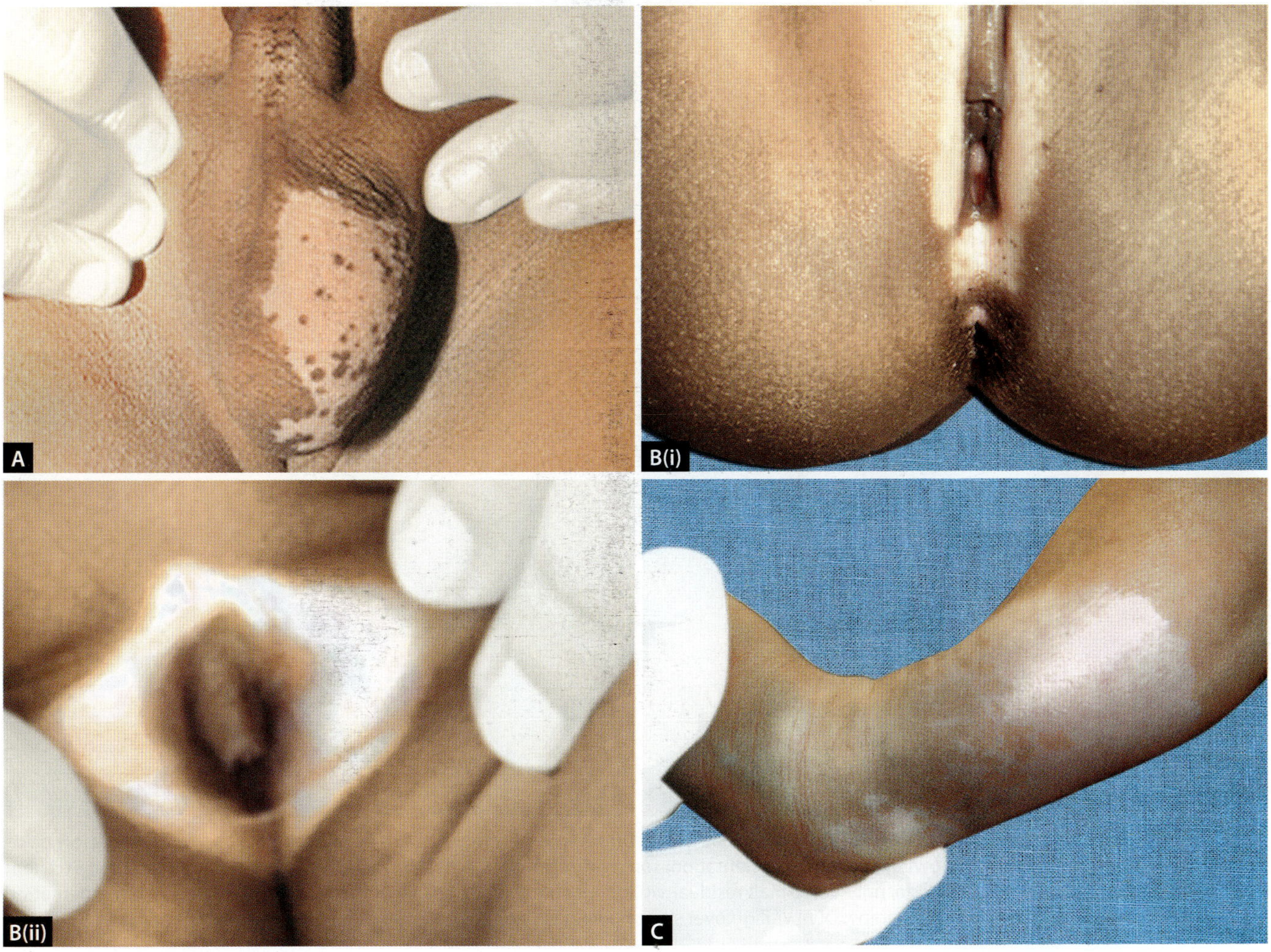

Figs. 4A to C: (A) Repigmentation over a scrotal patch in an 8-year-old boy; B(i) Vitiligo over genitalia in an young girl; B(ii) Vitiligo over vulva; (C) Newborn with congenital vitiligo.

"Each person must live their life as a model for others." —**Rosa Parks**

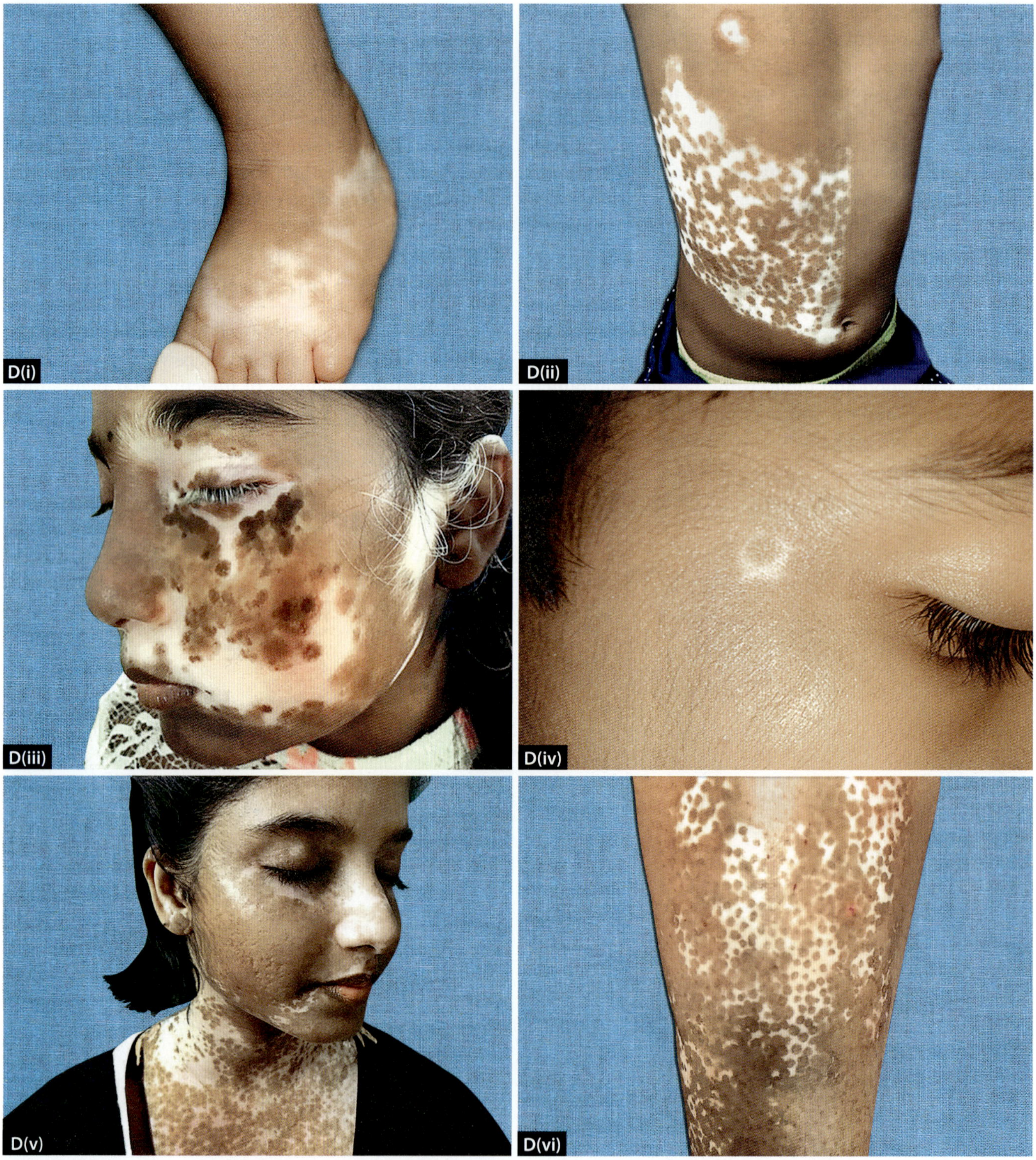

Figs. 4D(i) to (vi): D(i) Vitiligo over dorsum of foot in a small child; D(ii) Repigmenting vitiligo, note perifollicular repigmentation post-treatment; D(iii) Segmental vitiligo showing uneven repigmentation, some normal repigmentation and some overpigmentation; D(iv) Excellent repigmentation of a large patch of vitiligo, note very small residual vitiligo macule; D(v) Extensive vitiligo showing very good repigmentation with narrow-band ultraviolet B (NBUVB) therapy; D(vi) Vitiligo over shin showing very good repigmentation with NBUVB therapy.

"My philosophy of life is that if we make up our mind what we are going to make of our lives, then work hard toward that goal, we never lose somehow we win out." —**Ronald Reagan**

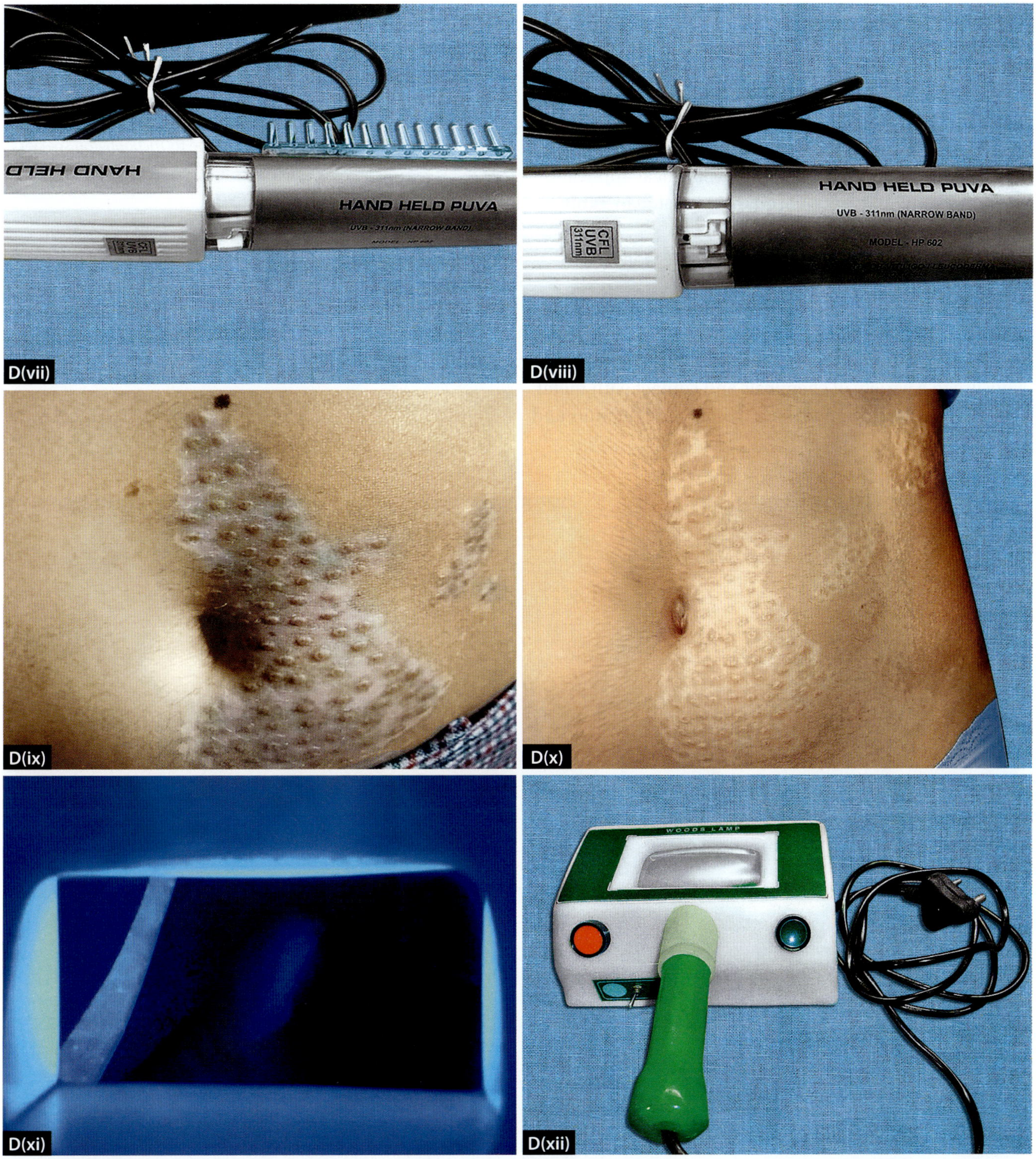

Figs. 4D(vii) to (xii): D(vii) Hand-held narrow-band ultraviolet B (NBUVB) 1 machine; D(viii) Close-up view; D(ix) Further color match following punch grafting; D(x) Vitiligo patch nicely repigmented post punch grafting; D(xi) Wood's lamp when lighted; D(xii) Wood's lamp machine.

black light from a high pressure mercury lamp fitted with a special filter (Wood's filter) made of nickel oxide and silica. The examination should be performed in a dark room and the light should be held 4–6 inches from the skin or hair to be examined and look for fluorescence. Before examination, any topical medicaments, oil, grease, and soap residues should be wiped away. Clinical application of Wood's lamp in various dermatoses is listed in **Table 1**.

Table 1: Clinical application of Wood's lamp in various dermatoses.

Disorder	*Wood's lamp fluorescence*
Tinea capitis	• Bluish-green due to *Microsporum* species • Dull blue due to *Trichophyton* species
Pityriasis versicolor	Yellow white or copper orange fluorescence
Erythrasma	Coral-red fluorescence
Vitiligo	Accentuation of bright-blue white fluorescence
Melasma—epidermal type	The epidermal pigmentation become more apparent
Porphyria (RBC/urine/teeth/blister fluid/feces)	Red-pink fluorescence

(RBC: red blood cell)

CHEMICAL (CONTACT) LEUKODERMA [FIGS. 4E(i) TO G]

Contact leukoderma is an acquired leukoderma that occurs as a result of repeated topical or systemic exposure to a variety of chemicals and contact with metal, leather, etc. These chemicals are mainly alkyl phenols and

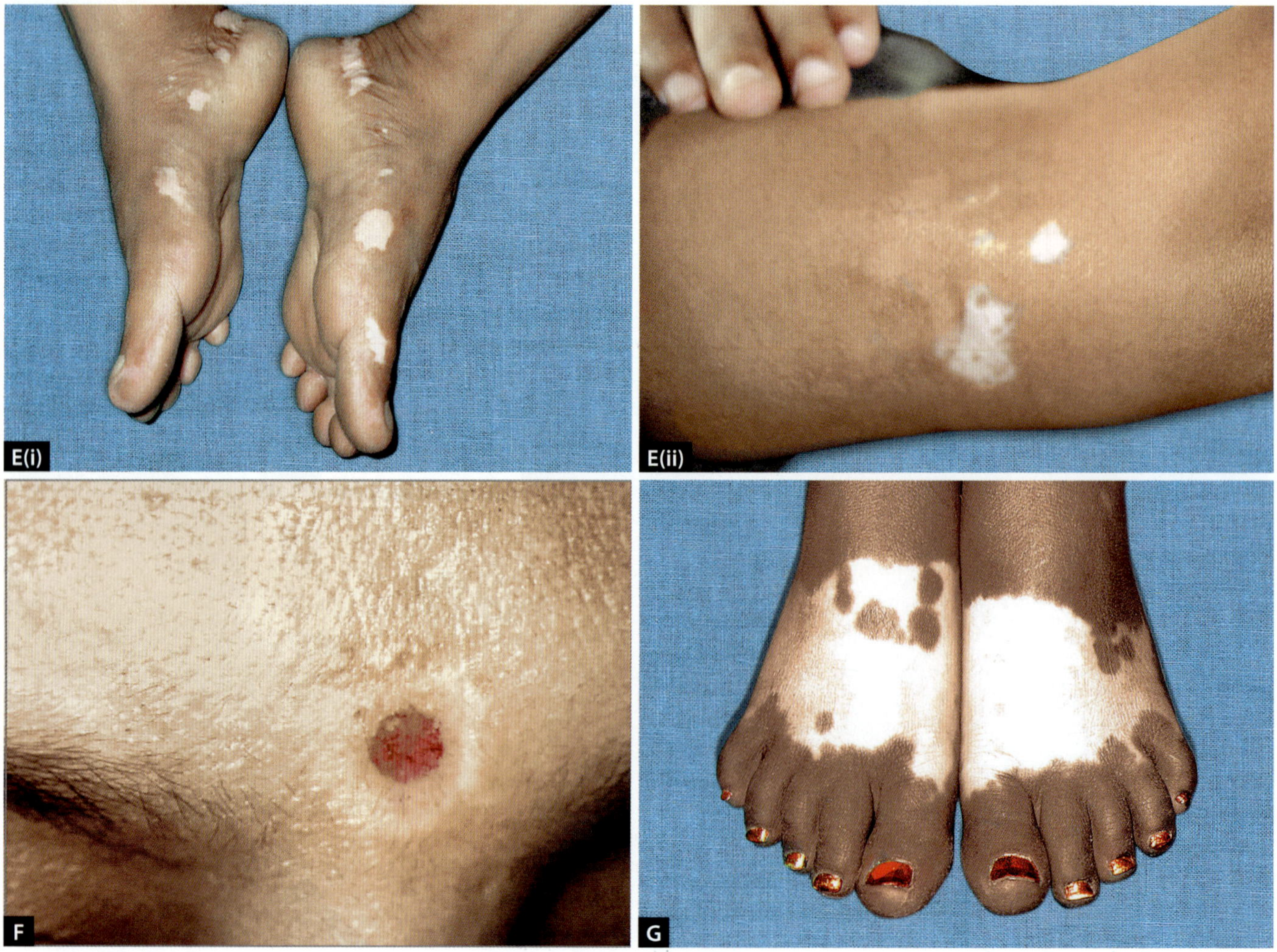

Figs. 4E(i) to G: E(i) Contact dermatitis to metal leading to depigmentation; E(ii) Focal vitiligo showing very good repigmentation; (F) Bindi leukoderma; (G) Footwear leukoderma.

"Transformation is a process, and as life happens there are tons of ups and downs. It's a journey of discovery there are moments on mountaintops and moments in deep valleys of despair." —**Rick Warren**

catechols. They are used in the manufacturing of plastics, resins, synthetic rubber, paints, petrolatum products, deodorants, pesticides, disinfectants, germicides photographic chemicals, printing ink, varnishes, etc. These chemicals are also present in certain objects of our daily use, e.g., footwear, plastic watch strap, purse, and bindis. Compounds of the phenolic group are thought to cause contact leukoderma by competitive inhibition of tyrosinase and release of toxic metabolites producing injury to the melanocytes. Injection of triamcinolone and botulinum toxin has also been implicated as a cause for contact leukoderma. This condition presents as well demarcated areas of depigmentation in the areas suspected to be in contact with a possible chemical implicated in the causation. Diagnosis is generally made by history and clinical examination. Treatment includes removal of the offending agent and educating the patient regarding the possible sources of the implicated chemicals. Topical application with corticosteroids and tacrolimus has shown beneficial effects.

HALO NEVUS [FIGS. 4H TO J(ii)]

Halo nevus is a benign melanocytic nevus in which a ring of hypopigmentation/depigmentation (1–5 mm) develops around the pigmented nevus. This hypopigmentation is due to immunologically mediated melanocytic damage. Majority of such nevi occurs in childhood and are mostly seen on the back. It classically presents as a ring of depigmentation around a dermal melanocytic nevus. Halo nevus is often seen in children having vitiligo. This halo phenomenon is also associated with compound and intradermal nevi, Spitz nevi, neurofibromas, melanomas, and congenital melanocytic nevi.

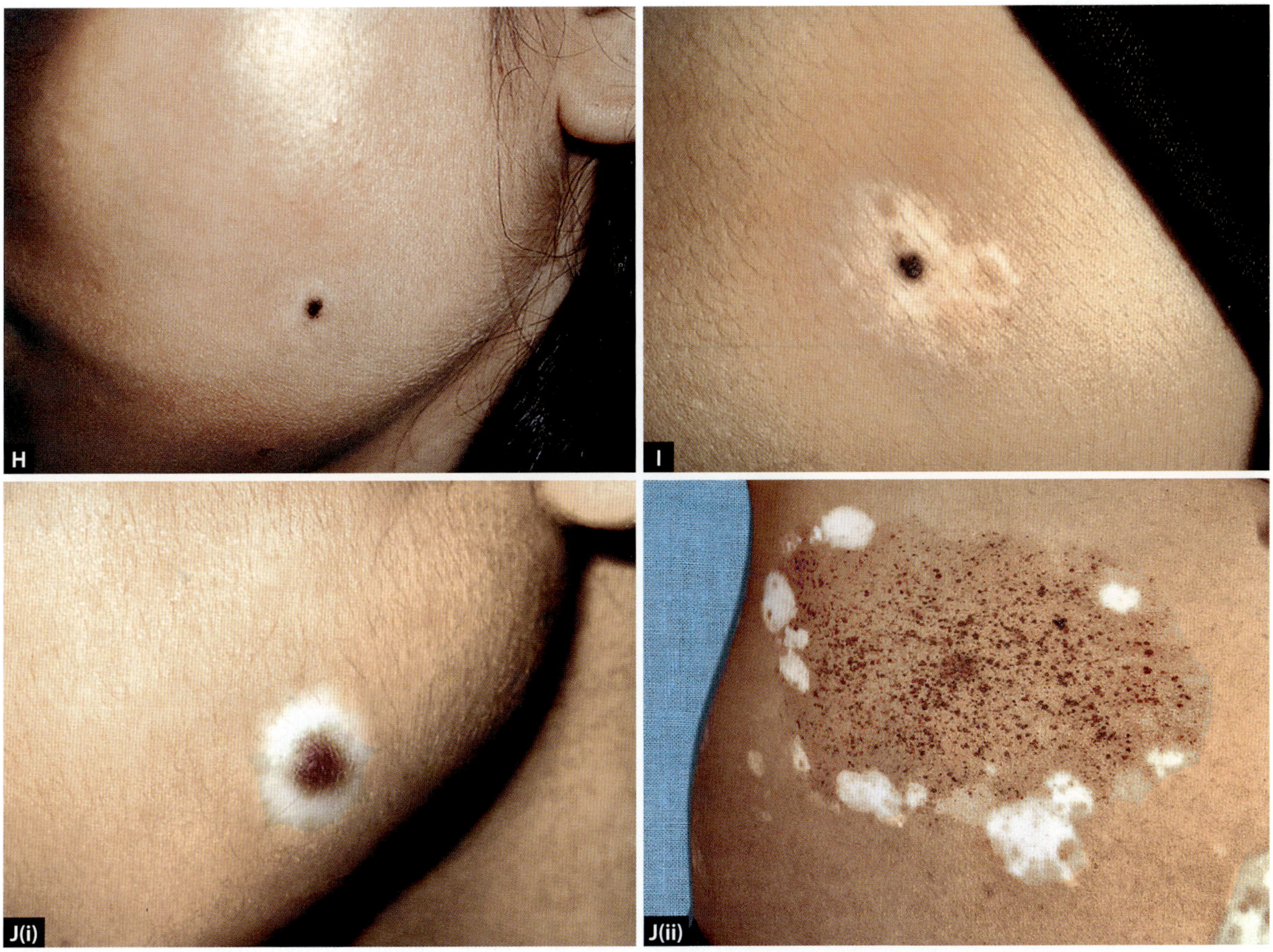

Figs. 4H to J(ii): (H) Halo nevus; (I) Close-up view of halo nevus; J(i) Halo nevus in a 6-year-old boy; J(ii) Halo phenomenon surrounding nevus spilus at the centre.

"Live life to the fullest, and focus on the positive." —**Matt Cameron**

Treatment

The nevi are usually benign and do not require excision. However, when the central melanocytic nevus looks atypical, it may require excision. Regular follow-up and observation is necessary.

IDIOPATHIC GUTTATE HYPOMELANOSIS (FIGS. 4K TO M)

It is a disorder which is more common in adults. The incidence of this condition increases with an increase in age. It is found occasionally in children with a female preponderance. It presents as about 5 mm to 1 cm sharply defined porcelain white macules which are asymptomatic and does not increase in size. These macules are most commonly located on the extensor aspect of the forearms and shins; however, lesions can also occur on the trunk. The pathogenesis remains unknown, although sun exposure is considered to be a triggering factor for this condition. The diagnosis is almost always clinical and the closest differential diagnosis is that of vitiligo. No treatment has been found to be effective for this disorder.

NEVUS DEPIGMENTOSUS (FIGS. 5 AND 6)

This is an isolated nevoid abnormality of skin presenting as circumscribed area of depigmentation usually present at birth, changing little thereafter. The lesions are often single but may be multiple, circumscribed and either rounded, dermatomal or in whorls and streaks resembling incontinentia pigmenti achromians of Ito. The condition is a fairly common congenital anomaly of skin. It has been recently considered as a forme fruste of pigmentary mosaicism.

Treatment

There is no specific treatment for this condition. The worried parents are to be told about the nature of this skin

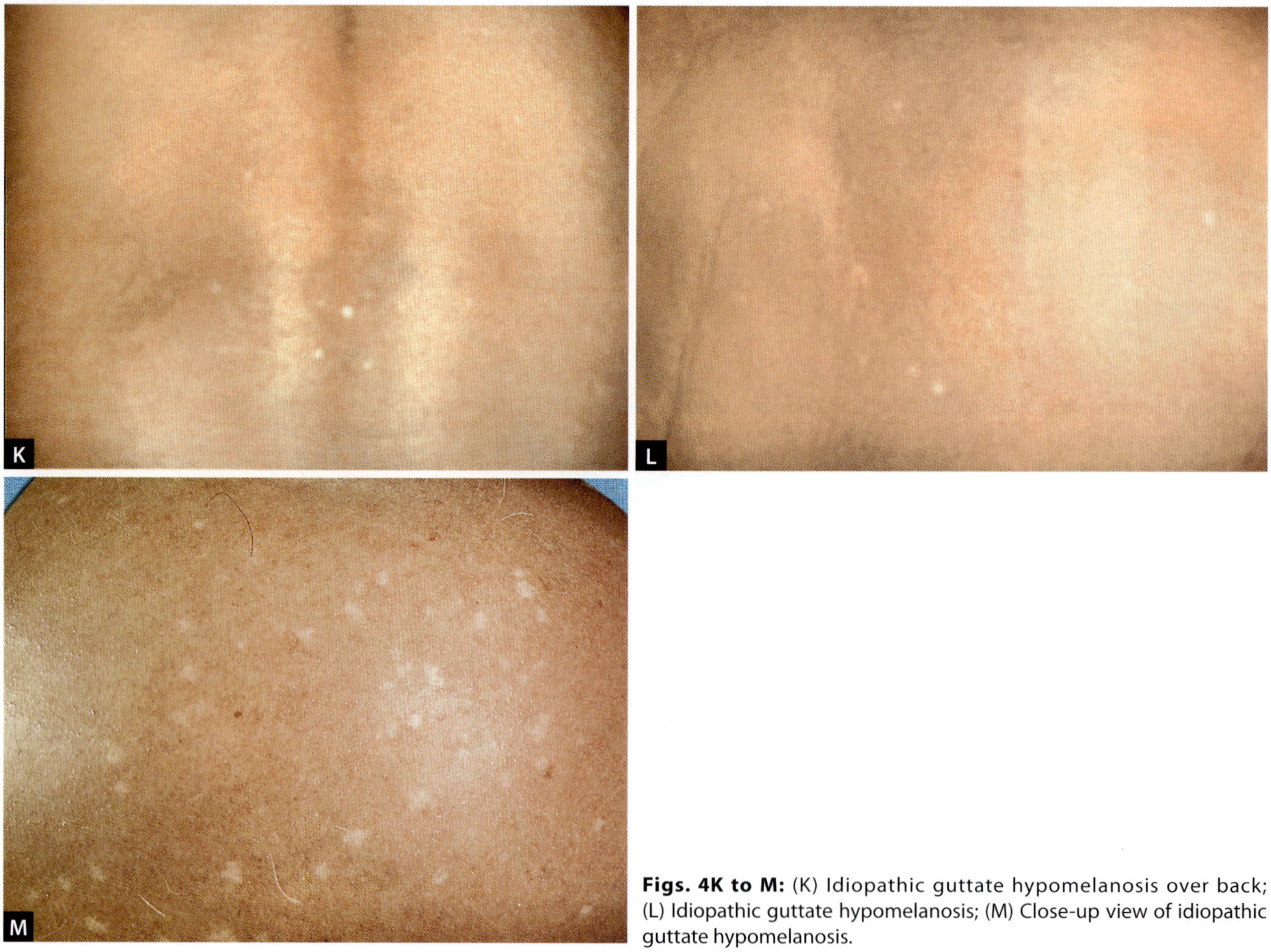

Figs. 4K to M: (K) Idiopathic guttate hypomelanosis over back; (L) Idiopathic guttate hypomelanosis; (M) Close-up view of idiopathic guttate hypomelanosis.

problem and that it is not leukoderma (meaning vitiligo) and that it will increase in size at par with the increase in body surface area with the growth and development of the child. And that appearance of new depigmented patches over other areas of the body is less likely. Reassurance and counseling of the parents form the cornerstone of management.

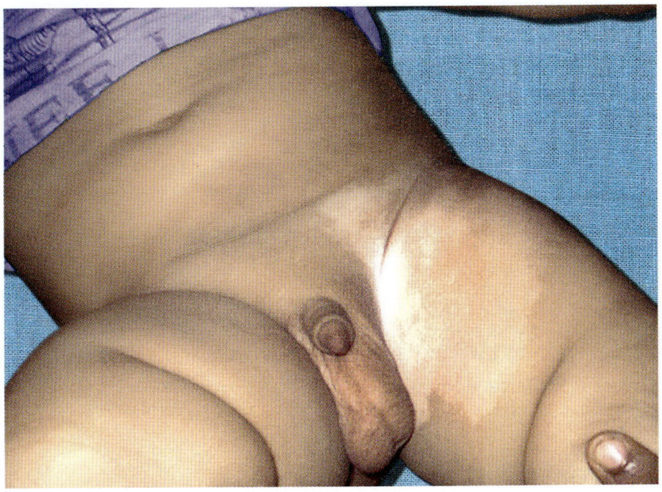

Fig. 5: Nevus depigmentosus, note irregular border.

NEVUS ANEMICUS (FIGS. 7A AND B)

Nevus anemicus is an uncommon congenital anomaly of the skin, and is seen as circumscribed rounded, oval, or linear area of pallor having a normal texture. Lesions may be single or multiple. Small blotches may be irregularly grouped. The margins of the lesion are ill-defined. Under diascopic pressure, the nevus becomes indistinguishable from the blanched surrounding skin. It occurs most commonly over the trunk. Nevus anemicus may be associated with various genetic syndromes such as neurofibromatosis type 1 (NF-1), tuberous sclerosis, and phakomatosis pigmentovascularis (PPV) type II to IV. Nevus anemicus should be differentiated from nevus

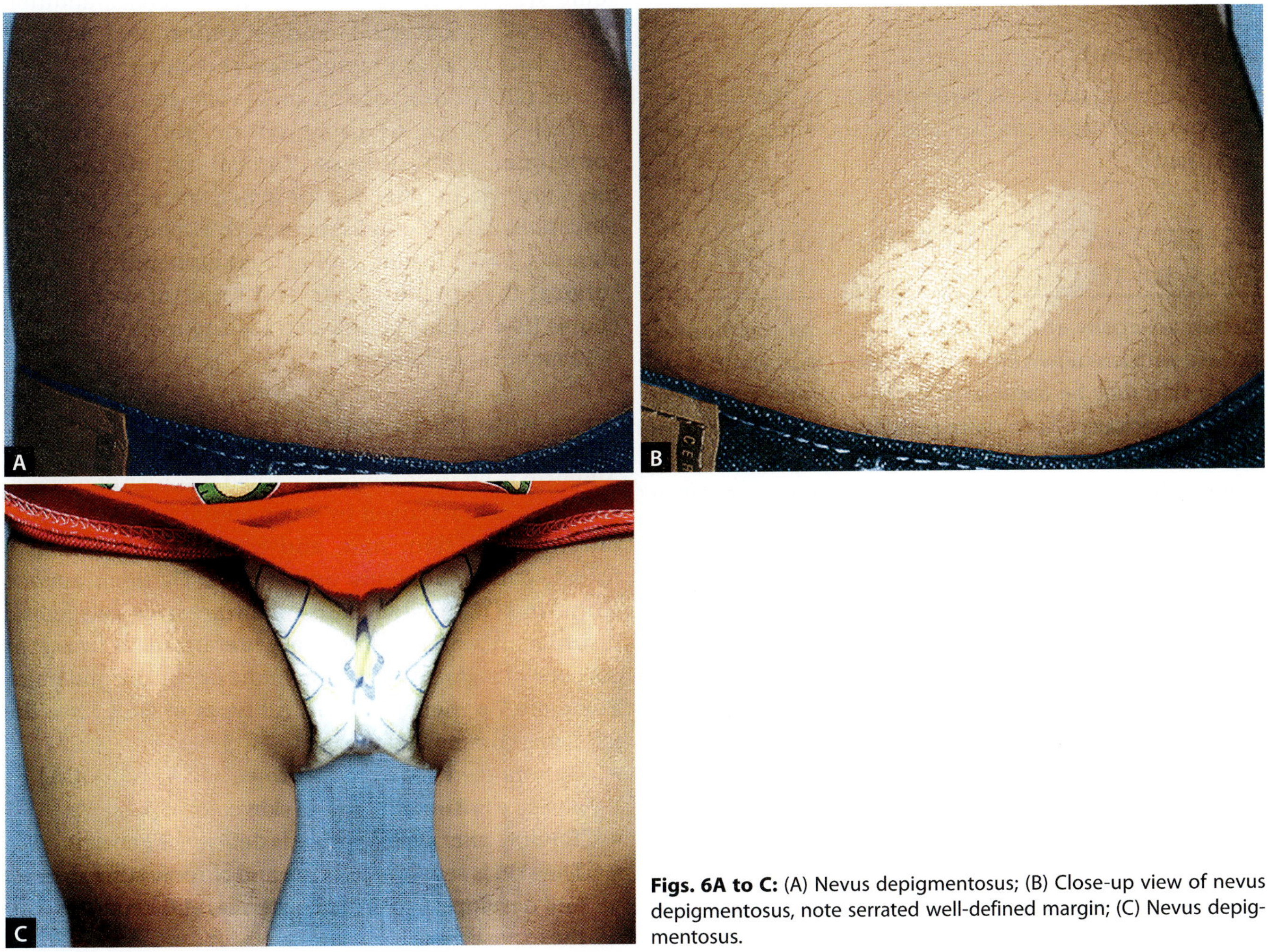

Figs. 6A to C: (A) Nevus depigmentosus; (B) Close-up view of nevus depigmentosus, note serrated well-defined margin; (C) Nevus depigmentosus.

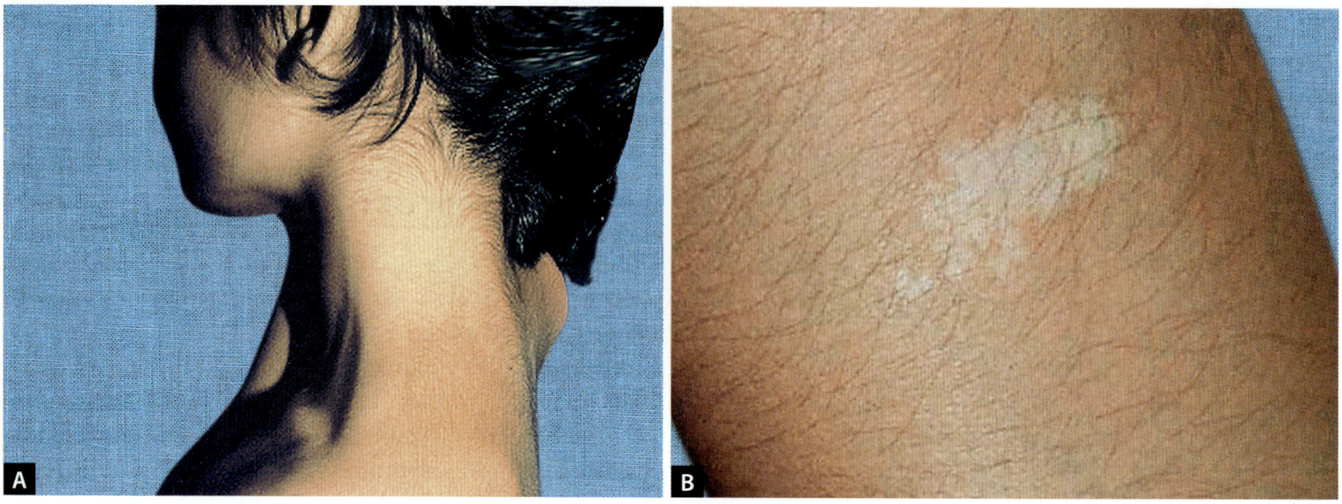

Figs. 7A and B: (A) Nevus anemicus over neck; (B) Nevus anemicus.

depigmentosus and vitiligo. Wood's lamp examination does not accentuate the hypopigmentation as compared to nevus depigmentosus and vitiligo.

Treatment

The condition needs to be explained to the children and parents. Reassurance and counseling are very important.

LICHEN SCLEROSUS ET ATROPHICUS (FIGS. 8A TO L)

Lichen sclerosus et atrophicus (LSA) is an uncommon disease with unknown etiology in which small white areas of the skin may be associated with an atrophic scarring over the perineum seen more commonly in adult female. The condition over the female genitalia is known as kraurosis vulvae. It occurs in pediatric age group as well in the form of ivory white patches, flat-topped papules over skin with follicular plugging and atrophy of the skin. LSA in childhood is associated with Koebner phenomenon. Anogenital region is commonly involved in children. Clinical features include itching, burning sensation with urination, and constipation. Often these are misdiagnosed as vitiligo.

Diagnosis

Histopathology of the skin confirms the diagnosis. Epidermis is atrophic with subepidermal vacuolization, hyalinized superficial dermis with band-like lymphocytic infiltrate.

Treatment

Mild to moderately potent topical steroids, emollient offer some symptomatic relief. Over genital areas, addition of topical antibacterials and/or anticandidal may be helpful to treat any associated secondary infection. Topical (2%) testosterone cream has also been advocated. Topical estrogen or progesterone gel is also used sometimes with success. Topical tacrolimus 0.1% has shown to be effective for active stage as well as in remission phase. Complications such as phimosis, meatal stenosis, labial fusion, and clitoral obliteration require surgical therapy. In severe and resistant cases, short course (2–4 weeks) of oral steroids and methotrexate for 6–12 months can be given.

ALBINISM (FIGS. 9 TO 12A)

Albinism is an uncommon inherited disorder of melanin synthesis characterized by a congenital lack of pigmentation of the skin, hair, and eyes. It occurs in two forms, oculocutaneous and ocular. Oculocutaneous albinism (OCA) is an autosomal recessive congenital disorder in which there is a generalized decrease or absence of pigment formation in the eyes, skin, and hairs. There are 7 variants of OCA. All types of OCA have the following common features:

- Generalized reduction (brown OCA, red OCA) or absence (all other types) of skin color
- Tanning after sun exposure is deficient or absent.
- The skin is sensitive to acute and chronic sun exposure and develops xerosis, pachyderma, and keratoses over the exposed parts.

"It is always important to know when something has reached its end. Closing circles, shutting doors, finishing chapters, it doesn't matter what we call it; what matters is to leave in the past those moments in life that are over." —**Paulo Coelho**

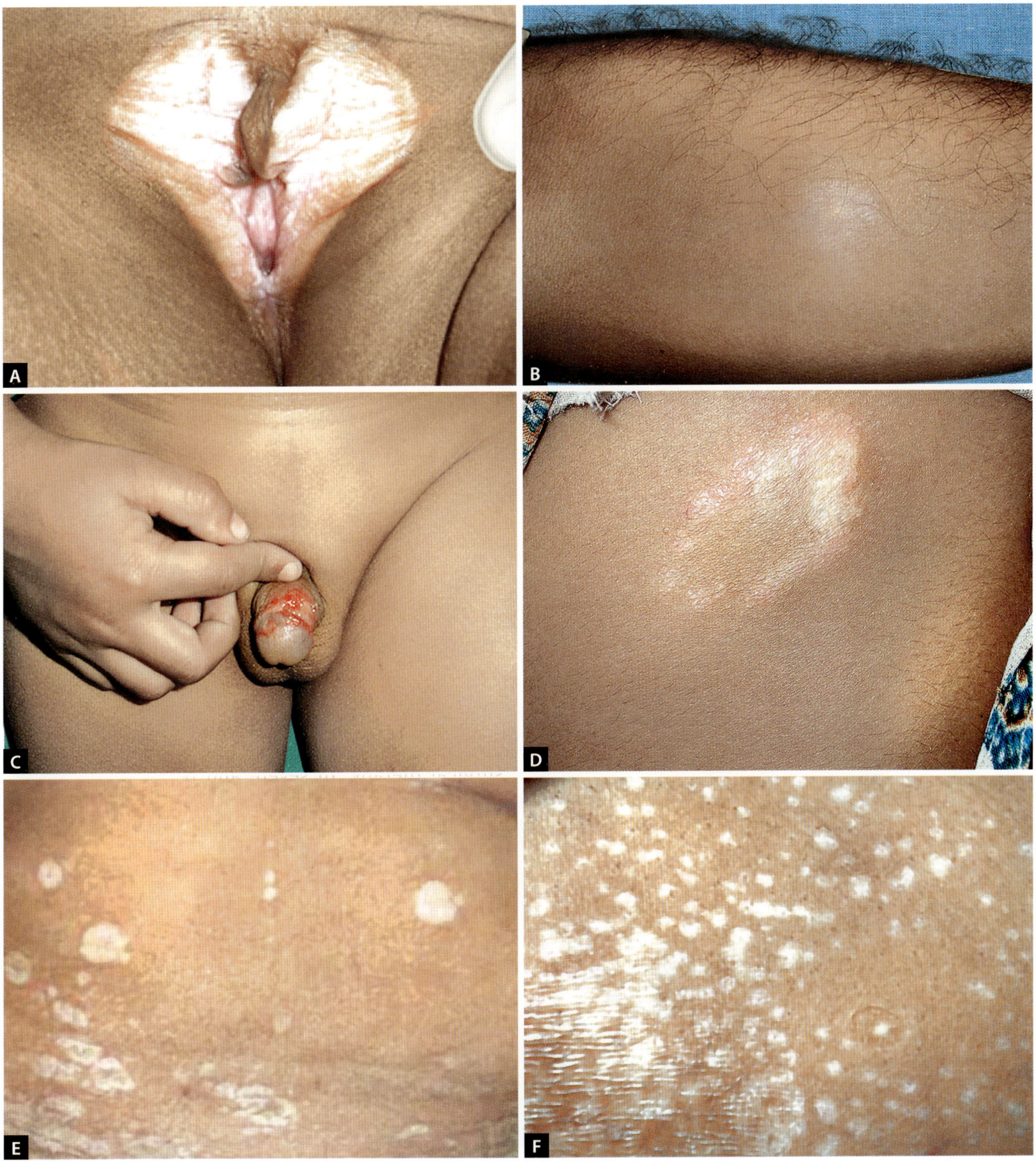

Figs. 8A to F: (A) Lichen sclerosus et atrophicus (LSA) over external genitalia in an young girl; (B) Milky white-sclerosed skin of LSA over thigh; (C) LSA with erosions over glans penis and prepuce in 3-year-old boy; (D) LSA lesion, note lilac border; (E) Lesions of LSA, note Koebner phenomenon; (F) LSA, note porcelain-white appearance of lesions.

"There is no real ending. It's just the place where you stop the story." —**Frank Herbert**

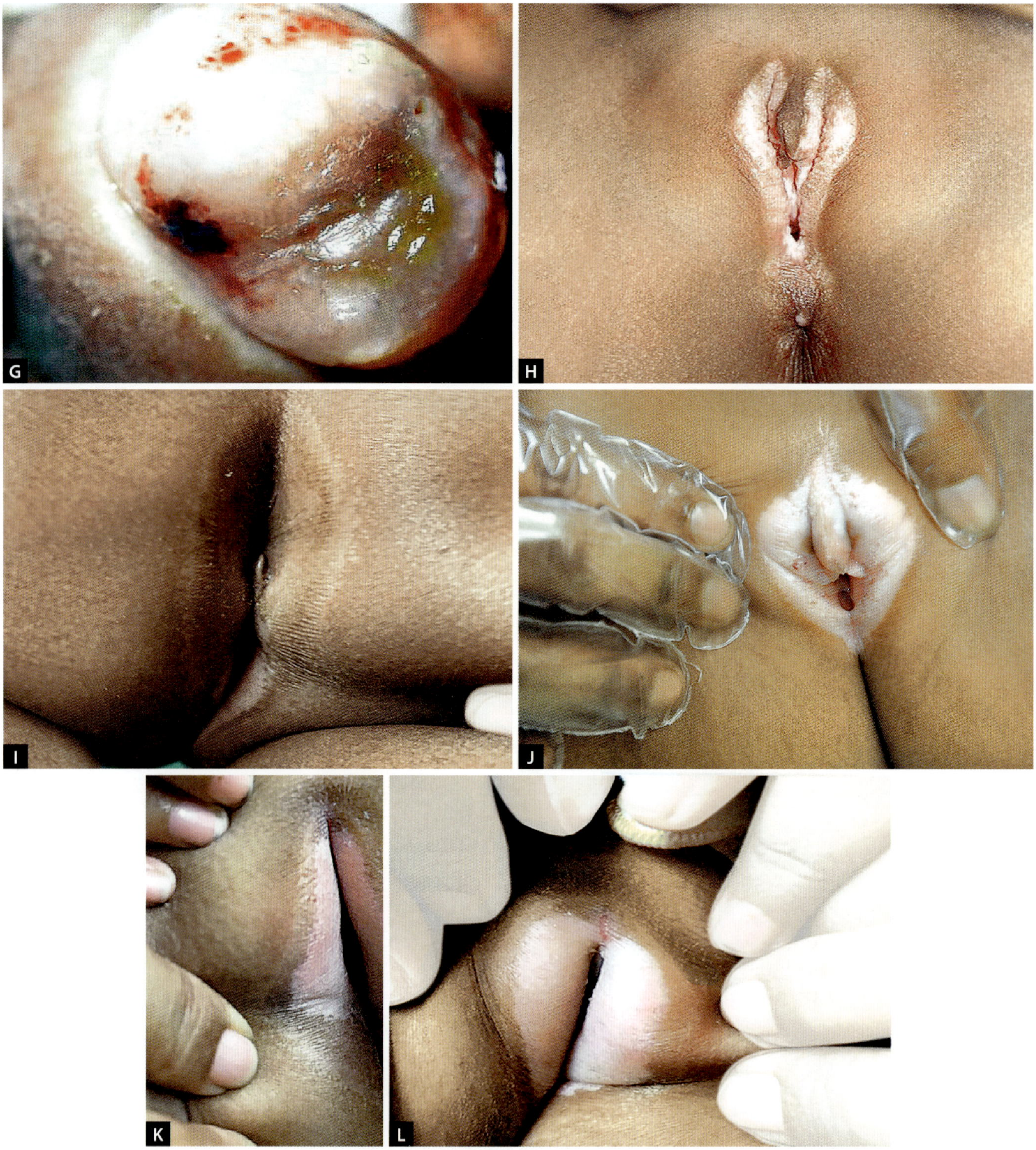

Figs. 8G to L: (G) Lichen sclerosus et atrophicus (LSA) over glans and prepuce in an adolescent male (balanitis xerotica obliterans); (H) LSA over vulva in a 9-year-old girl; (I) LSA perianal; (J) LSA vulva, visibly it appears indurated with hemorrhagic spots; (K) LSA vulva; (L) Same girl with vulvar LSA.

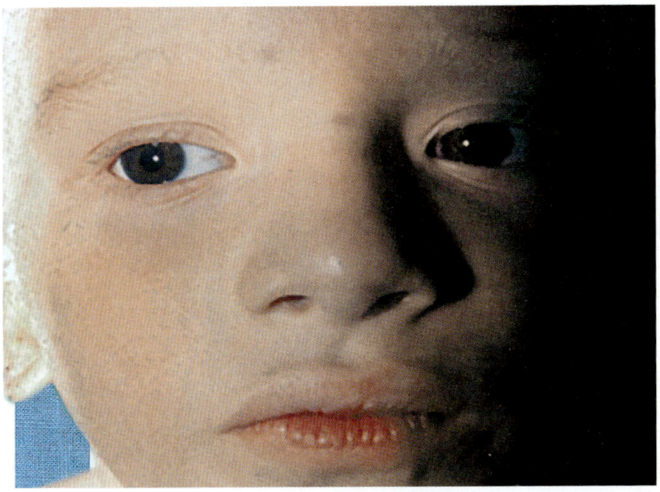

Fig. 9: Oculocutaneous albinism.

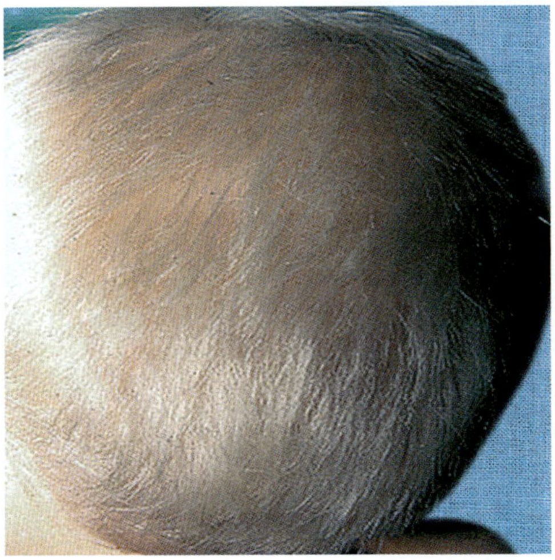

Fig. 10: White hairs in albinism.

- Translucent irides with nystagmus and hypopigmented ocular fundi.

Clinically, OCA manifests as generalized depigmented skin with white hairs all over the body from birth. Other anomalies include short stature, mental retardation, developmental anomalies, reduced fertility, and life expectancy.

Complications

Sun-induced damage of the skin results in premature senility, freckling, lentigines, actinic keratoses, and squamous cell carcinoma. Occasionally, melanoma also develops.

Management

Explaining the condition to the parents forms the crux of management protocol. The parents should be educated about exposing the affected children to sunlight as less as possible. An ophthalmological check-up is important. Sunscreens are to be used from the very infancy. In case of acute phototoxic reactions, topical steroids and antihistamines are to be used for 7–10 days to control it. If the reaction is severe, short (7–10 days) course of oral corticosteroids is helpful in providing symptomatic relief as well as enhancing the healing of the wounds. This is to be followed by regular use of sunscreens.

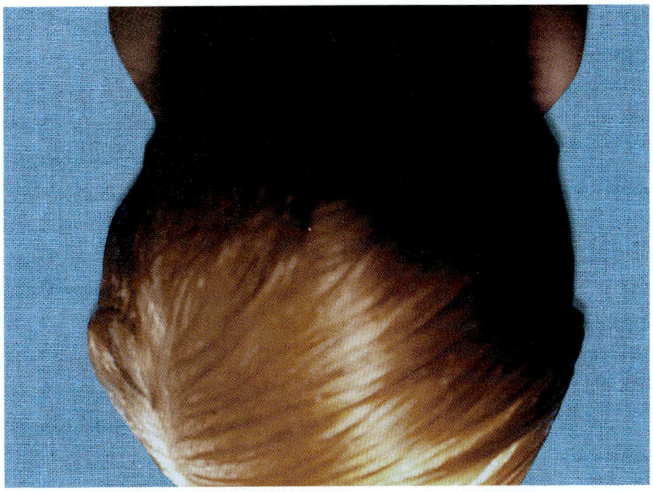

Fig. 11: White and brown hairs in albinism.

HERMANSKY–PUDLAK SYNDROME (FIG. 12B)

Hermansky–Pudlak syndrome (HPS) is an extremely rare autosomal recessive disorder which results in pigment dilution, platelet storage defect leading to bleeding diathesis, and lysosomal accumulation of ceroid-like material in reticuloendothelial system. Individuals will have varying amounts of skin pigment dilution (melanin). Eye problems include photophobia, strabismus, and nystagmus. HPS also impairs vision. The condition may be associated with granulomatous colitis and pulmonary fibrosis.

LICHEN STRIATUS (FIGS. 13A TO G)

Lichen striatus is a self-limiting inflammatory linear dermatitis of unknown origin. It is often associated with atopy. It usually occurs in children between the ages of 5 and 15 years and is more common in girls. Small pink, lichenoid papules, discrete at first but rapidly coalescing, appear suddenly and extend over the course of a week or month to form a dull red, slightly scaly, linear band 2 mm to 2 cm in width and often irregular. Occasionally, the bands broaden into plaques especially on the buttocks. The lesions may be only a few centimeters in length or may

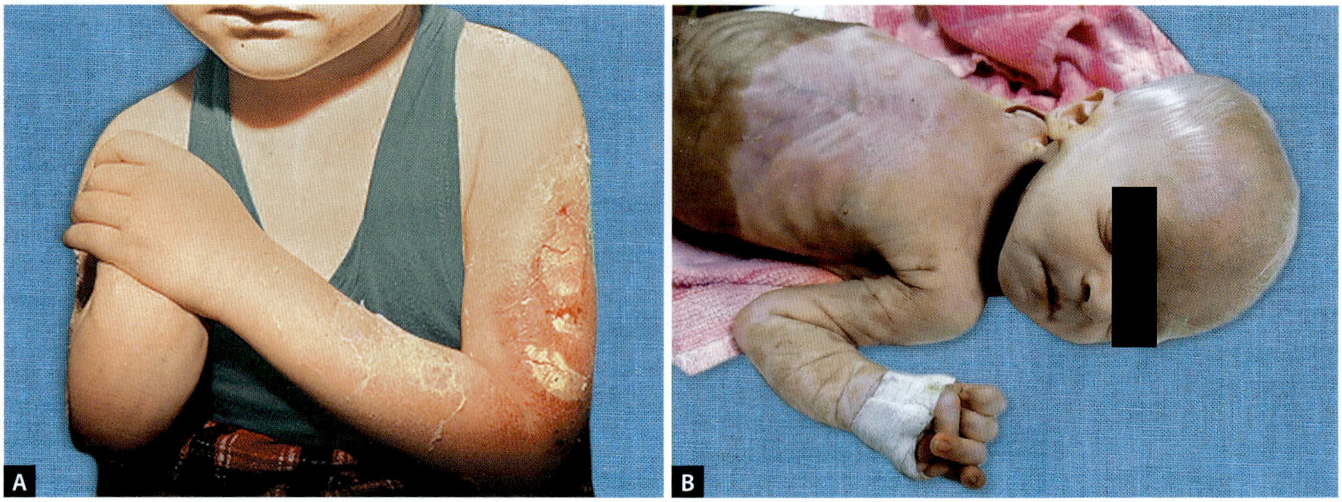

Figs. 12A and B: (A) Acute phototoxic reaction in an albino child; (B) Hermansky–Pudlak syndrome.

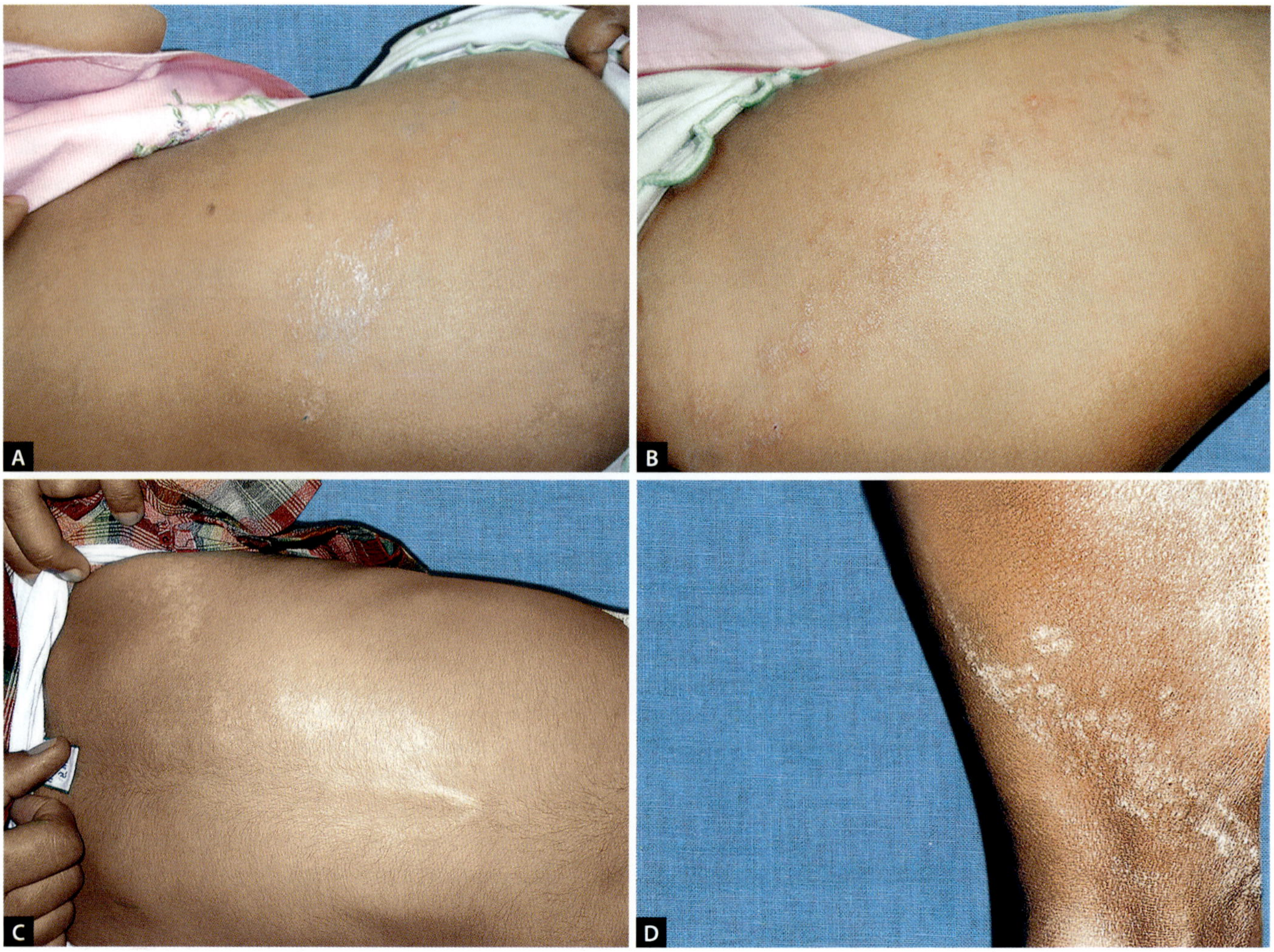

Figs. 13A to D: (A) Lichen striatus over thigh in a 3-year-old girl; (B) Same girl with lichen striatus; (C) Lichen striatus over back; (D) Hypopigmented linear streak over thigh in lichen stratus.

"Change is hard at first, messy in the middle and gorgeous at the end." —**Robin Sharma**

extend the entire length of the limb and may be continuous or interrupted. The lesions occur most commonly on one arm or leg or on the neck but may develop on the trunk. They may appear hypopigmented in dark-skinned people. Nail involvement in the form of longitudinal ridging, splitting, and onycholysis may occur. There are usually no symptoms, but pruritus may occur occasionally.

Natural History

The lesion reaches its maximum extent within 2–3 weeks. Spontaneous resolution can be expected within 3–6 months but some lesions may persist for over a year or two.

Differential Diagnosis

Epidermal nevi and inflammatory linear epidermal nevus may be confused clinically with lichen striatus but nevi persist indefinitely. Linear lichen planus and psoriasis can usually be differentiated clinically and histopathologically.

Treatment

Usually, the lesions resolve spontaneously. But it takes long time to do so, from 3 months to 2 years. Topical corticosteroids (mild or moderately potent) may hasten the healing process. If the lesions are symptomatic, i.e., mildly pruritic, oral antihistamines may be prescribed. The lesions are dry and, therefore, topical emollient application is helpful. Topical tacrolimus and retinoids have shown some improvement. Counseling is important.

IDIOPATHIC ERUPTIVE MACULAR HYPOMELANOSIS (FIG. 13H)

Idiopathic eruptive macular hypomelanosis is a newly described paraviral exanthem reported from India.

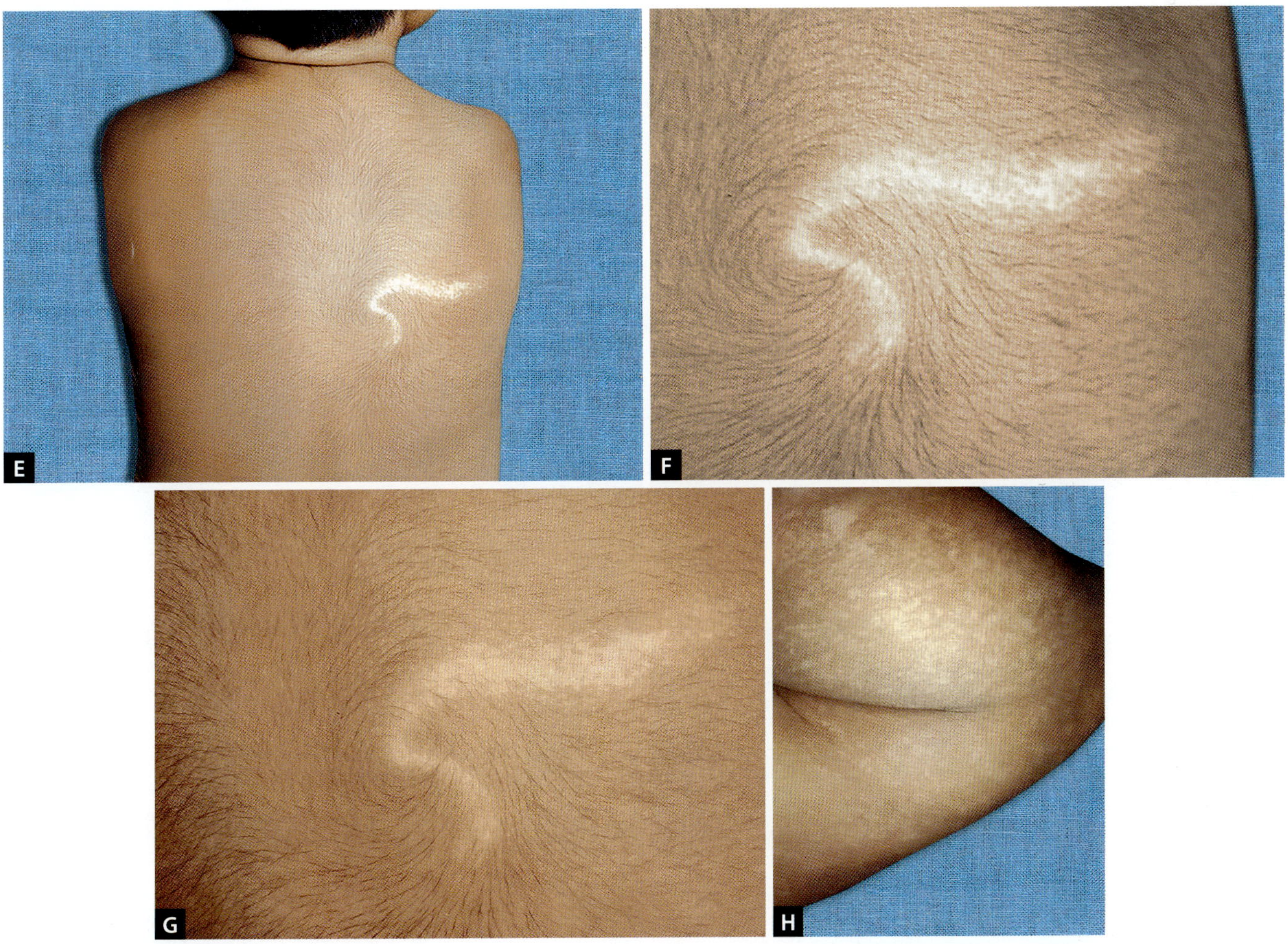

Figs. 13E to H: (E) Lichen striatus, note serpiginous whitish streak; (F) Close-up view, note serpiginous pattern; (G) Further magnified view, note lichenoid component; (H) Idiopathic eruptive macular hypomelanosis.

"Everything will be okay in the end. If it's not okay, it's not the end." —**John Lennon**

It is postulated to be caused by a viral infection because of several reasons: (1) A prodromal coryzal phase for 1–2 weeks preceding the onset of the eruption, (2) the eruptive nature with successive crops of lesions, (3) the fairly uniform sizes of lesions, (4) spontaneous resolution without active intervention, and (5) relatively young age of the children affected, thus indicating a primary infection rather than endogenous reactivation of a virus. We believe that it is a paraviral exanthem, which means a single viral etiology is yet to be identified. It is not clear why are there no reports of this condition from other ethnic groups and other countries apart from India so far. Involvement of pinna of both ears was found in many patients. Sometimes a tendency to coalescence of hypopigmented macules is observed. One reason might be that a hypopigmented rash would be more prominently noted in darker-skinned races. Another reason could be the self-limited course of the disease. Thus, many children with eruptive hypomelanosis might not be brought to medical attention. It is likely that a significant proportion of such children are seen only by primary care physicians and not referred to dermatologists or pediatricians because the rash is asymptomatic and self-resolving. We believe, many specialists may not be aware of this new clinical entity because of a paucity of published reports.

POSTINFLAMMATORY HYPOPIGMENTATION (FIGS. 14 AND 15)

Pigmented skin shows more of a pigmentary reaction following trauma or inflammation than nonpigmented or lightly pigmented skin. It is also not uncommon to see secondary hypopigmentation following eczema, pityriasis alba, sarcoidosis, leprosy, herpes zoster, pityriasis versicolor, or other common eruptions. It may also follow cryotherapy and the topical use of or intralesional injection of corticosteroids.

Natural History

The hypopigmentation resolves spontaneously in majority of the cases over a period of 3 months to 3 years.

Treatment

NBUVB therapy has shown good improvement in pityriasis rosea and pityriasis lichenoides chronica-induced hypopigmentation.

POSTINFLAMMATORY HYPERPIGMENTATION (FIGS. 16A TO F)

Postinflammatory hyperpigmentation is probably the most common cause of hyperpigmentation in all age groups. Postinflammatory hyperpigmentation develops following friction, trauma, boils, etc. It is more commonly seen in dark complexioned children and there is a tendency in some children to develop hyperpigmentation. This type of hyperpigmentation is more commonly seen in atopic individuals with papular urticaria. The condition may develop anywhere on the body. However, when it occurs over exposed parts, ultraviolet rays may accentuate the spot and/or delay their resolution.

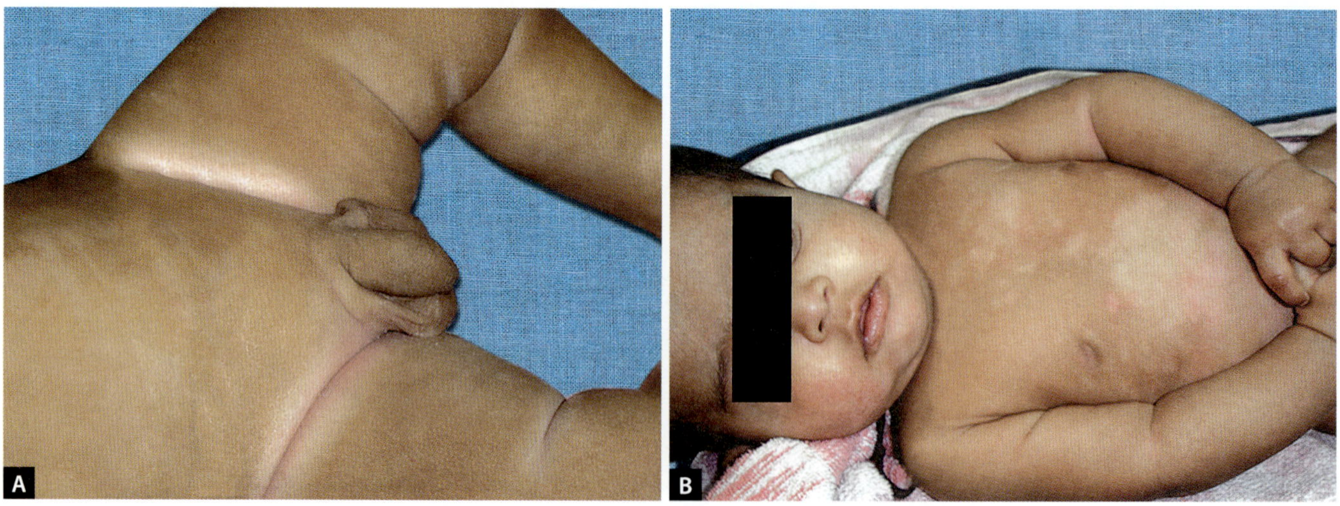

Figs. 14A and B: (A) Postinflammatory hypopigmentation following infantile seborrheic dermatitis; (B) Another view in the same infant.

"Stop worrying about the potholes in the road and enjoy the journey." —**Babs Hoffman**

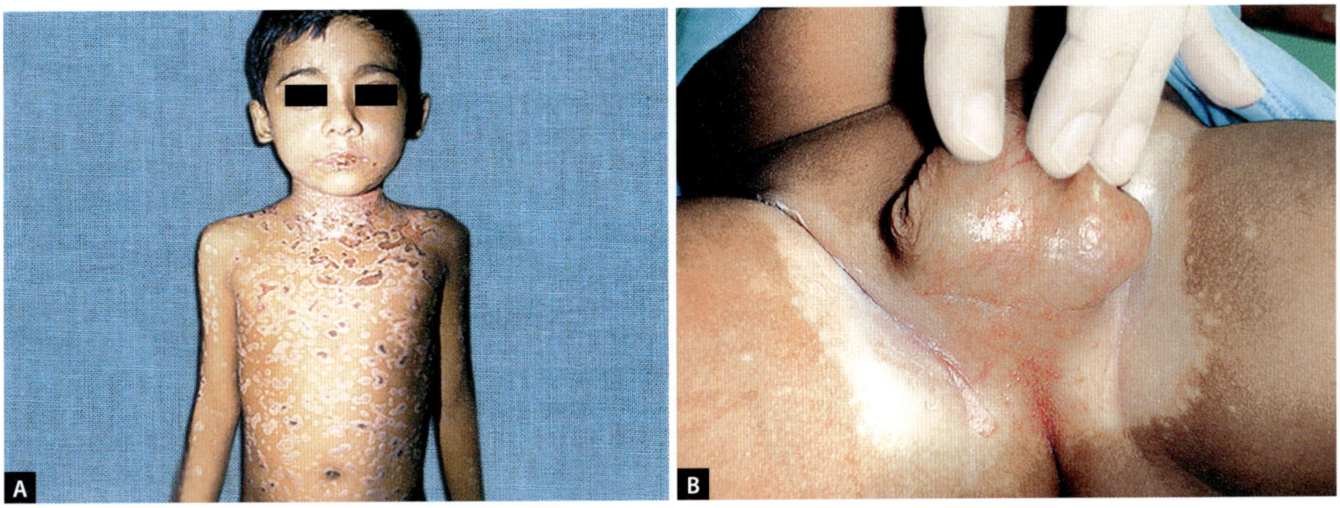

Figs. 15A and B: (A) Postinflammatory hypopigmentation (PIH) in a boy following Stevens–Johnson syndrome (SJS); (B) PIH in an infant with intertrigo.

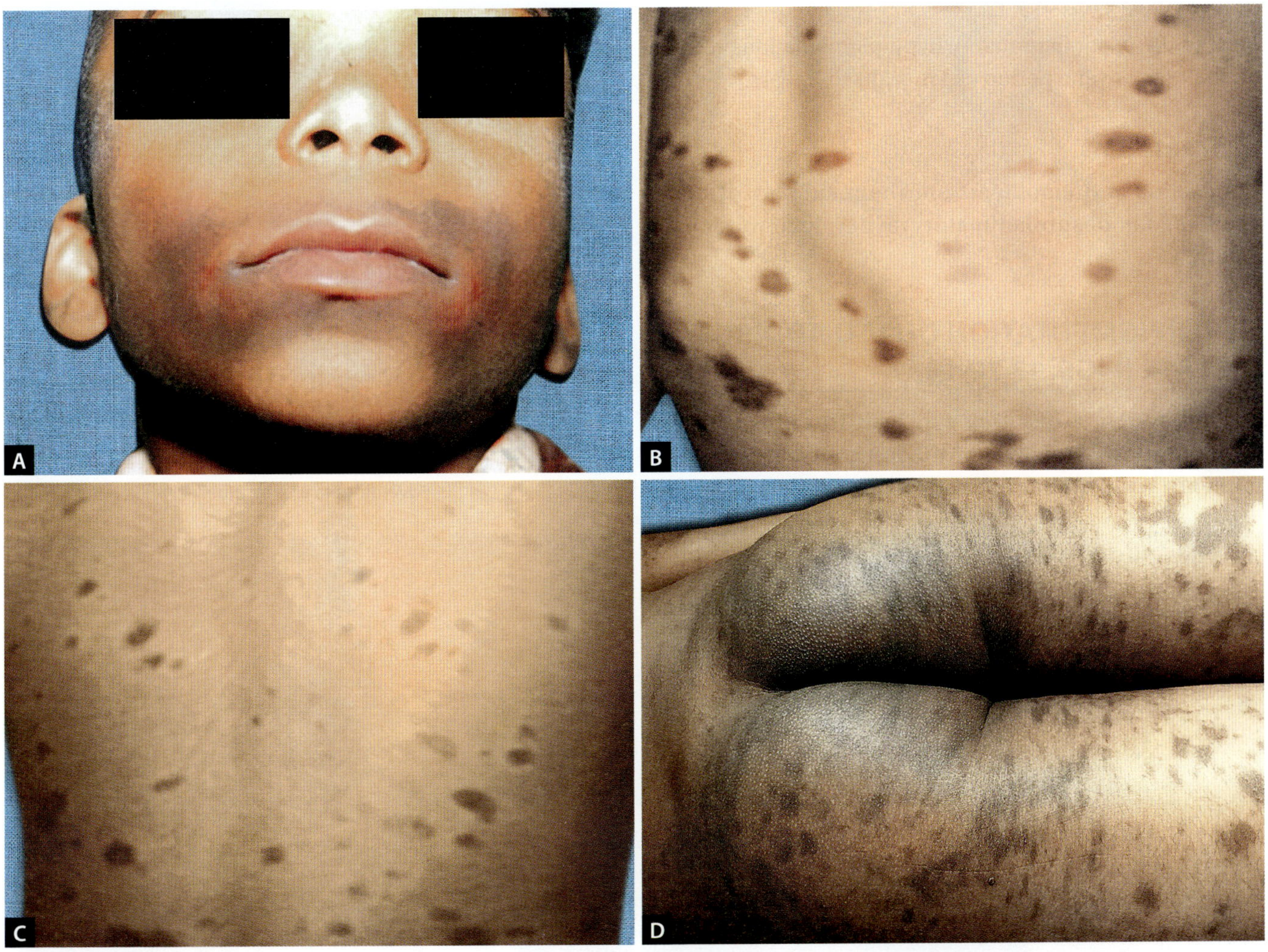

Figs. 16A to D: (A) Facial melanosis due to regular massage of mustard oil over face; (B) Postinflammatory hyperpigmentation following pityriasis lichenoides et varioliformis acuta (PLEVA); (C) Lesions over back in the same boy; (D) Postinflammatory hyperpigmentation following lichen planus.

"Any believable prediction will be wrong. Any correct prediction will be unbelievable." —**Kevin Kelly**

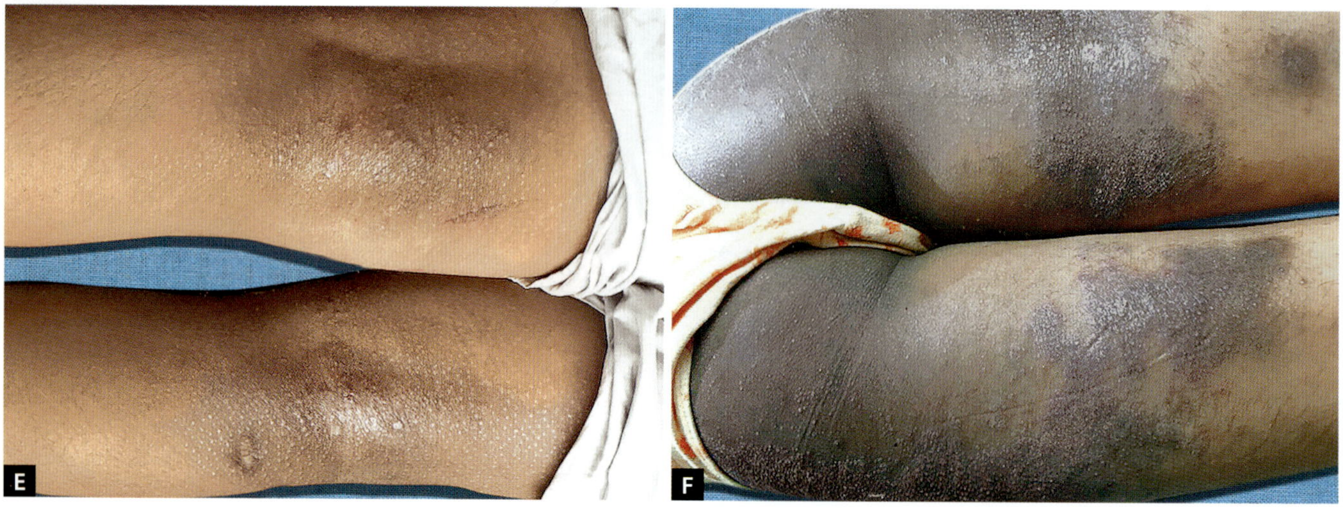

Figs. 16E and F: (E) Postinflammatory hyperpigmentation following atopic dermatitis (flexural); (F) Postinflammatory hyperpigmentation following posterior thigh dermatitis.

Natural History

Most of the postinflammatory hyperpigmentations resolve on their own over a period of 3 months to 2 years.

Treatment

Counseling and emollients are the main stay of management for postinflammatory hyperpigmentation in children.

HYPERPIGMENTATION DUE TO ADDISON'S DISEASE (FIGS. 17 TO 19A)

Several systemic diseases can lead to diffuse hyperpigmentation. However, Addison's disease usually presents with a characteristic type of pigmentation.

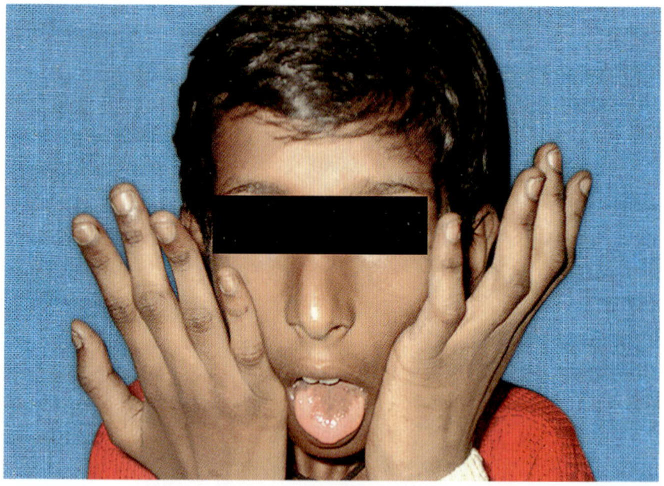

Fig. 17: Hyperpigmentation of Addison's disease over fingers and tongue.

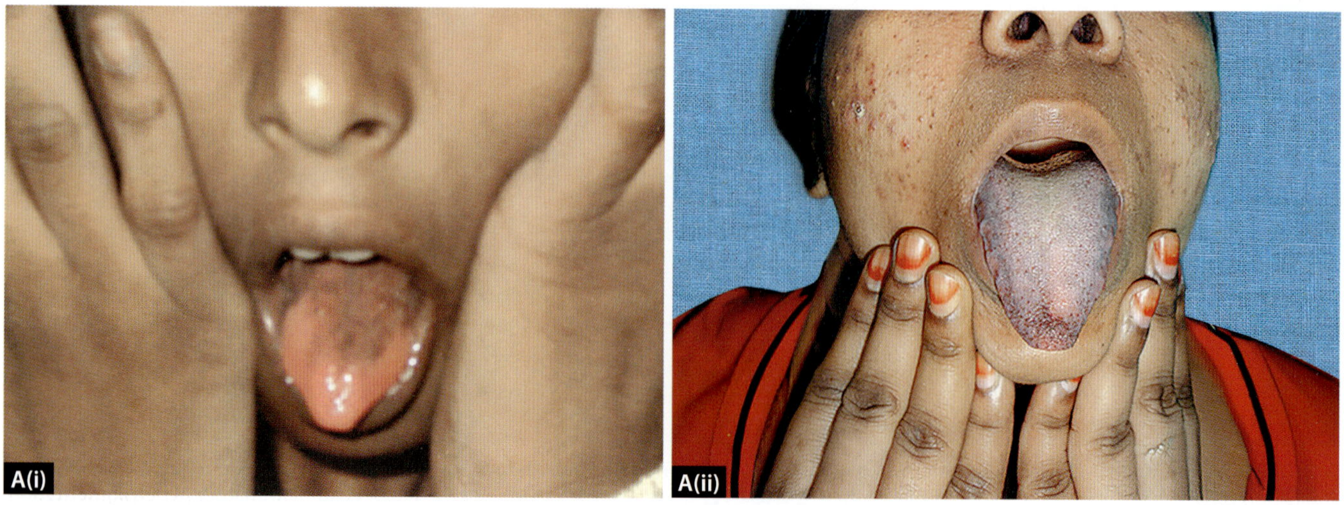

Figs. 18A(i) and (ii): A(i) Close-up view of tongue pigmentation; A(ii) Hyperpigmentation of tongue, finger joints in Addison's disease.

"I do not feel obliged to believe that the same God who has endowed us with sense, reason, and intellect has intended us to forgo their use." **—Galileo Galilei**

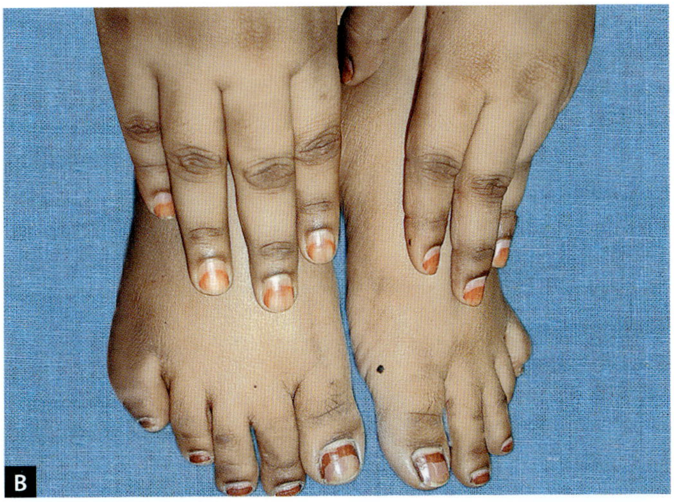

Fig. 18B: Hyperpigmentation over fingers and toes in a patient with Addison's disease.

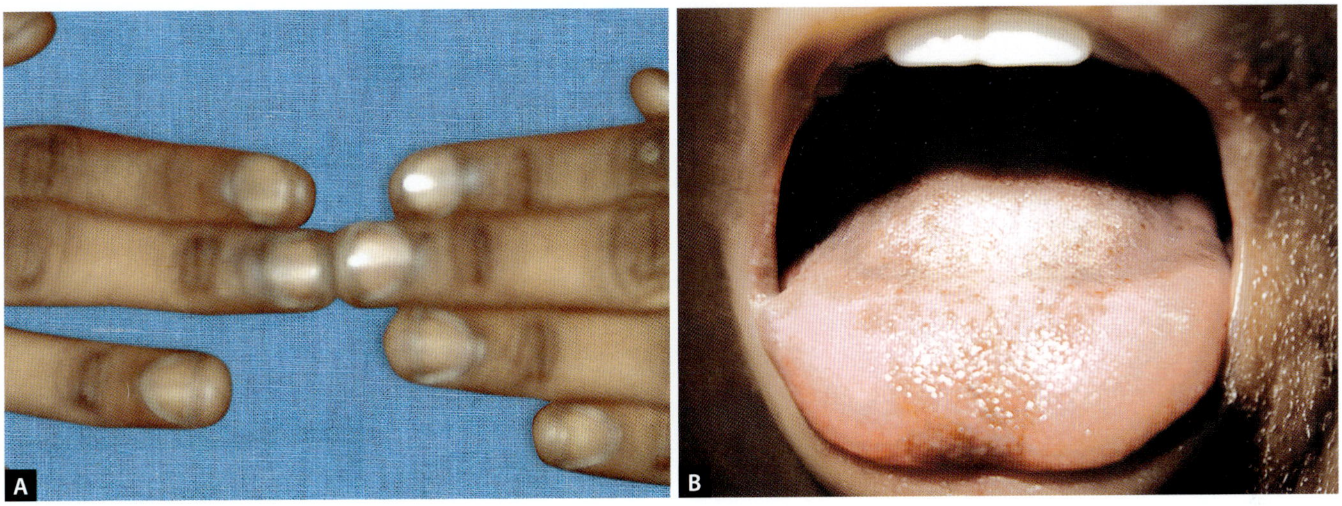

Figs. 19A and B: (A) Pigmentation of fingers and nails in Addison's disease; (B) Familial hyperpigmentation of tongue in a 7-year-old girl.

The pigmentation is diffuse in nature and prominent over the sun-exposed areas. Additional sites of involvement include the oral mucosa, palmoplantar creases, sites of friction or pressure, flexural areas, areola, and genitalia. This pigmentation is due to increased production of melanocyte-stimulating hormone (MSH) and adrenocorticotropic hormone (ACTH).

FAMILIAL HYPERPIGMENTATION OF TONGUE (FIGS. 19B TO E)

Familial hyperpigmentation of the tongue is a peculiar hyperpigmentation seen among various members of some of the families. It does not have a definite inheritance pattern and believed to be mostly sporadic in onset. It is mostly seen in individuals with skin type IV and V. There is either patchy or band-like hyperpigmentation over the dorsum of the tongue. There may be involvement of contiguous oral mucosa, e.g., gum and cheek.

The first author of this book (SD) and colleague described it for the first time in Indian literature.

Management

The condition needs to be explained properly to the parents/children and they are to be reassured.

HYPERPIGMENTATION OF KNUCKLE AND DORSAL ASPECT OF INTERPHALANGEAL JOINTS OF FINGERS IN ATOPICS (FIGS. 20 TO 22)

It is quite commonly seen and usually does not respond to any demelanising creams. Regular application of moisturizers helps to an extent.

"The whole problem with the world is that fools and fanatics are always so certain of themselves, and wiser people so full of doubts." **—Bertrand Russell**

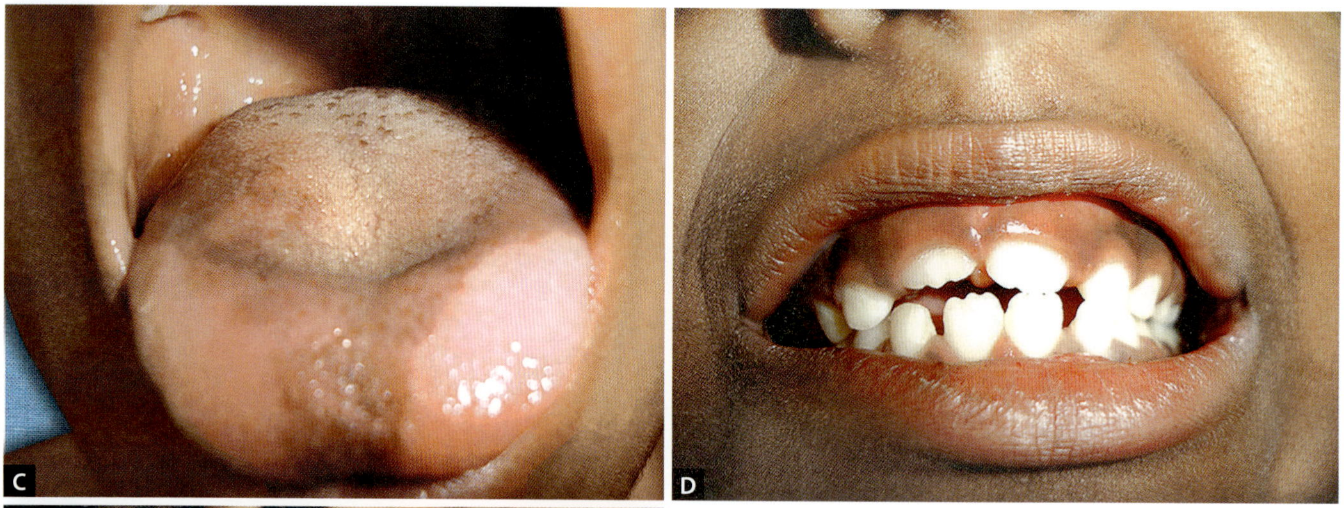

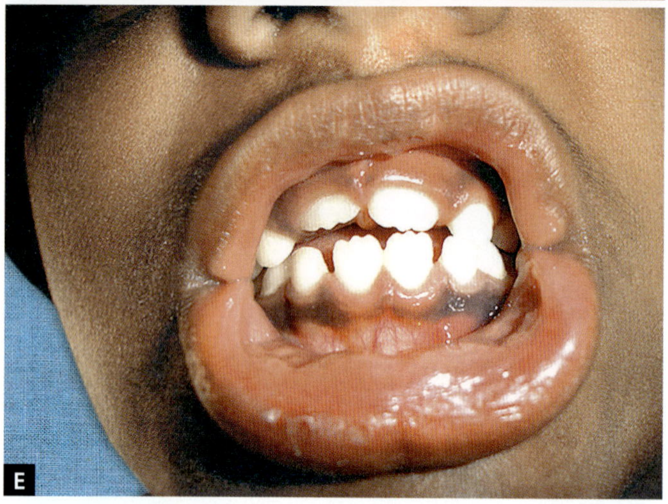

Figs. 19C to E: (C) Same girl, close-up view; (D) Familial hyperpigmentation over gum in a 4-year-old boy; (E) Same boy, close-up view.

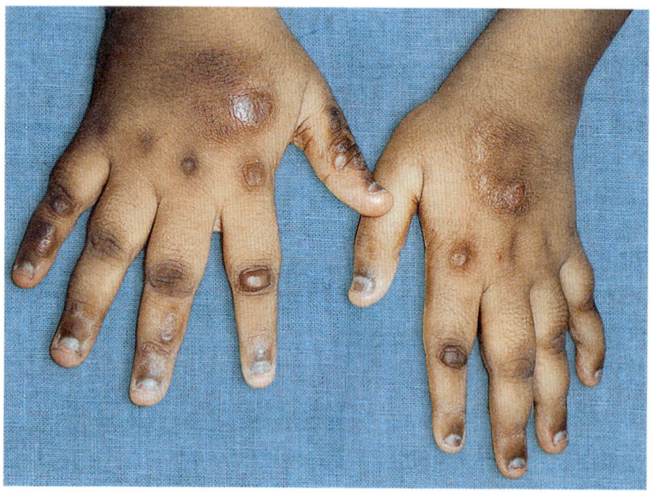

Fig. 20: Pigmentation over knuckles in atopics.

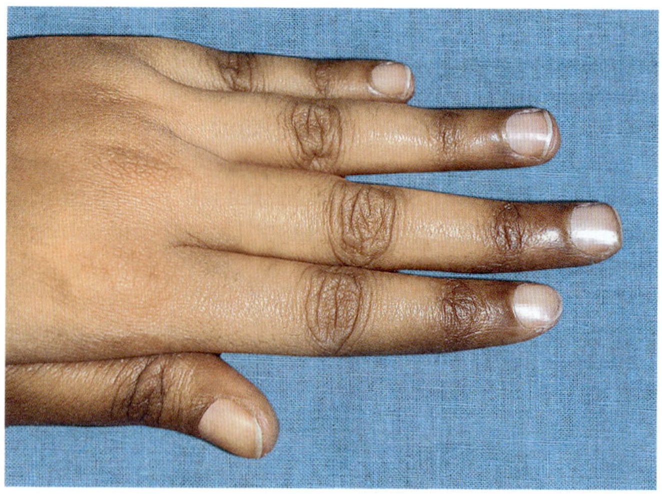

Fig. 21: Hyperpigmentation over fingers in atopics.

"You can avoid reality, but you cannot avoid the consequences of avoiding reality." —**Ayn Rand**

FANCONI ANEMIA AND HYPERPIGMENTATION (FIGS. 23A AND B)

Fanconi anemia (FA) is a rare genetic disease resulting in impaired response to DNA (deoxyribonucleic acid) damage. FA is characterized by bone marrow failure, acute myelogenous leukemia (AML), solid tumors, and developmental abnormalities. Classic features include abnormal thumbs, absent radius, short stature, diffuse hypermelanosis of skin, café-au-lait macules, abnormal facial features (triangular face and microcephaly), abnormal kidneys, and decreased fertility. Approximately 80% of patients ultimately develop bone marrow failure by the age of 20 years.

CARBON BABY SYNDROME (FIG. 23C)

Carbon baby syndrome, also known as universal acquired melanosis is a rare condition characterized by progressive and diffuse hyperpigmentation of the skin and mucous membrane, which later can become mottled. The onset of the condition can occur from 3 to 5 months of age. The etiology is still elusive. The proposed mechanism

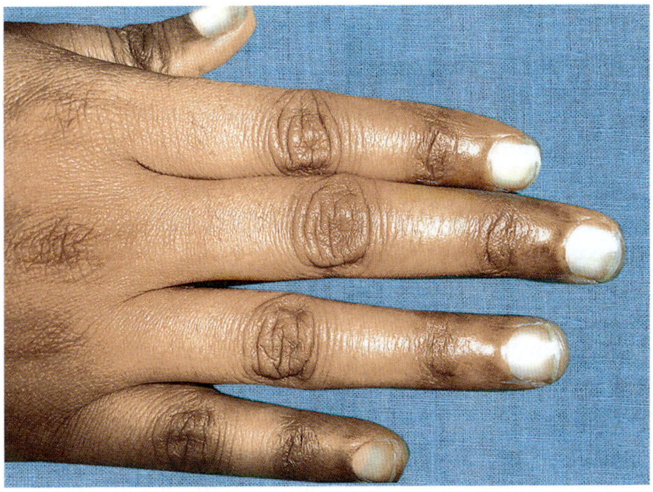

Fig. 22: Same patient.

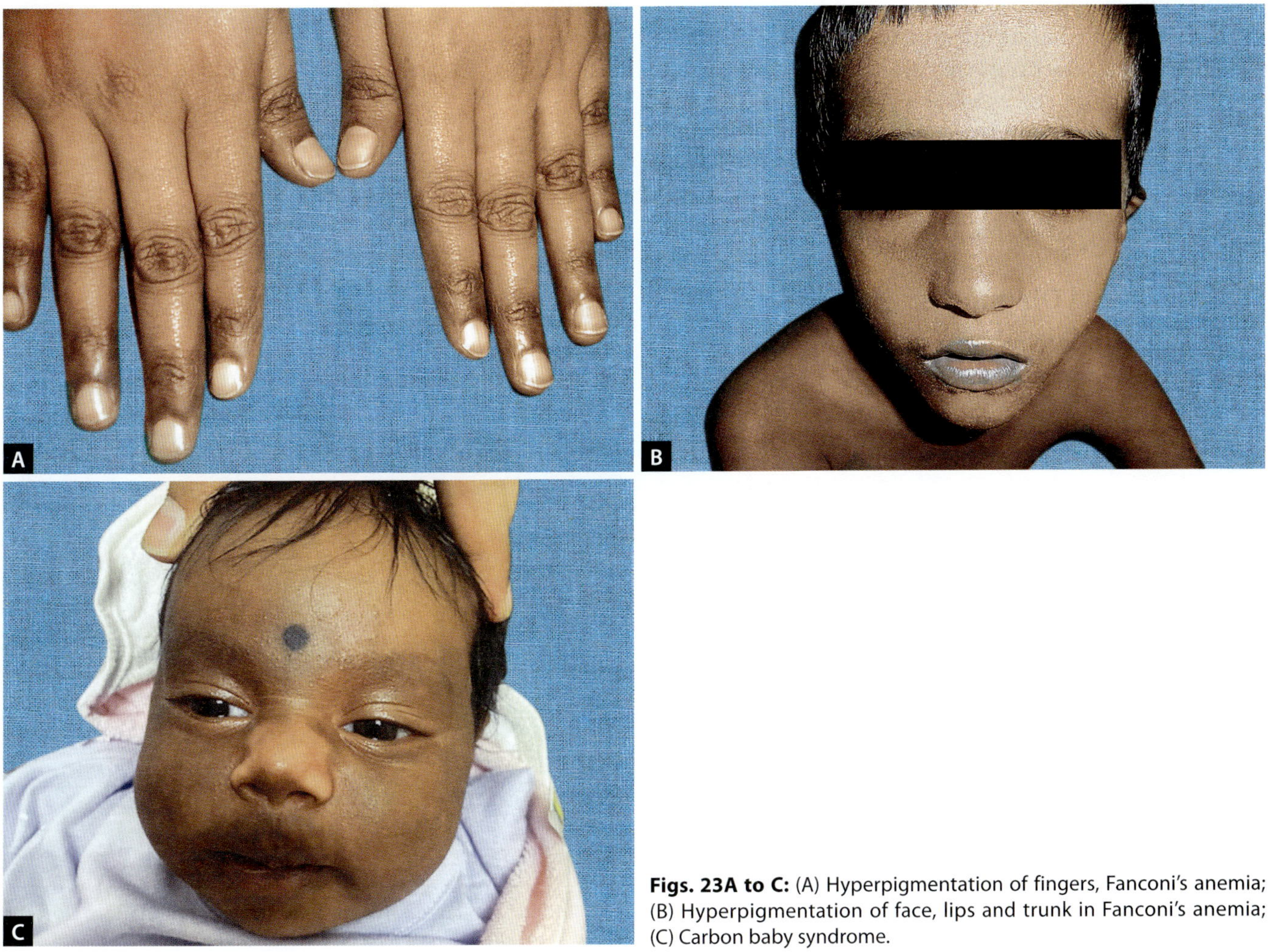

A

B

C

Figs. 23A to C: (A) Hyperpigmentation of fingers, Fanconi's anemia; (B) Hyperpigmentation of face, lips and trunk in Fanconi's anemia; (C) Carbon baby syndrome.

"There are no facts, only interpretations." —**Friedrich Nietzsche**

includes excessive production of beta-melanocyte-stimulating hormone, abnormal sensitivity of melanin towards normal and abnormal endocrine and nervous stimuli and probably could be associated with genetic mutation. Histopathologically there is diffuse melanin deposition throughout the epidermis with minimal dermal pigmentation without increase in the number of melanocytes. It is not associated with systemic manifestations.

IDIOPATHIC ERUPTIVE MACULAR HYPERPIGMENTATION (FIGS. 24 TO 26)

It is characterized by the development of asymptomatic macules over the neck, trunk, and proximal limbs. The age group affected is generally between 1 and 31 years. The following criteria should be fulfilled for the diagnosis of this condition.

- Eruption of brown, nonconfluent, asymptomatic macules on the trunk, neck, and proximal extremities in a child or adolescent patient.
- Absence of preceding inflammatory lesions
- No history of any drug exposure
- Histopathology shows basal layer hyperpigmentation of the epidermis and prominent dermal melanophages without visible basal layer damage or lichenoid inflammatory infiltrate.
- Normal mast cell counts

Differential Diagnoses

- Erythema dyschromicum perstans
- Lichen planus pigmentosus
- Mastocytosis
- Postinflammatory hyperpigmentation
- Drug-induced pigmentary changes

It is important to consider this condition in the differential diagnosis of the pigmentary disorders affecting the pediatric age group as it shows spontaneous resolution and no specific treatment is necessary.

DYSCHROMATOSIS HEREDITARIA (FIGS. 27 AND 28)

The term dyschromatosis denotes presence of both hypo- and hyperpigmentation. In this segment, we are focusing on two classical forms of dyschromatoses—dyschromatosis symmetrica hereditaria (DSH) and dyschromatosis universalis hereditaria (DUH).

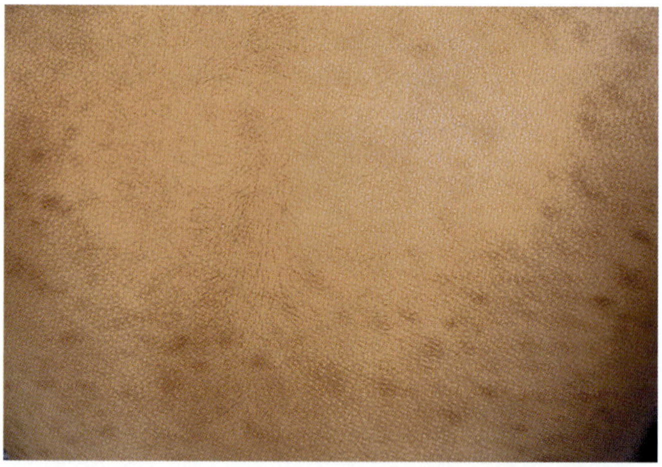

Fig. 25: Idiopathic eruptive macular hyperpigmentation, note innumerable ill-defined mildly hyperpigmented macules.

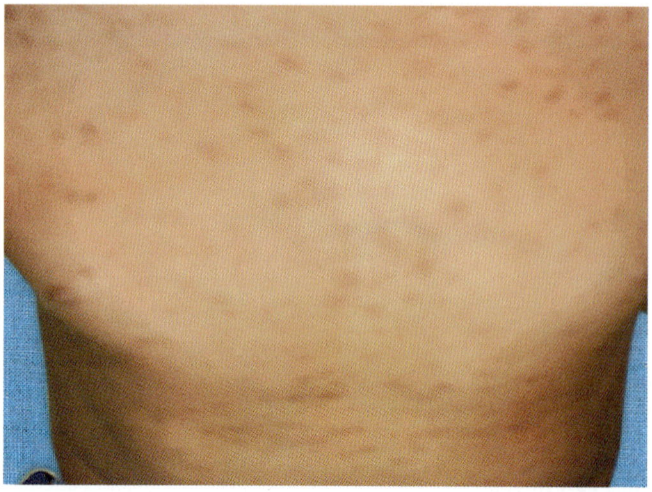

Fig. 24: Idiopathic eruptive macular hyperpigmentation.

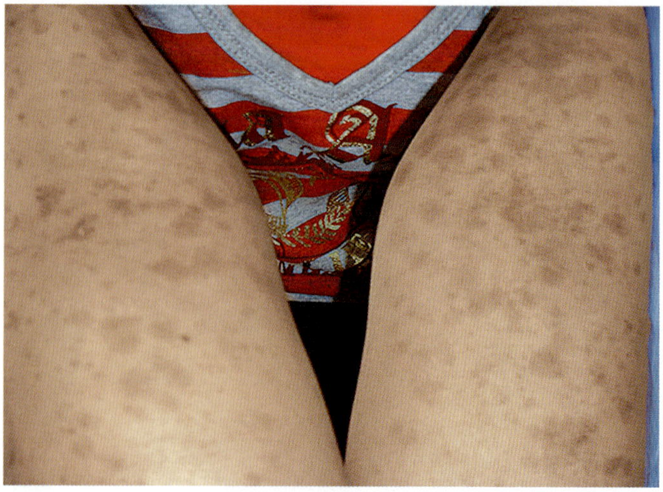

Fig. 26: Idiopathic eruptive macular hyperpigmentation, close-up view.

"Nothing in the world is more dangerous than sincere ignorance and conscientious stupidity." —**Martin Luther King Jr**

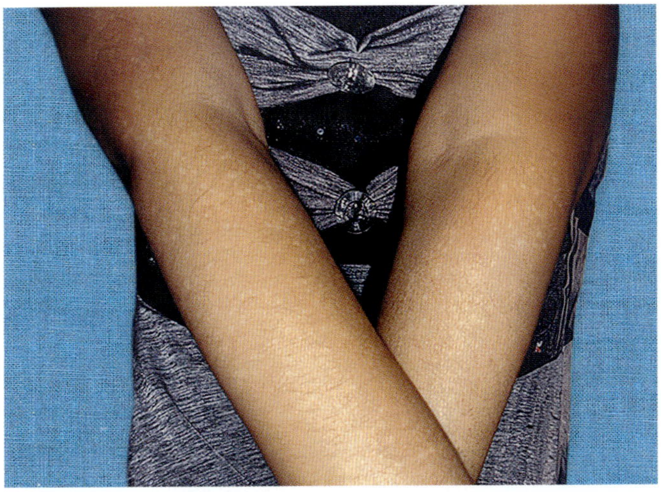

Fig. 27: Dyschromatosis hereditaria.

Dyschromatosis symmetrica hereditaria, also known as reticulate acropigmentation of Dohi, is autosomal dominant in inheritance and prevalent in Japanese. The underlying pathology is mutation of *DSRAD* gene which encodes double-stranded RNA specific enzyme adenosine deaminase, an RNA-editing enzyme. The disease usually starts by the age of 6 years and is characterized by small hyper- and hypopigmented macules, often mixed in a reticulate pattern, which increase in number and size and stabilize by adolescence. Thereafter, lesions persist indefinitely. Hyperpigmented macules darken following sun exposure. There is a predilection for distal extremities, especially for dorsa of the hands and feet with sparing of palms, soles, and mucous membrane. Histopathological section of hyperpigmented

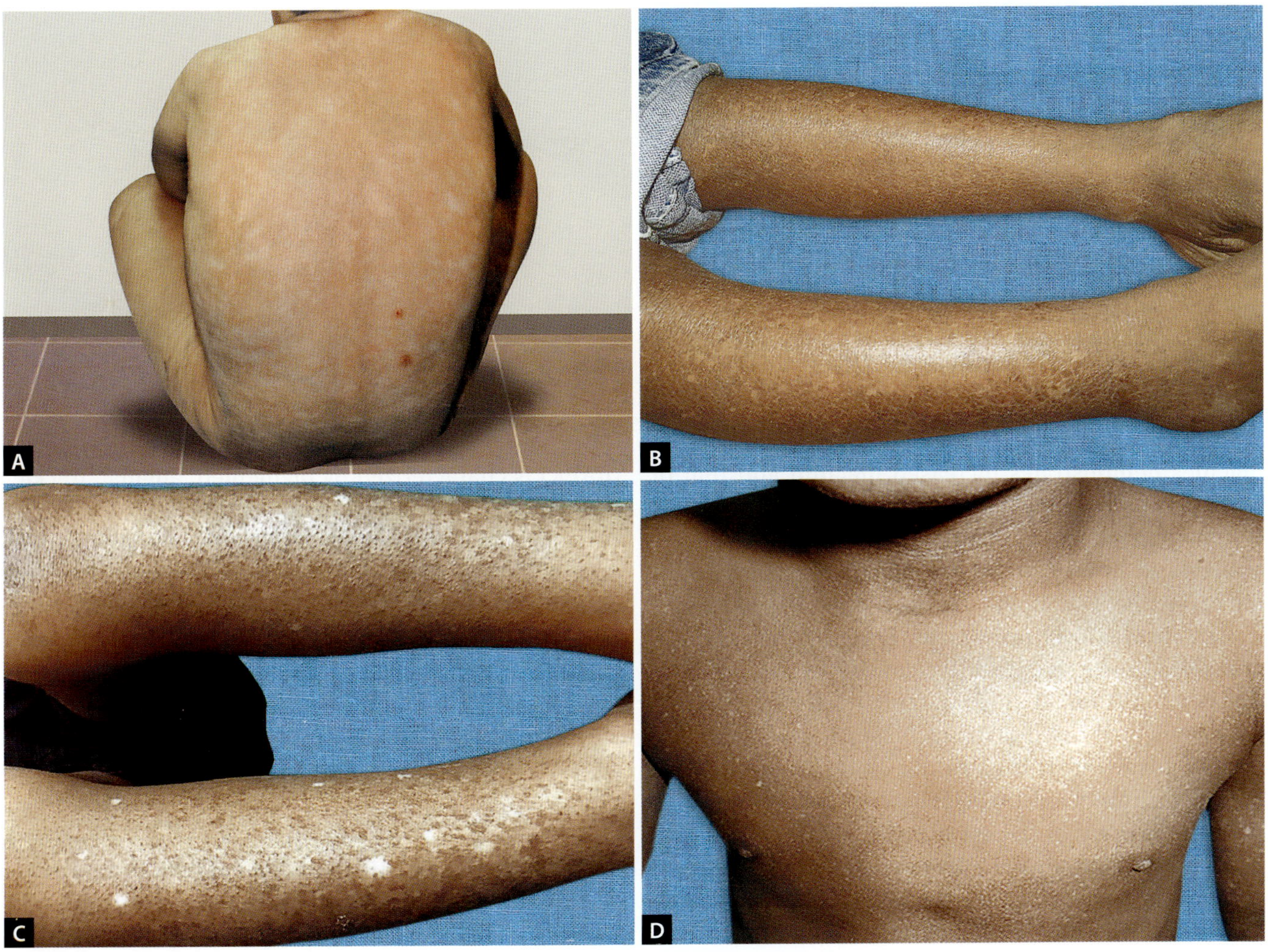

Figs. 28A to D: (A) Dyschromatosis hereditaria, lesions over back; (B) Dyschromatosis universalis hereditaria (localized over legs); (C) Dyschromatosis universalis hereditaria (localized over legs), another child; (D) Dyschromatosis universalis hereditaria (generalized over face and trunk).

"People demand freedom of speech to make up for the freedom of thought which they avoid." —**Soren Aabye Kierkegaard**

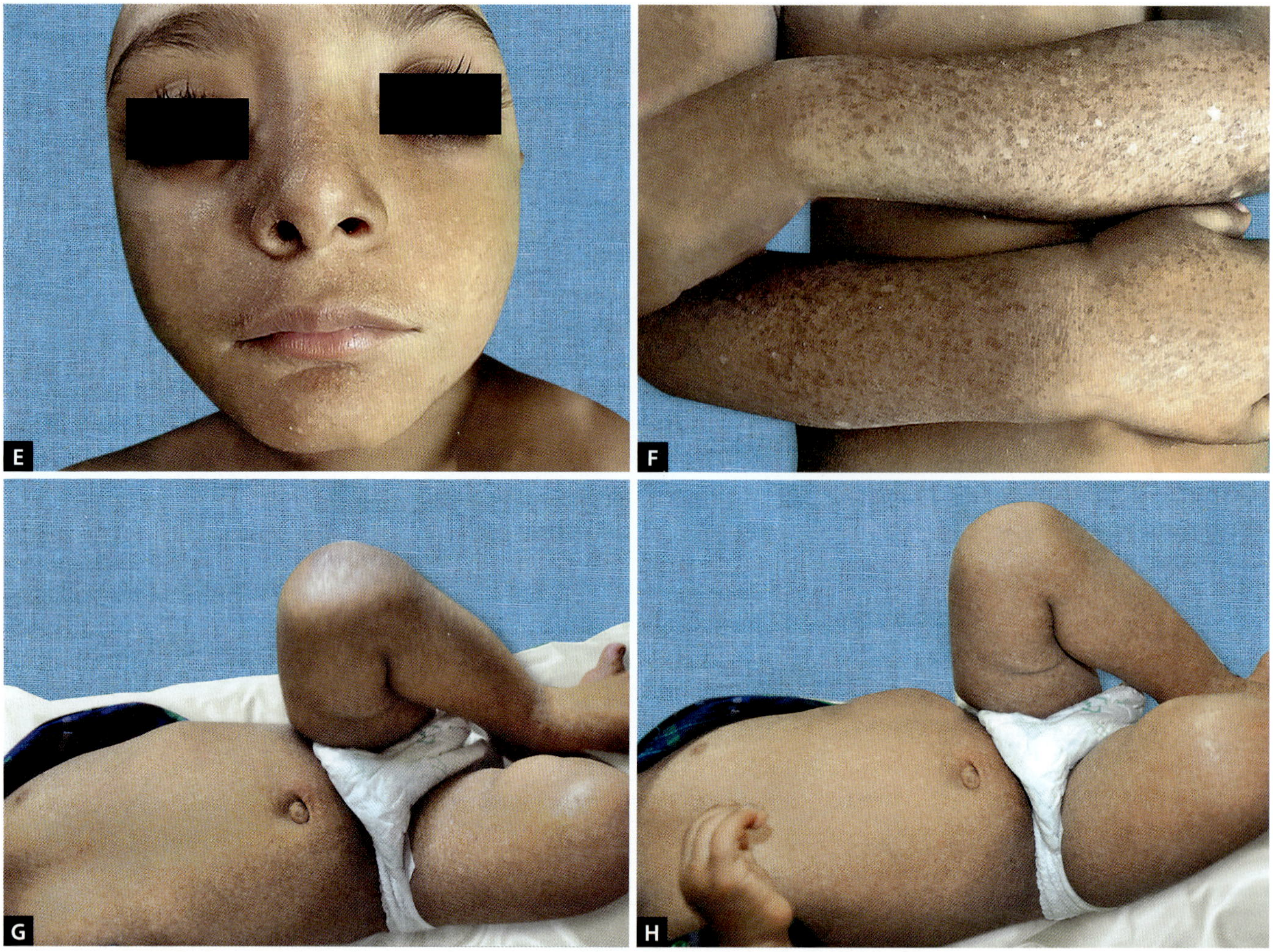

Figs. 28E to H: (E) Dyschromatosis universalis hereditaria (DUH), lesions over face; (F) Same boy, lesions over forearms; (G) DUH generalized; (H) Same child, another view.

macules demonstrates increased melanin and that of hypopigmented ones demonstrate decreased number of dopa-positive melanocytes. No satisfactory treatment is available till date. Different modalities that can be tried are topical steroid, PUVA, spilt thickness skin graft, and laser.

Dyschromatosis universalis hereditaria is a rare, autosomal recessive disorder caused by mutation in the gene *ABCB6*. It is characterized by hyper- and hypopigmented macules in reticulate pattern distributed mainly over the trunk. Palms, soles, and mucous membrane may show pigmentary changes. Lesions may become apparent by the age of 1 year. Like DSH, DUH is also prevalent in Japanese. Patient is otherwise healthy; uncommon associations are ocular and auditory defects, developmental delay, short stature, and seizure disorders.

These two disorders are mainly differentiated by the pattern of distribution. Among other important differentials, reticulate acropigmentation of Kitamura (RAPK) is characterized by pigmented, angular, freckle-like lesions with atrophy with predilection for dorsal hands and feet, but hypopigmented lesions are typically absent. Involvement of axilla and groin with break in dermatoglyphics in palm favors the diagnosis of this entity. In Dowling–Degos (DD) disease, reticulate pigmentation is chiefly distributed around flexures such as axilla, neck, inframammary and sternal area.

RETICULATE ACROPIGMENTATION OF KITAMURA (FIGS. 29 AND 30A)

Reticulate acropigmentation of Kitamura is a rare genetic pigmentary disorder. It is an autosomal dominant condition first described in Japan in 1943 by Kitamura and is largely documented in Asian countries. Familial cases are reported. Its onset is usually in infancy, and most commonly develops in the first and second decade of life. Initially, it starts as freckle-like pigmentation, both hypopigmentation and hyperpigmentation on the dorsum of the hands and feet, and later spreads to involve

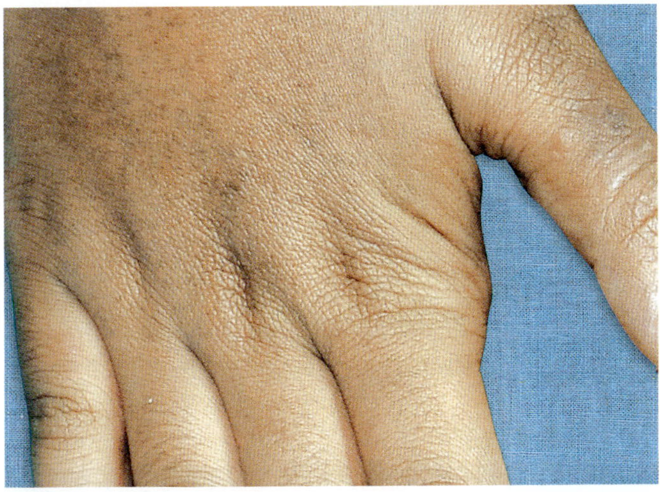

Fig. 29: Reticulate acropigmentation of Kitamura lesions over dorsum of hand.

both extensor and flexor aspect of upper and lower limbs including palms and soles. Rarely, it can involve the trunk. These lesions are slightly atrophic. Small pits are present on palms and soles causing break in the epidermal ridge pattern and this feature is diagnostic of RAPK.

Histologically shows epidermal atrophy, elongation, and increased melanin in the rete ridges. RAPK should be differentiated from acropigmentation of Dohi which has similar reticulate pigmentation. The presence of skin atrophy, pits, and break in the epidermal ridge pattern differentiates from acropigmentation of Dohi. The condition is progressive and the course of the pigmentation cannot be changed.

DOWLING–DEGOS DISEASES (FIGS. 30B AND C)

It is an autosomal dominant disease mostly seen in adults. However, rarely it may be seen in young adults

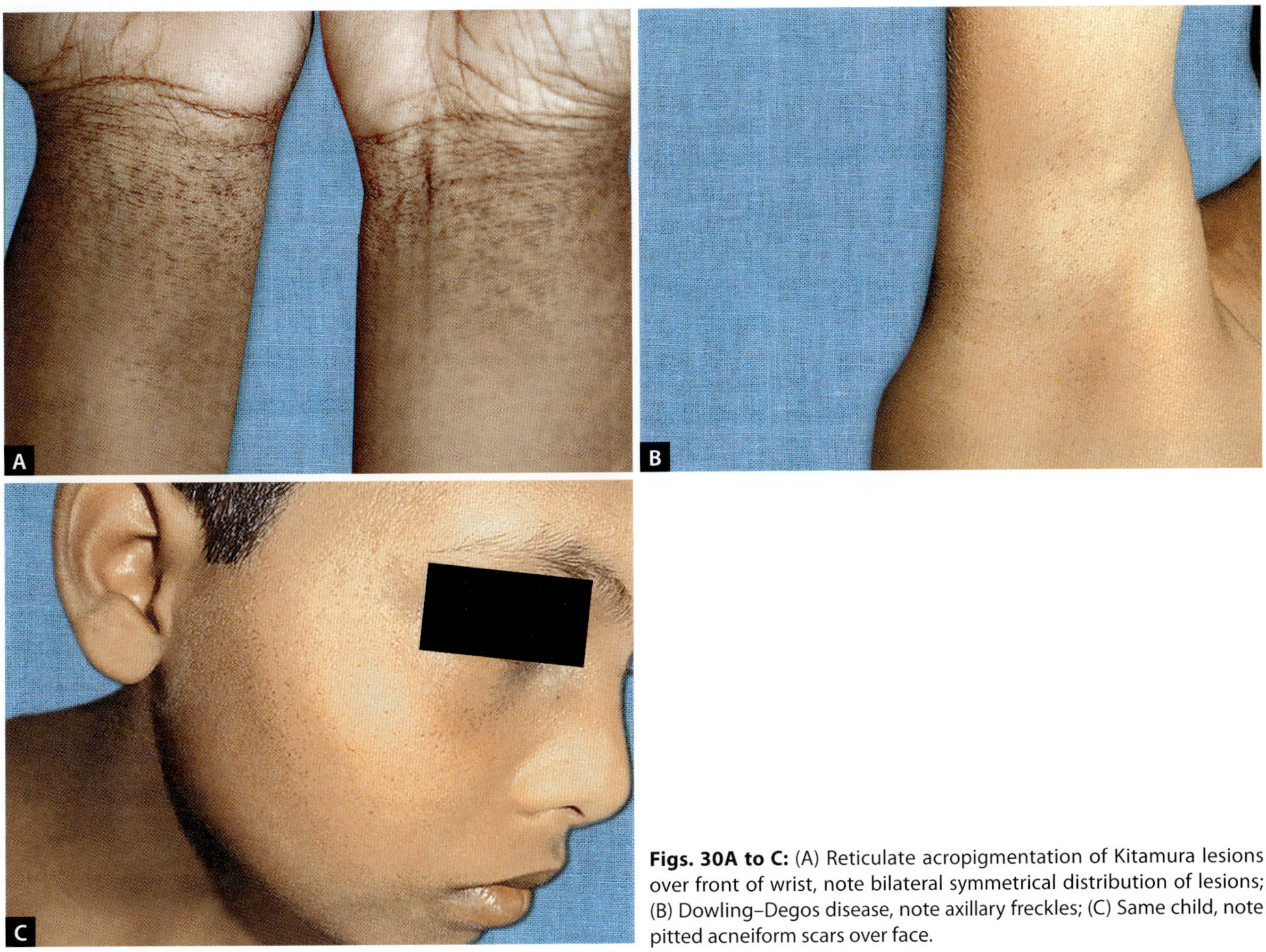

Figs. 30A to C: (A) Reticulate acropigmentation of Kitamura lesions over front of wrist, note bilateral symmetrical distribution of lesions; (B) Dowling–Degos disease, note axillary freckles; (C) Same child, note pitted acneiform scars over face.

"Not everything that can be counted counts, and not everything that counts can be counted." —**Albert Einstein**

or adolescents. It presents as reticulate brownish to black hyperpigmentation over intertriginous areas, e.g., axillae, groin, and inframammary region. There may be comedonal lesions and pitted acneiform scars over face. In some patients, there may be an overlap of features of Dowling-Degos disease and RAPK.

PIGMENTARY DEMARCATION LINES (FIGS. 31 TO 35)

Pigmentary demarcation lines (PDLs), also referred to as Futcher or Voigt lines, are abrupt transitions from deeper pigmented skin to lighter pigmented skin and represent natural variation of melanization. These are commonly seen in blacks and Japanese and are more common in

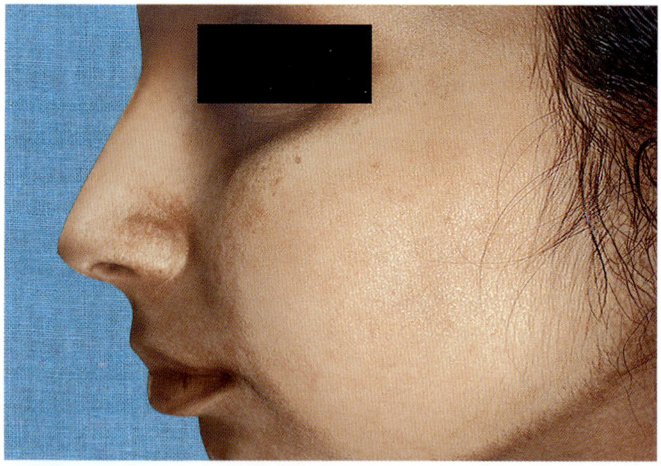

Fig. 33: Another view of pigmentary demarcation line over face (PDL G).

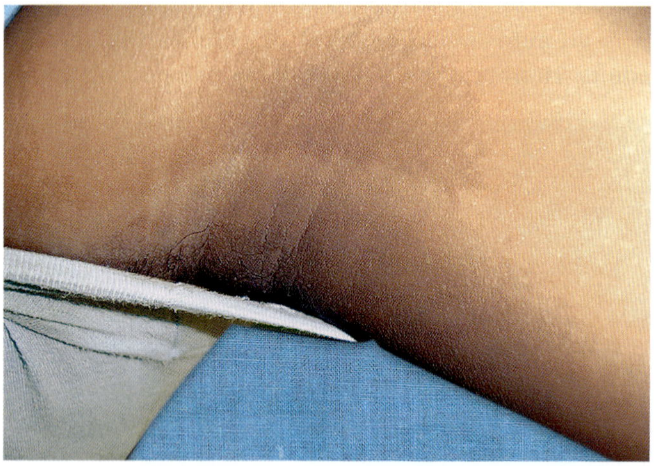

Fig. 31: Pigmentary demarcation line over upper arm adjoining axilla (PDL A) in a 17-year-old girl.

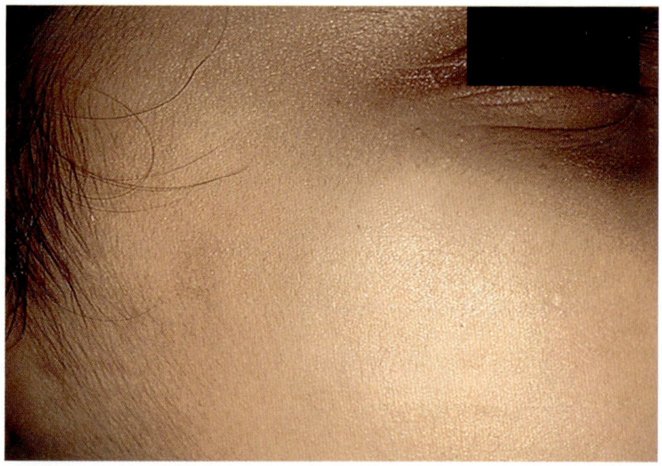

Fig. 34: Pigmentary demarcation line, face (PDL F).

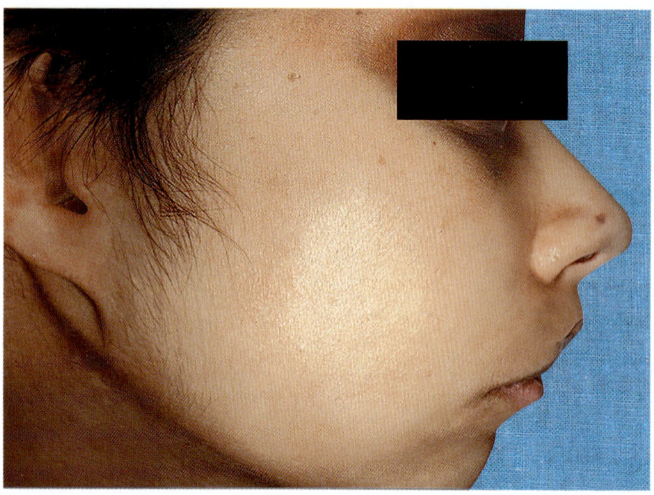

Fig. 32: Pigmentary demarcation line over face, note it merges with periorbital melanosis.

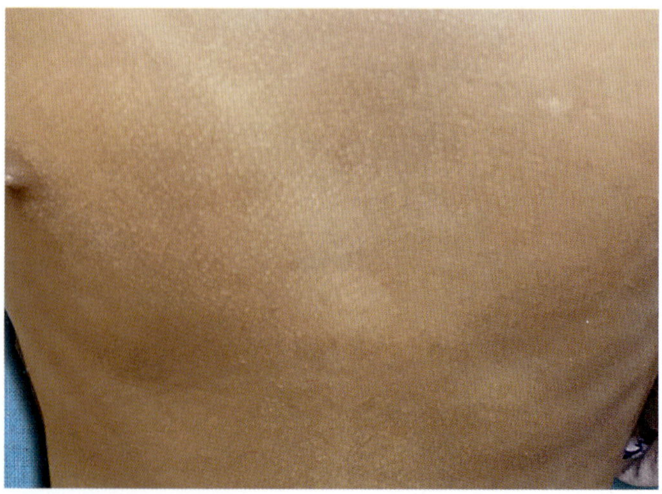

Fig. 35: Hypopigmented PDL over chest.

"Without deviation from the norm, progress is not possible." —**Frank Zappa**

females. About 79% of the black females have at least one PDL; on the other hand, it is encountered in only 15% of white females.

Eight PDLs have been described and labeled as A-H. A-E over trunk and limbs and F-H are facial patterns and are commonly described in Indians. The author and colleague described PDL F lines over face for the first time.

A — on the lateral aspect of the upper arm extending over the pectoral area
B — on the posteromedial portion of the lower limb
C — midsternal line, a vertical hypopigmented line in the pre- and parasternal area
D — on the posteromedial area of the spine
E — bilateral hypopigmented streaks, bands or lanceolate areas over the chest in the zone between the mid-third of the clavicle, and the periareolar skin.
F — "V"-shaped hyperpigmented lines between the malar prominence and the temple
G — "W"-shaped hyperpigmented lines between the malar prominence and the temple
H — linear bands of hyperpigmentation from the angle of the mouth to the lateral aspects of the chin.

Pigmentary demarcation lines usually appear around puberty and facial patterns may sometimes get revealed with some triggers such as pregnancy and acute ailments such as hepatitis and varicella. Genetic predisposition, hormonal influence, and cutaneous mosaicism are some of the suggested explanation for the occurrence of the PDLs.

Facial PDLs are of aesthetic concern and are often misdiagnosed as melasma, postinflammatory pigmentation, nevus of Ota, or melanocytic nevus. PDL over face was described in the literature for the first time by the first author of this book (SD) and colleague. None of the treatment modalities available such as chemical peeling, sunscreen, Kligman formulation, and intense pulse light give satisfactory and sustained result.

PIGMENTARY MOSAICISM (FIGS. 36 TO 39)

Pigmentary mosaicism is a term that describes varied patterns of pigmentation in the skin caused by genetic heterogeneity. The term encompasses a heterogeneous group of disorders which includes "hypomelanosis of Ito," "linear and whorled hypermelanosis," and segmental form of nevus depigmentosus and is characterized by patterned streaks of hypo- or hyperpigmentations. In a substantial number of cases, pigmentary mosaicism is observed alongside extracutaneous abnormalities typically involving the central nervous system and the musculoskeletal system. Also refer to Chapter 10 (Neurocutaneous Disorders).

WHAT'S NEW

- The novel drug, a decapeptide solution related to basic fibroblast growth factor (bFGF), comprises a sequence of amino acids derived from bFGF. This solution effectively stimulates both the growth and migration of melanocytes, leading to repigmentation. When

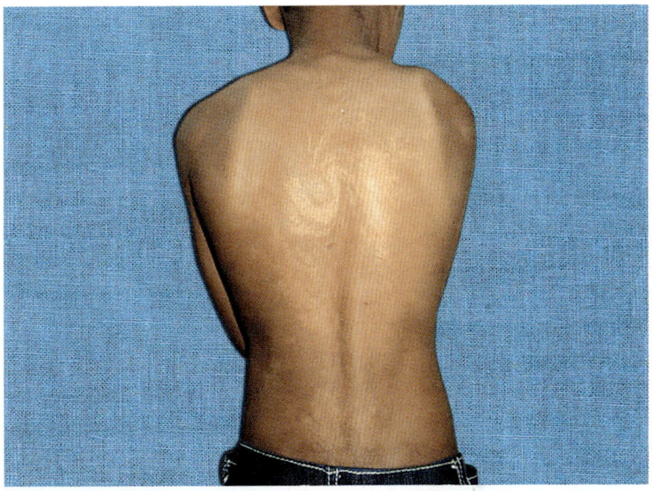

Fig. 36: Pigmentary mosaicism, note Blaschkoid pattern over the back (hypopigmented patches).

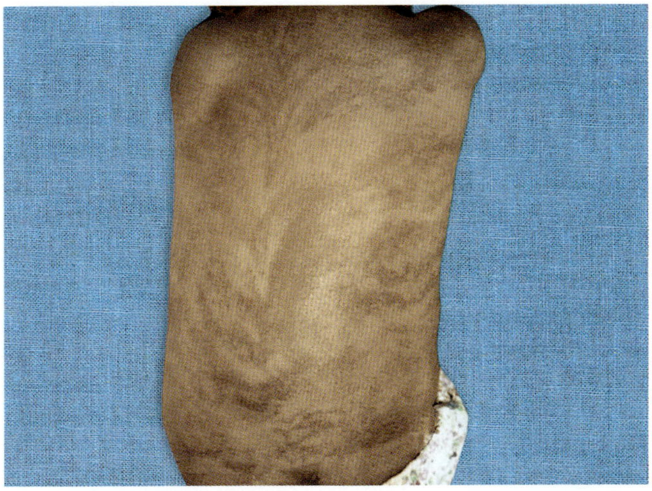

Fig. 37: Pigmentary mosaicism, note Blaschkoid pattern over the back (hyperpigmented patches).

"In theory, there is no difference between theory and practice. But in practice, there is." **—Yogi Berra**

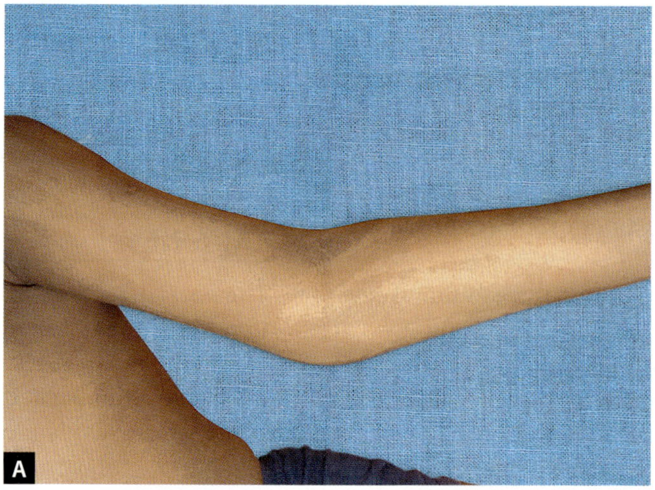

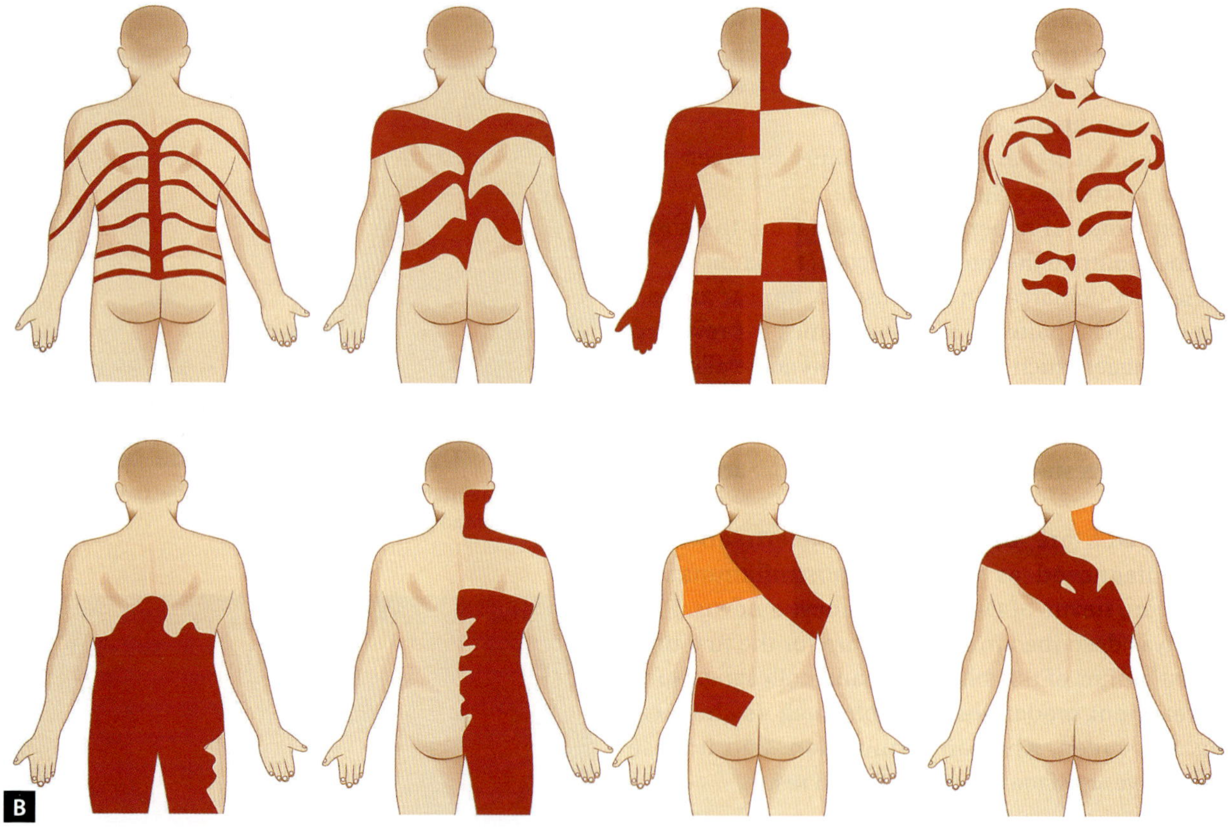

Figs. 38A and B: (A) Pigmentary mosaicism, note Blaschkoid pattern over the upper limbs; (B) Schematic diagram of pigmentary mosaicism.

applied topically once a day, it demonstrates positive outcomes. Notably, combining it with tacrolimus 0.1% ointment appears to enhance results.

- Piperine, a phytochemical derived from Piper nigrum, exerts its effects by promoting melanocyte proliferation and dendrite formation in vitro. Notably, its efficacy appears to be enhanced when combined with UV radiation (UVR).
- Dermoscopy in vitiligo: There are eight dermoscopic patterns that are identified in pediatric vitiligo. They are:
  1. Perifollicular pigmentation
  2. Reduced/absent pigment network
  3. Trichromic pattern
  4. Tapioca sago pattern
  5. Perifollicular depigmentation

"A friend is one soul abiding in two bodies." **—Aristotle**

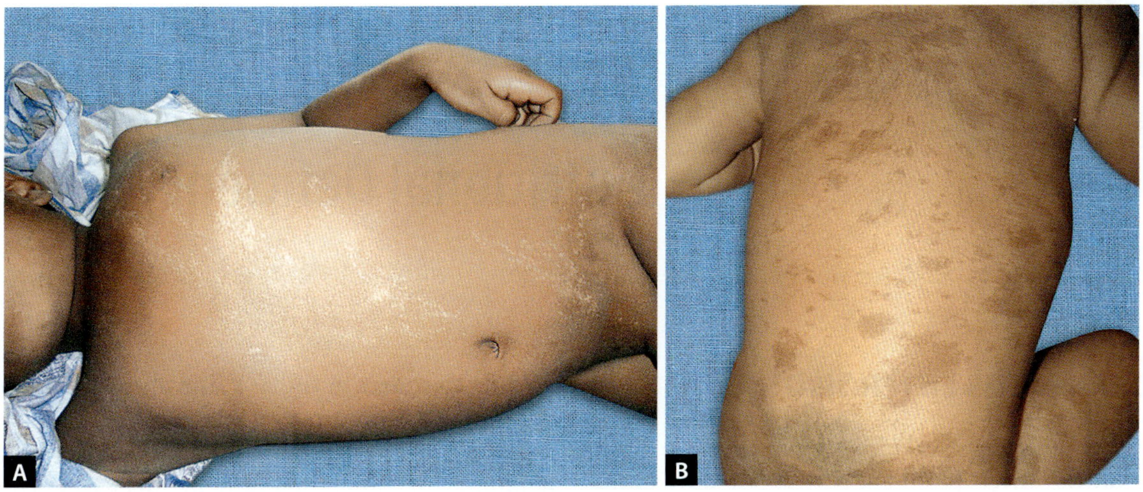

Figs. 39A and B: (A) Hypomelanosis of ito in a mosaic pattern; (B) Hyperpigmented macules in pigmentary mosaicism present in phylloid pattern.

6. Starburst appearance
7. Leukotrichia
8. Erythema

- In order of frequency, Trichrome was the most common pattern and amoeboid pattern was the least common.
- Acquired dermal macular hyperpigmentation (ADMH) serves as an inclusive term that encompasses various overlapping acquired dermal pigmentary disorders. These conditions include lichen planus pigmentosus, ashy dermatosis, erythema dyschromicum perstans, Riehl's melanosis, and pigmented contact dermatitis.

SUGGESTED READINGS

1. Ezzedine K, Silverberg N. A Practical approach to the diagnosis and treatment of vitiligo in children. Pediatrics. 2016;138(1):e20154126.
2. Kono M, Akiyama M. Dyschromatosis symmetrica hereditaria and reticulate acropigmentation of Kitamura: an update. J Dermatol Sci. 2019;93(2):75-81.
3. Kubasch AS, Meurer M. Okulokutaner und okulärer Albinismus [Oculocutaneous and ocular albinism]. Hautarzt. 2017;68(11): 867-75.
4. Soni B, Raghavendra KR, Yadav DK, Kumawat P, Singhal A. A clinic-epidemiological study of hypopigmented and depigmented lesions in children and adolescent age group in Hadoti region (South East Rajasthan). Indian J Paediatr Dermatol. 2017;18:9-13.
5. Raju SP, Kaur S, Loganathan E. Management of childhood vitiligo—a brief review. Pigment International. 2022;9(1):14-24.
6. Godínez-Chaparro JA, Roldán-Marín R, Soto-Mota A, Calzada-Mendoza CC. Dermatoscopic Patterns in Childhood Vitiligo and their Association with Reflectance Confocal Microscopy Findings. Dermatol Pract Concept. 2023;13(4):e2023306.
7. Shah S, Baskaran N, Vinay K, Bishnoi A, Parsad D, Kumaran MS. Acquired dermal macular hyperpigmentation: an overview of the recent updates. International Journal of Dermatology. 2023; 62(12):1447-57.

CHAPTER

12

Nutritional Deficiency Disorders

ACRODERMATITIS ENTEROPATHICA (FIGS. 1 AND 2)

Acrodermatitis enteropathica (AE) is an autosomal recessive disorder where male and female children are affected equally. It is caused by *SLC39A4* gene mutation leading to defect in dietary zinc absorption in the duodenum and jejunum. The classical triad of dermatitis, intractable diarrhea and alopecia which are the diagnostic hallmarks of AE, is seen only in 20% cases. The disease typically starts 4–6 weeks after weaning or earlier if the infants are not breastfed. However, zinc deficiency has also been found in premature babies who are exclusively breastfed. The disease is characterized by acral and periorificial vesiculobullous, pustular and eczematous eruptions, alopecia, nail dystrophy, diarrhea, glossitis, stomatitis, photophobia, and secondary infections of skin by bacteria or *Candida*. A low serum zinc level and a rapid response to zinc supplementation suggest the role of zinc malabsorption in the causation of the disease. The etiology of zinc malabsorption could be either lack of a zinc-binding ligand in the small intestine or trapping of zinc in the wall of the intestinal lumen.

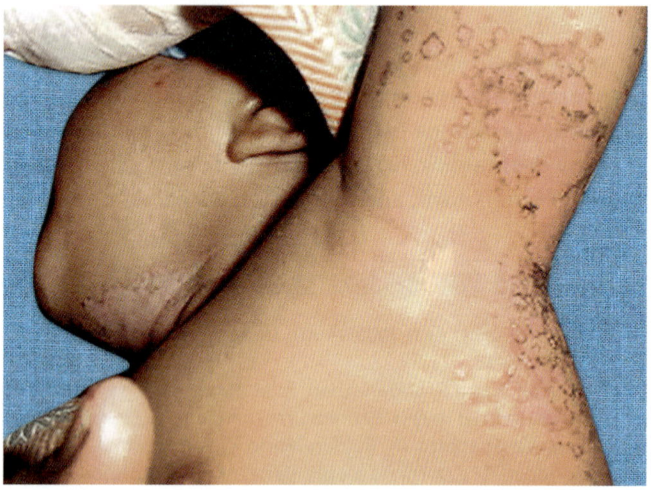

Fig. 1: Annular scaly eczematous lesions of acrodermatitis enteropathica (AE).

Diagnosis

The diagnosis of AE is based on the clinical features that include dermatitis localized around body orifices, buttocks, extensor surfaces of the major joints, scalp, fingers and

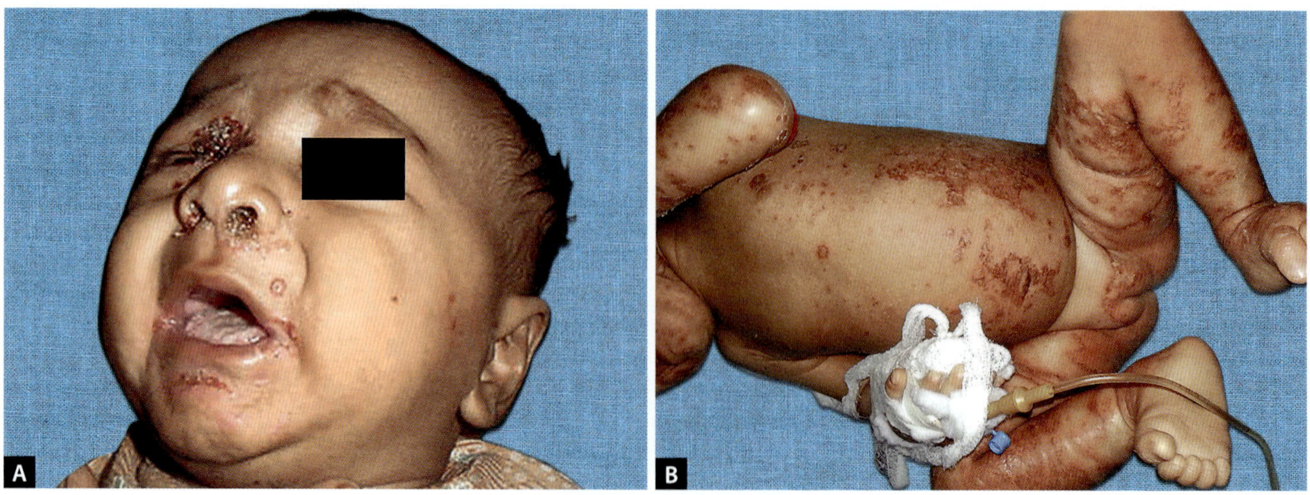

Figs. 2A and B: (A) Perioral lesions of acrodermatitis enteropathica (AE). (B) Eczematous brown scales of AE.

"Alone, we can do so little; together we can do so much." —**Helen Keller**

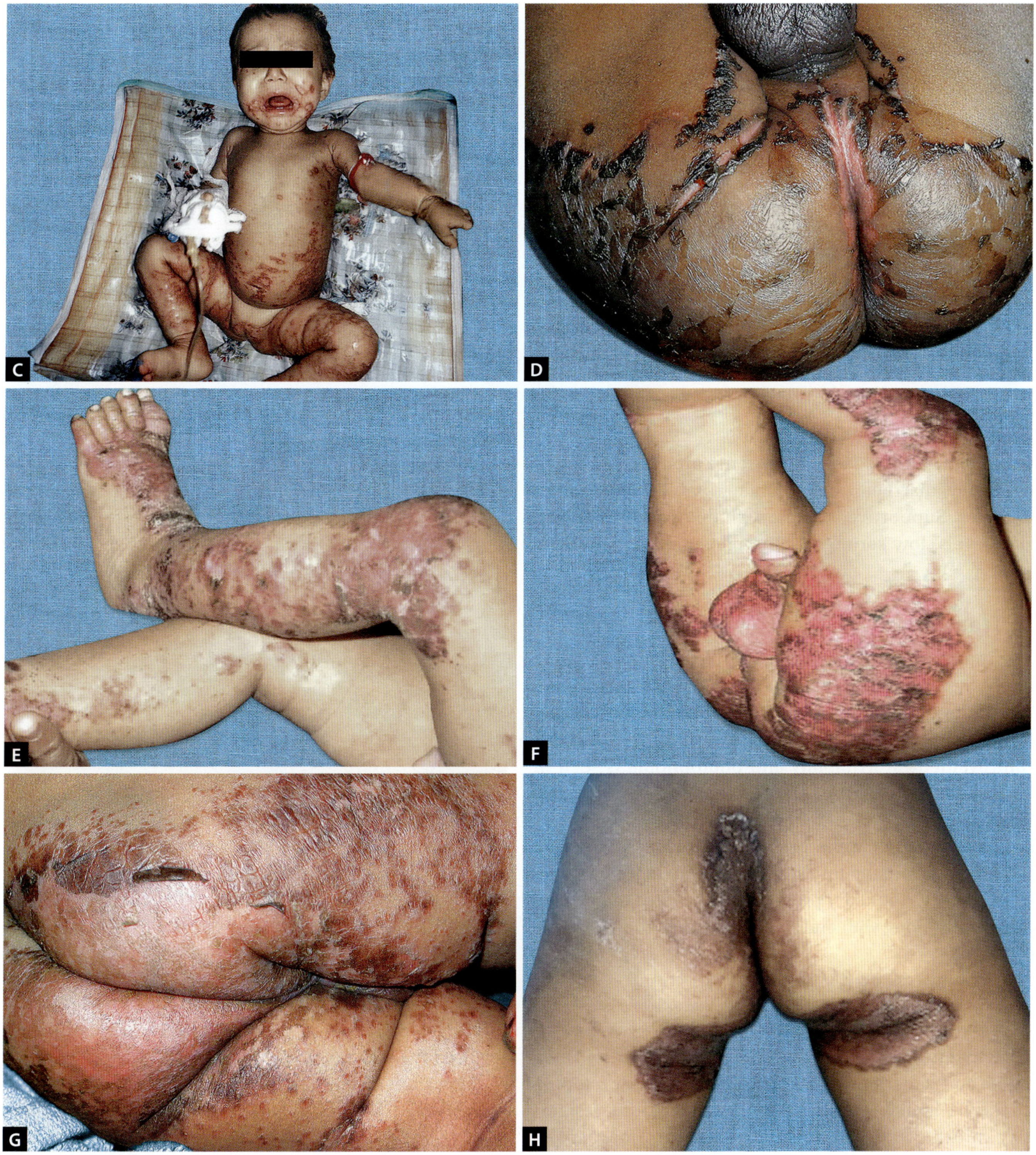

Figs. 2C to H: (C) AE, note acral, perioral involvement. (D) Severe perianal involvement. (E) Acral involvement on AE. (F) Involvement of buttocks in AE. (G) Close-up view. (H) Another 7-year-old with classical features of acrodermatitis enteropathica.

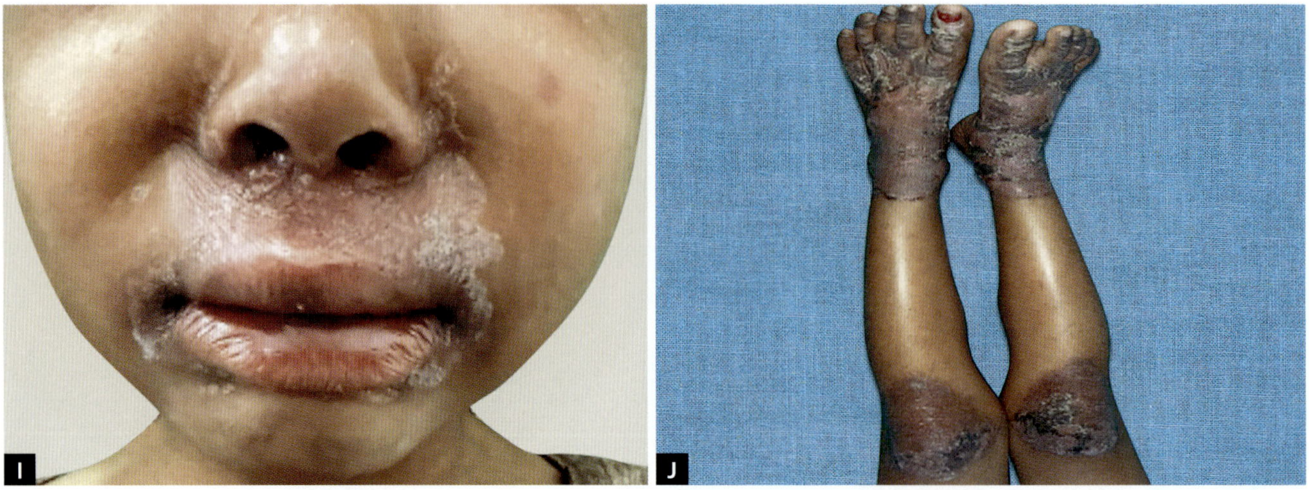

Figs. 2I and J: Same child with perioral and lower limb involvement.

toes, recurrent infections, recurrent paronychia and nail dystrophy, diarrhea, photophobia, irritability, and failure to thrive. Supportive laboratory findings are low serum zinc levels, low serum alkaline phosphatase, and lipid levels.

Treatment

Treatment of AE is essentially supplementation of zinc orally. Supplementation is done by zinc gluconate, acetate or sulfate 5 mg/kg/day in 2–3 divided doses (usually 50 mg/day for infants and 150 mg/day for older children). Improvement in irritability and photophobia is seen in 24–48 hours and diarrhea and skin lesions by 72–96 hours. Hair growth and weight gain usually starts after 3–4 weeks of therapy. Zinc supplementation is to be maintained life long. Various dietary sources of zinc are meat, fish, eggs, poultry, and dairy products. These need to be given adequately along with oral zinc supplementation.

PROTEIN–ENERGY MALNUTRITION (FIGS. 3 AND 4)

Protein–energy malnutrition (PEM), one of the most important causes of childhood mortality in developing countries, includes three related conditions—marasmus, kwashiorkor, and intermediate form marasmic-kwashiorkor. Marasmic babies are stunted, weigh <60% of their ideal body weight and present without hypoproteinemia or edema. Marasmus results from long-term deficiency of protein and calories, whereas kwashiorkor is mainly due to protein deficiency with relatively adequate caloric intake. But the recent

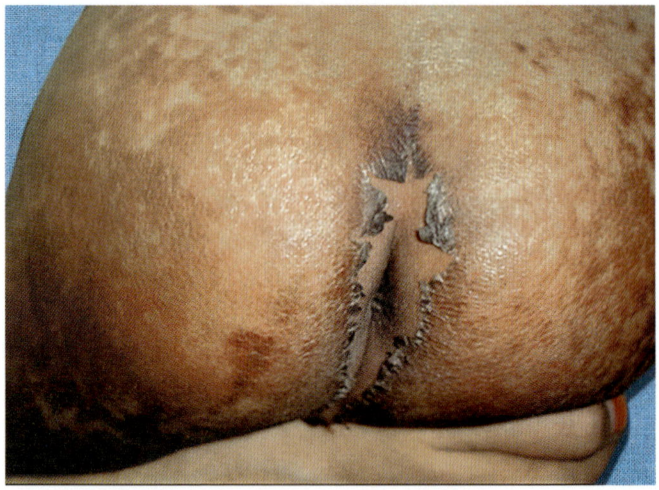

Fig. 3: Scaly eczematous lesions of kwashiorkor.

hypothesis suggests that the host's ability to cope up with the nutritional stress determines the outcome of PEM. In kwashiorkor, children weigh 60–80% of their expected body weight with features of hypoproteinemia and edema. Marasmic kwashiorkor, accounting for most of the undiagnosed cases of PEM, exhibits features of both the two severe forms of it.

Marasmus means wasting (derived from the Greek word *marasmos*). Cutaneous changes are infrequent, minimal, and are not classical. Loss of subcutaneous fat results in dry, wrinkled, thin, lax skin, and the characteristic "monkey facies". Hair are lusterless, fine, rough, and brittle. In adults, follicular hyperkeratosis may be a feature. Associated vitamin deficiency may give rise to angular cheilitis and atrophic glossitis. Owing to poor cell-mediated immunity, children are susceptible to a number of infections such as

"Twenty years from now you will be more disappointed by the things that you didn't do than by the ones you did do, so throw off the bowlines, sail away from safe harbor, catch the trade winds in your sails. Explore, Dream, Discover." —**Mark Twain**

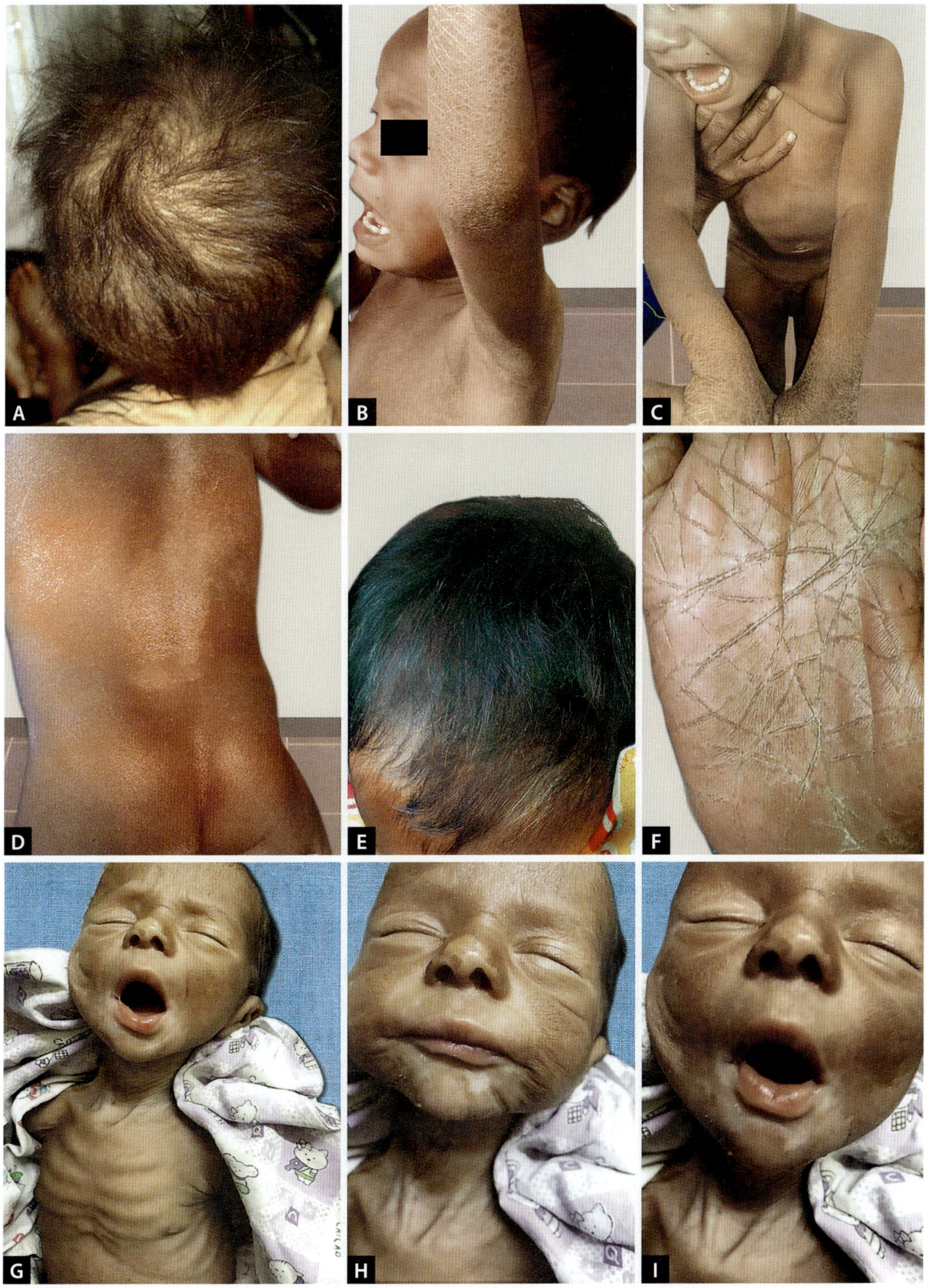

Figs. 4A to I: (A) Dry lusterless hairs with alopecia in kwashiorkor. (B) Dry lusterless skin of marasmus. (C) Skin in marasmus. (D) Dry lusterless hyperpigmented skin in marasmus. (E) Dry lusterless hairs of marasmus. (F) Dry palm of marasmus. (G) Marasmus, note sunken face, dry skin and pigmentation. (H) Close-up view of same infant. (I) Further magnification.

"I've missed more than 9000 shots in my career. I've lost almost 300 games. 26 times I've been trusted to take the game winning shot and missed. I've failed over and over and over again in my life. And that is why I succeed." —**Michael Jordan**

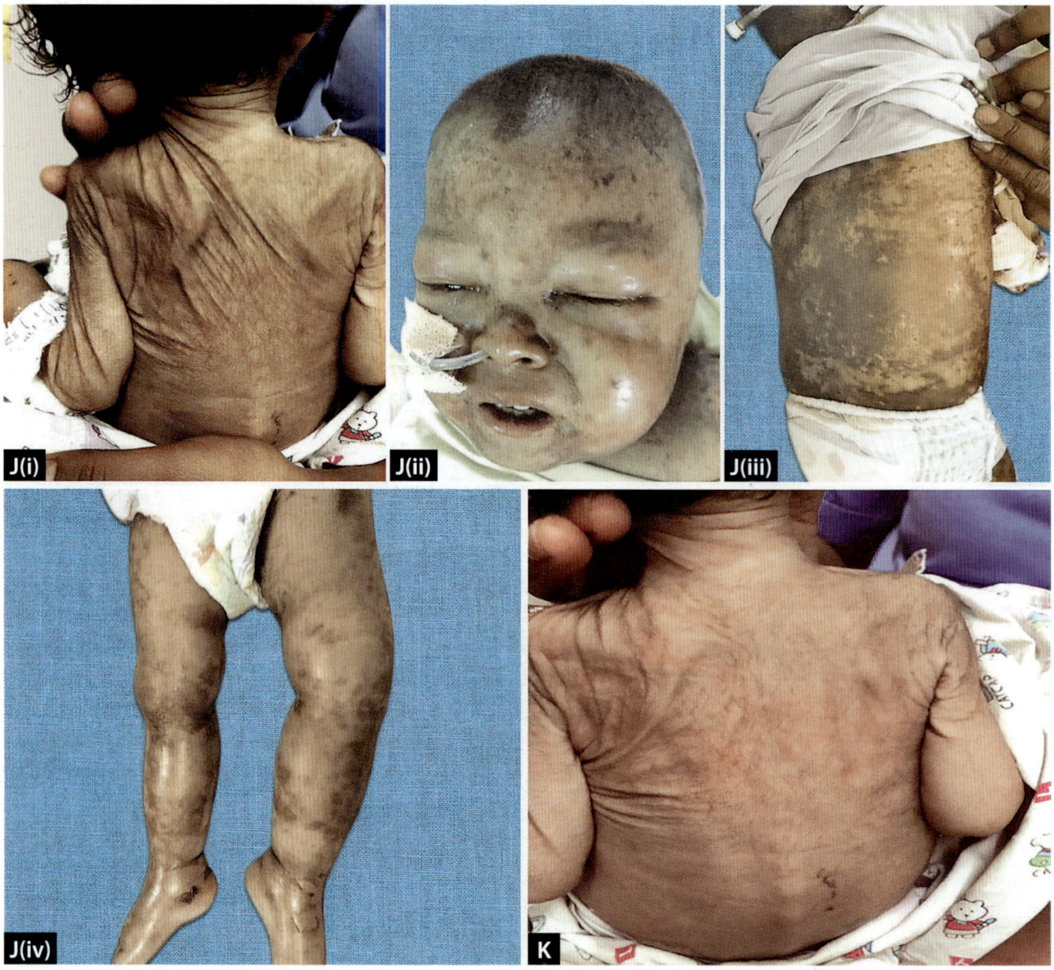

Figs. 4J(i) to K: J(i) Back, look wrinkled lusterless skin in marasmus. J(ii) Edematous face, pigmentation, and alopecia in kwashiorkor. J(iii) Same infant, trunk. J(iv) Same infant, lower limbs. (K) Close-up view of dry wrinkled skin on back in marasmic child.

cutaneous and systemic candidiasis, cancrum oris, and abscess which can complicate the condition.

Kwashiorkor, "the sickness of the deposed baby" is mainly a problem of underdeveloped and developing countries, but has also been reported from developed countries. In developed countries, nutritional ignorance, food allergen avoidance, and food faddism are the predisposing factors. The underlying pathophysiology is multifactorial. Protein deficiency is either qualitative or quantitative. The clinical manifestations can be explained by decreased production or production of structurally immature collagen, low cystine content of hair, low zinc level, impaired antioxidant status, and hypoproteinemia. Kwashiorkor is characterized by skin and hair changes, growth retardation, potbelly, and the hallmark sign, pitting edema which may become generalized and thus masking the wasting. It is seen between the age group of 6 months to 5 years and begins as erythema that blanches on pressure, rapidly followed by small dusky purple patches that do not blanch. Cutaneous lesions are seen in 20–40% of cases. They are hypopigmented in dark-skinned individuals and erythematous to purple on fair complexion. Perioral pallor may be the presenting sign. Characteristic cutaneous lesions are sharply demarcated, hyperpigmented patches with slightly raised edges distributed over the areas of friction or pressure. This gradually progresses leading to extensive desquamation and erosion with flexural fissuring, which is variously described as "flaky paint" or "crazy pavement" or "enamel paint" dermatosis. Hair changes are more prominent in kwashiorkor in comparison to marasmus. Hair is hypopigmented with various types of dyschromatosis, dry, lusterless, soft and easily pluckable. Alternate bands of pale and dark hair in a single strand reflecting the period of poor and good nutrition produces

"Strive not to be a success, but rather to be of value." —**Albert Einstein**

the striking "flag sign" of hair. Other associated skin findings and complications are same as that of marasmus. Anorexia, diarrhea, mental apathy, and irritability are the other presenting features.

Prognosis is good with optimal treatment which is mainly directed toward correction of nutritional deficiencies according to the degree of malnutrition and treatment of associated infection and infestations. During the acute phase, skin lesions are treated with emollient and topical zinc oxide paste. Breastfeeding should be encouraged as long as possible in developing countries. Mortality rate of untreated kwashiorkor may be as high as 30%.

PHRYNODERMA (FIGS. 5A AND B)

It develops as a result of vitamin A, B complex, C, E, and essential fatty acid deficiency. Vitamin A deficiency manifests as xerosis or generalized dryness of skin, xerophthalmia or dryness of eyes, and phrynoderma which is characterized by keratotic follicular papules resembling "toad skin" distributed on the dorsal and lateral areas of the extremities mainly the elbows, knees, and buttocks.

Diagnosis

Diagnosis is mainly clinical and confirmed by low serum level of vitamin A and other vitamins.

Management

Emollients, keratolytics, and topical retinoids have been useful apart from correction of nutritional deficiencies.

VITAMIN B$_2$ (RIBOFLAVIN) DEFICIENCY (FIGS. 6 AND 7)

The characteristic feature is cheilitis which presents as red glossy and slightly scaly lips usually associated with glossitis with loss of tongue papillae and mucositis. Other features are pruritic seborrheic dermatitis, conjunctivitis, keratitis, and photophobia. Riboflavin is a water-soluble vitamin abundant in animal products, green leafy vegetables, and yeasts. Daily requirement for children is 1–1.5 mg.

VITAMIN B$_{12}$ (CYANOCOBALAMIN) DEFICIENCY (FIGS. 8 TO 10)

Vitamin B$_{12}$ is sourced mostly from meat, poultry, and dairy products as it lacks endogenous synthesis. So the

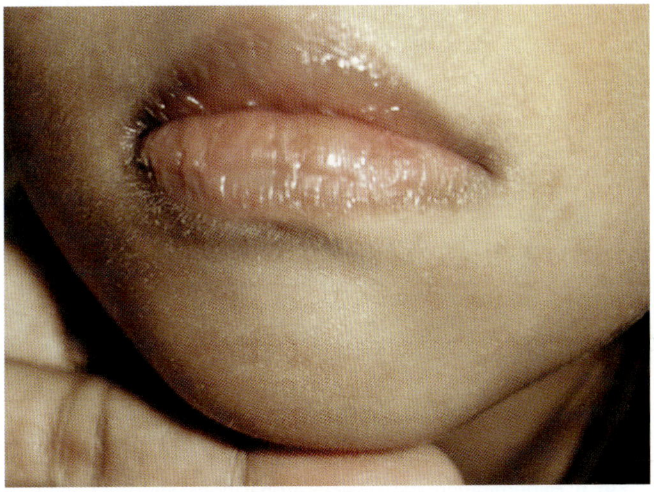

Fig. 6: Red lips of riboflavin deficiency.

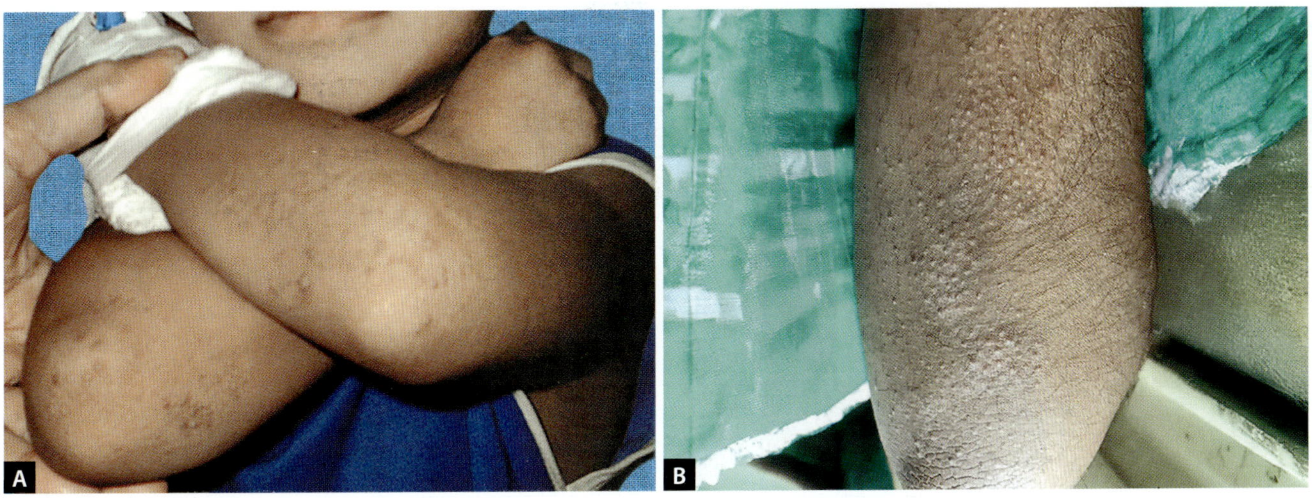

Figs. 5A and B: (A) Keratotic papules of phrynoderma over elbows. (B) Phrynoderma, note keratotic papules.

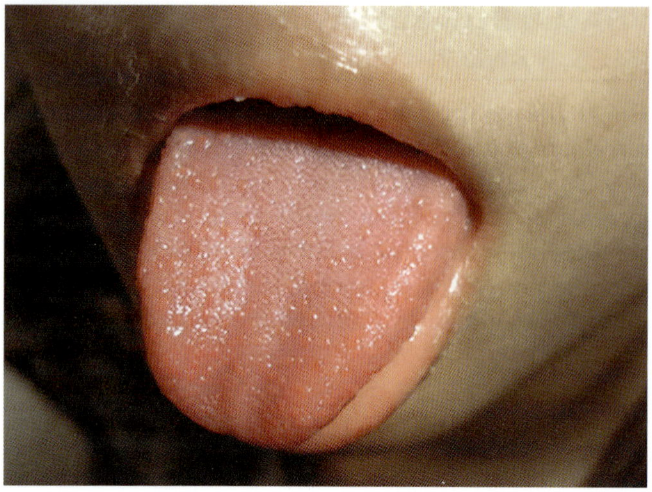

Fig. 7: Red tongue of riboflavin deficiency.

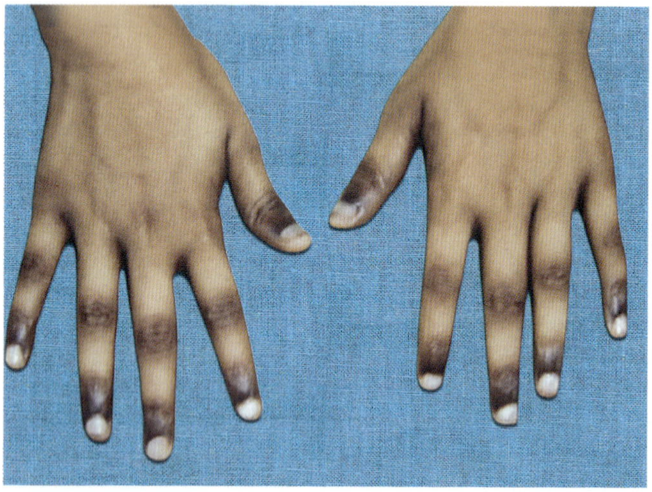

Fig. 8: Hyperpigmentation over interphalangeal joints of fingers.

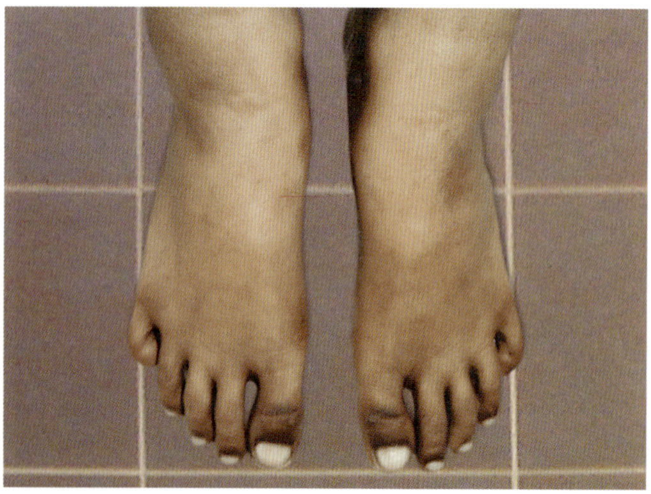

Fig. 9: Hyperpigmentation over the interphalangeal joints.

deficiency is more prevalent in vegans and vegetarians. Vitamin B_{12} deficiency presents usually with hematologic, gastrointestinal, neurologic, and less commonly, psychiatric, cardiovascular, and dermatological manifestations. Mucocutaneous presentations are usually addisonian-like hyperpigmentation over knuckles, palms, and soles which may be diffuse or symmetric, pallor, glossitis, angular stomatitis, and gray hair. Glossitis can initially be linear and later progress to red, painful tongue with atrophy of the filiform papillae (Hunter glossitis). Hair may be dry, brittle, thin, and lusterless. Three hypotheses proposed regarding pathophysiology of B_{12} deficiency-induced hyperpigmentation are: (1) decrease in reduced form of glutathione increasing the activity of tyrosinase; (2) defective melanin transfer between melanocytes and keratinocytes; and (3) disturbed melanin distribution due to megaloblastic changes in the keratinocytes. As this hyperpigmentation often resembles that seen in Addison's disease, hypocortisolemia should be ruled out. Again these signs are often nonspecific, subtle, or asymptomatic, thereby resulting in delayed diagnosis perpetuating morbidity. So increased index of suspicion of cutaneous clues, most characteristically of the virtually surrogate knuckle hyperpigmentation, may help early diagnosis and prompt management of vitamin B_{12} deficiency, thereby decreasing preventable morbidity.

The deficiency may result from inadequate intake (rare), lack of secretion, inhibition of the intrinsic factor by the stomach or abnormalities in the receptor site in the ileum.

Diagnosis

The confirmation is done by estimating serum vitamin B_{12} level.

Treatment

Treatment is by intramuscular injection of vitamin B_{12} or oral therapy.

PELLAGRA (FIGS. 11 AND 12)

Pellagra occurs due to the deficiency of niacin which is due to inadequate intake of nicotinic acid or its precursor tryptophan or ingestion of antinicotinic substances such as phenytoin and isoniazid.

Pellagra is classically described as a triad of dermatitis, diarrhea, and dementia. It is heralded by loss of appetite and a general feeling of weakness. Abdominal pain, depression, and photosensitivity are the other presenting

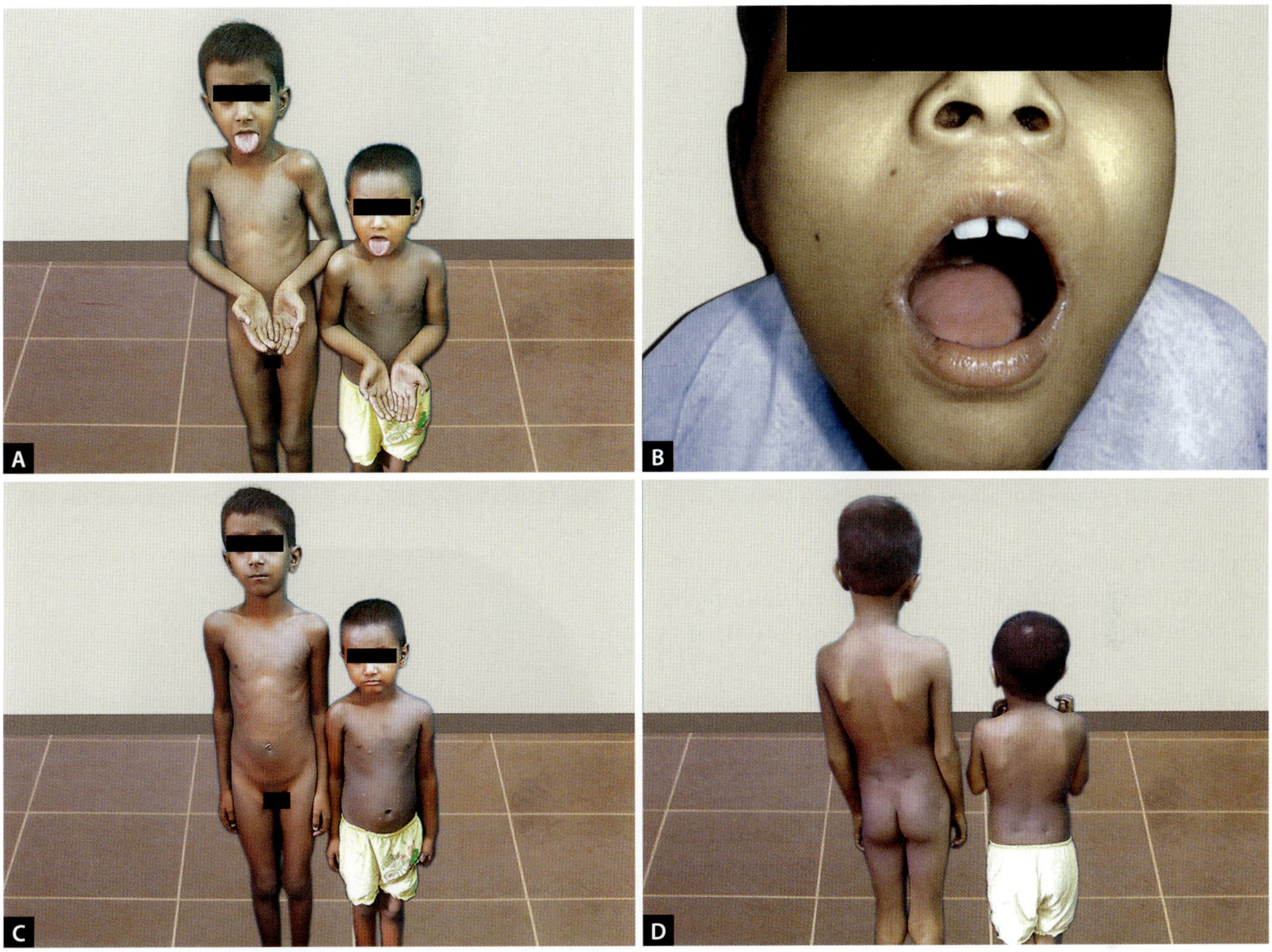

Figs. 10A to D: (A) Diffuse hyperpigmentation in two siblings due to vitamin B_{12} deficiency. (B) Hyperpigmentation of lips and tongue in cyanocobalamin deficiency. (C and D) Same siblings showing diffuse hyperpigmentation on the face, trunk, extremities and back.

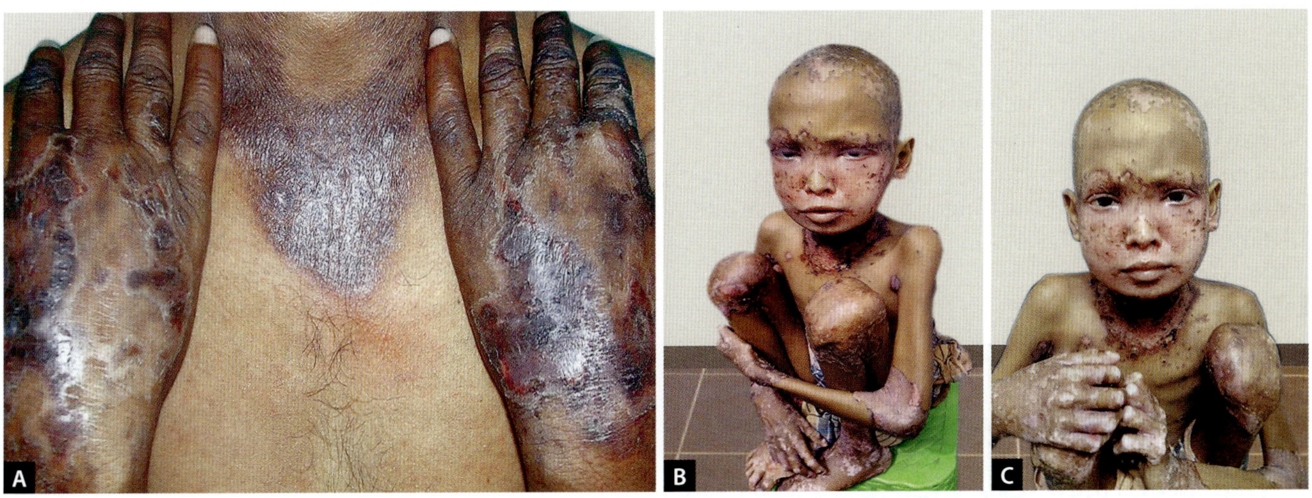

Figs. 11A to C: (A) Eczematous hyperpigmented patches of pellagra over front of neck and dorsum of hands. (B) Eczematous hyperpigmented patches extensively, bilateral symmetrical. (C) Same child—close-up view, note classical casal necklace.

"The most common way people give up their power is by thinking they don't have any." —**Alice Walker**

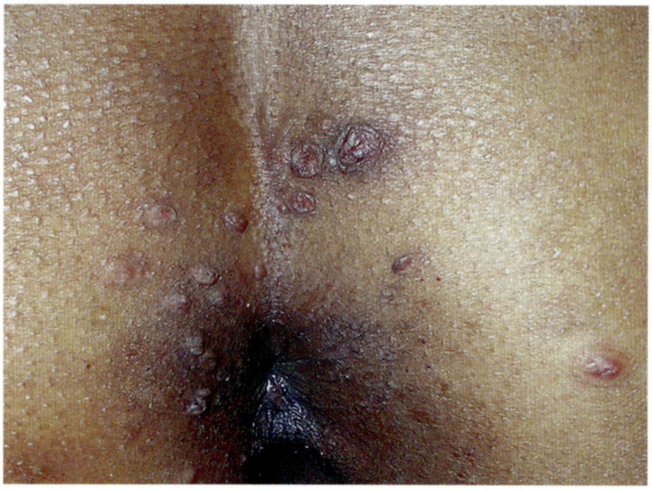
Fig. 12: Pellagra skin lesions around perianal area.

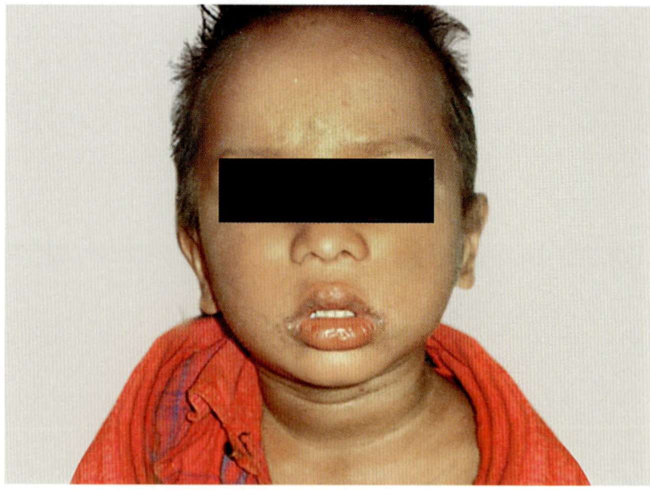
Fig. 13: Biotinidase deficiency, note mild dermatitis and dry skin.

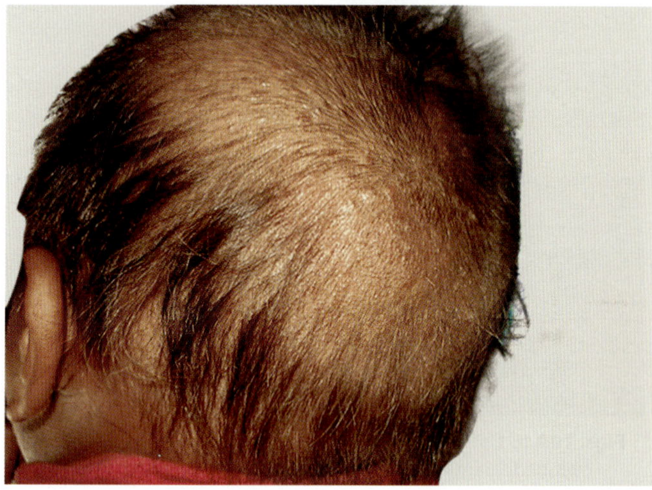
Fig. 14: Same girl, note lusterless brownish hairs and alopecia.

symptoms. In the later stages, central nervous symptoms predominate. Dementia, delirium, peripheral neuropathy, and posterolateral cord degenerative symptoms may occur.

Cutaneous manifestations include photosensitivity, symmetrically distributed erythematous, pruritic or asymptomatic scaly macules on areas of sun exposure, heat, friction, and pressure. The sites affected generally include face, neck, dorsa of hands, feet, inguinal and diaper areas. These areas present with well-demarcated areas of erythema and superficial scaling with or without vesiculation simulating sunburn, subsides with a dusky brown discoloration. The appearance when it occurs on the V area of the neck is described as Casal necklace, whereas on the hands and feet, it is described as pellagrous gloves and boots. On the nose, it presents as dull erythema with powdery white scales. Acute vesiculation, ulceration, exudation, cracking, and secondary infection are the complications encountered in this condition. The lesions resolve with atrophy and dyspigmentation.

Ulcers are noted on the tongue and fissuring is noted over the angle of mouth. The tongue appears red, swollen and dark, described as black tongue.

Treatment

Nicotinic acid 100–400 mg/day in addition to the other vitamin B supplements.

The disease is progressive and fatal, if untreated.

BIOTINIDASE DEFICIENCY (FIGS. 13 AND 14)

It is a rare, inherited metabolic disorder in which body is unable to use and recycle vitamin biotin due to deficiency of the enzyme biotinidase. Mode of inheritance is autosomal recessive. Mutation of the culprit *BTD* gene results in biotinidase deficiency. Biotinidase is responsible for release of biotin from protein in the diet such as egg, liver, and milk or recycle biotin during normal protein turnover in cells. Biotin or vitamin B_7 plays an important role in processing certain proteins, carbohydrates, and fats. Mutation in *BTD* gene is responsible for elimination or reduction of biotinidase activity leading to impaired separation or recycling of biotin. Profound biotinidase deficiency is characterized by <10% biotinidase activity, whereas in partial biotinidase deficiency, the activity of the enzyme is reduced between 10 and 30%. Profound biotinidase deficiency manifests as seizures, ataxia, hypotonia, breathing problem, delayed development, alopecia, skin rash (seborrheic dermatitis and psoriasis-like), candidiasis, and loss of hearing and vision. Partial

"The most difficult thing is the decision to act, the rest is merely tenacity." —**Amelia Earhart**

biotinidase deficiency, a milder variety of the disease manifests only in the presence of any stress such as infection. Treatment is lifelong supplementation of biotin 5–10 mg on regular basis as symptoms may recur at any time. Certain food such as raw egg should be avoided in these patients; due to high content of avidin which can further aggravate biotin deficiency. Supportive treatment should be offered to those patients with already established problem such as providing hearing aid for hearing problem.

SCURVY (FIGS. 15 TO 19)

Scurvy, caused by vitamin C deficiency, is less common in the pediatric population and is primarily seen in children with developmental and behavioral issues including autism, malabsorptive processes, iron overload due to multiple transfusions, chemotherapy, bone marrow transplant, and hemodialysis or diseases involving dysphagia such as celiac disease, Crohn's disease, and severe allergies to food product. A restricted/unbalanced diet is an important factor in causing scurvy as in cases of cerebral palsy where children subsist on predominant milk-based diets and boiled cow's milk is a very poor source of vitamin C. Preterm babies who are on prolonged total parenteral nutrition therapy are also prone to develop scurvy. Infantile incidence is uncommon as both breast milk and fortified formula are an adequate source.

Clinical manifestations in scurvy is largely due to impaired collagen synthesis and disordered connective tissue resulting in hemorrhage because of blood vessel fragility and defective wound healing which can occur in almost any organ leading to changes in the bone, skin, and mucous membranes within

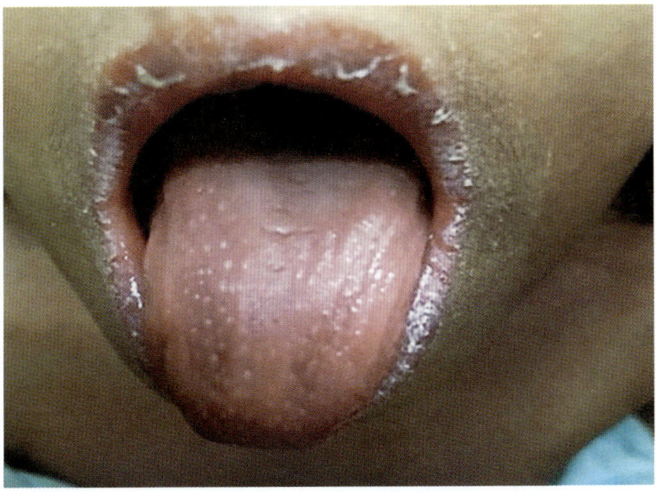

Fig. 15: Tongue in scurvy.

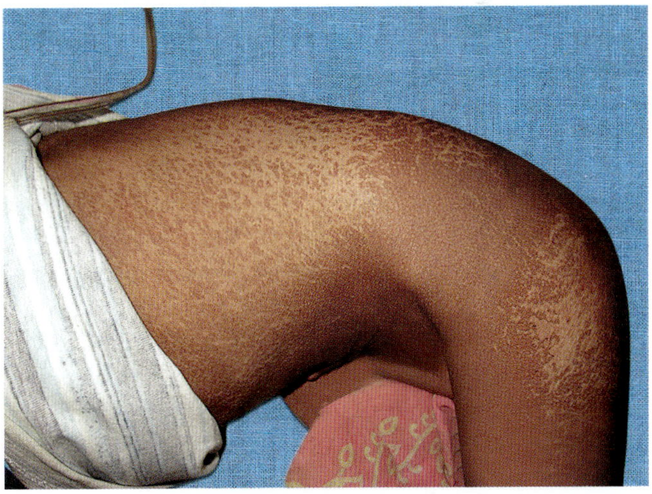

Fig. 17: Same child, view of back.

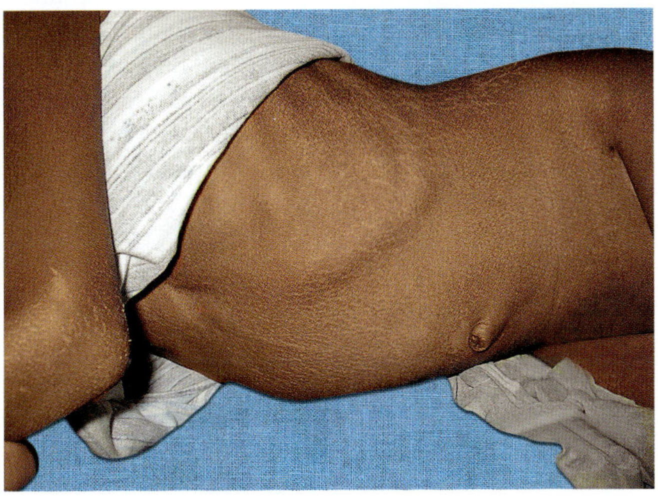

Fig. 16: Skin changes of scurvy, trunk.

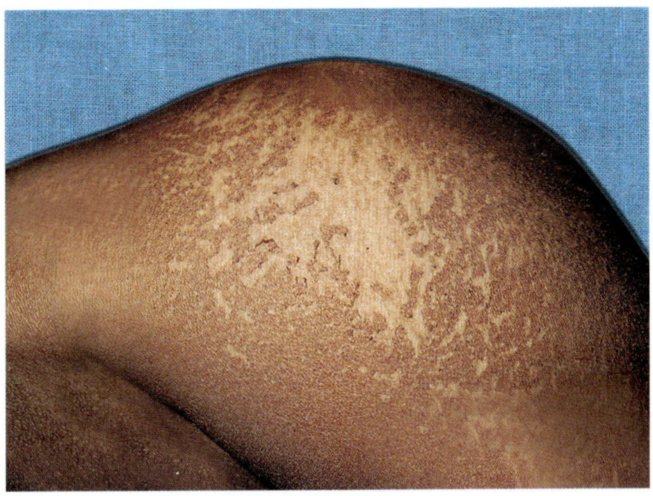

Fig. 18: Same child, close-up view.

"Team work is the ability to work together toward a common vision. The ability to direct individual accomplishments toward organizational objectives. It is the fuel that allows common people to attain uncommon results." —**Andrew Carnegie**

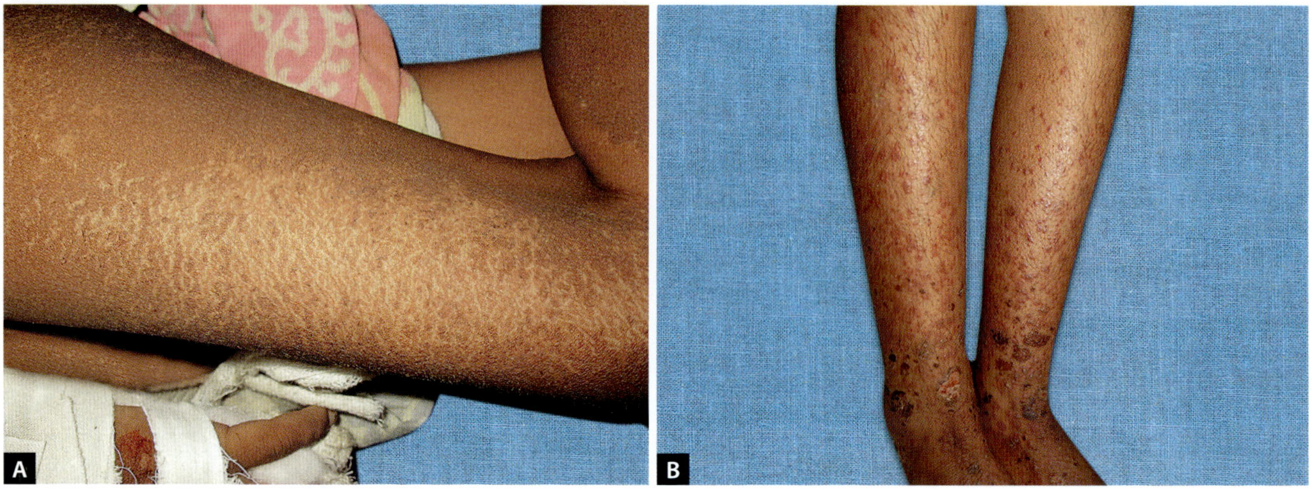

Figs. 19A and B: (A) Same child, back of thigh. (B) Note follicular hemorrhagic papules in scurvy.

1–3 months of depletion of the vitamin C pool in the body. The characteristic manifestations may be remembered by the four *H's* of *h*emorrhage, *h*yperkeratosis, *h*ypochondriasis, and *h*ematologic abnormalities. The most specific dermatological manifestations are follicular hyperkeratosis and perifollicular hemorrhage, with petechiae, ecchymoses, subungual or submucosal hemorrhages and coiled hair. These hemorrhagic skin lesions may coalesce and become palpable, especially on the lower extremities and resemble a systemic vasculitis. Oral symptoms include gingival hypertrophy and bleeding, receding gums leading to loosening of teeth, and dental caries. Abnormalities in the hair follicle (corkscrew or coiled hair with perifollicular hemorrhage) can be explained by the fragility of perifollicular collagen and abnormal disulfide bonding and keratin formation. Splinter hemorrhages on the nail and occasionally alopecia can also occur. Dermatological manifestations have to be differentiated from other pathologies presenting with purpura including immune thrombocytopenic purpura, Henoch-Schönlein purpura, disseminated intravascular coagulation, Rocky Mountain-spotted fever, meningococcemia, or hypersensitivity vasculitis. Mucosal involvement may mimic necrotizing gingivitis. Symmetric hyperpigmented rash on sun-exposed areas in niacin deficiency and alopecia, and lack of petechial and follicular findings in biotin and zinc deficiency easily distinguish them from scurvy.

Other features seen in pediatric population with scurvy includes scorbutic tongue, xerosis with exfoliation, musculoskeletal manifestations (bone pain, limb pain, swelling over long bones, pseudoparalysis, and progressive leg weakness and fractures), constitutional symptoms (lassitude and fatigue, failure to gain weight, loss of appetite, and irritability), and hypochromic microcytic anemia. Seizures and cardiorespiratory symptoms resulting in sudden death have also been reported.

The diagnosis of scurvy is based on history of poor dietary intake of vitamin C, classic clinical features and radiological findings (sclerotic and lucent metaphyseal bands, with periosteal reaction and adjacent soft-tissue edema), and response to treatment with vitamin C. Dermoscopy can aid in the diagnosis by confirming follicular purpura and corkscrew hair. Skin biopsy of the affected areas show similar findings in histopathology. The level of vitamin C in leukocytes is more accurate compared to serum vitamin C levels to assess deficient stores. Oral administration of vitamin C (100–300 mg to 1,000 mg/day) is adequate even in the most severe cases. Daily intake of fresh fruits and vegetables (grapefruits, oranges, lemons, limes, potatoes, spinach, broccoli, red peppers, and tomatoes) would provide a good source of vitamin C. Improvement of constitutional symptoms often occurs within 24 hours, with spontaneous bleeding improving over days to weeks. Corkscrew hair take up to a month to resolve, and complete resolution is usually seen by 3 months.

PYRIDOXINE (VITAMIN B_6) DEFICIENCIES AND ANGULAR STOMATITIS (FIGS. 20 AND 21)

Angular stomatitis also called as perlèche presents as inflammation and maceration of the angles of the mouth associated with fissuring and exudate. Angular cheilitis in children can result due to repeated lip licking,

"Don't judge each day by the harvest you reap but by the seeds that you plant." **—Robert Louis Stevenson**

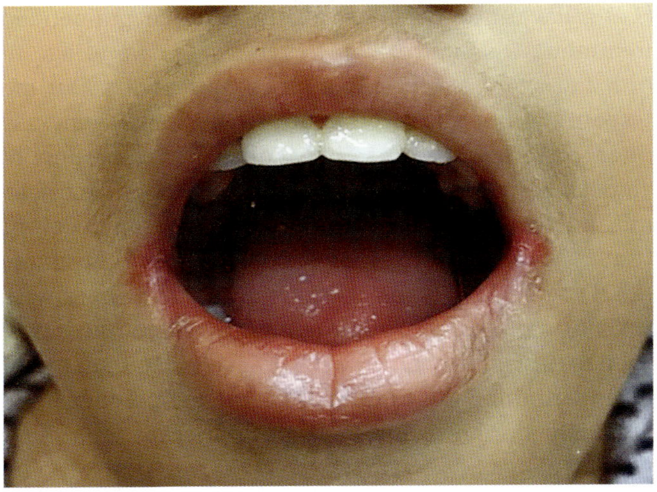

Fig. 20: Angular stomatitis.

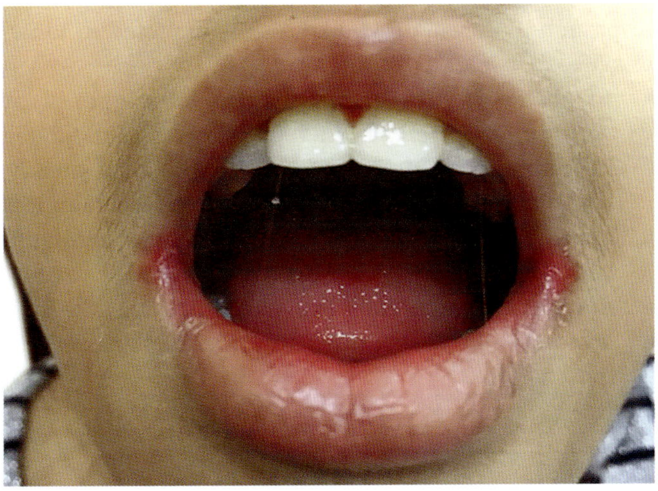

Fig. 21: Same child, close-up view.

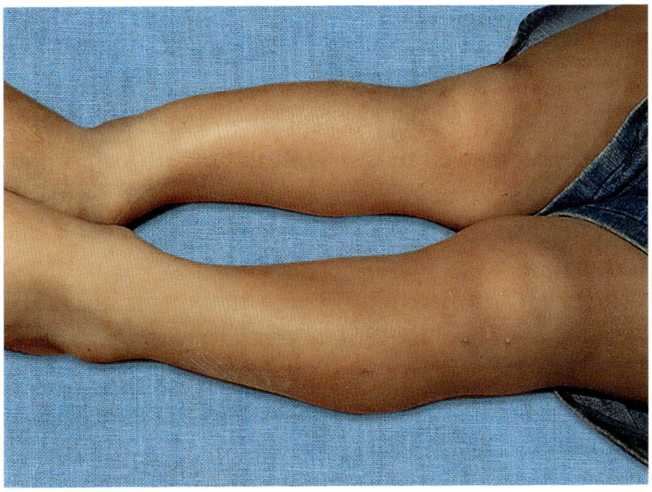

Fig. 22: Vitamin D-resistant rickets, note bowing of legs, dry xerotic skin.

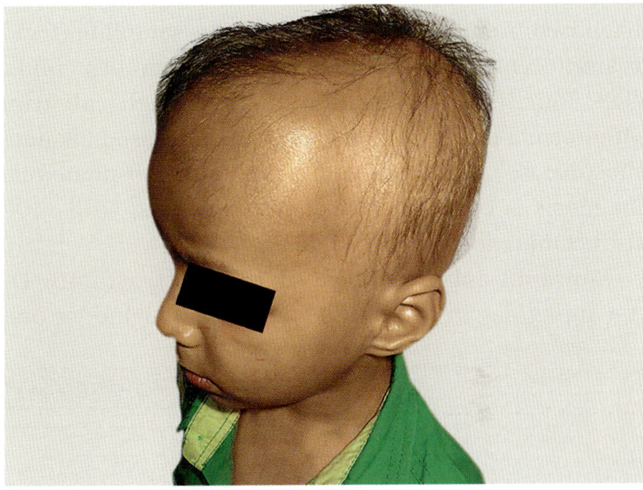

Fig. 23: Same child, note diffuse alopecia.

excessive salivation or drooling, dental malocclusion, and orthodontic appliances. It may not be always associated with nutritional or vitamin deficiency. Secondary infection with candidiasis can occur. Treatment consists of removal of predisposing factors, low-dose topical steroid, topical antibiotics, and topical antifungals. Recurrences are possible.

VITAMIN D RESISTANT RICKETS (FIGS. 22 AND 23)

Hereditary vitamin D-resistant rickets (HVDRR) is a rare autosomal recessive disorder resulting from inactivating homozygous or compound heterozygous mutations in the *VDR* gene, encoding the vitamin D receptor and is characterized by hypocalcemia, hypophosphatemia, secondary hyperparathyroidism, elevated alkaline phosphatase, and an increased serum 1, 25-dihydroxyvitamin D_3 level. It is also known as pseudovitamin D-deficiency type 2, vitamin D-dependent rickets type 2A (VDDR-2A), or rickets-alopecia syndrome.

Alopecia is found in many patients with HVDRR and may be the only obvious symptom in some cases. Presence of alopecia differentiates it from VDDR type 1. Approximately 80% of patients have early-onset alopecia, usually starting at birth, either totalis or universalis and the degree of alopecia is associated with the severity of the vitamin D resistance. Absence of scalp hair in newborns born in families with a prior history of the disease provides an initial clue to diagnose HVDRR. Vitamin D receptor (VDR) is composed of DNA-binding and ligand-binding domains (DBD and LBD respectively) for vitamin D_3, retinoid X receptor (RXR), and co-activators.

"The real opportunity for success lies within the person and not in the job." —**Zig Ziglar**

A ligand-independent action of the VDR has been proposed to be critical during hair follicle development. Mutations located on the DBD result in alopecia and severe rickets, whereas mutations on the LBD result in various degrees of rickets symptoms, with or without alopecia. Histopathological examination demonstrates thinning and hypoplastic hair follicles, with no specific scarring or inflammatory characteristics. The alopecia seen in HVDRR is clinically and pathologically indistinguishable from the generalized atrichia with papules found in patients with mutations in the *HR* gene.

McCune-Albright syndrome (MAS), linear nevus sebaceous syndrome, and nevus spilus have been shown to be associated with vitamin D-resistant hypophosphatemic rickets secondary to elevated circulating fibroblast growth factor 23 (FGF-23).

Hereditary vitamin D-resistant rickets can be diagnosed prenatally by chorionic villus sampling (CVS) or amniocentesis to detect defects in the unborn child's VDR. Biochemical alterations include high calcitriol with normal calcidiol, hypocalcemia, increased alkaline phosphatase, and phosphaturia and hypophosphatemia. Diagnosis is confirmed by genetic analysis, with >100 distinct mutations described till date.

Supraphysiological dose of 1,25$(OH)_2$ vitamin D_3 (1–6 μg/kg/day in two divided doses) and high dose oral (1–3 g/day) or intravenous calcium is the recommended treatment, essential before reaching 3 years of age in order to avoid potentially fatal complications. But the response of alopecia to this treatment regimen is generally poor, although there has been one previous report of alopecia responding to 1, 25$(OH)_2$ vitamin D_3. Cinacalcet, an allosteric modulator of calcium-sensing receptor (CaSR), with inhibitory effects on parathyroid hormone (PTH) secretion, when used as adjunctive therapy in HVDRR patients, restored their calcium and phosphate homeostasis, with normal PTH levels occurring over extended follow-up periods. Patients with alopecia are generally more resistant to calcitriol therapy than those without alopecia.

WHAT'S NEW

Approach to a case of AE like rash is depicted in **Flowchart 1**.

- *Extrinsic atopic dermatitis* can be triggered by *vitamin A deficiency*, which enhances Th2-mediated inflammation and activates mast cells. Consequently, *vitamin A supplementation* may be a viable treatment approach for preventing or managing atopic dermatitis in the future.
- Acrodermatitis metabolica enteropathica-like syndrome manifests with superficial scalded skin overlying

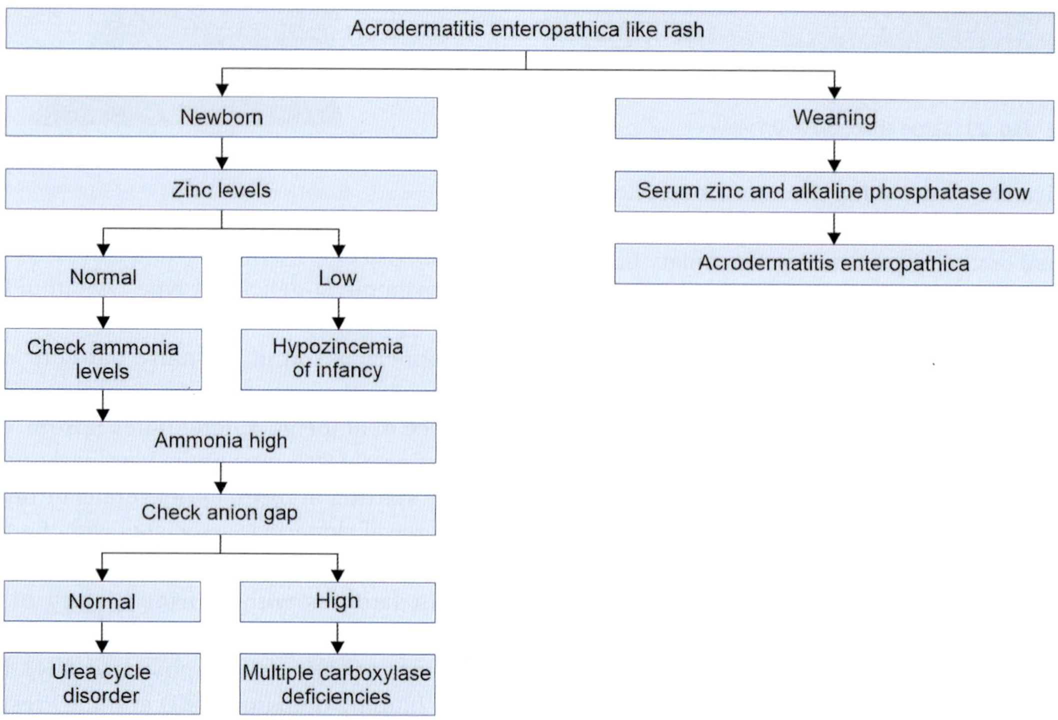

Flowchart 1: Approach to a case of acrodermatitis enteropathica like rash.

"Where there is no struggle, there is no strength." **—Oprah Winfrey**

erythematous tissues, along with symptoms such as stomatitis, cheilitis, and alopecia. This condition is associated with methylmalonic aciduria.

- *Cobalamin F (CblF) deficiency* is an autosomal recessive disorder caused by mutations in the *LMBRD1* gene. Clinically, it manifests as diffuse dyschromia affecting the palms and soles, along with hyperpigmentation of the fingernails, toenails, and graying of scalp hair. These features closely resemble those seen in dyskeratosis congenita and are accompanied by signs of *vitamin B_{12} deficiency*. As a result, CblF deficiency should be considered in the differential diagnosis of *diffuse reticulated dyschromia*. Unlike nutritional vitamin B_{12} deficiency, CblF deficiency necessitates lifelong replacement therapy.

SUGGESTED READINGS

1. Pandit VS, Udaya K. A study of neonatal dermatoses in a tertiary care center. Indian J Paediatr Dermatol. 2019;20:36-40.
2. Reginatto FP, Muller FM, Peruzzo J, Cestari TF. Epidemiology and predisposing factors for erythema toxicum neonatorumand transient neonatal pustular: a multicenter study. Pediatr Dermatol. 2017;34:422-6.
3. Yang H, Chen JS, Zou WJ, Tan Q, Xiao YZ, Luo XY, et al. Vitamin A deficiency exacerbates extrinsic atopic dermatitis development by potentiating type 2 helper T cell-type inflammation and mast cell activation. Clin Exp Allergy. 2020;50(8):942-53.
4. El Hadadi F, Mezni L, Ismaili N, Benzekri L, Senouci K. Acrodermatitis enteropathica-like eruption. JAAD Case Rep. 2022;24:20-3.
5. Altawil L, Alshihry H, Ahmed H, Shamseldin HE, Alkuraya F. Vitamin B12 deficiency secondary to cobalamin F deficiency simulating dyskeratosis congenita. JAAD Case Rep. 2020; 6(9):882-5.
6. Somasundaram A, Chiramel MJ, Sathishkumar D, Korula S. Skin as a Window to Diagnose Inborn Errors of Metabolism. Indian J Paediatr Dermatol. 2023;24(1):8-18.

"Hardwork beats talent when talent doesn't work hard." **—Tim Notke**

CHAPTER

13

Urticaria, Mast Cell, and Histiocytic Disorders

URTICARIA [FIGS. 1 TO 3E(v)]

Urticaria (hives and nettle rash) manifests as itchy transient erythematous and edematous eruptions over skin which lasts from few minutes to several hours. It disappears spontaneously leaving behind normal looking skin. Angioedema manifests as localized swelling of the skin and mucosa with stinging sensation. It lasts for 30 minutes to 24 hours. Similar to adults, urticaria in children can be classified into acute urticaria (<6 weeks) and chronic urticaria (>6 weeks). Both urticaria and angioedema can develop as a result of type I, III, or IV hypersensitivity reaction. Important causes of urticaria and angioedema in pediatric age group are viral infections, insect bites, some food items, drugs [antibiotics and nonsteroidal anti-inflammatory drugs (NSAIDs)] and physical factors, e.g., exercise and heat. Food dyes and additives are implicated in both acute and chronic urticaria.

Vaccination is by and large safe in children with a history of chronic urticaria. However, it is better to be avoided during acute episode of urticaria.

ANGIOEDEMA [FIGS. 3E(vi) TO (xi)]

Angioedema presents as acute, evanescent, circumscribed swelling of the deep dermis/subcutaneous or submucosal tissue or mucus membranes as a result of vascular leakage. It usually affects the distensible tissues such as the lips or eyes, most commonly, though lobes of the ears, external genitalia, or mucosa of mouth, tongue, larynx, or gastrointestinal tract can also be involved. Swelling that involves the upper airways is a cause of greater concern due to the potential of airway compromise. Laryngeal edema is a life-threatening condition and should be treated as a medical emergency. Tenderness or pain is absent or mild or can be very severe as in gastrointestinal angioedema which presents as acute abdomen. Various types of angioedema are given in **Table 1**.

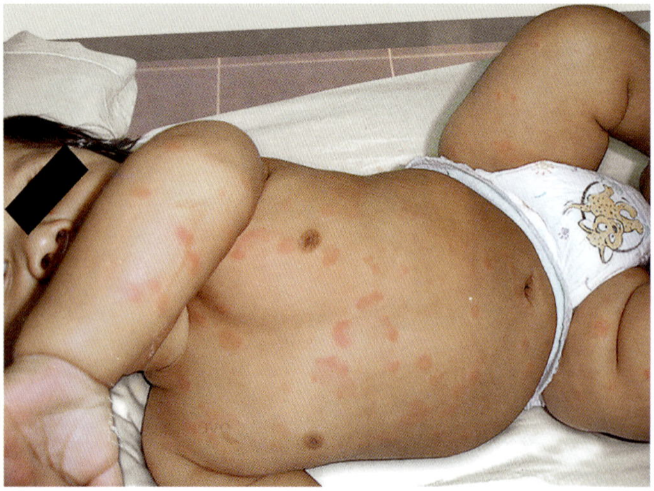

Fig. 1: Acute urticarial wheals in an infant.

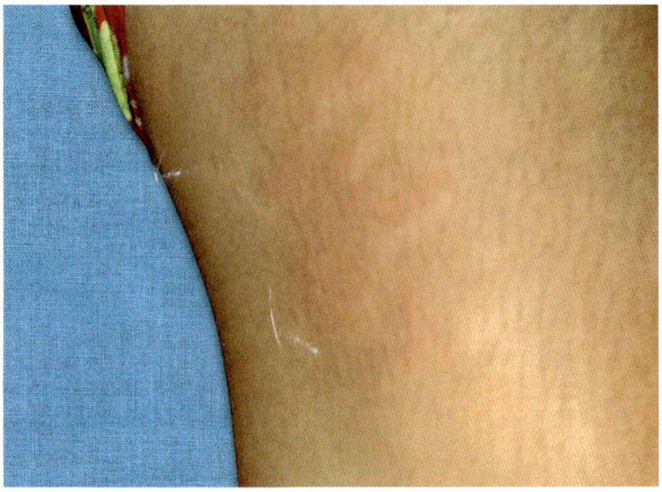

Fig. 2: Urticarial wheals.

"Set your life on fire. Seek those who fan your flames." —**Rumi**

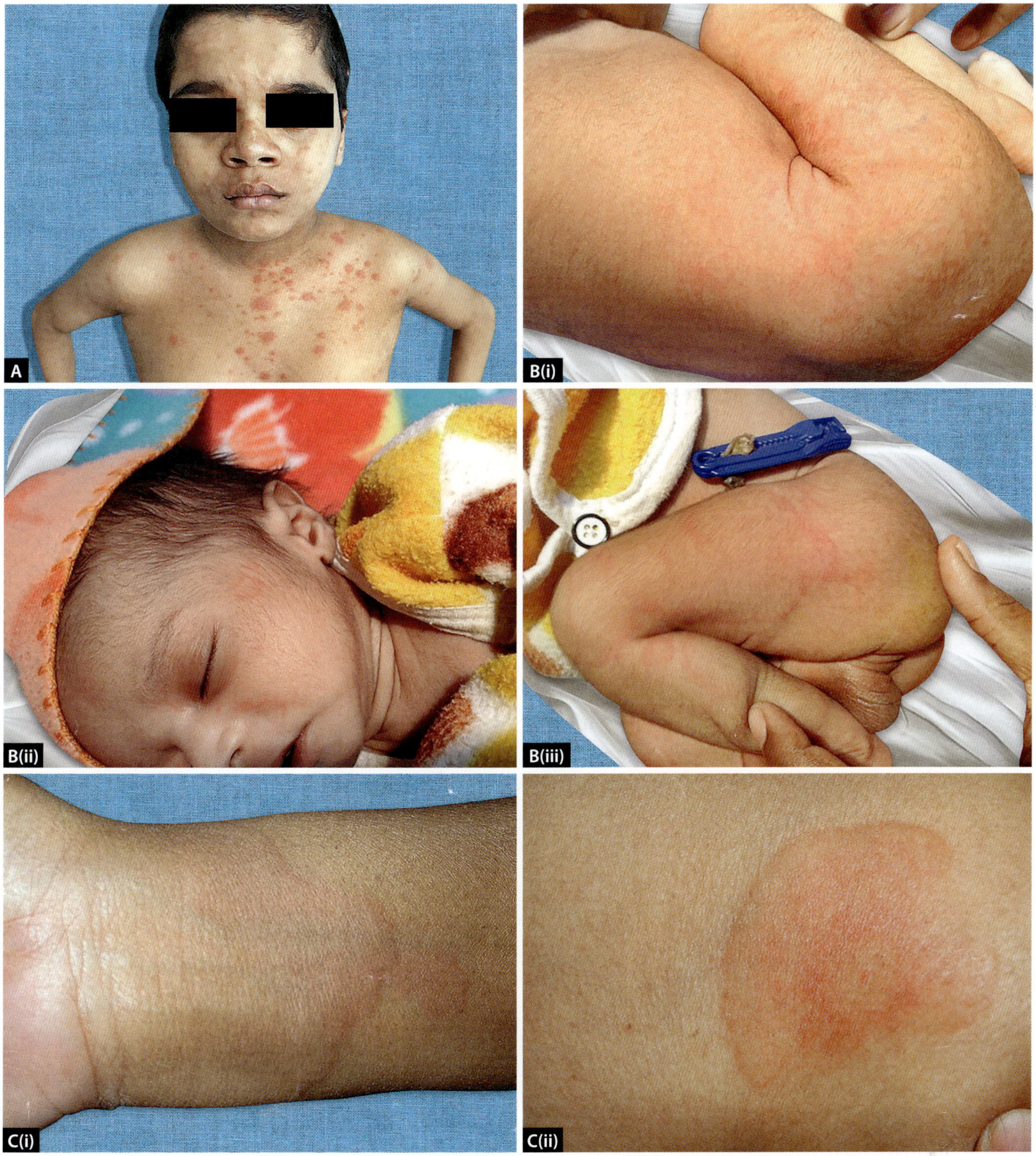

Figs. 3A to C(ii): (A) Urticaria in a school-going child; B(i) Urticaria in an infant; B(ii) Same infant, wheals over face; B(iii) Same infant, giant wheals; C(i) Urticarial hive, note pseudopodia-like extension; C(ii) Urticarial hive.

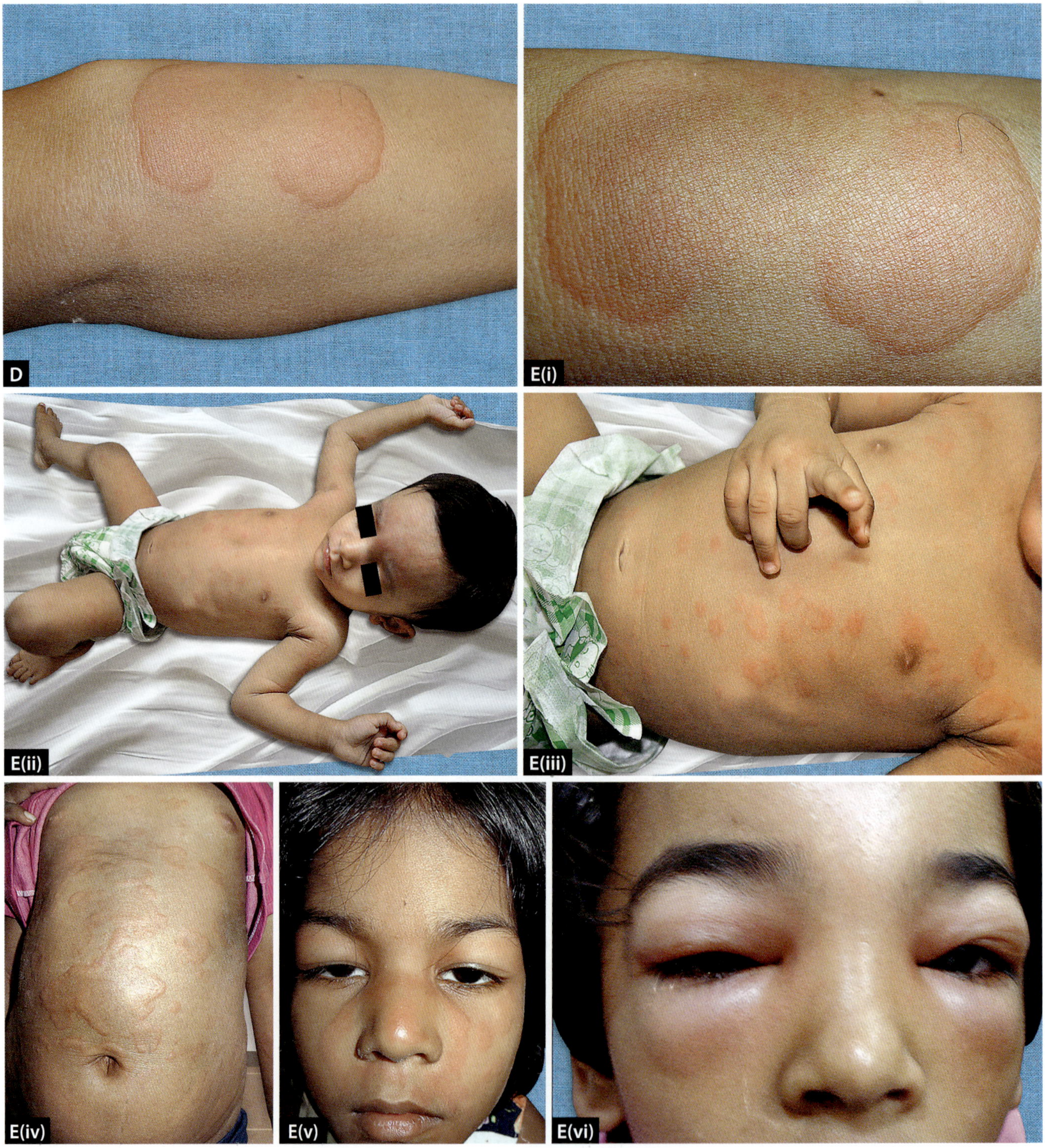

Figs. 3D to E(vi): (D) Various shapes and sizes of urticarial hives; E(i) Close-up view; E(ii) Acute urticaria in an infant; E(iii) Same infant, close-up view; E(iv) Acute urticarial wheals; E(v) Acute urticarial wheals in a 5-year-old girl; E(vi) Angioedema of eyelids.

"The greatest day in your life and mine is when we take total responsibility for our attitudes. That's the day we truly grow up." —**John C Maxwell**

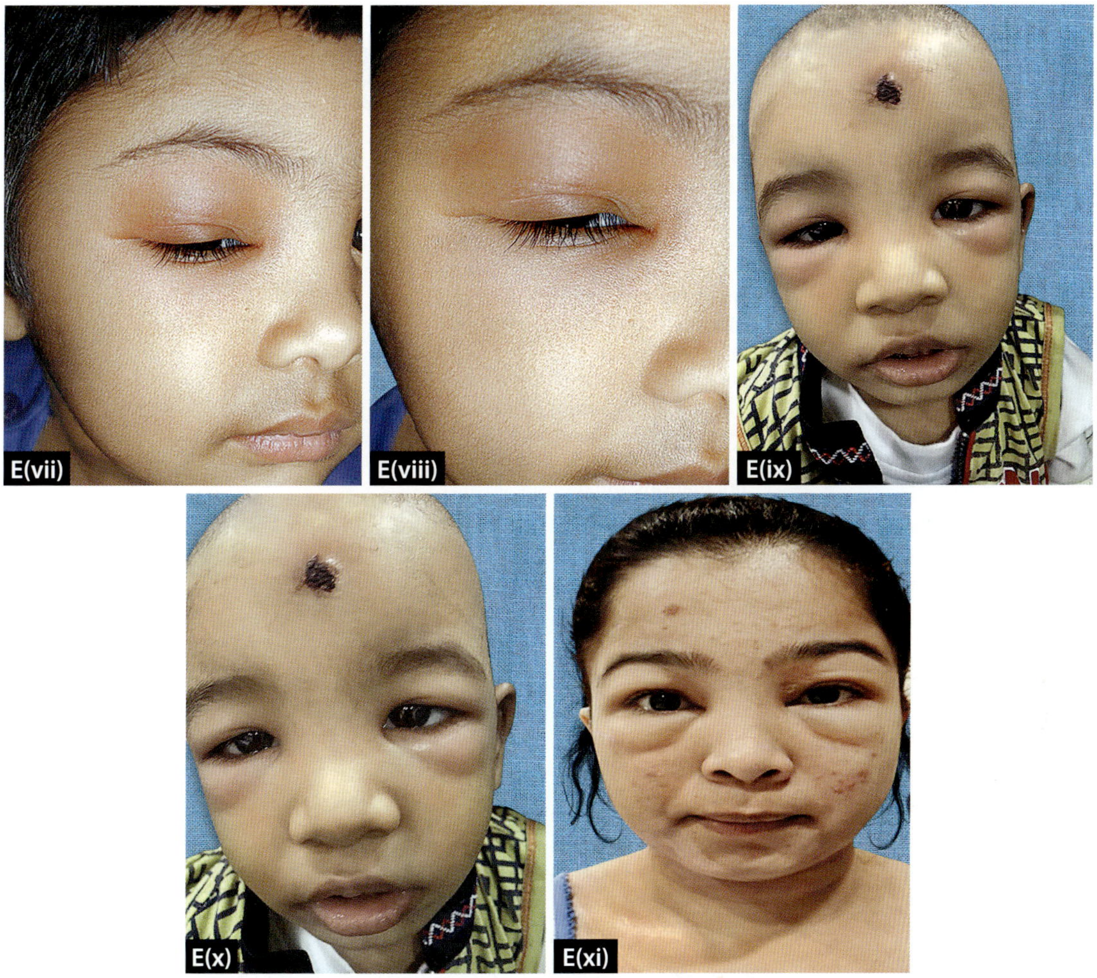

Figs. 3E(vii) to (xi): E(vii) Angioedema of eyelid; E(viii) Angioedema of eyelid, close-up view; E(ix) Angioedema in a 3-year-old boy; E(x) Same boy, close-up view; E(xi) Angioedema.

DERMOGRAPHISM [FIGS. 4A(i) TO (iii)]

This phenomenon involves the triple response of Lewis: (1) local erythema due to capillary vasodilatation, (2) edema, and (3) flare due to axon reflex-induced dilatation of arterioles.

It may arise from firm stroking of the skin. The response is normal but in 5% of normal people, this response is sufficiently exaggerated to warrant the term dermographism. Patients complain of wealing and itching at the sites of trauma, friction with clothing or scratching the skin. The itching is often disproportionately severe compared with wealing and is often most severe at night. Dermographism is not increased in chronic idiopathic urticaria nor is there any correlation with systemic disease or food allergy. Dermographism is usually idiopathic but sometimes may follow a drug reaction. Dermographism is usually demonstrated with firm stroking of the skin on the forearm. A linear itchy wheal develops in 10 minutes and persists for approximately 15 minutes.

Management

Oral antihistamines form the mainstay of treatment of urticaria and angioedema. Classical H_1 blockers have sedative and anticholinergic effects. There have been few pharmacokinetic studies of antihistamines in children. Most of the prescribing patterns are empirically based upon experience. By and large, the onset of action of most antihistamines is 30–60 minutes after ingestion. However, full action is not reached for 2–3 hours. Various antihistamines that are safe in children for urticaria and angioedema are highlighted in **Table 1**. There is little reason to choose one antihistamine over another except

"Life is not a problem to be solved, but a reality to be experienced." —**Soren Kierkegaard**

Table 1: Various types of angioedema.

Type of angioedema	Pathophysiology	Clinical features	Investigations	Treatment
Hereditary angioedema type 1	Low levels of functional C1-INH	• Initial manifestation occurs in children at median age of 4.8 years • Family history positive in 25% cases • Sudden attacks of angioedema occur every 2 weeks throughout patient's life, lasting for 2–5 days. No associated urticaria or itching • Mortality rate is high due to laryngeal edema • Factors that trigger attacks are minor trauma, surgery, sudden changes of temperature or sudden emotional stress, or sex hormone fluctuations and menses	• C1-INH levels low • C4 almost always low • C1/C3/C1q—normal	• Replacement therapy with concentrates or fresh frozen plasma • Antifibrinolytic tranexamic acid • Short-term prophylaxis can be obtained from stanozolol
Hereditary angioedema type 2	C1-INH within reference range or even increased levels of antigenic but nonfunctional C1-INH	Same as above	• C1-INH levels normal or raised but dysfunctional • C4 low • C1/C3/C1q—normal	Same as above
Hereditary angioedema type 3	C1-INH function and complement components are normal	• Seen more commonly in females • Criteria for diagnosis include—long history of recurrent attacks of skin swelling, abdominal pain or upper airway obstruction, absence of urticaria, familial occurrence, normal C1-INH and C4 concentrations and failure of treatment with antihistamines, corticosteroids, and C1-INH concentrate	Complement profile normal	Does not respond to C1-INH replacement, but may respond to danazol
Acquired angioedema type 1	Linked to an underlying lymphoproliferative disorder, complement activating factors, idiotype anti-idiotype antibodies or other immune complexes that destroy the function of C1-INH	Presentation is like hereditary angioedema but here it occurs in the fourth decade of life	• C1-INH and C4 levels—low • C1q levels are normal or low	• Replacement of C1-INH through fresh frozen plasma, plasma-derived C1-INH • Recombinant human C1-INH • Aminocaproic acid or tranexamic acid • Antiandrogens such as danazol
Acquired angioedema type 2	Autoantibodies directly inhibit the C1-INH function		• Same as AAE-1 • Autoantibody testing positive	• Same as above • But antiandrogens are ineffective • Systemic corticosteroids are temporarily given immunosuppressive therapy found to be effective • Plasmapheresis, B2-bradykinin receptor antagonist, and the kallikrein inhibitor are promising therapies for patients refractory to other treatments

Continued

"What we think determines what happens to us, so if we want to change our lives, we need to stretch our minds." **—Wayne Dyer**

Continued

Type of angioedema	*Pathophysiology*	*Clinical features*	*Investigations*	*Treatment*
Nonhistaminergic angioedema	Same as angioedema without urticaria	Swelling due to nonhistaminergic angioedema may occur anywhere including the face, arms, legs, genitalia, throat, and abdomen, although abdominal symptoms are far less common	Complement profile is normal	Antifibrinolytics such as tranexamic acid or epsilon aminocaproic acid is used
Idiopathic angioedema	Associated with swelling or hives that persists for longer than 6 weeks. It can be associated with thyroid dysfunction	Swelling can occur anywhere in or on the body and may be accompanied by urticaria	Complement profile is normal	Antihistamines are primarily used
Allergic angioedema	Characterized by hives or swelling or both in reaction to environmental factors such as food, insect bite, cold, heat, latex or drug	Swelling most commonly of the face and throat. Urticaria is often present. If the condition persists for >6 weeks, it is considered chronic idiopathic urticaria	Complement profile is normal	• Antihistamines for mild cases • Diphenhydramine 50 mg IV/IM for moderate cases + Inj hydrocortisone 200 mg IV or methylprednisolone 40–60 mg IV may reduce the possibility of relapse • For laryngeal swelling or airway obstruction, epinephrine (1:1000) should be administered IM at a dose of 0.01 mg/kg or 0.3 mg repeated every 10–15 minutes, if necessary • Intubation or tracheostomy, if necessary
ACEI-induced angioedema	Angioedema is caused by ACEI and swelling may occur few hours or years after first starting the medication	Swelling may occur anywhere, including the throat, face, lips, tongue, hands, feet, genitalia, and intestines. Urticaria is very rare	Complement profile is normal	Medication is either suspended or changed

(AAE: acquired angioedema; ACEI: angiotensin-converting-enzyme inhibitors; C1-INH: C1-esterase inhibitor)

for avoidance of adverse effects including sedation in school going children. However, usually chosen H_1 blockers are chlorpheniramine, cetirizine, hydroxyzine, and promethazine. They are to be advocated orally twice daily in syrup or tablet form. On an average, for cases of acute urticaria, 5–10 days and for chronic urticaria, 3–6 months' course is required. For resistant cases, H_2 blockers, viz., ranitidine is combined with H_1 blockers.

For school-going children or older children, a combination of nonsedating antihistamine during day time and sedating antihistamines at night time is preferred. For cases of anaphylaxis, and angioedema, adrenaline is to be given subcutaneously at a dose of 0.05 mg/kg/day in two divided doses. Hydrocortisone, methylprednisolone, or even dexamethasone can be used intramuscularly or intravenously for severe urticaria and angioedema. Reassurance and counseling parents form the cornerstone of management of urticaria and angioedema in infants and children.

URTICARIA MULTIFORME [FIGS. 4A(iv) AND (v)]

Urticaria multiforme is considered a morphologic subset of urticarial reactions. It is a common, benign hypersensitivity reaction mediated by histamine that

"Believe that life is worth living and your belief will help create the fact." **—William James**

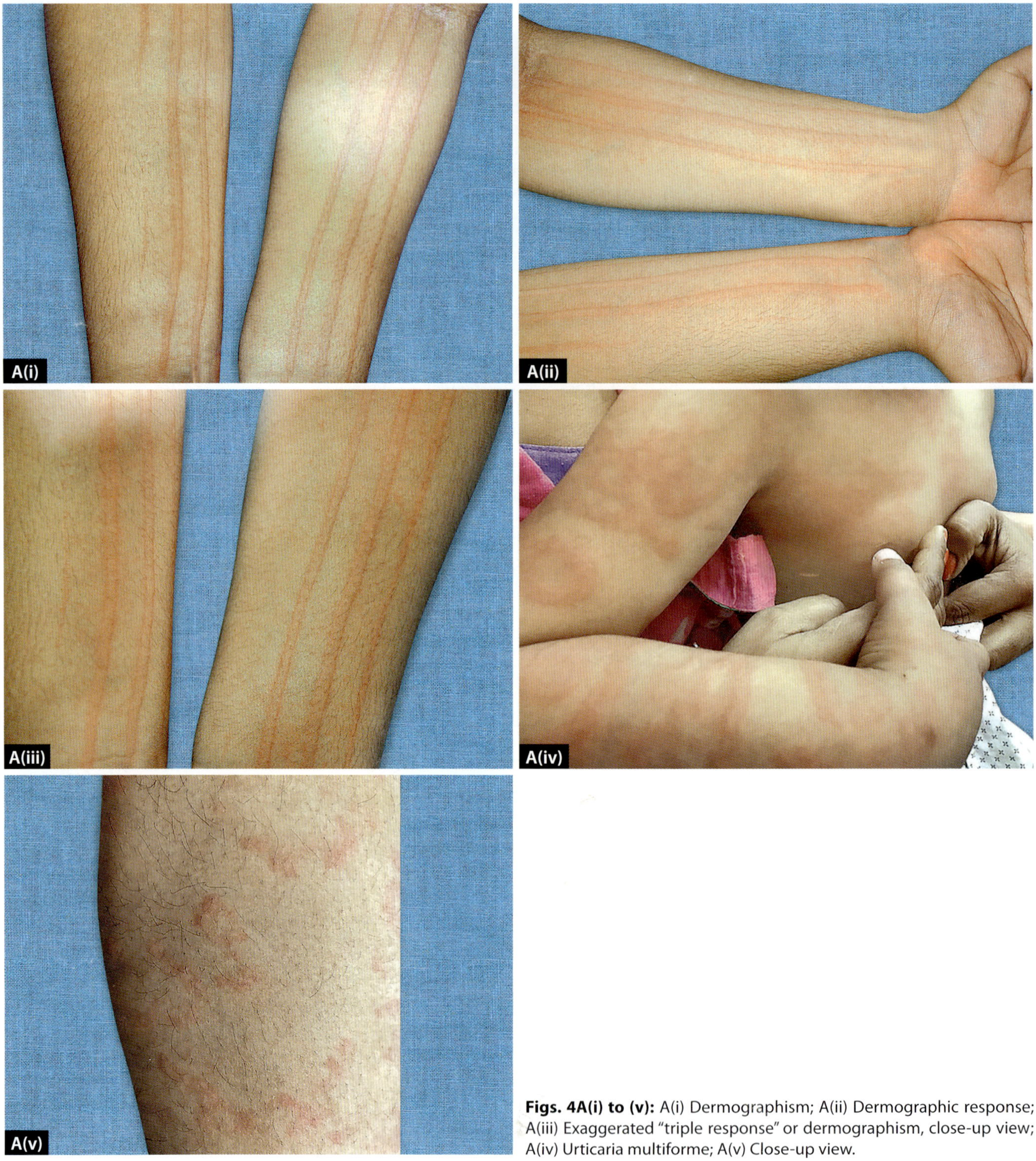

Figs. 4A(i) to (v): A(i) Dermographism; A(ii) Dermographic response; A(iii) Exaggerated "triple response" or dermographism, close-up view; A(iv) Urticaria multiforme; A(v) Close-up view.

predominantly affects children between 4 months and 4 years of age. It manifests mostly after a preceding illness, drug intake, or vaccination.

Culprit drugs reported are amoxicillin, topiramate, nitrofurantoin, aspirin, omeprazole, and reported vaccines include those against varicella, rotavirus, *Haemophilus influenzae*, diphtheria, tetanus, and pertussis. Child appears nontoxic and systemic findings are typically limited to a low-grade fever. Cutaneous findings include large polycyclic, annular, erythematous wheals on the face, trunk, and extremities. The wheals may develop an ecchymotic or dusky center with facial angioedema or acral edema. The lesions are acute, transient, blanchable, often pruritic but not painful. Dermographism is associated in 50% of the cases. It is most commonly misdiagnosed as erythema multiforme, serum sickness-like reaction, or urticarial vasculitis. Although the dusky appearance is in favor of erythema multiforme, there are no true target lesions, blistering, or necrosis of the skin and/or mucous membranes. Patients with urticaria multiforme respond well to antihistamines. But usually the cutaneous eruptions are self-limited and lasts about 1–2 weeks without any intervention. The lesions heal without postinflammatory hyperpigmentation or scarring.

MASTOCYTOSIS [FIGS. 4B(i) TO 9]

Mastocytosis is a clonal disease of hematopoietic stem cell characterized by proliferation and accumulation of mast cells in various organs such as skin, bone marrow, liver, spleen, and lymph nodes. Almost half of all cases of mastocytosis occur in children. The clinical picture ranges from mastocytoma to diffuse cutaneous mastocytosis but the most common presentation is urticaria pigmentosa.

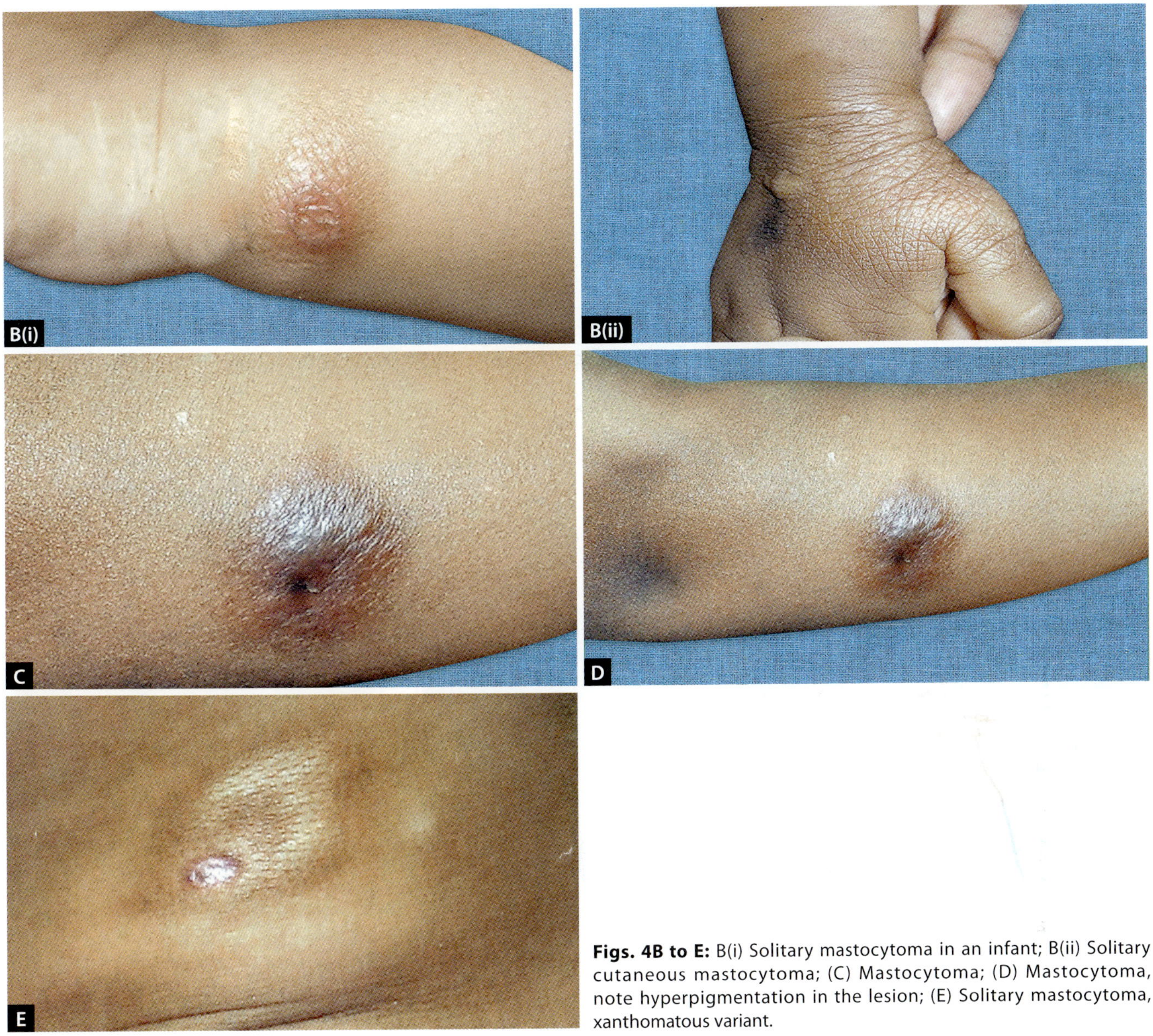

Figs. 4B to E: B(i) Solitary mastocytoma in an infant; B(ii) Solitary cutaneous mastocytoma; (C) Mastocytoma; (D) Mastocytoma, note hyperpigmentation in the lesion; (E) Solitary mastocytoma, xanthomatous variant.

"Too often we underestimate the power of a touch, a smile, a kind word, a listening ear, an honest compliment, or the smallest act of caring, all of which have the potential to turn a life around." —**Leo Buscaglia**

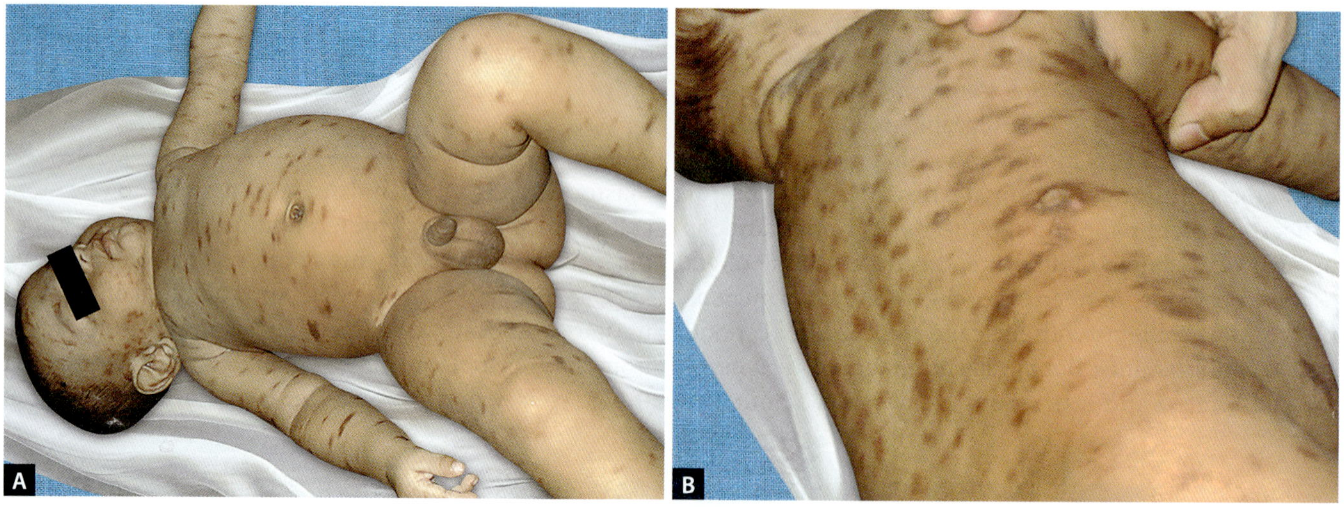

Figs. 5A and B: (A) Hyperpigmented infiltrated papules of mastocytosis; (B) Close-up view, mastocytosis lesions.

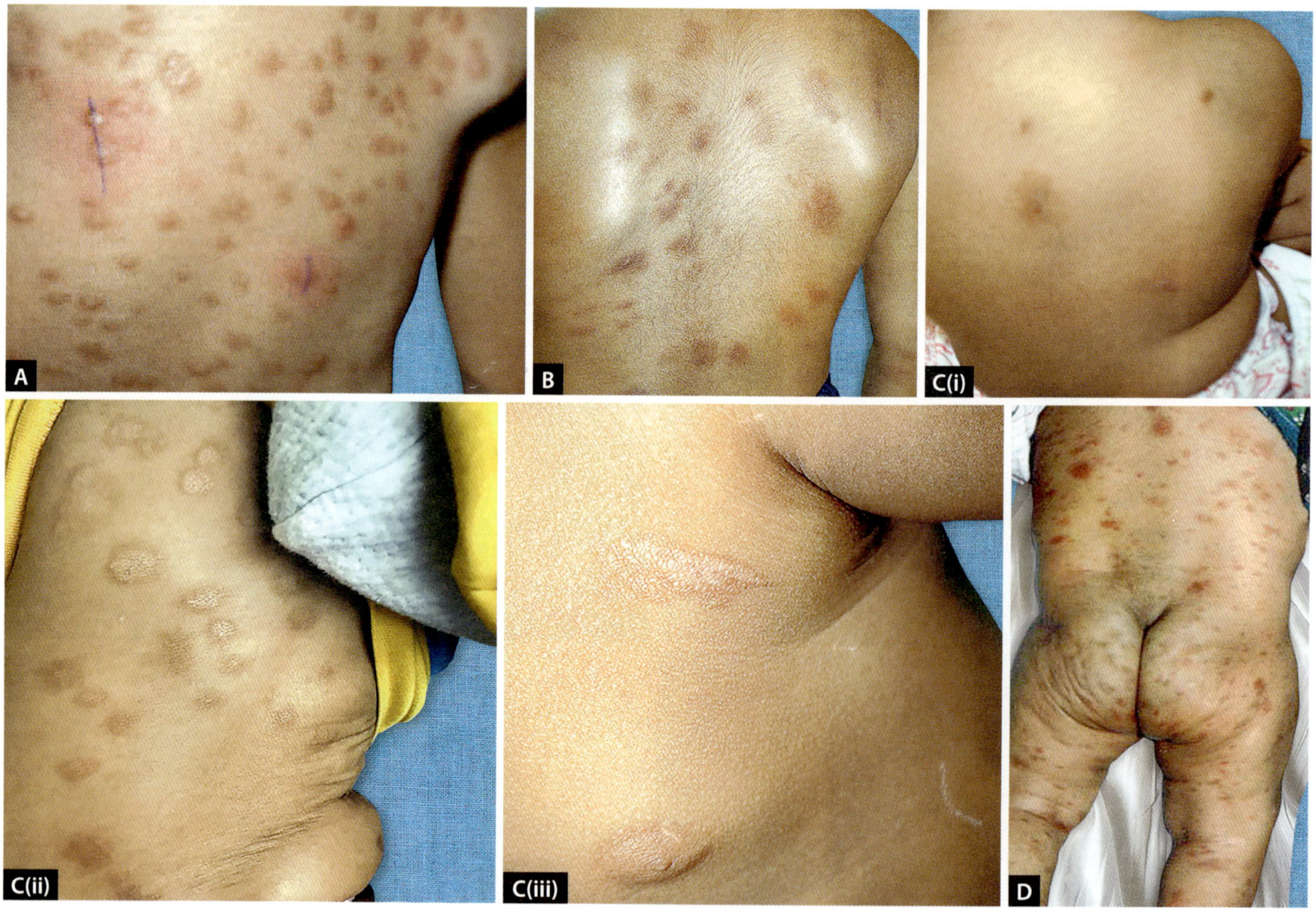

Figs. 6A to D: (A) Darier's sign demonstrated; (B) Multiple lesions of urticaria pigmentosa; C(i) Urticaria pigmentosa on back; C(ii) Mastocytosis after remission; C(iii) Mastocytosis-xanthomatous variant; (D) Mastocytosis in a 1-year-old infant.

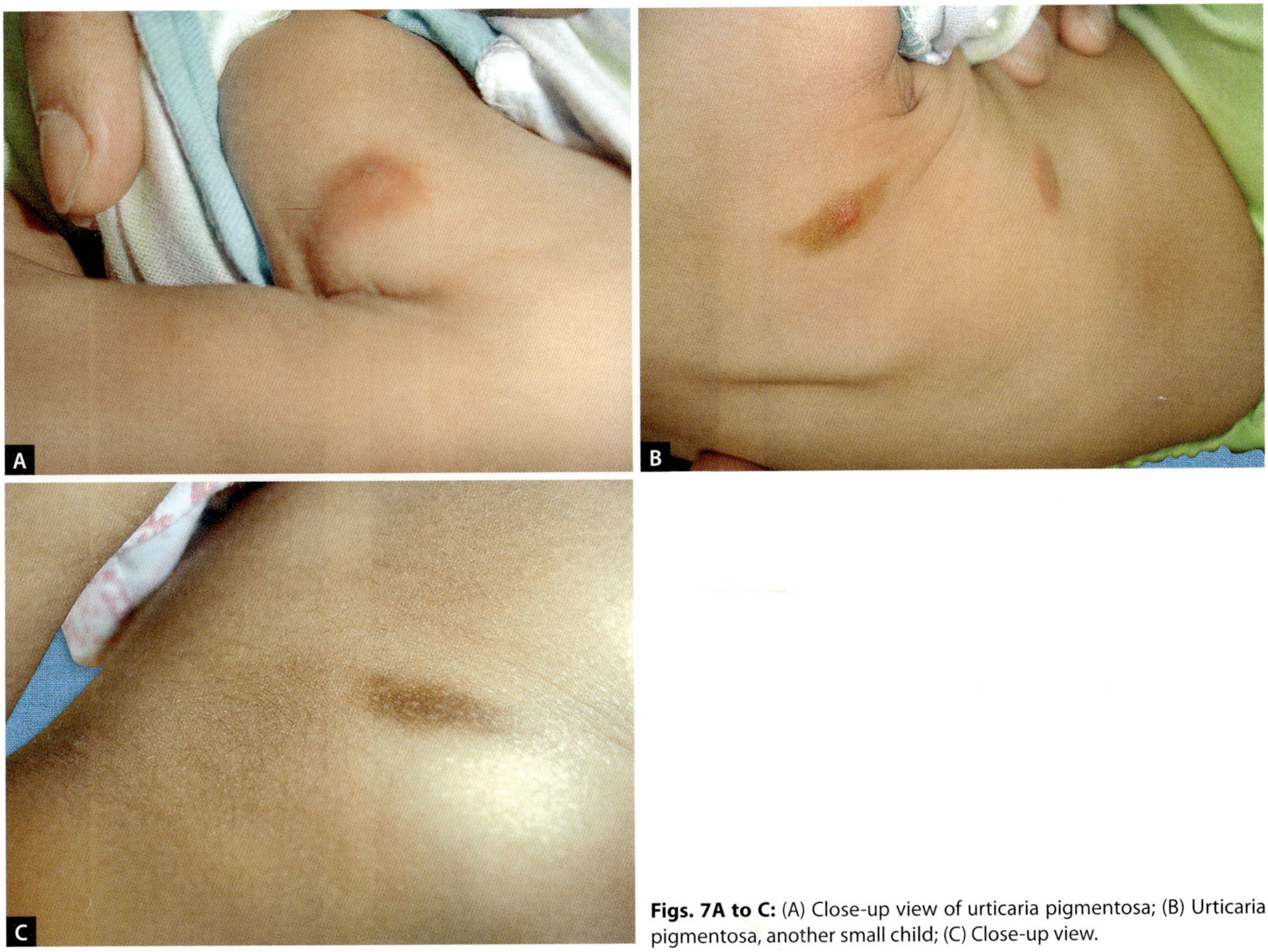

Figs. 7A to C: (A) Close-up view of urticaria pigmentosa; (B) Urticaria pigmentosa, another small child; (C) Close-up view.

Rarely xanthomatous variant can be seen. Around 50% of all childhood cases undergo resolution by puberty. Classification of mastocytosis is described in **Box 1**.

SOLITARY MASTOCYTOMA

In this disease, the lesions generally appear at birth or early in infancy, increase somewhat in size for several months, and eventually regress spontaneously, generally within a period of several years. With this form of mastocytosis, lesions are indeed solitary in most patients. However, sometimes many lesions may occur. Some patients have been reported to develop a generalized form of urticaria pigmentosa.

This disease can occur on any part of the body but are noted most commonly on the arms, wrist, trunk, and the neck. Clinically, they are seen as slightly elevated flesh-colored to light brown nodules or tan plaques. Sometimes, they can display a yellowish or pink hue. Generally, lesions are round or oval in shape and measure 1–5 cm in diameter. They may have a thick or rubbery quality with a smooth or pebbly peau d'orange (orange peel-like) consistency. Stroking or rubbing of lesions may at times produce symptoms or flushing or colic. Darier's sign is positive. Sometimes bullous lesions may be seen over the lesions of solitary mastocytoma developing as a result of trauma or friction.

Prognosis

Solitary mastocytomas have the most favorable prognosis among all forms of mastocytosis. In this disorder, the present symptoms are usually mild and spontaneous resolution within a period of several years is the rule (almost always before the age of 10 years). Unless the lesions are symptomatic and troublesome, surgical excision is usually not necessary.

"There is more to life than increasing its speed." —**Mahatma Gandhi**

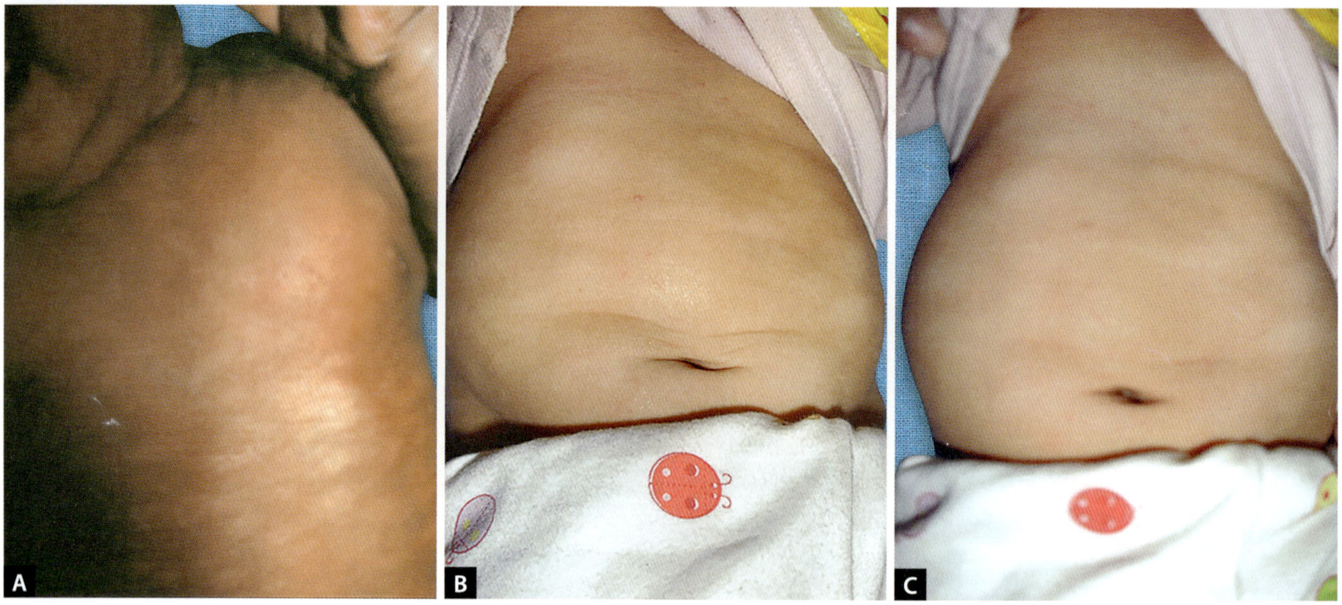

Figs. 8A to C: (A) Diffuse cutaneous mastocytosis; (B) Diffuse cutaneous mastocytosis, note thickened skin; (C) Same child, note infiltrated skin with leathery appearance.

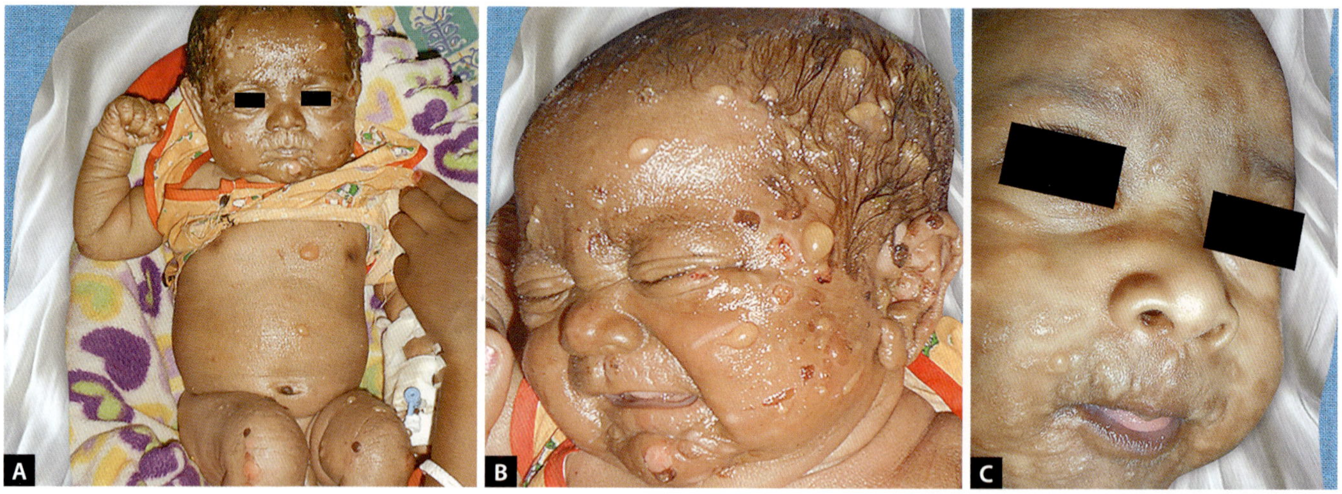

Figs. 9A to C: (A) A 5-month-old baby with diffuse cutaneous mastocytosis; (B) Same baby, note purse-string appearance of perioral skin; (C) Urticaria pigmentosa with bullous lesions.

URTICARIA PIGMENTOSA

It is the most common type of mastocytosis seen in children. In majority of cases, the onset is between birth and 2 years of age. The most common eruption consists of monomorphic, pigmented, maculopapular, or nodular lesions mainly on the trunk with a widespread symmetrical distribution. The lesions have a characteristic edge which is not absolutely sharp. The diagnosis is established by demonstrating gentle rubbing of the lesional skin that causes local itching, redness, and wheals (Darier's sign). Lesions may become confluent to form plaque-like areas. The principal symptom of urticaria pigmentosa is intense itching which is aggravated by rubbing and scratching. The pigmentation is due to melanin which is present in increased amounts in the basal layer. It has been estimated that 60% of infancy or childhood cases show blister formation. However, blister formation is not associated with a poor prognosis. Blistering usually subsides spontaneously after 2–3 years.

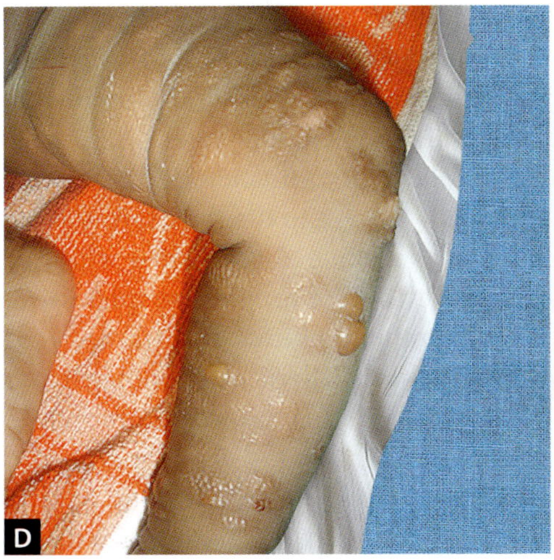

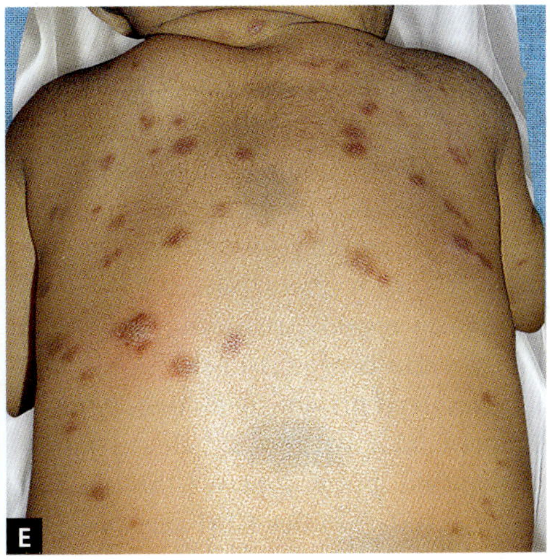

Figs. 9D and E: (D) Same baby, lesions over legs; (E) Telangiectasia macularis eruptiva perstans (note reddish hue over and around the lesions).

Box 1 | Updated WHO classification of mastocytosis 2016.

- *Cutaneous mastocytosis (CM):*
  - Maculopapular CM /urticaria pigmentosa (UP)
  - Diffuse CM (DCM)
  - Mastocytoma of skin
- *Systemic mastocytosis (SM):*
  - Indolent SM (ISM)
  - Smoldering SM (SSM)
  - SM with associated hematologic neoplasm (AHN)
  - Aggressive SM (ASM)
  - Mast cell leukemia (MCL)
- Mast cell sarcoma (MCS)

DIFFUSE CUTANEOUS MASTOCYTOSIS

In this rare mast cell disorder, there is diffuse mast cell infiltration; the skin has a yellowish thickened appearance and is of doughy consistency. The term pseudoxanthomatous mastocytosis has been given to certain forms of this group. Pigmentation is often absent, cutaneous folds are exaggerated, and the changes are mostly marked in the axillae and groins. In extreme cases, the skin becomes pachydermatous. Nodules and small dermal tumors may also be present. Pruritus is intense. A characteristic feature is the appearance of large hemorrhagic blisters following mild trauma or occurring spontaneously. Systemic symptoms include flushing, hemorrhage, nausea, vomiting, diarrhea, hypotension, dyspnea, headache, dizziness, irritability, tachycardia, abdominal pain, melena, sepsis, and overt shock leading to death. There may be systemic mast cell infiltration with hepatosplenomegaly. The prognosis is not good in such cases.

Diagnosis

Diagnosis of all types of mastocytoses is confirmed by histopathological examination of skin biopsy specimen. Special precautions must be taken while sending a skin biopsy for confirmation of diagnosis. The tissue must be preserved in alcohol and not formalin as it is routinely done.

Special staining for mast cell is to be done by stains such as toluidine blue or Giemsa.

Treatment

Treatment is usually symptomatic. Antihistamines form the backbone of treatment and must be given according to the age and body weight of the affected child. Conventional H_1 blockers, e.g., chlorpheniramine, promethazine, or hydroxyzine are of great help to control itching and urticarial response; cetirizine is also effective. Application of moderately potent topical steroids, intralesional triamcinolone acetonide, helps in resolution of these lesions. Maintenance therapy over a long period of time and regular follow-up of these children is necessary. Ultraviolet (UV) therapy may be used in adults and children above 6 years of age. Oral corticosteroids and epinephrine are given only if there is anaphylactic storm and in systemic mastocytosis. Other modes of therapy for systemic involvement include interferon-α therapy, cyclosporine, hydroxyurea, cladribine, and imatinib. Counseling and avoidance of triggers such as bathing in extremes of temperature, prevention of insect bites, and any physical trauma is necessary. Over the counter, cough medications should be avoided as they contain dextromethorphan and codeine which can activate mast cells.

"Our prime purpose in this life is to help others. And if you can't help them, at least don't hurt them." —**Dalai Lama**

LANGERHANS CELL HISTIOCYTOSIS (FIGS. 10 TO 13)

Langerhans cell histiocytosis (LCH), a rare neoplasm of hematopoietic myeloid precursor cells, is clinically characterized by spontaneously resolving lesions to a progressive life-threatening multisystem disorder. It is a neoplastic histiocytic disorder characterized by clonal proliferation of immature myeloid precursor cells and their accumulation in various organs of the body. The term histiocytosis-X was used previously to identify three related clinical entities of unknown etiology, characterized by histiocytic proliferation and comprises the triad of Letterer–Siwe disease, Hand–Schüller–Christian disease, and eosinophilic granuloma. At present, the above classification is obsolete. It commonly affects younger age group with a peak incidence at 1–4 years of age. Around 2% cases present in the neonatal age group. The exact etiopathogenesis of LCH is not known and proposed mechanisms include neoplastic responses. About 50% of cases have been associated with *BRAF-V600E* mutations and MAP2K pathway activity. In the year 2016, working group of the Histiocyte Society reclassified LCH into two major categories based on the extent of the disease: "Single system LCH (S-S LCH)" which is subclassified into unifocal and multifocal and "Multisystem LCH (M-S LCH)" with or without involvement/dysfunction of "risk organs." Approximately 30–56% pediatric cases with diffuse skin involvement may progress to multisystem disease.

Cutaneous lesions in LCH are varied and mimic various skin disorders, the most common being seborrheic dermatitis. The various morphological forms include scaly red papules, erythematous scaly dermatitis, vesiculopustules, petechiae, purpura, erosions and crusting, nodules, ulceration, otitis media, paronychia, and mucosal lesions. In neonates, LCH can present as vesiculopustular lesions, napkin dermatitis or nonspecific form that may delay the diagnosis. Any child with persistent diaper dermatitis not resolving with treatment, purpuric lesions should raise the suspicion of LCH. Systemic involvement includes respiratory (cough, tachypnea, pneumothorax), hepatosplenomegaly, lymphadenopathy, diabetes insipidus, growth hormone deficiency, gastrointestinal symptoms, bone pain, and hematological involvement such as anemia, pancytopenia, central nervous system involvement such as spasticity, seizures, encephalopathy, and ear infections. Mucosal involvement is seen more in disseminated form. They can present as gingival erythema, erosions, and hemorrhage. Purpuric nodules on the palms and soles serve as a poor prognostic sign. Congenital self-healing histiocytosis also known as "Hashimoto–Pritzker disease" presents with scaly papules and nodules with crater-shaped ulcers. Controversy exists about this entity as some authors believe that it is a part of LCH and regular follow-up is necessary to watch out for systemic involvement.

Natural History

The course is characteristically chronic. Prognosis depends upon the age of onset, duration of symptoms, and the degree of systemic involvement. Death may result from hemorrhage, anemia or infection, and systemic involvement.

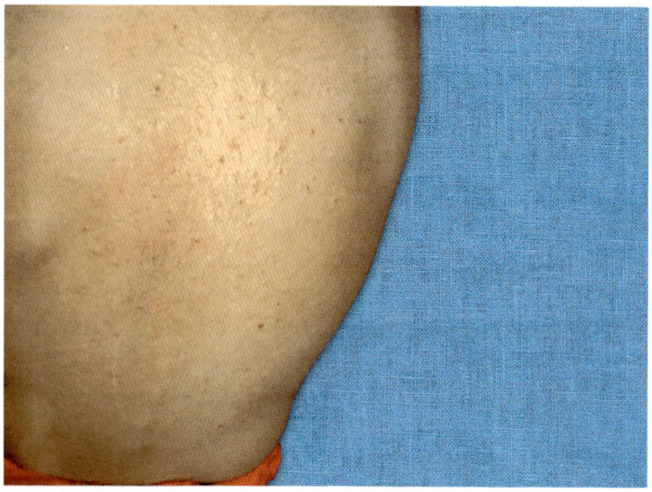

Fig. 10: Infiltrated red scaly papules of Langerhans cell histiocytosis over back.

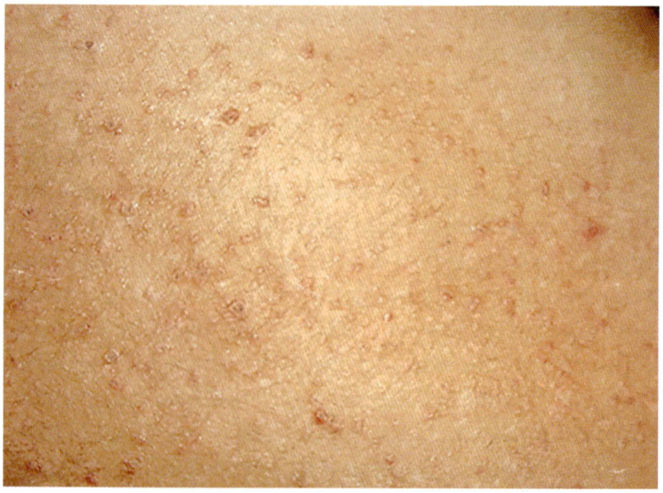

Fig. 11: Close-up view of the lesions.

"There are three constants in life...change, choice and principles." —**Stephen Covey**

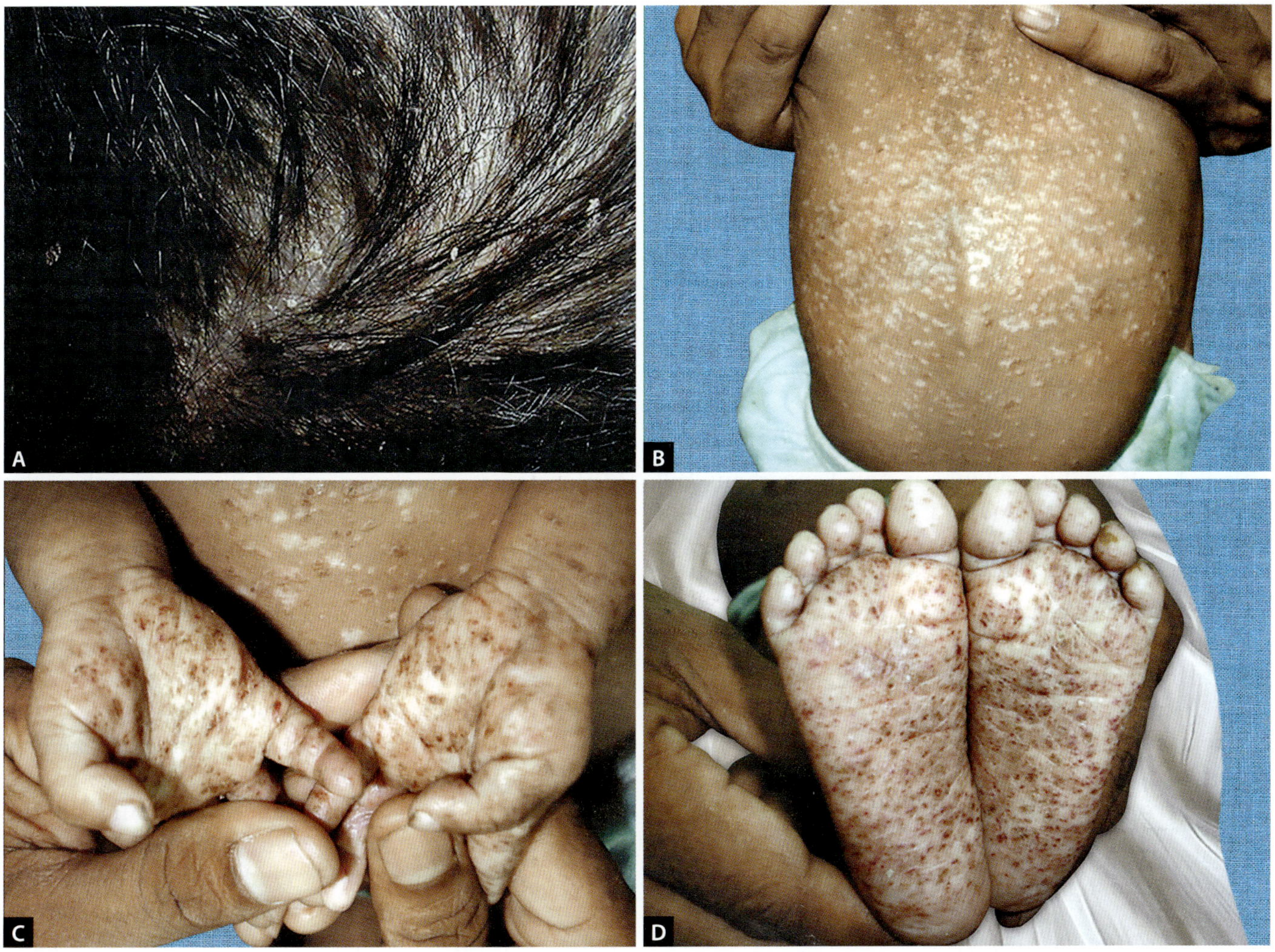

Figs. 12A to D: (A) Infiltrated lesions of histiocytosis over scalp; (B) Infiltrated papules and postinflammatory depigmentation over back in a child; (C) Purpuric macules over palms in an infant with Langerhans cell histiocytosis; (D) Same infant, purpuric macules over the soles.

Diagnosis

Langerhans cell histiocytosis is diagnosed clinically and confirmed by histopathology and immunohistochemistry (CD1a, S-100, and CD 207).

Management

Therapeutic regimens for LCH vary widely. Patients with diffuse systemic disease of the reticulohistiocytic system suffer impaired immunity and are susceptible to recurrent infections. Blood transfusions and antibiotics improve the long-term outlook for such patients. Immunosuppressive drugs in proper combination may give long-term remissions. Prednisolone at a dose of 2–4 mg/kg/day may result in complete clearing of lesions or long-term remissions for 1–2.5 years. Alkylating agents, viz., nitrogen

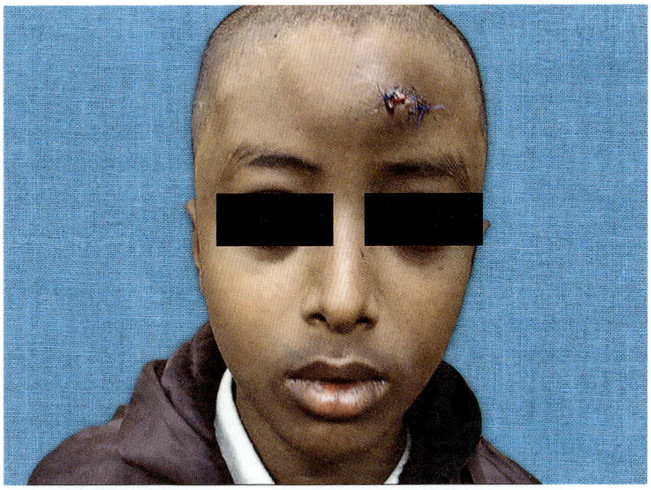

Fig. 13: Nodular lesions of Langerhans cell histiocytosis over the forehead.

mustard, chlorambucil, and cyclophosphamide, appear to be highly effective. Methotrexate, either alone or in combination with oral corticosteroids, is also an effective modality of treatment. Radiotherapy is effective for localized skeletal lesions. The overall prognosis of LCH had been so far depicted as "poor." However, the current data suggest that it may not be as unfavorable as it had been believed to be. Aggressive chemotherapy and good supportive care may not only provide long-term remission but may even render complete cure.

BENIGN CEPHALIC HISTIOCYTOSIS (FIG. 14)

This is a self-healing cutaneous non-Langerhans cell histiocytosis (NLCH) involving the head, neck, and face region. It is most common in children seen at 15 months of age with almost 45% of cases occurring under 6 months of age.

Clinically, it manifests as yellow brown macules and minimally elevated papules in a reticulate pattern. The less common affected sites include trunk, extremities, buttocks, and pubis.

Differential Diagnoses

- Flat warts
- Juvenile xanthogranuloma—micronodular type
- LCH
- Multiple melanocytic nevi
- Urticaria pigmentosa

The diagnosis is established by biopsy and using special stains.

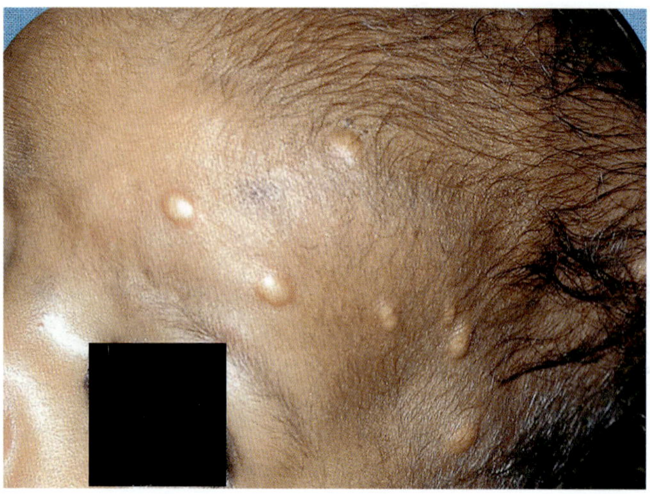

Fig. 14: Benign cephalic histiocytosis.

Internal involvement may occur when the condition leads to infiltration of the pituitary gland, and bones including spine, tibia, and skull.

Management

This condition is generally characterized by a benign course with spontaneous healing and residual atrophic pigmented scars. Treatment is unnecessary however close monitoring is warranted and follow-up is necessary to look for progression and internal involvement.

DERMATOFIBROMA (FIGS. 15 AND 16)

Dermatofibroma, also known as benign fibrous histiocytoma, is a circumscribed fibrous growth of the skin. It occurs more commonly in adolescence and rare in younger children. Trauma (insect bite reactions) acts as a predisposing factor. There is proliferation of fibroblastic spindle cells and histiocytic cells in dermis. Clinically presents as asymptomatic to painful slow growing, firm, indolent, red to brown nodules. The lesions measure 2–5 mm, rarely >15 mm occurring as giant lesion. They occur as single or multiple lesions, distributed more commonly on the extremities. Lateral pressure on the lesion produces dimpling on the surface known as "dimple sign." Clustering, eruptive and atypical variants have been described. Congenital type of dermatofibroma has been reported in literature. Multiple eruptive dermatofibroma has been associated with autoimmune diseases, immunosuppressant drugs, human immunodeficiency virus (HIV), hematological malignancies, and pregnancy. Diagnosis is mainly clinical but histopathological examination is confirmatory. There are numerous fibroblasts with increased collagen in dermis with proliferation of epidermis. Dermatofibroma persists for many years. Treatment is symptomatic. Painful lesions may be excised.

ERYTHEMA ANNULARE CENTRIFUGUM (FIG. 17)

Erythema annulare centrifugum (EAC) is a condition where annular erythematous lesions appear and spread centrifugally while showing central clearance at the same time. The inner border of the advancing edge may have a trailing scale. EAC is not a diagnosis by itself but a reactive erythema seen in many conditions. Of the major figurate erythemas, EAC is by far the most common and often a diagnosis of exclusion.

"Life is a series of natural and spontaneous changes. Don't resist them that only creates sorrow. Let reality be reality. Let things flow naturally forward in whatever way they like." —**Lao Tzu**

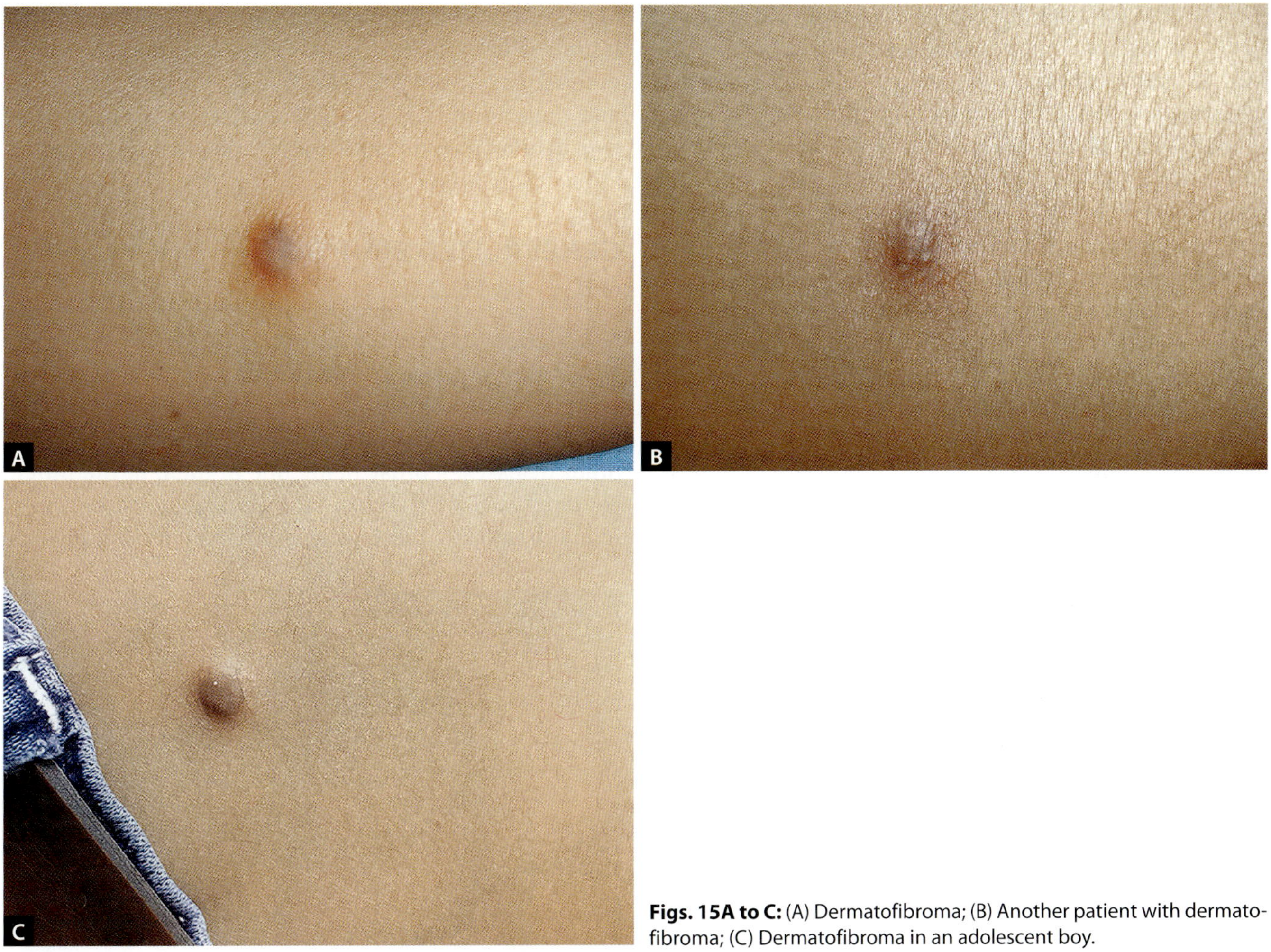

Figs. 15A to C: (A) Dermatofibroma; (B) Another patient with dermatofibroma; (C) Dermatofibroma in an adolescent boy.

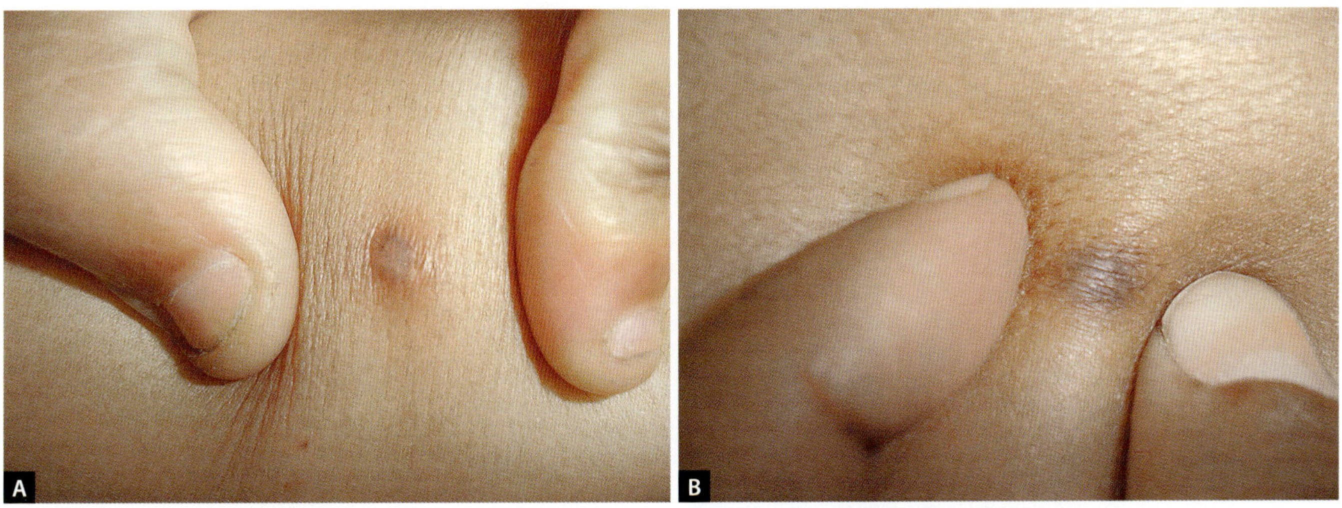

Figs. 16A and B: (A) Demonstration of "Dimple sign"; (B) Close-up view of "Dimple sign."

The term EAC was first used by Darier in 1916. It is seen in all age groups without gender-specific predisposition. The etiopathogenesis is yet unknown and in very few cases a causative agent can be identified. Some suggest that EAC may be the result of a hypersensitivity reaction to some agent. Some probable etiologic agents include fungal elements such as *Candida, Penicillium*, viruses such as poxvirus, HIV, varicella-zoster, parasites, and bacteria such as *Pseudomonas*. Other agents such as drugs (rituximab, salicylates, antimalarials, cimetidine, etc.) and food have also shown to be associated. Malignancy associated EAC is seen in solid tumors and lymphoproliferative disorders.

Histopathology of EAC shows an infiltrate comprising histiocytes, lymphocytes, and sometimes eosinophils around blood vessels of the superficial vascular plexus. The infiltrate has been described as "coat-sleeve appearance."

Erythema annulare centrifugum lesions are usually asymptomatic with annular or polycyclic shape that enlarge slowly reaching up to 10 cm in diameter while gradually clearing in the center. Pruritus may be present occasionally. When the lesion heals, post-inflammatory hyperpigmentation may be seen. Systemic involvement is exceedingly rare unless associated with malignancy. Since EAC is a diagnosis of exclusion, a thorough cutaneous and systemic examination is undertaken to find the cause. Once the diagnosis has been established, treatment is mainly directed towards symptomatic relief with topical emollients and antihistamines.

Topical steroids may be applied to the advancing edge. If an infectious etiology can be ascertained, then appropriate antimicrobial treatment can be started. Other lesions which can have an associated scaling need to be differentiated from EAC like annular variant of psoriasis and tinea corporis. Other differentials which need to be kept in mind include annular urticaria, pseudolymphoma, annular sarcoidosis, etc.

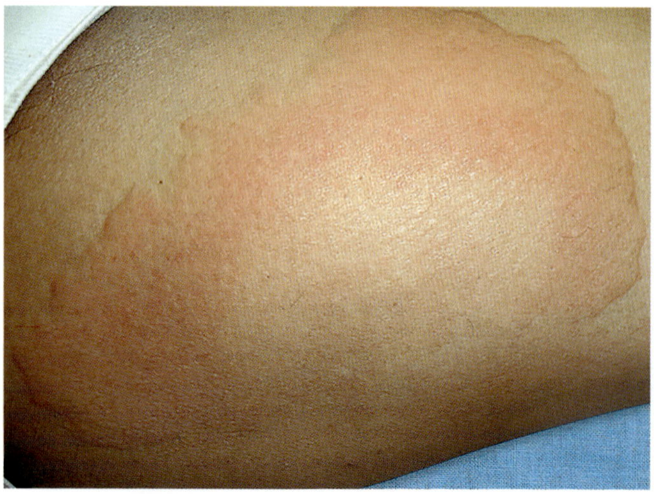

Fig. 17: Erythema annulare centrifugum, note large annular lesion with urticarial border.

GENERALIZED ERUPTIVE HISTIOCYTOSIS (FIGS. 18 TO 25)

Generalized eruptive histiocytosis (GEH) is a rare type of NLCH that presents usually as multiple asymptomatic, symmetric skin colored papules on the face, trunk, and arms with flexural sparing. The disease may mimic several other diseases, leprosy being one of them in the Indian context. Usually, it is seen in adults, but rarely, it may be seen in children. GEH presents as erythematous to brownish,

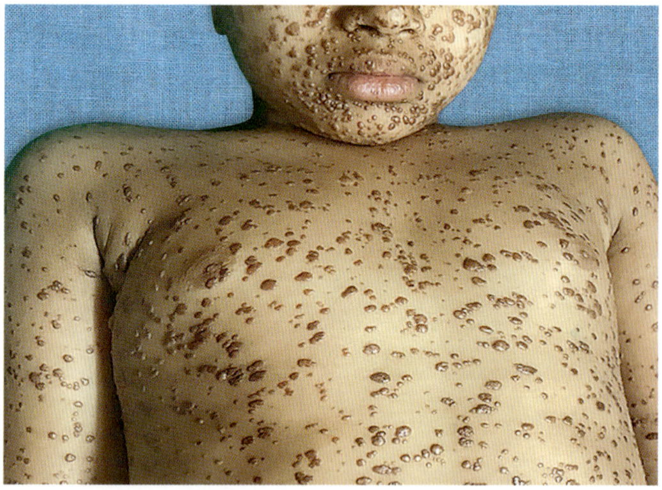

Fig. 18: Generalized eruptive histiocytosis in a 9-year-old boy.

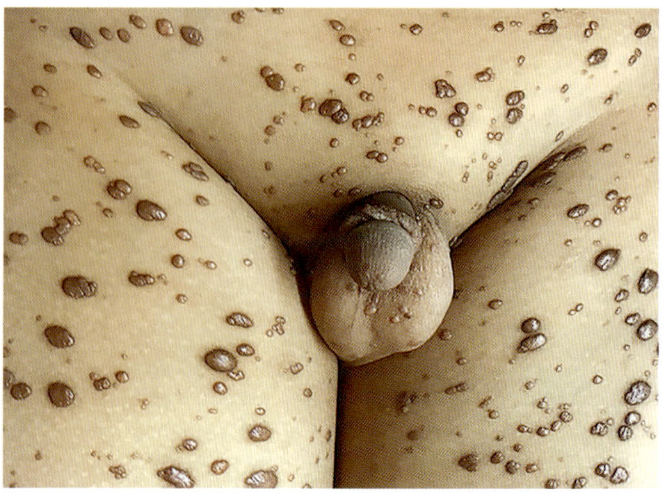

Fig. 19: Same boy lesions over groin and thighs.

"Only a life lived for others is a life worthwhile." **—Albert Einstein**

asymptomatic, symmetrically distributed papules on the face, upper extremities, and trunk with lesions occurring in crops. There is no extracutaneous involvement. It has been reported to be associated with acute monocytic leukemia and myelodysplastic syndrome. Histological evaluation shows dermal infiltration with monomorphic histiocytes. Electron microscopy demonstrates lack of Birbeck granules but have concentric laminated bodies. Immunohistochemistry is positive for CD68 lysozyme, alpha 1 antitrypsin, CD11b, HAM56, MAC387, CD14b, and Factor XIIIa. Antigen markers provide an important means to classify the disease. While some lesions regress spontaneously, majority persist for few decades. Various treatment options are psoralen and ultraviolet light therapy (PUVA), isotretinoin, intralesional triamcinolone injection for larger lesions, etc.

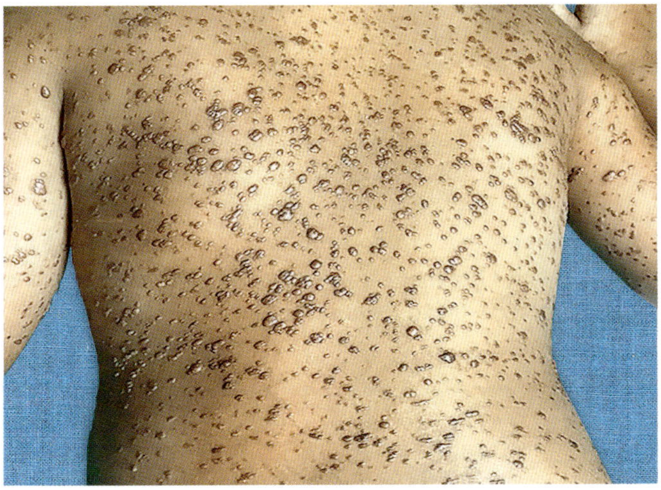

Fig. 20: Extensive lesions over back.

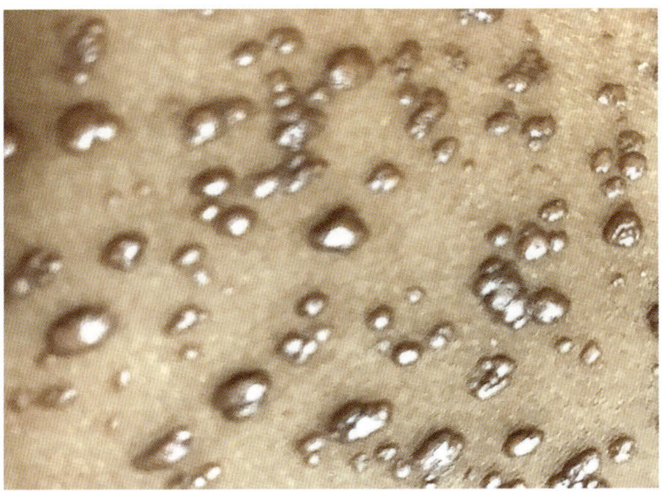

Fig. 21: Close-up view of lesions, note the xanthomatous appearance.

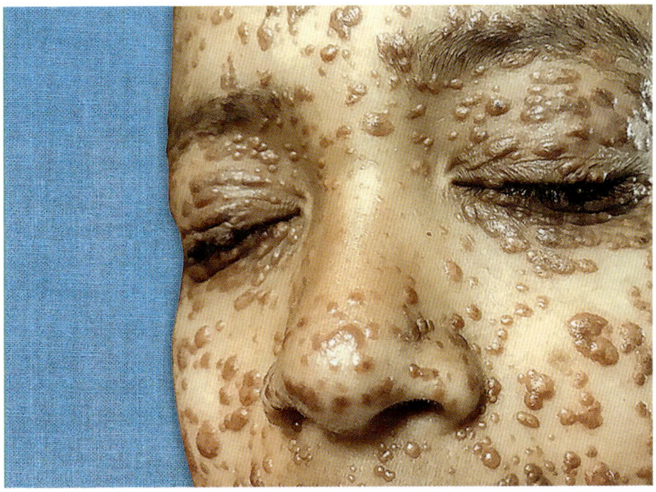

Fig. 22: Multiple lesions over face including eyelids.

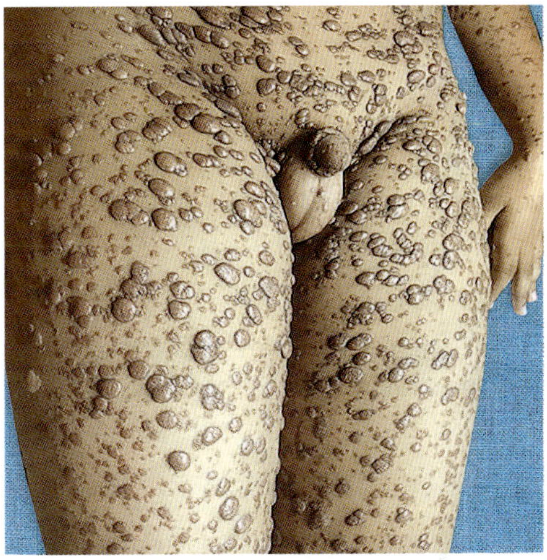

Fig. 23: Swarming of lesions over lower abdomen, groin, and genitalia in a 11-year-old boy.

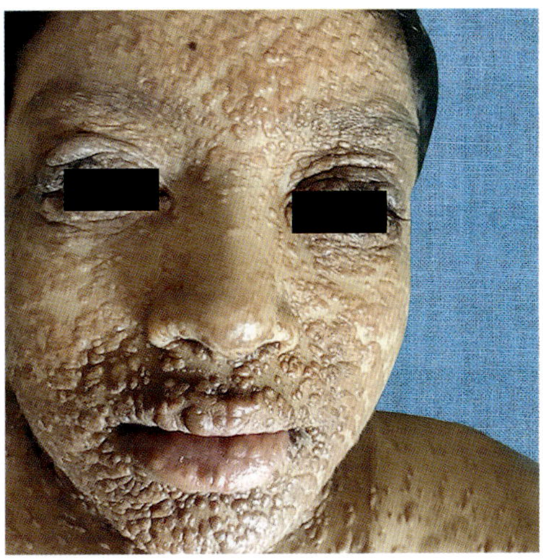

Fig. 24: Same boy, extensive grouped lesions on face.

"If you think education is expensive, try ignorance." —**Andy McIntyre**

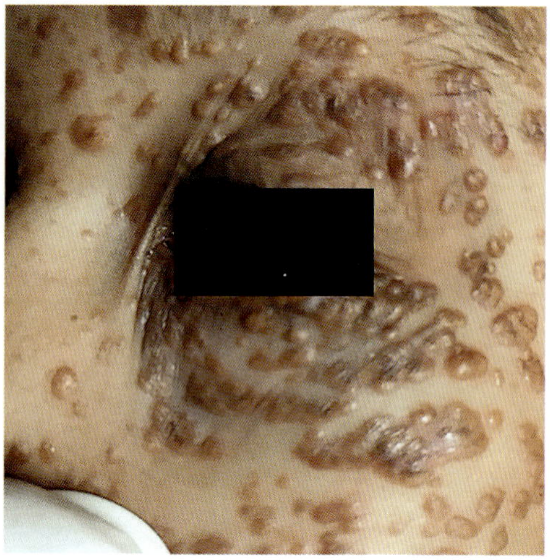

Fig. 25: Same boy, close-up view of eyelid, studded with lesions.

WHAT'S NEW

- SIP/SAIP/SIDerP guidelines for the management of pediatric urticaria:
  Patient started with second generation antihistamine at standard dose
  ⇩ If inadequate control after 4 weeks or earlier
  Patient <12 years of age → Increase the dose up to fourfold the standard dosage for age
  If patient >12 years of age → Omalizumab can be used as an add on to antihistamines
  ⇩ If inadequate control after 6 weeks or earlier, if symptoms are intolerable
  If child <12 years → Leukotriene receptor antagonist OR Omalizumab (>6 years of age) OR Cyclosporine as an add on drug to antihistamines
  If child >12 years of age → Increase antihistamine dose up to fourfold the standard dosage OR Leukotriene receptor antagonist OR Cyclosporine as an add on to antihistamines.
- Berotralstat, the first orally administered non-steroidal therapy for hereditary angioedema, has gained approval for both adults and pediatric patients over 12 years of age. Its mechanism of action involves inhibiting kallikrein, leading to a reduction in bradykinin production.
- Dabrafenib, a targeted inhibitor specifically designed for mutant BRAF, serves as a viable treatment option for pediatric Langerhans cell histiocytosis with BRAF V600 mutation. It can be administered either as a monotherapy or in combination with trametinib, a mitogen-activated protein kinase inhibitor. This approach effectively addresses the aberrant signaling pathways associated with the disease.

SUGGESTED READINGS

1. Allen CE, Merad M, McClain KL. Langerhans cell histiocytosis. N Engl J Med. 2018;379(9):856-68.
2. Jenkinson HA, Lundgren AD, Carter MC, Diaz LZ, Levy ML. Management of a neonate with diffuse cutaneous mastocytosis: case report and literature review. Pediatr Dermatol. 2019; 36(4):486-9.
3. Krooks J, Minkov M, Weatherall AG. Langerhans cell histiocytosis in children: diagnosis, differential diagnosis, treatment, sequelae, and standardized follow-up. J Am Acad Dermatol. 2018;78(6):1047-56.
4. Kudryavtseva AV, Neskorodova KA, Staubach P. Urticaria in children and adolescents: an updated review of the pathogenesis and management. Pediatr Allergy Immunol. 2019; 30(1):17-24.
5. Chang J, Cattelan L, Ben-Shoshan M, Le M, Netchiporouk E. Management of pediatric chronic spontaneous urticaria: a review of current evidence and guidelines. J Asthma Allergy. 2021;14:187-99.
6. Lee A. Berotralstat: First Approval. Drugs. 2021;81:405-9.
7. Whitlock JA, Geoerger B, Dunkel IJ, Roughton M, Choi J, Osterloh L, et al. Dabrafenib, alone or in combination with trametinib, in BRAF V600–mutated pediatric Langerhans cell histiocytosis. Blood Advances. 2023;7(15):3806-15.

"Nothing ever becomes real unless it is experienced." —**John Keats**

CHAPTER

14

Metabolic Disorders

ALKAPTONURIA (FIGS. 1A AND B)

Alkaptonuria is a rare, autosomal recessive disorder of homogentisic acid (HGA) metabolism, an intermediate product of phenylalanine and tyrosine metabolism. The basic defect is in the mutation of homogentisate dioxygenase (*HGD*) gene located on chromosome 3q21–q23 which leads to excessive urinary excretion of HGA and deposition of the same in connective tissue all over the body including cartilage, tendon, heart valve, and urinary tract.

Clinical Features

Dark urine, which turns black on standing in alkaline pH may be the initial presentation in many cases but not always. Urinary pH due to ascorbic acid is the major determinant of oxidation. Some patients with acidic urine never present with dark urine on standing. Other initial presentations may be black cerumen and pigmentation of axillary skin along with staining of undergarments due to ochronotic pigment deposition in sweat gland.

Adult patients present with evident ochronotic discoloration of sclera, conjunctiva, cartilage of ear, tympanic membrane and cartilage of nose and hand. Variable degree of deafness and tinnitus are attributed to HGA-induced inhibition of lysyl oxidase, enzyme responsible for collagen cross linking. In many cases involvement of larynx and trachea shows no symptoms. Blue-gray pigmentation of skin affects ear, tip of the nose, extensor tendons of hands, palmoplantar, and mucosal surface.

Ochronotic axial arthropathy, radiologically characterized by early calcification of intervertebral disc followed by decreased joint space is the most disabling late manifestation. Among other systems, aortic valve, prostate and kidney involvement are worth mentioning.

Investigations

Histopathology is characterized by deposition of yellow-brown, large, irregular ochre bodies composed of degenerated collagen and ochronotic pigment in reticular dermis.

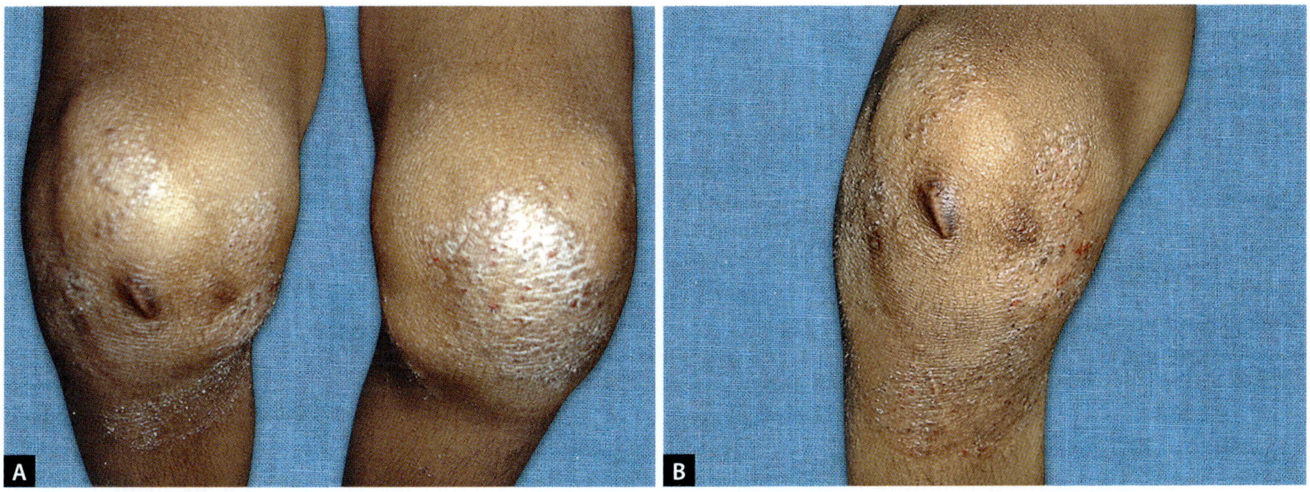

Figs. 1A and B: (A) Scaly eczematous plaques of alkaptonuria over knees; (B) Close-up view of lesion, alkaptonuria.

"When life is too easy for us, we must beware or we may not be ready to meet the blows which sooner or later come to everyone, rich or poor."

—Eleanor Roosevelt

Differential Diagnosis

Differential diagnoses include exogenous ochronosis (pigmentation due to exogenous drugs and chemicals), Addison's disease, hemochromatosis, argyria, cutaneous porphyrias, photosensitivity pigmentation, and pellagra.

Treatment

Treatment is mainly supportive with restriction of high protein, high phenylalanine and high tyrosine-containing diet, supplementation of large amount of dietary vitamin C and proper follow-up for articular and cardiac involvement in future.

ADDISON'S DISEASE (FIGS. 2A AND B)

It is a condition when the adrenal glands fail to produce the hormone cortisol adequately and sometimes the production of aldosterone is also affected. It affects males and females equally. It is also referred to as adrenal insufficiency or hypocortisolism.

Deficiency of cortisol can occur in one of the following ways:

- *Primary adrenal insufficiency*: Most cases are caused by gradual destruction of the outer layer of the adrenal glands by the body's own immune mechanism. Adrenal insufficiency occurs when at least 90% of the adrenal cortex has been destroyed. As a result, often both glucocorticoid (cortisol) and mineralocorticoid (aldosterone) hormones are lacking.
- *Polyendocrine deficiency syndrome type 1*: It occurs in children, and adrenal insufficiency may be accompanied by:
  - Underactive parathyroid glands
  - Slow sexual development
  - Pernicious anemia
  - Chronic candida (yeast) infections
  - Chronic active hepatitis
  - Hair loss (in very rare cases)
- *Polyendocrine deficiency syndrome type 2*: It is often called Schmidt's syndrome, usually affects young adults and is characterized by:
  - An underactive thyroid gland
  - Slow sexual development
  - Diabetes
  - Vitiligo
- *Tuberculosis*: In this infection the adrenal glands can be completely destroyed resulting in deficiency of cortisol.
- Secondary adrenal insufficiency can occur in case of exogenous corticosteroid administration leading to hypothalamic-pituitary-adrenal axis suppression, surgical removal of the adrenal glands, surgical removal of hypothalamus or pituitary and radiation therapy in cases of pituitary gland tumors.

Clinical Features

The symptoms of adrenal insufficiency usually begin gradually. Characteristics of the disease are:

- Chronic, worsening fatigue
- Muscle weakness
- Loss of appetite
- Weight loss
- Nausea
- Vomiting
- Diarrhea
- Low blood pressure that falls further when standing, causing dizziness or fainting (orthostatic hypotension).
- Hypoglycemia, which is more severe in children than in adults.

Symptoms of a crisis include:

- Sudden penetrating pain in the lower back, abdomen, or legs
- Severe vomiting and diarrhea
- Dehydration
- Low blood pressure
- Loss of consciousness

Left untreated, an Addisonian crisis can be fatal.

Cutaneous Manifestations

Hyperpigmentation—diffuse hyperpigmentation with accentuation of the sun-exposed areas, sites of trauma, axillae, perineum, nipples, palmar creases, melanocytic nevi, mucous membranes, hair and nails.

Loss of ambisexual hair can occur in postpubertal women. Rarely there can be fibrosis and calcification of cartilage including ear.

There can be associated findings of mucocutaneous candidiasis and vitiligo.

Diagnosis

A diagnosis of Addison's disease is made by laboratory tests such as adrenocorticotropic hormone (ACTH) stimulation test and corticotropin-releasing hormone (CRH) stimulation test. The aim of these tests is first to determine whether levels of cortisol are insufficient and then to establish the cause. X-ray examination of the

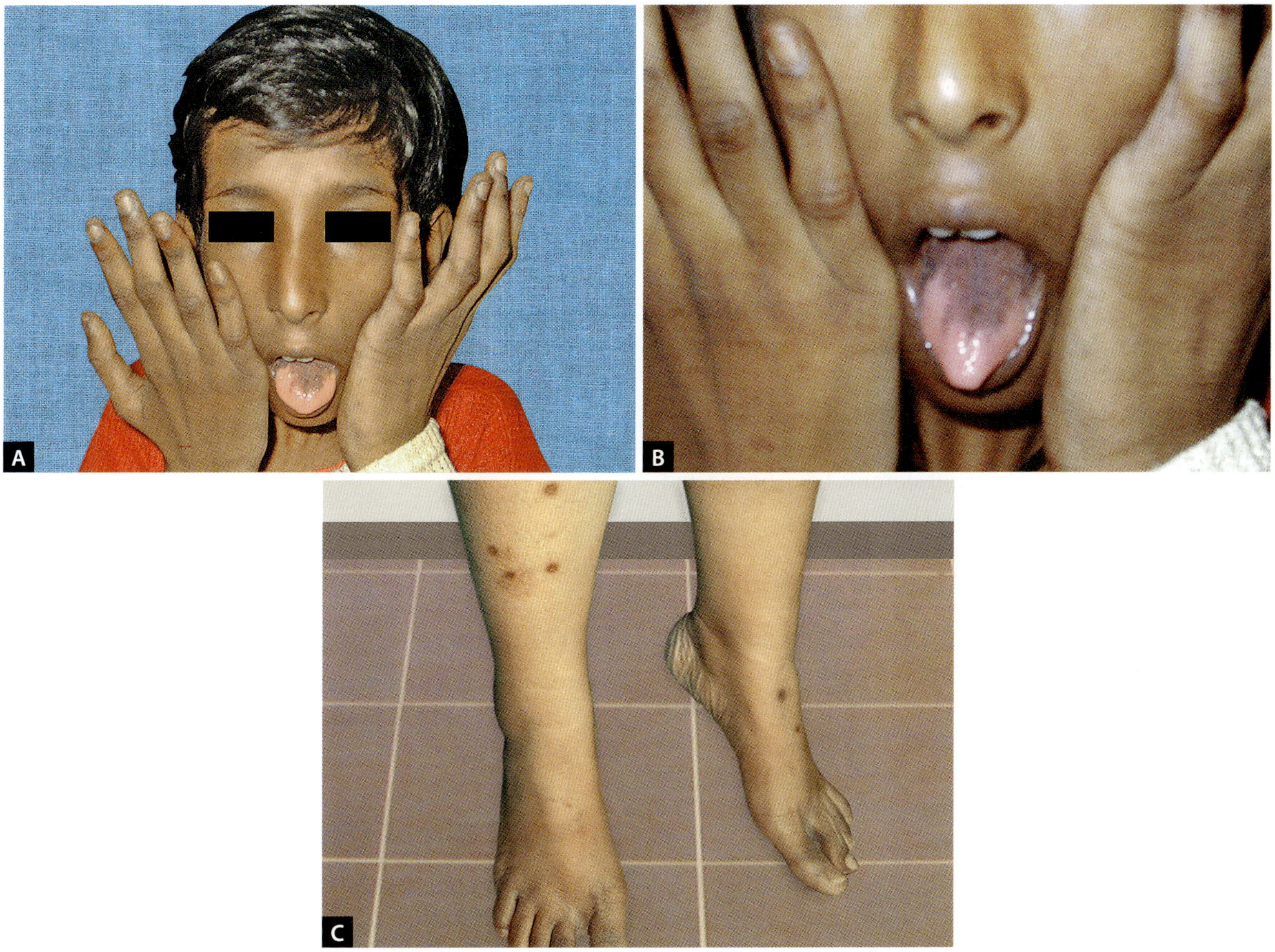

Figs. 2A to C: (A) Hyperpigmentation of Addison's disease; (B) Addison's disease, close-up view; (C) Diabetic dermopathy.

adrenal and pituitary glands also are useful in helping to establish the cause. CT scan, tuberculin testing and assay of pituitary hormones may also be helpful in diagnosing the condition.

Treatment

Cortisol is replaced orally with hydrocortisone tablets, a synthetic glucocorticoid, taken once or twice a day. If aldosterone is also deficient, it is replaced with oral doses of a mineralocorticoid called fludrocortisone acetate, which is taken once a day. Patients receiving aldosterone replacement therapy are usually advised to increase their salt intake. Because patients with secondary adrenal insufficiency normally maintain aldosterone production, they do not require aldosterone replacement therapy. The doses of each of these medications are adjusted to meet the needs of individual patients.

During an Addisonian crisis, low blood pressure, low blood glucose, and high levels of potassium can be life-threatening. Standard therapy involves intravenous injections of hydrocortisone, saline, and dextrose. This treatment usually brings rapid improvement. When the patient can take fluids and medications by mouth, the amount of hydrocortisone is decreased until a maintenance dose is achieved. If aldosterone is deficient, maintenance therapy also includes oral doses of fludrocortisone acetate.

DIABETIC DERMOPATHY (FIG. 2C)

This condition is extremely uncommon in the pediatric age group and is associated with diabetes.

It is characterized by the presence of red brown papules <1–2 cm in size which regress slowly to produce slightly depressed atrophic pigmented macules. These may persist or may clear to leave normal skin. The pretibial skin is the most commonly affected site. The other sites affected include arms, thighs, and trunk. Generally, no treatment is effective for this condition.

"We make a living by what we get, but we make a life by what we give." —**Winston Churchill**

NECROBIOSIS LIPOIDICA DIABETICORUM (FIGS. 2D AND E)

This is a condition which follows but sometimes may precede the diagnosis of diabetes in children. It is generally located in the pretibial area, trunk, upper limb, face, and scalp in a decreasing order of occurrence at these sites. It presents as an asymptomatic erythematous papule or nodule or plaque with a raised rim and a depressed center which has a waxy atrophic appearance. The color may vary from brown to yellowish orange. The center may sometimes show ulceration.

Treatment is generally required when there is ulceration or an expanding edge is present. High potency topical steroids and intralesional steroids have been tried. Skin grafting may also be another option.

CUSHING'S DISEASE [FIGS. 2F TO H(iii)]

This condition occurs due to excess glucocorticosteroid production. Increased production can be due to increased ACTH production from pituitary adenoma. It can also result from micronodular adrenal hyperplasia, adrenal carcinoma, adrenal adenoma, and ectopic ACTH secretion. Cushing's disease may also occur due to the exogenous administration of steroids.

Clinical Features

It is characterized by weight gain, growth retardation, delayed sexual maturation, fatigue and weakness, menstrual irregularities, and emotional labilities. Hypertension and osteopenia can also be a manifestation. Nodular adrenal hyperplasia can be associated with myxomatous tumors of heart, skin, and breast. It can also be a part of the CARNEY complex (lentigines, epithelioid blue nevi, and pigmented schwannomas).

Cutaneous features include moon facies and buffalo hump with truncal obesity. Plethoric facies and broad purple striae are seen most commonly. Striae may be present at the sites of skin tension with skin fragility and poor wound healing. Purpura with minimal trauma is noted. Hyperpigmentation, hypertrichosis, acneiform eruption, and acanthosis nigricans are the other cutaneous manifestations.

Investigations

Twenty four hours urine cortisol levels, plasma cortisol levels, low-dose dexamethasone suppression test, salivary cortisol levels, ACTH, CRH levels aid in the diagnosis.

Treatment

Treatment of the underlying etiology leading to increased ACTH production is important in the management of Cushing's disease.

DIABETIC BULLA (FIGS. 2I AND J)

Bullosis diabeticorum, also known as bullous disease of diabetes and diabetic bullae, is a rare, distinct, spontaneous, noninflammatory, blistering condition of unknown etiology occurring in the setting of diabetes mellitus. It is rarely seen in children. Cantwell and Martz named the condition in 1967, Krane first reported this condition

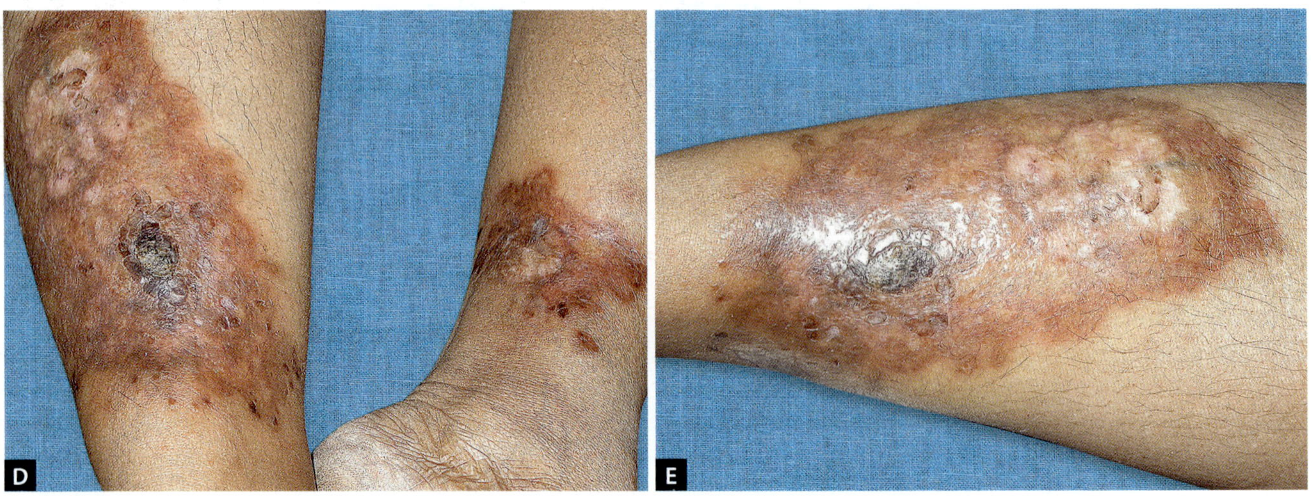

Figs. 2D and E: (D) Necrobiosis lipoidica diabeticorum; (E) Necrobiosis lipoidica diabeticorum, close-up view.

"All life is an experiment. The more experiments you make the better." **—Ralph Waldo Emerson**

in 1930. The exact etiology of bullosis diabeticorum is unknown but it is thought to be multifactorial in origin. It has been reported to occur in approximately 0.5% of diabetic patients of the adult US population and one recent Indian study showed occurrence in 2% of the diabetic population, however, the data on its occurrence

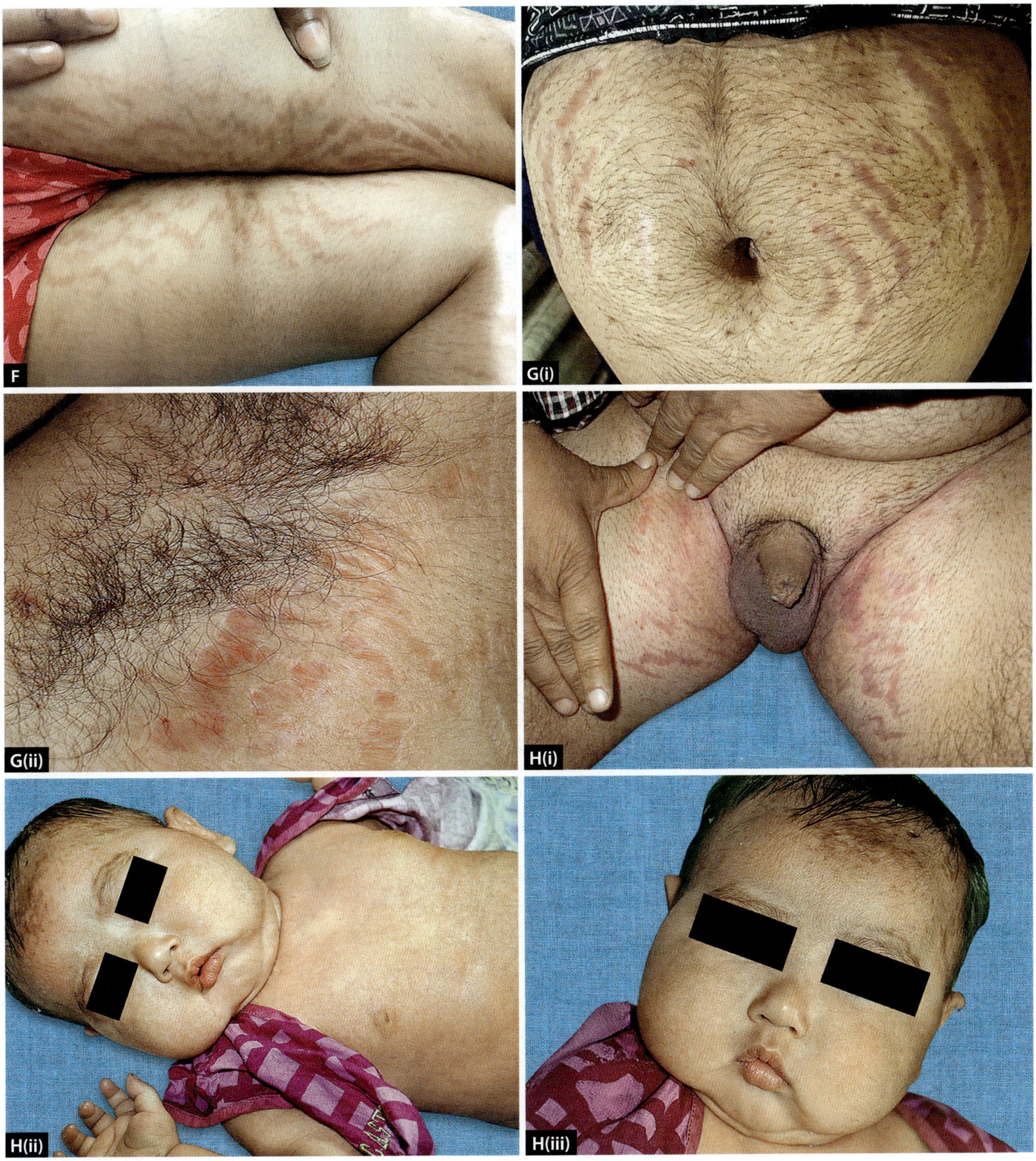

Figs. 2F to H(iii): (F) Cushing's disease in an 17-year-old girl, note the stretch marks over thighs; G(i) Cushing's disease in an 18-year-old girl, note swollen abdomen, stretch marks over abdomen and hypertrichosis; G(ii) Same patient, note atrophic scars over axilla; H(i) Same patient, atrophic scars over thighs; H(ii) Steroid-induced iatrogenic Cushing's syndrome in a 5-month-old baby; H(iii) Same baby, close-up view.

"My mission in life is not merely to survive, but to thrive; and to do so with some passion, some compassion, some humor, and some style." **—Maya Angelou**

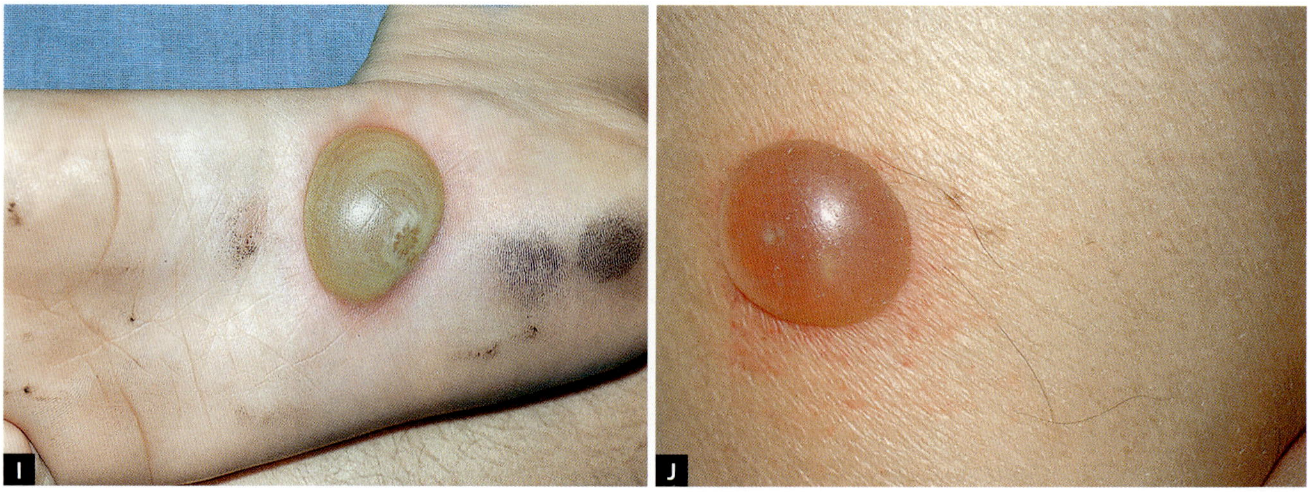

Figs. 2I and J: (I) Diabetic bullae over sole; (J) Diabetic bullae.

in children is lacking. There is a male preponderance of the disease with a male-to-female ratio of 2:1 and the age range varies from 17 to 84 years.

The blisters have a propensity to be large and often have an asymmetrical shape. Although they are much more common over the acral areas and are more common on the lower extremities, nonacral sites (e.g., trunk) may also be involved.

XANTHOMA (FIGS. 3 TO 5A)

Xanthomas are yellowish tumors of the skin which contain lipid-laden histiocytes. They are usually associated with an abnormality of lipid metabolism, and detection of such abnormality helps to rule out any systemic involvement in such cases. Poorly soluble lipids are transported in serum by lipoproteins. Abnormalities in lipid transport and metabolism may result in elevation in serum triglycerides and/or cholesterol. The deposition of these lipids in skin and soft tissue results in development of xanthomas. Various primary dyslipoproteinemias have been enlisted in **Table 1**. Various systemic diseases which may trigger hyperlipoproteinemia are poorly controlled diabetes mellitus, hypothyroidism, fulminant hepatic necrosis, etc.

Various types of xanthoma may point toward a particular type of hyperlipidemia. Plane xanthomas present as soft yellowish plaques on any site but with special predilection for old scars or traumatized areas in the past. Xanthelasma is basically a plane xanthoma over the eyelids. It is usually associated with hypercholesterolemia in about half of the cases. Diffuse lesions may be seen on the trunk, face, neck, etc. Tuberous xanthomas arise as yellow nodules on the extensor surfaces of the extremities and buttocks. They may coalesce to cover large areas. However, they never get adhered to underlying soft tissue structures as in cases of tendinous xanthoma. Eruptive xanthomas develop suddenly as 1–4 mm diameter yellow-red papules over extensor surfaces of the extremities, buttocks and bony prominences. They appear in crops or showers and are usually associated with markedly elevated triglycerides. Tendinous xanthomas present as smooth asymptomatic nodules on ligaments, tendons, and other deep soft tissue structures. They are usually several centimeters in size and occur most commonly on the ankles, knees, and elbows.

Differential Diagnosis

Xanthomas must be differentiated from xanthogranulomas which are not associated with derangement of lipid metabolism.

Treatment

Xanthoma is treated by chemical cautery with 40–60% trichloroacetic acid or silver nitrate solution. The other modalities are electrodesiccation or laser therapy. Very big tuberous or tendinous xanthomas can be excised under local anesthesia. Control of hyperlipidemia is done by judicious use of various lipid lowering agents, correction of associated systemic diseases, if any, and by strict dietary regimens.

"Once you say you're going to settle for second, that's what happens to you in life." —**John F Kennedy**

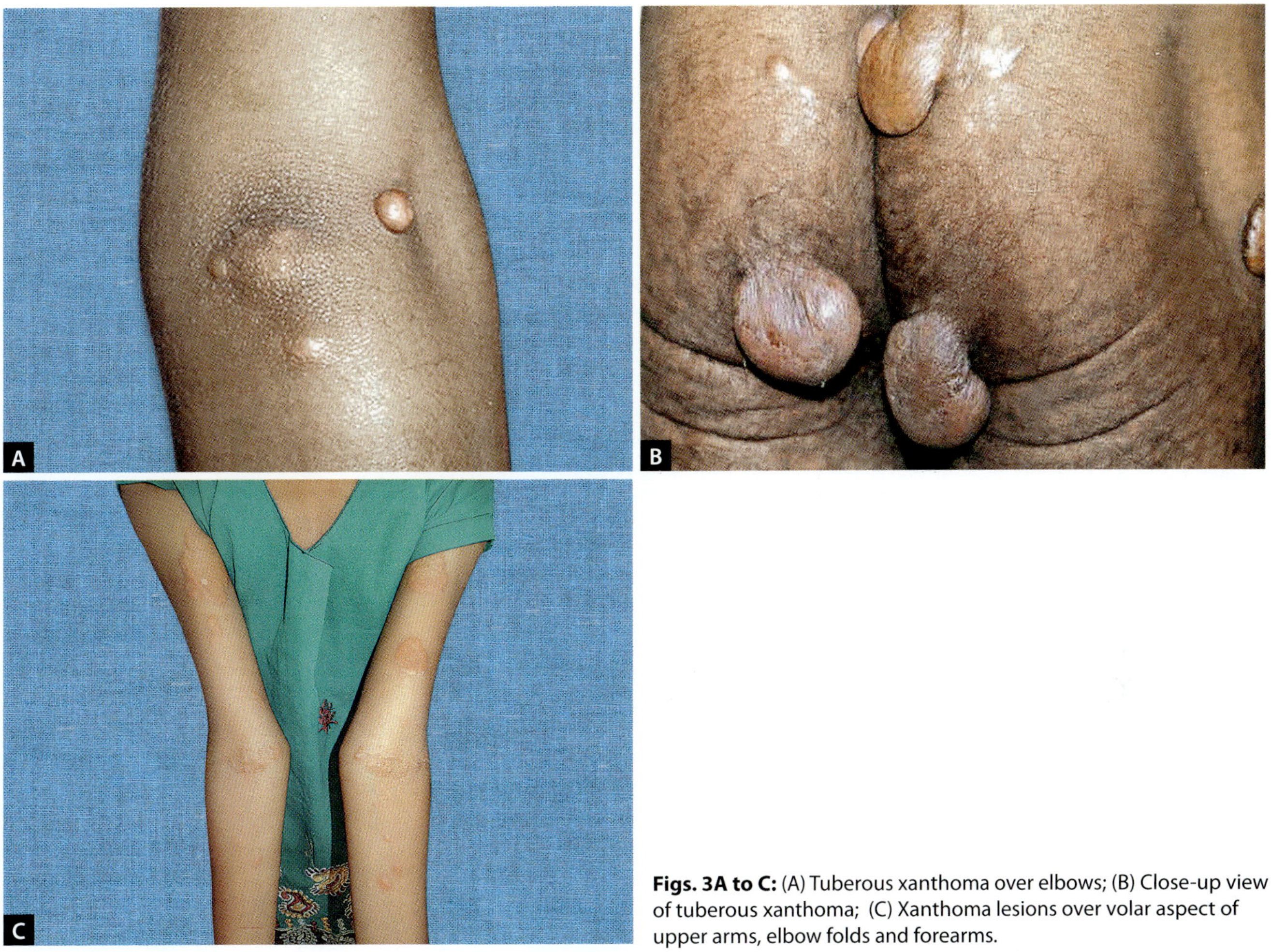

Figs. 3A to C: (A) Tuberous xanthoma over elbows; (B) Close-up view of tuberous xanthoma; (C) Xanthoma lesions over volar aspect of upper arms, elbow folds and forearms.

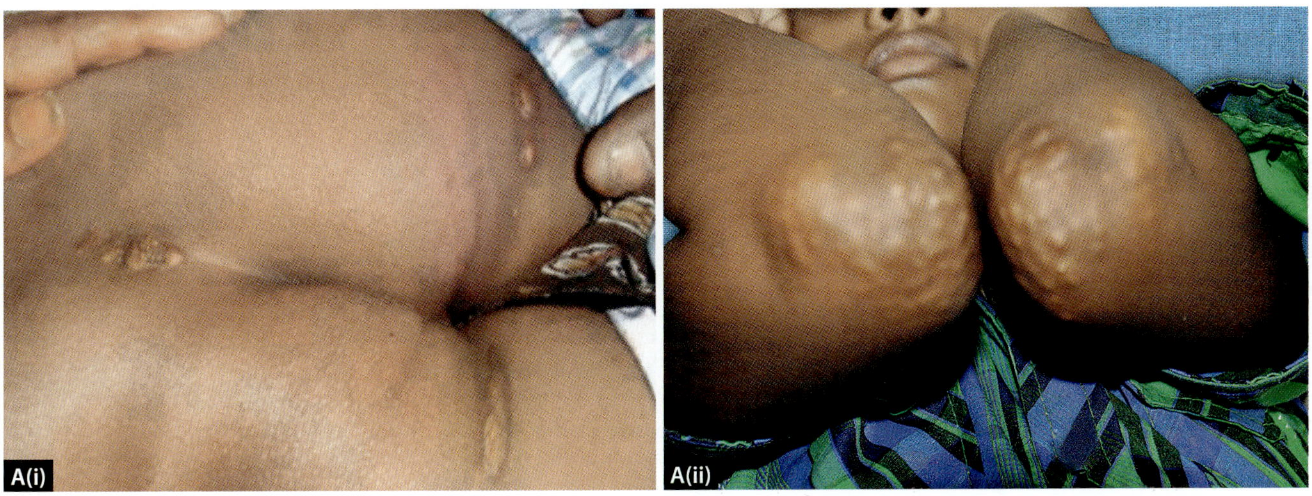

Figs. 4A(i) and (ii): A(i) Plane xanthoma over the natal cleft; A(ii) Xanthoma over elbows in a 4-year-old boy.

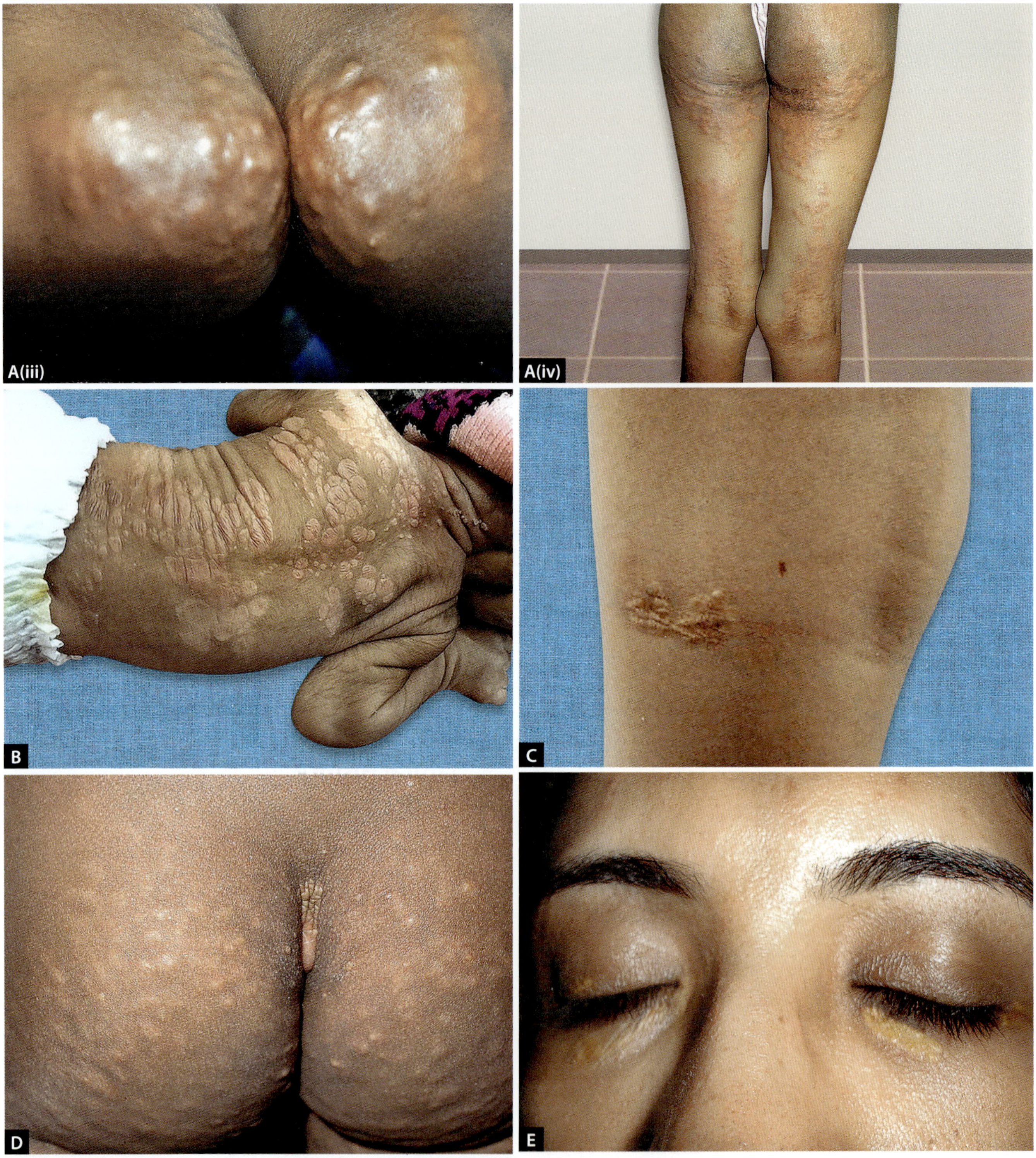

Figs. 4A(iii) to E: A(iii) Xanthoma over elbows, close-up view; A(iv) Extensive xanthomas over buttock, flexor of thighs and legs in a 7-year-old girl; (B) Extensive plane xanthomas over back of an infant; (C) Xanthoma over popliteal fossa; (D) Xanthoma over buttocks in a 7-year-old boy; (E) Xanthelasma in an 18-year-old girl.

"Literature adds to reality, it does not simply describe it. It enriches the necessary competencies that daily life requires and provides; and in this respect, it irrigates the deserts that our lives have already become." **—CS Lewis**

Table 1: Correlations of lipoprotein defects, inheritance and clinical presentations of xanthomas.

Type (prevalence)	Pattern	Chol	TG	Inheritance	Possible mechanism	Clinical presentation	Age of detection	Secondary diseases
I (rarest)	Chyl	+	+++	AR	LDL defect of deficiency	Eruptive xanthomas (60–70%), abdominal pain, hepatosplenomegaly, lipemia retinalis, creamy plasma, pancreatitis	Early childhood	Pancreatitis, diabetes
IIa (common)	LDL	+++	+ or N	AD	LDL receptors nonfunctional	Tendinous xanthomas (40–50%), xanthelasmas (20–25%), corneal, arcus (10–15%), tuberous xanthomas, atherosclerosis	Early childhood in homozygotes	Hypothyroidism, nephrotic syndrome
IIb (common)	LDL, VLDL	+++	+ or N	AD	VLDL overproduction	Some, abnormal GTT		Hepatic disease
III (relatively common)	IDL	++ (variable)	+ (variable)	AR	Homozygous apoprotein E2, decreased remnant clearance, overproduction of VLDL	Xanthomas (75–80%; tuberous, palmar, tendinous, eruptive), abnormal GTT, hyperuricemia, atherosclerosis, obesity	Adult	Hepatic disease, dysglobulinemia, uncontrolled diabetes
IV (most common)	VLDL	+	++	AD	Carbohydrate induced	Atherosclerosis, abnormal GTT, eruptive or tuberous xanthomas	Adult	Hypothyroidism, diabetes, pancreatitis, glycogen storage disease, nephrotic syndrome, multiple myeloma
V (uncommon)	Chyl, VLDL	+	++	AR	Overproduction of VLDL, defect in metabolism of VLDL	Abdominal pain, obesity, xanthomas (eruptive), hepatosplenomegaly	Young adult	Insulin dependent diabetes, pancreatitis, alcoholism

(Chol: cholesterol; TG: triglycerides; Chyl: chylomicrons; LDL: low density lipoprotein; VLDL: very low density lipoprotein; IDL: intermediate density lipoprotein; AR: autosomal recessive; AD: autosomal dominant; GTT: glucose tolerance test; N: normal)

JUVENILE XANTHOGRANULOMA (FIGS. 5B TO H)

Juvenile xanthogranuloma represents a benign, self-limiting disease of non-Langerhans cell histiocytosis characterized by accumulation of lipid-laden macrophages. It mostly occurs in infants, children and occasionally adults, and it is characterized by one or several (occasionally numerous) red to yellow nodules located on the skin and other organs.

Typically the lesions are present at birth (20%) or during the first 6–9 months of life, and may persist or continue to erupt for years. They run a benign course, often increasing in number until about 1–1½ years of age and then involute spontaneously. They may be several hundred in number. They may range from several millimeters to 1 cm or more in diameter, and frequently they have a discrete, firm or rubbery consistency. On occasion, large juvenile xanthogranulomas may measure from 4 to 10 cm in diameter.

Natural History

The vast majority (90% or more) of patients with juvenile xanthogranuloma are self-limiting. Rare cases lasting until adulthood have been reported. Generally those that have their onset after the 1st year of life manifest complete healing usually within 1–5 years. Lesions may also occur in the lung, pericardium, central nervous system, liver, spleen, and testes.

Systemic Associations

There have been patients with a combination of juvenile xanthogranulomas and café au lait spots or neurofibromatosis who developed chronic myelogenous leukemia or acute myelomonocytic leukemia. Patients with this association, therefore, should be checked periodically for the possibility of an associated leukemia.

Treatment

Explaining the condition and counseling of the parents is necessary.

"Anyone who stops learning is old, whether at twenty or eighty. Anyone who keeps learning stays young. The greatest thing in life is to keep your mind young."
—Henry Ford

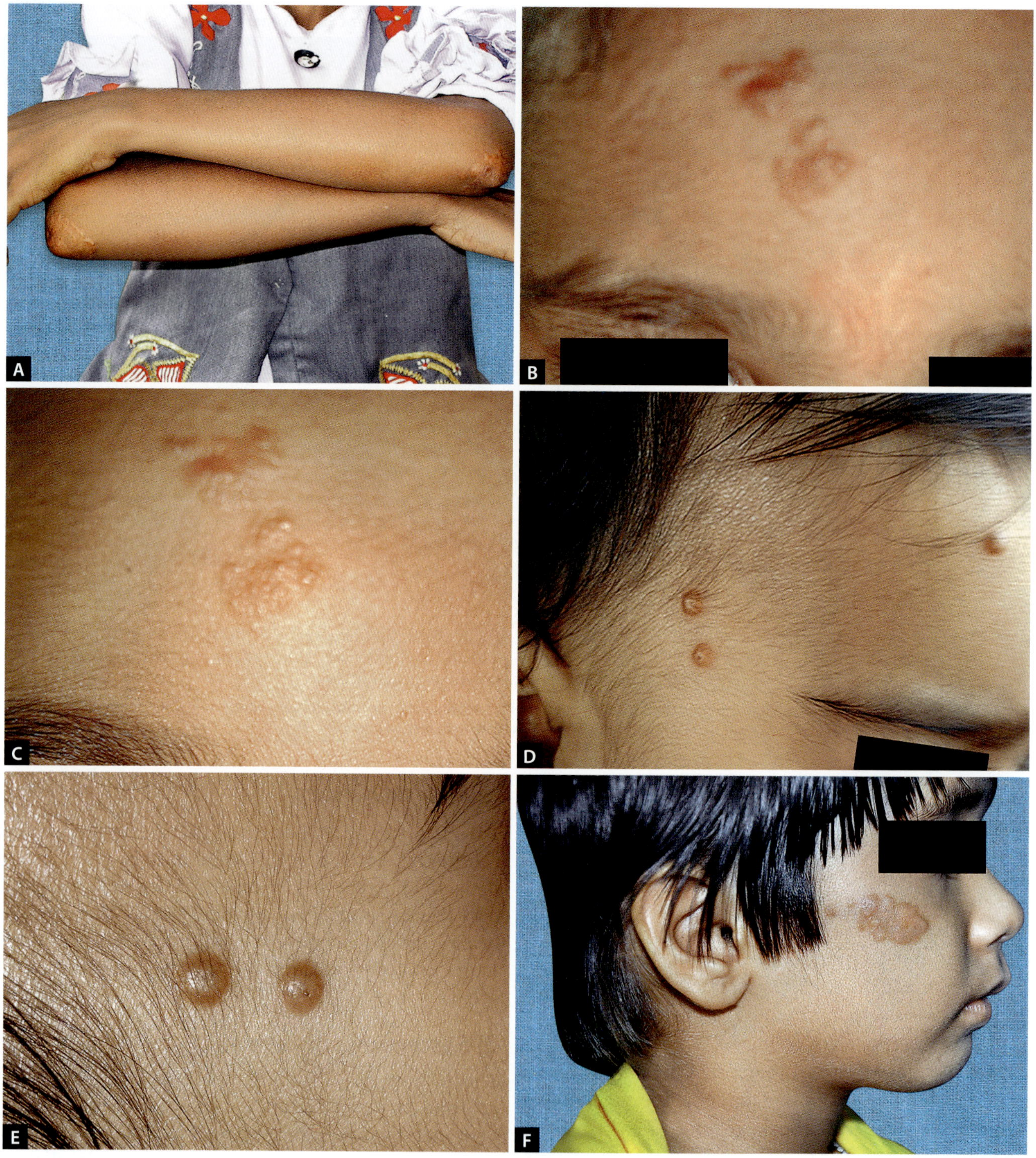

Figs. 5A to F: (A) Plane xanthoma over the elbows in a 5-year-old girl; (B) Juvenile xanthogranuloma (JXG) lesions over forehead; (C) JXG, close-up view; (D) JXG, classical lesions; (E) Juvenile xanthogranuloma (JXG), close-up view; (F) JXG in a 3-year-old girl.

PORPHYRIA

Porphyria is a group of diseases of heme biosynthesis in which a metabolic product porphyrin is synthesized which affects various organs such as skin, gastrointestinal tract, liver, neurological system, etc. The heme biosynthesis pathway is described in **Flowchart 1**. The various types of porphyrias are listed in **Box 1**.

"Many of life's failures are people who did not realize how close they were to success when they gave up." **—Thomas A Edison**

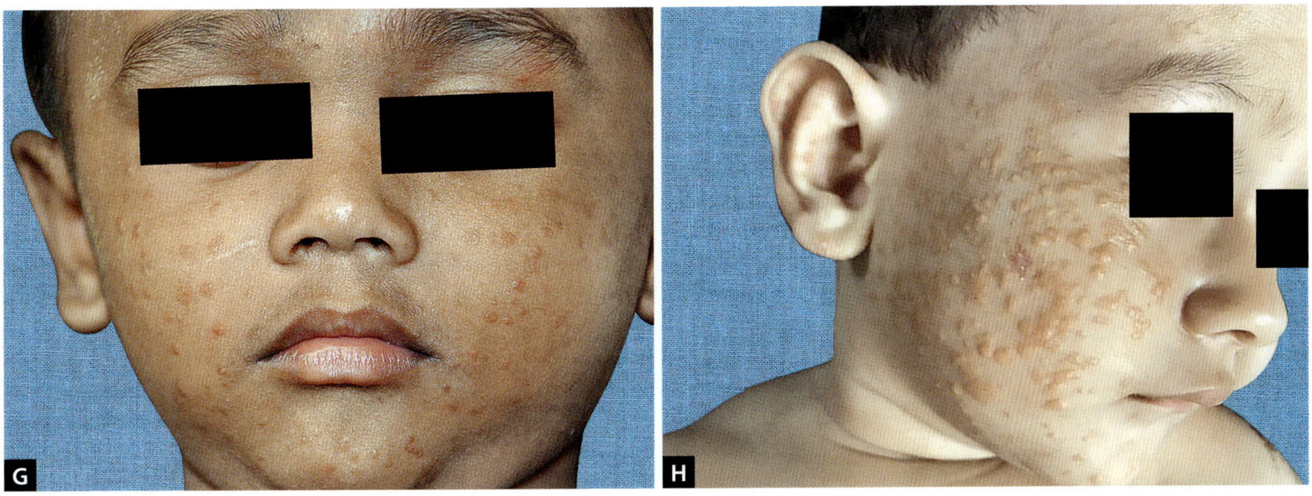

Figs. 5G and H: (G) Extensive Juvenile xanthogranuloma (JXG) over face in an infant; (H) Extensive JXG over face in a 1-year-old boy.

Glycine + Succinyl CoA

↓ Pyriodxal phosphate — ALA synthase

δ aminolevulinic acid

1. ↓ ALA dehydratase

Porphobilinogen

2. ↓ Porphobilinogendeaminase

Hydroxymethylbilane

3. Uroporphyrinogen III synthase → **Uroporphyrinogen III** | Spontaneous → **Uroporphyrinogen I**

Uroporphyrinogen III

4. ↓ Uroporphyrinogen decarboxylase

Coproporphyrinogen III

5. ↓ Coproporphyrinogen oxidase

Harderoporphyrinogen

6. ↓ Coproporphyrinogen oxidase

Protoporphyrinogen

7. ↓ Protoporphyrinogen oxidase

Protoporphyrin IX

8. ↓ Ferrochelatase Fe^{++}

Heme

Uroporphyrinogen I

↓ Uroporphyrinogen decarboxylase

Coproporphyrinogen I

1. ALA dehydratase deficiency porphyria
2. Acute intermittent porphyria
3. Congenital erythropoietic porphyria
4. Porphyria cutanea tarda and hepatoerythropoietic porphyria
5. Hereditary coproporphyria
6. Harderoporphyria
7. Porphyria variegata
8. Erythropoietic protoporphyria

Flowchart 1: Heme biosynthesis pathway.
(ALA: aminolevulinic acid)

Box 1 | Classification of porphyria.

Acute porphyrias
- Acute intermittent porphyria
- Plumboporphyria (aminolevulinic acid dehydratase deficiency porphyria)

Cutaneous porphyrias
- *Porphyria cutanea tarda:*
  - Type I (sporadic)
  - Type II (familial)
  - Type III (familial)
  - Type IV (toxic)
- *Erythropoietic porphyrias:*
  - Congenital erythropoietic porphyria (Günther's disease)
  - Erythropoietic protoporphyria
  - Congenital erythropoietic coproporphyria
- Hepatoerythropoietic porphyria

Mixed porphyrias
- Variegate porphyria
- Hereditary coproporphyria (harderoporphyria)

CONGENITAL ERYTHROPOIETIC PORPHYRIA (GUNTHER'S DISEASE) (FIGS. 6 TO 9A)

It is an extremely rare disease characterized by appearance of red urine during infancy, severe photosensitivity, hemolytic anemia and splenomegaly. Photosensitivity is frequently absent in the neonatal period but generally becomes apparent during the first few years of life. Recurrent vesiculobullous eruptions on sun-exposed areas of the skin eventually results in mutilating ulcerations, scarring, and loss of acral tissue, such as ears, tip of the nose, distal phalanges, and nails. Other common

"Our greatest happiness does not depend on the condition of life in which chance has placed us, but is always the result of a good conscience, good health, occupation, and freedom in all just pursuits." —**Thomas Jefferson**

clinical features include hypertrichosis, conjunctivitis, keratitis, brown stained teeth that fluoresce under exposure to Wood's light, hyperpigmentation, hemolytic anemia, growth retardation, and bone fragility. The biochemical disturbance in this disorder is due to the deficiency of an enzyme uroporphyrinogen cosynthetase III, resulting in marked overproduction of uroporphyrin I and coproporphyrin I in circulating erythrocytes and bone marrow cells. Prenatal diagnosis is possible by means of analysis of amniotic fluid and cells. Splenomegaly is the constant feature of this entity. Hemolytic anemia is also a very important feature. The color of the urine may vary from faint pink to burgundy or port-wine, depending on the concentration of uroporphyrin derived from the oxidation of uroporphyrinogen.

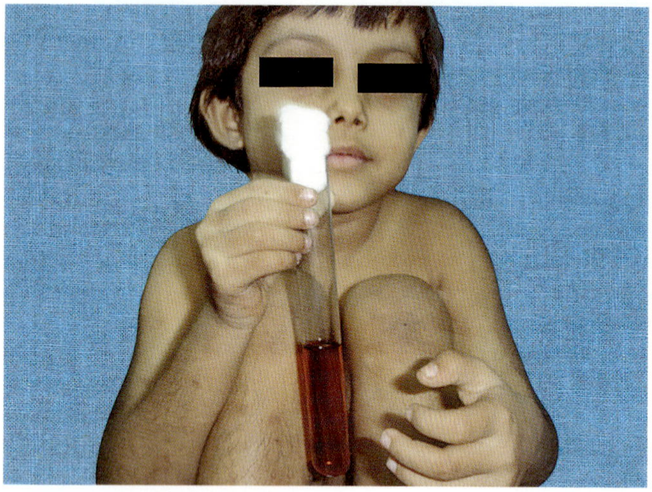

Fig. 6: Scarring, hypertrichosis, and red urine in a 4-year-old girl.

Prognosis

The prognosis of erythropoietic porphyria is poor, with few patients surviving till fourth or fifth decade. Death is frequently related to the associated hemolytic anemia.

Treatment

Treatment consists of avoidance of sunexposure and application of broad spectrum sunscreens. Oral

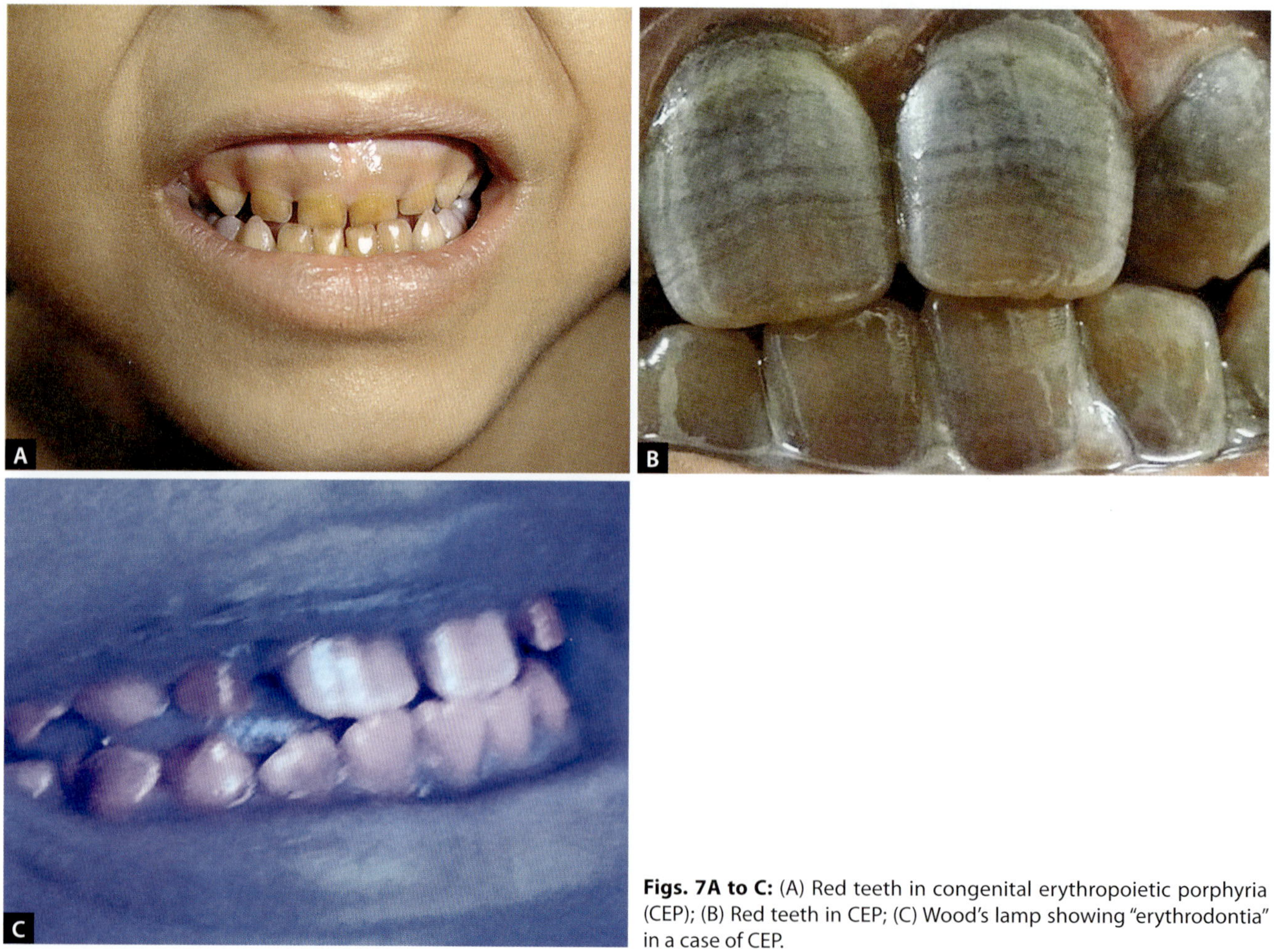

Figs. 7A to C: (A) Red teeth in congenital erythropoietic porphyria (CEP); (B) Red teeth in CEP; (C) Wood's lamp showing "erythrodontia" in a case of CEP.

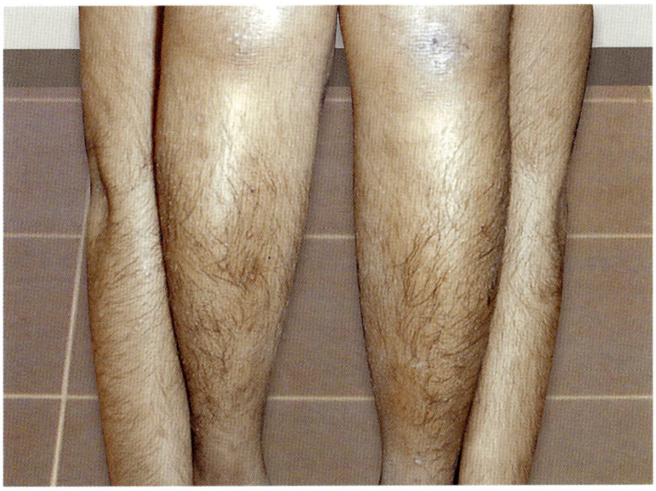

Fig. 8: Hypertrichosis over forearms and legs in congenital erythropoietic porphyria.

beta-carotene, in doses of 30–150 mg/day has been an effective photoprotective agent. Counseling of the parents is of paramount importance.

ERYTHROPOIETIC PROTOPORPHYRIA (FIGS. 9B TO E)

Erythropoietic protoporphyria is the most common cutaneous type of porphyria in children caused by loss of function mutation in *FECH* (ferrochelatase) gene. It presents as autosomal dominant, autosomal recessive or X-linked dominant type. It presents at infancy or in childhood between 1 and 6 years of age. There is photosensitivity from early age. Clinical features include itching, burning after exposure to sunlight, edematous and erythematous papules, papulovesicular, urticarial,

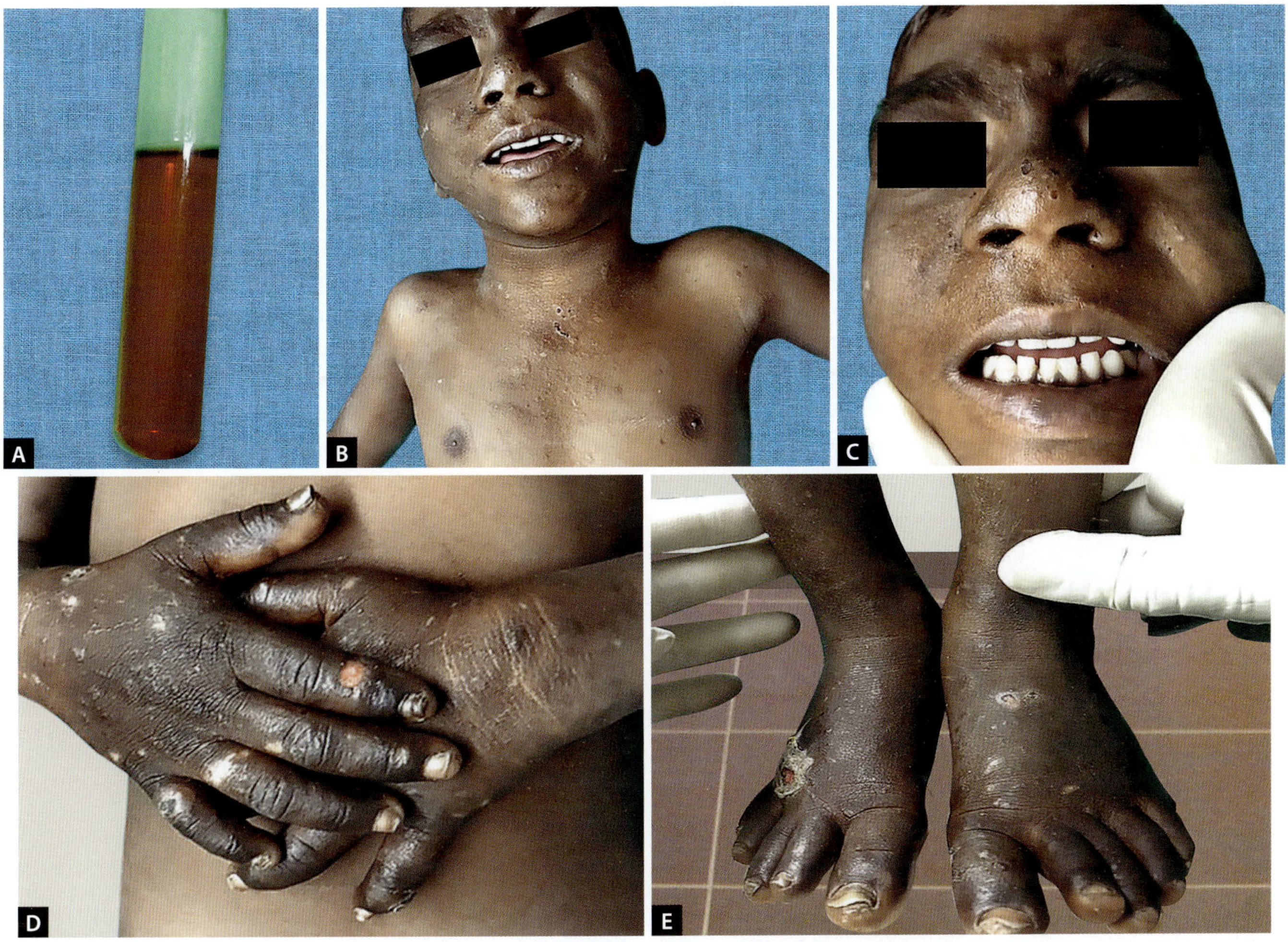

Figs. 9A to E: (A) Red urine in congenital erythropoietic porphyria; (B) Erythropoietic protoporphyria, note photosensitivity-related pigmentation, pock-like scars over face, neck, and upper chest; (C) Same boy, close-up view of face; (D) Hands showing radiodermatitis-like changes; (E) Feet and lower legs showing similar changes like hands.

"Communication is a skill that you can learn. It's like riding a bicycle or typing. If you're willing to work at it, you can rapidly improve the quality of every part of your life." —**Brian Tracy**

eczematous and petechial eruptions, superficial linear to shallow circular scarring, hypopigmentation and hyperpigmentation involving face, dorsum of hands, and photoexposed parts. Nails show photo-onycholysis. Systemic features include anemia, hypersplenism, cholecystitis, cholelithiasis, and hepatic abnormalities. Differential diagnoses include polymorphic light eruption, solar urticaria, and hydroa vacciniforme. There is an increased free protoporphyrin level in erythrocytes, plasma, bone marrow, liver, feces, and skin but not in urine. Management of erythropoietic protoporphyria includes photoprotection with sun protective clothing and broad-spectrum sunscreens. Transfusion may be helpful in hemolytic anemia.

PORPHYRIA CUTANEA TARDA

Porphyria cutanea tarda (PCT) is the most common cutaneous porphyria and has a higher incidence rate in HIV-infected children as compared to other children. Several reports have shown HIV infection to be an independent risk factor for PCT in contrast to the earlier belief of it being a coincidental association with PCT.

Porphyria cutanea tarda is a disorder of heme synthesis and is characterized by reduced activity of the enzyme uroporphyrin decarboxylase in the hepatocytes (acquired form) or in both erythrocytes and hepatocytes (familial form). Direct immunofluorescence study in PCT is characterized by IgG, IgA ± IgM, C3 in the walls of the papillary dermal blood vessels and along the dermoepidermal junction. For persons with PCT, avoiding sun exposure and other porphyrinogenic precipitants is important.

Phlebotomy and low-dose chloroquine or hydroxychloroquine are specific forms of treatment for PCT. Hydroxychloroquine has been described in both short-term high-dose and longer-term low-dose regimens. Though high-dose treatment (250 mg TDS for 3 days) results in rapid clinical and biochemical remission, it is associated with flu-like symptoms and hepatotoxicity. Low-dose hydroxychloroquine regimens of 200 mg twice weekly have been shown to be effective in producing clinical remission and reducing porphyrin.

FABRY'S DISEASE (FIGS. 10A AND B)

This is an X-linked recessive disorder where the primary metabolic defect is deficiency of a α-galactosidase A which normally catabolizes the accumulated glycosphingolipid. The characteristic cutaneous lesions of Fabry's disease or angiokeratoma corporis diffusum appear between 5 and 13 years of age, as symmetrical clusters of punctate macules or papular dark red angioectasias which do not blanch with pressure. They usually appear in the area between the umbilicus and knees, number in thousands and tend to cluster in the iliosacral areas, around the umbilicus and over the scrotum, buttocks, posterior thorax, and thighs. They become little hyperkeratotic with time. Hands and feet are usually spared. Majority of the patients may have pinpoint macular purplish spots on the lips, particularly near the vermilion border of the lower lip. Heterozygous females show clinical manifestations in 20% cases

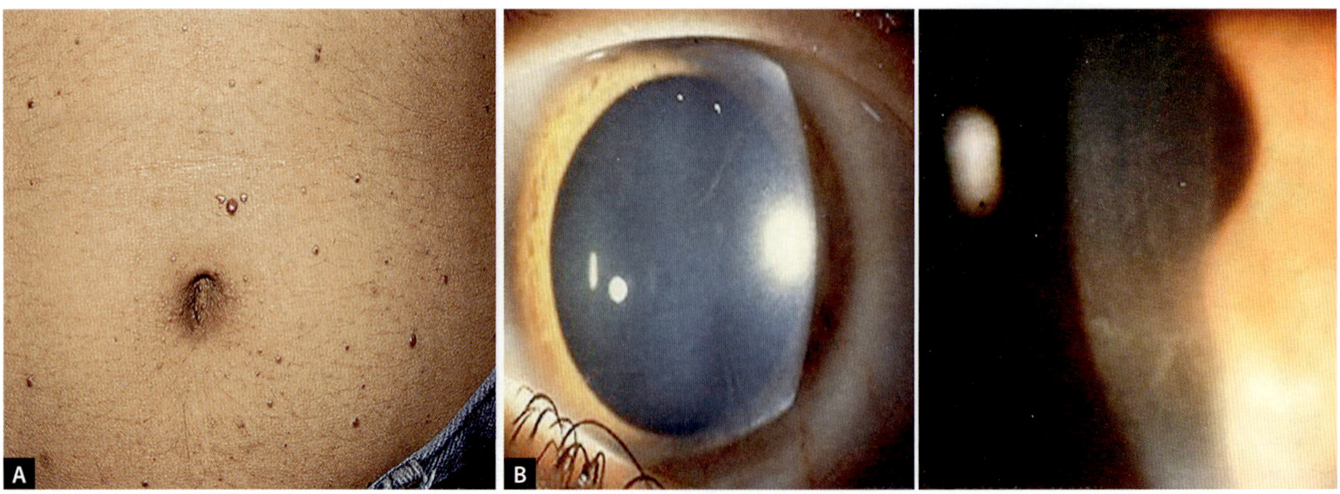

Figs. 10A and B: (A) Angiokeratoma lesions in Fabry's disease; (B) Cornea verticillata, note corneal deposit and a faint golden-brown whorl pattern.

"Today is life the only life you are sure of. Make the most of today. Get interested in something. Shake yourself awake. Develop a hobby. Let the winds of enthusiasm sweep through you. Live today with gusto." —**Dale Carnegie**

but have milder form of the disease. In childhood, the eruptions are accompanied by recurrent episodes of fever, pain and paresthesia of hands and feet. Paralysis, scant body hair, hypohidrosis, ankle and pedal edema are common.

Systemic Associations

Patients are often hypertensive and susceptible to cerebrovascular accidents, coronary artery disease, and renal disease. Neurological complications, diarrhea, colitis, proctitis, arthritis, cataracts and corneal opacities are the other manifestations. Corneal opacities result from deposition of sphingolipid in a peculiar spoke-like fashion and is known as cornea verticillata **(Fig. 10B)**.

Treatment

Treatment is generally supportive. Laser therapy may be helpful for angiokeratoma. Painful crises may be managed with phenytoin or carbamazepine. Enzyme replacement therapy using human recombinant α-galactosidase has resulted in symptomatic improvement. However, best hope in future lies in gene therapy.

FARBER'S DISEASE (FIG. 11)

Farber's disease is an autosomal recessive disease of lipid metabolism associated with a deficiency of a lysosomal acid ceramidase and tissue accumulation of ceramide. The disease clinically manifests as subcutaneous nodules near the joints and over pressure points, along with progressive, painful and deformed joints. Hoarseness due to laryngeal involvement can lead to aphonia, feeding and respiratory difficulties, failure to thrive, and intermittent fever. Symptoms usually appear between the age of 2 weeks and 4 months.

Diagnosis

The diagnosis can be established by demonstration of the deficiency of an enzyme acid ceramidase in cultured skin fibroblast or in white blood cells. Prenatal diagnosis can be done by measurement of the enzyme in cultured amniotic cells.

Prognosis

The disease often leads to death within the first few years.

Treatment

There is no specific treatment. Systemic corticosteroids may provide some relief in childhood onset cases.

LESCH–NYHAN SYNDROME (FIGS. 12 AND 13)

This is an X-linked recessive disorder of purine metabolism, caused by deficiency of hypoxanthine-guanine phosphoribosyltransferase (HPRT) which leads to an overproduction of uric acid. Mental retardation, choreoathetotic movements, self-mutilation, and gout-like manifestations of hyperuricemia are the chief clinical features. Self-mutilation is characterized by loss of tissue around the mouth and fingers as a result of compulsive self-destructive biting of these areas. Heterozygous females are asymptomatic.

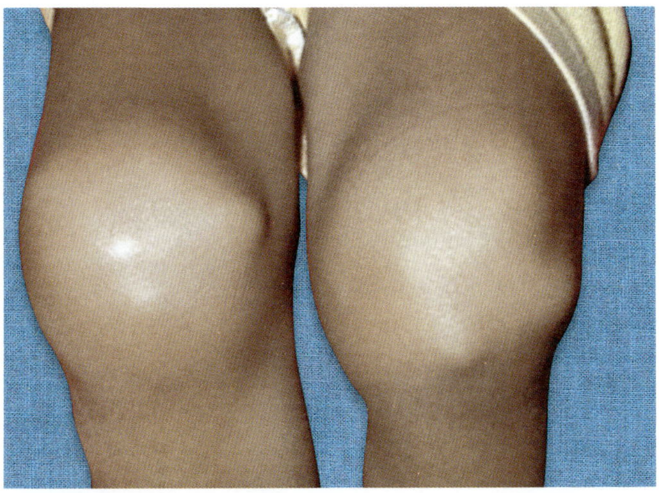

Fig. 11: Subcutaneous nodules around knees in Farber's disease.

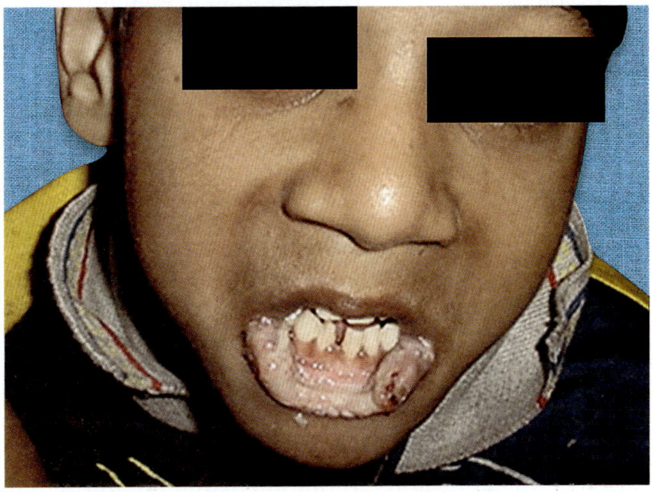

Fig. 12: Mutilated lower lip in Lesch–Nyhan syndrome.

"The secret of success is learning how to use pain and pleasure instead of having pain and pleasure use you. If you do that, you're in control of your life. If you don't, life controls you." —**Tony Robbins**

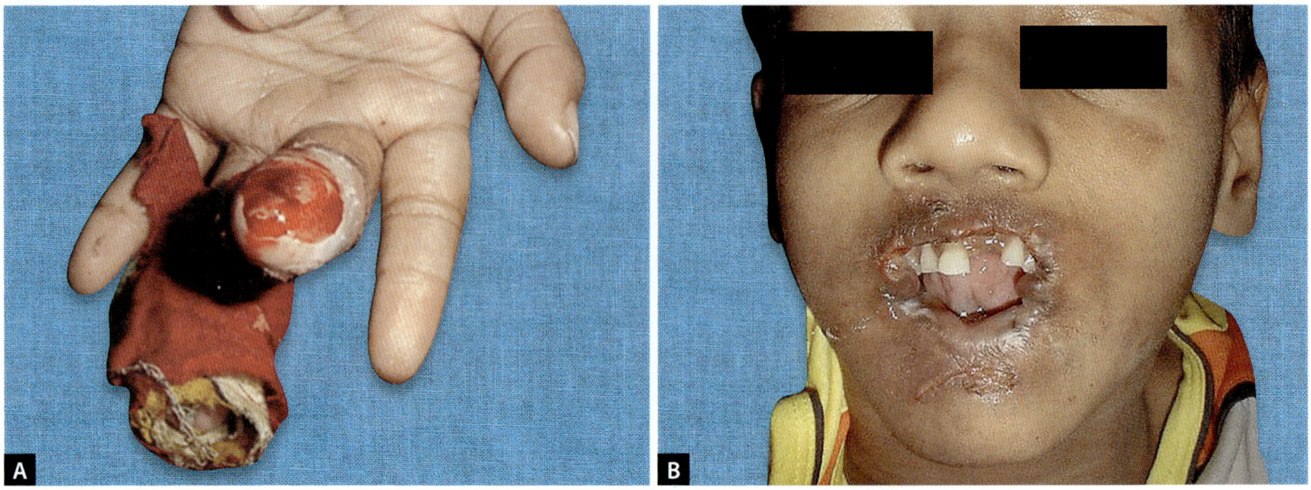

Figs. 13A and B: (A) Mutilated fingers in Lesch–Nyhan syndrome; (B) Another child with Lesch–Nyhan syndrome, note mutilated lips.

Management

Treatment is with allopurinol (in dosages of 100–300 mg/day in divided doses; >10 years, 600–800 mg/day) to control uric acid levels, tophaceous deposits, nephropathy, and gouty arthritis. Hand bandages and elbow splints are used to control the self-mutilating behavior of the patients. Lip biting may require extraction of deciduous teeth but permanent teeth should be spared as lip biting diminishes with age. Counseling parents is important.

CALCIPHYLAXIS (FIGS. 14 TO 16)

Calciphylaxis, also referred to as calcific uremic arteriolopathy or calcifying panniculitis is a rare disorder with the majority of cases occurring in middle aged to elderly women with end-stage renal disease (ESRD). Vascular and soft tissue calcifications may be present in pediatric ESRD patients. However, calcification of cutaneous arterioles leading to skin necrosis is extremely rare. Other risk factors include obesity, diabetes mellitus, hypercalcemia, hyperphosphatemia, an elevated calcium-phosphate product, secondary hyperparathyroidism, and a variety of hypercoagulable states. It results from calcification of tunica media and fibrotic changes in intima of the cutaneous arterioles along with thrombotic occlusion. Clinically, it presents with painful violaceous nodules or plaques, retiform purpura, and deep, stellate, or wedge-shaped ulcers and cutaneous gangrene. Adipose-rich areas (trunk, breasts, abdominal pannus, flanks, buttocks and proximal lower extremities) are frequently involved, however, distal lesions presenting as digital and penile necrosis have also been reported. Vasculopathy may also

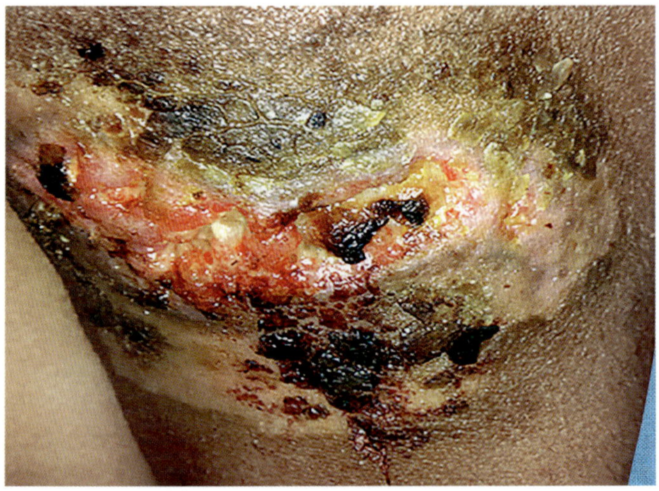

Fig. 14: Calciphylaxis, note infiltrated necrosed skin.

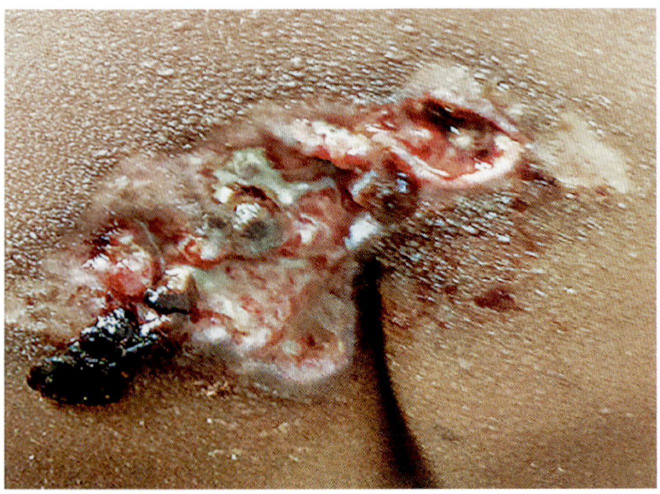

Fig. 15: Calciphylaxis, note thrombosis.

"In three words I can sum up everything I've learned about life: it goes on." —**Robert Frost**

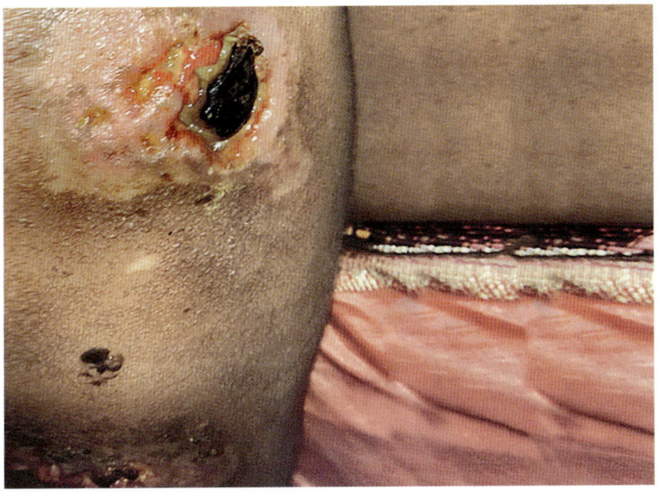

Fig. 16: Cutaneous necrosis seen in calciphylaxis.

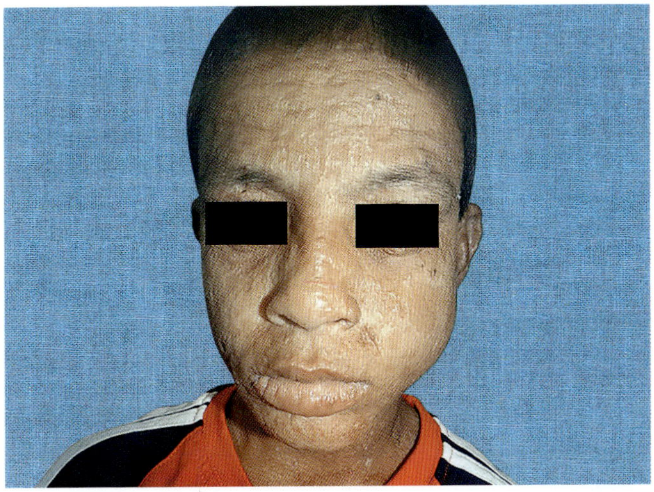

Fig. 17: Lipoid proteinosis in a 9-year-old boy.

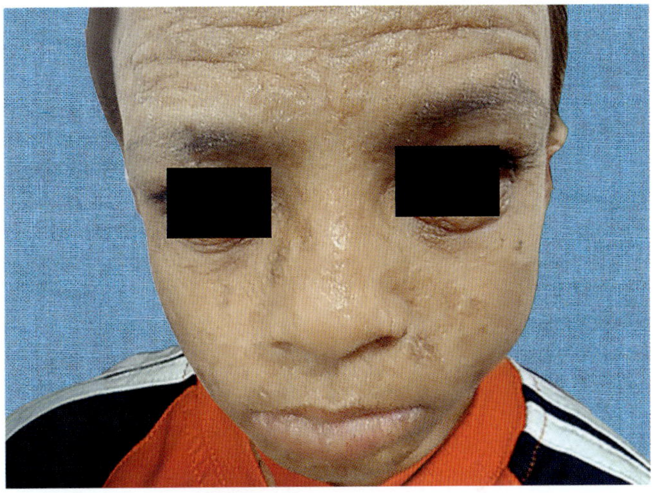

Fig. 18: Same boy, close-up view of face; note waxy infiltrated skin.

affect visceral organs and skeletal muscle. The prognosis is poor with a mortality rate of 60–80%. Death occurs within months of diagnosis, with sepsis being the leading cause. Treatment includes optimization of the calcium dysregulation and reversing microoclusive processes that potentiate calciphylaxis. Supportive management (low-calcium dialysate, paricalcitol, and sevelamer—a phosphate binder) may benefit children with secondary hyperparathyroidism. Systemic corticosteroids are of no benefit. Bisphosphonates have been shown to be effective in treating patients with calciphylaxis. Sodium thiosulfate (STS) may play a role in chelating calcium from tissue deposits. In the pediatric population, parathyroidectomy in combination with medical management may be the best treatment option in stopping the progression of disease.

In the pediatric population, an increased risk of calciphylaxis in boys with ESRD and secondary hyperparathyroidism; frequent acral, distal, and visceral involvement; worse prognosis in acral necrosis; and increased resistance to medical treatment compared to the affected adult population has been noticed.

LIPOID PROTEINOSIS (FIGS. 17 TO 23)

This is also known as hyalinosis cutis et mucosae. It is a rare autosomal recessive disorder, characterized by deposition of hyaline material in the mucosa, skin and various organs. There is mutation of the gene encoding extracellular matrix protein 1 *(ECM1)*. The symptoms of the disease vary greatly from individual-to-individual. They may include hoarse voice in early childhood, infiltration and scarring of the skin, easily damaged skin with poor wound healing, dry, wrinkly skin, and beading of the papules around the eyelids (eyelid beading sign). All of these are results of a general thickening of the skin and mucous membrane; in some cases there is cerebral calcification in the medial temporal lobes which can lead to epilepsy and neuropsychiatric abnormalities. There may be calcification of corpus callosum also.

Lipoid proteinosis is progressive till early third decade of life and thereafter the disease process stabilizes. However, there is gradual thickening and nodularity of the vocal cords and epiglottis leading to increase in hoarseness and aphonia. Thickening of tongue and infiltration of the frenulum makes the patient unable to protrude the tongue.

Currently, there is no cure for this disease although there are ways to individually treat many of its symptoms. The discovery of the mutations of the *ECM1* gene has

"We have always held to the hope, the belief, the conviction that there is a better life, a better world, beyond the horizon." —**Franklin D Roosevelt**

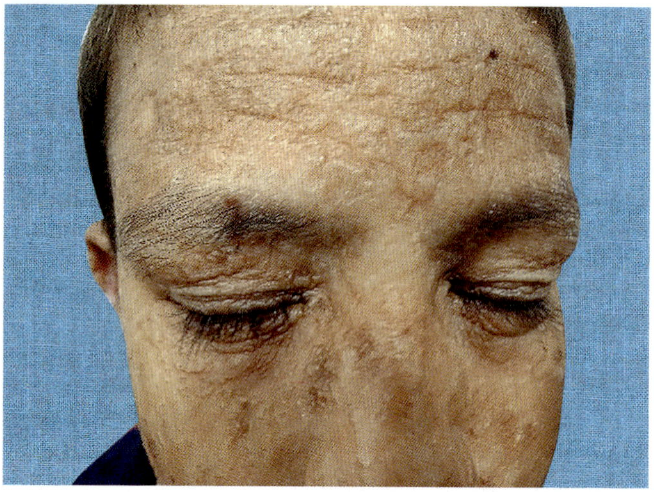

Fig. 19: Close-up view of face, waxy skin, pockmarks, and deep scars.

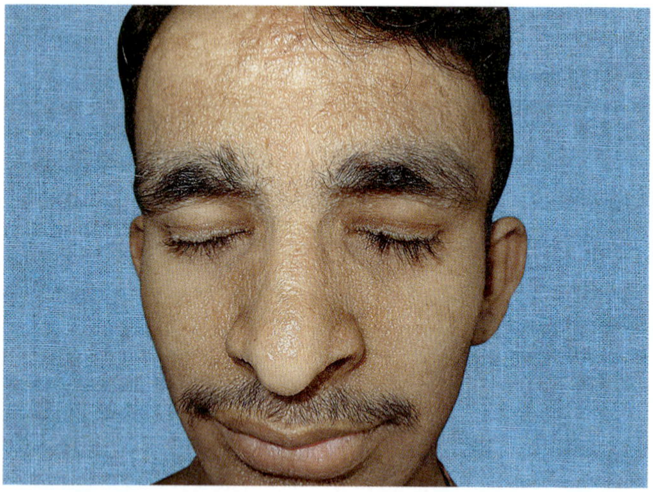

Fig. 20: Close-up view of eyelids, note "eyelid-beading sign".

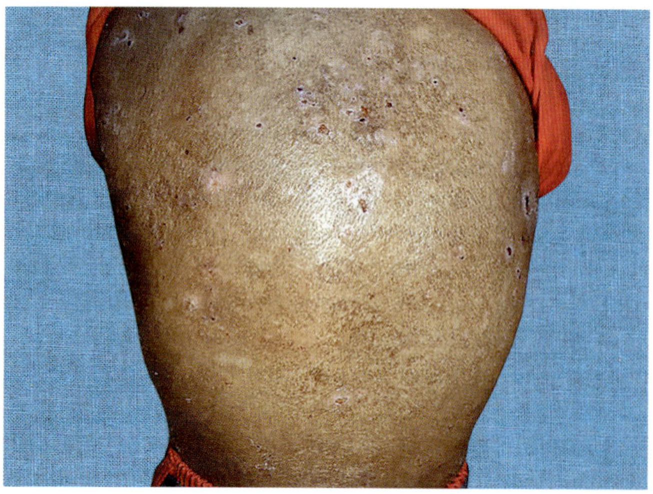

Fig. 21: Infiltrated skin and scars over back.

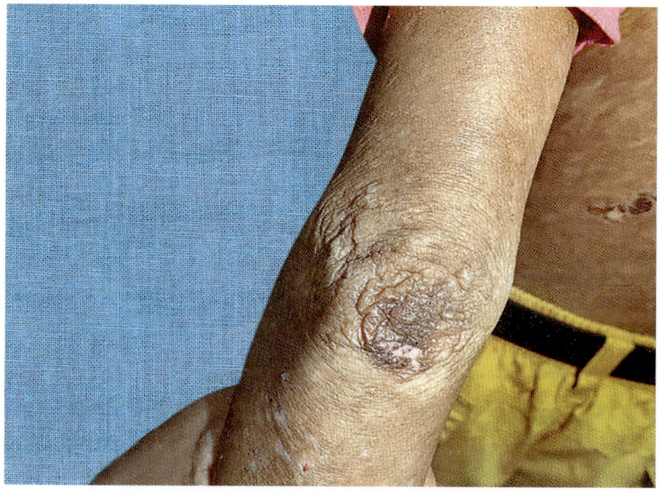

Fig. 22: Waxy infiltration of skin over elbow and arm.

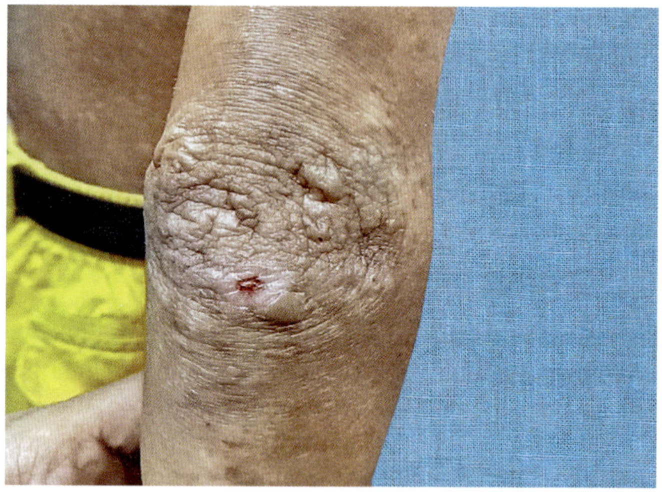

Fig. 23: Close-up view of elbow scars.

opened the possibility of gene therapy or a recombinant *ECM1* protein for this condition.

LIPODYSTROPHY

Lipoatrophy and lipodystrophy are used interchangeably. Lipodystrophy means absence of fat at certain places and compensatory accumulation of fat over other areas. Lipodystrophies are a group of disorders characterized by an abnormality in the fat resulting in partial or generalized loss of fat. Decrease in fat reserve reduces the levels of adipokines, including adiponectin and leptin. These are required to maintain the normal glucose and lipid metabolism. Leptin is responsible for satiety and it protects organs such as liver from damage due to intrahepatic fat accumulation.

Lipodystrophies are classified into congenital and acquired depending on the age at onset. Based upon the extent of body area involved, it can be classified as localized, partial body and whole body. There are various congenital partial and generalized lipodystrophy. Similarly, there are different types of acquired localized and acquired generalized lipodystrophy.

MULTIPLE SULFATASE DEFICIENCY (FIG. 24)

Multiple sulfatase deficiency is an autosomal recessive, progressive multisystem lysosomal storage disorder. It presents at variable age and has wide clinical presentation. There is low levels of at least two sulfatase enzymes and is caused by biallelic mutation in the *SUMF1* gene resulting in accumulation of glycosaminoglycans and sulfated lipids. Based on the age of onset, progression and disease severity, it can be classified into neonatal, infantile, and juvenile type of multiple sulfatase deficiency. Neonatal type is the most severe variant presenting at birth and death occurring within first 2 years of life. Clinically multiple sulfatase deficiency is characterized by progressive neurological deterioration, leuko-dystrophy, developmental regression, mental retardation, seizures, organomegaly, skeletal and heart abnormalities, progressive hearing loss, hepatosplenomegaly, dysostosis multiplex, poor growth, dysmorphic facies, coarse facial features, upper respiratory infections, and cardiac hypertrophy. Cutaneous features include ichthyosis-like presentation. Genetic counseling is important.

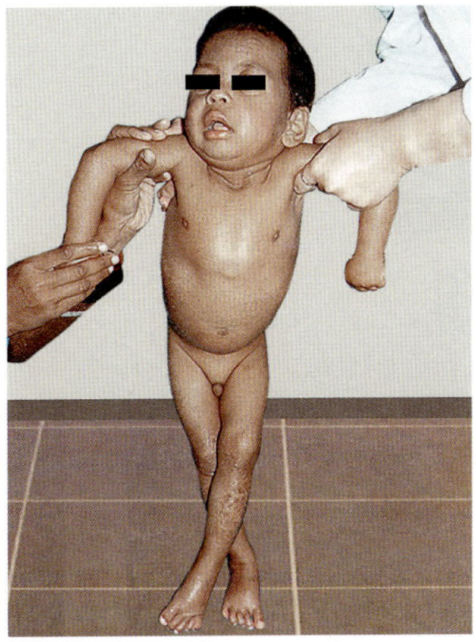

Fig. 24: Multiple sulfatase deficiency, note ichthyotic skin over legs.

WHAT'S NEW

- *Cutaneous features of peroxisomal disorders*:
  - CHILD syndrome: Presents as ichthyosiform erythroderma along blaschoid lines, ipsilateral limb defects and internal organ defects
  - Mevalonic aciduria: Presents with edema along with a morbilliform rash.
  - Refsum's disease: Presents with ichthyosis along with systemic manifestations such as nystagmus, arrythmias, deafness, retinitis pigmentosa
  - Hyperoxaluria: Livedo racemose like eruptions on legs
- *Holocarboxylase deficiency*: It presents with ichthyosis and collodion membrane with a characteristic tomcat odor of urine
- *Cutaneous manifestations of lysosomal storage disorders*:
  - Gaucher's disease: Type 2 presents with cutaneous features such as ichthyosis and collodion baby
  - Schindler's disease: Type 2 presents with cutaneous features in the form of angiokeratoma corporis diffusum
  - Mucopolysaccharidoses: Presents with ivory white papules and nodules in reticular pattern between the angle of scapula, chest and thighs and extensive Mongolian spots
  - GM1 gangliosidosis: Presents with hirsutism, extensive Mongolian spots and angiokeratomas.

SUGGESTED READINGS

1. Barthel A, Benker G, Berens K, Diederich S, Manfras B, Gruber M, et al. An update on Addison's disease. Exp Clin EndocrinolDiabetes.2019;127(2-03):165-75.
2. Lala SM, Naik H, Balwani M. Diagnostic delay in erythropoietic protoporphyria. J Pediatr. 2018; 202: 320-3.e2.
3. Lause M, Kamboj A, Faith EF. Dermatologic manifestations of endocrine disorders. TranslPediatr. 2017;6(4):300-12.
4. Oza VS, Stringer T, Campbell C, Hinds B, Chamlin SL, Frieden IJ, et al. Congenital-type juvenile xanthogranuloma: a case series and literature review. Pediatr Dermatol. 2018;35(5):582-7.
5. Vernon HJ. Inborn errors of metabolism: advances in diagnosis and therapy. JAMA Pediatr. 2015;169(8):778-82.
6. Somasundaram A, Chiramel MJ, Sathishkumar D, Korula S. Skin as a Window to Diagnose Inborn Errors of Metabolism. Indian Journal of Paediatric Dermatology. 2023;24(1):8-18.

"The best way to predict the future is to create it." —**Abraham Lincoln**

CHAPTER

15

Collagen Vascular Diseases and Vasculitis

DISCOID LUPUS ERYTHEMATOSUS (FIGS. 1 TO 7B)

Discoid lupus erythematosus (DLE) presents as erythematous indurated plaques, with adherent scales, on removal of which patulous follicular openings are seen. The lesions are mostly distributed over head and neck area with most of the lesions being on the face. The lesions are usually bordered by hyperpigmented margins. On healing, the lesions produce hypo- or depigmented scars. An important sanctuary site for the lesions is scaphoid fossae of the external ears. Ultraviolet light is understood to play a significant role in perpetuation of the lesions and the distribution of the lesions over the photoexposed areas.

Discoid lupus lesions are the most common skin lesions of childhood systemic lupus erythematosus (SLE). However, DLE lesions may occur without SLE as well. About 15–20% of patients with DLE eventually go on to develop SLE. Generalized lesions in DLE are at risk for SLE.

Management

Topical corticosteroids, chloroquine or hydroxychloroquine and sunscreens are the main treatment modalities for DLE. Moderately potent steroids, e.g., fluticasone, mometasone are prescribed for lesions over face, head and neck. Potent steroids, e.g., clobetasol propionate or betamethasone dipropionate cream/ointments are used for lesions over trunk and extremities. The average dose of hydroxychloroquine for children is 5–10 mg/kg/day. Various sunscreens with SPF 15 or more are useful in preventing the sun induced aggravation of DLE lesions.

LUPUS ERYTHEMATOSUS [FIGS. 7C TO E(iv)]

Lupus erythematosus (LE) is an autoimmune condition that has a wide range of manifestations including the mild form involving the skin to devastating multisystem involvement. The manifestations of LE

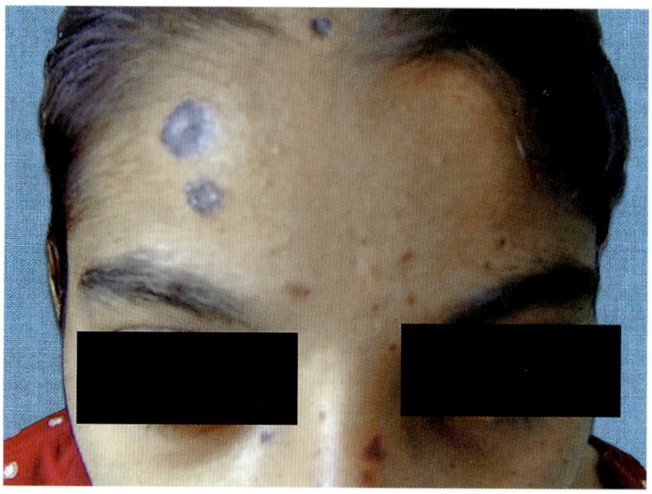

Fig. 1: Discoid lupus erythematosus (DLE) lesions over forehead.

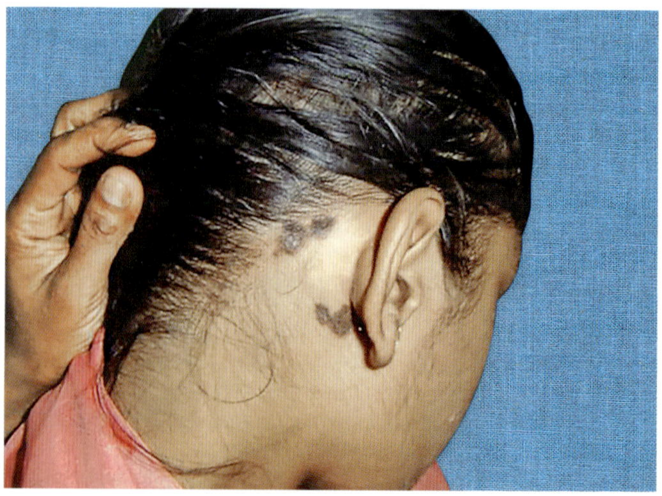

Fig. 2: Discoid lupus erythematosus (DLE) lesions over retroauricular area.

"The way to get started is to quit talking and begin doing." —**Walt Disney**

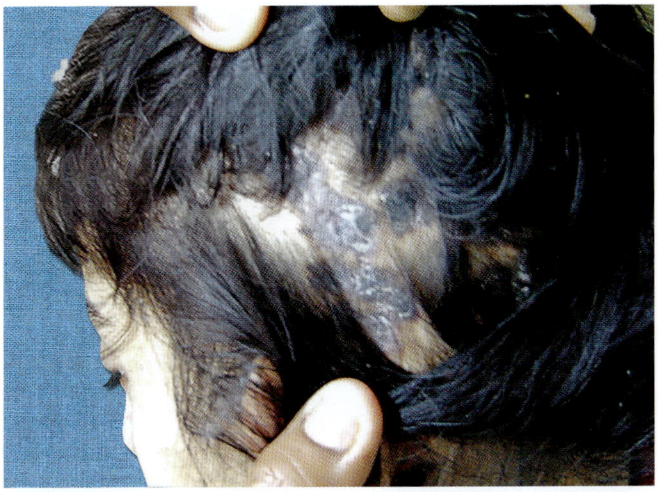

Fig. 3: Discoid lupus erythematosus (DLE) lesions over scalp.

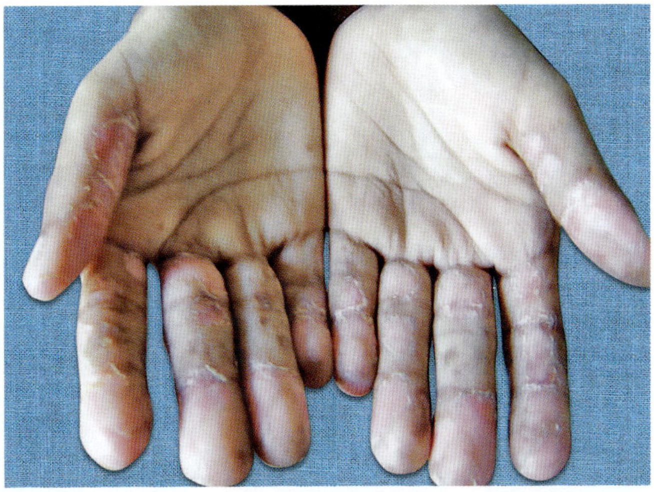

Fig. 4: Discoid lupus erythematosus (DLE) lesions over the palms.

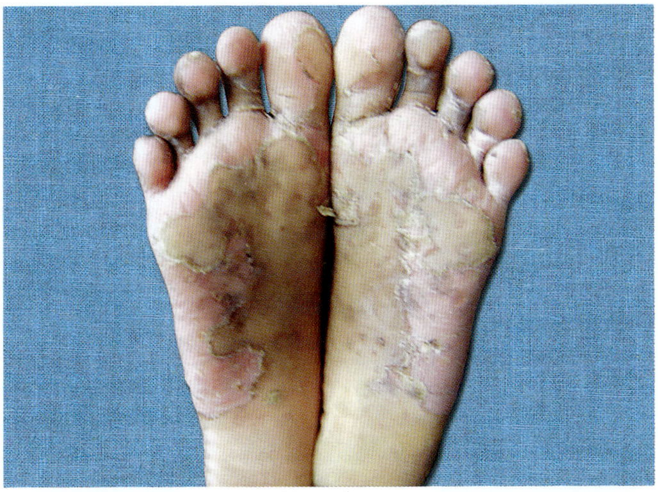

Fig. 5: Discoid lupus erythematosus (DLE) lesions over the soles.

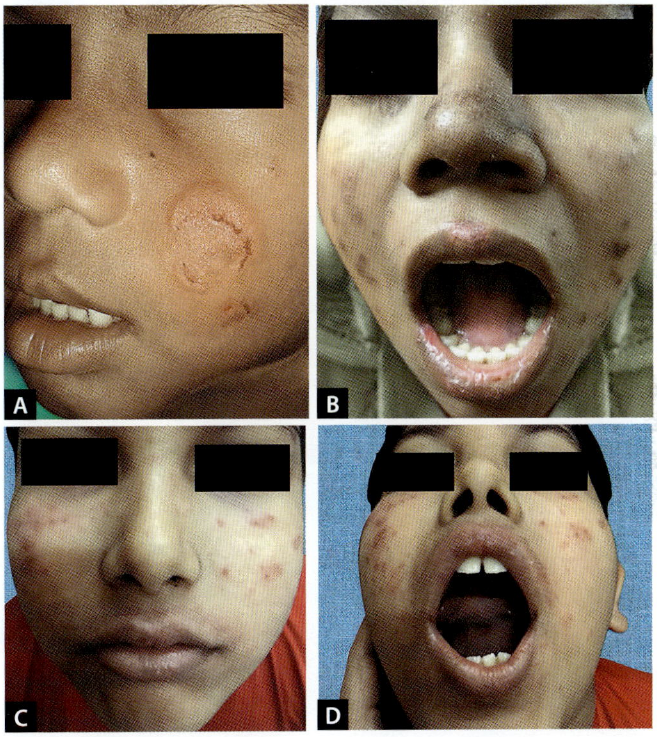

Figs. 6A to D: (A) Discoid lupus erythematosus (DLE) lesion over face in a 4-year-old boy; (B) Disseminated DLE lesions over face and lips; (C) Multiple DLE lesions over face; (D) Same boy, oral cavity.

can be divided into specific type showing interface dermatitis and nonspecific lesions which do not show the characteristic histological findings.

Pediatric SLE is more acute and severe than adult SLE. There is a higher frequency of renal, neurologic, hematologic involvement with fever and lymphadenopathy in pediatric SLE. Juvenile SLE is seen under 16 years of age. In 2012, the Systemic Lupus International Collaborating Clinics (SLICC) revised and validated the American College of Rheumatology criteria **(Table 1)**. According to the criteria, for diagnosing SLE the patient must have biopsy proven lupus nephritis with antinuclear antibody (ANA) or double stranded DNA (dsDNA) antibodies or the patient has to satisfy four of the criteria (including at least one clinical and one immunological criteria).

The LE-specific lesions include three recognized subtypes:

1. *Acute cutaneous lupus erythematosus (ACLE)*: (i) Localized, indurated erythematous lesions (malar rash) and (ii) widespread indurated erythema.
2. *Subacute cutaneous lupus erythematosus (SCLE)*: (i) Papulosquamous and (ii) annular-polycyclic forms.

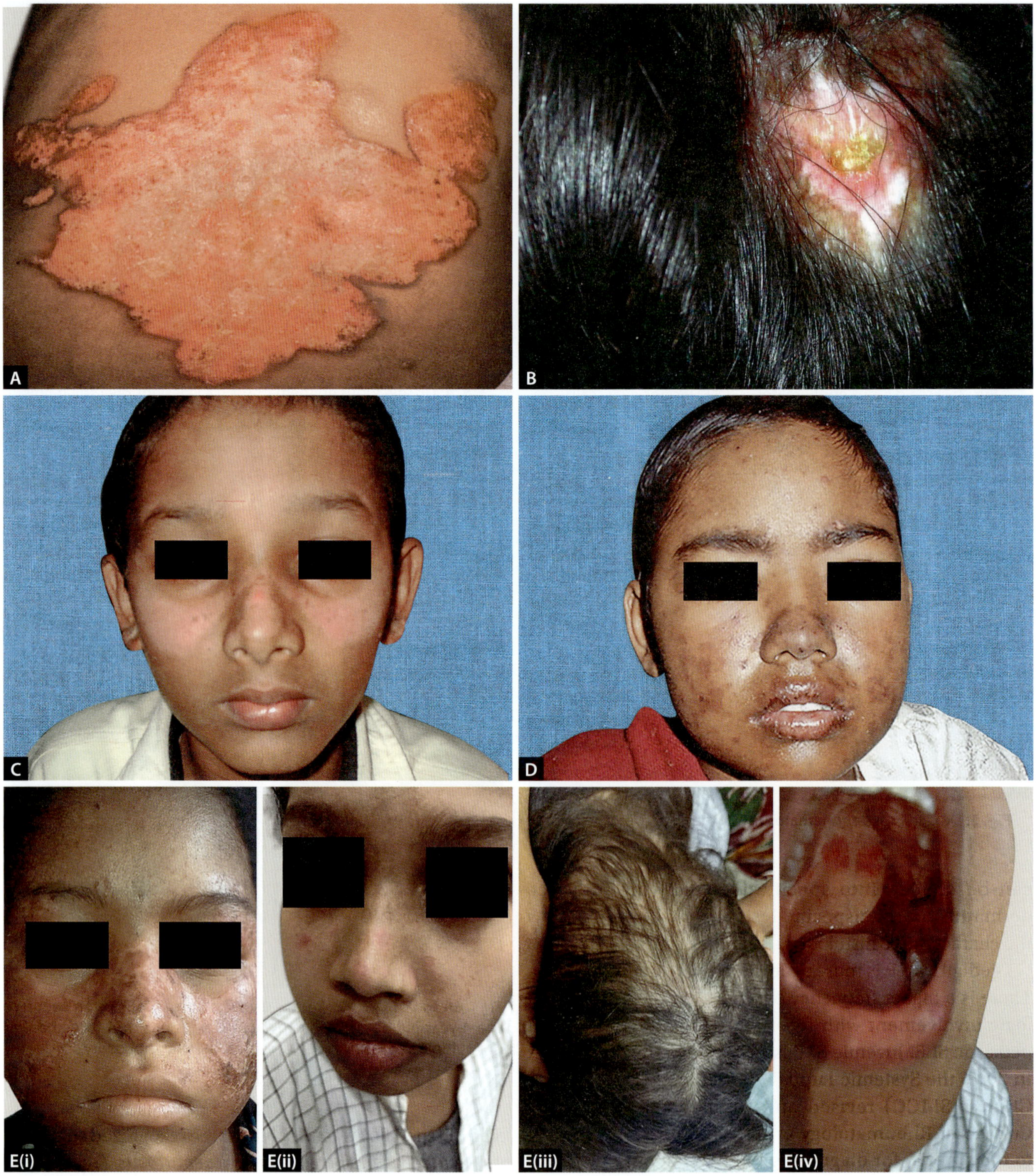

Figs. 7A to E(iv): (A) Large-sized discoid lupus erythematosus (DLE) lesion over back, note hyperpigmented border; (B) DLE over scalp with scarring alopecia; (C) Butterfly erythema over the face in systemic lupus erythematosus (SLE); (D) Erythematous scaly papules and scars over the face and lips; E(i) Butterfly malar rash of SLE in a 7-year-old girl; E(ii) Malar rash in a patient of SLE; E(iii) Lupus hair in the same patient; E(iv) Palatal ulcers in same patient.

"Your life does not get better by chance, it gets better by change." **—Jim Rohn**

Table 1: SLICC criteria for diagnosis of SLE.

Clinical criteria	Immunological criteria
• Acute or subacute cutaneous lupus • Chronic cutaneous lupus • Oral/Nasal ulcers • Nonscarring alopecia • Inflammatory synovitis with physician-observed swelling of two or more joints (or) tender joints with morning stiffness • Serositis • *Renal:* Urine protein/creatinine (or 24 hours urine protein) representing at least 500 mg of protein/24 hour or red blood cell casts • *Neurological:* Seizures, psychosis, mononeuritis multiplex, myelitis, peripheral or cranial neuropathy, cerebritis (acute confusional state) • Hemolytic anemia • Leukopenia (< 4,000/mm^3 at least once) or lymphopenia (< 1000/mm^3 at least once without other cause) • Thrombocytopenia (< 100,000/mm^3) at least once	• ANA above laboratory reference range • Anti-dsDNA above laboratory reference range • Anti-Sm • Antiphospholipid antibody • Low complement (C3, C4, CH50) • Direct Coombs test in the absence of hemolytic anemia

(ANA: antinuclear antibody; Anti-dsDNA: anti-double stranded DNA; SLE: systemic lupus erythematosus; SLICC: Systemic Lupus International Collaborating Clinics)

3. *Chronic cutaneous lupus erythematosus (DLE)*: (i) Localized DLE, (ii) generalized DLE, and (iii) hypertrophic DLE.

Pathogenesis of Cutaneous Lupus Erythematosus

This condition is postulated to have multifactorial etiology. Apoptosis, necrosis, and chemokine production appear to mediate the recruitment and activation of autoimmune T-cells and interferon-producing plasmacytoid dendritic cells, which subsequently release more effector chemokines, thus amplifying chemokine production and leukocyte recruitment which in turn mediates an inflammatory process leading to the manifestations of cutaneous lupus. Ultraviolet ray exposure has been accepted as the single most remarkable trigger for the initiation of this inflammatory cascade.

Chronic Cutaneous Lupus Erythematosus

This group has the earliest age of disease onset with a mean age of 9.9 years and the boys to girls ratio is by and large 1:1.1. Also when compared to other patients of cutaneous lupus erythematosus, this group is least likely to have a family history of autoimmune diseases and lowest rates of laboratory abnormalities in hematological, urinary and autoantibody abnormalities.

Discoid Lupus Erythematosus

The common sites affected are the face including the lips, ears, "V" region of the neck and extensor aspects of arms and forearms. Other areas that can also be affected include the scalp, eyelids, trunk, palmoplantar skin and the inguinal regions. This presents with erythematous plaque with central atrophy and peripheral rim of hyperpigmentation with adherent scaling at the center. Keratotic spikes similar in appearance to carpet tacks may be seen on the under surface of the scale removed from classical DLE lesions (carpet tack sign/tin tack sign) **(Figs. 1 to 3)**. The first author (SD) and colleague has reported the largest series of DLE in India and has seen a good number of such cases in children. The distinction between localized DLE with involvement above the neck and generalized DLE has prognostic implications as the risk of developing SLE is 20% in generalized DLE versus 5% in the localized type.

Hypertrophic Type

This type clinically resembles hypertrophic lichen planus or keratoacanthoma and may also present as a verrucous papule. This type is marked by its chronicity and poor response to treatment.

Lichenoid Discoid Lupus Erythematosus

This variant has morphological resemblance to lichen planus.

Lupus Erythematosus Telangiectoides

This variant is marked by the abundant telangiectasia along with discoid plaques.

Lupus Erythematosus Linearis

This type has been described mostly in children where there is presence of linear lesions mainly affecting the face and neck area.

Pigmented Lupus Erythematosus

It has been described in Indian patients with asymptomatic slate gray facial pigmentation with ANA positivity and histological features of DLE.

Lupus Erythematosus Panniculitis

It generally presents with a firm depressed painless nodular lesion on the face, trunk, and proximal extremities. As the name suggests there is involvement of the deeper

"They always say time changes things, but you actually have to change them yourself." —**Andy Warhol**

dermis and subcutaneous tissue leading to lipoatrophy, scarring, and disfigurement.

Chilblain Lupus Erythematosus

It is characterized by edema, redness and tenderness of the tips of the fingers, toes, nose and earlobes. The familial form has been associated with *TREX1* gene mutation.

Lupus Erythematosus Tumidus

This presents more often as a solitary than multiple tumid, succulent skin colored to erythematous plaque with patulous follicular openings predominantly affecting the face. This variant is the most photosensitive and most responsive to treatment.

Rowell's Syndrome

The entity Rowell's syndrome is controversial. Some authors believe it to be a part of SLE and not a subtype of LE. Rowell and coworkers described the occurrence of erythema multiforme in association with LE. Zeitouni et al. proposed three major and three minor criteria to diagnose the condition. The major criteria consist of the presence of LE (systemic, discoid or subacute), EM-like lesions and speckled pattern of ANA. The minor criteria include chilblains, anti-Ro and/or anti-La antibodies and positive RF. All three major criteria and at least one minor criterion are required to establish the diagnosis of Rowell's syndrome.

Investigations

The tests include complete blood count, erythrocyte sedimentation rate (ESR), liver and renal function tests and urine analysis. The serological tests include ANA, anti-dsDNA antibodies, and C3 and C4. Biopsy from the skin lesion and direct immunofluorescence from a photoprotected uninvolved skin yields better results.

Treatment

- *Photoprotection*: A broad-spectrum sunscreen forms one of the pillars of management. Strict chemical and physical sunscreens should be propounded for use by the patients.
- *Topical therapy*: This forms the mainstay of treatment when the lesions are few. Topical calcineurin inhibitors, topical steroids, and retinoids have been used with good response. Intralesional triamcinolone acetonide and cryotherapy are the other modalities which can also be used.
- *Systemic therapy*: Antimalarials are the single most important drug in the systemic management of chronic cutaneous lupus erythematosus. They exert their effect by their photoprotective and anti-inflammatory action. The standard dose range of hydroxychloroquine is 200–400 mg/day (adults: 6–6.5 mg/kg ideal body weight per day; children: <5 mg/kg ideal body weight per day). Clinical improvement is usually seen in 4–6 weeks. Ocular toxicity is the most dreaded complication and an ophthalmological evaluation is necessary before the initiation of therapy.
- Oral steroids, prednisolone is usually prescribed at a dose of 0.5–1 mg/kg/day. The dose may be tapered once clinical improvement is evident.
- Methotrexate, thalidomide, clofazimine, dapsone, and sulfasalazine have been tried at various occasions with variable response.
- Physical and surgical measures that have been tried include laser therapy, cryotherapy, surgical excision, and dermabrasion.

SUBACUTE CUTANEOUS LUPUS ERYTHEMATOSUS [FIGS. 7F(i) TO G(iii)]

Subacute cutaneous lupus erythematosus differs from chronic cutaneous lupus erythematosus. SCLE does not scar and the lesions do not show atrophy. Immunologically it is characterized by the presence of anti-Ro/La antibodies. It generally affects women of the middle age group. Rarely, it may be seen in children. The author has seen few cases of SCLE in children **(Fig. 4)**. Two clinical variants have been described: (1) papulosquamous variant and (2) the annular polycyclic subtype. Rare forms include exfoliative erythroderma, acral distribution of annular form, pityriasiform, and exanthematous variant. Patients with SCLE can develop DLE or lesions of ACLE or LE nonspecific lesions such as cutaneous vasculitis, Raynaud's phenomenon, or livedo reticularis during the course of their disease. More recently, LE gyratum repens has been described as a rare annular variant of SCLE. SCLE can be induced by drugs such as thiazides, antiepileptics, calcium channel blockers, angiotensin-converting enzyme (ACE) inhibitors, terbinafine, and nonsteroidal anti-inflammatory drugs (NSAIDs).

Treatment

It is generally the same as in case of chronic cutaneous lupus erythematosus. If the patient is unresponsive to the use of topical mediations and antimalarials, other drugs in the form of dapsone, clofazimine, and thalidomide can be tried.

ACUTE CUTANEOUS LUPUS ERYTHEMATOSUS

It generally presents as a localized or generalized form which is photosensitive and transient. Of all adult and pediatric patients of SLE, malar rash is the most common specific cutaneous manifestation and is seen in approximately 80% of cases.

Localized Acute Cutaneous Lupus Erythematosus

This condition presents with malar rash which is defined as bright erythema involving the malar regions and nose symmetrically in a butterfly distribution **(Fig. 5)**. The rash has a tendency to wax and wane with disease activity.

Generalized Acute Cutaneous Lupus Erythematosus

It presents with a typical morbilliform rash **(Figs. 6A to D)**. TEN-like ACLE presents with bullous lesions and sheets of epidermal detachment without involvement of the oral mucosa, eyes, and genitalia. The immunology and biopsy findings help in establishing a diagnosis.

Lupus Erythematosus Nonspecific Lesions

Lupus erythematosus nonspecific skin lesions are seen in association with active SLE. The LE nonspecific lesions include cutaneous vasculitis, photosensitivity, livedo reticularis, Raynaud's phenomenon, alopecia (nonscarring), sclerodactyly, anetoderma, leg ulcers, papulonodular mucinosis, calcinosis cutis, LE nonspecific bullous lesions, and rheumatoid nodules. Livedo reticularis is associated with the presence of vasculitis and antiphospholipid antibody syndrome (APS). The majority of these lesions do not correspond to vasculitis but to thrombotic vasculopathy. Nonscarring alopecia is a manifestation which presents with thin, dry, lusterless, brittle hair also known as lupus hair. Mucosal involvement in SLE is generally asymptomatic. Oral, nasal, genital, and conjunctival mucosa may be involved. Painless ulceration of the hard palate, mucosal erosions, gingivitis, and erythema may occur during flare of disease activity.

Bullous Lupus Erythematosus

Bullous LE occurs in the presence of active SLE and often may be accompanied by lupus nephritis. The bullae are usually seen on the face, neck and upper trunk, and heal with milia.

Treatment

The treatment of cutaneous lesions seen in LE has been discussed earlier. Dapsone is effective for the treatment of bullous LE.

NEONATAL LUPUS ERYTHEMATOSUS (FIGS. 7H TO J)

Neonatal lupus erythematosus (NLE) is an autoimmune condition affecting approximately 1–2% of neonates born to mothers with autoantibodies of SLE or Sjögren syndrome, occurring due to the passive transmission of antibodies to SSA/Ro and SSB/La. The most serious complication of NLE is complete heart block. About 10% have an associated cardiomyopathy at the initial diagnosis or develop it later.

Role of Antibodies in the Pathogenesis

The incidence of congenital complete heart block appears to be more common in offspring of women with high titers of anti-SSA/Ro and anti-SSB/La compared with mothers with low titers. It has also been found that antibodies with a specificity for the 52 kD component of the SSA/Ro protein (Ro52) are more frequently found and are present at higher concentrations in the serum of children with congenital heart block and their mothers. The role of antibodies in predicting the cutaneous manifestations of NLE has, however, been conflicting in various studies. Although the pathogenesis is not fully understood, it has been postulated that heart block results from binding of anti-SSA/Ro and/or anti-SSB/La antibodies to fetal cardiac tissue, leading to autoimmune injury of the atrioventricular (AV) node and its surrounding tissue. In addition to inducing tissue damage, anti-SSA/Ro and/or anti-SSB/La antibodies may inhibit calcium channel activation or the cardiac L- and T-type calcium channels themselves which are crucial for the action potential propagation and conduction in the AV and sinoatrial (SA) nodes.

"Harmony makes small things grow, lack of it makes great things decay." —**Sallust**

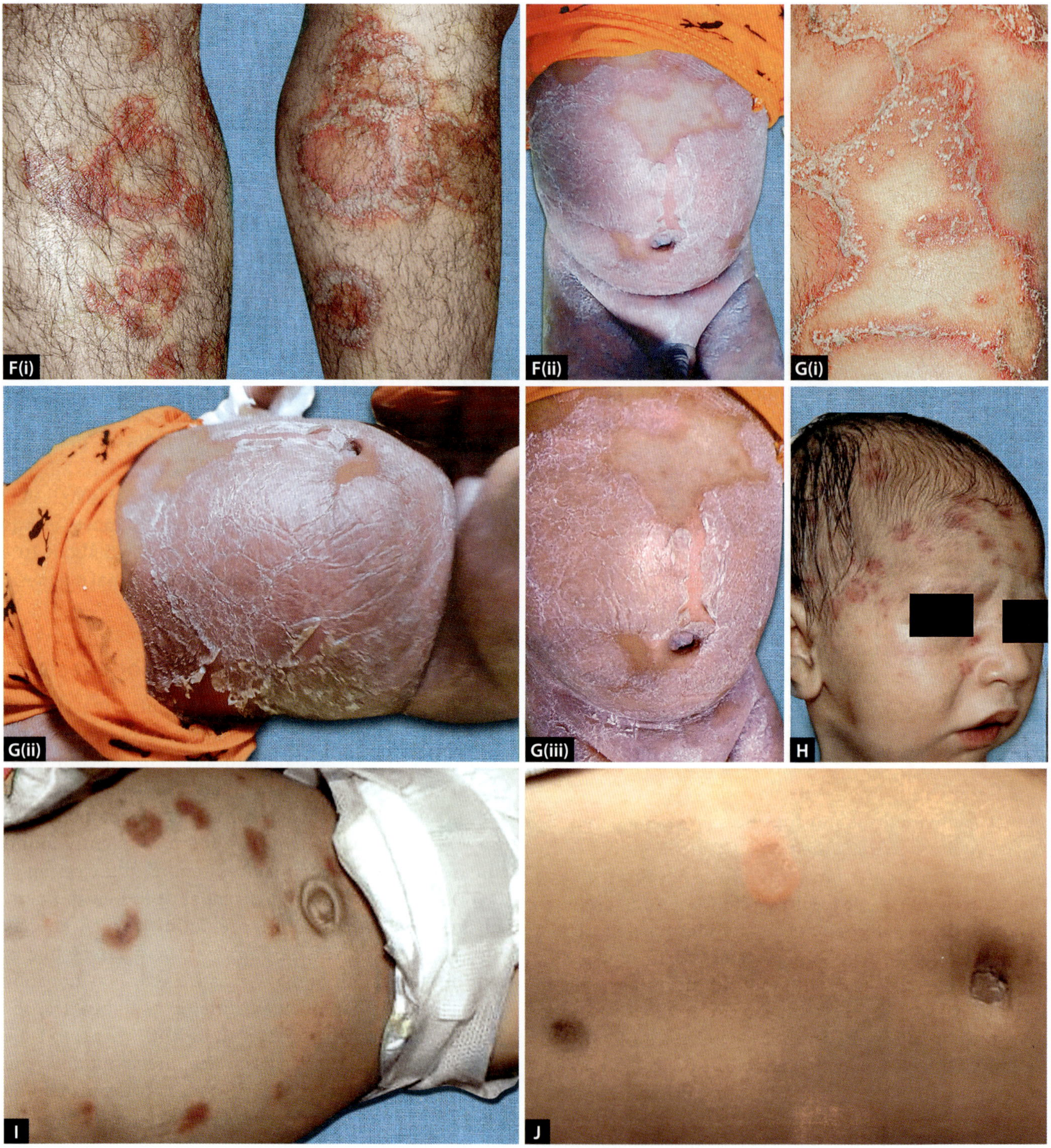

Figs. 7F(i) to J: F(i) Annular and psoriasiform lesions of subacute cutaneous lupus erythematosus (SCLE); F(ii) SCLE with annular and psoriasiform lesions; G(i) Close-up view of SCLE lesions; G(ii) Close-up view of trunk lesions; G(iii) Psoriasiform lesions, close-up view; (H) Neonatal lupus erythematosus (NLE) lesions over face; (I) Same child, lesions on trunk; (J) Cutaneous lesion of NLE.

Other Factors

There have been reports of development of classical cutaneous manifestations of NLE in the absence of complete heart block when other antibodies such as U1RNP have been present in the absence of anti-Ro/La. Genetic factors in the infant, in particular the HLA alleles

*DQB1*02, DRB1*03*, and a polymorphism in the promoter region of the gene for tumor necrosis factor alpha may also play a role in the disease manifestation in a neonate. Maternal-fetal microchimerism may contribute to complete heart block in NLE.

Clinical Features

Cutaneous Manifestations

The rash of NLE is that of SCLE presenting as annular erythematous scaly plaques with scaling or psoriasiform lesions. There is a typical erythematous to a dusky rash periorbitally giving rise to "Raccoon eye" appearance. The rash is noted at birth in some cases, but may not develop until after exposure to UV light. The rash is usually self-limiting and almost always resolves by 6–8 months of age because the half-life of immunoglobulin G (IgG) antibodies is approximately 21–25 days.

Cardiac Manifestations

Neonatal lupus erythematosus is responsible for 80–95% of all cases of congenital complete heart block diagnosed in utero or in the neonatal period. Second-degree block detected in utero and first- or second-degree heart block found in infants at birth, can progress to complete heart block. The involvement of SA node may occur in 3–4% of fetuses giving rise to dysrhythmias, which is generally not permanent. Other cardiac abnormalities reported include arrhythmias, conduction defects, congestive cardiac failure due to cardiomyopathy and on rare occasions myocarditis. There have also been reports of endocardial fibroelastosis in the absence of anti-Ro/La antibodies.

Other Systemic Involvement

Hepatic involvement in the form of asymptomatic transaminitis and hepatitis have been noted. Hematological manifestations include anemia, neutropenia, thrombocytopenia, and aplastic anemia on rare occasions. Neurologic manifestations in the form of hydrocephalus and neuropsychiatric manifestations have also been reported. An unique radiological finding in NLE is chondrodysplasia punctata and stippling of the epiphyses.

Diagnosis

The diagnosis of NLE is made when a fetus or newborn of a mother with anti-SSA/Ro and/or anti-SSB/La, or possibly anti-RNP antibodies develops heart block and/or the typical rash or hepatic or hematologic manifestations in the absence of other explanation.

Prenatal Screening

Prenatal screening for anti-SSA/Ro and anti-SSB/La antibodies is warranted for women who are known to be at risk of having a pregnancy complicated by NLE. Performing weekly pulsed Doppler fetal echocardiography from the 18th through the 26th week of pregnancy and then every other week until 32 weeks should be strongly considered. The most vulnerable period for the fetus is reported to be during the period from 18 to 24 weeks' gestation. Complete heart block (and usually second-degree block) results in fetal bradycardia that can be detected by routine fetal auscultation, ultrasonography (sonogram), or echocardiography.

Differential Diagnoses

- Urticaria
- Erythema marginatum
- Dermatophyte infection (tinea corporis)
- Seborrheic dermatitis
- Annular erythema of infancy

Treating Fetal Heart Block

Complete heart block is irreversible even with glucocorticoid therapy. Second-degree heart block may be reversible, but it also may progress to complete heart block despite therapy. Fluorinated glucocorticoids such as dexamethasone and betamethasone, which are not inactivated by placental 11β-hydroxysteroid dehydrogenase, may suppress the associated pleuropericardial effusion or hydrops and may improve outcomes. However, usage of oral corticosteroids in the mother during pregnancy to reduce the risk of complete heart block increase the chances of cleft palate in the fetus.

Preventive treatment with hydroxychloroquine has been recommended by some authors whereas the treatment with oral corticosteroids and intravenous immunoglobulin (IVIg) has been condemned by others.

Course and Outcome

The rash of NLE is generally temporary and subsides without any scarring or dyspigmentation in about 6–8 months. Infants with noncardiac manifestations of NLE should at least have an ECG, and possibly an echocardiogram, since first-degree block is clinically silent and can progress postnatally. Most of the surviving infants at a later stage require a pacemaker. These children also run the risk of developing various other autoimmune conditions such as pauciarticular and polyarticular onset juvenile idiopathic arthritis, psoriasis, thyroid disease, iritis, type 1 diabetes mellitus, and nephrotic syndrome.

DERMATOMYOSITIS (FIGS. 8 TO 11)

Juvenile dermatomyositis (JDM) has some special features apart from the classical ones such as heliotrope erythema around the eyes and Gottron's papules over the dorsal aspect of fingers overlying the middle and distal interphalangeal joints. The additional features are widespread cutaneous and extracutaneous vasculitis, telangiectatic eruptions and calcinosis cutis. Deposition of calcium in the skin is seen over joints mostly. However, on chest X-ray one can find extensive calcification in the skin over anterior chest wall. Periungual telangiectasia is a characteristic feature of JDM. Other features of JDM include oral ulcers, limb edema, xerosis, poikiloderma, and lipodystrophy. Rarely they can manifest as flagellate erythema.

The course of JDM is variable. It can have a very insidious nonspecific onset such as fever, anorexia, malaise, abdominal pain, and gradual development of rash. In other situations, the onset of the disease can be explosive with fever, profound weakness, and severe multisystemic involvement.

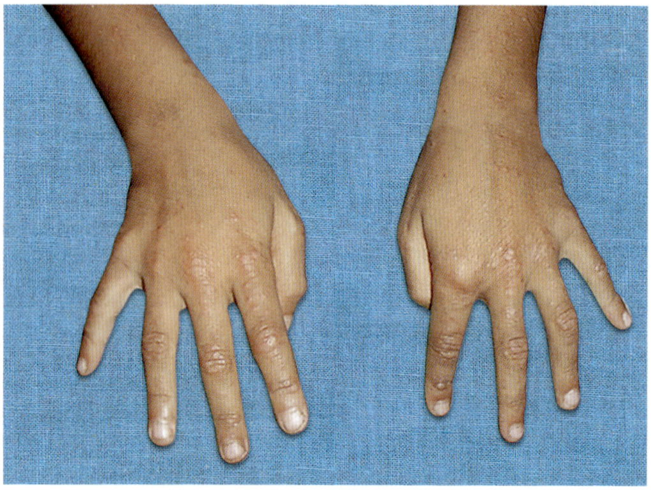

Fig. 8: Erythematous Gottron's papules over interphalangeal joints of fingers.

Management

Acetylsalicylic acid and other NSAIDs are helpful in reducing muscle tenderness, pain, and inflammation. With corticosteroids, the mortality has been reduced to < 10% from 33%. For acutely ill patients, hospitalization is advised. Most childhood forms of dermatomyositis require high dosage of oral corticosteroids. Prednisolone 2–3 mg/kg/day is the initial dose. The progression of the disease is measured by estimating muscle enzyme levels. Once the disease activity is brought down, gradually over the next 10–12 months various cytotoxics are used as steroid sparing agents while steroids are being tapered. Azathioprine (1–3 mg/kg/day), methotrexate (1 mg/kg/week) or cyclosporine (2.5–5 mg/kg/day) may be used; oral antimalarial agents have been used in controlling cutaneous manifestations. Localized small plaques of calcinosis frequently disappear spontaneously. In severe

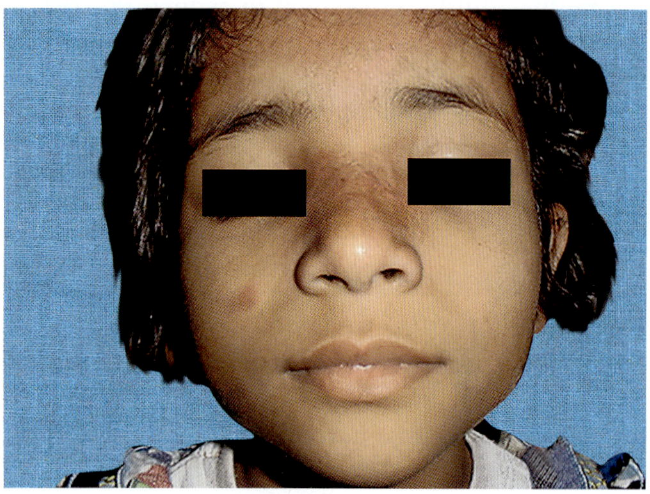

Fig. 9: Erythematous papular lesions of dermatomyositis over the face.

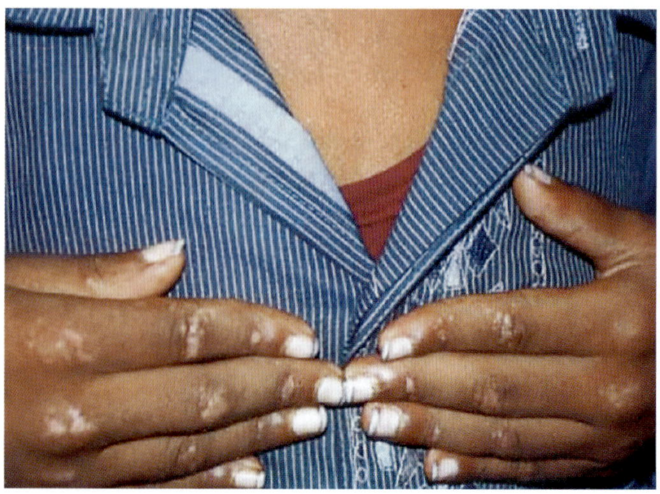

Fig. 10: Resolving Gottron's papules.

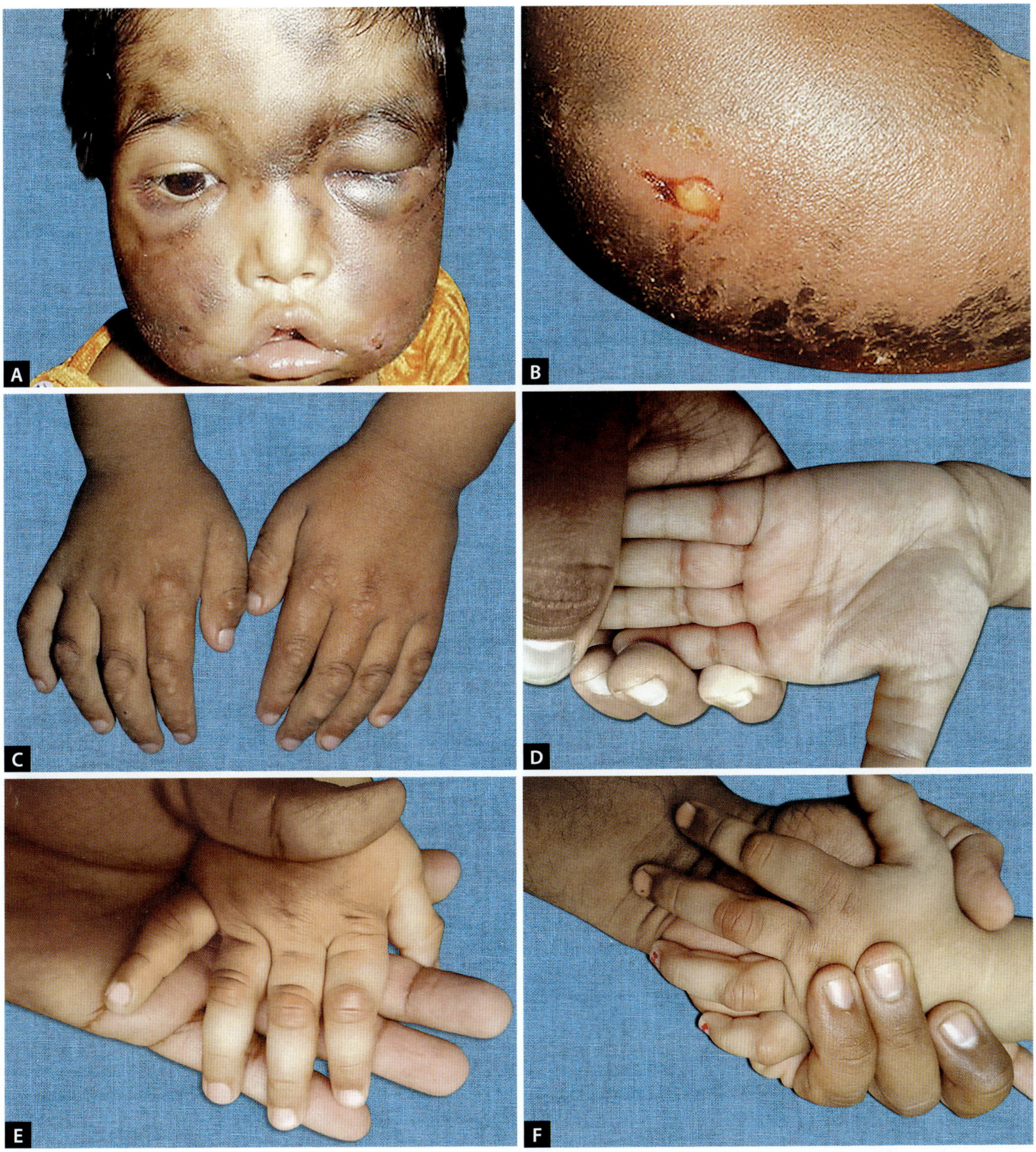

Figs. 11A to F: (A) Hyperpigmentation, swelling, heliotrope rash and scarring in dermatomyositis; (B) Hyperpigmentation, ulceration, and calcinosis of childhood dermatomyositis; (C) Gottron's papules; (D) A 5-month-old baby presenting with palmar erythema in dermatomyositis; (E) Same baby, violaceous discoloration (Gottron sign) on the knuckles; (F) Same baby, close-up view.

and extensive calcinosis, diet low in calcium, phosphorus in conjunction with aluminum hydroxide gel (15–30 mL four times per day) may lower serum phosphorus and aid in the subsidence of cutaneous calcification.

Progressive Systemic Sclerosis (Figs. 12A to D)

The clinical features are essentially the same as that in adults. However, Raynaud's phenomenon is less

"Luck is what happens to you when fate gets tired of waiting." —**Gregory David Roberts**

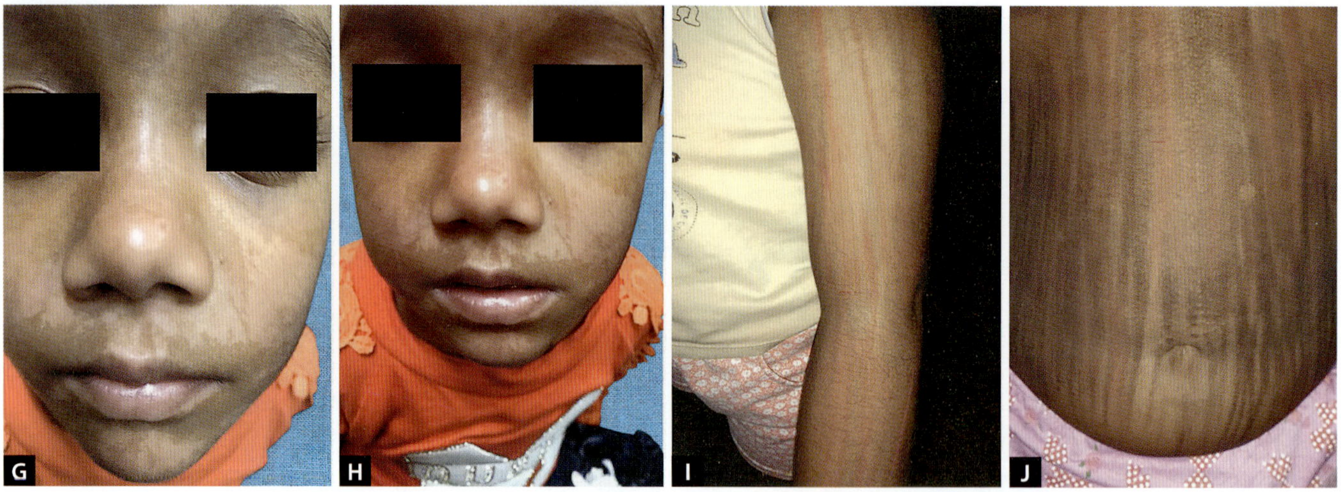

Figs. 11G to J: (G) Pigmentary changes in childhood dermatomyositis; (H) Same baby, close-up view; (I) Flagellate erythema in childhood dermatomyositis; (J) Flagellate erythema over trunk in childhood dermatomyositis.

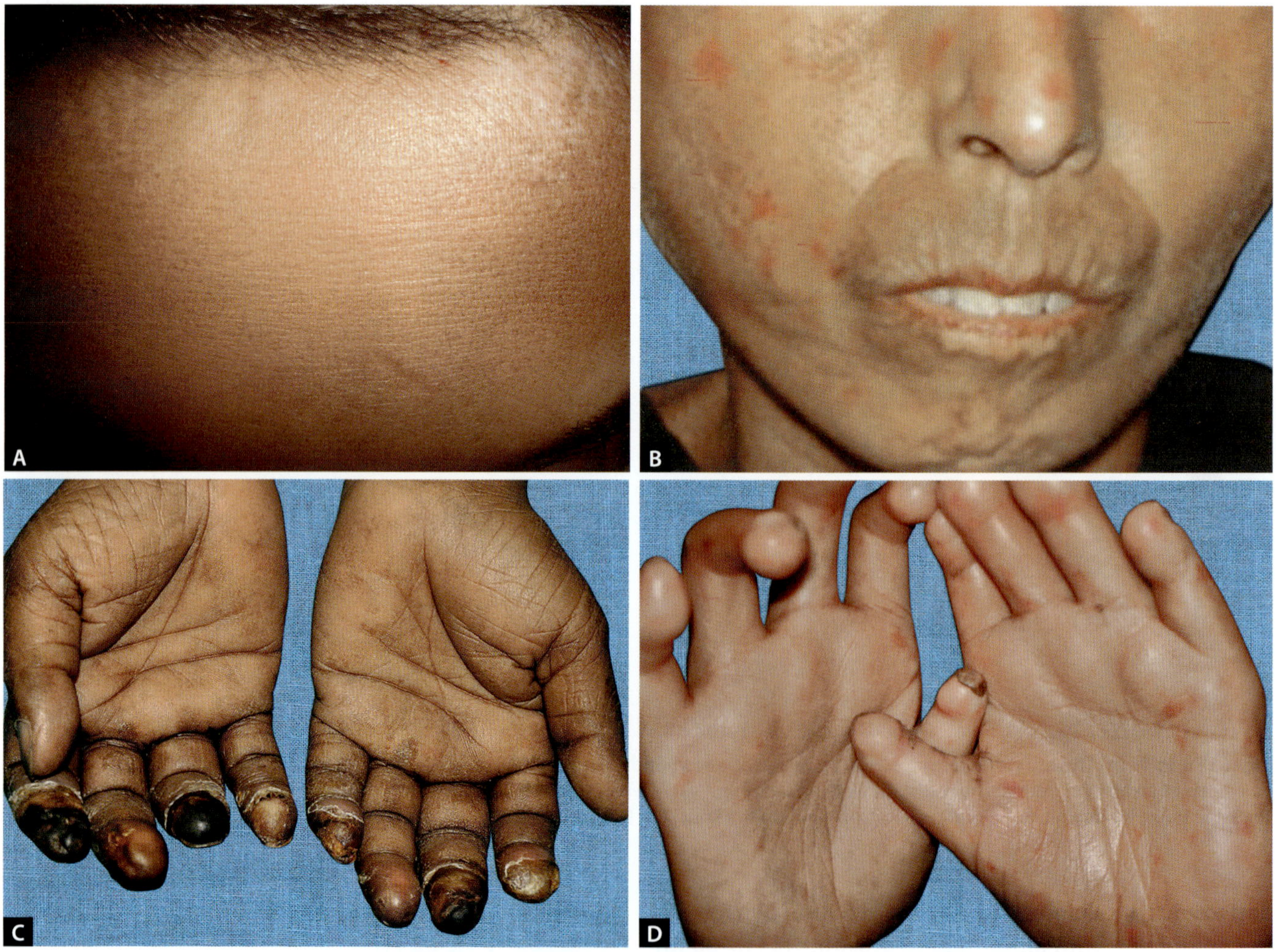

Figs. 12A to D: (A) Salt and pepper depigmentation over forehead in scleroderma; (B) Pinched mask facies, telangiectasia, microstomia; (C) Acrosclerosis with terminal tuft resorption in scleroderma; (D) Sclerodactyly, palmar telangiectasia.

Table 2: Proposed criteria for diagnosis of juvenile systemic sclerosis.

Major criterion (required):	
Proximal (to MCP/MTP joints) skin sclerosis/induration of the skin	
Minor criteria (at least two required):	
Cutaneous	Sclerodactyly
Peripheral vascular	Raynaud's phenomenon
	Nailfold capillary abnormalities
	Digital tip ulcers
Gastrointestinal	Dysphagia
	Gastroesophageal reflux
Cardiac	Arrhythmias
	Heart failure
Renal	Renal crisis
	New onset arterial hypertension
Respiratory	Pulmonary fibrosis (HRCT/radiograph)
	Decreased DLCO
	Pulmonary arterial hypertension
Neurologic	Neuropathy
	Carpal tunnel syndrome
Musculoskeletal	Tendon friction rubs
	Arthritis
	Myositis
Serologic	Antinuclear antibodies
	SSc selective autoantibodies [anticentromere, anti-topoisomerase I (Scl 70), anti-fibrillarin, anti-PM-Scl, anti-fibrillin or anti-RNA polymerase I or III]

(HRCT: high-resolution computed tomography; MCP/MTP: metacarpophalangeal/metatarsophalangeal; SSc: systemic sclerosis)

Source: Zulian F, Woo P, Athreya BH, Laxer RM, Medsger TA Jr, Lehman TJ, et al. The Pediatric Rheumatology European Society/American College of Rheumatology/European League against Rheumatism provisional classification criteria for juvenile systemic sclerosis. Arthritis Rheum. 2007;57:203-12.

frequent and renal disease is rare. The course of systemic sclerosis in childhood is slower and the disability and visceral involvement is usually less severe than in adults. The proposed criteria for juvenile systemic sclerosis is described in **Table 2**.

Management

The management is mainly supportive. Avoidance of factors which can lead to vasospasm, viz., tension, fatigue, stress, cold exposure or intake of cold drink/food is important. Rest and limited movements are advised if joint involvement is significant. Nifedipine is often prescribed in doses 5–10 mg two to three times per day for few months to reduce Raynaud's phenomenon and subsequent sclerosis of fingers and toes. Other drugs such as D-penicillamine, colchicine, etc., are reported to be effective but their efficacy is not uniform and toxicities limit their widespread use. For gastrointestinal symptoms such as reflux and regurgitation, frequent small feeds, antacids, and elevation of head end are done. Systemic corticosteroids have limited role, as they do not alter the course of the disease. However, they may be used in specific situations, e.g., debilitating arthritis not controlled by NSAIDs, patients with early edematous stage of scleroderma, in severe recurring digital ulcerations and acute toxic phase of the disease.

MORPHEA (FIGS. 12E TO G)

Morphea refers to localized or circumscribed scleroderma. It can be localized or focal, linear morphea, or fronto-parietal (en coup de sabre) with or without hemiatrophy of the face. Of total cases, 15% begin below the age of 10 years, in which the linear lesions predominate. The lesions usually present as hyperpigmented indurated shiny plaque(s) of variable size(s) and shape(s). Linear lesions are usually seen on the extremities or trunk.

Childhood onset occurs in 3% of all cases of scleroderma, 80% are associated with morphea and 20% with systemic sclerosis.

A severe mutilating form of morphea involves the dermis, fat, fascia, muscle and even bone, usually starts before the age of 14 years. The condition may develop from liner morphea and is known as pansclerotic morphea.

Natural History

In pediatric age group, morphea tend to regress spontaneously in a good number of patients by 3–5 years. The lesions usually tend to subside leaving residual hyperpigmentation. Linear morphea, en coup de sabre and facial hemiatrophy tend to persist for long time.

Treatment

Topical potent corticosteroids, e.g., clobetasol propionate or betamethasone dipropionate once daily for 4–6 weeks may bring about resolution of lesions. Intralesional triamcinolone acetonide 40 mg/mL at every 3–4 weeks' interval for 2–3 sittings is usually able to melt the morphea plaques. However, follow-up of the lesions is important. Other modalities for the treatment of morphea are antimalarials, colchicine, phenytoin sodium,

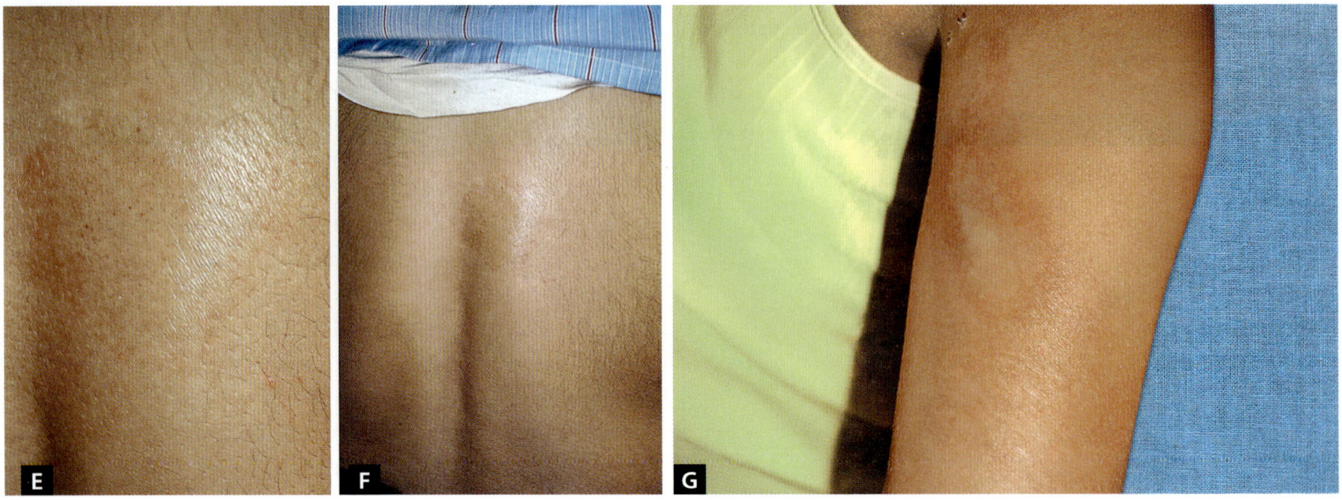

Figs. 12E to G: (E) Hyperpigmented indurated shiny plaque of morphea; (F) Plaque of morphea over back; (G) Morphea along with porcelain-whitish plaque at the centre.

methotrexate, cyclosporine, etc. The first line of therapy for linear morphea involving joints are oral steroids with methotrexate.

LINEAR MORPHEA (FIGS. 12H TO K)

Linear morphea is characterized by discrete, indurated linear band which usually presents as a single, unilateral lesion involving the extremities, face or scalp. Lesions may follow Blaschko's lines. En coup de sabre is a type of linear morphea which appears specifically on the face and frontoparietal scalp. In en coup de sabre a linear depressed groove is often associated with zone of alopecia and it resembles a saber wound or cut on the frontoparietal scalp. The groove may spread downward into cheek, nose and upper lip, and sometimes, it may involve the mouth, gum, chin or neck. The variety of coup de sabre represents a mild form of progressive facial hemiatrophy (the Parry-Romberg syndrome) which is a slowly progressive atrophy of the soft tissue of the corresponding half of the face and one half of the body, accompanied at times by contralateral Jacksonian epilepsy, trigeminal neuralgia, alopecia, enophthalmos or atrophy of the ipsilateral half of the upper lip, gum, and tongue.

EN COUP DE SABRE AND FACIAL HEMIATROPHY [FIGS. 12L(i) TO N]

Parry-Romberg syndrome is characterized by slowly progressive unilateral atrophy of facial subcutaneous fat, muscle, skin, cartilage, and bone. The condition typically presents during the first or second decade of life and then stabilizes. Apart from unilateral facial atrophy it presents with ipsilateral enophthalmos and deviation of the mouth and nose toward the affected side. Neurologic abnormalities occur in 15% of patients and include focal seizures, visual loss due to involvement of the retina and optic nerve, facial pain due to trigeminal neuralgia, and migraine. The pathogenesis of facial hemiatrophy is not clear. Trauma, infection with virus, immunologic abnormality, cranial vascular malformation, connective tissue disorder, and disturbance of fat metabolism can be a possibility. In addition, facial hemiatrophy may be congenital in nature. It is difficult to differentiate from scleroderma of the "en coup de sabre" type. Facial hemiatrophy is distinguished by a more extensive involvement of the lower face with only slight cutaneous sclerosis. Management needs a long-term follow-up of somatic disorders and prevention of psychological problems. Treatment is symptomatic and mainly consists of plastic surgery after the disease activity has stopped. Surgical options used are grafts (dermal and dermal-fat grafts), local or free-flap surgery, and injection of autologous tissue, lipofilling, paraffin, silicone, or polyalkylimide gel or poly-L-lactic acid. Medical management for facial hemiatrophy tried are topical/ intralesional steroids, antimalarials, topical vitamin E preparations, and topical vitamin D analogs.

NECROTIZING VASCULITIS (FIGS. 13 AND 14)

It is a histopathological description of a host of diseases affecting the skin and various other organ systems.

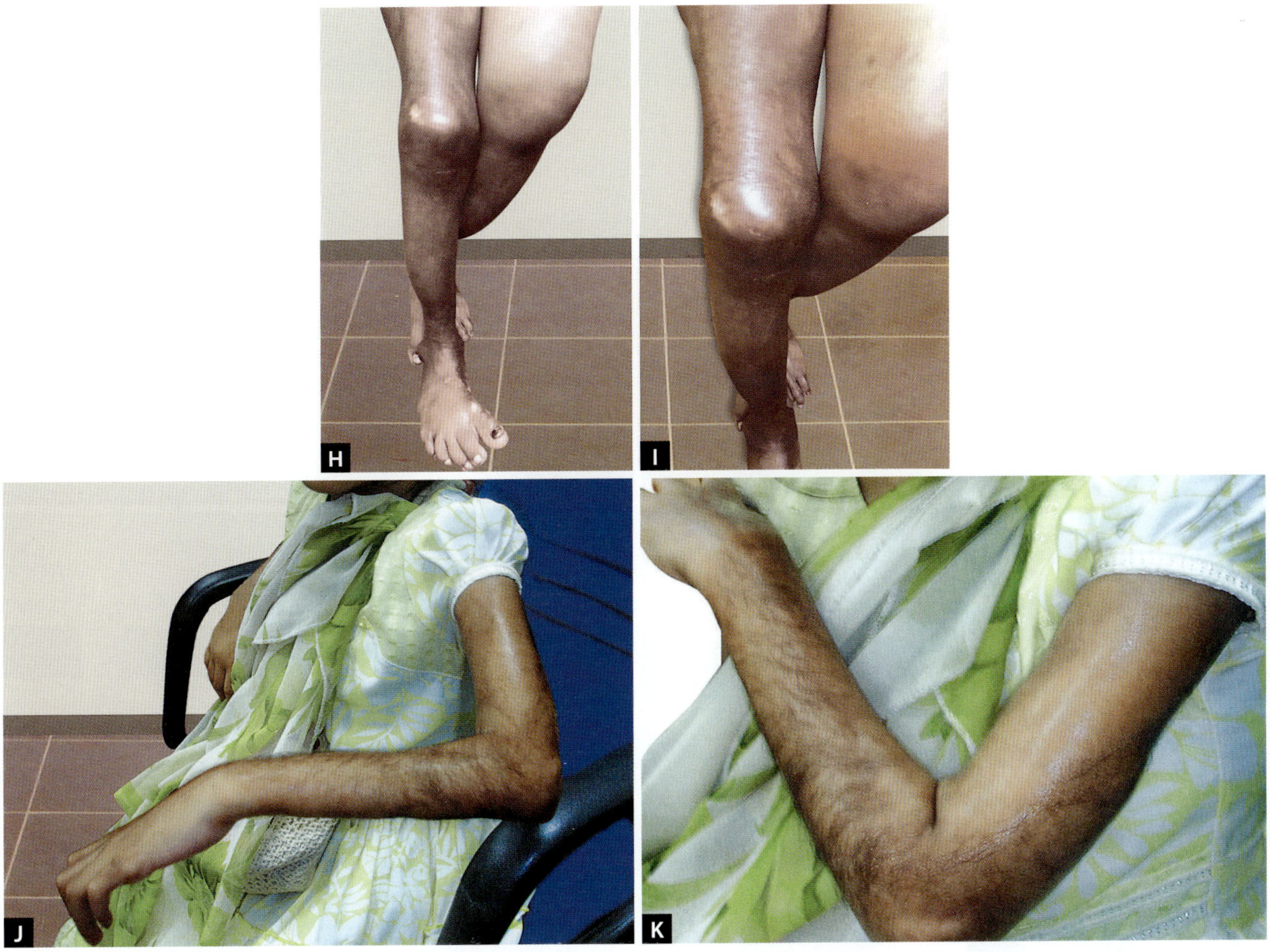

Figs. 12H to K: (H) Pansclerotic morphea of right lower limb in a 6-year-old girl; (I) Same girl, close-up view; (J) Linear scleroderma; (K) Same patient, close-up view.

The cutaneous lesions are quite varied in morphology, e.g., purpura, papule, plaques, vesicle, pustules ulcer, etc. Necrotizing vasculitis is seen in association with granulomatosis with polyangiitis, allergic granulomatosis (Churg-Strauss syndrome) and lymphomatoid granulomatosis.

LIVEDOID VASCULOPATHY (FIGS. 15 TO 17)

Also known as atrophie blanche, presents as a smooth, ivory-white plaque of sclerosis stippled with telangiectasia and surrounded by hyperpigmentation. The condition mostly occurs over lower legs or feet in adult women. However, it can occur in pediatric age group as well. It is seen in association with nevus flammeus and several other vascular disorders.

It is important to try to establish the type, etiology, and associated systemic involvement in vasculitis. Management of vasculitis is, therefore, a teamwork involving various specialists in different fields of pediatric medicine, e.g., pediatric internists, neurologists, cardiologists, gastroenterologists, nephrologists, ophthalmologists, etc.

Treatment

Systemic corticosteroids are the treatment of choice for all types of vasculitis depending upon the degree, severity and extent of skin involvement, systemic involvement, etc. Oral prednisolone 1–4 mg/kg/day may be used in mild-to-moderate cases and IV methylprednisolone as pulse therapy in severe cases or cases with multisystem involvement. Various steroid sparing agents used are azathioprine, cyclophosphamide, methotrexate, cyclosporine, etc. In children in whom steroids are contraindicated, dapsone or colchicine are used as substitutes.

"Notice the small things. The rewards are inversely proportional." —**Liz Vassay**

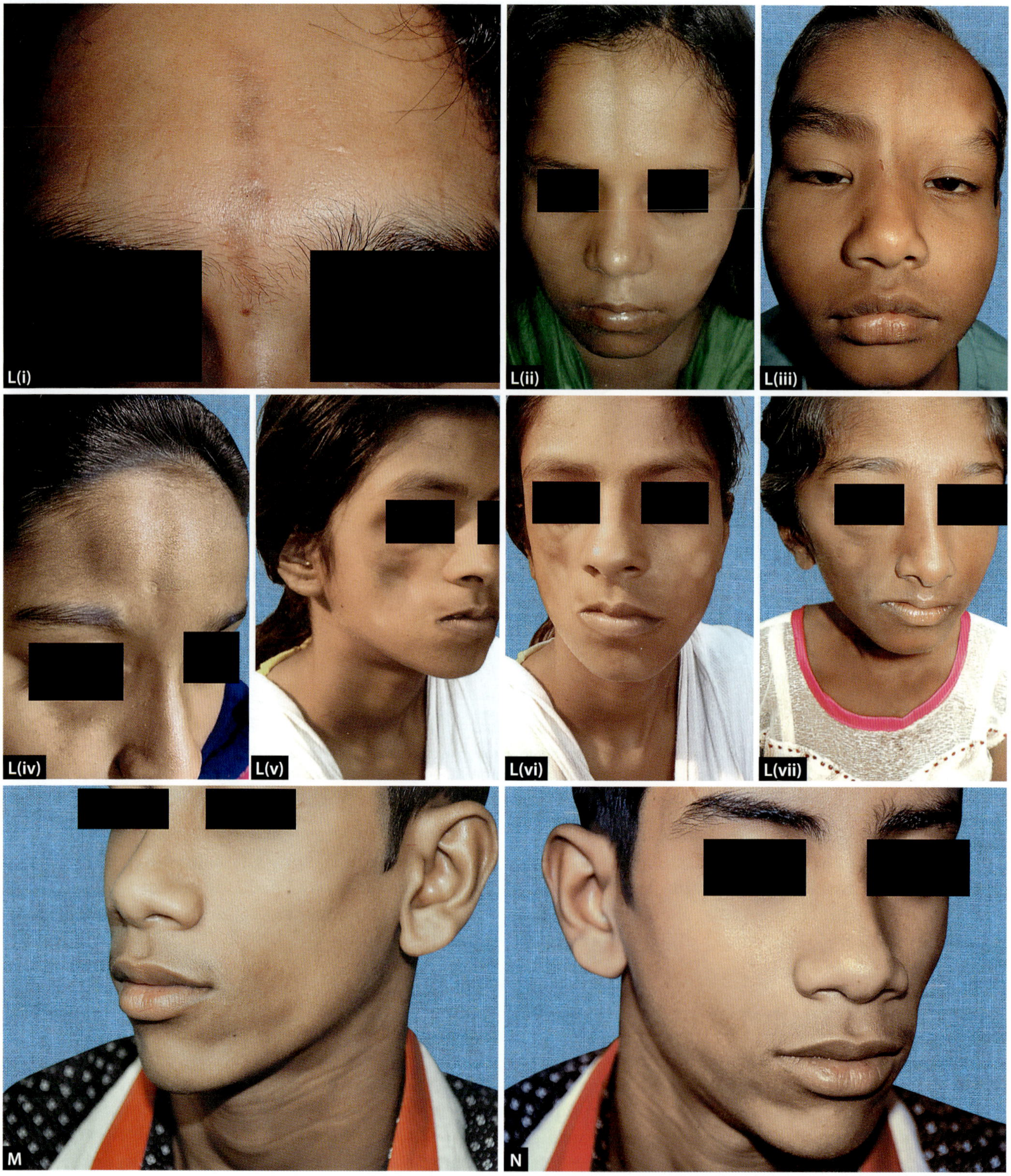

Figs. 12L(i) to N: L(i) En coup de sabre; L(ii) En coup de sabre in a 10-year-old girl; L(iii) En coup de sabre in a 9-year-old boy; L(iv) Same deformity in a 16-year-old girl; L(v) Facial hemiatrophy of right side; L(vi) Same girl, another view; L(vii) Parry–Romberg syndrome, another girl; (M) Facial hemiatrophy in a 16-year-old boy; (N) Same boy, close-up view.

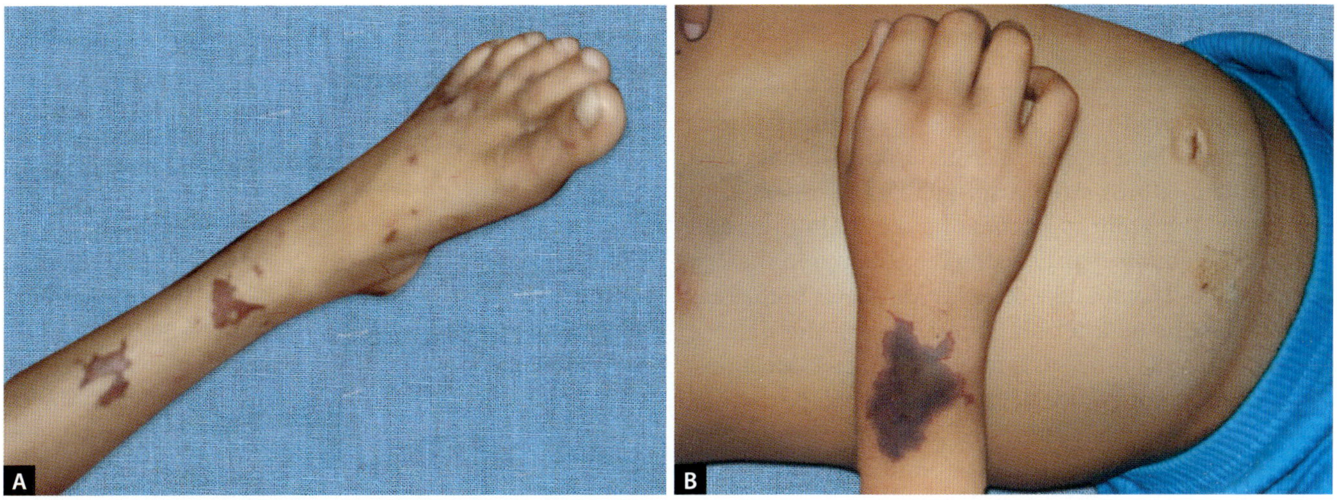

Figs. 13A and B: (A) Cutaneous necrosis in systemic leukocytoclastic vasculitis; (B) Same child, another view.

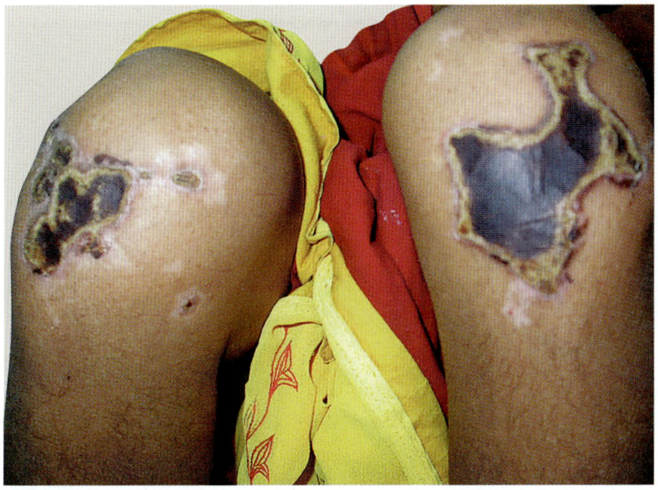

Fig. 14: Case of necrotizing vasculitis.

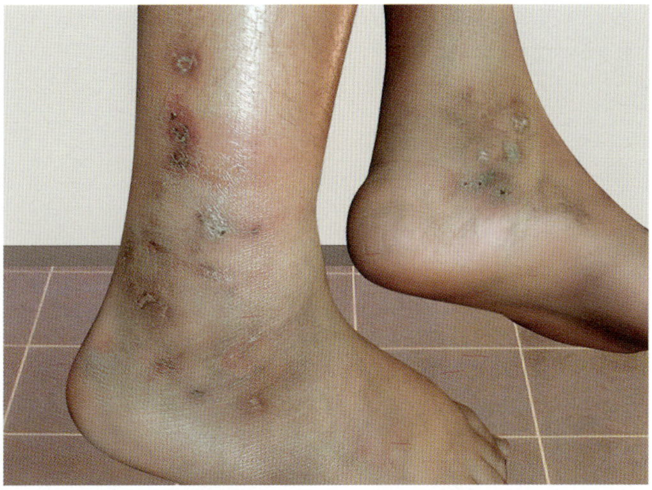

Fig. 15: Livedoid vasculopathy.

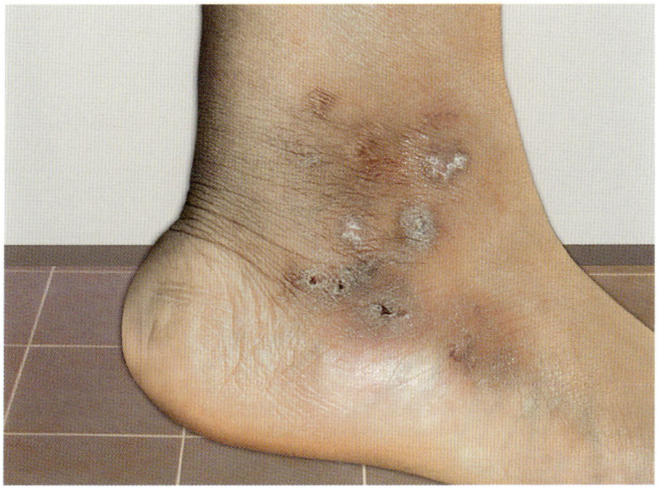

Fig. 16: Close-up view of livedoid vasculopathy.

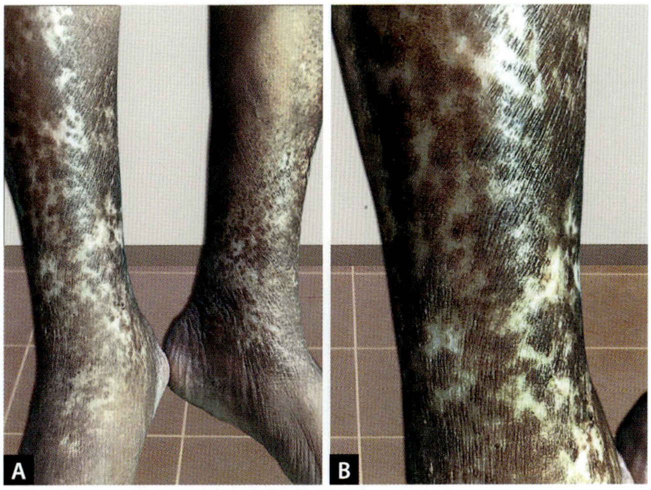

Figs. 17A and B: (A) Porcelain white skin in healed livedoid vasculopathy; (B) Same patient, close-up view.

"If you want to have clean ideas, change them as often as your shirt." —**Francis Picabia**

POLYARTERITIS NODOSA (FIGS. 18A TO D)

Polyarteritis nodosa (PAN) is a systemic disorder characterized by a severe necrotizing inflammation of small and medium sized arteries. It is manifested in two forms, the adult type affecting older children and adults; the infantile type affecting the children in the first 2 years of life. The infantile disease type affects both sexes equally, begins as a febrile illness and as the disease progresses, cardiac arteritis leads to aneurysms, infections, cardiomegaly, congestive heart failure, renal, peripheral artery, and nervous system involvement resulting in hypertension, abnormal urinary findings, peripheral ischemia, neuritis, paralysis, and seizures.

Natural History

The disease is almost always fatal, death resulting from cardiac decompensation. This fact distinguishes infantile PAN from Kawasaki's disease, though many authorities believe the latter to represent a variant of infantile PAN. In the adult type of PAN, there is a male predominance and is manifested by crops of subcutaneous nodules along the course of the superficial arteries of the trunk and extremities, with fever, arthritis, abdominal pain, Raynaud's phenomenon, hypertension, peripheral neuropathy, and myocardial infarction. Cutaneous manifestations are seen in half of the cases, are limited to the lower extremities and range from livedo reticularis, purpura, urticaria and bullae to maculopapular eruptions, necrotic vesicles, pustules,

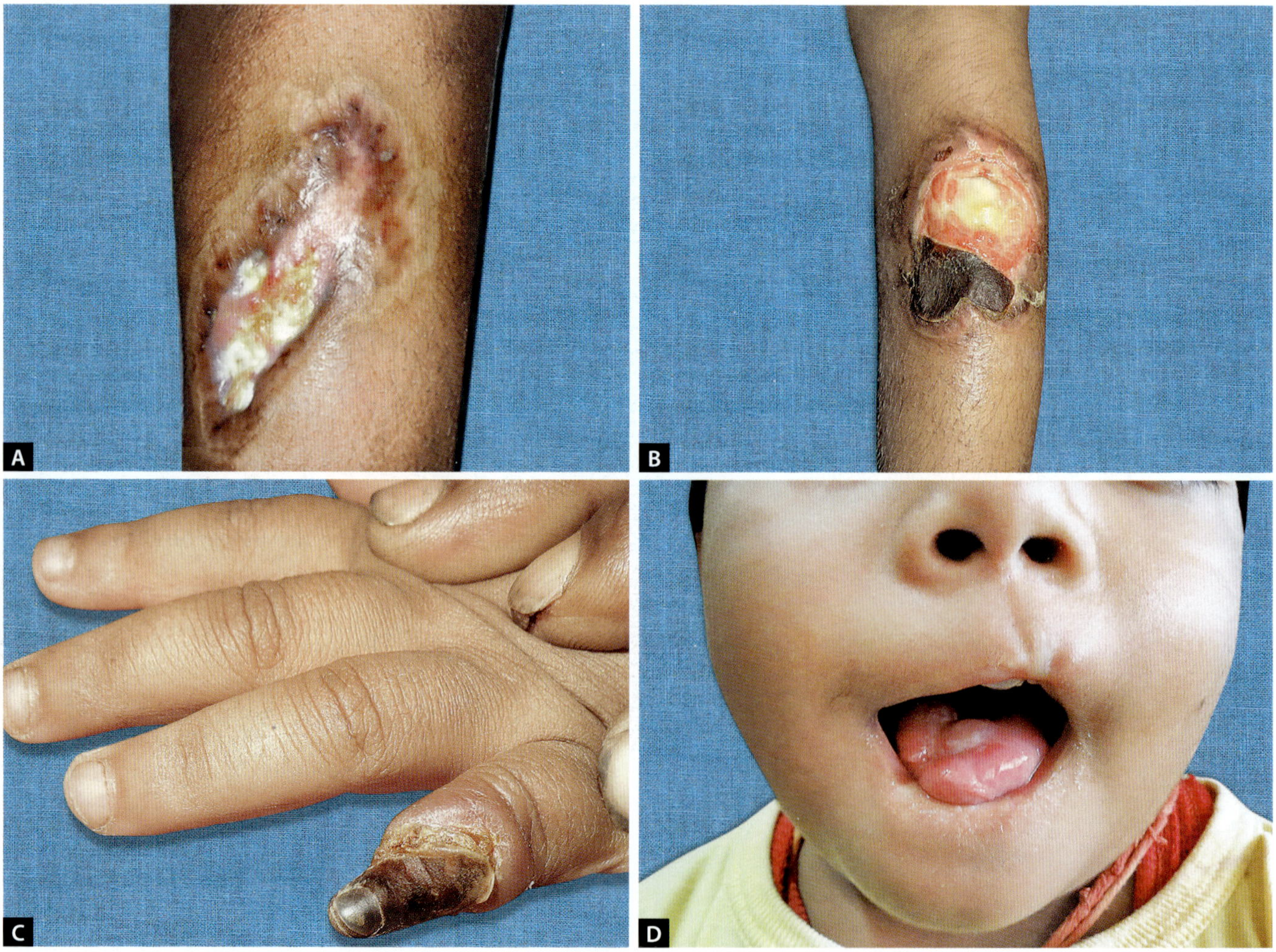

Figs. 18A to D: (A) Necrotic ulcer over leg of cutaneous polyarteritis nodosa (PAN); (B) Necrotic ulcer over knee in PAN; (C) Gangrene of little finger in PAN; (D) Gross destruction of tongue and perioral region in a case of PAN.

"I feel like this: whatever is in your path and in your heart, you need to do." **—J Cole**

subcutaneous nodules and ulceration. Ecchymoses and peripheral gangrene of fingers and toes are the other cutaneous manifestations. Benign cutaneous periarteritis nodosa is a clinical variant in which cutaneous lesions predominate and there is no visceral involvement. The term "nodosa" refers to the focal involvement of blood vessels manifesting as nodular lesions.

Prognosis

The prognosis of polyarteritis has improved with present day therapy.

Management

Supportive treatment and corticosteroids in the dose of 1–2 mg/kg/day of prednisolone or its equivalent forms the mainstay of therapy. When systemic corticosteroids fail, immunosuppressive agents may be used as steroid sparing agents; azathioprine or cyclophosphamide may be used. Other modalities of management include IV gamma globulin, methotrexate, plasma exchange, infliximab, etanercept, adalimumab and rituximab. Aspirin and NSAIDs have been tried in cutaneous PAN without systemic involvement.

PITYRIASIS LICHENOIDES (FIGS. 19A TO D)

Pityriasis lichenoides is a distinctive cutaneous eruption seen in children and young adults characterized by crops of macules, papules, or papulovesicles that tend to develop central necrosis and crusts soon after they arise. The disorder appears in two forms, an acute form seen mainly in children and young adults and a chronic form (commonly noted in adolescents and young adults).

Etiology

A number of theories have been proposed concerning the etiology of pityriasis lichenoides, but all are

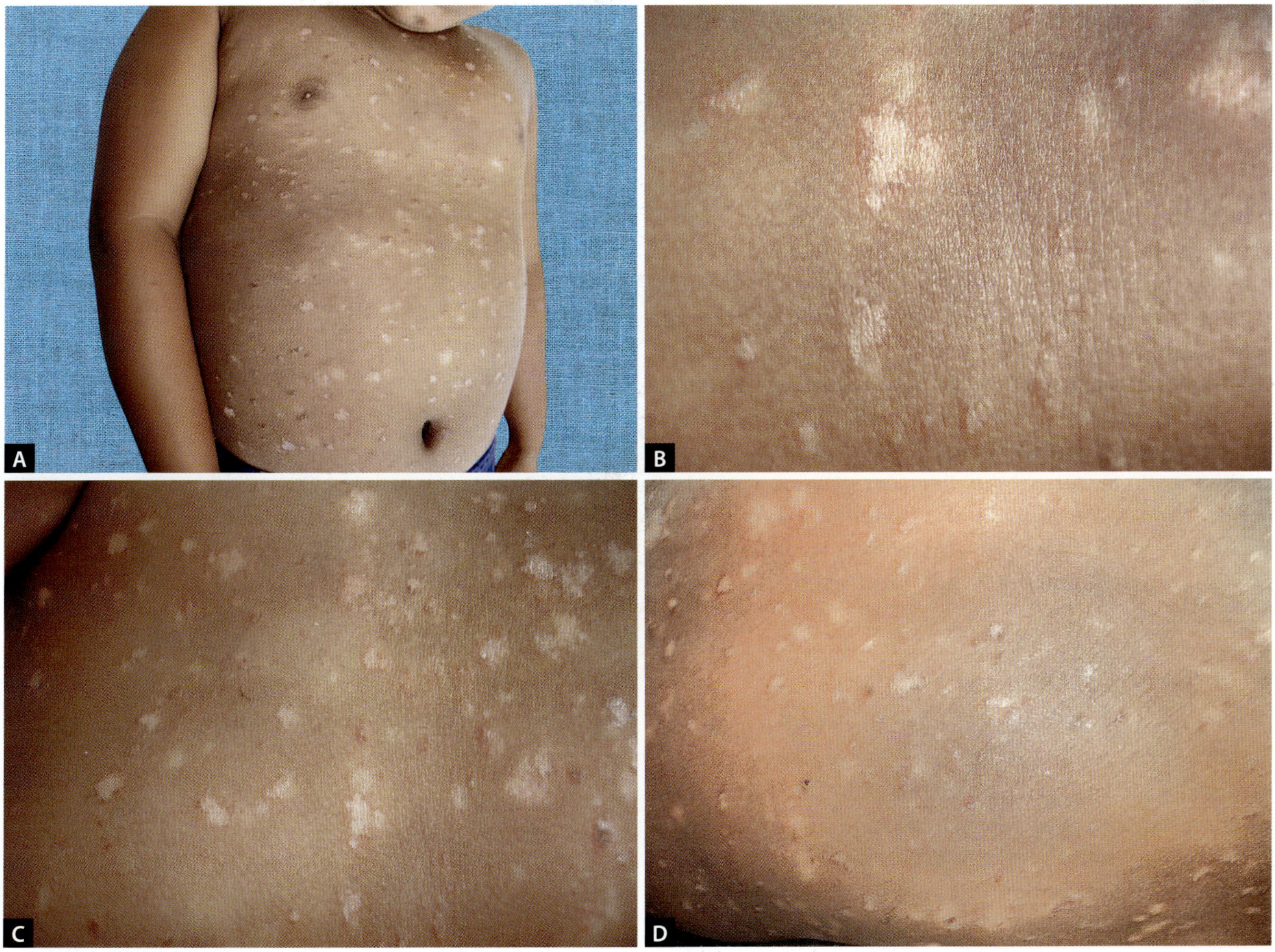

Figs. 19A to D: (A) Pityriasis lichenoides chronica (PLC) in a 5-year-old boy; (B) Close-up view of PLC; (C) PLC; (D) PLC, close-up view.

"Indifference and neglect often do much more damage than outright dislike." **—JK Rowling**

unsubstantiated. The clinical and histologic features suggest a vasculitis. Some authors suggest an autoimmune process, a hypersensitivity reaction triggered by various etiologic factors, or an exanthem of viral or rickettsial etiology.

Clinical Features

Acute pityriasis lichenoides (pityriasis lichenoides et varioliformis acuta, PLEVA) is a polymorphous eruption that usually begins as symmetrical 2–3 mm, oval or round, reddish brown macules and papules. The papules occur in successive crops and rapidly evolve into vesicular, necrotic, and sometimes purpuric lesions. These develop a fine crust and gradually resolve, with or without a varioliform scar. Occasionally temporary hypopigmentation or hyperpigmentation may result. Although the eruption is usually the first manifestation of the disease, occasionally fever and constitutional symptoms may precede or accompany cutaneous eruption. Lesions may involve the entire body but are most pronounced on the trunk, thighs, and upper arm, especially the flexural surfaces. The face, scalp, palms, soles and mucous membrane are frequently spared. The prognosis is generally good.

Chronic pityriasis lichenoides (pityriasis lichenoides chronica) may begin de novo or may evolve from pityriasis lichenoides acuta. The course of chronic pityriasis lichenoides is variable and may last for 6 months to several years. It begins with smooth and slightly firm, reddish papules that measure several millimeters to a centimeter in diameter. Scales when present are adherent, are slightly thicker in the center, and can be detached by gentle scraping to reveal a shiny brown surface (a diagnostic feature of this disorder.) Over a period of several weeks the individual papules recede, the skin separates spontaneously and a hyperpigmented or hypopigmented macule results and eventually fades without residual scar.

Differential Diagnosis

In the early stages pityriasis lichenoides may be mistaken for chicken pox, arthropod bites, impetigo, pityriasis rosea, allergic vasculitis, or scabies. Chronic forms may be confused with psoriasis, lichen planus, and secondary syphilis. The duration of the eruption (when in crops), the presence of macules and papules interspersed with vesicular, crusted, or hemorrhagic lesions with or without varioliform scarring and subsequent hypopigmentation help to differentiate pityriasis lichenoides from other conditions. When the diagnosis remains in doubt, histopathologic examination of a skin biopsy specimen usually substantiates the proper diagnosis.

Treatment

Antipruritics, nonsteroidal anti-inflammatory agents, and lubricants may be helpful in ameliorating the symptoms, and topical corticosteroids, tar preparations, sun exposure, ultraviolet light, and PUVA phototherapy have been effective for the treatment of persistent or chronic forms of the disorder. Tetracycline in high doses (2 g/day for older children and adults) and erythromycin (30–50 mg/kg/day, with a maximum of 1 or 2 g/day for older children and adults) for several weeks to 2 months are frequently helpful, particularly in the acute forms of the disorder. Methotrexate, in dosages of 7.5–20 mg weekly, has resulted in improvement in persistent cases. NBUVB therapy is beneficial in pityriasis lichenoides chronica.

ANTIPHOSPHOLIPID ANTIBODY SYNDROME (FIGS. 20 AND 21)

The APS is an autoimmune condition characterized by recurrent thromboembolic events. The exact incidence of its occurrence in the pediatric age group in Indian population is not known. Due to the higher incidence of infections in this age group there is a higher incidence of APL antibodies (APLAs) while the patients are asymptomatic, thereby making the establishment of diagnosis challenging. Secondary APS is associated with underlying SLE. Due to the higher incidence of positivity of APLAs in children, it

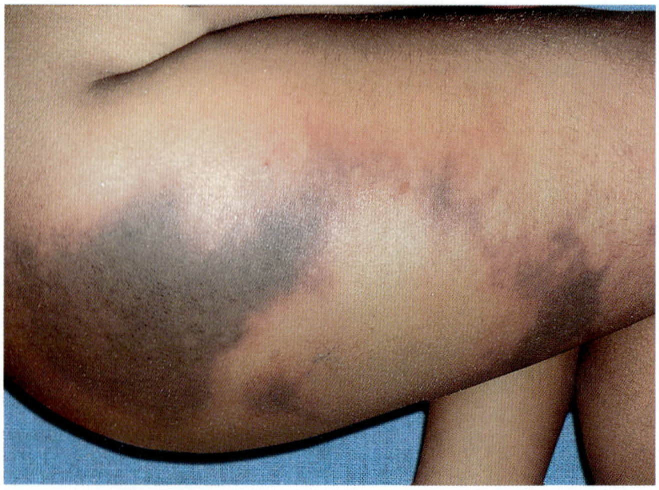

Fig. 20: Antiphospholipid antibody syndrome.

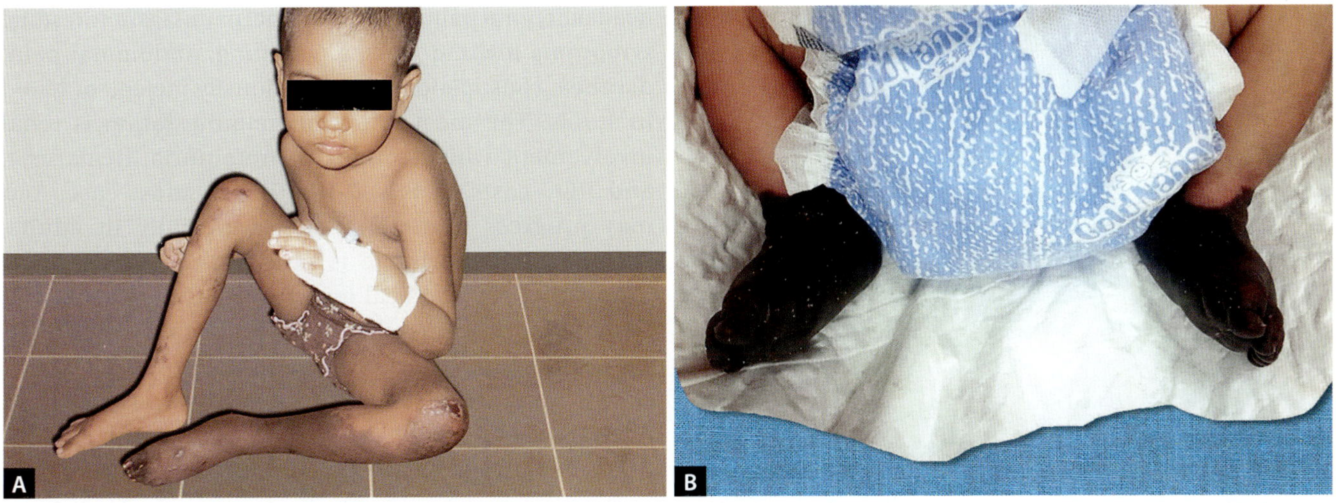

Figs. 21A and B: (A) A 5-year-old girl with antiphospholipid antibody syndrome (APS); (B) Gangrene of both feet in APLA syndrome.

is advised to conduct the diagnostic tests twice. Varying cutaneous features and lack of adequate awareness regarding the presenting signs and symptoms in pediatric population makes the diagnosis difficult. There are no guidelines for the management of this condition in children, and it is extrapolated from the guidelines used in the adults. Early detection of this condition helps in reducing morbidity and improving the care and management of the patient.

Antiphospholipid antibodies are defined as a group of antibodies directed against epitopes on plasma proteins that are uncovered by binding of these proteins to anionic phospholipids on plasma membranes. The most commonly used tests, to detect APL, include lupus anticoagulant (LAC), anticardiolipin (ACL) antibodies, and anti-β_2-glycoprotein I (GPI) antibodies. An accurate data on the true prevalence of the APS is unavailable due to the paucity of guidelines and disease detection criteria. The prevalence of anticardiolipin antibodies in various thrombotic conditions has been reported to be between 25.5 and 51.5%. Noncutaneous features include thrombotic events in the form of pulmonary thromboembolism, strokes, retinal vein, and artery thrombosis. Hematological abnormalities include thrombocytopenia, autoimmune hemolytic anemia, and leukocytopenia. Neurologic manifestations include headaches, seizures, and chorea.

Thrombosis has been attributed as the major clinical feature of APS with recurrence of thrombosis occurring in almost 20% of patients. A very small group of people with APLAs develop multiple clots in different organ systems throughout the body within a matter of days. This is called catastrophic APS syndrome.

APS manifesting in children with only cutaneous manifestation is generally rare. Cutaneous manifestations include gangrene, ulceration, livedo reticularis, thrombophlebitis, necrotic purpura, Raynaud phenomenon, leukocytoclastic vasculitis (LCV), Degos-like ulceration and pyoderma gangrenosum-like ulceration. Raynaud phenomenon and livedo reticularis represent the most common skin manifestations.

Children with catastrophic APS are managed with intravenous anticoagulation and plasmapheresis. The long-term management of APS has been advised with oral warfarin sodium.

HENOCH–SCHÖNLEIN PURPURA (FIGS. 22 TO 25)

It is a small vessel vasculitis affecting the skin, joint, gastrointestinal tract, and kidneys. Infections such as Group A streptococci, mycoplasma, EBV, varicella virus, parvovirus B_{19}, *Campylobacter*, *Helicobacter pylori*, *Bartonella henselae*; vaccination with typhoid, cholera, measles, yellow fever vaccine; insect bites, drugs such as penicillins, macrolides, and aspirin have been implicated. The triggers cause IgA immune complex deposition in the tissues. Children between the age of 4 and 8 years are commonly affected. Crops of lesions occur chiefly on the lower extremities that start as palpable purpura, becomes hemorrhagic in a day and starts fading in a few days. In 40% cases the cutaneous lesions are preceded by mild fever,

"And when they played they really played. And when they worked they really worked." —**Dr Seuss**

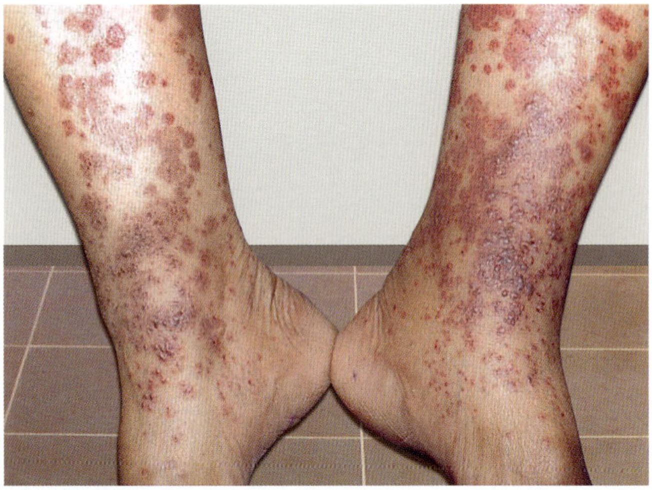

Fig. 22: Henoch–Schönlein purpura (HSP) over lower legs and ankle.

headache, joint pain, and abdominal pain. Gastrointestinal symptoms include nausea, vomiting, abdominal pain, diarrhea, constipation, and occasionally melena or blood in stools. The most important manifestation is renal involvement which produces proteinuria, hematuria, and RBC casts. It is self-limiting in most cases but may progress to renal failure especially in adults. Pulmonary hemorrhage is rare but can be fatal. On histopathology, classical features of LCV are seen with immunofluorescence demonstrating deposition of IgA, C3 in the vessel walls of the lesional and perilesional skin. Though a self-limiting condition lasting from 6 to 16 weeks, about 5–10% will have recurrence or persistence. Dapsone, colchicine can improve cutaneous lesions. Corticosteroids are useful in abdominal pain,

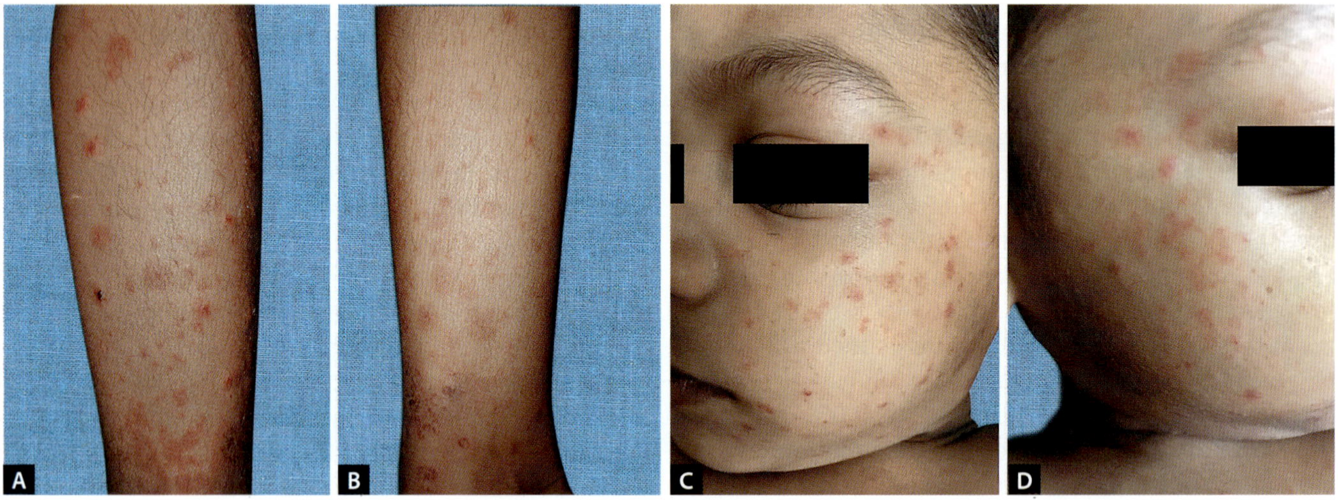

Figs. 23A to D: (A) Palpable purpura of Henoch–Schönlein purpura (HSP); (B) Same child, another view; (C) HSP over face; (D) Same child, another view.

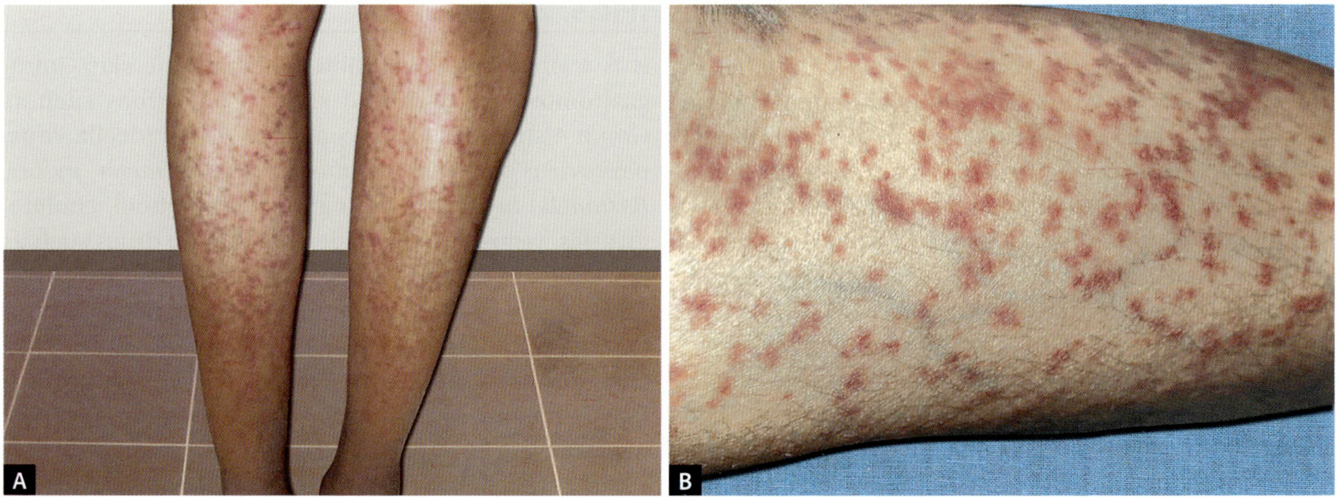

Figs. 24A and B: (A) Henoch–Schönlein purpura in an adolescent girl; (B) Close-up view of lesions.

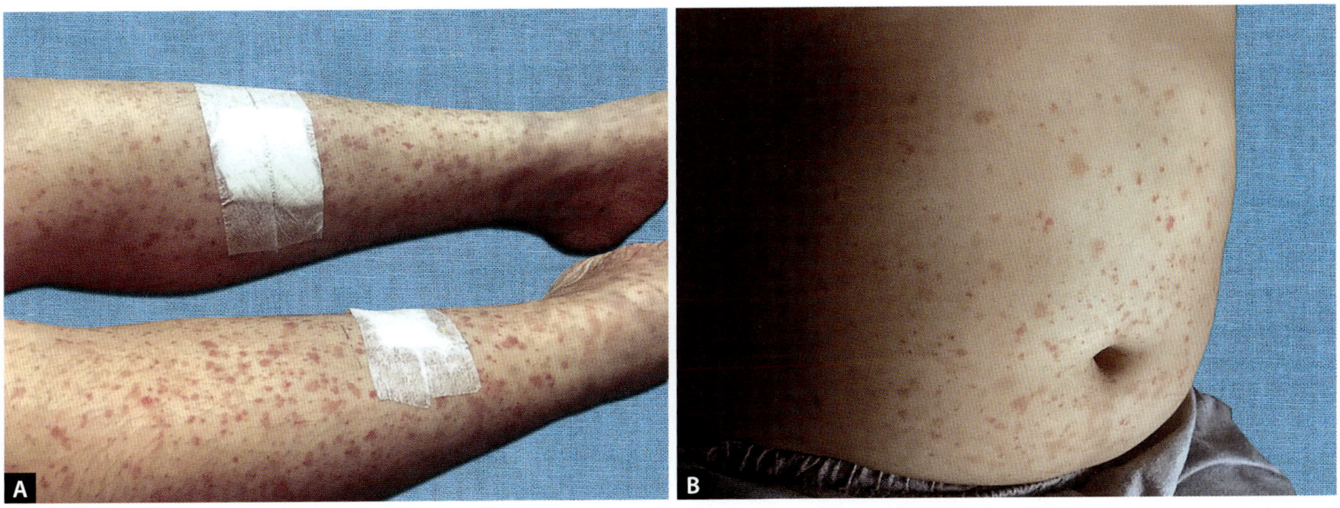

Figs. 25A and B: (A) Henoch–Schönlein purpura (HSP) over legs; (B) HSP over trunk.

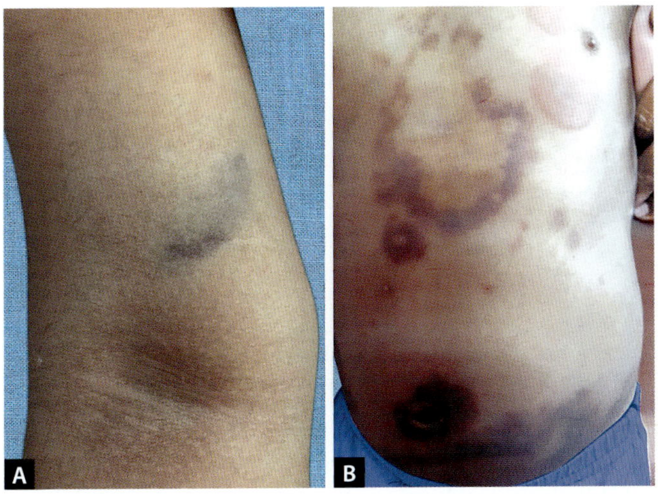

Figs. 26A and B: (A) Lesions of acute hemorrhagic edema of infancy; (B) Same baby, trunk lesions.

however, their role in renal disease is controversial. IVIg has been tried with some success in patients with abdominal pain. All children with HSP should be followed up for 6 months as systemic involvement can occur later even though the skin lesions have subsided.

ACUTE HEMORRHAGIC EDEMA OF INFANCY (FIGS. 26A AND B)

Acute hemorrhagic edema of infancy (AHEI) is an acute, benign small vessel LCV, mainly occurring in males between the ages of 3 months and 2 years. Exact etiology is unknown. But triggering factors include prior bacterial or viral infections mostly upper respiratory tract and urinary infection, drugs and vaccination. Painless nonpitting edema of the face and scrotum may be the first clinical sign of AHEI. Then there is appearance of nonpruritic annular purpuric plaques with well-defined borders and central vascular patterns, called as medallion-like lesions. These ecchymotic or cockade or targetoid lesions mainly affect the extremities, face, and ears. The trunk is usually spared and mucosal involvement is rare. Overall general condition is good and the child appears nontoxic. Skin biopsy shows features of LCV with fibrinoid necrosis and neutrophilic infiltration of the vessel wall. Differential diagnoses of AHEI include HSP, meningococcemia, and erythema multiforme, urticarial vasculitis, Sweet's syndrome, and drug eruption. But HSP is the foremost contender. Age of onset of AHEI (2–24 months) is lower when compared to HSP (4–7 years); again clinically distinguished by skin lesions (medallion-like lesions with edema in AHEI vs. smaller purpuric lesions in HSP). There is no effective treatment for AHEI and symptomatic care has been advocated. There is a need of recognizing this benign disorder early to avoid unnecessary investigations and medications and to properly counsel the parents to alleviate their anxiety and apprehension. Spontaneous recovery usually occurs within 1–3 weeks without any scars. Relapse of the disease may occur.

IDIOPATHIC THROMBOCYTOPENIC PURPURA (FIGS. 27 AND 28)

Idiopathic thrombocytopenic purpura (ITP) is known as autoimmune or immune thrombocytopenia. It is

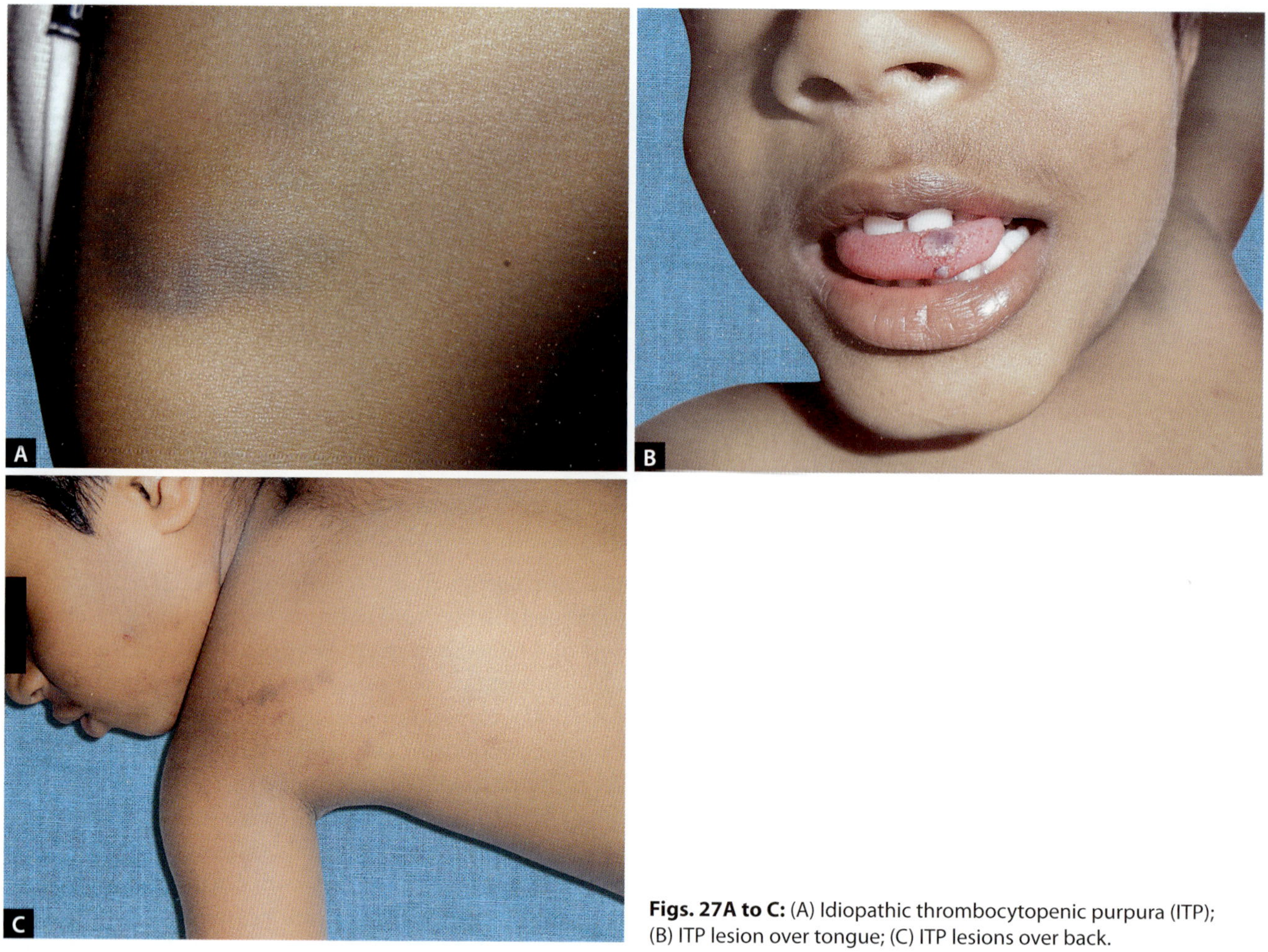

Figs. 27A to C: (A) Idiopathic thrombocytopenic purpura (ITP); (B) ITP lesion over tongue; (C) ITP lesions over back.

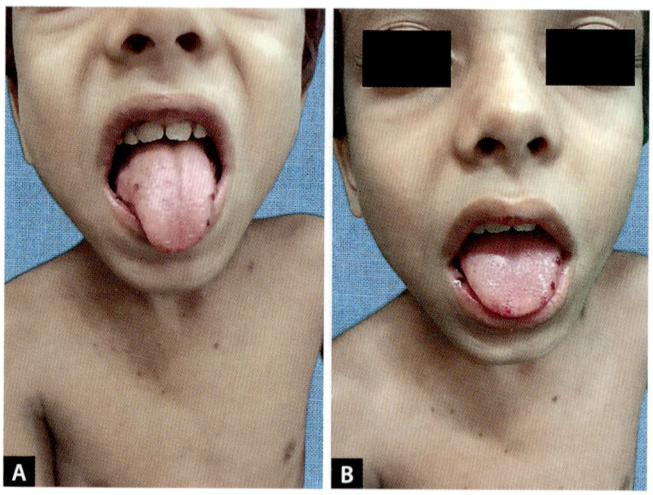

Figs. 28A and B: (A) Idiopathic thrombocytopenic purpura (ITP), note hemorrhagic spots over tongue; (B) Same child, close-up view.

no longer known as idiopathic. It has an incidence of 6.4 per 100,000 children. ITP is mediated by platelet autoantibodies that accelerate platelet destruction and inhibit their production. It is a diagnosis of exclusion. Primary ITP occurs in the absence of secondary cause. Secondary thrombocytopenia occurs following viral illness, drug intake, recent immunization, and primary immunodeficiency disorder.

Idiopathic thrombocytopenic purpura occurs at any age. It is more common in boys than girls. In children most cases are acute in onset. It is manifested by bleeding tendency that correlate with the severity of thrombocytopenia. Clinically presents with sudden onset of purpura without trauma, petechiae, ecchymoses, gingival bleeding, and hemorrhagic bullae on the oral mucosa. Complication such as intracranial hemorrhage may be fatal. Cutaneous features may mimic child abuse and should be differentiated from ITP. Investigation showing isolated thrombocytopenia indicates ITP.

Majority of children achieve spontaneous remission. These children should be regularly followed-up.

Treatment modalities include IVIg, oral steroids, immunosuppressants, and chemotherapeutic agents. Splenectomy is the definitive treatment of ITP when it is refractory to medical measures.

ECCHYMOSIS (FIGS. 29A TO C)

Also known as "bruise", represents an area of skin discoloration larger than 1 cm. They may be painful to touch. Usually ecchymosis will change colors and disappear as the blood collected in the skin gets reabsorbed. The progression of color changes occur like red to purple, black to blue, and brown. Ecchymoses are common over arms and legs since they are most likely to be injured. Bruising can also occur when one sustains injury over a bone, especially over wrist or ankle. Some young girls and boys are more prone to develop ecchymoses on slightest trauma, sometimes even too trivial to remember. However, if there is recurrent ecchymoses in a child, underlying coagulation defect/disorder needs to be ruled out.

ERYTHEMA ELEVATUM DIUTINUM (FIGS. 30A TO C)

Erythema elevatum diutinum (EED) is a rare chronic dermatosis mainly affecting adults. Children are rarely affected. Characteristic skin lesions are asymptomatic (pain is occasional), plum colored erythematous nodules, and plaques of variable size distributed symmetrically over extensors of extremities particularly over the joints, dorsal hands and feet, knees and elbows, buttocks (rarely back) and Achilles tendon; Occasionally face, pinnae of ears may be affected. The initial soft lesions eventuate to become fibrotic and develop atrophic scarring. Characteristic histologic features of LCV with some fibrin deposition and eosinophilic infiltrate in the upper and mid-dermis are seen in early lesions while capillary proliferation, inflammatory infiltrate of macrophages, plasma cells, and lymphocytes, and perivascular eosinophilic fibrosis are hallmark features of chronic lesions. Clinicopathologic correlation is important for the diagnosis as EED lesions

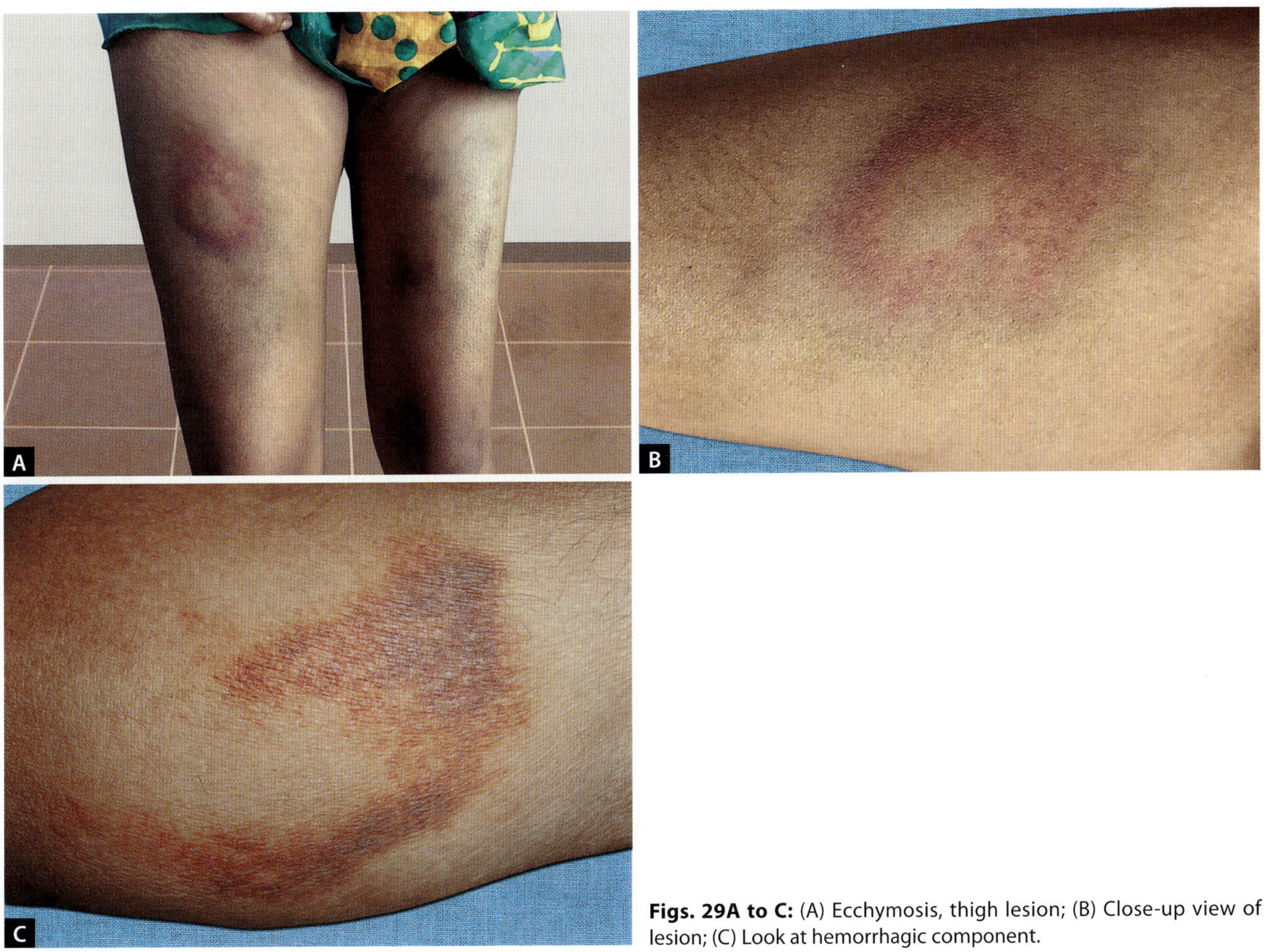

Figs. 29A to C: (A) Ecchymosis, thigh lesion; (B) Close-up view of lesion; (C) Look at hemorrhagic component.

"Courage and cheerfulness will not only carry you over the rough places in life, but will enable you to bring comfort and help to the weak-hearted and will console you in the sad hours." —**William Osler**

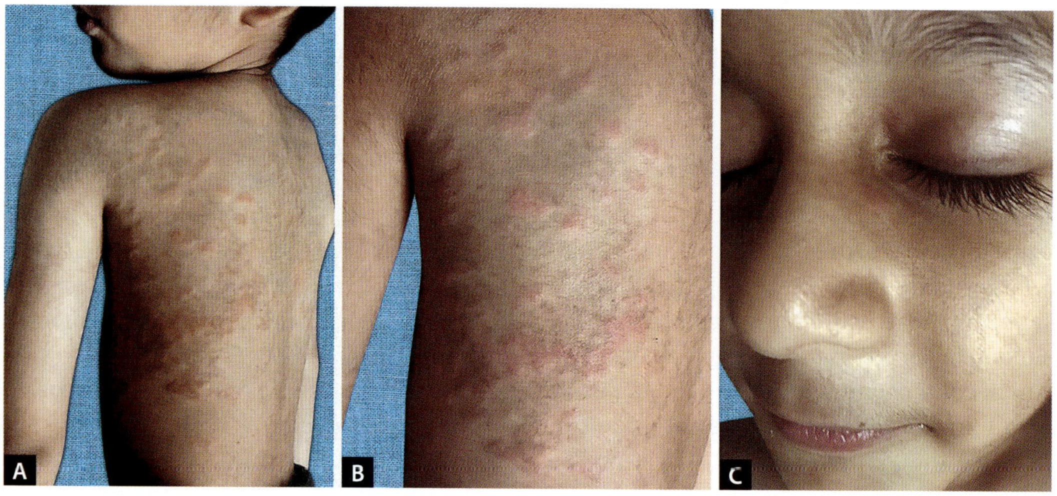

Figs. 30A to C: (A) Infiltrated lesions of erythema elevatum diutinum (EED) over back in a 7-year-old boy; (B) Same boy, close-up view of lesions; (C) Lesions over face.

may sometimes mimic cutaneous sarcoidosis, leprosy, DLE or psoriasis. Histologically it may be difficult to differentiate other forms of small vessel vasculitis and Sweet's syndrome. The etiopathogenesis of EED remains obscure and has been attributed to Arthus-like immune complex reaction and ensuing fibrin deposition. It has been reportedly associated with a number of autoimmune diseases (rheumatoid arthritis, celiac and inflammatory bowel disease, diabetes mellitus), infections (syphilis, *Streptococcus*, hepatitis, HIV infection), malignancies (multiple myeloma, B-cell lymphoma, breast carcinoma, myelodysplasia), monoclonal gammopathies, hypergammaglobulinemia, pyoderma gangrenosum, and relapsing polychondritis. IgA monoclonal gammopathy is found in a significant number of EED patients and some workers even advocate routine immunoelectrophoresis testing for it. Dapsone has remarkable therapeutic effect and remains mainstay of the treatment. However, resurgence is common on its discontinuation. Sulfapyridine, colchicine or cyclosporine are also found useful. Potent topical or intralesional corticosteroids are useful for the limited disease. Systemic corticosteroids generally are not effective.

DEGOS DISEASE IN INFANTS AND CHILDREN (FIGS. 31A TO C)

Degos disease, or malignant atrophic papulosis (MAP), is a rare thrombo-obliterative vasculopathy manifesting as a primary dermatological disorder in most cases. It has two variants: Cutaneous MAP is manifested in the skin alone, whereas systemic MAP affects the gastrointestinal tract, central nervous system, lungs, and other internal organs. Some patients who present with only cutaneous symptoms at first may develop systemic symptoms several years later. The exact pathology is not clear, although three most suggested hypotheses about the pathophysiology of the disease are vasculitis, coagulopathy and primary dysfunction of the endothelial cells. It starts as pale-rose round edematous papules, sometimes preceded by slight burning. Sites affected are trunk and limbs sparing face, palms, and soles. The lesions eventually progress to ulceration followed by porcelain white scarring with peripheral livid red and telangiectatic rim. MAP has been treated by several medical treatments, including antiplatelet agents (aspirin, dipyridamole, and clopidogrel), anticoagulants (heparin and warfarin), and immunosuppressants (corticosteroids, azathioprine, and methotrexate). No treatment has shown satisfactory response except eculizumab. It is a potentially life-threatening disease. The prognosis highly depends on the associated systemic involvement.

WHAT'S NEW

- *Anifrolumab*, a human monoclonal antibody that specifically targets the type I interferon receptor, has been linked to rapid clinical improvement in patients with *DLE*. This improvement is attributed to anifrolumab's selective inhibition of type I interferon signaling, a well-known factor associated with DLE disease activity.

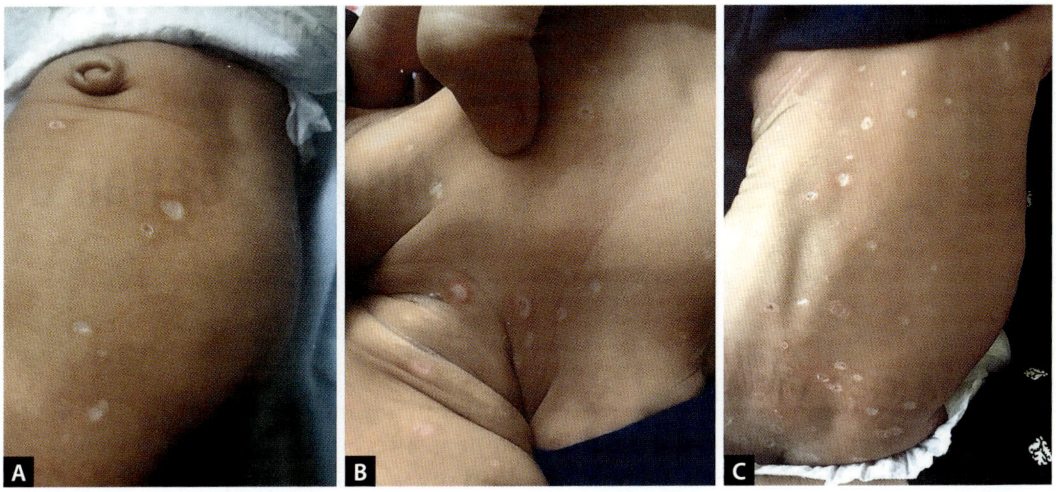

Figs. 31A to C: (A) Porcelain white macules of Degos disease in a 2-month-old infant; (B) Close-up view of lesions, note rim of erythema around a few lesions; (C) Same baby, note necrotic appearance of lesions over the back.

- *Baricitinib in JDM: Baricitinib*, a *Janus kinase inhibitor (JAKi)*, has shown promise in the treatment of *JDM*, a systemic vasculopathy characterized by weakness and rash with minimal adverse effects particularly in cases that are refractory to other treatment modalities.
- *Efficacy of topical ruxolitinib for cutaneous dermatomyositis*: While oral *ruxolitinib*, a *JAKi*, has been used for refractory adult and pediatric dermatomyositis, there has been limited investigation into the use of *topical ruxolitinib* for cutaneous manifestations. Topical treatment has the benefits of decreased mean plasma concentrations with low incidence of adverse events. Topical ruxolitinib presents with minimal adverse effects such as folliculitis, diarrhea and eosinophilia and therefore, can be considered as a safer alternaltive to oral ruxolitinib.

SUGGESTED READINGS

1. Cooper N, Ghanima W. Immunethrombocytopenia. N Engl J Med. 2019;381(10):945-55.
2. Li SC. Scleroderma in children and adolescents: localized scleroderma and systemic sclerosis. Pediatr Clin North Am.2018;65(4):757-81.
3. Tarvin SE, O'Neil KM. Systemic lupus erythematosus, Sjögren syndrome, and mixed connective tissue disease in children and adolescents. Pediatr Clin North Am. 2018;65(4):711-37.
4. Shaw KS, Rajeh A, Le T, Kahn PJ, Oza VS, Arkin LM, et al. Anifrolumab for Adolescent Discoid Lupus Erythematosus. JAMA Network Open. 2023;6(10):e2338200.
5. Kim H, Dill S, O'Brien M, Vian L, Li X, Manukyan M, et al. Janus kinase (JAK) inhibition with baricitinib in refractory juvenile dermatomyositis. Annals of the rheumatic diseases. 2021;80(3):406-8.
6. Lanis A, Kim H, Lu S, Tsai WL, Kaneshiro A, Ehrlich A, et al. Efficacy of topical ruxolitinib for cutaneous dermatomyositis. JAAD Case Reports. 2024;45:24-6.

CHAPTER 16

Diseases of Hair and Nail

ALOPECIA AREATA (FIGS. 1 TO 4)

Alopecia areata (AA) is a common disorder seen in children characterized by localized loss of hair. It presents as a circumscribed, bald, smooth patch often noticed by chance by the parents. Exclamation-mark hairs may be present at its margin. Subsequently, the initial patch may regrow or further new patches may appear after an interval of 3–6 weeks. Hairs regrown initially are often gray. It is frequently associated with atopy, autoimmunity, and family history of hypertension. It should be differentiated from tinea capitis and trichotillomania.

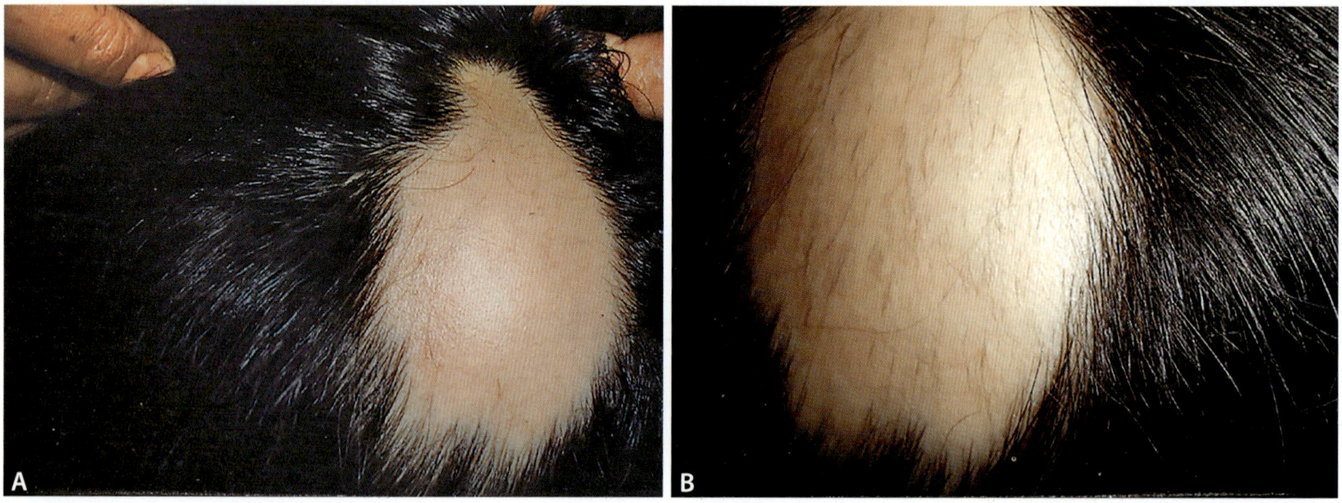

Figs. 1A and B: (A) Patch of alopecia areata over the scalp in a 10-year-old boy; (B) Growth of hairs in an alopecia areata (AA) patch.

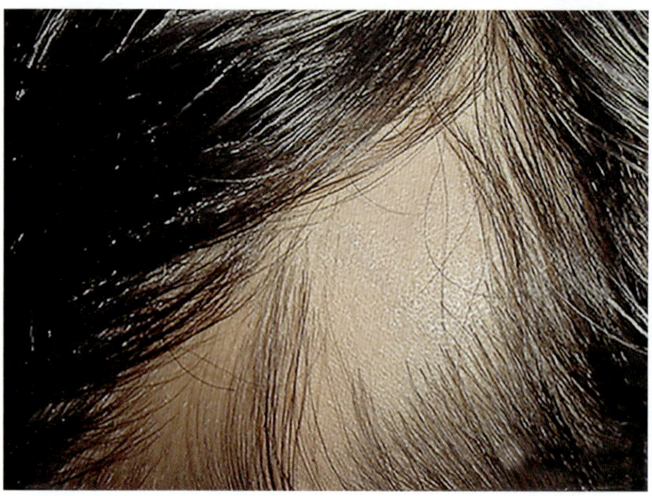

Fig. 2: Patch of alopecia areata (AA), note regrowth of hairs.

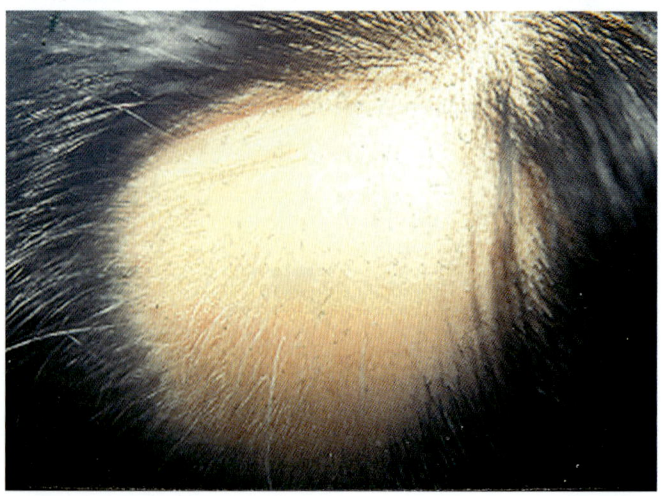

Fig. 3: Regrowth of hairs (gray in color) in a patch of alopecia areata (AA).

"Life is pure adventure, and the sooner we realize that, the sooner we will be able to treat life as art." —**Maya Angelou**

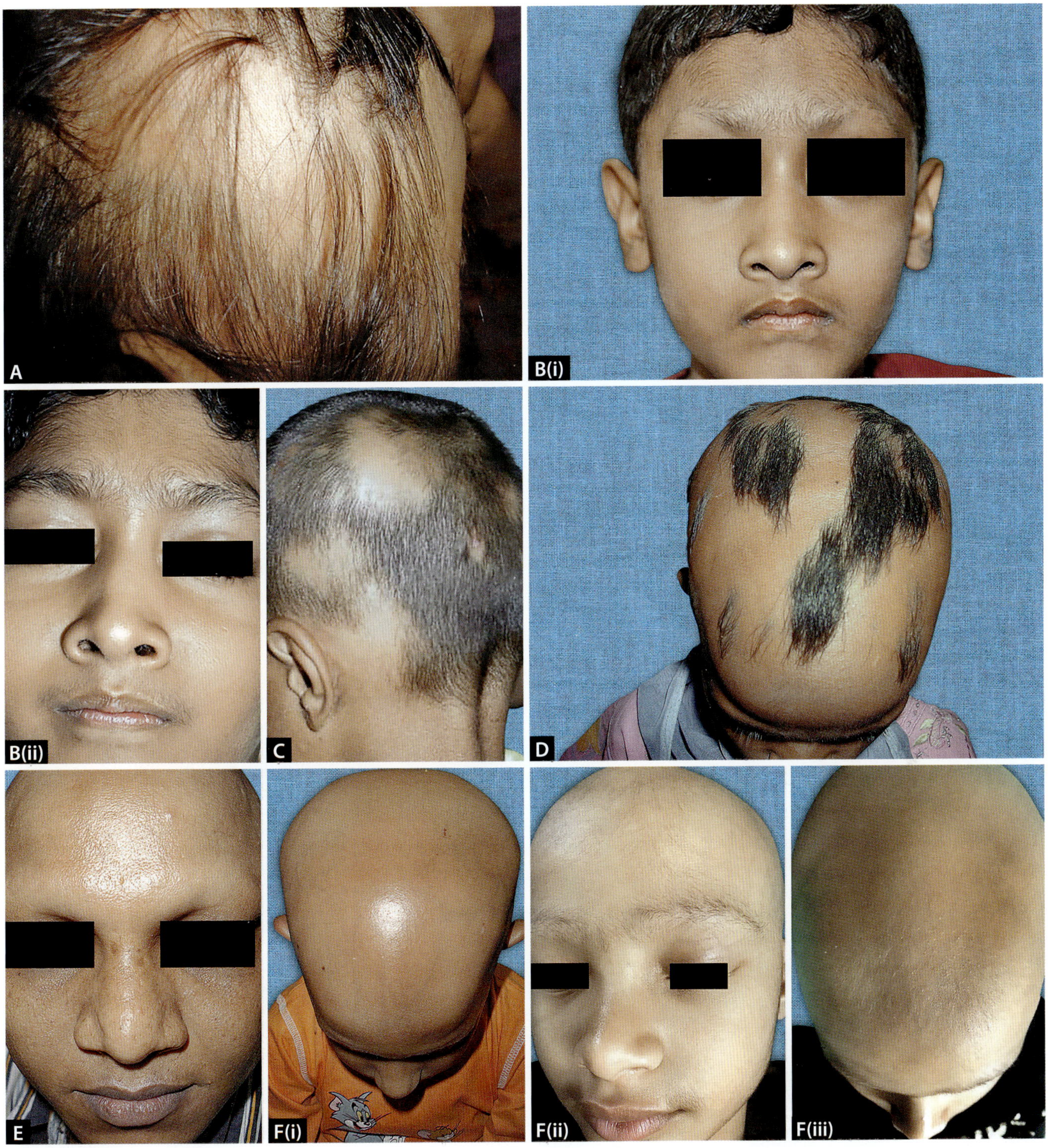

Figs. 4A to F(iii): (A) Ophiasis involving occipital region of scalp in a 9-year-old boy; B(i) Alopecia areata (AA) of eyebrows; B(ii) Same boy after treatment for 6 months; (C) Multiple patches of AA over scalp; (D) Extensive alopecia areata, almost going to alopecia totalis; (E) Alopecia universalis in a 17-year-old boy; F(i) Alopecia totalis in a 4-year-old boy; F(ii and iii) Alopecia totalis.

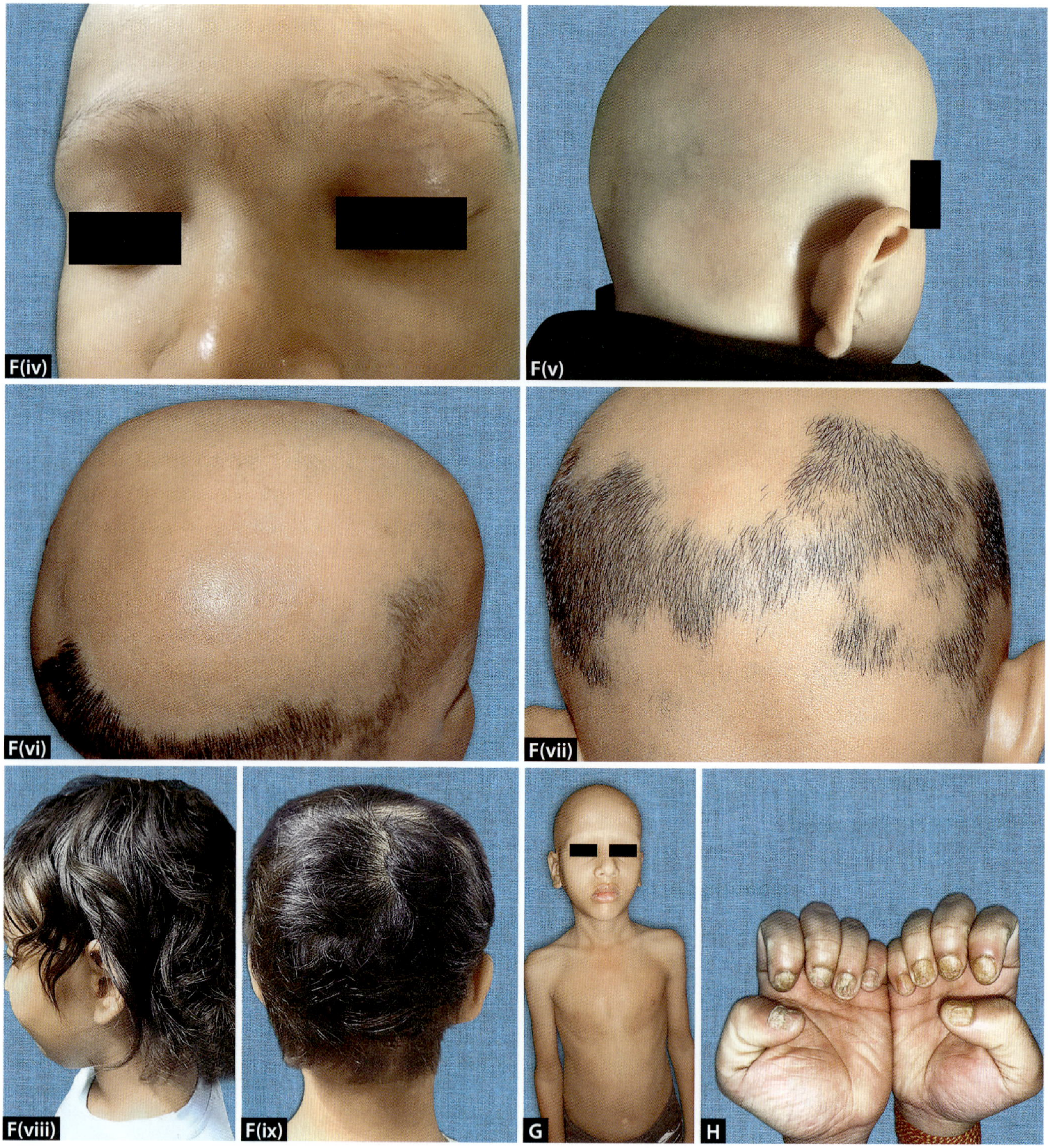

Figs. 4F(iv) to H: F(iv) Alopecia totalis (AT), regrowth of eyebrows with oral cyclosporine; F(v) AT, occipital area; F(vi) Good regrowth of hairs over occipital area with cyclosporine; F(vii) Further regrowth; F(viii) A 7-year-old girl with AT, treatment with cyclosporine A (CsA) rotationally—after 2 years; F(ix) Same girl, occipital area; (G) Alopecia universalis; (H) Sandpaper nails in adolescent with alopecia areata (AA) totalis.

Natural History

The course of the disease is unpredictable and new patches may appear when old patches start growing hair spontaneously. The newly grown hair may be gray or white but usually repigment by 2–6 months. Bad prognostic signs are early age at onset, large size and number of patches, band-like involvement over occipital region (ophiasis), sisaipho (ophiasis inversus), extensive involvement (alopecia totalis and universalis), or associated systemic autoimmune diseases (thyroiditis, lupus erythematosus, Down syndrome, pernicious anemia, and ulcerative colitis).

Treatment and Prognosis

Treatment consists of application of moderately potent topical corticosteroid for 4–6 weeks, intralesional triamcinolone acetonide injection every 3–4 weeks for 2-3 months. (this therapy is not preferred in younger children). Other modalities of treatment for extensive and recalcitrant AA include photochemotherapy (PUVA), cyclosporine, dithranol, topical minoxidil, or diphencyprone. Recently, newer therapies such as Janus kinase (JAK) inhibitors (tofacitinib) have shown promising results. Counseling forms the main stay of management.

Course of AA is unpredictable having spontaneous remission and relapse and the plethora of treatment modalities shows lack of adequate efficacy. In childhood, AA is a matter of concern due to its bad prognosis, associated atopy, psychological impact, and poor response to therapy. Localized AA can be treated with topical agents or reassurance as in many patients, it resolves without treatment. Children <10 years of age are generally treated with topical steroids, with second-line options including topical anthralin, topical minoxidil, and topical retinoids. In selected cases, systemic therapy is considered. In children older than 10 years apart from the above-mentioned therapies, intralesional steroids, contact immunotherapy such as squaric acid dibutyl ester or excimer laser can also be considered. Other treatment options include topical and systemic tacrolimus, tumor necrosis factor alpha (TNF-α) inhibitors, topical latanoprost, and topical 5-fluorouracil. Oral cyclosporine A (CsA) has been used as third line of management in alopecia areata. Its documented adverse effect of hypertrichosis by prolongation of anagen phase of hair growth cycle can add to its use in AA. Safety and efficacy of CsA in pediatric age group has been proven in atopic dermatitis and psoriasis. Attributing to decreased sensitivity to CsA, higher clearance, and decreased bioavailability, children are less susceptible to CsA-induced nephropathy than adults.

SCARRING ALOPECIA (FIGS. 5A TO C)

This is also known as cicatricial alopecia. This is the end result of a number of inflammatory processes in and around the pilosebaceous units. This type of alopecia develops as a result of irreversible destruction of hair follicular tissue and consequent permanent scarring with loss of hair on the affected areas. It is commonly seen in adults over the age of 20 years, less in children. This disease may be the result of a developmental defect (aplasia cutis); inflammatory changes of infective origin, like viral or fungal infection; physical trauma (irradiation, trichotillomania practiced over a long period of time, thermal or caustic burns); neoplastic disorders; various dermatoses such as (lichen planus, lupus erythematosus, localized or systemic scleroderma); or various dermatological conditions, e.g., keratosis pilaris atrophicans, folliculitis decalvans, dissecting cellulitis of the scalp, acne keloidalis, pseudopelade, and alopecia mucinosa.

Treatment

It is extremely difficult to induce regrowth of hair over the patches of scarring alopecia. Intralesional injection of triamcinolone acetonide (10 mg/mL) is of some help in selected cases. Hair transplant may show some result in few cases. Cosmetic camouflage is useful.

PSEUDOPELADE OF BROCQ (FIG. 5A)

Pseudopelade of Brocq is a slowly progressive cicatricial alopecia without clinically evident folliculitis and no marked inflammation. It is uncommon in children. It is often noticed by a parent as a small bald patch. The progression of the patches is very slow. The affected patches are smooth, soft, and slightly depressed and are round or oval in shape.

Treatment

The response to treatment is usually not very exciting. Infiltration of triamcinolone acetonide in a 2.5 mg/mL concentration into active areas at 6–8 weeks interval may be temporarily beneficial. Autografting or surgical expansion techniques can be considered.

"The woods are lovely, dark and deep. But I have promises to keep, and miles to go before I sleep." —**Robert Frost**

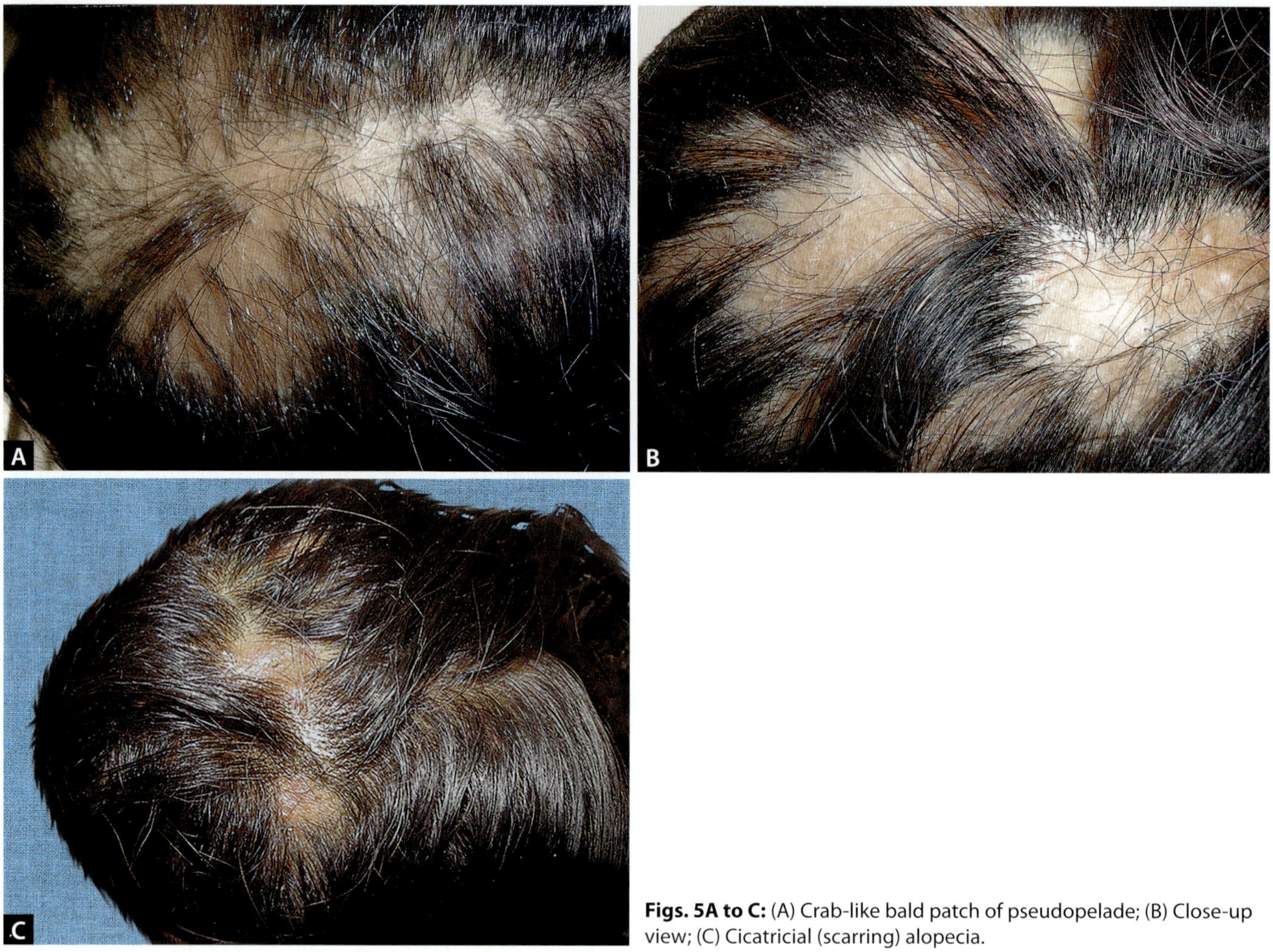

Figs. 5A to C: (A) Crab-like bald patch of pseudopelade; (B) Close-up view; (C) Cicatricial (scarring) alopecia.

SEBORRHEIC ALOPECIA (FIGS. 6A AND B)

Seborrheic alopecia is a type of inflammatory alopecia seen in adults and adolescent age group. It is less commonly seen in children. This condition is related to the excess production of sebum that promotes hair loss and accelerates ongoing hair loss. Seborrheic alopecia is often associated with symptoms such as flakiness, itching, trichodynia, and a greasy scalp.

5-alpha reductase is an enzyme which converts testosterone into dihydrotestosterone. Increased levels of 5-alpha reductase or an imbalance of hormones in the body can lead to an increased sebaceous gland activity. The severity of the disease will depend on the amount of circulating hormones and the number and sensitivity of receptors present in the scalp. It also depends on how much of the hormone is captured by these enzymes.

The regions of the scalp commonly affected by seborrheic alopecia are the temporal, frontal, and crown regions. The levels of 5-alpha reductase are much higher in the hair follicles in these regions as compared to the rest of the scalp. This predisposition is common to both men and women. The main difference is that the number of receptors is less in women as compared to men and thus they have less seborrhea and greasy scalp. Women may also have seborrheic alopecia due to hormonal and gastrointestinal causes. Androgenic alopecia may be worsened by seborrhea and thus it is not easy to understand which of the two play a greater role, especially in men.

Thus, androgenetic alopecia and seborrheic alopecia are often present together in the same patient. The mechanism by which sebum causes alopecia is as follows. The principle components of sebum are cholesterol, triglycerides, squalene, sphingosine, free fatty acids, etc. These cause acidification of the sebum and scalp pH. This leads to altered metabolism in the corneocytes. Also, the

"It is confidence in our bodies, minds and spirits that allows us to keep looking for new adventures, new directions to grow in, and new lessons to learn—which is what life is all about." —**Oprah Winfrey**

sphingosine component of sebum alters the bacterial growth leading to a state of inflammation and dermatitis which ultimately leads to alopecia.

TRICHOTILLOMANIA (FIGS. 6C TO J)

Trichotillomania is defined as an irresistible urge to pull out hair and a sense of relief after the hairs have been plucked. Hair pulling and plucking is most commonly from the scalp. Most of the children pull hair from the vertex, but temporal, occipital, and frontal hair loss in children may be more prominent on the side of manual dominance.

In most of the cases of trichotillomania, the hair pulling is associated with habitual disorders or situational stress. In very few cases, it is a manifestation of severe obsessive compulsive neurosis. The parents and the adolescent girls or boys often deny pulling their hair. It presents as a nonscarring patchy loss of hair with presence of broken hair at different lengths. It can be associated with perifollicular hemorrhages. Trichotillomania could be associated with nail biting, thumb sucking, nose picking, learning disability, and iron deficiency anemia. Differential diagnoses include AA, tinea capitis, tractional alopecia, and alopecia mucinosa.

Management

Treatment is basically supportive, psychological evaluation and behavior modification. For mild cases, moderately potent topical corticosteroid lotion may be helpful to reduce the inflammation or irritation. Addition of antihistamine may also reduce the itching sensation. In severe cases, the patient may need treatment with oral fluoxetine or pimozide and a thorough counseling by a psychiatrist. N-acetylcysteine in dose of 60 mg/kg/day has been tried in children with good results.

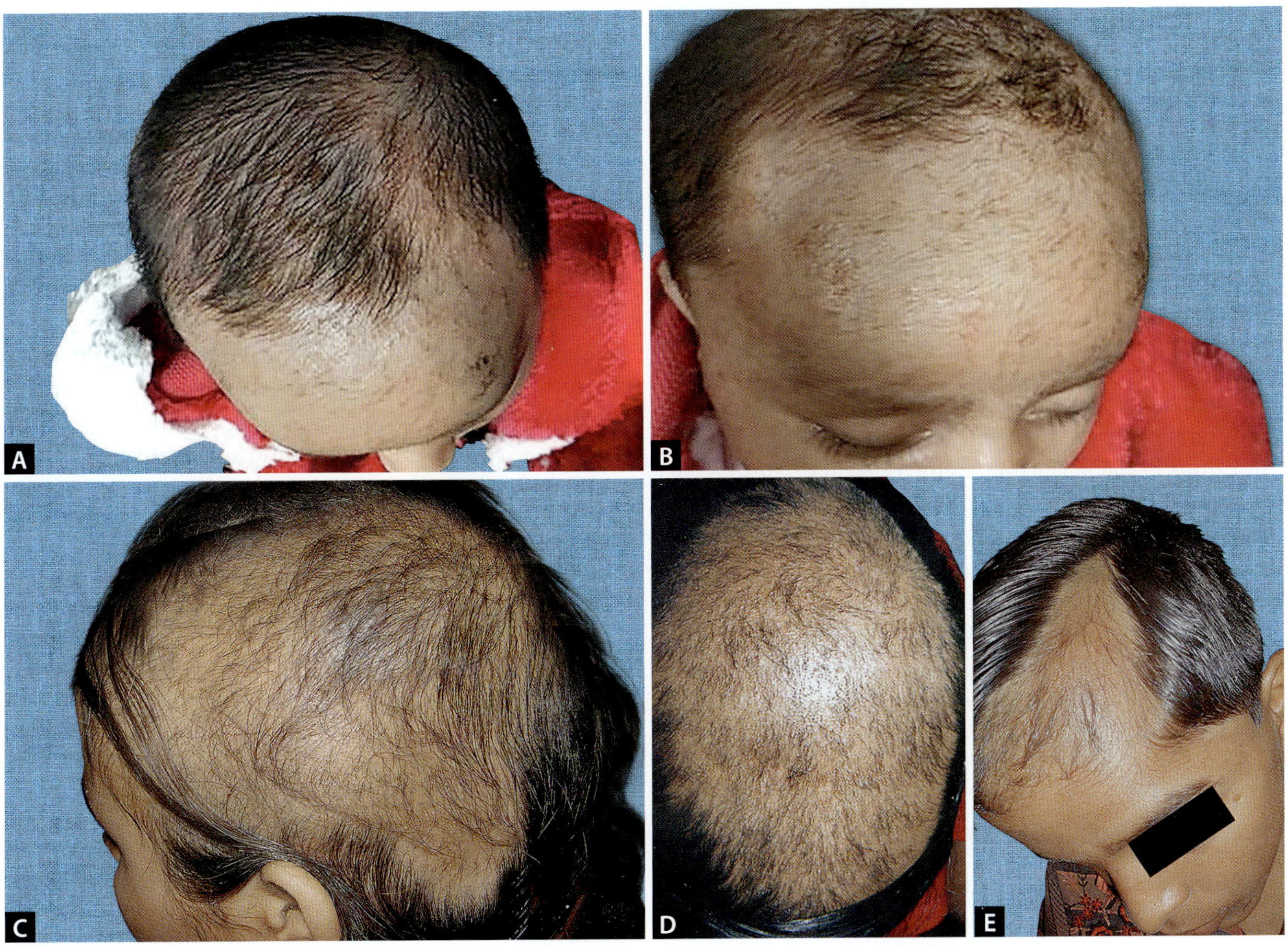

Figs. 6A to E: (A) Seborrheic alopecia; (B) Same baby, another view; (C) Trichotillomania (TTM); (D) TTM, close-up view; (E) TTM in a boy.

"Wisdom is not a product of schooling but of the lifelong attempt to acquire it." **—Albert Einstein**

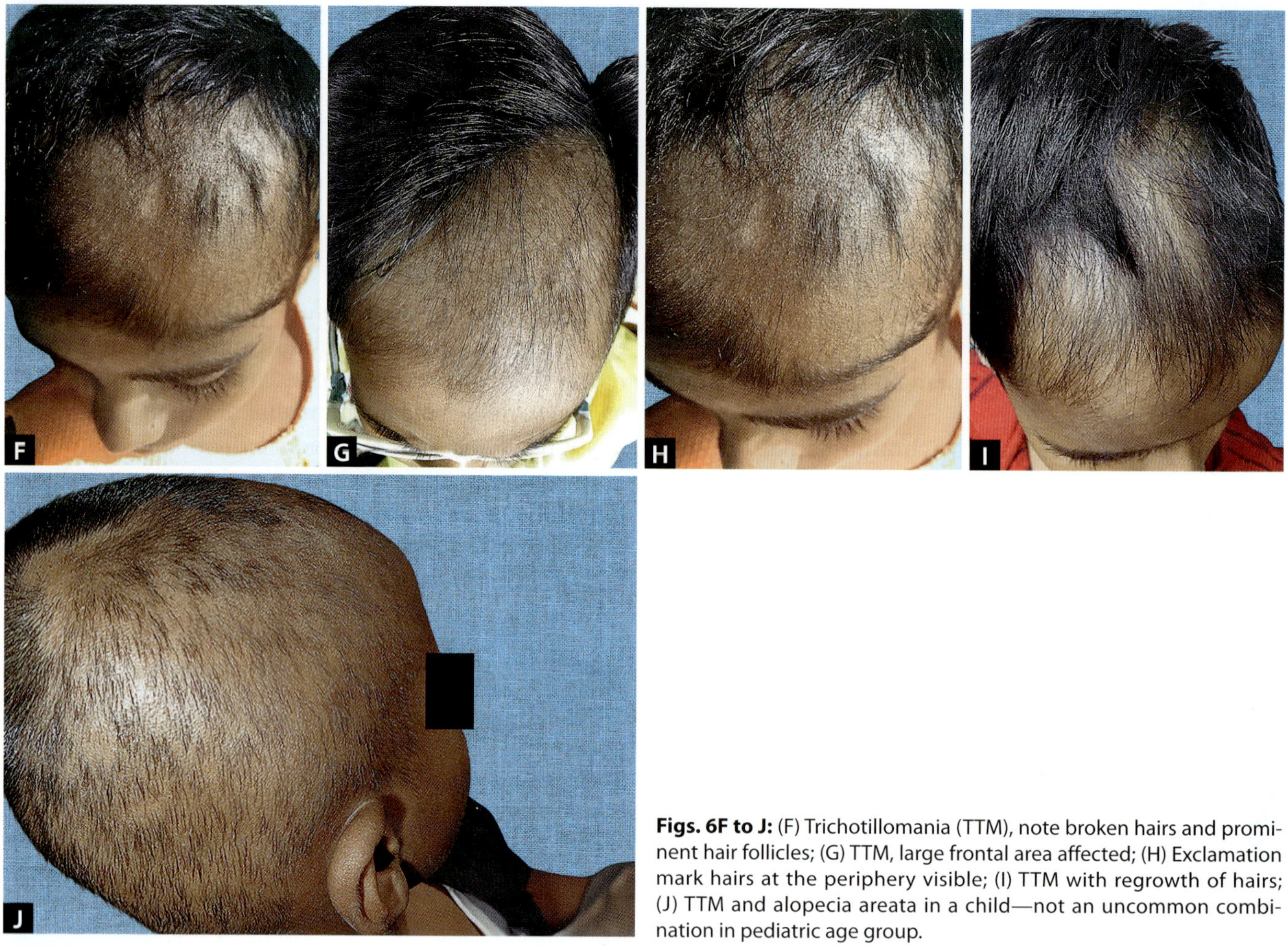

Figs. 6F to J: (F) Trichotillomania (TTM), note broken hairs and prominent hair follicles; (G) TTM, large frontal area affected; (H) Exclamation mark hairs at the periphery visible; (I) TTM with regrowth of hairs; (J) TTM and alopecia areata in a child—not an uncommon combination in pediatric age group.

OCCIPITAL ALOPECIA (FIGS. 7A AND B)

The scalp hair is shed during the fifth month of intrauterine life. After having regrown, the hairs enter telogen in a wave from front to back, starting about 12 weeks before term. After shedding of the telogen hairs from the frontal and parietal areas, the roots again enter the anagen phase in the similar wave from front to back. The roots in the occipital area do not enter telogen until term, and therefore conspicuous alopecia appears at this site. It is certainly not due to friction with the pillow over the occipital area, as it is believed to be. Counseling of the parents, particularly the anxious mothers, is very important after explaining the condition to them.

WOOLLY HAIR (FIGS. 8A TO I)

Woolly hair is tightly coiled hair occurring over the entire scalp in an individual not of negroid origin. It can be hereditary woolly hair, familial woolly hair, symmetrical, circumscribed or woolly hair nevus. In woolly hair, there is no change of color.

There are two important syndromes/diseases associated with woolly hair which are described here.

Naxos Disease

It is autosomal recessive in inheritance. Features are woolly hair, diffuse nonepidermolytic palmoplantar keratoderma, and right ventricular cardiomyopathy which produces arrhythmia.

Carvajal Syndrome

It is autosomal recessive in inheritance. Features are striate palmoplantar keratoderma with woolly hair and dilated cardiomyopathy principally affecting the left ventricle. There is defect in desmoplakin gene.

"We are just an advanced breed of monkeys on a minor planet of a very average star. But we can understand the Universe. That makes us something very special." —**Stephen Hawking**

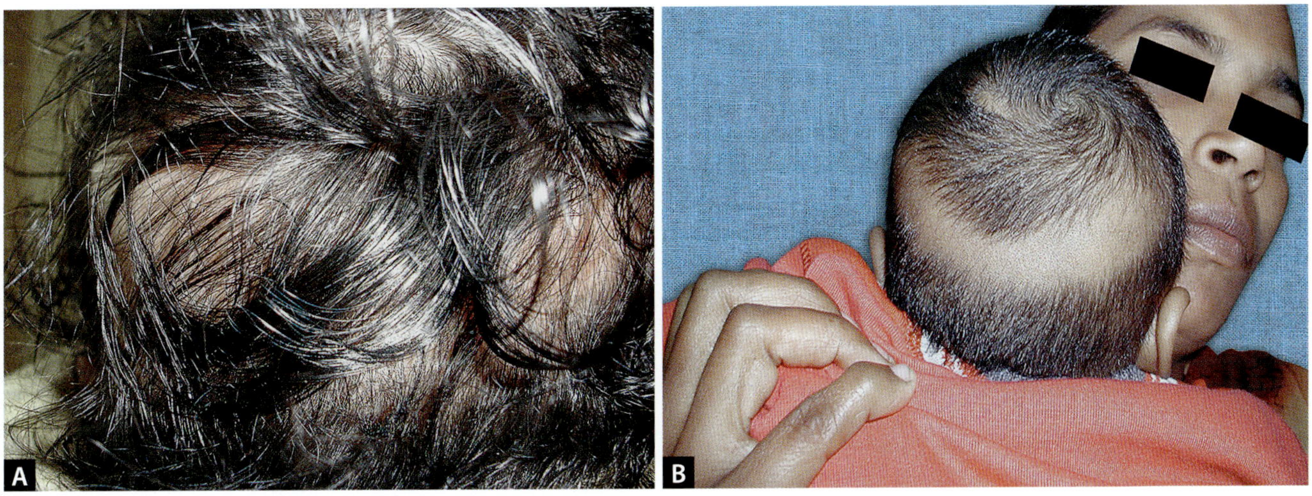

Figs. 7A and B: (A) Neonatal occipital alopecia; (B) Occipital alopecia in a newborn.

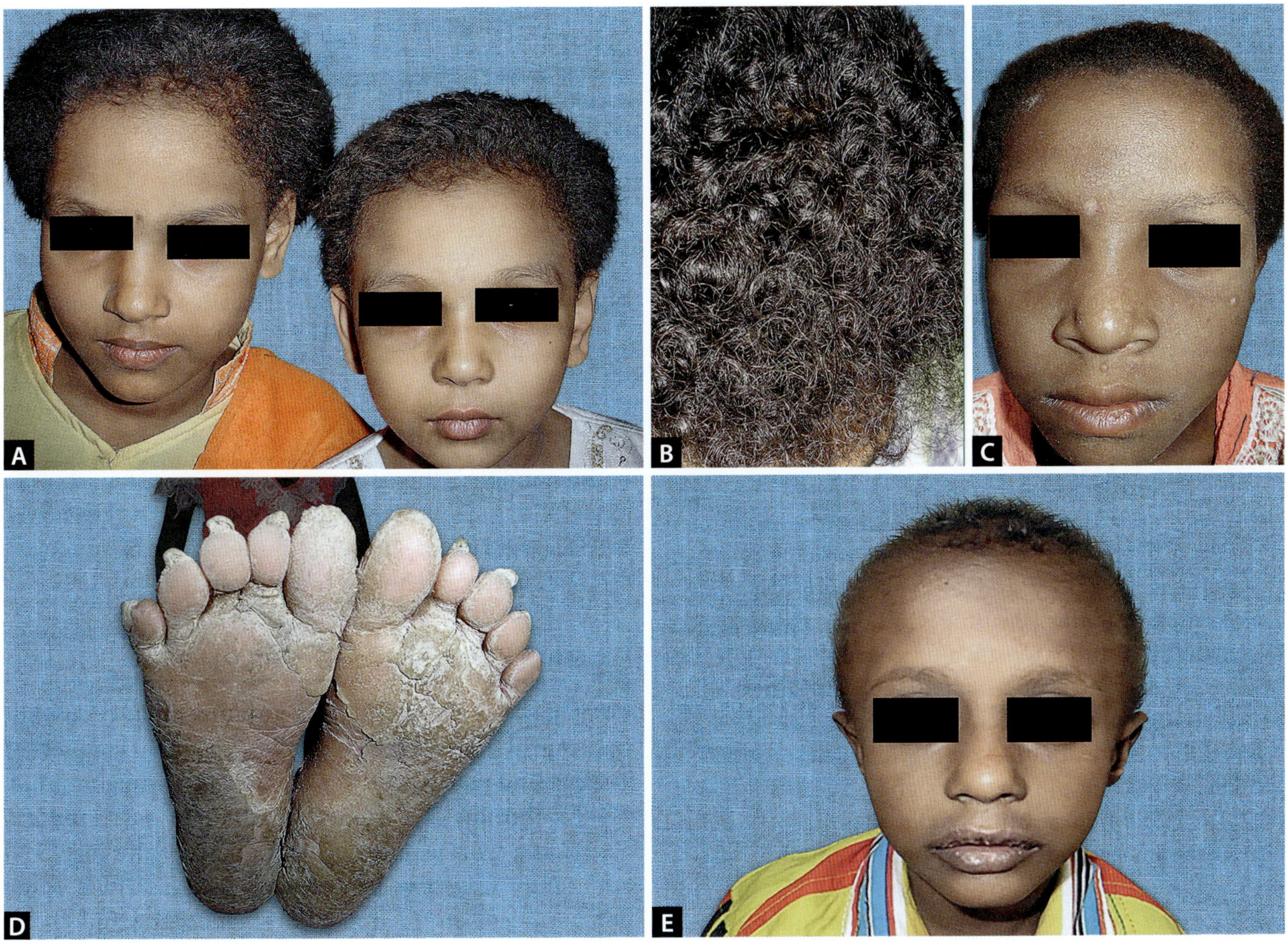

Figs. 8A to E: (A) Siblings with woolly hair; (B) Close-up view of woolly hair; (C) Naxos disease, woolly hair; (D) Naxos disease, plantar keratoderma; (E) Naxos disease, woolly hair.

"Travel isn't always pretty. It isn't always comfortable. Sometimes it hurts, it even breaks your heart. But that's okay. The journey changes you; it should change you. It leaves marks on your memory, on your consciousness, on your heart, and on your body. You take something with you. Hopefully, you leave something good behind." —**Anthony Bourdain**

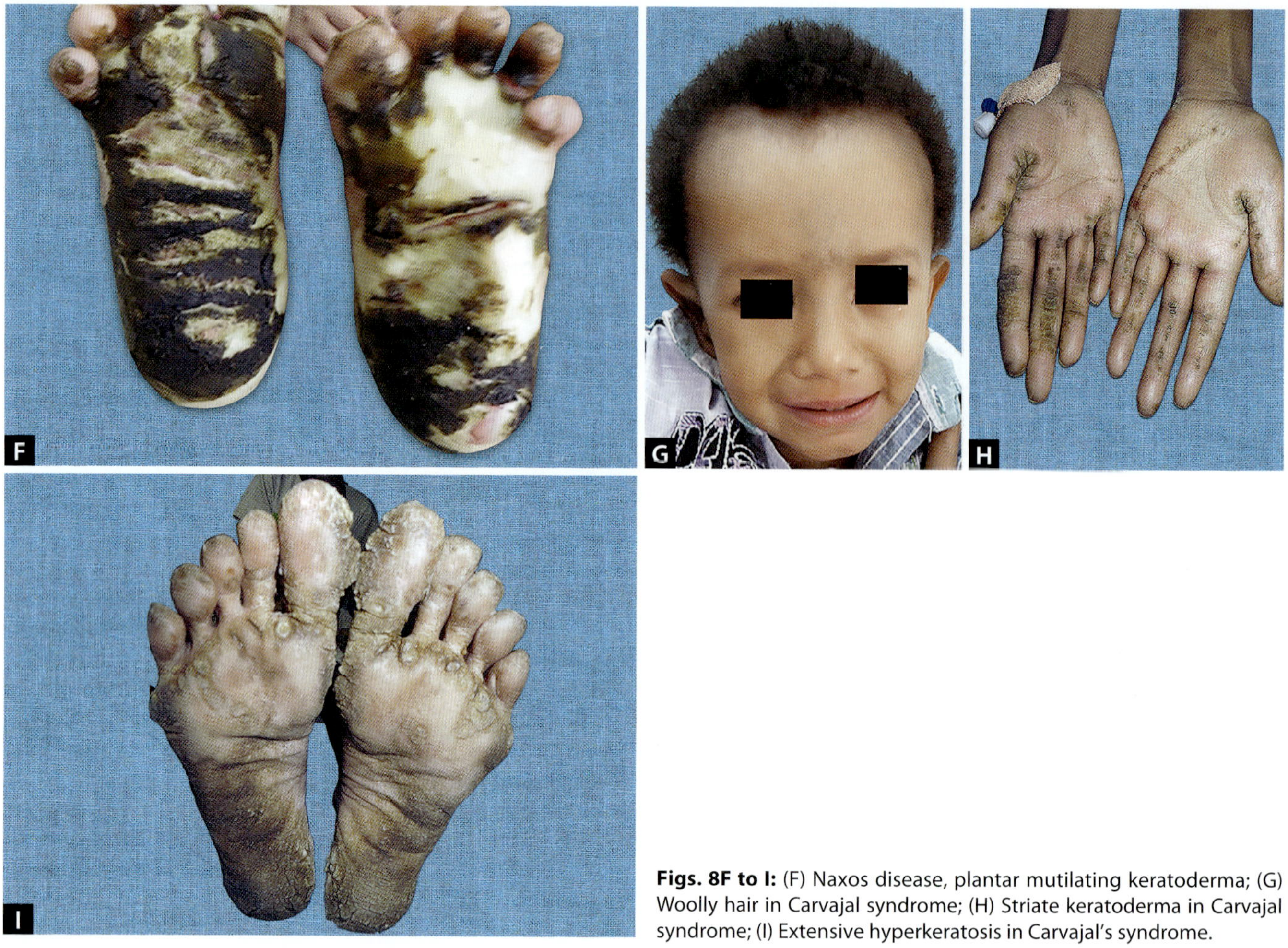

Figs. 8F to I: (F) Naxos disease, plantar mutilating keratoderma; (G) Woolly hair in Carvajal syndrome; (H) Striate keratoderma in Carvajal syndrome; (I) Extensive hyperkeratosis in Carvajal's syndrome.

MONILETHRIX (BEADED HAIR) (FIGS. 9A TO G)

Monilethrix (beaded hair) is a rare autosomal dominant disorder affecting both sexes equally. It is characterized by increased fragility and alopecia, microscopically appearance of nodes (beading) on hair and internodal fragility. The disorder mostly affects scalp hair. However, body hair may also be affected. The condition often becomes apparent late in childhood or during adult life. Associated abnormalities reported are retardation of growth and development, syndactyly, keratosis pilaris, trichorrhexis nodosa, brittle nails, cataracts, or dental abnormalities. A tendency to improvement or remission may occur at puberty or during pregnancy. In some patients, the hair disorder may persist throughout life. Hair do not grow beyond 1–2 cm in length because of breakage resulting in stubby appearance. There is no effective therapy for this condition.

Pseudomonilethrix

In this condition, there is irregular beading of hair shaft as opposed to the regular beading in monilethrix. The nodes here may also be artefactual as the defect can be produced by crushing a hair between two glass slides as well.

PIEBALDISM (FIGS. 10A TO F)

Piebaldism is transmitted as an autosomal dominant trait. Patches of skin totally devoid of pigment are present at birth and usually remain unchanged throughout life. Most common is a frontal median or paramedian, associated with a mesh of white hair (white forelock) and rarely this may be the only lesion. Often white patches occur on the upper chest, abdomen and limbs, bilaterally but not necessarily symmetrical. There are islands of pigmentation within the depigmented patch, sometimes may be surrounded by a narrow border of

"Twenty years from now you will be more disappointed by the things you didn't do than by the ones you did do. So throw off the bowlines. Sail away from the safe harbor. Catch the trade winds in your sails. Explore. Dream. Discover." —**Mark Twain**

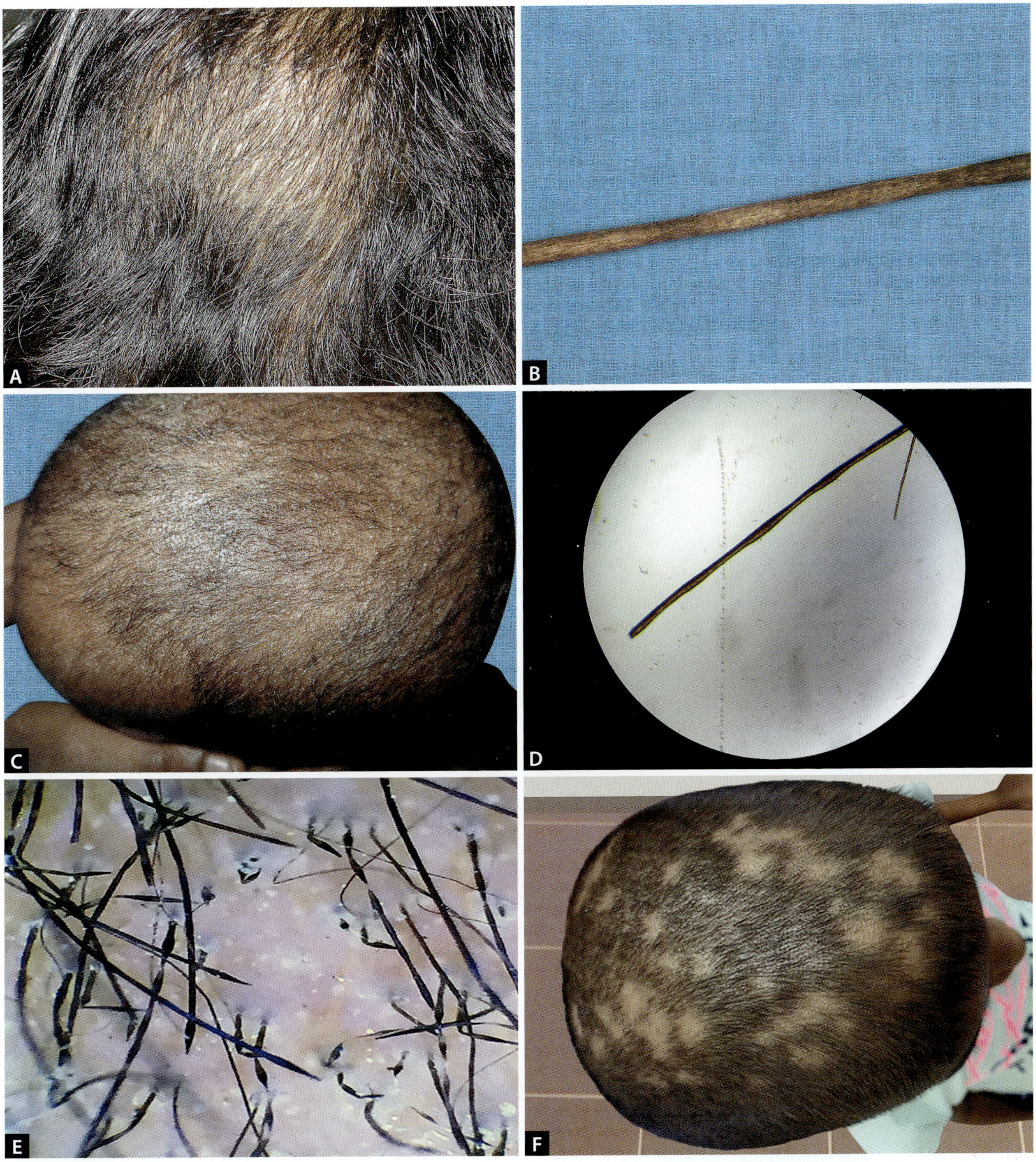

Figs. 9A to F: (A) Monilethrix; beaded hair shafts that break easily. The hairs are often unremarkable at birth and become abnormal during the first year of life; (B) Light microscopic feature of hair in monilethrix; (C) Fragile hair of monilethrix; (D) Light microscopy of hair showing beaded appearance; (E) Dermoscopy shows beaded hairs at regular intervals and "regularly bended ribbon sign"; (F) Tinea capitis gray patch.

"Because in the end, you won't remember the time you spent working in the office or mowing your lawn. Climb that goddamn mountain." —**Jack Kerouac**

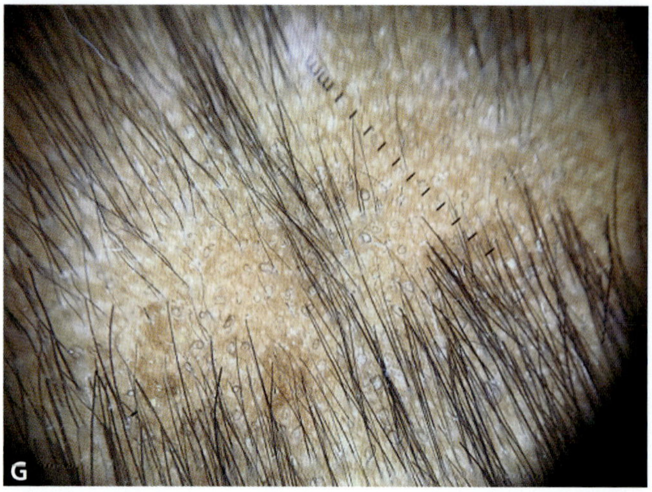

Fig. 9G: Comma hair and coiled hair on dermoscopy.

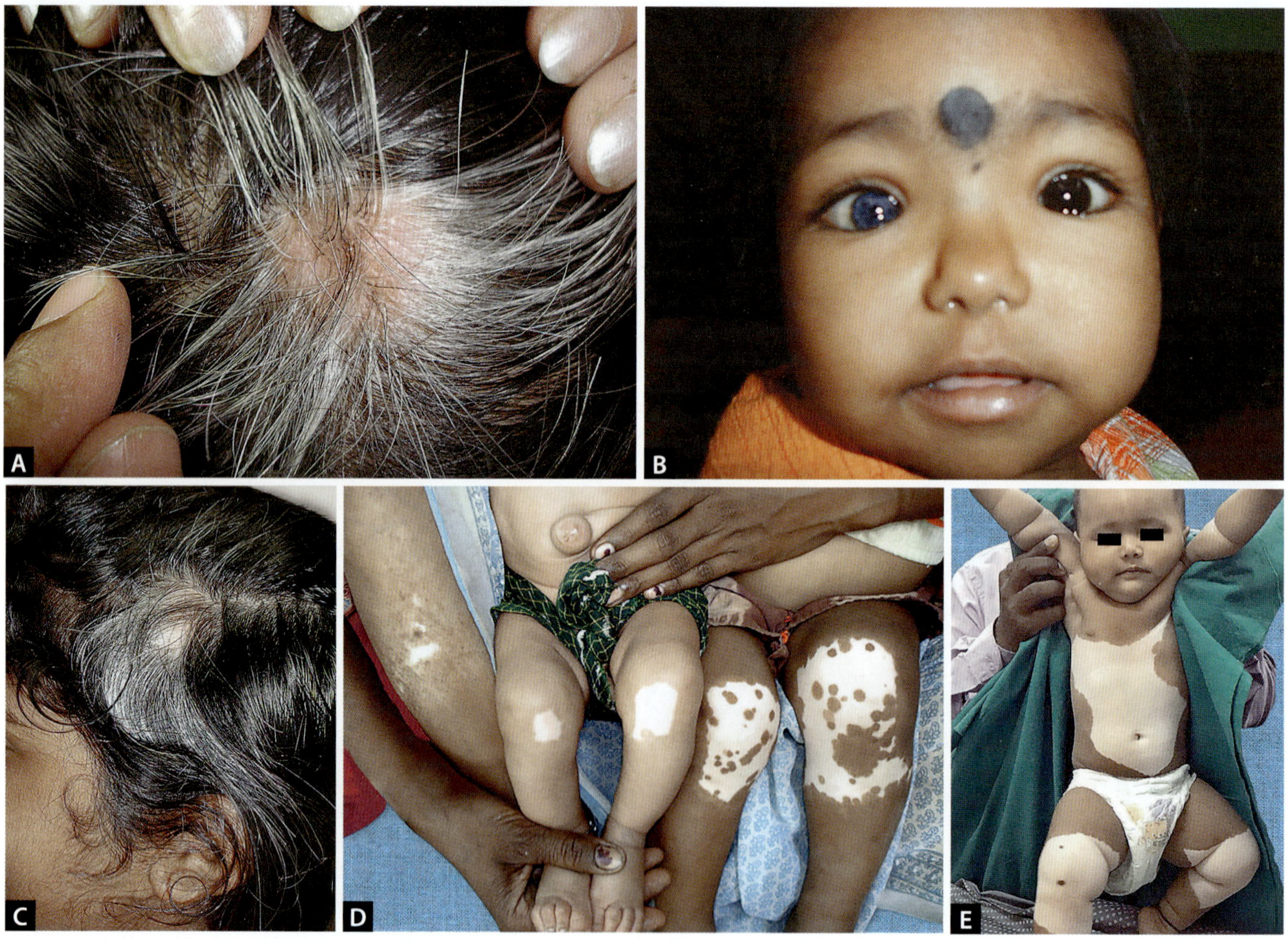

Figs. 10A to E: (A) Piebaldism; (B) Heterochromia iridis in child with Waardenburg syndrome; (C) Piebaldism, note tuft of white hairs; (D) Piebaldism in mother and siblings; (E) Piebaldism.

"To my mind, the greatest reward and luxury of travel is to be able to experience everyday things as if for the first time, to be in a position in which almost nothing is so familiar it is taken for granted." **—Bill Bryson**

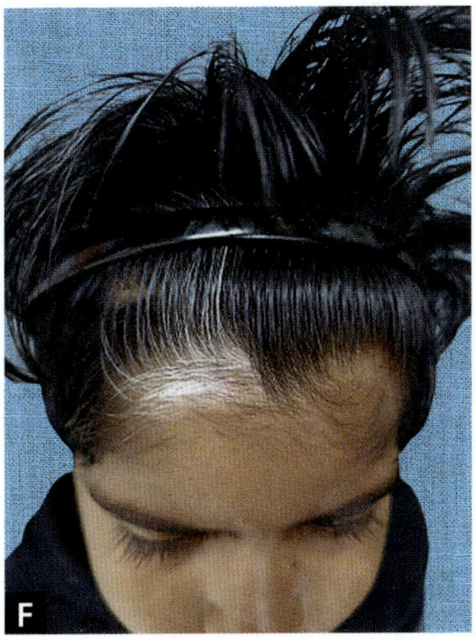

Fig. 10F: Piebaldism.

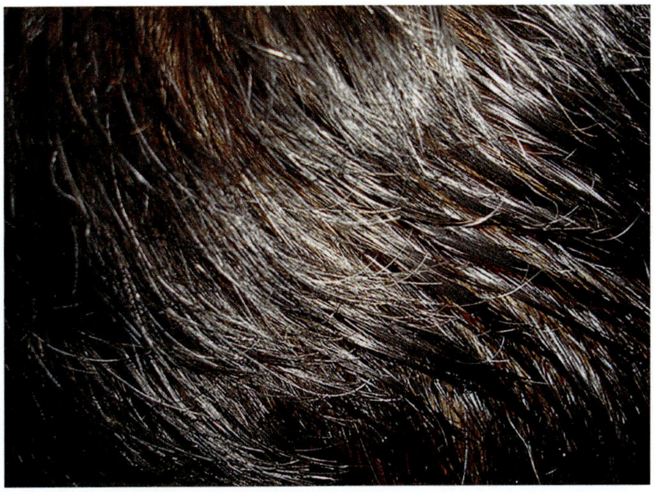

Fig. 11: Scattered white hairs all over scalp in premature canities in a 5-year-old girl.

hyperpigmentation. In vitiligo, the lesions appear later in life and their configuration and distribution are different. In piebaldism, there is almost invariably a white forelock.

Most patients with piebaldism are healthy and have a normal life expectancy.

Natural History

Various associated disorders found are heterochromia iridis, mental retardation, ataxia, motor incoordination, Hirschsprung's disease, recurrent pyogenic infections, and hepatosplenomegaly.

Waardenburg syndrome is a rare autosomal dominant disorder characterized by congenital deafness, lateral displacement of medial canthi, broad nasal root, white forelock, heterochromia iridis, and piebaldism-like skin depigmentation.

Treatment

Treatment of piebaldism consists of cosmetic camouflaging of depigmented patches. For prevention of sun-induced damage of the depigmented patches, regular use of sunscreen is a must and areas around eyes and eyelids are best protected by dark glasses.

PREMATURE CANITIES (PREMATURE GRAYING) (FIGS. 11 TO 12B)

Premature graying of hair probably has a genetic basis and occasionally occurs as an isolated autosomal dominant condition. The association between premature graying of hair and certain organ specific autoimmune disorders is well-documented. Premature graying may be an early manifestation of pernicious anemia, hyperthyroidism, hypothyroidism, and all autoimmune diseases that have a genetic predisposition. In Book syndrome, an autosomal dominant trait, premature graying is associated with premolar hypodontia and palmoplantar hyperhidrosis. The premature ageing syndromes, progeria and Werner syndrome may have premature graying as a prominent feature. Premature canities is becoming a growing concern in young children. In children, premature canities is more commonly associated with nutritional deficiency. More than five gray hair warrants investigation in children.

Management

Counseling is the cornerstone of management for cases of premature canities. For idiopathic cases, calcium pantothenic acid supplementation may be helpful. The children and the parents are to be told clearly that plucking of gray hair does not lead to an increase in the number of new gray hair and that it is a myth. Parents must also be counseled that presence of upto 5 gray hair is considered as normal.

PITYRIASIS AMIANTACEA (TINEA AMIANTACEA) (FIG. 12C)

Pityriasis amiantacea is an inflammatory scaly reaction of the scalp often without any evident cause. Usually, this disease is seen in children or adolescents in whom crusts are firmly adherent and asbestos-like. This disease is unrelated to fungal infection of scalp and probably represents a form of seborrhea or psoriasis of the scalp. This disorder is often persistent and resistant to therapy, when seen as a manifestation of psoriasis.

"Travel far enough, you meet yourself." —**David Mitchell**

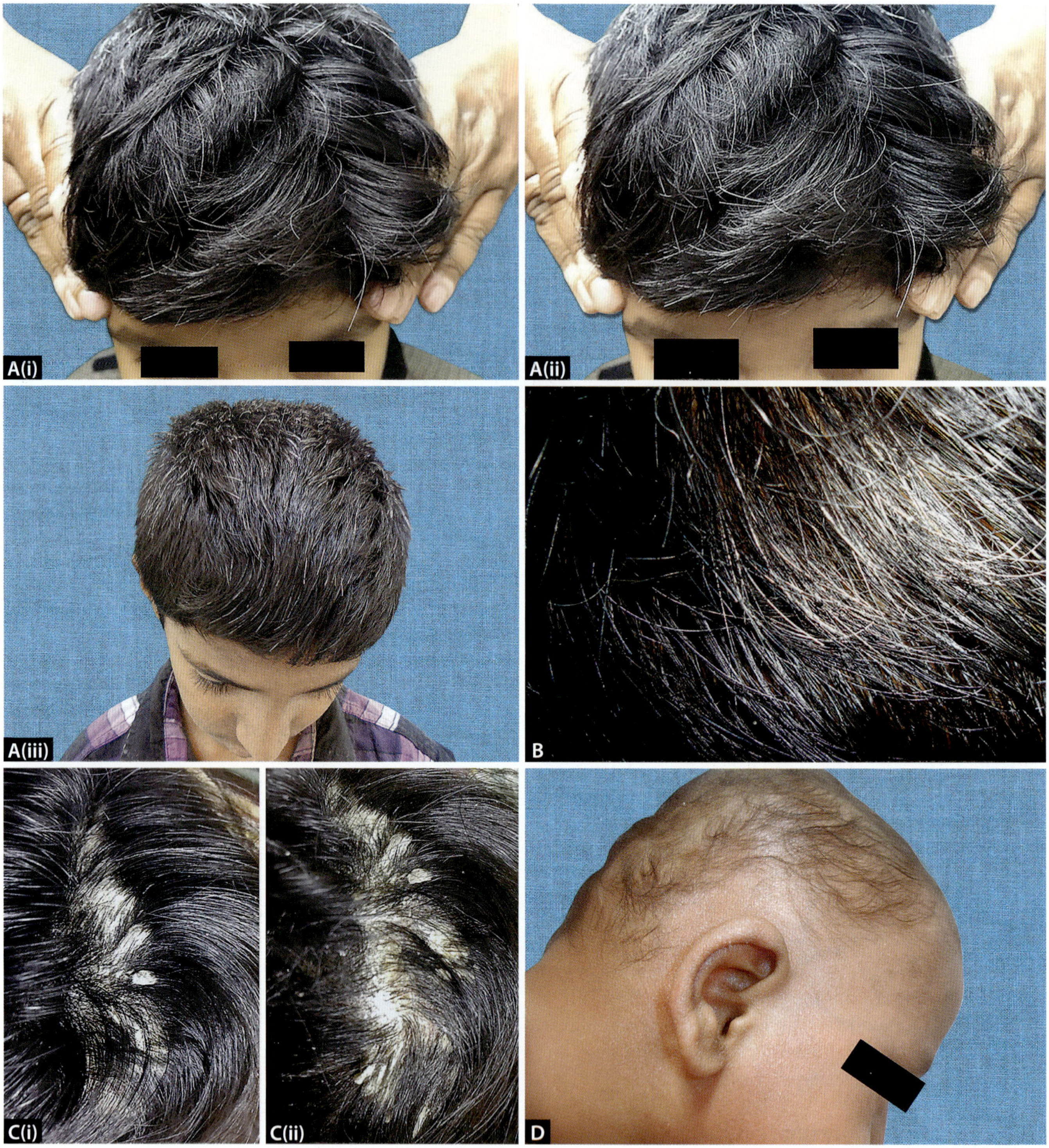

Figs. 12A(i) to D: A(i) Premature canities in a 4-year-old girl; A(ii) Same girl, close-up view; A(iii) Premature canitis in a 7-year-old boy; (B) Close-up view of hairs in premature canities; C(i) Pityriasis amiantacea in a 10-year-old girl; C(ii) Same girl, close-up view; note asbestos-like scales; (D) Neonatal hairs.

Treatment

Soaking of the scalp with lukewarm coconut or olive oil helps the thick crust to become soft. Daily application of coal tar shampoo over 2–3 months helps to resolve the lesions gradually.

NEONATAL HAIR (FIG. 12D)

Postnatal hair is divided into terminal and vellus hair. Vellus hair are very fine, lightly pigmented, and predominantly found on the face and arms. Terminal hair is thick, coarse, dark and found on scalp, eyebrows, and eyelashes. New follicles are not formed after birth.

The first crop of terminal hair is in anagen phase at birth but within few days, physiological conversion to telogen occurs. There is increased shedding of hair in the first 4 months. The shedding may be sudden or gradual and is generally completed before the first 6 months. The hair extends from the frontal hair margin up to the eyebrows and later gets converted to vellus hair in the first year of life.

Premature infants are covered with lanugo hair which is generally shed within the first month of life.

ANAGEN EFFLUVIUM (FIGS. 12E AND F)

Telogen hair is generally shed thereby making anagen hair loss abnormal, with the exception of loose anagen syndrome and AA. The most commonly recognized cause of anagen loss is exposure to radiotherapy or chemotherapy. Diminution of metabolic activity in the hair matrix results in increased shedding to the extent of about 90% scalp hair being lost. The hair loss starts within days to weeks of the insult. If exposure is persistent or particularly toxic, then anagen may be interrupted.

In general, chemotherapy induced hair loss is generally reversible when the therapy is stopped, whereas in case of radiotherapy induced hair loss, the rate of regrowth depends on the dose, intensity, and depth of penetration of the radiation. The resultant growth of hair may differ in color, curl, or texture.

Other causes of anagen loss include loose anagen syndrome, AA, and boric acid exposure or exposure to other toxic metals. Mercury exposure may lead to acrodynia characterized by a constellation of symptoms including pain in abdomen, extremities and joints, pink scaly palms and soles, headache, photophobia, irritability, hyperhidrosis, and hair loss. The diagnosis is made by measuring mercury levels in urine, blood, or hair.

Arsenic and thallium toxicity have also been implicated in anagen effluvium. Very severe protein malnutrition may also result in anagen effluvium. Colchicine and ingestion of some organic plants can also result in anagen effluvium.

Management is generally directed toward withdrawing the trigger for the loss of hair.

ANDROGENETIC ALOPECIA [FIGS. 12G(i) TO I]

This is a condition which represents the common baldness and is characterized by miniaturization of the dermal papillae and corresponding matrix. There is a decrease in the anagen and increase in telogen.

The initial presentation of this condition can be seen immediate postpuberty phase. It presents with thinning of hair of bilateral temporal area and the central parietal area in both boys and girls.

The investigations in a girl with suspected patterned hair loss should include evaluation for any signs of hirsutism, acne, and acanthosis nigricans. Blood investigations include thyroid function tests, free testosterone, and dehydroepiandrosterone sulfate. Attempts should also be made to rule out the possibility of polycystic ovarian disease in a girl. Noninvasive procedure such as trichoscopy using a dermatoscope is being increasingly preferred than biopsy to determine the hair diameter diversity and to demonstrate miniaturization of hair follicle. Biopsy of the scalp reveals terminal to vellus hair ratio of 3:1 in children as opposed to 4:1 in adults.

Management: In male children, topical minoxidil lotion 2% is the mainstay of treatment and can be increased to up to 5% strength. Finasteride is not recommended for use below 18 years of age.

In females, 2–5% minoxidil remains the mainstay of treatment. They can also benefit from treatment of underlying polycystic ovarian disease using hormonal therapy. Spironolactone has been used with good response in the Western countries.

TELOGEN EFFLUVIUM

Telogen effluvium is a common cause of diffuse hair loss in children. This type of hair loss occurs very commonly after any prolonged episode of fever, typhoid, chickenpox, after any surgical procedure, and autoimmune disorders

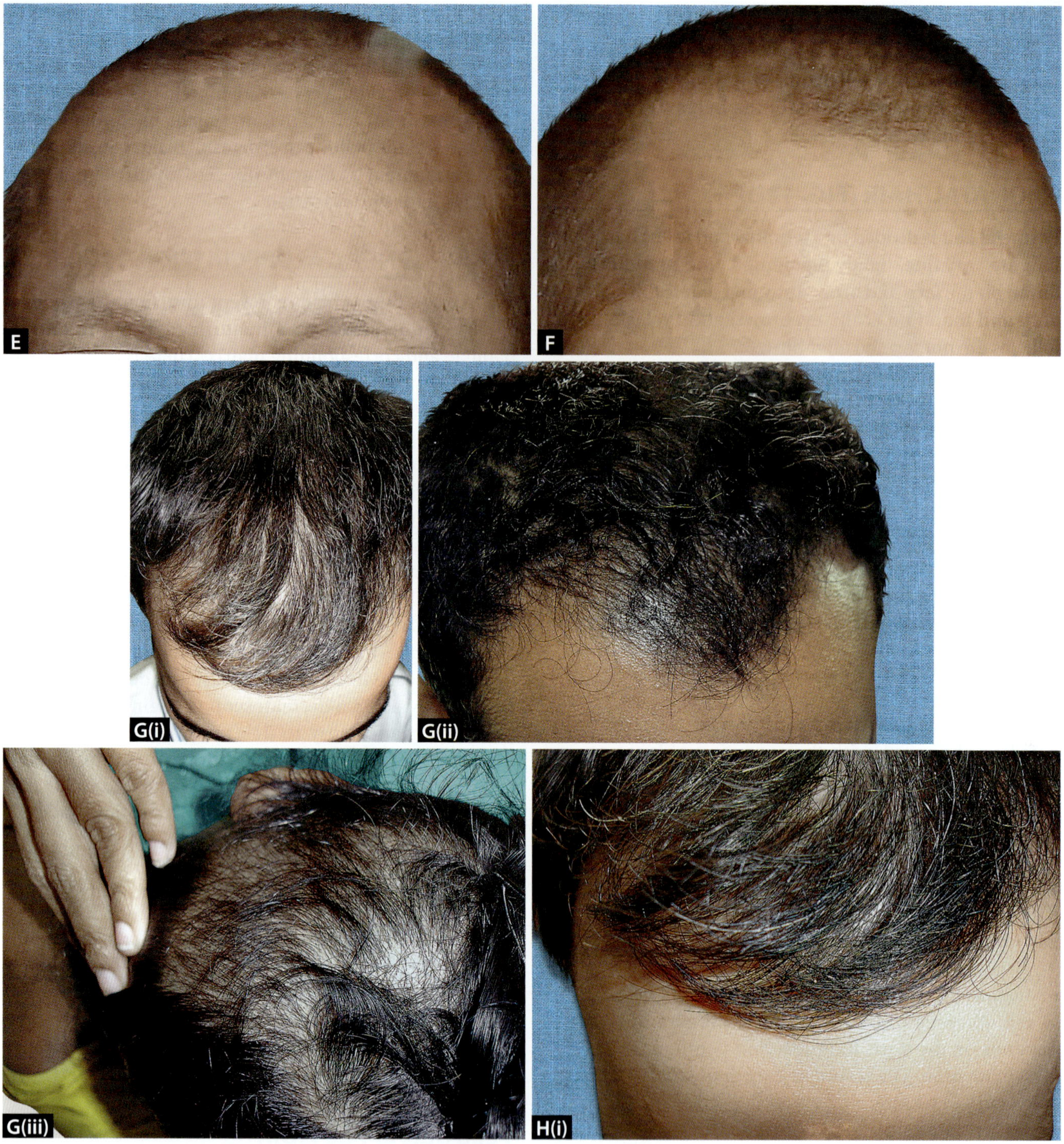

Figs. 12E to H(i): (E) Anagen effluvium; (F) Close-up view of anagen effluvium; G(i) Androgenetic alopecia (AGA) in an 18-year-old boy; G(ii) AGA in a boy; note frontal baldness; G(iii) AGA in a boy; note occipital baldness; H(i) Same boy with AGA, note frontal recession.

such as hypothyroidism. There is an abrupt shift from anagen to telogen phase with shedding occurring for 3–4 months. Within few months, hair usually regrow back to normal. Reassurance is important.

ACQUIRED PROGRESSIVE KINKING OF THE HAIR [FIGS. 12J(i) AND (ii)]

Acquired progressive kinking of the hair encompasses various conditions characterized by acquired curling

"To conquer fear is the beginning of wisdom." **—Bertrand Russell**

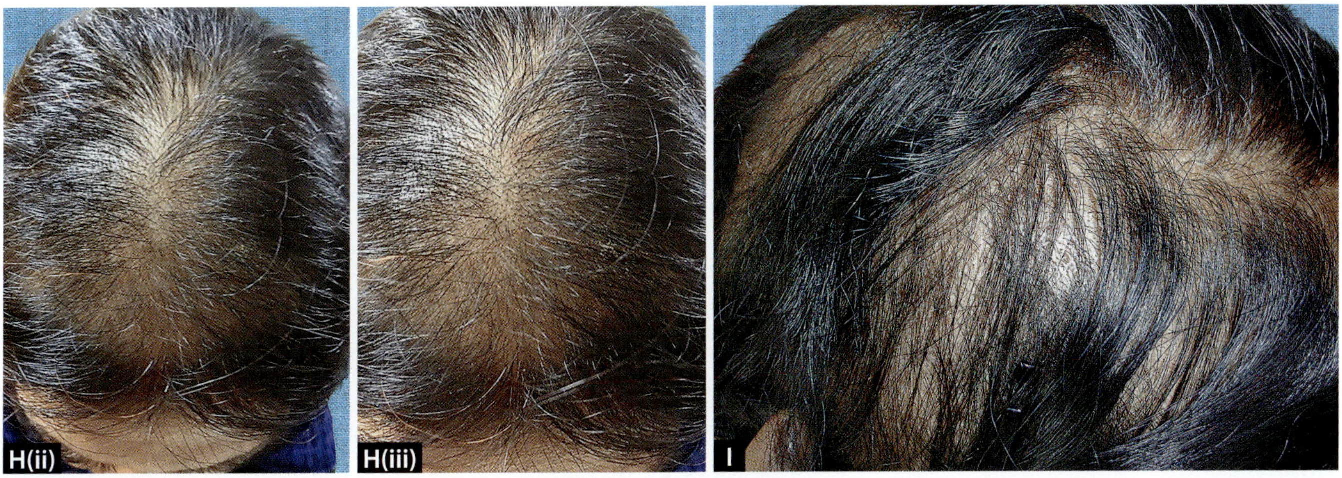

Figs. 12H(ii) to I: H(ii) Androgenetic alopecia (AGA) in a girl of 18 years; H(iii) Same girl, close-up view; (I) AGA in a girl, note diffuse thinning of hairs.

of the hair. Most commonly, this condition presents in young males and is characterized by the presence of short curly, lusterless, frizzy hair in the frontotemporal region and vertex of the scalp with subsequent progression to androgenetic alopecia. Localized and diffuse forms that are not associated with hair thinning have also been described.

PILI TORTI [FIGS. 12K(i) AND (ii)]

It is an autosomal dominant condition characterized by a flattened shaft and twisting of the hair along its own axis, about 180° with four to five twists in the same direction at irregular intervals, giving the hair a spangled appearance. Most commonly, pili torti is associated with ectodermal abnormalities such as keratosis pilaris, nail dystrophy, and dental anomalies.

The hair may be abnormal or sparse at birth or may be normal and progressively become brittle and fragile during infancy. Body hair may also be sparse. It may sometimes present after puberty as patchy alopecia of the scalp, eyebrows, and eyelash.

Acquired pili torti-like condition has been reported with anorexia nervosa, malnutrition, at the edge of cutaneous lupus erythematosus lesions, and oral retinoid therapy. Other disorders which can have pili torti as an association include Menkes disease, Laron syndrome, Bazex-Dupré-Christol syndrome, and hypotrichosis with juvenile macular dystrophy, ectodermal dysplasias, mitochondrial disorders, and urea cycle defects.

Pili torti associated with hearing loss is seen in Björnstad syndrome and therefore a screening for hearing loss is recommended in all these patients.

Light microscopy reveals groups of twisted flattened hair. At present, there is no effective therapy for this condition.

PILI ANNULATI

This condition is also known as ringed hair and is characterized by hair shafts that are banded by alternating light and dark color when seen in reflected light. It is inherited as autosomal dominant condition or may be sporadic. The major defect is the presence of air-filled cavities within the hair shaft at regular intervals giving rise to scattering of light which thereby becomes visible as a bright band. On microscopic evaluation, these air-filled cavities are seen as black regions. It is not associated with systemic abnormalities.

TRICHORRHEXIS NODOSA

As the name suggests, this condition is characterized by the formation of nodes in the hair shaft leading to fragility and breaking of the hair shaft. It can be congenital or acquired. The acquired forms are a result of physical or chemical trauma. It may present at birth or within couple of months of life. It has a female preponderance.

Macroscopically, these hair are characterized by white nodes which represent areas of cuticular disruption, and are placed at regular or irregular intervals along the hair shaft. The cortical fibers splay outward and fracture, giving the node the microscopic appearance of two brooms or paintbrushes thrust together end-to-end by their bristles. A primary congenital form of trichorrhexis nodosa is inherited as an autosomal dominant trait in some

"Don't grieve. Anything you lose comes round in another form." — **Rumi**

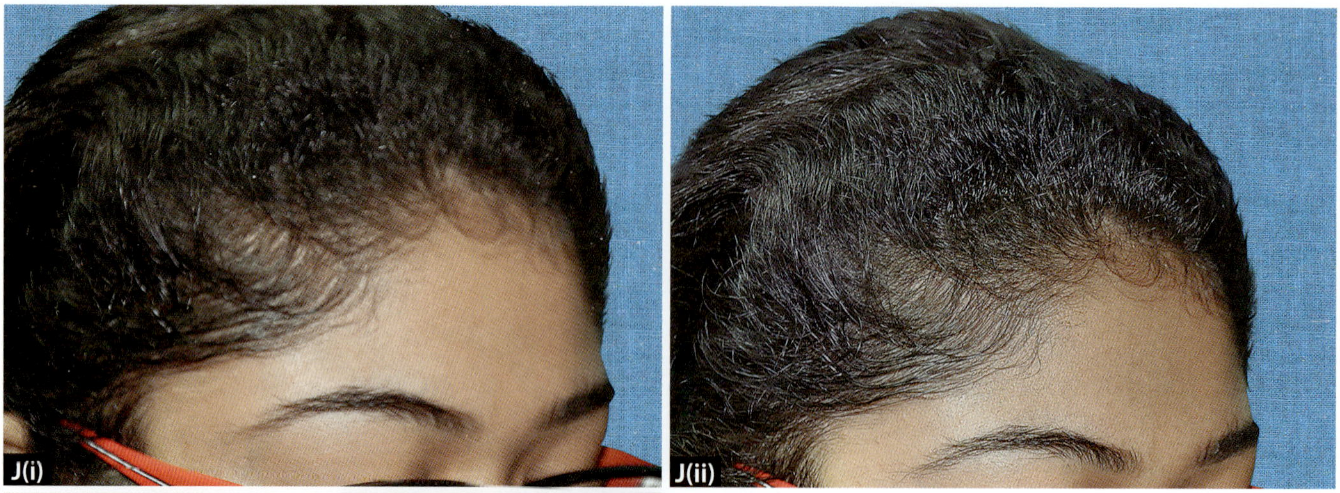

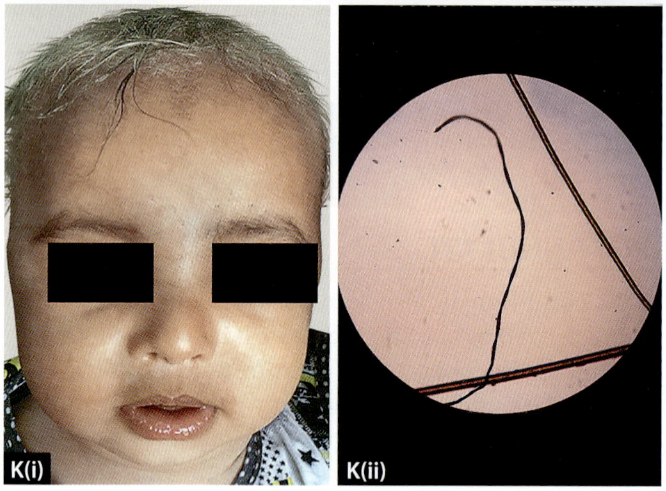

Figs. 12J(i) to K(ii): J(i) Acquired progressive kinking of hairs; J(ii) Same girl, close-up view of hairs; K(i) Menkes disease showing hypopigmented, brittle hair, note the steel wool appearance; K(ii) Microscopy of hair of same child showing pili torti.

families. It has been described in association with hypothyroidism, trichohepatoenteric syndrome, and biotinidase deficiency.

Clinical features: The patient presents with the nodes in the hair or history of failure to grow hair and easy breakability. Congenital trichorrhexis nodosa is apparent at a younger age and may be associated with other symptoms such as mental retardation, motor defects, growth failure, and seizures. Other associated symptoms may include nail and skin changes (ichthyosis), photosensitivity, ocular dystrophy, and infertility. It has also been seen in association with Menkes disease, Netherton syndrome, argininosuccinic aciduria, and oculodental digital dysplasia. Acquired trichorrhexis nodosa has three clinical patterns namely distal, localized, and proximal.

Dermoscopy shows breakage in hair shafts at multiple levels, producing an appearance suggestive of the ends of two brushes aligned in opposition, resembling "thrust paint brushes."

Differential diagnosis:

- Piedra
- Trichorrhexis invaginata
- Monilethrix
- Menkes kinky hair disease
- Trichomycosis axillaris and pubis
- Seborrheic dermatitis

Investigations:

- Dermoscopy and light microscopy reveals the classical paint brush fracture appearance.
- Tests should be performed to rule out trichothiodystrophy (TTD).

Management: The treatment should be aimed at avoiding chemical and physical trauma. Underlying metabolic disorders need to be treated accordingly.

"A journey is best measured in friends rather than miles." —**Tim Cahill**

TRICHORRHEXIS INVAGINATA [FIGS. 12L(i) AND (ii)]

It is also known as bamboo hair. It generally presents in infancy as sparse and short brittle hair. The defect is generally abnormal keratinization of hair shaft in the keratogenous zone allowing invagination of the distal portion into the proximal part, giving rise to a ball in socket-like deformity. Fracture of the shaft is commonly noted on dermoscopy along with golf tee or tulip-shaped end of the hair. Trichorrhexis invaginata is characteristic feature of Netherton syndrome. Eyebrow hair examination is very conclusive for Netherton syndrome. Other hair shaft abnormalities associated with Netherton syndrome are trichorrhexis nodosa and pili torti.

The sulfur levels are normal which helps in differentiating from TTD. As the abnormal hair may be seen only in some sections of the scalp, it is important to undertake multiple site examination.

There is no specific treatment for trichorrhexis invaginata. Spontaneous improvement with age is generally seen. PUVA therapy and retinoids have been reported to be useful in a few cases.

UNCOMBABLE HAIR SYNDROME [FIG. 12M(i)]

This condition is generally seen in infancy up to puberty. The patients generally complain of slow growing, silvery blond hair having a spun glass appearance which is unruly and unmanageable. The condition is autosomal dominant with incomplete penetrance but sporadic cases have also been noted. There are no reported associations or abnormalities. Premature keratinization of the inner root sheath has been implicated in the etiopathogenesis of this disorder. Electron microscopy reveals longitudinal grooving and the cross section appears triangular. The condition improves with age. Biotin supplements and regular use of hair conditioners have been found to be useful in management of this disorder.

LOOSE ANAGEN SYNDROME [FIGS. 12M(ii) AND (iii)]

It is an autosomal dominant condition but can be sporadic in few cases. The presenting complaints include sparse brittle hair, patches of dull matted hair, and easy pluckability. There is a strong female preponderance and the condition manifests at an age <6 years. These hair have malformed hair bulbs, absent root sheath, and ruffled cuticle giving rise to the floppy sock appearance. The main structural defect lies in the inner root sheath. Loose anagen syndrome has been divided into three types: A, B and C. Type B presents with patches of unruly hair, whereas types A and C present with increased shedding in clinically normal hair. The diagnosis is made when there is easy pluckability of 3–10 hair per hair pull or percentage of all hair obtained on hair pull (50% suggested). The differential diagnosis includes woolly hair nevus for type B and short anagen syndrome for type A. This condition remains elusive to treatment.

TRICHOTHIODYSTROPHY [FIG. 12M(iv)]

Trichothiodystrophy is a group of rare recessively inherited multisystem neuroectodermal disorders with

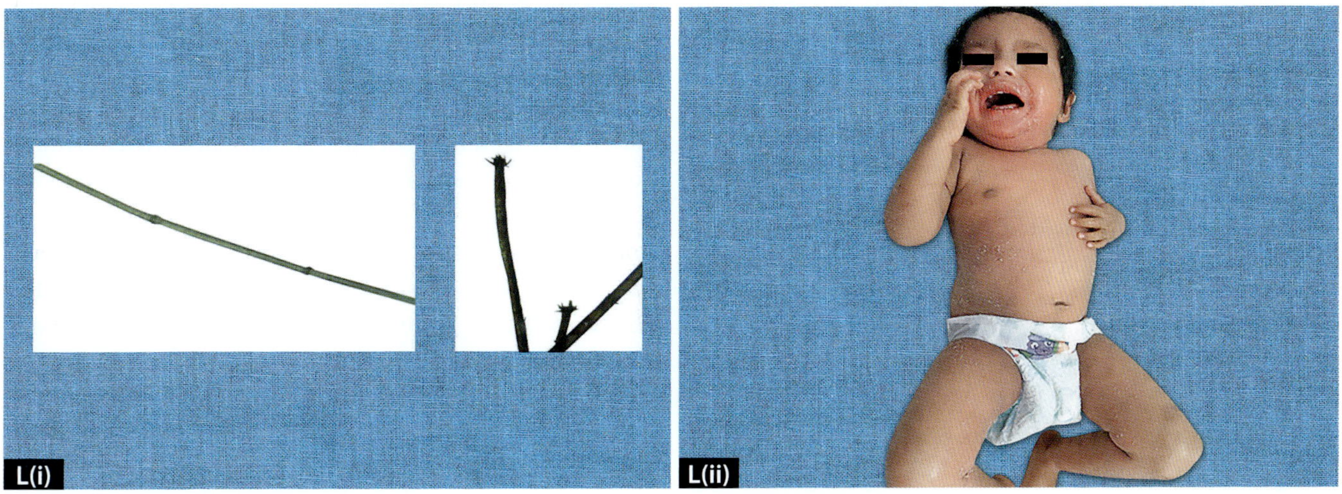

Figs. 12L(i) and (ii): L(i) Hair in trichorrhexis invaginata, bamboo hair; L(ii) Netherton's syndrome.

"Our mind is capable of passing beyond the dividing line we have drawn for it. Beyond the pairs of opposites of which the world consists, other, new insights begin." —**Hermann Hesse**

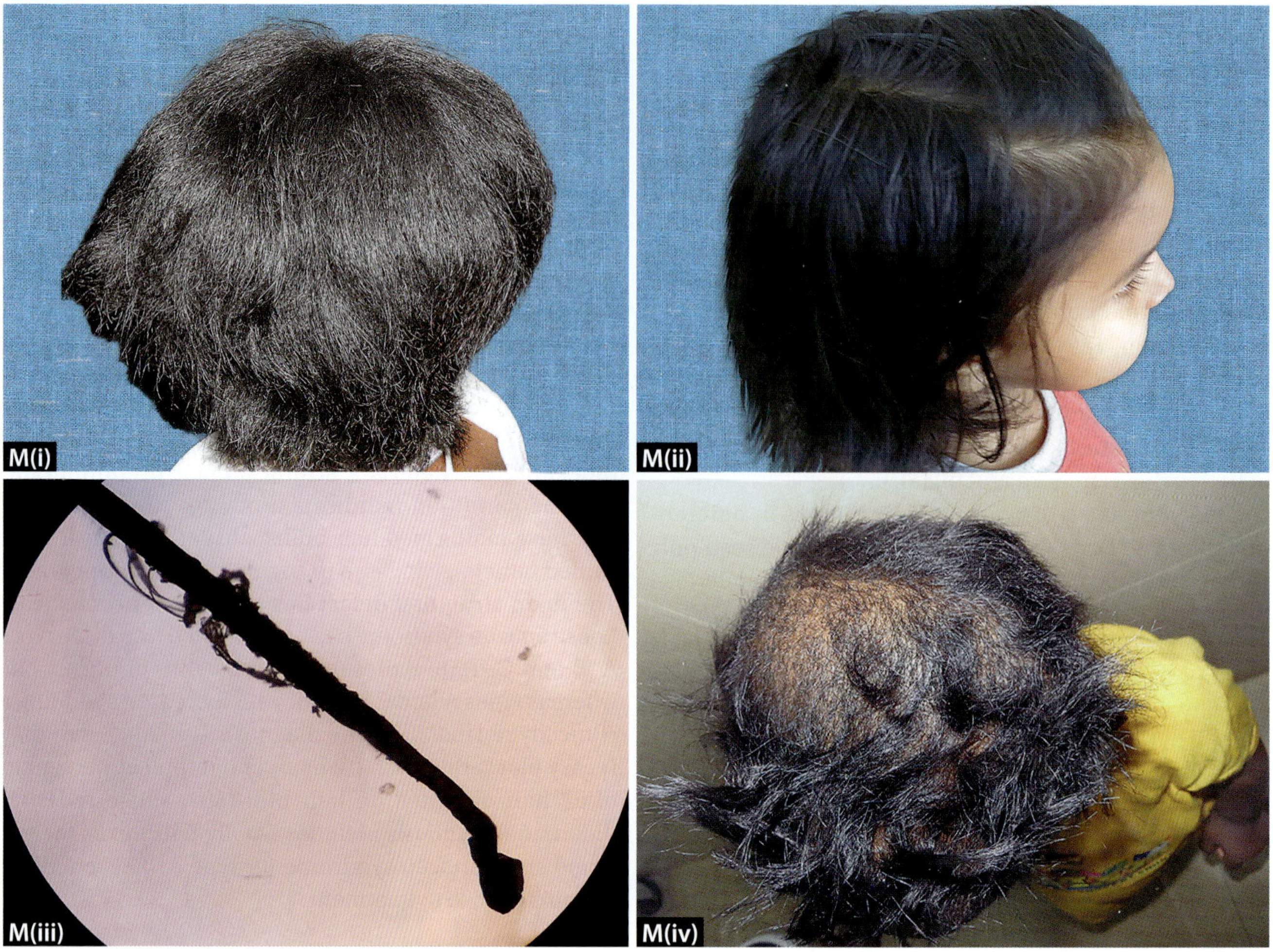

Figs. 12M(i) to (iv): M(i) Uncombable hair; M(ii) Loose anagen hair syndrome; M(iii) Microscopy of hair in loose anagen hair showing ragged cuticles and floppy sock appearance; M(iv) Trichothiodystrophy.

characteristic feature of brittle, sulfur-deficient hair (tricho, hair; thio, sulfur; dys, faulty; trophe, nourishment) caused by a defect of DNA repair and transcription. Clinical features can be described using several acronyms such as PIBIDS, IBIDS, and BIDS for photosensitivity, ichthyosis, brittle hair, intellectual impairment, decreased fertility, and short stature. TTD clinically presents either as photosensitive or nonphotosensitive classical forms. The majority of all photosensitive TTD exhibits mutations in one of the three subunits *[ERCC3 (XPB), ERCC2 (XPD),* and *GTF2H5 (p8/TTD-A)]* of the DNA repair/transcription factor IIH (TFIIH), whereas mutations in *MPLKIP, RNF113A,* and *GTF2E2* are observed in nonphotosensitive patients.

Trichothiodystrophy consists of a wide spectrum of clinical features varying degrees of severity, the most common being brittle hair or hair shaft abnormalities (96%), intellectual impairment or developmental delay (86%), short stature (73%), and ichthyosis (65%). The diagnostic feature is the presence of brittle, sparse, and dry hair (scalp, eyebrows, and eyelashes) due to low sulfur and cysteine content (10–50% of normal) and consists of alternating light and dark bands, called tiger tail pattern, under polarized microscopy. Trichoschisis, trichorrhexis nodosa-like fractures, and ribboning may also be present. Newborns may present with erythroderma or a collodion-like membrane, and may have low birth weight and congenital cataracts. Ichthyosis in TTD is related to downregulation of liver X receptor (LXR) responsive genes (*ABCA12* and *ABCG1*) that play a critical role in skin lipid homeostasis. Nail abnormalities include ridging, splitting, hypoplasia, koilonychia, and dystrophic nails. Thickening of the palms and soles are also present in some individuals. Characteristic facial features (microcephaly, protruding ears, and micrognathia) and short stature are

"What a distressing contrast there is between the radiant intelligence of the child and the feeble mentality of the average adult." —**Sigmund Frued**

seen in many patients. Other clinical findings include physical and mental retardation, hearing loss, decreased fertility, dental caries, proneness to infections, particularly respiratory infections, which can be life-threatening, bone abnormalities (osteosclerosis and osteopenia), hematological features (anemia, neutropenia, β-thalassemia trait), signs of premature aging, and in about half of the reported cases, cutaneous photosensitivity. Severely affected individuals may survive only into infancy or early childhood. It has to be differentiated from CS, XP, Menkes disease and Netherton syndrome. TTD patients do not appear to be at increased risk for skin cancer, unlike patients with xeroderma pigmentosum and XP/CS.

Clinical diagnosis made on the presence of "tiger-tail" bands of hair shafts under polarized light microscopy and other clinical features can be confirmed by cellular tests for defective DNA repair and subsequent mutational analysis. There is no cure. Multidisciplinary approach and genetic counseling form the basis of treatment. Infections should be treated aggressively and sun protection should be advised in those patients who are photosensitive.

TEMPORAL TRIANGULAR ALOPECIA [FIGS. 12M(v) TO (vii)]

Temporal triangular alopecia, also called as congenital triangular alopecia (Brauer Nevus), is a benign, circumscribed, nonscarring alopecia presenting at birth or can be acquired during the first decade of life. The exact etiology is not known, though mosaicism may play a role. Clinically, it presents as smooth bald patch with few vellus hair within the affected bald patch or central localized hair tuft distributed on the frontotemporal region. These vellus hair can be seen through magnification or trichoscopy. Alopecia patches can occur on other parts of the scalp apart from temporal region. The alopecia patch is triangular, oval, or lancet-shaped with base of the patch directed forward. It is usually unilateral in distribution, but bilateral can be seen in 20% cases. Diagnosis is mainly clinical. Trichoscopy shows follicular openings with short vellus hair. Temporal triangular alopecia has been associated with congenital heart diseases, Down syndrome, Klippel–Trénaunay syndrome, Turner syndrome, phakomatosis pigmentovascularis, woolly hair nevus, epilepsy, and bone and teeth abnormalities. Differential diagnosis includes AA, tinea capitis, trichotillomania, and aplasia cutis. It persists unchanged throughout life. Minoxidil has shown good improvement but relapse is common. Follicular unit transplant of hair has shown some consistent result in selected cases.

MENKES KINKY HAIR DISEASE [FIGS. 12M(viii) TO (x)]

Menkes kinky hair disease is a rare X-linked recessive disorder of copper metabolism leading to multisystem involvement and progressive neurodegeneration. The affected gene locus is Xq13.3. This rare lethal disease affects males without any racial predilection. Patients usually manifest at around 2–3 months of age and die at around 3–4 years due to respiratory failure secondary to infection. Basic defect is impaired intestinal copper transport leading to low-serum copper and ceruloplasmin level. Generally, a preterm or term baby presents with nonspecific features such as hypoglycemia, hypothermia, seizures, failure to thrive, difficulty in feeding, jaundice,

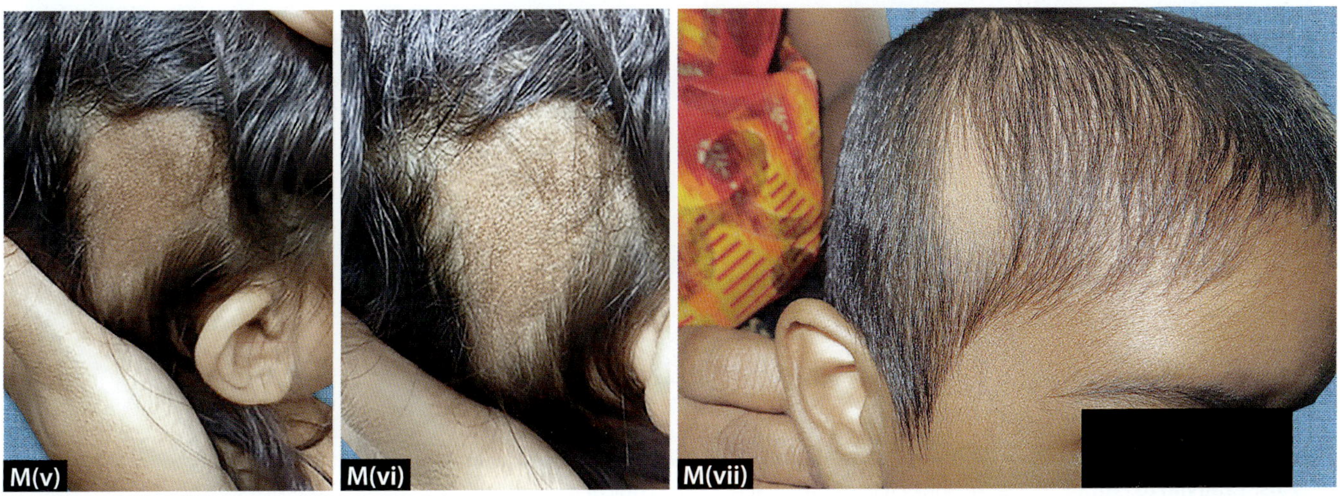

Figs. 12M(v) to (vii): Temporal triangular alopecia.

"Knowledge comes from learning. Wisdom comes from living." —**Anthony Douglas Williams**

and urinary diverticula. Progressive hypotonia and loss of previously obtained milestones point toward neurodegenerative nature of the disease. Gliosis and demyelination of cerebrum and cerebellum explain neurodegeneration. Most striking manifestation is short, sparse, coarse, silvery white twisted hair of scalp, eyebrows, and eyelashes. The entity is named after Menkes who first described the entity. Pili torti is the most common hair shaft defect described in this condition. Several hair shaft abnormalities have been documented like trichoclasis, trichoptilosis, and trichorrhexis nodosa. Simple light microscopy of hair clinches the diagnosis. Skeletal abnormalities such as spurring of the long bones, infantile cortical hyperostosis, and metaphyseal widening are reported. Close differentials are Netherton syndrome and TTD. Besides light microscopy of hair, magnetic resonance imaging is important to see the degree of insult to brain. Treatment is generally symptomatic and supportive.

PILOMATRICOMA [FIG. 12M(xi)]

Pilomatricoma or calcifying epithelioma of Malherbe, is a benign, slow-growing tumor of the skin arising from hair follicle matrix cells developing usually within the first two decades of life. Activating mutations in beta-catenin in the Wnt-signaling pathway appear to be involved in the pathogenesis of these tumors while adenomatous polyposis coli (*APC*) gene mutations have been identified in patients with multiple pilomatricomas. It occurs most often on the head or neck and rarely at other sites (trunk and extremities) presenting as single, sharply demarcated, firm, deep seated skin-colored to bluish asymptomatic papules or nodules. Multiple or noncephalic lesions have been associated with numerous syndromes (Turner, Gardner, Rubinstein-Taybi, and Kabuki), myotonic dystrophy, trisomy 9, spina bifida, sarcoidosis, and gliomatosis cerebri. Pilomatricoma variants include

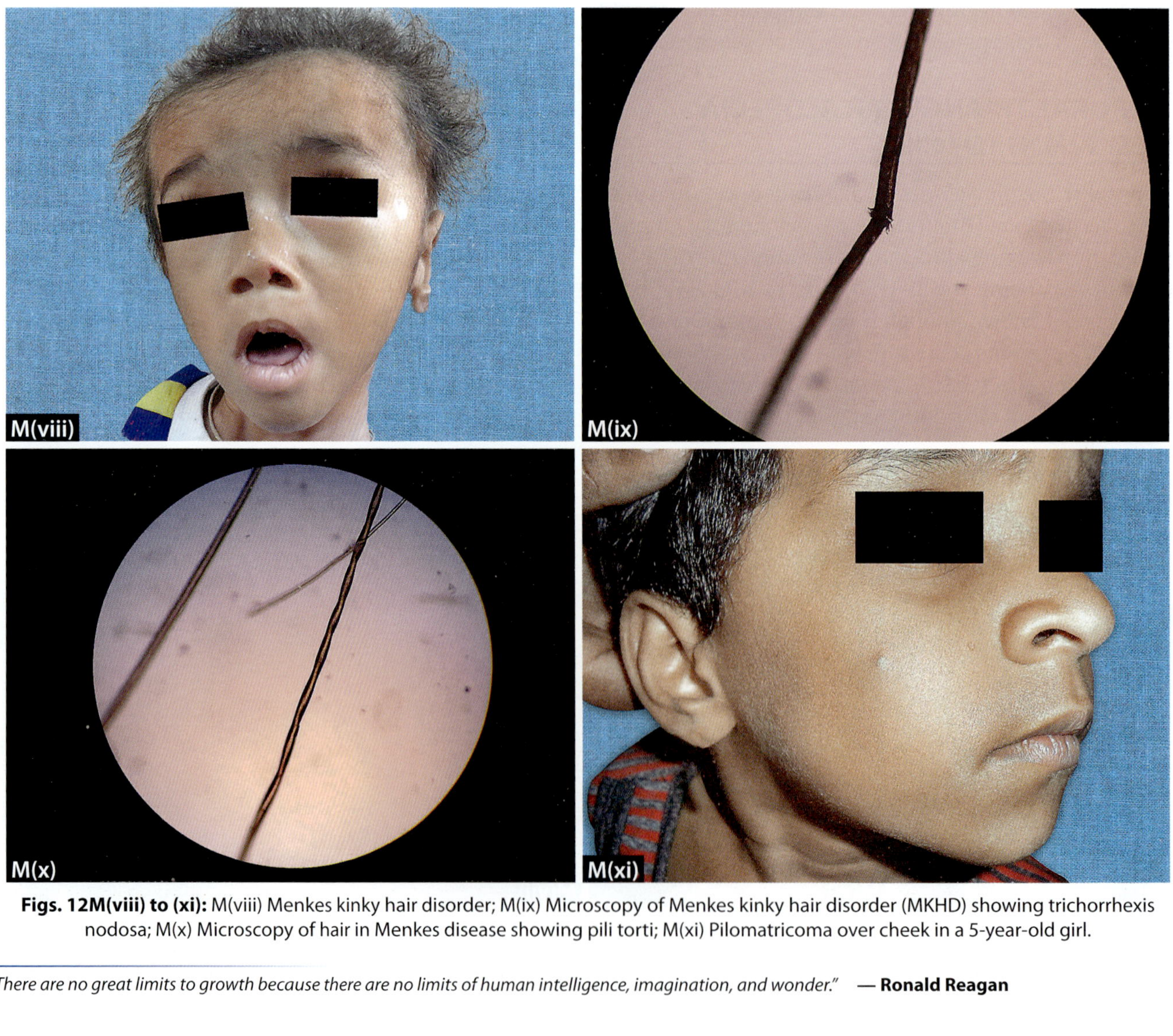

Figs. 12M(viii) to (xi): M(viii) Menkes kinky hair disorder; M(ix) Microscopy of Menkes kinky hair disorder (MKHD) showing trichorrhexis nodosa; M(x) Microscopy of hair in Menkes disease showing pili torti; M(xi) Pilomatricoma over cheek in a 5-year-old girl.

"There are no great limits to growth because there are no limits of human intelligence, imagination, and wonder." — **Ronald Reagan**

cystic appearing, perforating, anetodermic, proliferating, pigmented, pilomatricomal horn, and pilomatrix carcinoma (very rare).

The triad of basaloid cells, squamous cells, and characteristic shadow or ghost cells on fine-needle aspiration cytology (FNAC) is confirmatory of pilomatricoma. The definitive treatment is complete excision with clear margins. Recurrence is very rare. In case of multiple pilomatricomas, the presence of familial or associated conditions should be considered.

HYPERTRICHOSIS

Hypertrichosis refers to a generalized or localized nonandrogen-dependent excessive hair growth in males or females without evidence of masculinization or menstrual abnormalities **(Fig. 12N)**.

Congenital Hypertrichosis (Fig. 12O)

Congenital hypertrichosis encompasses the following conditions.

Hypertrichosis lanuginosa: It is an inherited condition in which lanugo hair persist throughout life or there is excess lanugo hair covering the entire body. Spontaneous loss of hair has been noted in childhood, others which persist have remained same until adulthood. Due to increased hairiness, various descriptive terms like "monkey men," "dog face," and "human skye terriers" have been used. Sporadic, autosomal dominant and autosomal recessive inheritance have been documented. The associations include glaucoma, missing teeth, and skeletal abnormalities.

Ambras syndrome: This condition has vellus hair than lanugo hair. It predominantly affects the face, ears, and shoulder area. The affected patients have dysmorphic facies and the condition is persistent.

X-linked dominant hypertrichosis: This condition affects males more than females and presents with increased growth of terminal hair in a generalized distribution which improves after puberty. Females show asymmetric hypertrichosis due to the lyonization effect.

Generalized hypertrichosis ***(Fig. 12P)***: Cornelia De Lange syndrome is an autosomal dominant condition which presents with overgrowth of eyebrows, lashes, synophrys, thin upper lip, saddle nose, cyanotic hue along the eyes, nose, and mouth along with recurrent gastrointestinal upset, upper respiratory tract infection, and seizures.

Hypertrichosis with gingival hyperplasia: It is an autosomal dominant condition presenting with increased body and facial hair along with gingival hyperplasia. It begins at puberty but sometimes may be present at birth or infancy. There is delayed tooth eruption with pebbling of the gums which interferes with chewing, respiration, and speech. There can be history of periodontal abscess formation. Debulking of the gum is generally helpful.

Nevoid hypertrichosis ***(Fig. 12Q)***: It is a rare congenital disorder characterized by growth of terminal hair in a circumscribed patch present at or soon after birth. Though the lesion is typically solitary, reports are there with multiple patches developing after puberty. Patches in multiple nevoid hypertrichosis may be linear, round, in check-board pattern or may follow Blaschko's line. The

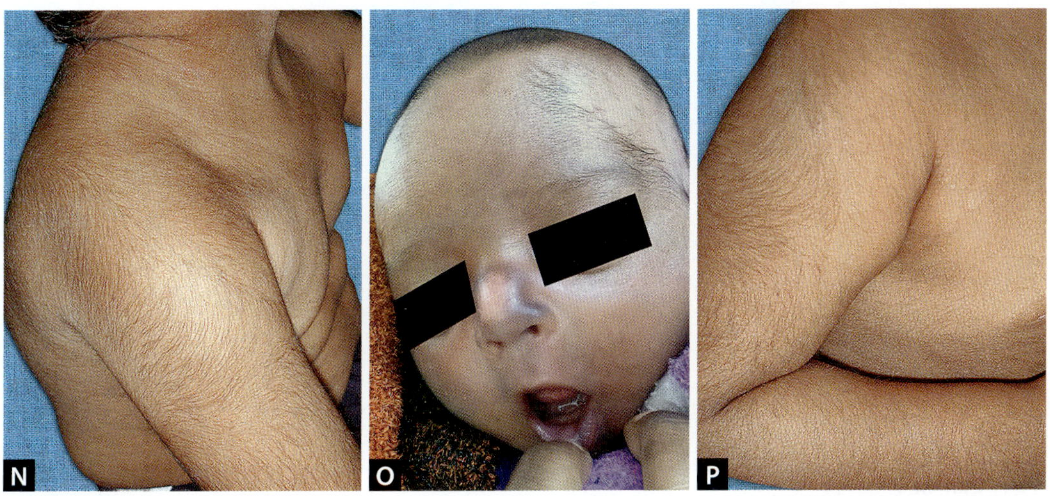

Figs. 12N to P: (N) Close-up view of hypertrichosis; (O) Neonatal hypertrichosis; (P) Generalized hypertrichosis.

"To expect the unexpected shows a thoroughly modern intellect." **—Oscar Wilde**

color of the terminal hair may be normal or hypopigmented. In primary nevoid hypertrichosis, the affected area is normally pigmented and there is no associated cutaneous or extracutaneous abnormality. Several systemic associations including partial lipodystrophy, scoliosis, vascular abnormalities, and hemihypertrophy have been reported with secondary nevoid hypertrichosis. Among the cutaneous associations, lipoma, dermoid cyst, and sacral dimple are worth mentioning. It is advised that any case of nevoid hypertrichosis must be investigated to rule out underlying systemic association. Histopathology reveals normal epidermis with increased number of hair follicle in the dermis. Important clinical differentials are smooth muscle hamartoma, congenital melanocytic nevus, and Becker's nevus. Histopathological differentiation from congenital melanocytic nevus should be made. The cutaneous lesion may persist for life or may spontaneously resolve. The underlying pathology may be explained by "twin spotting" phenomenon which comprise of two different clones of cells in a background of normal cells. Genetic mutations of this so called twin spot manifest phenotypically as paired nevoid cutaneous abnormalities.

Idiopathic Hypertrichosis [Figs. 12R(i) and (ii)]

It is a condition generally affecting girls where there is presence of excess body hair in a male pattern distribution in the absence of clinical evidence of endocrine or metabolic disorders. This condition occurs due to the hyperstimulation of the hair follicles in genetically predisposed individuals with normal androgen levels. When hirsutism is observed in postpubertal girls without other signs of virilization, endocrine abnormalities are unlikely. Endocrine disorders should be ruled out when there are signs of masculinization. The various endocrine abnormalities include exaggerated adrenarche, adrenal hyperplasia, Cushing's disease, hyperprolactinemia, and polycystic ovarian disease.

Investigations in these patients include assays of 17-ketosteroids levels, free testosterone levels, dehydroepiandrosterone sulfate levels, cortisol assay, luteinizing hormone (LH): Follicle-stimulating hormone (FSH) ratio, and ultrasound of the pelvis to look for any ovarian dysfunction.

Treatment

Hypertrichosis is overgrowth of hair with respect to age and site and is not androgen dependent. Treatment is directed toward removal of unwanted excess hair and avoidance of offending medicines in case of drug-induced hypertrichosis. Available therapeutic modalities are bleaching, trimming, shaving, plucking, waxing, depilatory creams, topical eflornithine (13.9%), and electrosurgical epilation. Different types of laser like long-pulse Nd:YAG (neodymium-doped yttrium aluminum garnet), diode, ruby, long and short-pulse alexandrite lasers, and intense pulsed light sources give encouraging results. Skin type is the determining factor in selection of laser.

DRUG-INDUCED HYPERTRICHOSIS [FIGS. 12S(i) AND (ii)]

Hypertrichosis refers to excessive hair growth independent of androgen excess that is abnormal for the age, sex, or race of an individual, or for a particular area of the body.

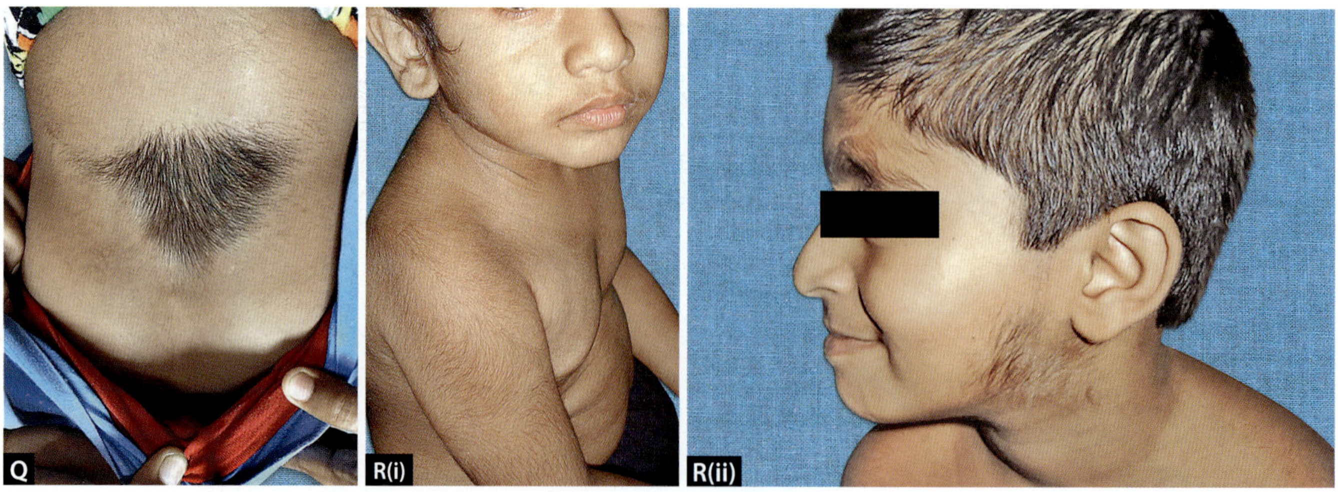

Figs. 12Q to R(ii): (Q) Nevoid hypertrichosis; R(i) Idiopathic hypertrichosis in a 6-year-old boy; R(ii) Hypertrichosis over cheek.

"Intelligence is the ability to adapt to change." —**Stephen Hawking**

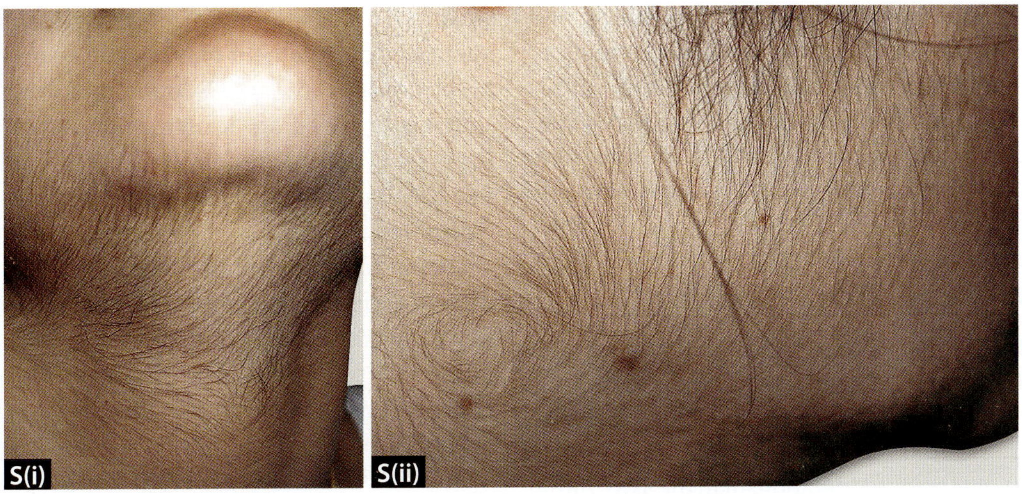

Figs. 12S(i) and (ii): S(i) Drug (cyclosporine) induced hypertrichosis; S(ii) Close-up view of cyclosporine induced hypertrichosis.

Acquired hypertrichosis is commonly related to medication usage and can either be generalized or localized.

Drugs most often implicated in the cause of acquired generalized hypertrichosis are minoxidil, cyclosporine, phenytoin, and diazoxide. Other drugs include antibiotics (streptomycin), corticosteroids, benoxaprofen, vasodilators (prostaglandin E1), spironolactone, acetazolamide, phenytoin, CsA, mycophenolate mofetil, psoralen, hexachlorobenzene, chelators (penicillamine), interferon-alpha, fenoterol, epidermal growth factor receptor (EGFR) inhibitors (cetuximab, panitumumab, erlotinib, and gefitinib), and omeprazole. Even exposure to medications such as minoxidil in utero may predispose to congenital generalized hypertrichosis. Clinically, it presents with reversible, slow growth of terminal hair over the forehead, temples, flexors, and trunk. Minoxidil-induced hypertrichosis is seen in 70% of treated children appearing weeks to months after the commencement of treatment over the cheeks, upper lip, and chins but can also appear in other areas of the body such as shoulders and extremities. It regresses within months of ceasing the medication. This diffuse hypertrichosis reaction depends on various factors such as higher amount or concentration of application, excessive systemic absorption, and high sensitivity of the follicular apparatus to minoxidil. It affects hair growth through various plausible mechanisms such as increased duration of the anagen growth phase, agonistic effects on adenosine triphosphate (ATP)-sensitive potassium channels, and prostaglandin stimulation in the dermal papillae. Diffuse hair growth following cyclosporine is seen in 60% of treated children within the first 6 months of therapy, is more common in children and adolescents compared with adults, and is more common in children being treated for graft-versus-host disease. It resolves several months after stopping treatment. Diazoxide causes hypertrichosis in 50–100% of children. Acetazolamide causes hypertrichosis mainly on the back and legs of children while penicillamine causes lengthening and coarsening of the hair on the trunk and the limbs. In case of phenytoin, hypertrichosis may occur after 2–3 months of use and resolves within 1 year of discontinuation in most children. Cortisone induces hypertrichosis after prolonged administration, most marked on the forehead, the temples and sides of the cheeks but also on the back and extensors of the limbs.

Acquired localized hypertrichosis (ALH) has been described following PUVA therapy, topical corticosteroids, tacrolimus, creams containing mercury or iodine, anthralin, and prostaglandin F-2α analogs (latanoprost and bimatoprost) presenting as hypertrichosis, hyperpigmentation, and epidermal hyperplasia at a site of friction. Rarely, ALH has been observed after vaccination with measles, Bacillus Calmette-Guérin (BCG), and pentavalent vaccine (containing adjuvants such as aluminum hydroxide and aluminum phosphate). The exact phenomenon is unknown, but prolonged exposure to antigen results in the production of various cytokines by the immune system. These cytokines can also affect nonimmune system cells such as those in the hair follicles and promote localized hair growth.

Various treatment modalities are present for removal of unwanted hair and it depends on the degree of hypertrichosis and the psychosocial needs of the child. Bleaching, trimming, waxing, physical and chemical

"Quiet people have the loudest minds." —**Stephen Hawking**

depilatories, electrolysis, intense pulsed light therapy, and laser hair removal are used for hair removal in children. When a precipitating cause is apparent, removal of this stimulus will result in resolution of the unwanted hair growth. Psychological counseling for the more severe, generalized cases or those that pose a difficult cosmetic problem may be required.

HIRSUTISM [FIGS. 12T(i) TO (iii)]

Hirsutism is excess growth of terminal hair in women in a male sexual pattern and is androgen dependent. It is characterized by excessive hair growth in the sex-hormone dependent areas. It is usually caused by androgen overproduction or increased metabolism in the skin. Along with hirsutism other features of virilization or masculinization due to androgen excess may be manifested like enlargement of the phallus or clitoris, deepening of voice, male type of body structure, temporal loss of hair, and menstrual irregularities (in postpubertal females).

A child may develop hirsutism due to prenatal or postnatal exposure to androgens. Exposure to androgens during the first trimester (e.g., in congenital adrenal hyperplasia) will lead to virilization of the female fetus. Postnatal causes may include early gonadarche, polycystic ovarian disease, adrenal hyperandrogenism, androgen-producing gonadal tumors causing precocious puberty.

Clinically, the child will have manifestations depending upon the onset and extent of exposure to androgens. Females exposed to androgens during intrauterine life will have ambiguous genitalia with fusion of the labia. With postnatal exposure, there will be accelerated growth with advanced bone age, increased weight gain, hypertension, hirsutism, enlargement of testis and breast, oily skin with acne, increased axillary and pubic hair, irregular menstrual spotting or bleeding. If congenital adrenal hyperplasia is present, then depending upon the enzymatic defect, salt wasting symptoms can occur along with features of virilization.

Precocious puberty may be central (true) or peripheral. Central causes include hypothalamic or pituitary lesions such as astrocytoma, craniopharyngioma, ependymoma, glioma, etc. Peripheral causes include ovarian androgen-producing tumors, testicular tumors, adrenal hyperandrogenism, etc. Drugs may also cause hirsutism-like anabolic steroids, methyl dopa, metoclopramide, phenothiazines, etc.

If a child presents with hirsutism along with other features of androgen excess, then a thorough and complete workup must be carried out. Hormonal profile, karyotyping, GnRH stimulation test, adrenocorticotropic hormone (ACTH) stimulation test, magnetic resonance imaging of the hypothalamic-pituitary area, bone-age radiograph, ultrasonography of the ovaries, and other relevant investigations. Treatment should include supportive measures such as shaving, epilation, bleaching, and depilatories. Specific treatment directed toward the cause of the hirsutism may be tried and the patient followed up regularly.

Treatment of hirsutism is challenging. Obese patients should be advised to reduce weight, thereby reducing insulin resistance and levels of androgen and LH while increasing sex hormone-binding globulins. Idiopathic,

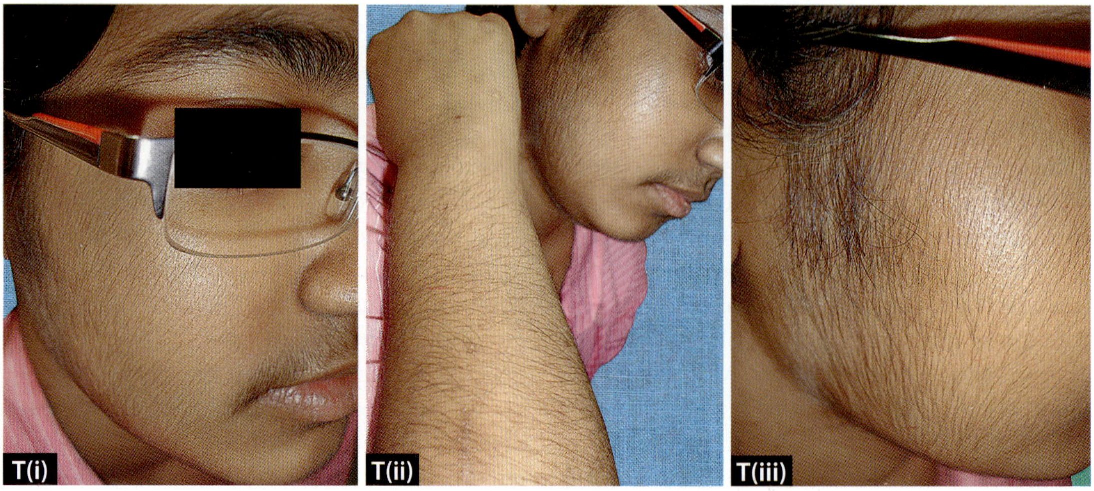

Figs. 12T(i) to (iii): T(i) Hirsutism in a 14-year-old girl; T(ii) Same girl, note hair growth over face and forearm; T(iii) Close-up view.

"The voice of the intellect is a soft one, but it does not rest until it has gained a hearing." —**Sigmund Freud**

familial, and racial hirsutism with normal hormonal level is treated as for hypertrichosis. In other cases, treatment should be individualized and is directed toward the underlying causes. Various drugs used to treat hirsutism either alone or in combination are spironolactone (100 mg/day), oral contraceptives, cyproterone acetate (2 mg/day), ethinylestradiol (35 μg/day), gonadotropin-releasing hormone (GnRH) agonists such as leuprolide, antiandrogens such as flutamide (250 mg/day followed by 125 mg/day), and finasteride (2.5–5 mg/day). Insulin sensitizer, metformin gives encouraging result in polycystic ovarian syndrome. Hirsutism associated with congenital adrenal hyperplasia can be managed successfully with very low-dose dexamethasone (<0.3 mg/day). Idiopathic hirsutism with high testosterone level is treated either by ovarian suppression with cyclical oral contraceptive pills (OCPs) or by adrenal suppression with low-dose dexamethasone (0.5–1 mg/day at bed time). Surgical resection of underlying ovarian or adrenal tumor improves hirsutism due to it.

SILVERY GRAY HAIR SYNDROMES

It comprises of three different entities which have many overlapping clinical features and microscopy of hair often comes handy in making a specific diagnosis of the conditions.

Griscelli Syndrome (Figs. 13A to D)

Griscelli syndrome is a rare autosomal recessive silvery gray hair disorder characterized by pigmentary dilution of skin and hair, with cellular and humoral immunodeficiency. It was described by Griscelli and Prunieras in 1978. Children characteristically present with silvery hair at birth or in early infancy. It can be associated with

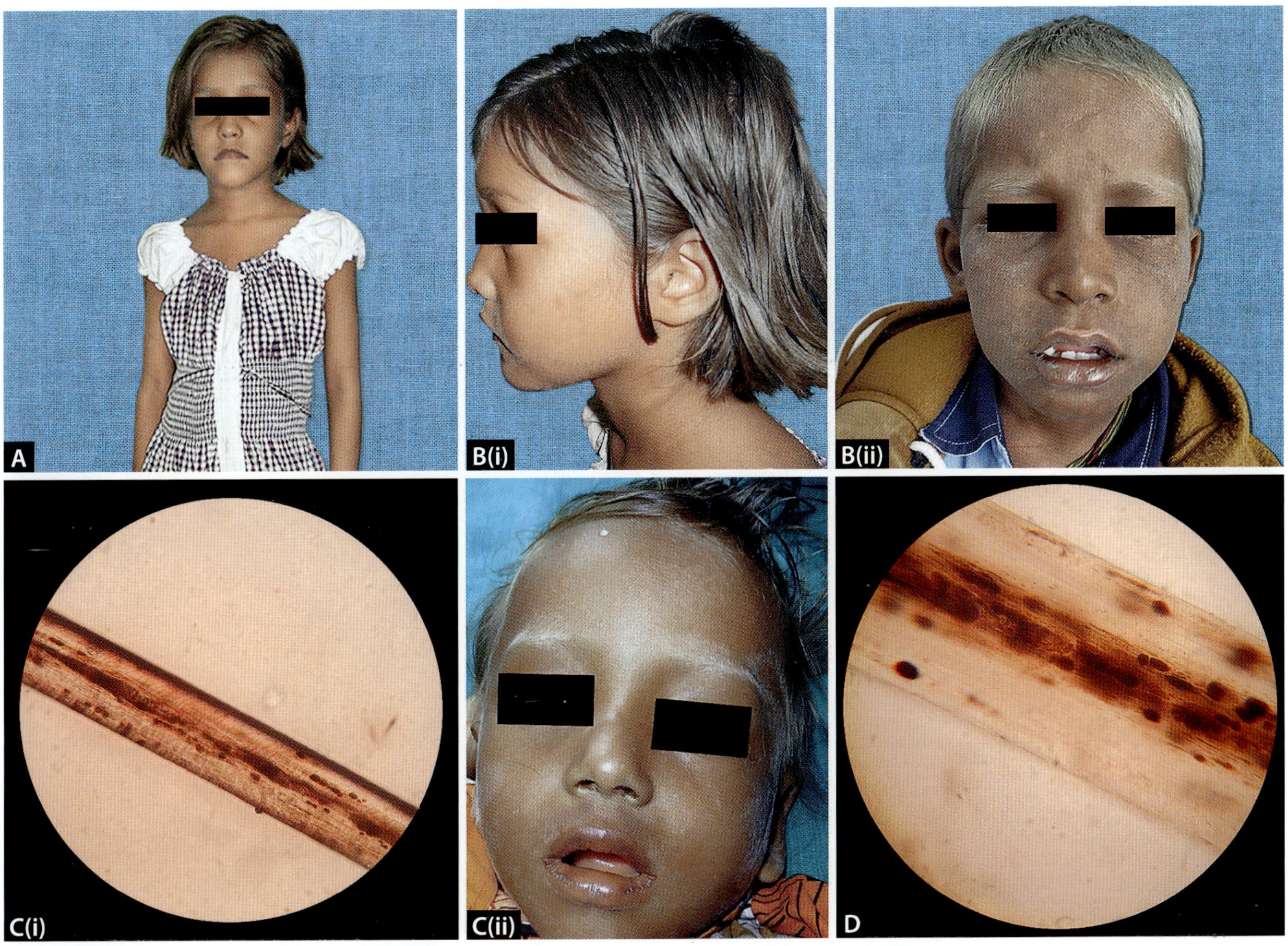

Figs. 13A to D: (A) Griscelli syndrome, note color of skin and hair; B(i) Griscelli syndrome, close-up view; B(ii) Griscelli syndrome in a 9-year-old boy; C(i) Griscelli syndrome, light microscopy of hair; C(ii) Griscelli syndrome in a 2-year-old boy; (D) Higher magnification of hair microscopy showing irregular pigment clumps.

"Knowledge with action converts adversity into prosperity." —**APJ Abdul Kalam**

hypopigmentation of skin. There are recurrent episodes of fever, hepatosplenomegaly, lymphadenopathy, pancytopenia, and neurological impairment. There are three types of Griscelli syndrome. Type 1 Griscelli syndrome results from *MYO5A* mutations. It is associated with severe neurological involvement with no immunodeficiency. Type 2 is associated with hemophagocytosis and immunodeficiency and is due to mutation in *RAB27A*. Type 3 Griscelli syndrome involves only skin and hair and results in mutation in the gene-encoding melanophilin (*MLPH*). The diagnosis is made by microscopic examination of hair shaft. Light microscopy shows irregular clumping of melanin in the hair shaft. It should be differentiated from other silvery gray hair syndromes. Prognosis is grave. Treatment is bone marrow transplantation.

Chédiak–Higashi Syndrome [Figs. 14A(i) to E(i)]

Chédiak–Higashi syndrome (CHS) is characterized by silvery sheen to hair and skin. There is intense hyperpigmentation of face and acral areas, especially on sun-exposed areas such as ears and nose. Other features are photophobia, iris pigmentation, strabismus, recurrent infections of skin and lungs, hepatosplenomegaly, lymphadenopathy, pancytopenia, jaundice, and neurological deterioration. Peripheral smear shows giant granules within phagocytes. Hair shaft examination shows small melanin pigment arranged in a regular pattern like a band inside the hair shaft. This disorder is fatal. Children usually die by 6 years of age. Treatment of choice is bone marrow transplantation.

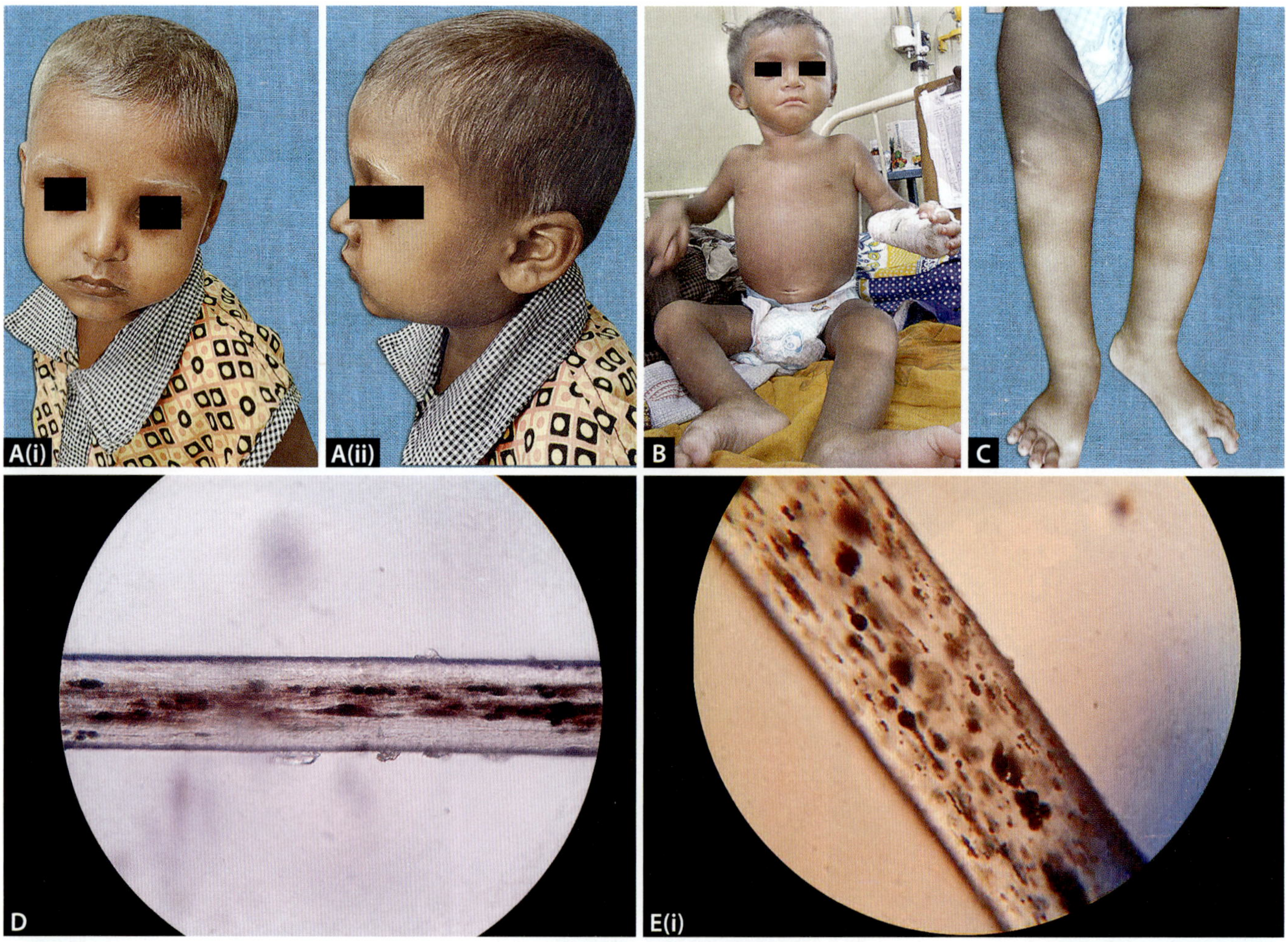

Figs. 14A(i) to E(i): A(i) Chédiak–Higashi syndrome (CHS); A(ii) Same boy, another view; (B) CHS; (C) CHS, note bronze pigmentation of skin over thigh and legs; (D) CHS, light microscopy of hair; E(i) Higher magnification showing pigment clumps in a regular pattern.

"Everything that is made beautiful and fair and lovely is made for the eye of one who sees." —**Rumi**

Elejalde Syndrome [Fig. 14E(ii)]

Elejalde syndrome is characterized by silvery gray hair with severe neurological involvement, seizures, hypotonia, and ocular abnormalities. There is no immunodeficiency or hemophagocytosis in this condition. Light microscopy of hair shaft shows large, irregularly distributed melanin pigments resembling Griscelli syndrome. It is now thought that Griscelli type 1 could be Elejalde syndrome. Management is bone marrow transplantation.

CUTIS VERTICIS GYRATA [FIGS. 14F TO H(ii)]

This entity implies hypertrophy and folds or furrow on the scalp usually in an anteroposterior direction. There is a definite male preponderance with onset before 30 years in most of the cases. Vertex is the most common site to get involved with normal hair. Number of folds varies from 2 to 20. Biopsy reveals normal or increased collagen with hypertrophy of sebaceous glands. Both X-ray and computed tomography (CT) scan are almost equally effective to detect this pathological entity. Surgical excision followed by grafting or scalp reduction can be tried in severe cases or in case of facial involvement. Causes of cutis verticis gyrata can be summarized as follows:

- *Idiopathic*
- *Hereditary*: Familial, pachydermoperiostosis, Ehlers–Danlos syndrome, Turner syndrome, Klinefelter syndrome, tuberous sclerosis, plexiform neurofibromatosis, associated with mental retardation, fragile X syndrome, and insulin resistance syndrome
- *Traumatic*
- *Inflammation*: Chronic folliculitis, and dissecting cellulitis of scalp
- *Endocrinal*: Myxedema and acromegaly
- *Neoplastic*: Leukemia
- *Others*: Syphilis, amyloidosis, melanocytic nevi.

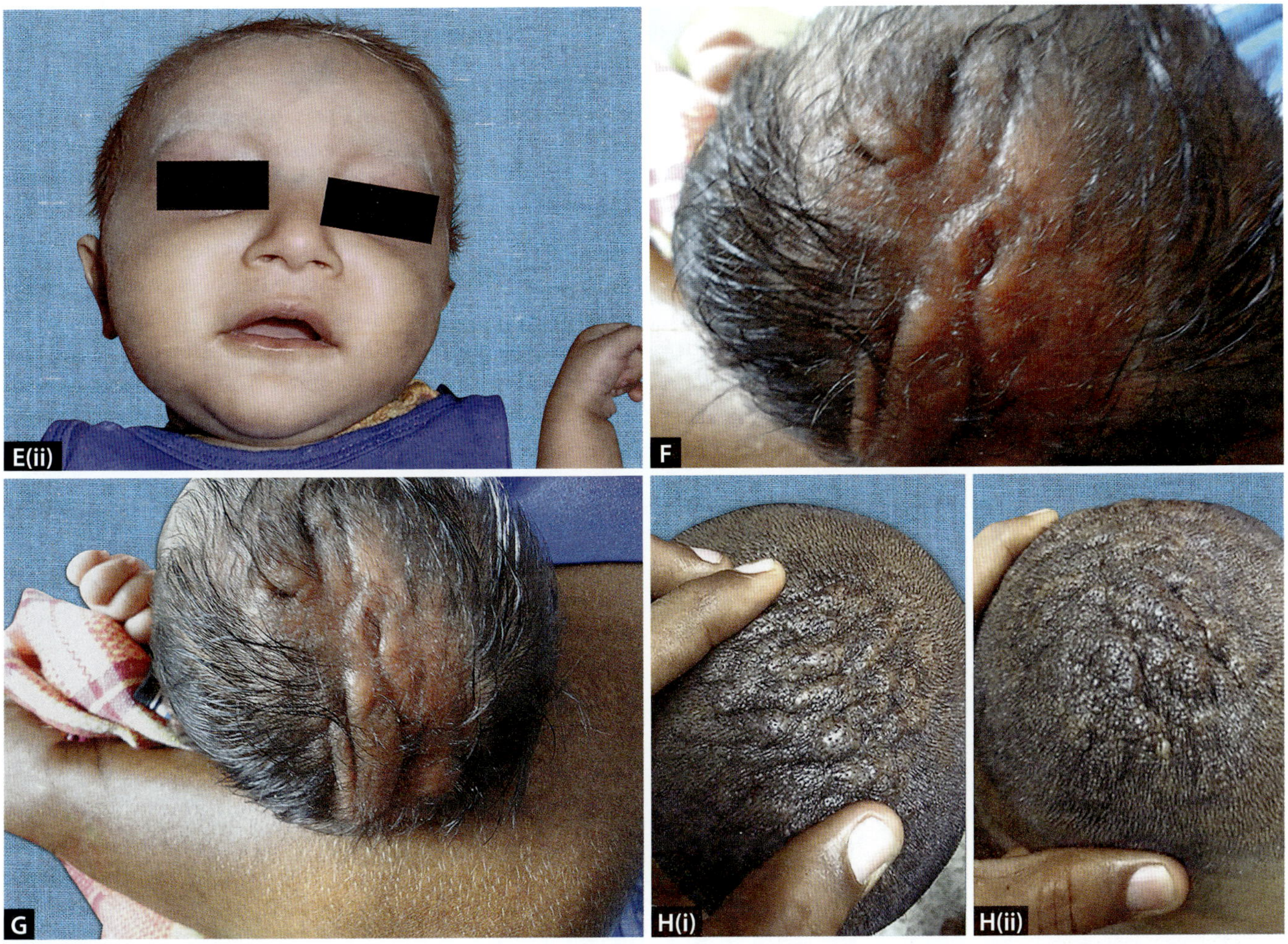

Figs. 14E(ii) to H(ii): E(ii) Elejalde syndrome in an infant; (F) Cutis verticis gyrata; (G) Close-up view; H(i) Close-up view of cutis verticis gyrata; H(ii) Cutis verticis gyrata of the scalp.

"There is a candle in your heart, ready to be kindled. There is a void in your soul, ready to be filled. You feel it, don't you?." —**Rumi**

CONGENITAL ATRICHIA [FIGS. 14H(iii) AND I]

Atrichia congenita without ectodermal defects (isolated form) is a rare autosomal recessive condition characterized by the shedding of scalp hair between 1 and 6 months of age, after which no growth occurs. Eyebrow, eyelash, and body hair may also be sparse or absent; patients may have a few pubic and axillary hair. It may occur either in isolation or with associated defects. Isolated congenital alopecia has been reported to occur in both sporadic and familial forms. In the isolated familial form, inheritance is usually autosomal recessive, although dominant or irregular dominant inheritance has occurred in some families. The gene locus for familial cases is on chromosome 8p21-22 and mutation of the human hairless (HR) gene on chromosome 8p21-22 produce the clinical picture of atrichia congenita. Human HR gene is a homologue of the murine hairless gene and encodes a zinc-finger transcription factor protein that is expressed in the brain and the skin.

MARIE UNNA HEREDITARY HYPOTRICHOSIS (FIG. 14J)

Marie Unna hereditary hypotrichosis (MUHH) is an autosomal dominant disorder characterized by a distinctive pattern of hair loss. It was first described by Marie Unna in a German family. It usually occurs as an isolated hair abnormality. Mutation of the *U2HR* gene, located in chromosome 8p21 is responsible for MUHH. Clinically, it presents with sparse or absent hair at birth, later there is regrowth of coarse, unruly hair in childhood and progressive, nonscarring loss of hair again at or nearing puberty. Eyebrow loss and presence of wiry, twisted hair is important for diagnosis. Other ectodermal structures are normal. Diffuse follicular hyperkeratosis with milia-like facial lesions may be present. Multiple anagen hair are extractable on gentle hair pull. Light microscopy of the hair shaft shows deeply pigmented, variations in shaft diameter, twisted and bent at odd angles that make it stand from the head. Histopathologically, there are reduced numbers of follicles with mild-to-moderate inflammatory infiltrate. There is no fibrosis and scarring. Differential diagnoses are alopecia universalis, congenital atrichia with papular lesions, hereditary hypotrichosis simplex, and localized autosomal recessive hypotrichosis. Hereditary hypotrichosis simplex is characterized by normal hair growth at birth, but there is hair loss without hair shaft abnormalities. Autosomal recessive hereditary hypotrichosis is associated with sparse hair, woolly hair **(Figs. 14K and L)**, skin fragility, palmoplantar keratoderma, and cardiomyopathy. There is no effective treatment available for MUHH and counseling should be done.

ERUPTIVE VELLUS HAIR CYST (FIG. 14M)

Eruptive vellus hair cysts are developmental defects of vellus hair follicle with occlusion at the follicular level. It presents as 1–2 mm skin-colored to variably pigmented follicular papules, most commonly occurring on the anterior chest. The exact etiology of it is not known. An autosomal pattern of inheritance has been suggested. The cysts are commonly seen between 4 and 18 years of age, but can occur at any age. Clinically, the lesions are follicular, round or dome-shaped papules. The lesions are by and large asymptomatic. The cysts resolve spontaneously over a period of a few months to years. However, application of

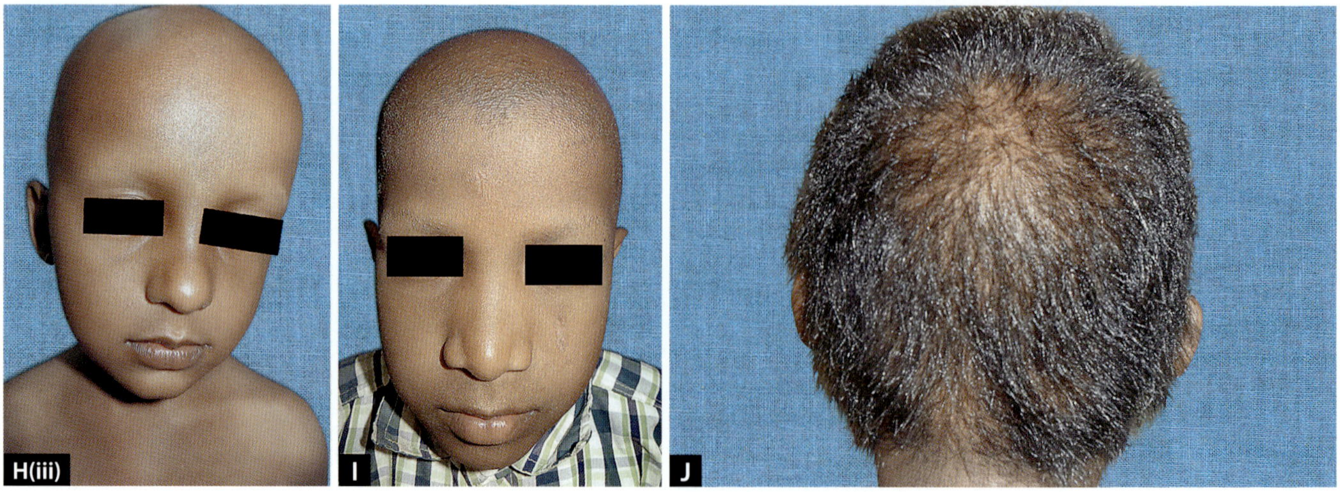

Figs. 14H(iii) to J: H(iii) and (I) Congental atrichia; (J) Marie Unna hereditary hypotrichosis.

"When you were born, you cried and the world rejoiced. Live your life so that when you die, the world cries and you rejoice." **—Saint Kabir Das**

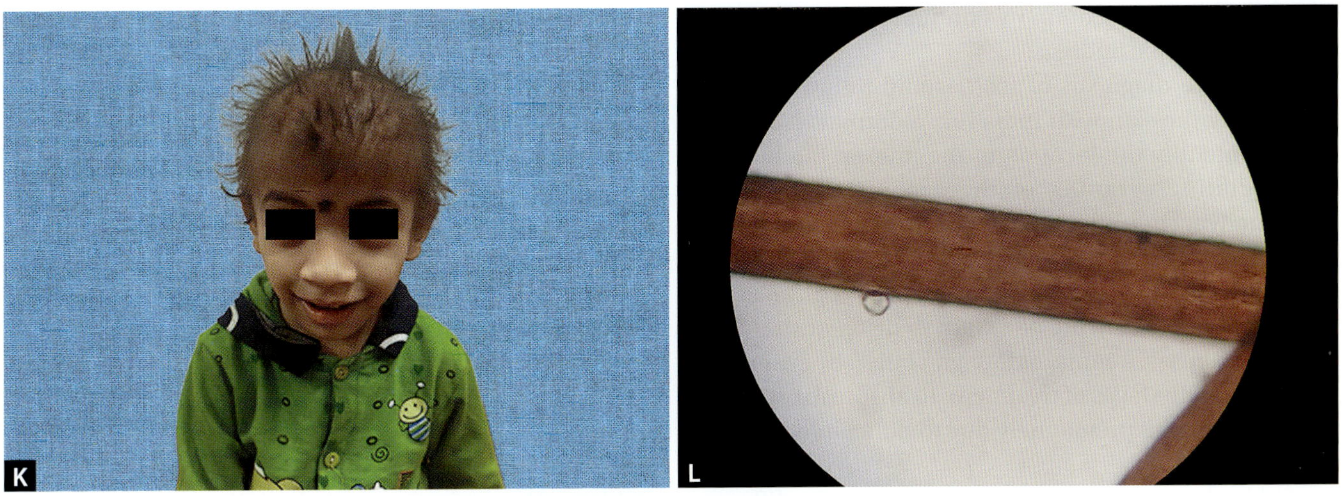

Figs. 14K and L: (K) Woolly hair; (L) Trichoscopy of woolly hair.

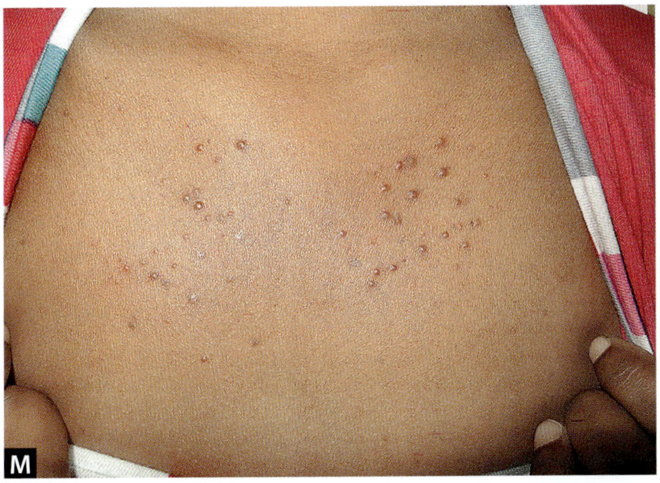

Fig. 14M: Eruptive vellus hair cyst.

topical tretinoin, electrodesiccation, CO_2 laser therapy has been tried for quick cosmetic outcome.

DERMOSCOPE

Also known as dermoscopy or epiluminescence microscopy, dermoscope allows for inspection of skin lesions unobstructed by skin surface reflections. The dermoscope consists of a magnifier, a light source (polarized or nonpolarized), a transparent plate, and sometimes a liquid medium between the instrument and the skin. When the images or video clips are digitally captured or processed, the instrument can be referred to as a digital epiluminescence dermatoscope.

This technique is useful to dermatologists in distinguishing benign from malignant lesions, especially in the diagnosis of melanoma.

There are three main modes of dermoscopy:

1. Nonpolarized light, contact
2. Polarized light, contact
3. Polarized light, noncontact

Polarized light allows for visualization of deeper skin structures, while nonpolarized light provide information about the superficial skin. Most modern dermatoscopes allow the user to toggle between the two modes, which provide complementary information.

With doctors who are experts in dermatoscopy, the diagnostic accuracy for melanoma is significantly better than those who do not have any specialized training. Thus, there is considerable improvement in the sensitivity (detection of melanomas) as well as specificity (percentage of nonmelanomas correctly diagnosed as benign), compared with naked eye examination. As compared to diagnostic accuracy with naked eye examination, dermatoscopy increases the sensitivity by 20% and specificity by 10%. By using dermatoscopy, the specificity is increased, reducing the frequency of unnecessary surgical excisions of benign lesions.

- The typical application of dermatoscopy is early detection of melanoma.
- Digital dermatoscopy (videodermatoscopy) is used for monitoring skin lesions suspicious of melanoma. Digital dermatoscopy images are stored and compared to images obtained during the patient's subsequent visit. Suspicious changes in such a lesion are an indication for excision. Skin lesions, which appear unchanged overtime, are considered benign.
- Aid in the diagnosis of skin tumors such as basal cell carcinomas, squamous cell carcinomas, cylindromas, dermatofibromas, angiomas, seborrheic keratosis,

and many other common skin tumors have classical dermatoscopic findings.

- Aid in the diagnosis of scabies and pubic louse. By staining the skin with India ink, a dermatoscope can help identify the location of the mite in the burrow, facilitating scraping of the scabetic burrow. By magnifying pubic louse, it allows for rapid diagnosis of the difficult to see small insects.
- Aid in the diagnosis of warts. By allowing a physician to visualize the structure of a wart, to distinguish it from corn, calluses, trauma, or foreign bodies. By examining warts at late stages of treatment, to ensure that therapy is not stopped prematurely due to difficult to visualize wart structures.
- Aid in the diagnosis of fungal infections. To differentiate "black dot" tinea, or tinea capitis (fungal scalp infection) from AA.
- Aid in the diagnosis of hair and scalp diseases, such as AA, female androgenic alopecia, monilethrix, Netherton syndrome, and woolly hair. Dermoscopy of hair and scalp is called trichoscopy.
- Determination of surgical margin of hard to define skin cancers. Examples would be Bowen's disease, superficial basal cell carcinomas, and lentigo malignas. These tumors have very indistinct margins. By allowing the surgeon to correctly identify the true extent of the tumor, the need for repeat surgery is decreased.

PUNCTATE LEUKONYCHIA (FIGS. 15 TO 17)

Punctate leukonychia is a condition mostly seen in children. The cause is repeated minor trauma to the nail matrix causing disturbance in nail matrix keratinization. The incomplete keratinization of the nail matrix leads to

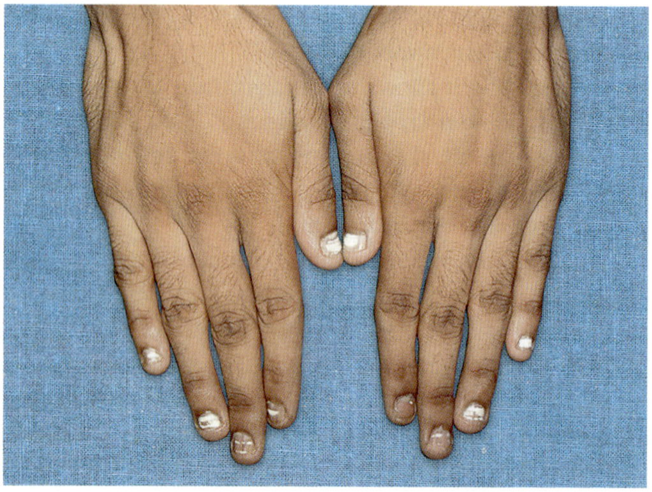

Fig. 15: Punctate leukonychia over multiple nails.

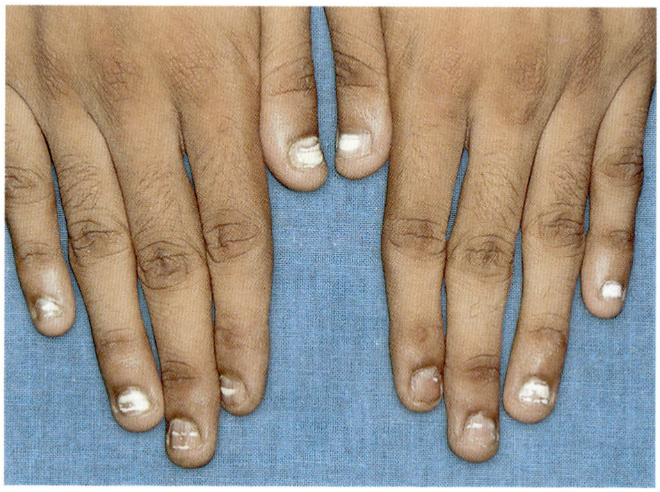

Fig. 16: Punctate leukonychia, close-up view.

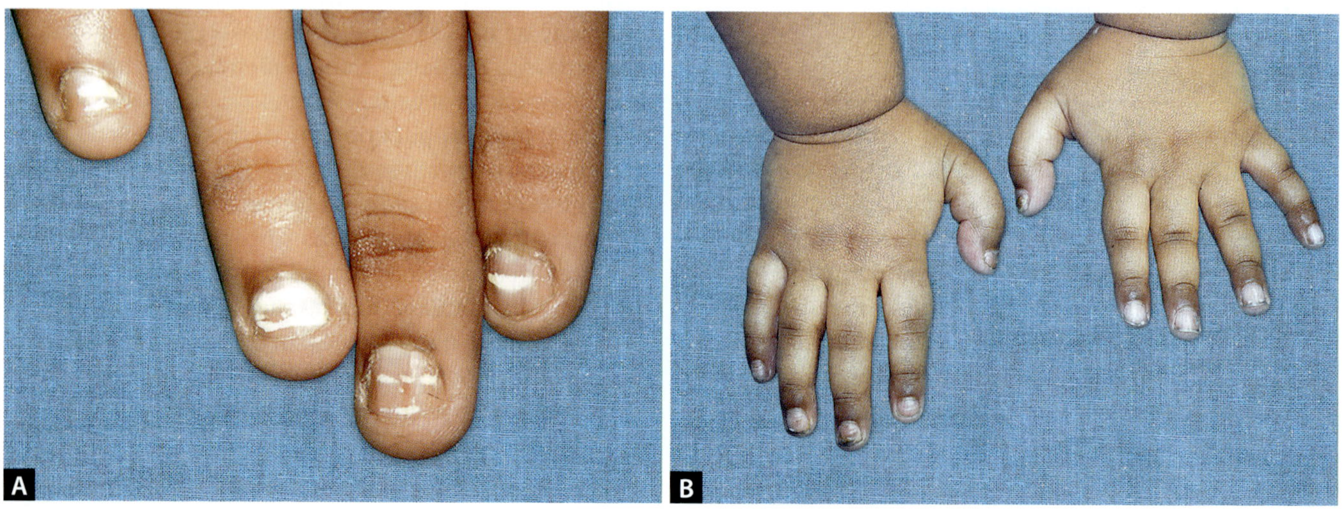

Figs. 17A and B: (A) Close-up view of punctate leukonychia; (B) Punctate leukonychia.

the formation of parakeratotic cells in the matrix which appear as white spots in the nail plates. The condition usually involves multiple finger nails with a variable number of white opaque spots which tend to grow out with the growth of the nail. The condition is often believed to be due to calcium deficiency. However, there is no scientific documentation for this. Punctate leukonychia spontaneously regresses by avoiding trauma.

TOTAL LEUKONYCHIA (FIG. 18A)

White discoloration of the nails may be either because of defect in the nail plate or nail bed. The nail plate defect causing total leukonychia is an inherited condition in which all nails become porcelain white. In subtotal leukonychia, the proximal two-third of the nails is white and the distal part remains pink.

Nail bed pallor may result from anemia, edema, or vascular impairment.

YELLOW NAIL SYNDROME (FIG. 18B)

It is a distinct entity characterized by yellow thickened nail, lymphoedema, and respiratory disorders. Nails grow very slowly (<0.2 mm/week). Other important nail changes are absent lunulae, absent cuticle, and increased curvature, both transversely and longitudinally. Adults are more commonly affected and involvement of all of the nails is a common feature. Among the respiratory disorders, pleural effusion, pulmonary tuberculosis, chronic sinusitis, and chronic bronchitis are worth mentioning. Other important systemic associations are malignancies such as mycosis fungoides, autoimmune diseases such as rheumatoid arthritis, drugs such as D-penicillamine therapy, and immunodeficiency state. Treatment of underlying respiratory disease or malignancy results in the resolution of nail changes though spontaneous clearance is also reported. Different treatment modalities such as oral zinc, oral and topical vitamin E, oral antifungal have shown encouraging results.

BEAU'S LINE [FIG. 18C(i)]

These are the transverse depression in the nail plate which begin at the cuticle and progress distally as the nail grows out. Beau's line denotes temporary arrest of the growth of nail matrix and analogous to Pohl-Pinkus constriction in the hair. It is commonly found bilaterally, though unilateral involvement is also reported. Involvement of thumb and great toe nail is most severe. Time passed since insult can be determined from the distance between the leading edge of the depression and proximal nail fold. Beau's line of local cause can be suspected if margin of the same corresponds with proximal nail fold, whereas margin following lunulae is suggestive of systemic cause. Important local causes are trauma, paronychia, eczema, and hand-foot-mouth disease. Among the systemic causes childbirth, mumps, measles, pneumonia, zinc deficiency, Kawasaki disease, renal failure, and drugs such as retinoids. Beau's lines are usually seen after 4–6 weeks post-hand-foot-mouth disease.

KOILONYCHIA [FIGS. 18C(ii) TO (iv)]

This entity can be described as loss of normal contour of nail; nail becomes either flat or concave with everted edge. Thinning of nail is not a rule; it may be thickened, softened, or even normal. Finger nail is affected more frequently than toe nail. A majority of cases are idiopathic. Familial cases are also reported. Some of the inherited disorders with associated koilonychia are focal dermal dysplasia, incontinentia pigmenti, LEOPARD syndrome, and monilethrix. Koilonychia is common in Sherpas and Tibetans due to chronic cold exposure and hypoxemia. Dermatological causes such as lichen planus, psoriasis, Raynaud's phenomenon, acanthosis nigricans, and AA should be kept in mind. Koilonychia is an important marker of iron deficiency anemia even before the appearance of clinical and biochemical sign of anemia. Other systemic associations are hemochromatosis, ischemic heart disease, thyroid disorders, acromegaly, malnutrition, pellagra, and porphyria.

NAIL PITTING [FIGS. 18J(ii) TO (vii)]

Nail disorders comprise of approximately 10% of all dermatologic conditions. Among them pitting are most commonly encountered. Pits are superficial depressions within the nail plate with varying morphology and distribution. It indicates a defect in the uppermost layer of the nail plate, which arises from the proximal nail matrix. Clusters of parakeratotic cells in the stratum corneum disrupt the process of normal keratinization. As the nail plate grows outward, these parakeratotic foci are exposed and there is gradual sloughing of these cells leaving a depression within the nail plate. Common causes include psoriasis, lichen planus, vitiligo, AA, eczema, chronic renal failure, and idiopathic. Types of pitting include:

- Irregular pitting is seen in psoriasis (shallow and small <1 mm)

"The two most powerful warriors are patience and time." —**Leo Tolstoy**

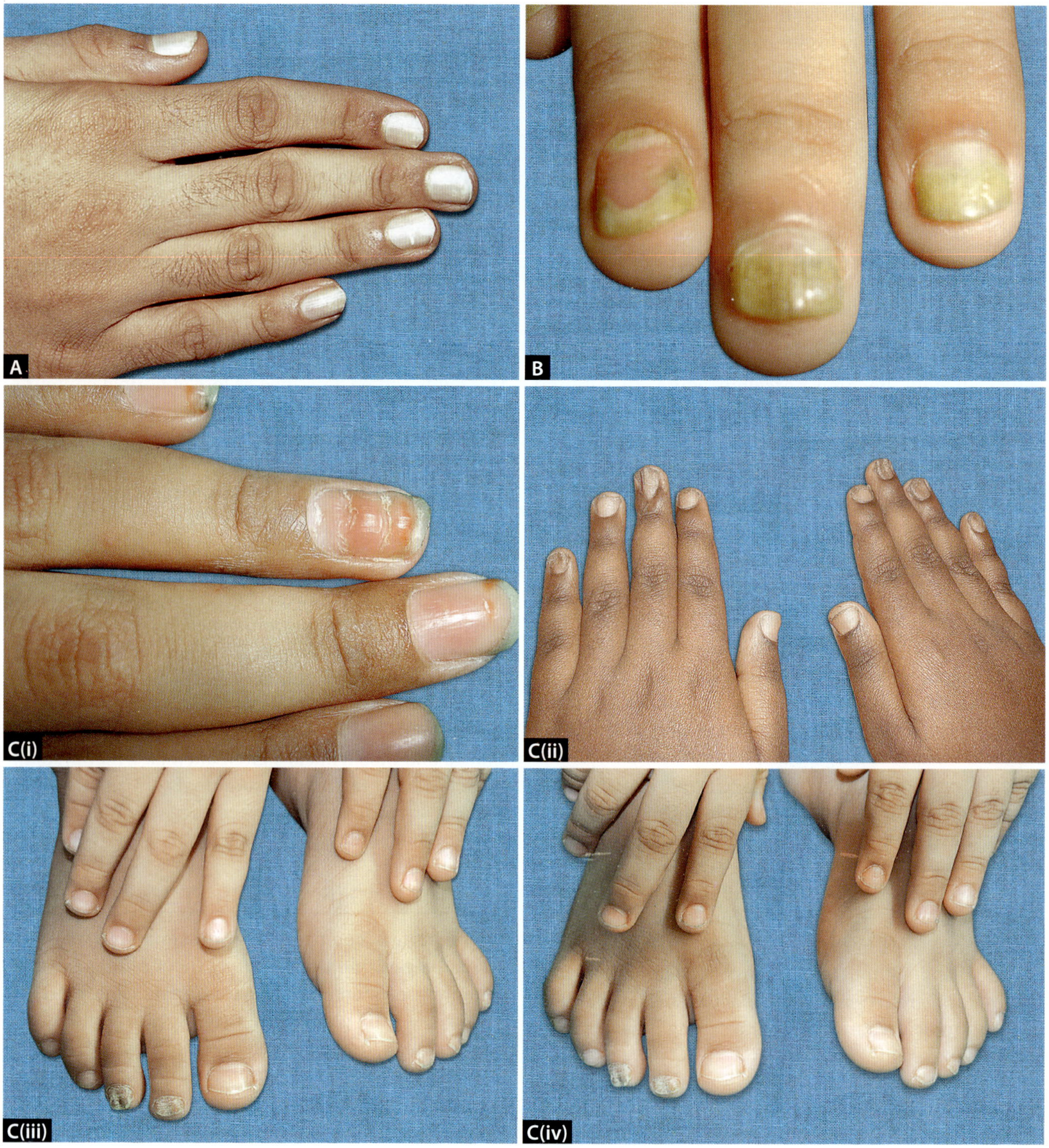

Figs. 18A to C(iv): (A) Total leukonychia; (B) Yellow nails; C(i) Beau's line; C(ii) Koilonychia and pitting of nails; C(iii) Koilonychia of two toe nails; C(iv) Close-up view of same nails.

- *Geometric pitting*: Multiple small superficial pits are seen in AA.
- *Coarse pitting and cross ridging*: Very irregular pits are seen in eczematous dermatitis.
- *Elkonyxis*: Very large pits are seen in syphilis, Reiter's disease, after trauma or isotretinoin therapy.
- *Rosenau's depression*: Small-pitted craters found on the middle and ring finger in diabetes mellitus.

"We can easily forgive a child who is afraid of the dark; the real tragedy of life is when men are afraid of light." —**Plato**

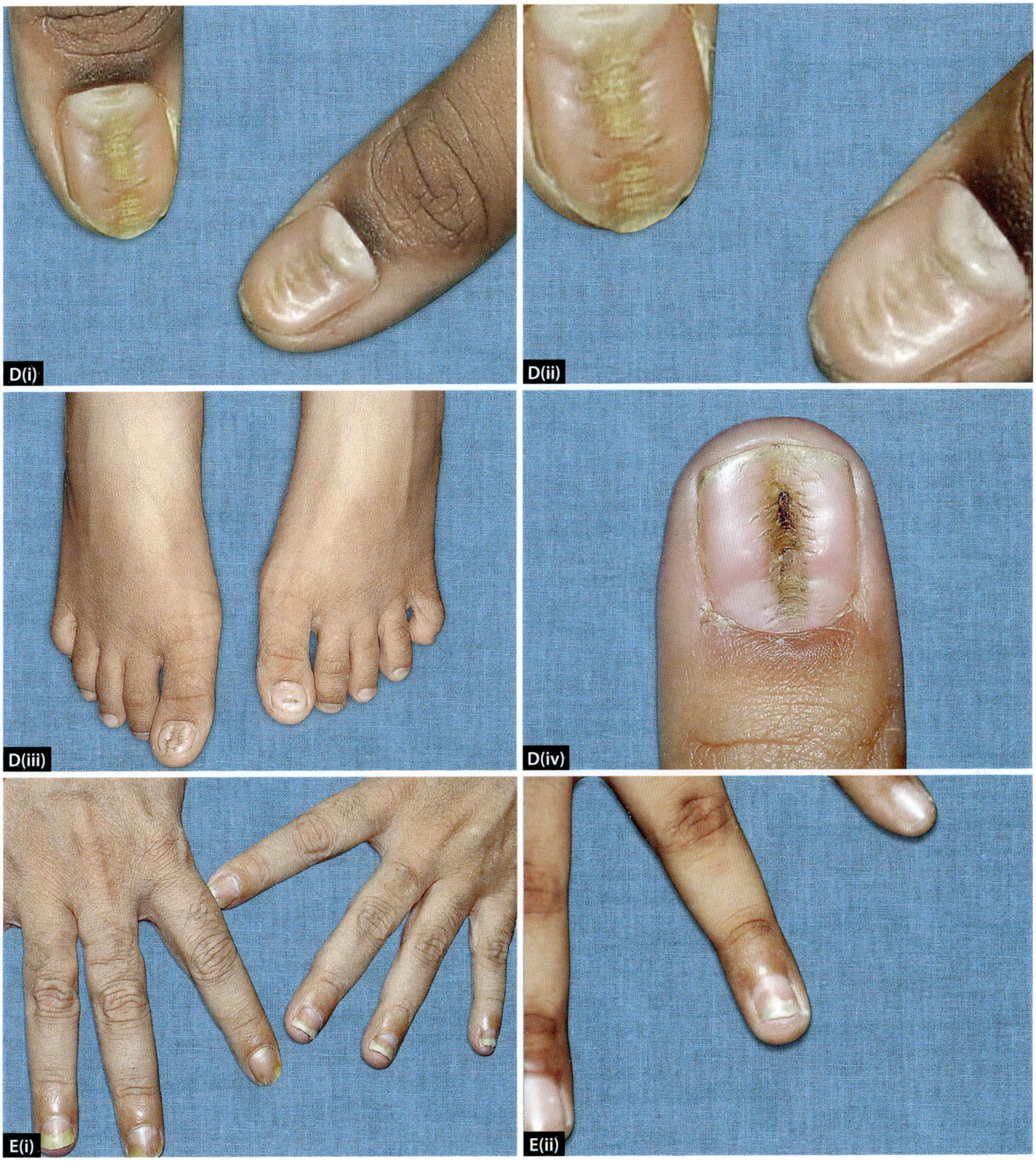

Figs. 18D(i) to E(ii): D(i) Median nail dystrophy; D(ii) Same patient, close-up view; D(iii) Median nail dystrophy—toe nails; D(iv) Median nail dystrophy—close-up view of a finger nail; E(i) Onycholysis, multiple nails; E(ii) Onycholysis, close-up view.

Isolated nail involvement with >20 pits are suggestive of having a psoriatic etiology. Pitted nail grows faster as compared to a normal nail. Pitting is occasionally helpful to diagnose a case for psoriatic arthritis, in the absence of other definitive markers, especially where it is the only cutaneous manifestation of psoriasis.

"Sometimes the easiest way to solve a problem is to stop participating in the problem." **—Jonathan Mead**

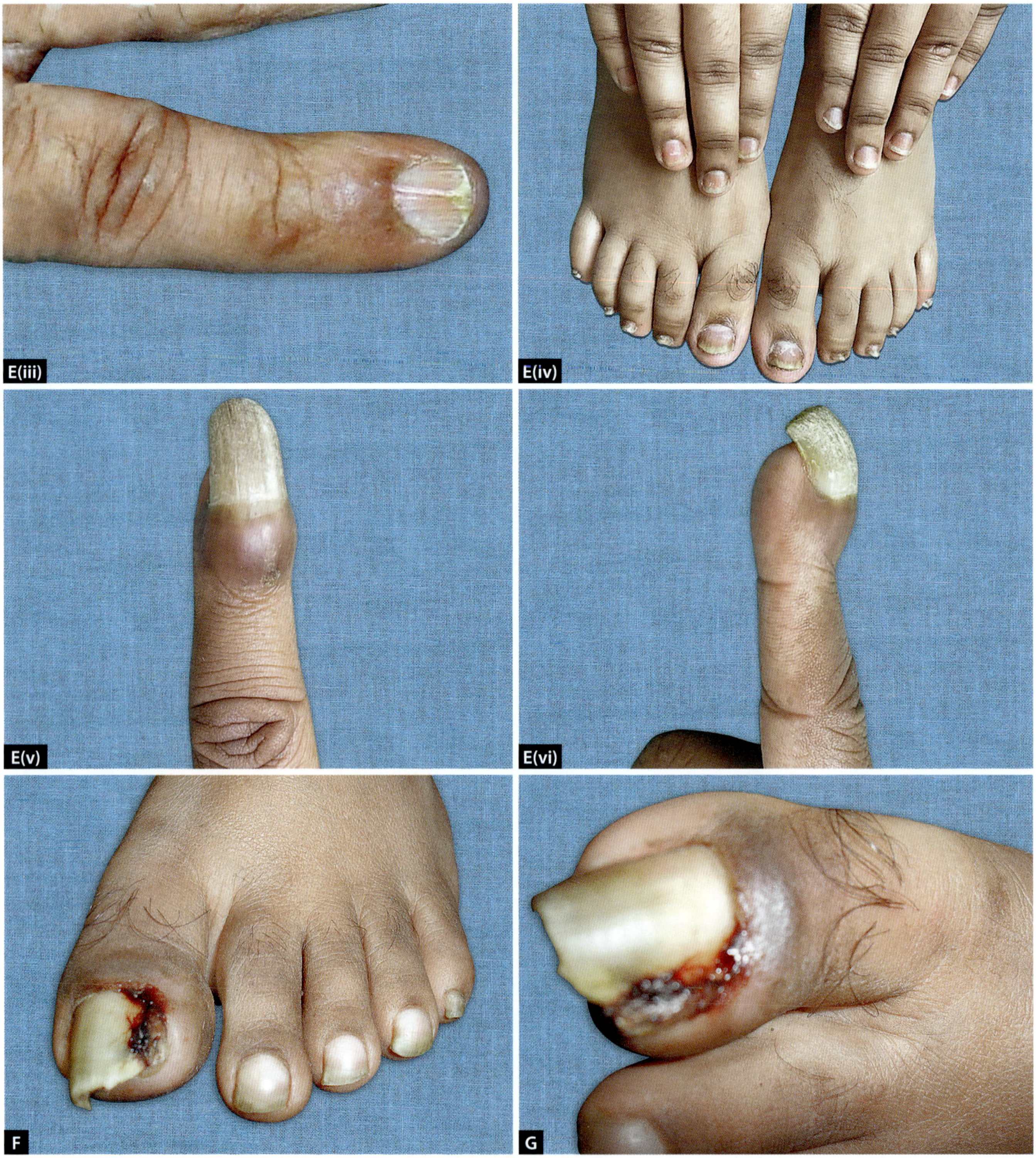

Figs. 18E(iii) to G: E(iii) Terminal onycholysis; E(iv) Onycholysis, note separation of nail plate from nail bed; E(v and vi) Onychogryphosis; (F) Ingrown toe nail; (G) Close-up view.

"The function of Freedom is to free someone else." —**Toni Morrison**

ONYCHOGRYPHOSIS [FIGS. 18E(v) AND (vi)]

The term onychogryphosis denotes excessive thickening and increased curvature of nail plate. This condition is most commonly seen in elderly and great toe nail is most frequently affected. Neglect in terms of lack of cutting nail for long period is supposed to be the most common cause. Other important causes are trauma, onychomycosis, peripheral vascular disease, psoriasis, Darier's disease, pachyonychia congenita, ectodermal dysplasia, atopic erythroderma, and neurological disorders.

MEDIAN NAIL DYSTROPHY (DYSTROPHIA UNGUIS MEDIANA CANALIFORMIS) (FIG. 18D)

This entity represents a midline canal or split in the nail plate which starts from the cuticle and extends to the growing free edge. Lateral extensions of the split toward the edge of the nail resemble inverted fir tree. This rare entity usually affects thumb nails symmetrically. Most probable underlying cause is damage to nail matrix. Though several causes have been reported starting from familial, tumor growth such as papilloma of matrix, drug such as isotretinoin; but main cause is repeated trauma. In children, it may be caused by repeated thumb sucking also called as habit tic deformity.

ONYCHOLYSIS [FIGS. 18E(i) TO (iv)]

Onycholysis is the separation of nail plate from nail bed. Usually, it starts from distal free edge and progresses proximally, whereas proximal onycholysis (onychomadesis) also occurs. Important local causes are occupational trauma, chronic exposure to irritants, and untreated hand dermatitis with secondary infection such as *Candida* and *Pseudomonas*. Cosmetic procedures such as manicure, use of nail polish base coat, nail hardeners, and artificial nail in females make them more susceptible. Vaginal candidiasis is an important source of transfer of infection to nail causing onycholysis. Other dermatological causes worth mentioning are psoriasis, lichen planus, atopic dermatitis, pemphigus vulgaris, leprosy, and syphilis. Among the systemic causes, hyperthyroidism, anemia, scleroderma, porphyria, and peripheral vascular disease should be kept in mind. Photo-onycholysis may occur following therapy with tetracycline, psoralen, chloramphenicol, fluoroquinolones, and thiazides, whereas chemotherapeutic drugs and retinoids cause non-photodependent onycholysis.

INGROWN TOE NAIL (ONYCHOCRYPTOSIS) (FIGS. 18F TO H)

Ingrown toe nail is characterized by lateral growth followed by embedding of nail edge into the nail fold leading to pain, inflammation, and granulation tissue formation. Ingrown toe nail is rare in elderly; it mainly affects hallux of young adults with congenital malalignment of great toe nail. Predisposing factors are trauma, ill-fitting shoes, and aggressive or improper trimming of lateral edge of nail. Isotretinoin- or indinavir-induced periungual granulation tissue should be kept in differential diagnosis. Prevention through patient education is an important aspect of management. Other treatment modalities are soaking of foot in warm soap water, lifting of lateral nail plate with cotton or dental floss, and surgical removal of lateral portion of nail plate. Chemical, surgical, or laser ablation of nail matrix prevents recurrences.

HABIT TIC DEFORMITY [FIGS. 18I AND J(i)]

This entity represents one of the self-induced nail abnormality due to nervous habit of pushing back the midportion of the cuticle of the thumb with the index finger of the affected hand. Thumb nail plate shows multiple transverse grooves and central longitudinal depression. Median nail dystrophy of Heller is considered to be a variant of this deformity.

PTERYGIUM UNGUIS (FIG. 18K)

The term "pterigion" literally denotes wing. This defect occurs as a result of focal destruction of nail matrix which leads to attachment of proximal nail fold epithelium to nail bed epithelium; ultimately both of the epithelia grow out distally. Finger nails are affected more commonly than toe nails. Though classically seen in lichen planus, other important causes are leprosy, toxic epidermal necrolysis, pemphigus foliaceus, cicatricial pemphigoid, sarcoidosis, porokeratosis, and peripheral vascular disease. In this regard, another term should be highlighted, i.e., pterygium inversum unguis. It is a different entity where distal portion of nail bed gets adhered to ventral surface of nail plate. Though can occur following repeated trauma such as typing and manicuring; most common acquired causes are systemic sclerosis and systemic lupus erythematosus.

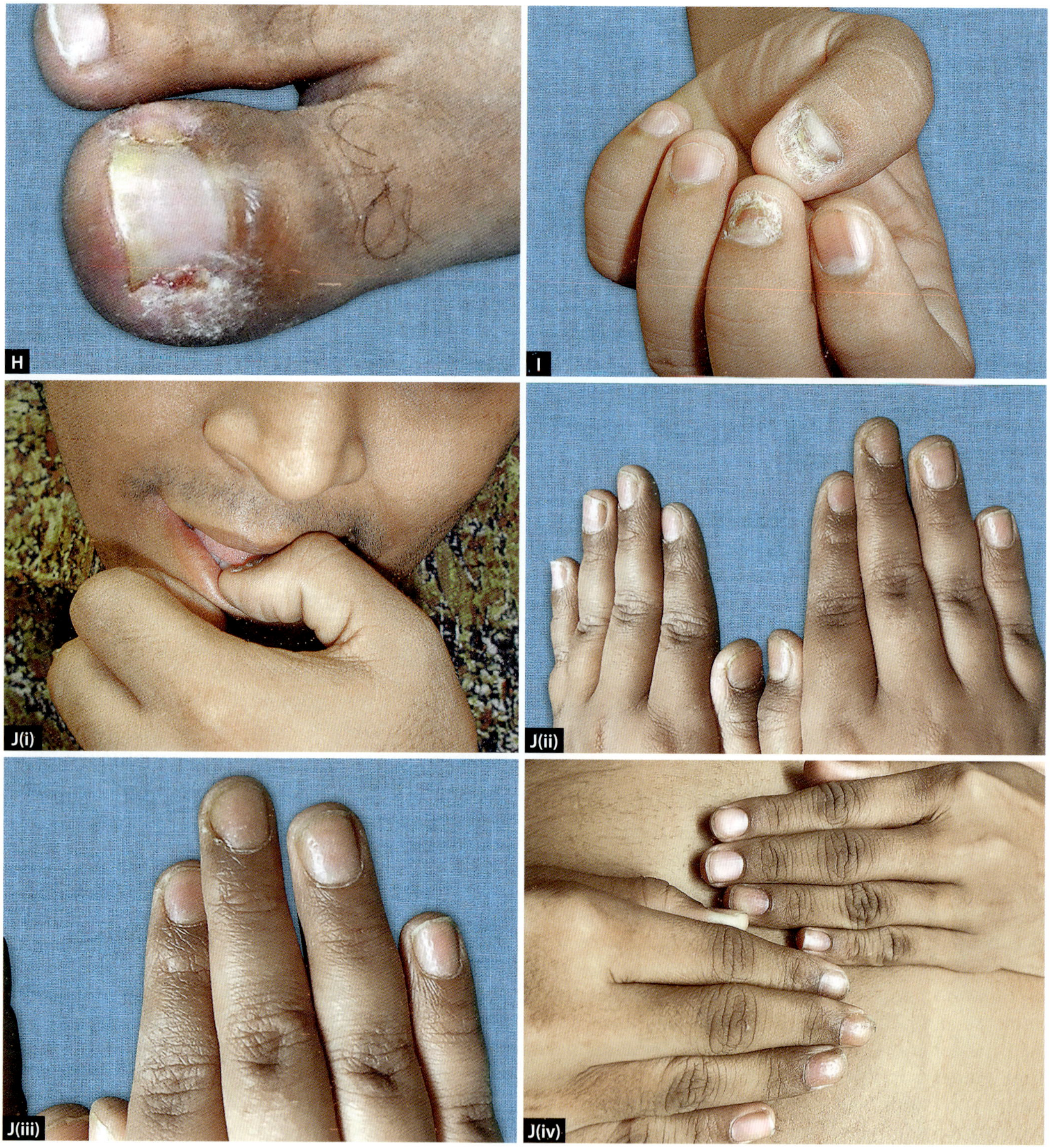

Figs. 18H to J(iv): (H) Ingrown toe nail, different presentation; (I) Habit tic dystrophy of nail; J(i) Habit tic nail dystrophy (demonstration); J(ii) Pitting of the finger nails; J(iii) Nail pitting of finger nails, close-up view; J(iv) Nail pitting.

MELANONYCHIA STRIATA (FIGS. 18L TO N)

This nail discoloration represents linear streaks of black or brown pigmentation affecting nails of one or more digits. Melanonychia results from either activation or hyperplasia of normally quiescent melanocytes. The most common cause is racial mainly in blacks

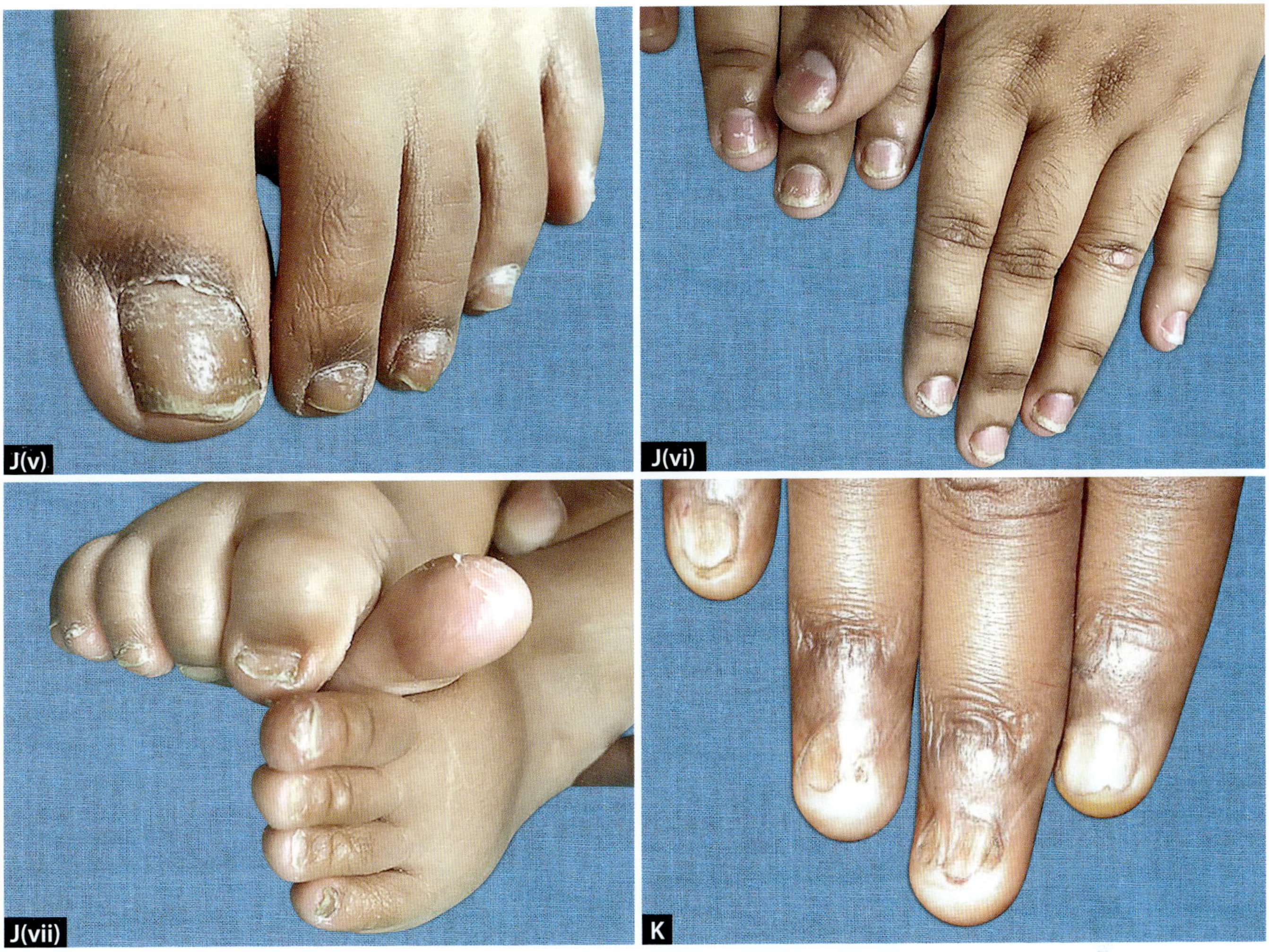

Figs. 18J(v) to K: J(v) Close-up view of toe nail pitting; J(vi) Psoriasis of nails showing pitting, punctate leukonychia and onycholysis; J(vii) Nail in lichen planus, note thinning of nail plate, pitting; (K) Pterygium unguis.

followed by drugs such as minocycline, zidovudine, and antimalarials. Other important causes are trauma, postinflammatory hyperpigmentation following lichen planus, onychomycosis, vitamin B_{12} and folic acid deficiency, hyperthyroidism, Cushing syndrome and nonmelanocytic tumor of nail apparatus such as onychomatricoma and Bowen's disease. Longitudinal melanonychia of a single nail should raise suspicion of nail matrix tumor, most importantly malignant melanoma. Signs suggestive of malignant melanoma are triangular shape (broader proximally), blurred lateral border of the band, heterogeneity in pigmentation and pigmentation of nail fold, and finger tip due to radial growth of subungual melanoma (Hutchinson's sign). Longitudinal melanonychia in children is usually benign in nature. They should be followed up and biopsy should be ordered only when there is widening, darkening of the lesion or development of other signs suggesting malignant transformation (adult type melanoma).

MUEHRCKE'S NAILS (FIG. 19)

Muehrcke's nails present as paired white bands parallel to lunula in the nail bed with pink discoloration between two white lines. They are commonly associated with hypoalbuminemia. The nail changes may disappear on correction of hypoalbuminemia, if associated.

TWENTY NAIL DYSTROPHY (FIGS. 20A TO E)

Twenty nail dystrophy (TND), also known as trachyonychia (rough nails), is a self-limiting spontaneously occurring idiopathic condition of the nails involving all 20 nails (fingers and toes). All the nails may not be affected. It is characterized by ridging, pitting, thickening increased curvature, discoloration of the nail plates without any

"An inch of time is an inch of gold but you can't buy that inch of time with an inch of gold." —**Chinese Proverb**

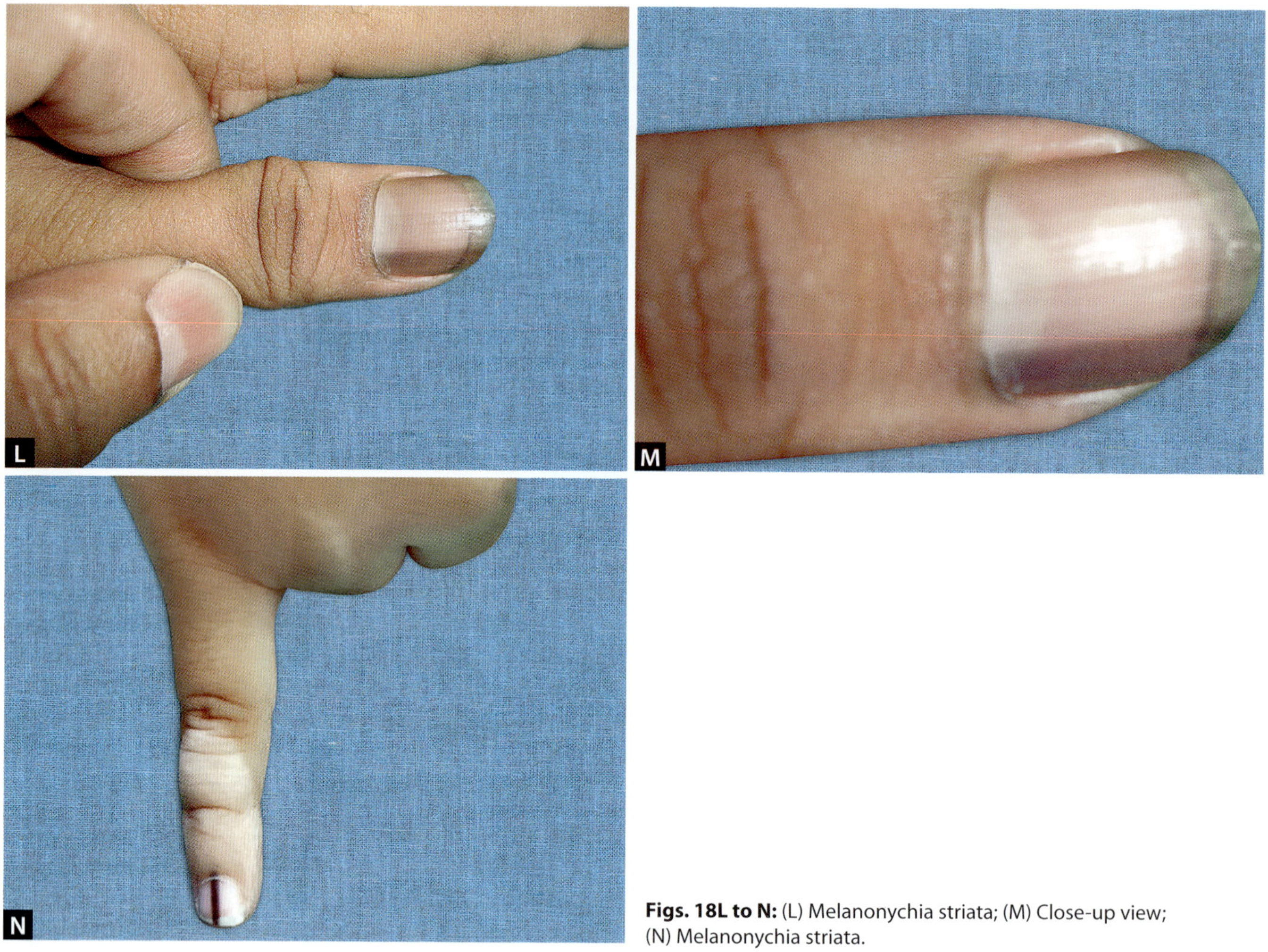

Figs. 18L to N: (L) Melanonychia striata; (M) Close-up view; (N) Melanonychia striata.

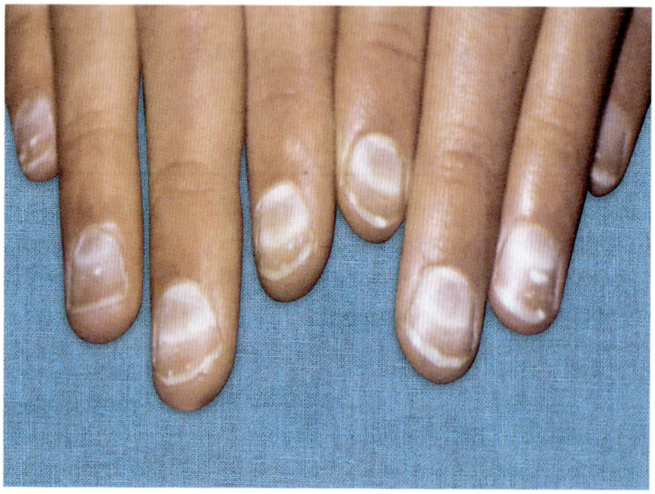

Fig. 19: White bands of Muehrcke's nails.

changes in the nail folds or cuticle. Nail biopsy has revealed eczematous change in some nail matrix and psoriasiform in others. The condition classically occurs in childhood and a significant number of cases resolve spontaneously in few years which may vary from 1 to 10 years. Counseling forms the cornerstone of management. Secondary trachyonychia has been associated with AA, vitiligo, lichen planus, psoriasis, and atopic dermatitis. Different modalities of treatment includes 0.1% tazarotene gel, PUVA therapy, intralesional triamcinolone, systemic retinoids, cyclosporine, and methotrexate.

NAIL SHEDDING OR ONYCHOMADESIS (FIGS. 21 TO 23)

Necrolysis in Stevens-Johnson syndrome and TEN, not only causes shedding of skin but can also cause shedding of nails. Onychomadesis also occurs in hand-foot-mouth disease and a host of other conditions where it may be periodical. It starts as formation of a horizontal depression over the nail plate called "Beau's line" followed by gradual proximal separation of nail plate from nail bed and shedding.

"Life, if well lived, is long enough." —**Seneca**

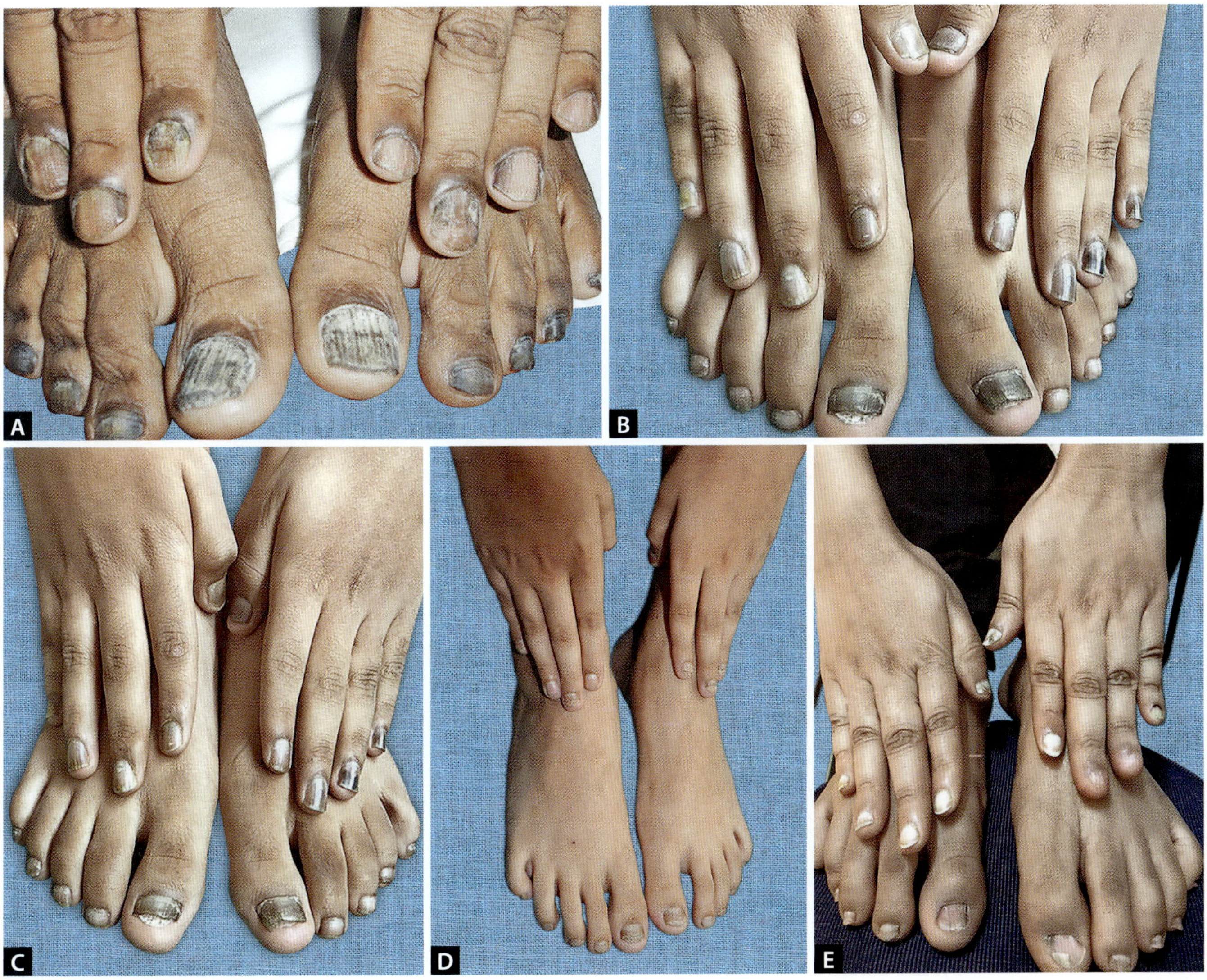

Figs. 20A to E: (A) Thickening along with total dystrophy of nails in twenty nail dystrophy (TND); (B) Close-up view of TND; (C) TND, look at dystrophy of all 20 nails; (D) TND, another patient; (E) Spontaneous resolution of TND after 8–10 years.

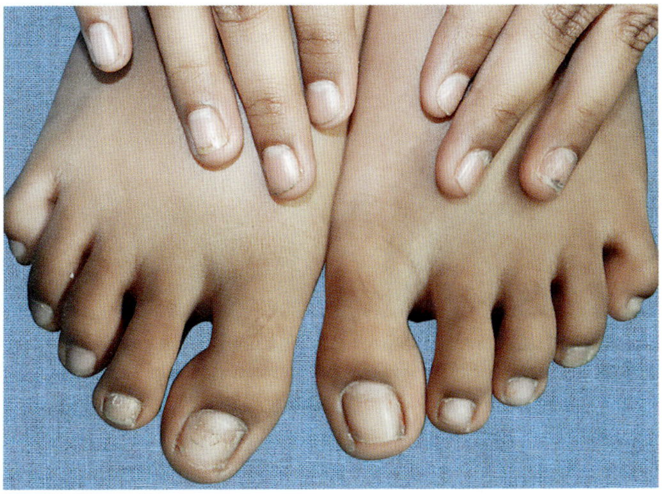

Fig. 21: Nail shedding in Stevens–Johnson syndrome.

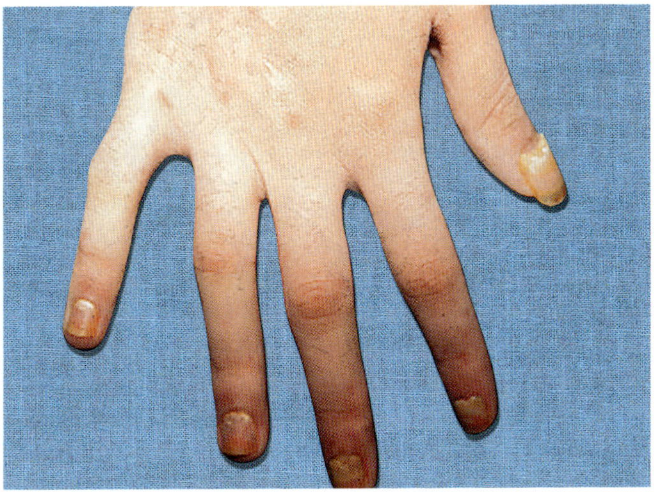

Fig. 22: Close-up view of nail shedding inStevens–Johnson syndrome.

"You are only here for a short visit. Don't hurry, don't worry. And be sure to smell the flowers along the way." —**Walter Morgen**

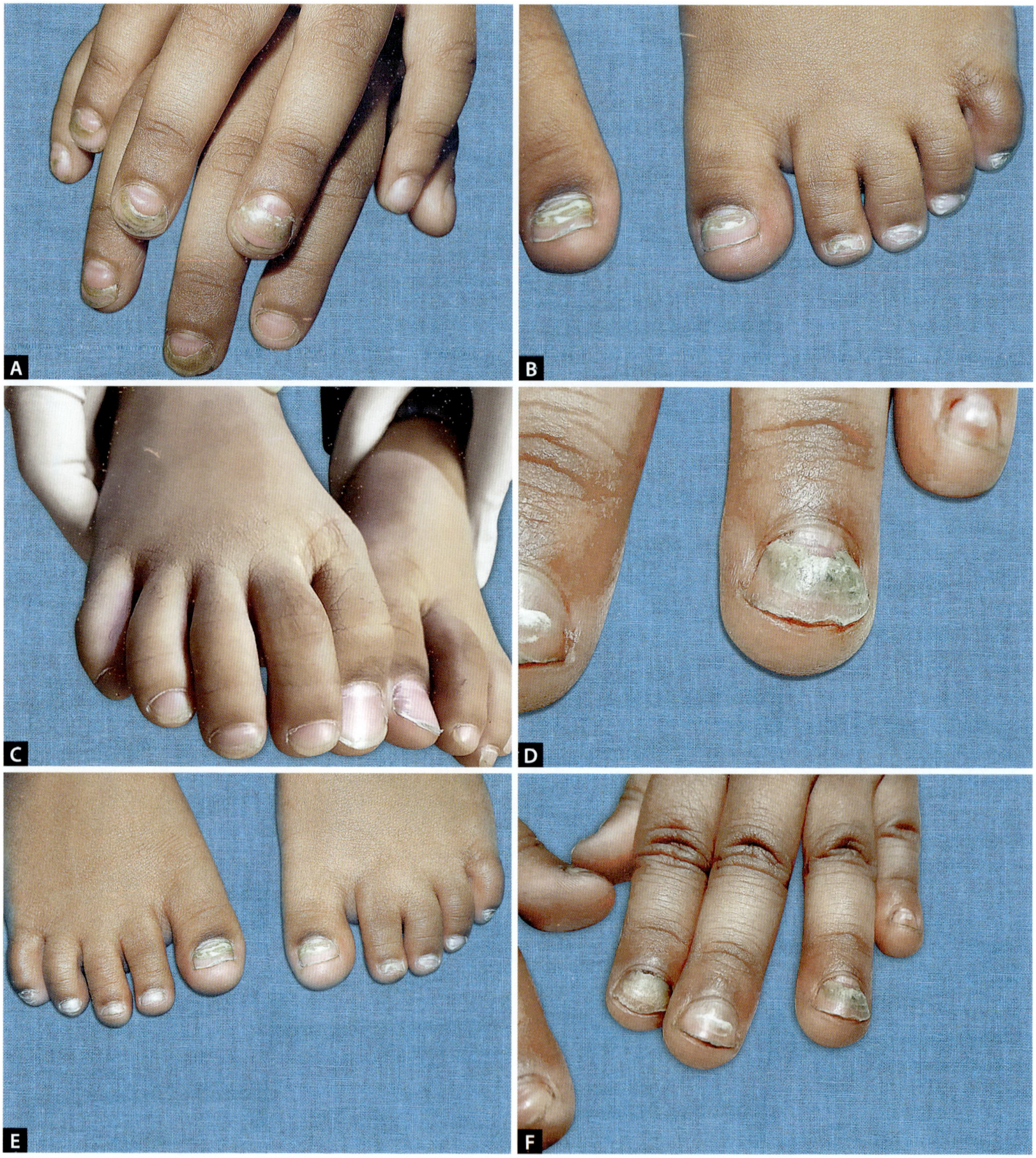

Figs. 23A to F: (A) Onychomadesis; (B) Onychomadesis, note layer of nail peeling off; (C) Onychomadesis; (D) Onychomadesis, close-up view. (E) Onychomadesis, very common after few weeks' of hand–foot–mouth disease (HFMD); (F) Onychomadesis, close-up view.

It may take 3–6 months for the fingernails and 6–12 months for toenails to grow to their full size. No additional treatment for growth of nails is required.

ONYCHOMYCOSIS (FIGS. 24 TO 26)

Onychomycosis is a broad term encompassing all fungal infections of the nail. It is much less common in pediatric population compared to adults, but it is possible that the disease is underrecognized and underreported. Cosmetic disfigurement is often the reason for seeking treatment since the nails appear dry, lusterless with debris beneath the nail plate, and pain due to pressure on the underlying nail bed from the deformed nail. The most common organism is *Trichophyton rubrum*. Candidal onychomycosis can also occur in neonates and infants if the infection is acquired intrauterine or vaginally.

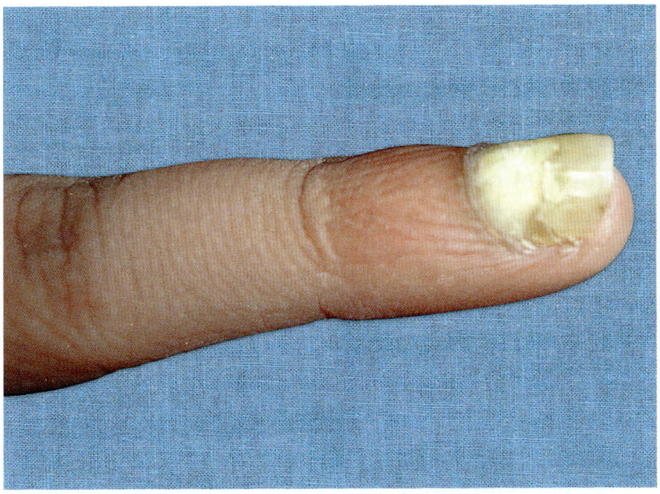

Fig. 24: White superficial onychomycosis.

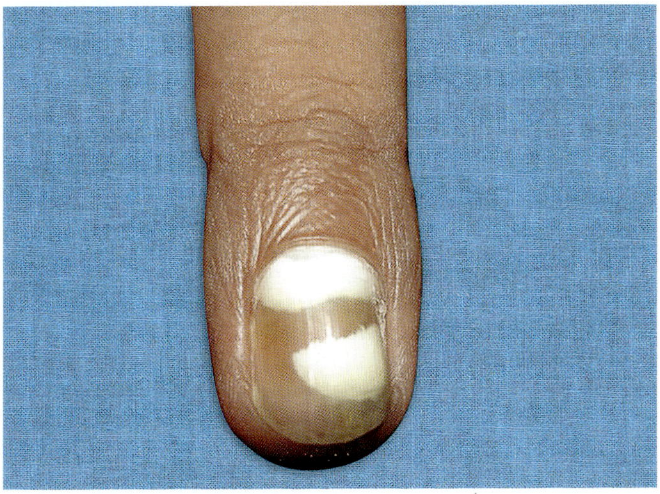

Fig. 25: Close-up view.

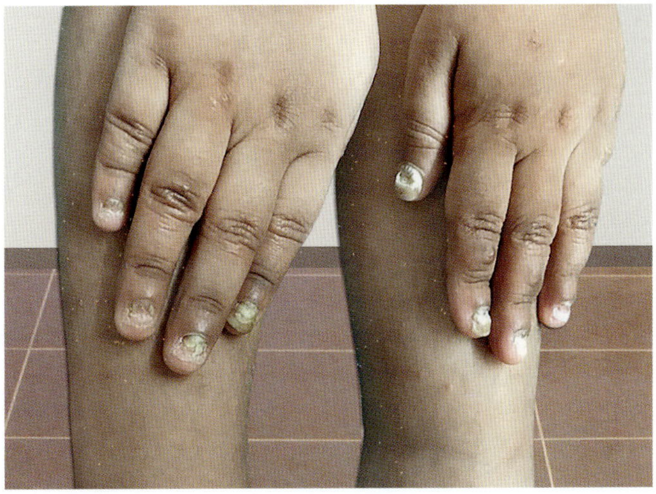

Fig. 26: Onychomycosis due to dermatophyte, note destruction of nail plates.

Some predisposing factors include dermatophytic infection in the family, Down syndrome, diabetes mellitus, and immunosuppression. Clinically, the toe nails are more commonly involved and the presentation is asymmetrical. Associated findings of tinea pedis and tinea corporis may be present. The nails are dry, thickened, scaly, and lusterless.

Onychomycosis must be differentiated from psoriasis, lichen planus, trachyonychia, and pachyonychia congenita. A KOH preparation usually establishes the diagnosis and culture will help to determine the species. Treatment can be tried with systemic and topical antifungals. Manual debridement and filing of nails can be done to remove pressure points causing pain.

CHRONIC PARONYCHIA (FIGS. 27A AND B)

Chronic paronychia, not uncommon in children, is an inflammatory dermatosis involving the nail folds present for >6 weeks. It is differentiated from acute paronychia by the natural history and absence of marked edema, pain, and pustule formation. It results from chronic manipulation, inflammation, or infection. Clinically, there is transverse ridging of the nail plate, loss of cuticle, and mild proximal/lateral periungual infection. Association with *Candida albicans* infection is usually present. Chronic paronychia may also be associated with inflammatory skin diseases such as atopic dermatitis and psoriasis. In the pediatric age group, finger sucking is the most common cause, leading to maceration of the digits and increasing the risk of transmission of oral flora to the hyponychium and nail folds. Repeated or persistent paronychia in infants

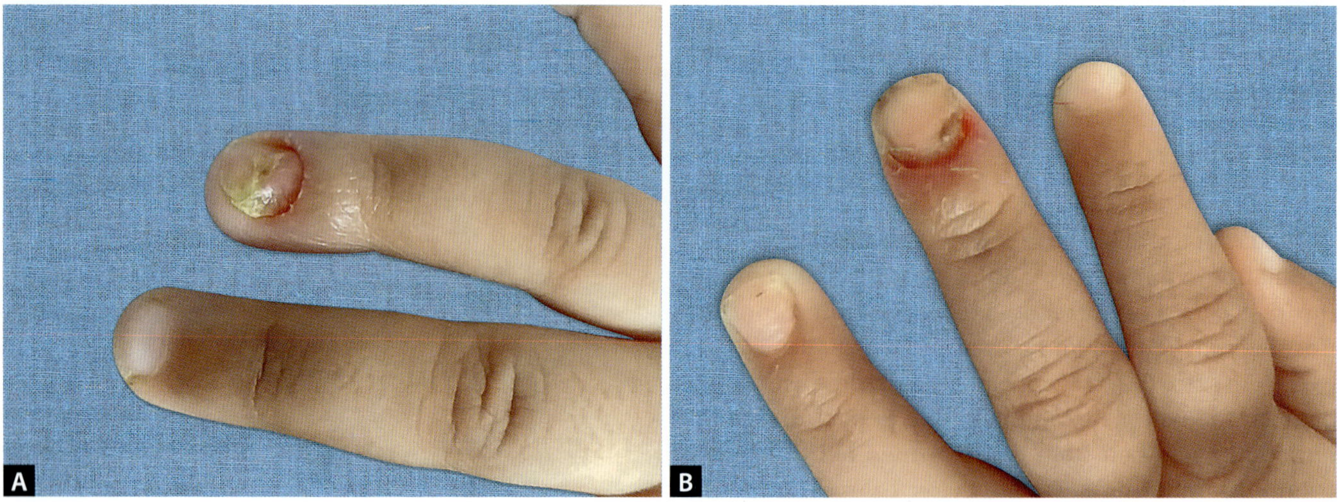

Figs. 27A and B: Chronic paronychia, note thickening and loss of cuticle of posterior nail folds.

might represent a serious underlying disorder such as endocrine diseases, immunodeficiency syndromes, and systemic diseases such as histiocytosis X, acrodermatitis enteropathica, and reactive arthritis.

Acute flares occur over a long period of time. Nail plate may take several months to grow properly. Attempts at reducing moisture of the affected digit are the first step in treatment and preventing recurrences. Topical antifungal such as clotrimazole applied twice daily when *Candida* is suspected is effective. Topical clindamycin solution kills bacteria, has a bitter taste to discourage further sucking, and has alcohol propylene glycol vehicle that dries out residual moisture and thus can be helpful. Topical steroids in combination with antimicrobials is useful when the inflammation of the nail folds is significant, which is slow to settle on antimicrobial therapy alone. Oral fluconazole and itraconazole may be helpful in severe or resistant involvement. Oral antibiotics if used should cover oral flora. Acute painful flares can be managed by compression, drainage, and/or oral antimicrobial therapy. Herpetic whitlow should be considered in the differential diagnosis if standard treatments are not effective.

WHAT'S NEW: PEDIATRIC ANDROGENETIC ALOPECIA

Androgenetic alopecia predominantly affects post-pubertal individuals and is the leading cause of adult hair loss. Its occurrence in children is seldom discussed, lacking substantial data on incidence. Tosti et al., observed a 'female pattern' of AGA in prepubertal children, while adolescent boys may exhibit a similar pattern, particularly in certain populations. Family history often correlates with AGA occurrence in both genders. Adolescents with AGA frequently manifest other skin conditions, and some females may exhibit elevated androgen levels. Diagnosis typically relies on clinical examination, with trichoscopy aiding in confirmation. Therapeutic options for AGA in children remain unapproved, though some adult treatments have shown efficacy.

SUGGESTED READINGS

1. Castelo-Soccio L. Diagnosis and management of hair loss in children. Curr Opin Pediatr. 2016;28(4):483-9.
2. Kranseler JS, Sudbury R. Alopecia areata. Update on management. Indian J Paediatr Dermatol. 2017;18;261-6.
3. Rudramurthy P, Lokanatha H.Chédiak-Higashi syndrome: a case series from Karnataka, India. Indian J Dermatol. 2015;60:524.
4. Singal A, Bisherwal K.Disorders of nail in infants and children. Ind J Pediatr Dermatol. 2019;20:101-11.
5. Solís-Arias MP, García-Romero MT. Onychomycosis in children: a review. Int J Dermatol. 2017;56(2):123-30.
6. Griggs J, Burroway B, Tosti A. Pediatric androgenetic alopecia: A review. J Am Acad Dermatol. 2021;85(5):1267-73.
7. Gomes TF, Soares RO. Pediatric androgenetic alopecia: an updated review. J Dtsch Dermatol Ges. 2023;21(1):19-25.
8. Barton VR, Toussi A, Awasthi S, Kiuru M. Treatment of pediatric alopecia areata: A systematic review. J Am Acad Dermatol. 2022;86(6):1318-34.
9. Singal A, Bisherwal K. Disorders of nail in infants and children. Ind J Pediatr Dermatol. 2019;20:101-11.
10. Bellet JS. Pediatric Nail Disorders. Dermatol Clin. 2021; 39(2):231-43.

"I have no special talent. I am just passionately curious." —**Albert Einstein**

CHAPTER

17

Acne, Rosacea, and Hidradenitis Suppurativa

INTRODUCTION

Acne is a chronic inflammatory condition of the pilosebaceous apparatus which manifests as comedones, inflammatory papules, nodules, and pustules.

VARIOUS TYPES OF ACNE

- Neonatal acne
- Infantile acne
- Juvenile acne
- Senile acne
- *Occupational acne*:
  - Chloracne
  - Chemical acne
- Mechanical acne
- Acne excoriée des jeunes filles
- Acne conglobata
- Acne fulminans
- Pyoderma faciale
- Acne with solid facial edema
- Pyogenic arthritis, pyoderma gangrenosum, acne (PAPA) syndrome
- Synovitis, acne, pustulosis, hyperostosis, osteitis (SAPHO) syndrome
- *Acne with associated endocrinological abnormalities*: Polycystic ovarian disease and congenital adrenal hyperplasia
- *Acneiform eruptions*:
  - Steroid folliculitis
  - Drug-induced acne
  - Gram-negative folliculitis
  - Radiation acne
  - Tropical acne
  - Acne aestivalis
  - Pseudoacne of nasal crease
  - Apert syndrome

ACNE VULGARIS (FIGS. 1 AND 2)

Acne vulgaris (vulgaris means common) is basically a disease of oily skin which manifests for the first time in

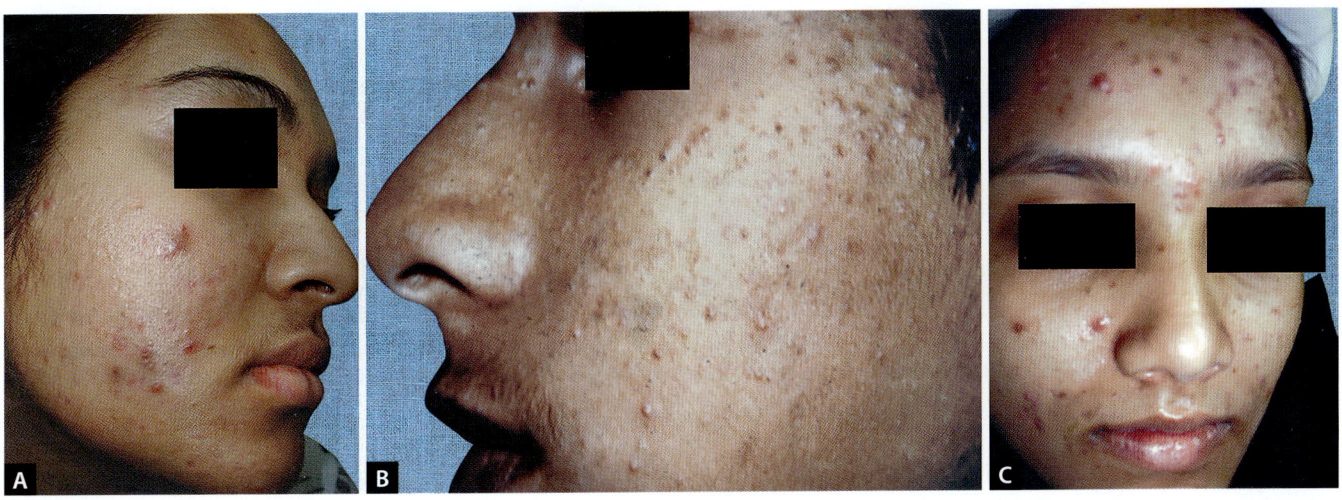

Figs. 1A to C: (A) Inflammatory papules and nodules of acne vulgaris. (B) Erythematous papules and comedones in acne vulgaris. (C) Lesions of acne vulgaris in a young girl.

"A wise owl sat on an oak, the more he saw the less he spoke, the less he spoke the more he heard. Why aren't we like the wise old bird?" —**Charles M Schulz**

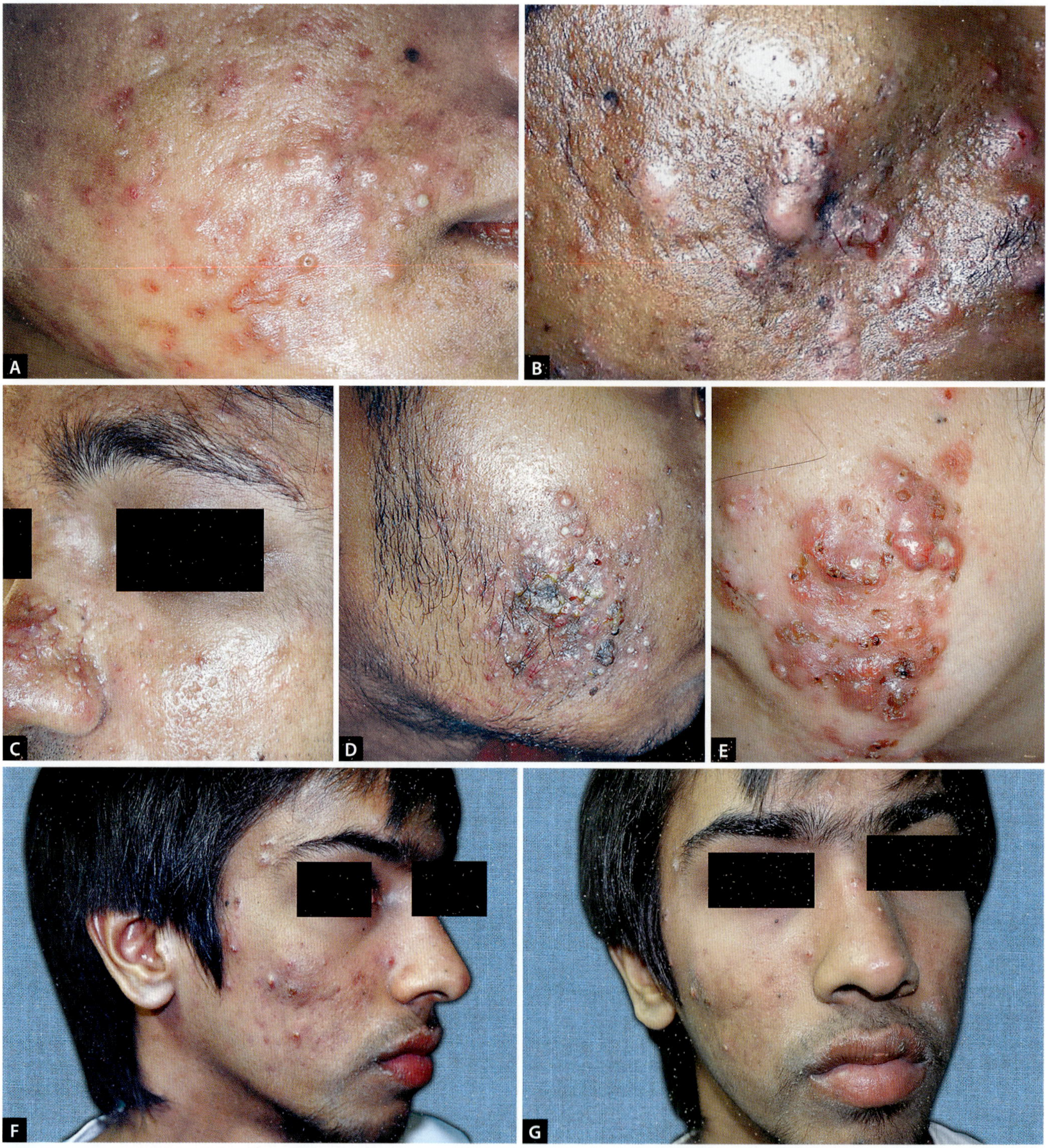

Figs. 2A to G: (A) Close-up view of severe acne. (B) Keloidal lesions in acne. (C) Acne scars. (D) Papules, nodules and pustules of severe acne. (E) Nodulocystic acne, close-up view. (F) Moderately severe acne treated with oral isotretinoin. Note the presence of dry face, exfoliation and red lips. (G) Same boy, front view.

adolescence. Faulty keratinization of pilosebaceous duct, infection by *Propionibacterium acnes*, and increased androgen hormonal activity are incriminated in the pathogenesis of acne. Majority of lesions are seen over the face and to some extent over back and upper arms. Lesions are in the form of comedones (open or black and closed or white), inflammatory erythematous papules, nodules, and pustules. In very severe cases big cysts, abscess, or intercommunicating sinus tracts can be seen. The lesions heal with ice-pick scars or pox-like scars. However, scarring is more common when the lesions are fiddled. Large hypertrophic scars are seen in nodulocystic lesions. Patients with acne often have an oily skin and seborrhea and increased dandruff due to colonization of the scalp by *Pityrosporum* yeast.

Management

The management of acne vulgaris is divided into topical therapy, systemic therapy, acne surgery, and counseling. For topical treatment, various antibacterial and anti-inflammatory agents include benzoyl peroxide (2–10%), erythromycin (2%), clindamycin (1%), and azelaic acid (10%, 20%). Various comedolytic agents are topical tretinoin (0.025%, 0.05%, 0.1%), adapalene (0.1%), and tazarotene (0.05%).

Various systemic drugs are used in moderate-to-severe acne. These are tetracycline (250–500 mg 6 hourly) and doxycycline (100 mg daily) for 8–12 weeks. Erythromycin (250 mg 6 hourly) and azithromycin (500 mg daily for 3 days every week) are also useful for long-term control of inflammatory acne. Isotretinoin, a vitamin A derivative, is useful for severe nodulocystic acne. It is given at a dose of 0.5–1 mg/kg/day for 3–4 months. In adolescent girls with evidence of excess androgen hormone, antiandrogens such as cyproterone acetate and spironolactone may be useful. Comedo expression is the simplest surgical procedure by which both black and white comedones can be expressed out. The topical medication subsequently works better. For acne scars, various surgical techniques practiced are punch elevation, microdermabrasion, dermarollers, lifting of scars by injection of fillers, laser surgery, etc. Since adolescent boys and girls with acne suffer from lot of stress and stigma, their counseling and reassurance is an important aspect of management of acne.

ACNEIFORM ERUPTIONS [FIGS. 3A(i) TO C]

Acneiform eruption is a specific subset of dermatosis that resembles acne vulgaris and is characterized by follicular papules and pustules. Drug-induced acneiform eruption is typified by monomorphic pattern, lack of comedones, unusual location beyond the seborrheic areas, an unusual age of onset, resistance to conventional therapy, and temporal relationship with drug therapy. The commonly implicated drugs are as follows:

- *Hormones*:
  - Corticosteroids
  - Testosterone and anabolic steroid
  - Oral contraceptives
- *Halogens*:
  - Iodinated radiopaque contrast media
  - Potassium iodide
  - Bromides (propantheline bromide)
- *Immunomodulators*: Cyclosporine, sirolimus
- *Neuropsychotherapeutic drugs*:
  - Antiepileptic medications
  - Lithium
  - Aripiprazole
  - Tricyclic antidepressants
  - Selective serotonin reuptake inhibitors
- *Antitubercular drugs*:
  - Isoniazid
  - Rifampicin
  - Ethionamide
- *Vitamins*: B_1, B_6, B_{12}
- *Cytostatic drugs*:
  - Actinomycin D
  - Azathioprine
  - Thiouracil
- Epidermal growth factor receptor inhibitors including monoclonal antibodies (cetuximab and panitumumab) and tyrosinase kinase inhibitors (Gefitinib)
- *Miscellaneous*:
  - Dantrolene
  - Quinidine
  - Antiretroviral therapy
  - Psoralen and ultraviolet A (PUVA) therapy

Treatment

Apart from reassurance and counseling, no treatment is required for this condition. Topical benzoyl peroxide 2.5% gel and topical retinoids have been useful for acneiform eruptions.

PERIORAL DERMATITIS (FIGS. 3D TO G)

Perioral dermatitis is a benign eruption characterized by erythematous papules, pustules, and scaling around the mouth. It can also affect perinasal and periocular regions; hence, it is called periorificial dermatitis. The etiology is multifactorial such as use of mid-high

"You cannot fail at being yourself." —**Wayne Dyer**

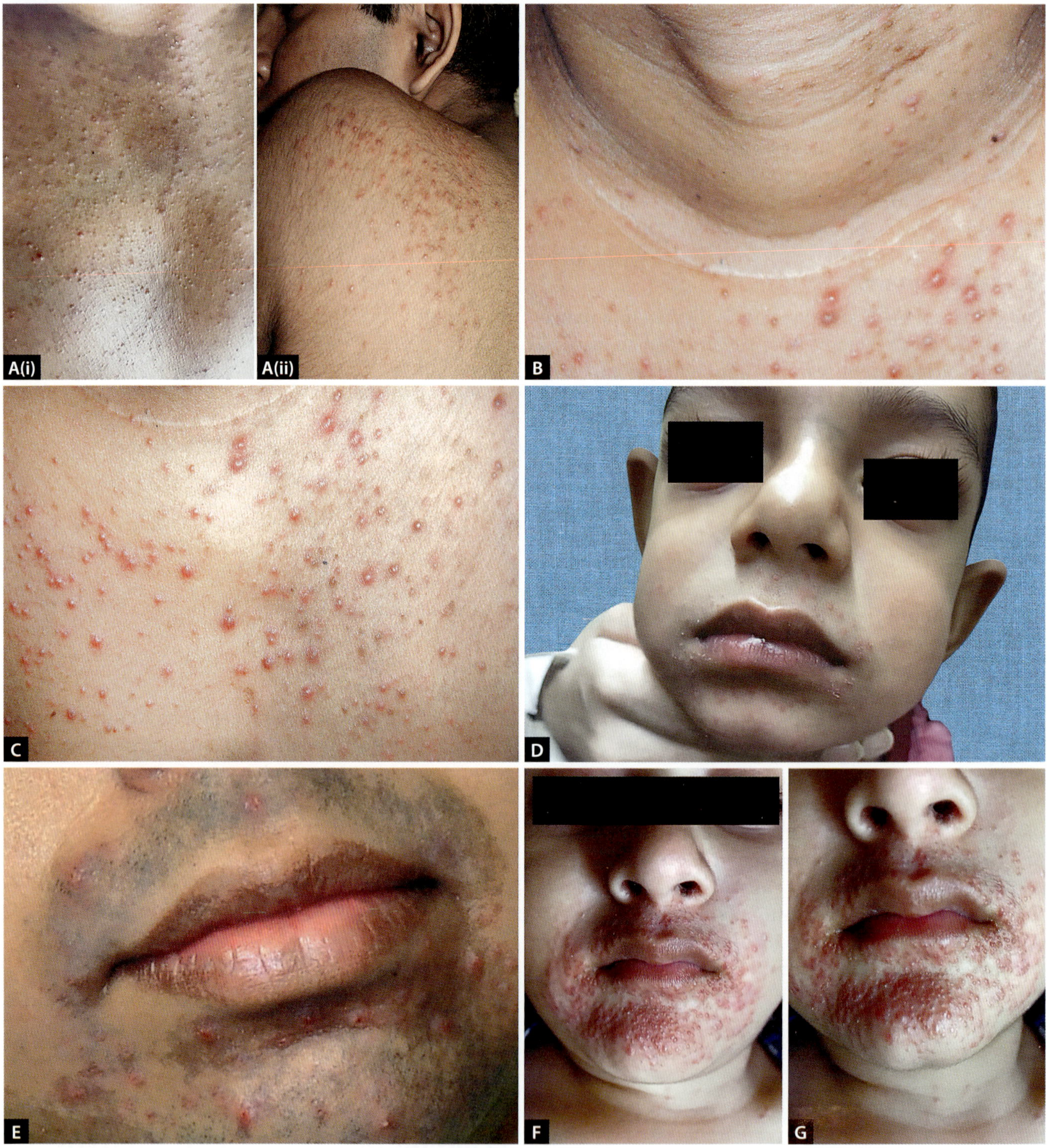

Figs. 3A(i) to G: A(i) Acneiform eruptions over back. A(ii) Acneiform eruptions over back in an adolescent boy (potent topical steroid induced). (B) Acneiform eruptions (from oral steroids for few months). (C) Close-up view of acneiform lesions. (D) Perioral dermatitis in a 3-year-old girl, note inflammatory acneiform papules. (E) Close-up view of perioral dermatitis. (F) Perioral dermatitis in a 5-year-old girl. (G) Same girl, close-up view.

"The first and greatest victory is to conquer self." —**Plato**

potency corticosteroids, nasal and inhaled corticosteroids, atopic dermatitis, lip-licking, infections due to *Candida albicans*, fusiform bacteria and *Demodex* mites, fluorinated toothpaste, chewing gum, dental fillings, moisturizers, and physical sunscreens. Perioral dermatitis is characterized by papulopustular eruption over an erythematous base which classically involves perioral and periorbital regions. As the disease evolves, fine but prominent scaling becomes evident. Following improvement after few weeks, erythema persists. Itching is not a prominent feature. Patients usually complain of uncomfortable burning sensation of the affected area. Lesions typically spare a narrow zone of approximate 5 mm around the vermilion border of the lip in case of perioral involvement. Treatment is frustrating for the physician. Perioral dermatitis is usually self-limiting once the inciting factor is removed. The first line of treatment is topical antibiotics (metronidazole, erythromycin, sulfur-based products). Topical tacrolimus and pimecrolimus are also effective. In severe and recalcitrant cases, oral antibiotics such as erythromycin or tetracyclines for 6–8 weeks and low-dose acitretin (0.2 mg/kg/day) may be effective.

In this regard, dermatologist should also keep in mind that periorificial granulomatous dermatitis is a distinct entity from perioral dermatitis seen in prepubertal children. This entity is clinically characterized by grouped papules in perioral, periorbital, and perinasal areas and histologically by sarcoidal granuloma. Treatment options are the same as perioral dermatitis.

ACNE EXCORIÉE (FIGS. 4A TO D)

Acne excoriée is a form of acne most frequently seen in adolescent girls and often associated with various degrees of emotional stress. The condition can be occasionally

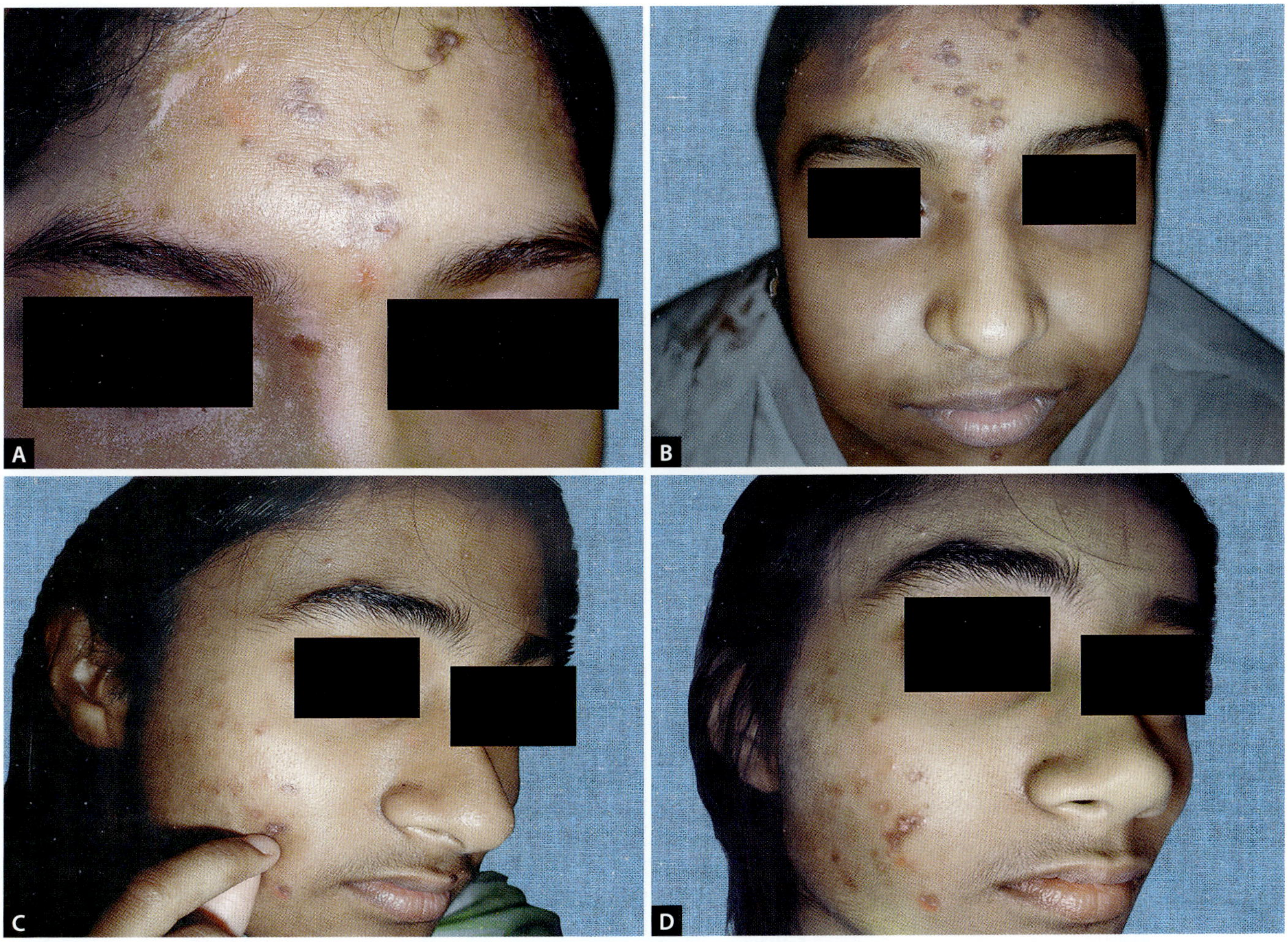

Figs. 4A to D: (A) Acne excoriée—note excoriated papules, postinflammatory hyperpigmentation. (B) Acne excoriée in a 16-year-old girl. (C) Demonstration of excoriation. (D) Lesions of acne excoriée in the same girl.

"Watch what you say, and whatever you say, practice it." —**Soyen Shaku**

seen in boys. Excoriating or squeezing of acne lesions may vary from mild irritation to severe scarring and occasional gross mutilation. In the mild forms, a simple counseling and local therapy may be all that is required to control the situation. In severe forms, intensive psychiatric therapy may be required to control the underlying psychiatric basis of this disorder.

ACNE KELOIDALIS NUCHAE [FIGS. 4E TO H(ii)]

Acne keloidalis nuchae is a condition seen commonly in the African-American people of the younger age group, over the occipital scalp and posterior neck. It is characterized by follicular papules and pustules which later become keloidal. It is a misnomer as there is no relation to acne, and histopathology does not reveal keloid formation. Unlike acne, it is never characterized by the presence of comedones.

Etiopathogenesis

Although the etiology is not clear, it has been postulated to be a result of chronic irritation caused by the curly hair inciting an inflammatory response. Close shaving and chronic irritation have been implicated in the formation as well. Chronic low-grade infection and an autoimmune hypothesis have also been suggested.

It generally affects the younger age group ranging from 14 to 25 years and has a male preponderance.

Clinical Features

The lesions are characterized by skin-colored to erythematous firm, dome-shaped papules located in the occipital area or the nape of neck. Occasional pustules may also be seen. In the late stages, there can be keloidal plaques arranged in a band-like distribution. Scarring alopecia eventually ensues.

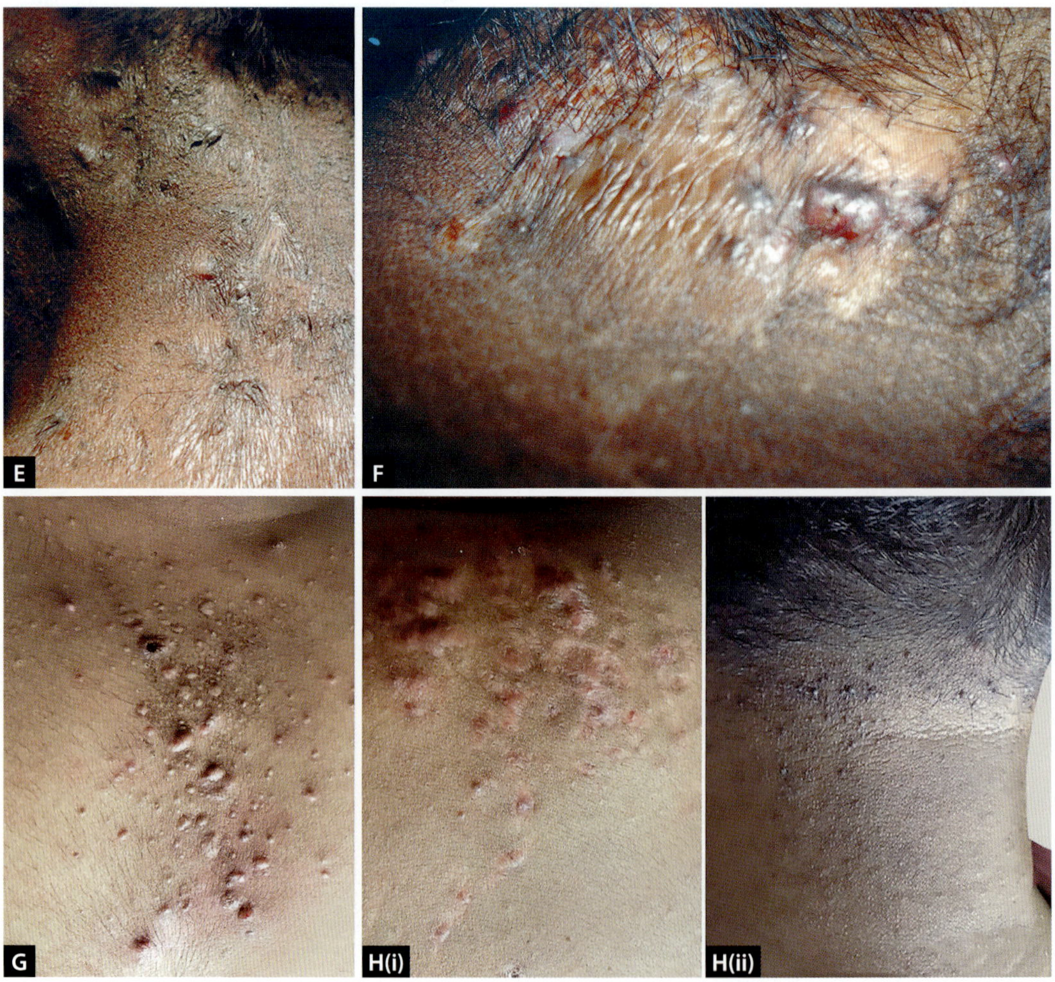

Figs. 4E to H(ii): (E) Acne keloidalis nuchae. (F) Close-up view. (G) Acne cheloidalis (back). H(i and ii) Acne keloidalis (nape of the neck).

"What you seek is seeking you." —**Rumi**

Differential Diagnosis

- Folliculitis decalvans
- Dissecting cellulitis of the scalp
- Hidradenitis suppurativa
- Acne conglobata

Investigations

Bacterial culture is recommended in case of secondary infection.

Management

Intralesional triamcinolone acetonide, 5-fluorouracil, and immunotherapy can be given.

Cryotherapy and radiotherapy have also proven to be successful. Oral retinoids may also be tried.

ROSACEA (FIGS. 5 AND 6)

Rosacea is commonly confused with acne, a condition seen in late adolescence to adult age. The lesions are essentially the same as those of acne vulgaris, but comedone formation is usually absent. Basic lesions are erythematous papules, pustules and telangiectasia. Erythema is more pronounced as compared to acne vulgaris and pustules are plenty in number. Patients often complain of hot flushes over the face aggravated by hot drinks and hot and spicy food. Alcohol can aggravate the condition and photosensitivity is a usual feature. Localized lymph-edema leads to the formation of a bulbous swelling of the nose known as rhinophyma.

Treatment

Treatment of rosacea includes both topical and systemic agents. Topical metronidazole (0.75–1.5%) is a good anti-inflammatory and antibacterial agent. It is applied in either gel or cream form. Topical clindamycin (1%) and azelaic acid (10%) are also useful. Regular application of sunscreens with an SPF of 15 or more should be emphasized as the condition may aggravate on

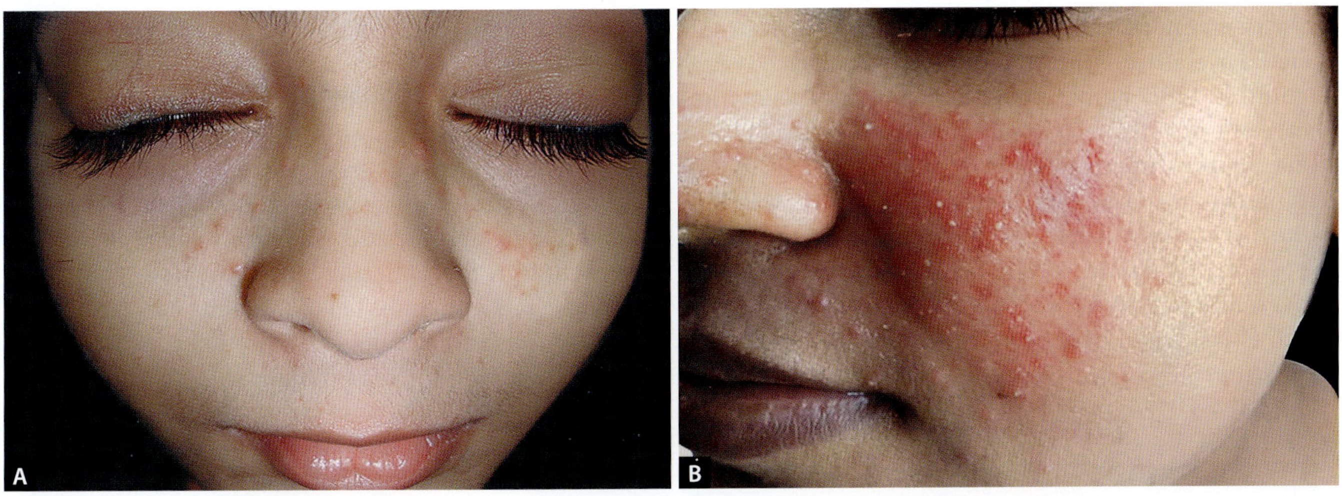

Figs. 5A and B: (A) Rosacea. (B) Rosacea—note flushing, erythematous papules and pustules.

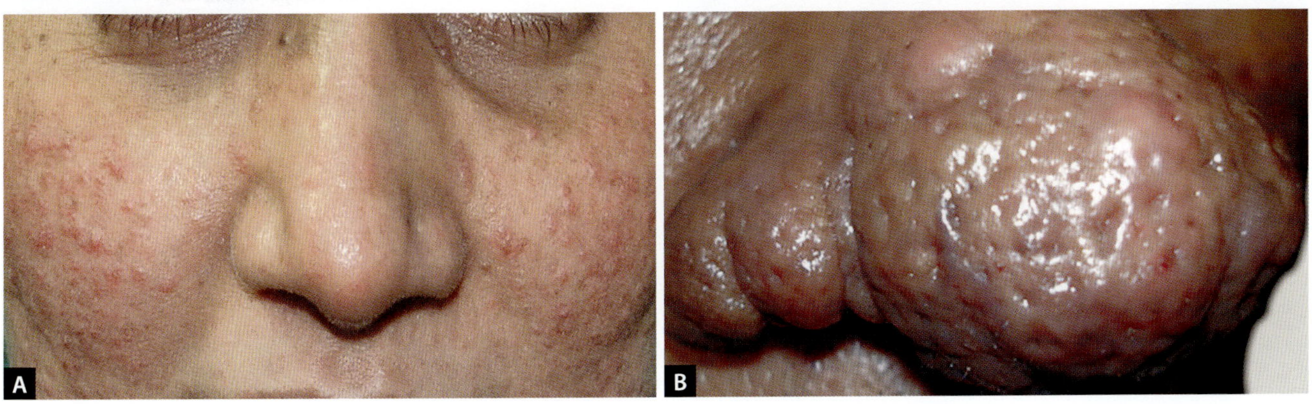

Figs. 6A and B: (A) Steroid-induced rosacea (history of potent steroid application over face for many months). (B) Rhinophyma.

"It surprises me how disinterested we are today about things like physics, space, the universe and philosophy of our existence, our purpose, our final destination. It's a crazy world out there. Be curious." —**Stephen Hawking**

exposure to sunlight. Calamine lotion application may also help for the same reason.

Various systemic agents useful for rosacea are tetracycline, doxycycline, and metronidazole. The dose and duration are more or less the same as in the case of acne vulgaris. Various food and drinks are to be restricted as they can aggravate rosacea by causing vasodilatation. These are hot tea, coffee, hot food, cold drinks, and tonics containing alcoholic beverages. Reassurance and counseling of the patients are extremely useful. Pediatric rosacea often persists into adulthood.

Role of Rifaximin in Rosacea

Rosacea is characterized by persistent erythema of the convexities of face. Other manifestations are telangiectasia, flushing, erythematous papules and pustules, and occasionally phymatous changes. Dysregulation of innate and adaptive immunity, neurovascular changes, chronic inflammation, and infections play an important role in the pathogenesis of rosacea. A new insight into the pathogenesis was suggested after the observation that there is an increased prevalence of small intestinal bacterial overgrowth (SIBO) in patients with rosacea than in controls. SIBO perpetuates rosacea by increasing the release of cytokines such as tumor necrosis factor (TNF)-alpha, suppressing interleukin-17, and augmenting the Th1-mediated immune response. This observation led to the use of a new therapeutic weapon for management of rosacea, Rifaximin. It is a semisynthetic antibiotic derived from a naturally occurring chemical Rifamycin which is produced by a bacterium called *Streptomyces mediterrane*. It was initially introduced for the treatment of traveler's diarrhea. It has demonstrated efficacy in irritable bowel syndrome and inflammatory bowel disease. Rifaximin acts in rosacea by suppressing gut flora. When given in a dose of 400 mg three times daily for a period of 10–14 days, it led to significant improvement of skin lesions in patients with rosacea with coexistent SIBO. Common side effects associated are nausea, vomiting, bloating, urgency to defecate, fluid retention, allergic reaction, and rarely pseudomembranous colitis. Safety during pregnancy is yet to be established and it is not usually recommended in children below 12 years of age.

HIDRADENITIS SUPPURATIVA (FIGS. 7 AND 8)

Hidradenitis suppurativa is a chronic suppurative and cicatricial disease of the apocrine sweat glands in the axillary, inguinal, and anogenital regions. Coagulase-positive staphylococci, streptococci, *Escherichia coli*, *Bacillus proteus*, or *Pseudomonas aeruginosa* are partly implicated though hidradenitis suppurativa is not a true infection.

In the early stages of hidradenitis suppurativa, sections of the skin show keratinous obstruction of the apocrine duct and dilatation, and associated inflammatory changes leading to painful abscess formation. As the process becomes more chronic, there is fibrosis and scarring with destruction of the apocrine gland, eccrine gland, and pilosebaceous apparatus. In the healing stage, one sees deep tortuous invaginations of the epidermis filled with keratin and representing the sinus tracts.

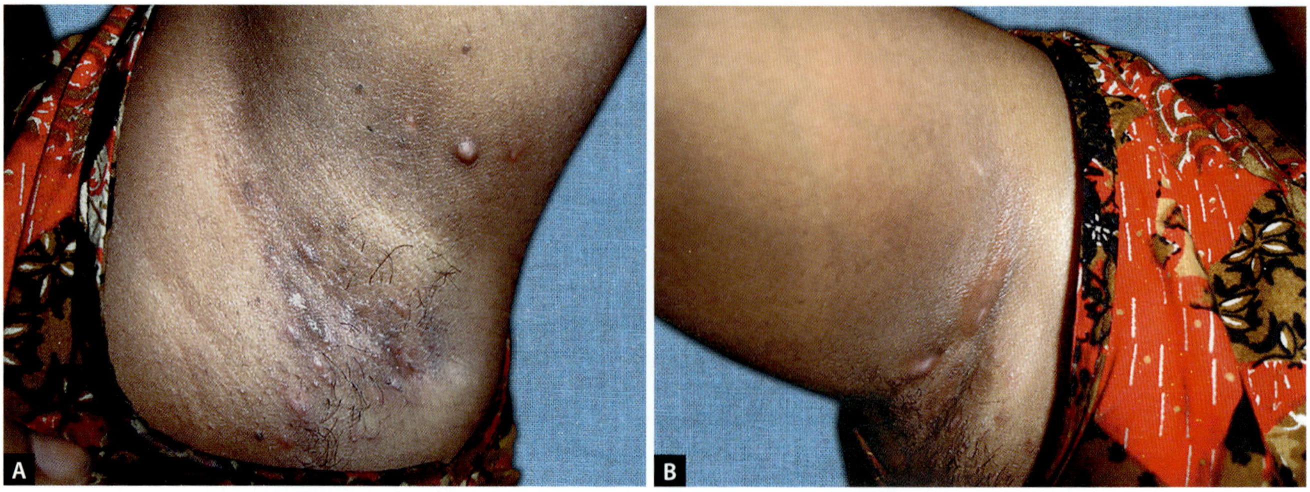

Figs. 7A and B: (A) Papules and nodules of hidradenitis suppurativa. (B) Close-up view of lesions.

"Nothing ever exists entirely alone. Everything is in relation to everything else." **—Buddha**

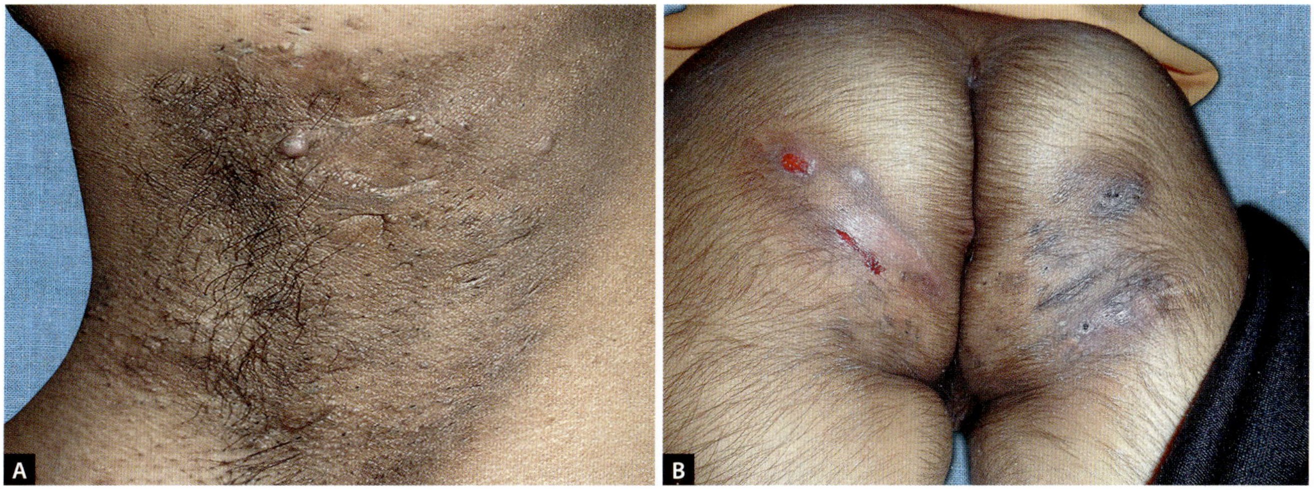

Figs. 8A and B: (A) Hidradenitis over axilla. (B) Hidradenitis suppurativa in an 18-year-old boy.

Treatment

Optimal therapy for hidradenitis suppurativa depends on early and accurate diagnosis. Long-term antibiotics are to be given to control the infection. Though different treatment modalities are available for this chronic, suppurative, cicatricial follicular disease, permanent cure is difficult. Treatment options can be broadly classified into medical and surgical. Among the topical measures, maintenance of local hygiene with antibacterial soap, chlorhexidine solution, or benzoyl peroxide wash; use of topical aluminum chloride or botulinum toxin A if there is excessive sweating; and prophylactic use of topical antibiotics such as clindamycin have some preventive value. Though the concept is well appreciated that hidradenitis suppurativa is not a true infection and bacterial infection, if any, is a secondary phenomenon, oral antibiotics are still considered to be important treatment modalities. Tetracyclines, sulfamethoxazole/trimethoprim, dapsone, and clindamycin plus rifampicin combination are useful in this group.

A short course of oral prednisolone or intralesional triamcinolone can be used to control acute flare.

Oral retinoids such as isotretinoin/acitretin shows some encouraging result. The prerequisites are that the drug has to be used in high dose and for 1 year or more. In females, cyproterone acetate, spironolactone, and oral contraceptive pills and in males or postmenopausal women, finasteride are proved to be a welcome adjuvant.

Other useful therapies are cyclosporine, infliximab, etanercept, adalimumab, botulinum toxin A, fractionated CO_2 laser, and photodynamic therapy.

Incision and drainage of abscesses in recalcitrant cases can be considered. Total excision of the affected region is required early in the disease. The use of broad-spectrum antibiotics controls infection and elimination of the local factors might reverse the process, but in the chronic phase surgery remains the only curative mode of therapy. Repeated incision and drainage of abscesses and incomplete excision of infected tracts, however, are often harmful since they permit extension of the infections and an increase in fibrosis and tract formation. Advanced cases, therefore, have a more negative outlook. In such cases, excision followed by coverage with a split thickness skin graft is useful.

PITYROSPORUM FOLLICULITIS (FIGS. 9 AND 10)

The condition is typically described as itchy dome-shaped follicular papules and occasional pustule distributed over shoulder, chest, and upper back in adolescents/young adults. Face and scalp might be involved. Central whitish-yellow color often represents compact keratin. Hot and humid weather, occlusion, and excess sebum production are some known triggers. Organ transplant recipients and patients on antibiotic therapy (tetracycline/doxycycline therapy in particular) are at risk. Alteration of normal skin flora following tetracycline/doxycycline therapy contributes to the formation of lesions. Close differentials include acne vulgaris and other superficial folliculitis, irritant folliculitis, gram-negative folliculitis, and drug-induced folliculitis. Cutaneous candidiasis and miliaria rubra should also be considered. Diagnosis can be confirmed by yellow-green fluorescence in Wood's lamp examination and demonstration of *Pityrosporum* yeast in potassium hydroxide preparation or biopsy. A prompt response to antifungal drugs is another indirect evidence of *Pityrosporum* playing a central role; 2.5% selenium sulfide shampoo is generally effective. Among oral antifungals, fluconazole 400 mg once and itraconazole 200 mg/day for 5–7 days are given. Relapses are common. In those cases, oral antifungals might be needed for few weeks/months with proper monitoring of liver and kidney functions.

Oral tetracycline or doxycycline has no role. Topical tretinoin has shown some response. Oral isotretinoin may be useful in some cases.

Natural History

The condition resolves spontaneously over a number of years. Reassurance and counseling are important.

FOX–FORDYCE DISEASE (FIGS. 11A TO C)

Fox–Fordyce disease is a rare, chronic disease of apocrine gland-bearing areas commonly affecting young women in the age group of 13–35 years. Preponderance in women may be attributed to hormonal component, as symptoms rarely present before puberty. The disease is characterized by intensely pruritic, small, firm, discrete, conical, flesh-colored or slightly pigmented follicular papules distributed chiefly in axillae, areola, and pubis though other apocrine gland-bearing areas such as umbilicus,

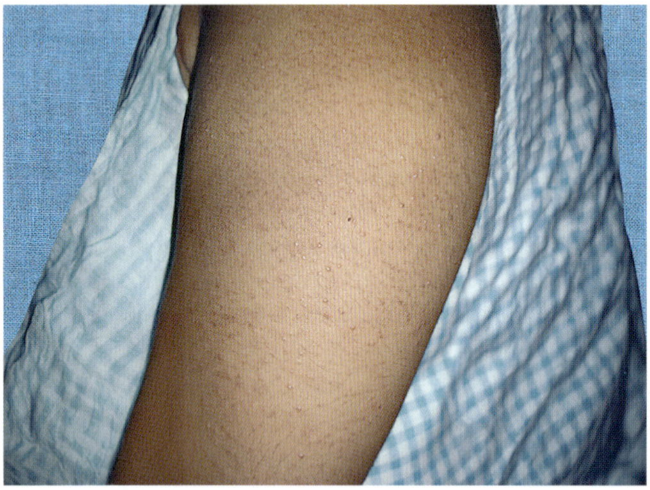

Fig. 9: Pityrosporum folliculitis in a 9-year-old girl.

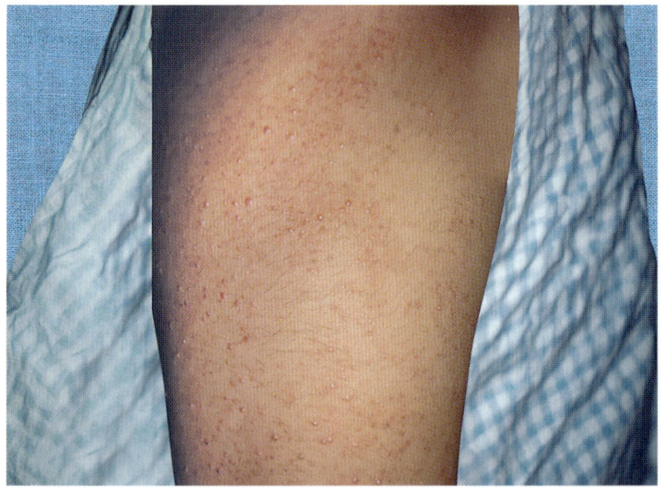

Fig. 10: Same girl, close-up view of lesions.

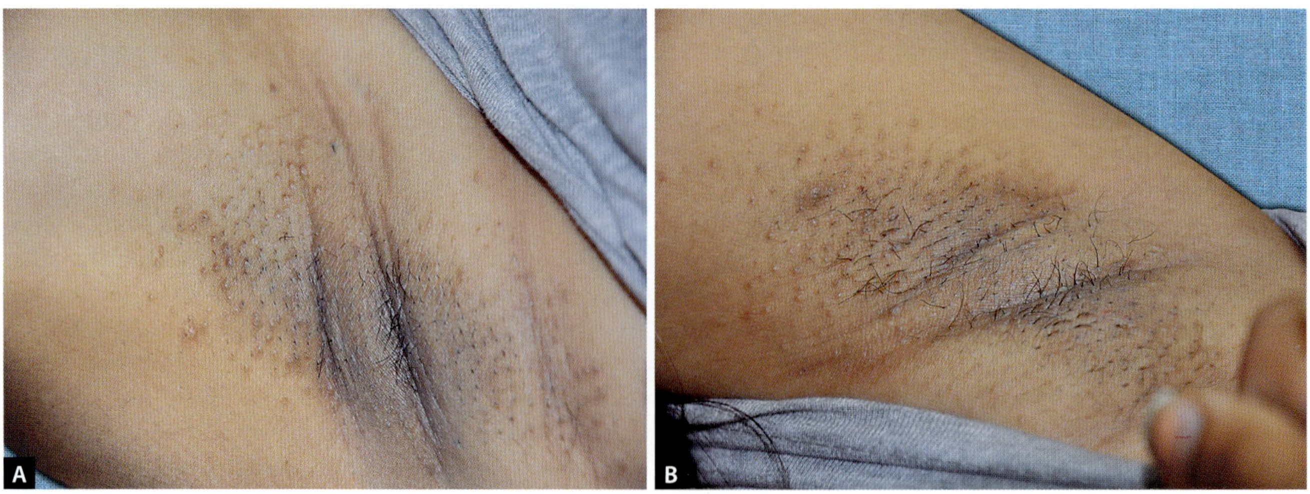

Figs. 11A and B: (A) Intensely itchy papules of Fox–Fordyce disease in a 16-year-old girl. (B) Fox–Fordyce disease, axilla—most common site.

"Either you run the day, or the day runs you." **—Jim Rohn**

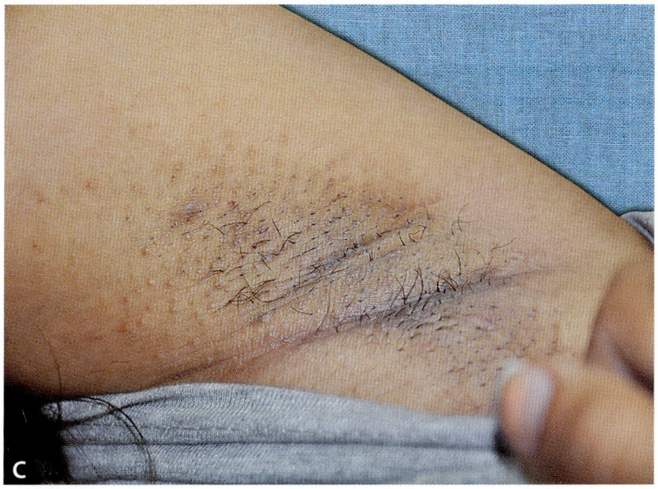

Fig. 11C: Same girl, close-up view. Note dome-shaped shinny papules.

labia majora, perineum, medial thigh, and hairy chest may be involved. Intense paroxysmal pruritus aggravated by the agents which increase apocrine sweat such as physical, emotional stress, and intradermal injection of medications is typical of this entity. But usually apocrine sweat and odor become absent in case of extensive lesions. Sparse hair of the affected areas may be due to excessive scratching. The pathogenesis of this disorder is not fully understood. Reports of familial cases indicate that the role of genetic factors could not be underestimated. Patients usually improve during pregnancy and after menopause; endocrinal factors may have some role. Important histological findings are lymphocytic infiltrate around the upper third of hair follicles and upper dermal blood vessel, infundibular spongiosis at the entrance of apocrine duct, and presence of foam cells. Various treatment modalities have been tried; none proved to be satisfactory starting from topical steroid and calcineurin inhibitors, intralesional steroid, oral retinoids, and phototherapy. Electrocoagulation, excision, and liposuction of the affected area have some favorable outcome.

SUGGESTED READINGS

1. Ashton R, Weinstein M. Acne Vulgaris in the Pediatric Patient. Pediatr Rev. 2019;40(11):577-89.
2. Cotton CH, Chen SX, Hussain SH, Lara-Corrales I, Zaenglein AL. Hidradenitis Suppurativa in Pediatric Patients. Pediatrics. 2023;151(5):e2022061049.
3. Choi E, Ooi XT, Chandran NS. Hidradenitis suppurativa in pediatric patients. J Am Acad Dermatol. 2022;86(1):140-7.
4. Layton AM, Ravenscroft J. Adolescent acne vulgaris: current and emerging treatments. Lancet Child Adolesc Health. 2023;7(2):136-44.

"With confidence you have won before you have started." —**Marcus Garvey**

CHAPTER

18

Adverse Drug Eruptions

INTRODUCTION

Various adverse cutaneous drug reactions (ACDRs) can be classified as follows:

- *Nonimmune cutaneous reactions*: Photosensitivity eruptions, pigmentary changes, warfarin necrosis of skin, pruritus, etc.
- *Immune-mediated cutaneous reactions*: It can be either—
  - Mild or benign: Maculopapular eruptions, urticarial rash, angioedema, and fixed drug eruptions (FDEs).
  - Severe rash: Vasculitis, acute generalized exanthematous pustulosis (AGEP), drug reaction with eosinophilia and systemic symptoms (DRESS), Stevens–Johnson syndrome (SJS), and toxic epidermal necrolysis (TEN)

Drug reactions can also be divided considering dose relatedness, timing, and patient susceptibility (DoTS). Dose relatedness points to the doses above, below, or within the common therapeutic range (toxic, hypersusceptibility, and collateral adverse reactions). The significance of time relatedness considers time between first use and the appearance of the adverse reaction and hence are—immediate, first dose, early, intermediate, late, and delayed. Several factors that enhance the susceptibility to the adverse reactions are—genetic, age, gender, physiological changes, exogenous drugs, and diseases.

EPIDEMIOLOGY AND THE ROLE OF RISK FACTORS

Adverse cutaneous drug reactions are now quite common, and some can be lethal and life threatening. Reactions to different drugs affect almost about 3% of patients admitted in the hospital. Reaction rates from different studies show a range from 0 to 9.5% and are more for antimicrobials and for anti-HIV (human immunodeficiency virus) drugs. In a study by the author and co-workers on adverse drug reaction (ADR) in patients up to 18 years of age showed that 26% patients had a maculopapular rash, 22% had FDE, 20% erythema multiforme (EM), 12% TEN, 10% SJS, 6% urticaria, and 4% erythroderma. Cotrimoxazole was the most common antibacterial responsible for eruptions and antiepileptics were the most common drugs implicated in EM, TEN, and SJS. Asian studies have shown younger age group to be affected more than older age children.

The risk of reaction increases with the number of drugs taken, age of the patient, and viral infections. Patients at risk are those with transplants, HIV infection, and those suffering from collagen vascular diseases. Drugs with higher molecular weight and structural complexity are likely to produce a higher incidence of drug reactions. Genetic ability of an individual to detoxify toxic metabolites predisposes to the development of drug reaction. HLA (human leukocyte antigen) genes *HLA-B*1502* predisposes to carbamazepine-associated SJS and TEN and *HLA-B*5701* to abacavir hypersensitivity syndrome.

ETIOPATHOGENESIS

The exact pathogenesis of drug reactions in many cases is unknown. Drug eruptions due to hypersensitivity reaction relies on an immune mechanism. Reactions on account of nonimmunological mechanism are more common. Drugs may behave as haptens by combining with peptides and hence become immunogenic. Immunologic reactions result from IgE-dependent, immune complex-initiated, cytotoxic, or cellular immune mechanisms. Gell and Coombs classification of immunological reactions delineates four types of immunological reactions:

- *Type I*: Acute IgE-mediated reactions cause mast cell degranulation as in anaphylactic and urticarial reactions.
- *Type II*: Cytotoxic reactions occur due to antibodies binding to cell surface antigens, with subsequent complement fixation leading to production of

"The best and most beautiful things in the world cannot be seen or even touched; they must be felt with the heart." **—Hellen Keller**

anaphylatoxin (C5a), polymorphonuclear leukocyte aggregation, and tissue injury by hydrolytic neutrophil enzymes as in immune cytopenias.

- *Type III*: In immune complex reactions, antigen–antibody complexes are produced and accumulate in tissues as in vasculitis.
- *Type IV*: In cell-mediated or delayed hypersensitivity reactions, T-lymphocyte sensitization is brought about by a hapten–protein complex as in contact dermatitis, maculopapular eruptions, DRESS, SJS/TEN, AGEP, and FDE.

Nonimmunologic reactions occur in the form of nonimmunologic activation of effector pathways, overdosage, cumulative toxicity, interactions between drugs, and metabolic alterations. Drugs release mediators from mast cells and precipitate anaphylaxis or urticaria. Some drugs may activate complement in absence of antibody. Phototoxic reaction starts when the drug/chromophore absorbs radiation to elicit a reaction.

Severe cutaneous adverse reactions encompass DRESS or drug-induced hypersensitivity syndrome (DIHS) and SJS/TEN. Pharmacogenetic studies now point to an association between HLA alleles and drug hypersensitivity. HLA typing has significantly reduced the incidence of abacavir hypersensitivity on account of its association with *HLA-B*5701*. Being aware of the interlink between HLA alleles and these syndromes, including abacavir-hypersensitivity reaction, allopurinol DRESS/DIHS and SJS/TEN, and SJS/TEN with amine anticonvulsants help in prevention through screening. *HLA-B*5701* routine genetic screening test to prevent abacavir hypersensitivity provides the initiation for further such tests. The role of genetic screening to identify patients at potential risk for severe cutaneous ADR is now well established. These maybe fatal and idiosyncratic as in the cases of SJS and TEN overlap and DRESS. Advanced research in genomics have identified genes that have increased propensity to cause ADR specific to drug and phenotype.

Common offending drugs are variable in diverse ethnic populations. SJS and TEN are mostly found to be precipitated by nonsteroidal anti-inflammatory drugs (NSAIDs) and sulfonamides in the Western literature whereas carbamazepine is found to be the major implicated agent for SJS in Southeast Asia. The role of carbamazepine in the west is more in causation of DIHS. Allopurinol often plays the causal role in SJS but has no obvious ethnic bias. Susceptibility to nevirapine hypersensitivity has been noted in Caucasian, Australians having *HLA-DRB1*0101* with high CD4+ T-cell counts and carbamazepine hypersensitivity and *HLA-B*1502* has been observed in Han Chinese and allopurinol-induced severe cutaneous adverse reactions are positive for *HLA-B*5801*.

Considering the linkage of *HLA-B*1502* and carbamazepine, *HLA-B*1502* allele was found in 100% of people with carbamazepine-induced SJS/TEN, and only 3% of carbamazepine-tolerant people in a study from Taiwan. The same was further substantiated in cohort of Chinese descent originating from different geographic regions. This association was not found among people with European descent. The allele hence is ethnically relevant. Allele with functional effect in the pathogenesis of reaction will be observed consistently in populations. The variability of Chinese and European population may be due to the fact that pharmacogenetic studies have positive results in a population with a high incidence of such an allele. *HLA-B*1502* allele is 4.8–12.8% in Southeast Asians in contrast to 0–0.1% noted in white people. The increased susceptibility of disease from genetic polymorphism is influenced by the prevalence as noted in *HLA-B*1502* having lower incidence in Caucasians.

Stevens–Johnson syndrome is mostly polygenic. Polymorphisms in the proapoptotic gene *Fas-L*, the *toll-like receptor 3* gene and the IL-4 receptor/IL-13 signaling pathway are documented in most studies. Screening for *HLA-B*1502* in a high-risk population has a 100% sensitivity and 97% specificity for carbamazepine-induced overlapping SJS and TEN. A high-resolution genetic testing using a sequence-specific primer assay for this allele from blood or buccal swabs is now in vogue.

*HLA-B*5801* allele, in comparison to *HLA-B*1502*, is equally distributed in ethnic groups. The allele maybe established by high-resolution, sequence-based HLA genotyping which is quite an expensive method.

Stevens–Johnson syndrome and its association with HLA-B molecules indicate an obvious role in its causation. This presents the drug to CD8 cells resulting in clonal expansion of CD8 cytotoxic lymphocytes. This cytotoxic effector response leads to apoptosis of keratinocytes. These pathways are not specific to overlapping SJS and TEN. It has been found that granulysin, a cytolytic protein from CD8 cells, is present in blister fluid in significant levels and correlates with disease activity.

DIAGNOSTIC WORKUP

The drug history forms the cornerstone in the diagnosis and allergology examination and tests further substantiate

"The Wound is the place where the light enters you." —**Rumi**

it. Skin prick test, intradermal and patch tests are common forms of allergy tests. Specific IgE level is a popular in vitro method for immediate reaction detection. Basophil activation test and lymphocyte proliferation assays also add to the investigation basket. Some cases need provocation tests for a complete workup.

On completion of a thorough clinical history, patients with drug allergy are tested. An accurate medication history, details of recent medication, over-the-counter medicines, herbal and homeopathic preparations, and vaccines or contrast media have to be documented. A common feature of nonimmunological reactions is that in many cases, symptoms appear 24–48 hours after drug intake; the time of onset of symptoms is vital in the evaluation process. Characteristic time lag between initiation of drug and reaction are: 4–14 days for maculopapular eruptions, 7–21 days for SJS/TEN, 14–48 days for DRESS, and FDE and generalized exanthematous pustulosis often occur early (within 48 hours).

On the basis of the drugs suspected, patients may undertake skin tests such as prick tests, intradermal tests, in vitro tests, and allergen challenges. Topical medications usually need patch tests for confirmation. Patients having severe drug reaction such as TEN are not subjected to drug challenge for the risk of fulminant nature of the drug reaction and complications.

The laboratory findings in serious drug-induced cutaneous eruptions are eosinophil count >1,000/μL, lymphocytosis with atypical lymphocytes, and abnormal liver function test. Tests for IgE are available for the drugs such as penicillins, cephalosporins, peptide and protein drugs (insulin). In some patients receiving antiretroviral therapy, the need for HLA typing before initiating abacavir is routinely recommended. Skin tests such as intradermal tests with delayed-reading and cutaneous patch tests can be useful in some cases. Patch test for drug is easily executed with almost any available drug. Intradermal tests have the advantage of higher sensitivity but has technical and procedural complexities. The use of intradermal and patch tests for confirmation of nonimmunological reactions to beta-lactams has yielded a sensitivity of 2.6% as a positive reaction to patch tests in 8 of 298 patients tested with phenoxymethylpenicillin. In some studies, 37.8% and 9% positive results were noted which points to the fact that sensitivity of skin test is low as with beta-lactam-induced exanthems. The usefulness of the patch testing was again established in reactions by cardio-vascular or antiepileptic drugs in similar studies.

Drug provocation tests are useful on account of the fact that intradermal or patch testing has low sensitivity; some patients are given the drug to confirm a causal association. Provocation testing is a useful method; however, a very careful administration in a specialized center is recommended. This test is generally not recommended and contraindicated in cases of severe eruptions.

In vitro diagnostic tests such as the lymphocyte transformation test banks on the principle—T cells can proliferate when exposed to a specific antigen. This theory has been utilized to detect T-cell sensitization to a drug. This test has sensitivity rates of 60–70% and relatively low specificity (85%). Role of dendritic cells in amoxicillin-specific lymphocyte proliferation studies showed dendritic cells improved lymphocyte transformation test sensitivity.

Skin biopsy from the acute reaction site with immunohistochemistry data help in the investigation of the immunologic mechanisms involved and not the drug involved. Mononuclear cell infiltrate, composed mainly of activated T cells-expressing DR antigens and CD69 activation markers, is a usual finding.

MACULOPAPULAR ERUPTIONS (FIGS. 1A TO G)

Maculopapular eruptions are also known as morbilliform or exanthematous eruptions. It is one of the most common types of drug eruptions encountered in pediatric age group. It is mediated by type IV hypersensitivity reactions. The average time lag between initiation of drug and reaction is 7–10 days but the onset of rash may be as late as second or third week. The eruption may develop much earlier in case of rechallenge. They present as widespread exanthematous macules and papules and usually resolve by 7–14 days with desquamation.

Differential Diagnosis

Various viral exanthems often resemble maculopapular drug rash. Involvement of mucosae and conjunctiva, and leukocytosis are features suggestive of viral exanthem. In drug-induced cases, eosinophilia in peripheral blood is usually observed.

Drugs Responsible

Drugs commonly responsible for maculopapular eruptions are penicillin, ampicillin, amoxicillin, carbamazepine, cotrimoxazole, chlorpromazine, antitubercular agents, NSAIDs, etc.

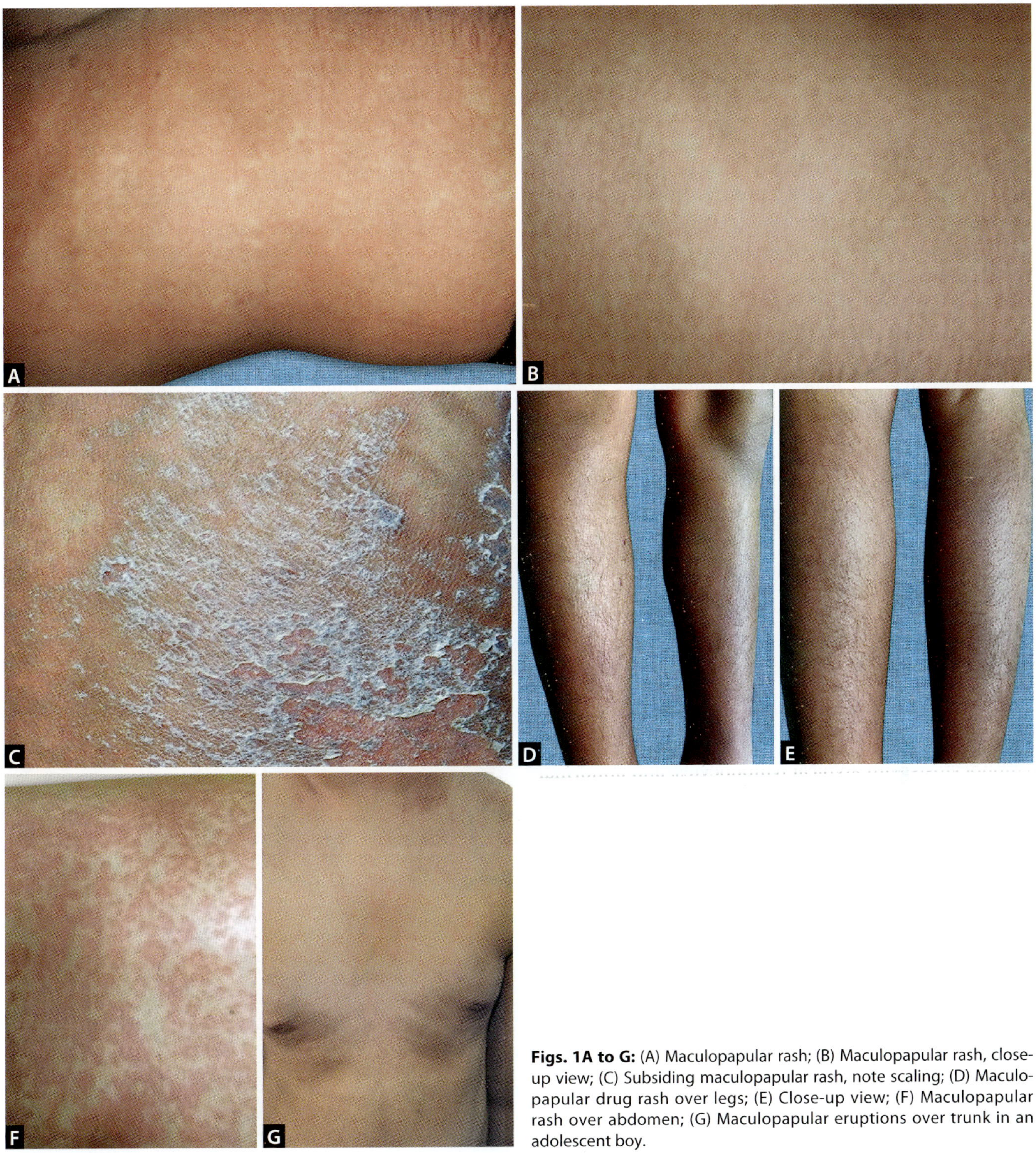

Figs. 1A to G: (A) Maculopapular rash; (B) Maculopapular rash, close-up view; (C) Subsiding maculopapular rash, note scaling; (D) Maculopapular drug rash over legs; (E) Close-up view; (F) Maculopapular rash over abdomen; (G) Maculopapular eruptions over trunk in an adolescent boy.

Treatment

Withdrawal of the drug usually leads to resolution of rash. However, if the patient is on life-saving drugs and one of them is suspected, the drug can be continued with monitoring. When maculopapular eruptions present as a part of serum sickness, withdrawal of the incriminated/suspected drug is mandatory. For associated itching, oral antihistamine is prescribed. Topical calamine lotion/

"Dreamers can't be tamed." —**Paulo Coelho**

emollients can be used. The rash subsides with fine branny scales which ultimately leave behind hypo- or hyperpigmentation. The rash may recur on rechallenge.

FIXED DRUG ERUPTION (FIGS. 2 TO 4)

Fixed drug eruption is a characteristic type of drug eruption presenting as itchy, well-defined, hyperpigmented macules/patches ranging from several millimeters to 10 cm. There is a halo of erythema surrounding the dark central area. On taking the same or chemically similar drug(s), the rash relapses at the same sites which were previously affected suggesting a reactivation of the hypersensitivity. Apart from the skin, mucosae can also be involved in FDE. The common sites affected are lips and genitalia. Atypical forms of FDE include generalized bullous, linear, nonpigmenting, cellulitis-like, psoriasiform-type, FDE with pigmentary loss, and erythema dyschromicum perstans-like FDE.

Generalized bullous FDE is a severe form and probably represents a rare variant and thought to be variant of SJS/TEN. There are well-demarcated blisters and erythematous macules. Constitutional symptoms are mild with absence of mucosal erosions and systemic involvement. As compared to SJS/TEN, it has a better prognosis. In linear FDE, lesions occur in a linear or dermatome pattern probably as an immune response to previously subclinical herpes zoster infection presenting as an isotopic phenomenon. This linear variant has been reported with levofloxacin and trimethoprim. Sometimes the characteristic feature of hyperpigmentation of FDE is not seen and this variant is called nonpigmenting FDE

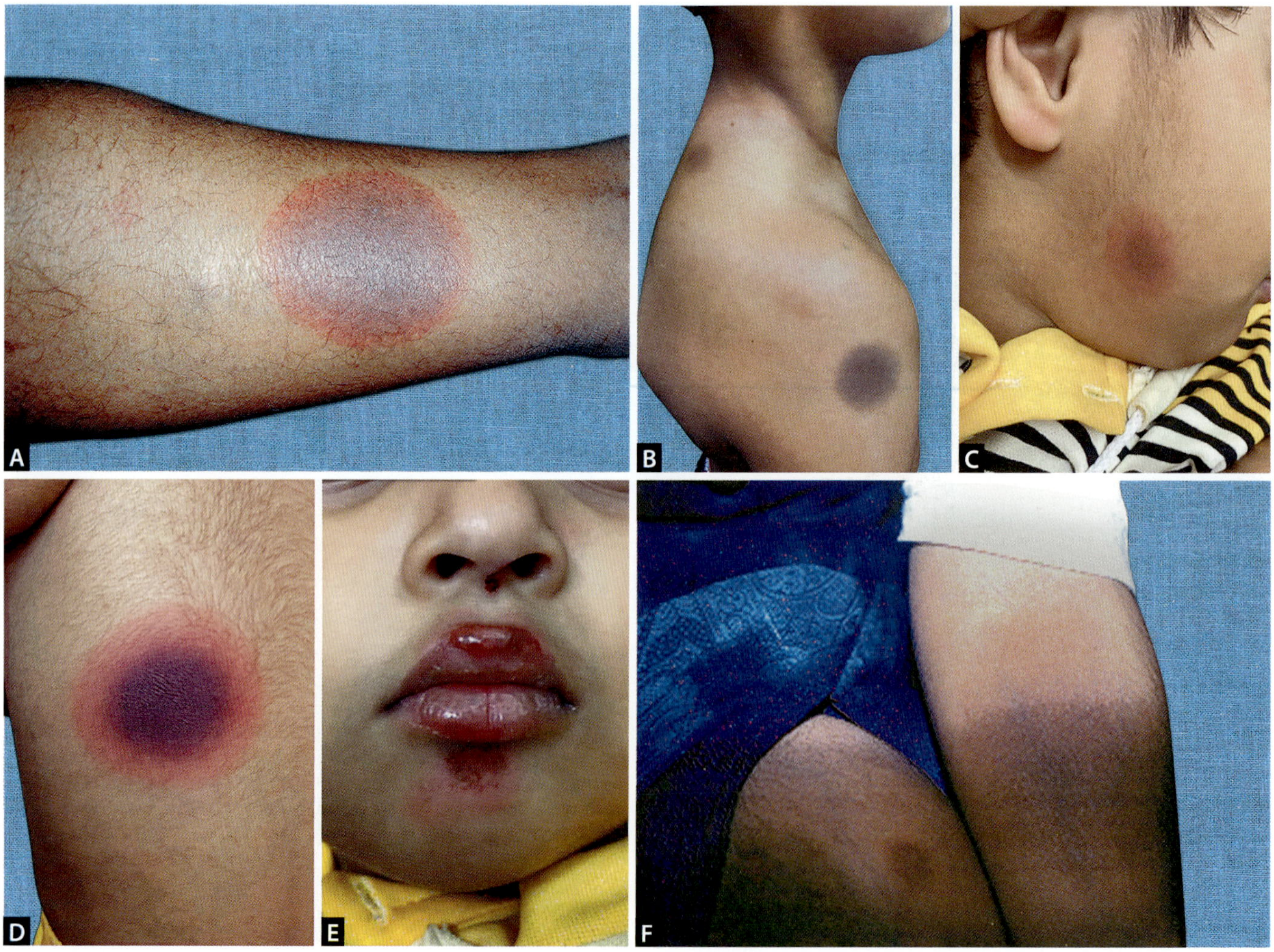

Figs. 2A to F: (A) Fixed drug eruption (FDE), note central hyperpigmentation within rim of erythema; (B) Hyperpigmented patch of subsided FDE; (C) Acute FDE, note peripheral erythema; (D) Same boy with back lesion of acute FDE, note central violaceous/blackish color and peripheral rim of erythema; (E) Mucocutaneous involvement in the same boy; (F) Hyperpigmented patch of FDE.

"Happiness is the Highest form of health." —**Dalai Lama**

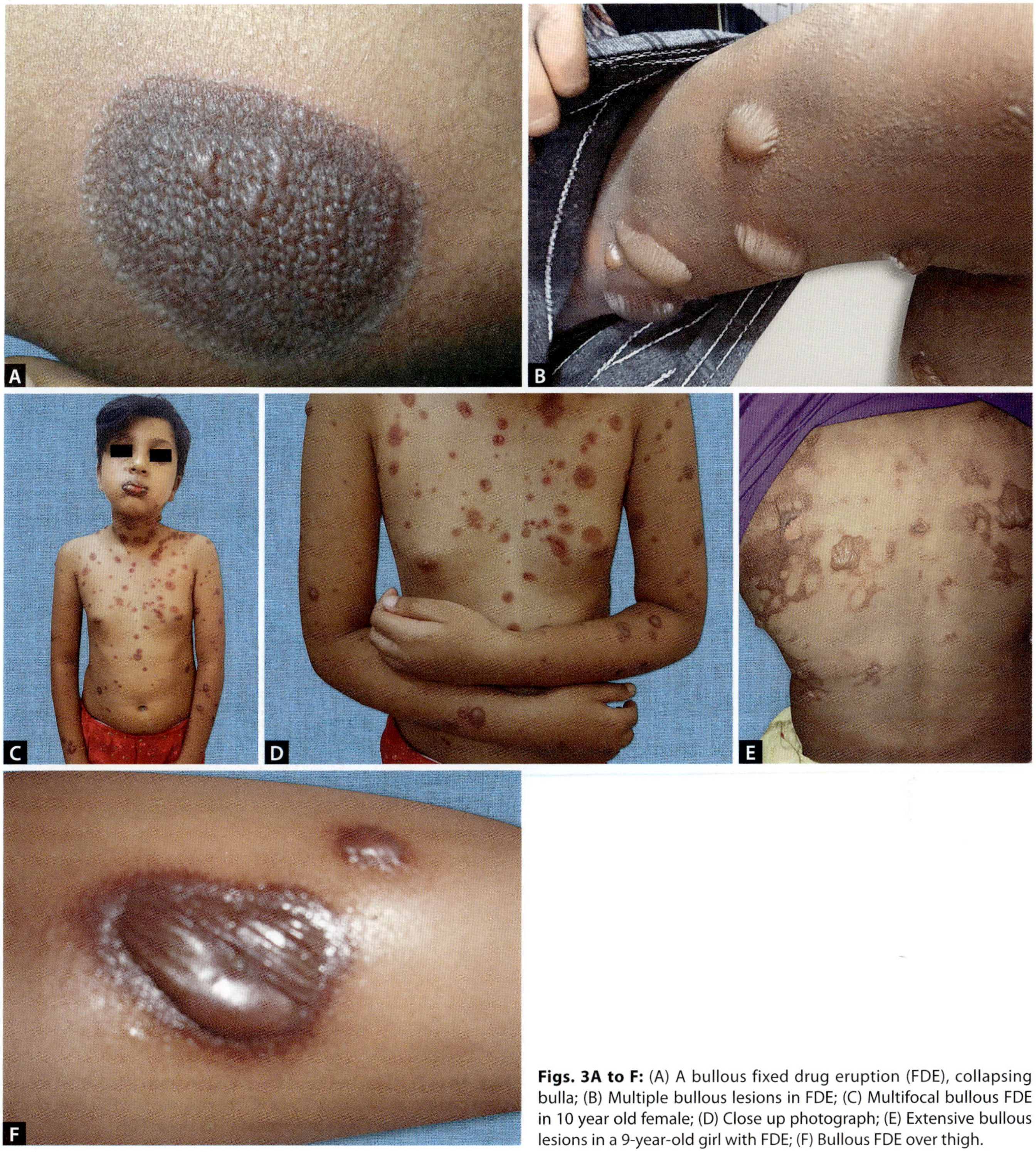

Figs. 3A to F: (A) A bullous fixed drug eruption (FDE), collapsing bulla; (B) Multiple bullous lesions in FDE; (C) Multifocal bullous FDE in 10 year old female; (D) Close up photograph; (E) Extensive bullous lesions in a 9-year-old girl with FDE; (F) Bullous FDE over thigh.

where the lesions fade in 2–3 weeks leaving no residue. In FDE with pigmentary loss, the lesions heal with hyperpigmentation and eventually develop depigmentation in the middle of the lesion which could be due to post-inflammatory changes or to destruction of melanocytes.

Drugs Responsible

Common drugs causing FDE include sulfonamides, tetracyclines, metronidazole, tinidazole, fluoroquinolones, barbiturates, NSAIDs, etc. Oral rechallenge is usually done with half the strength of a single dose of a drug.

"Nothing in the world is ever completely wrong. Even a stopped clock is right twice a day." —**Paulo Coelho**

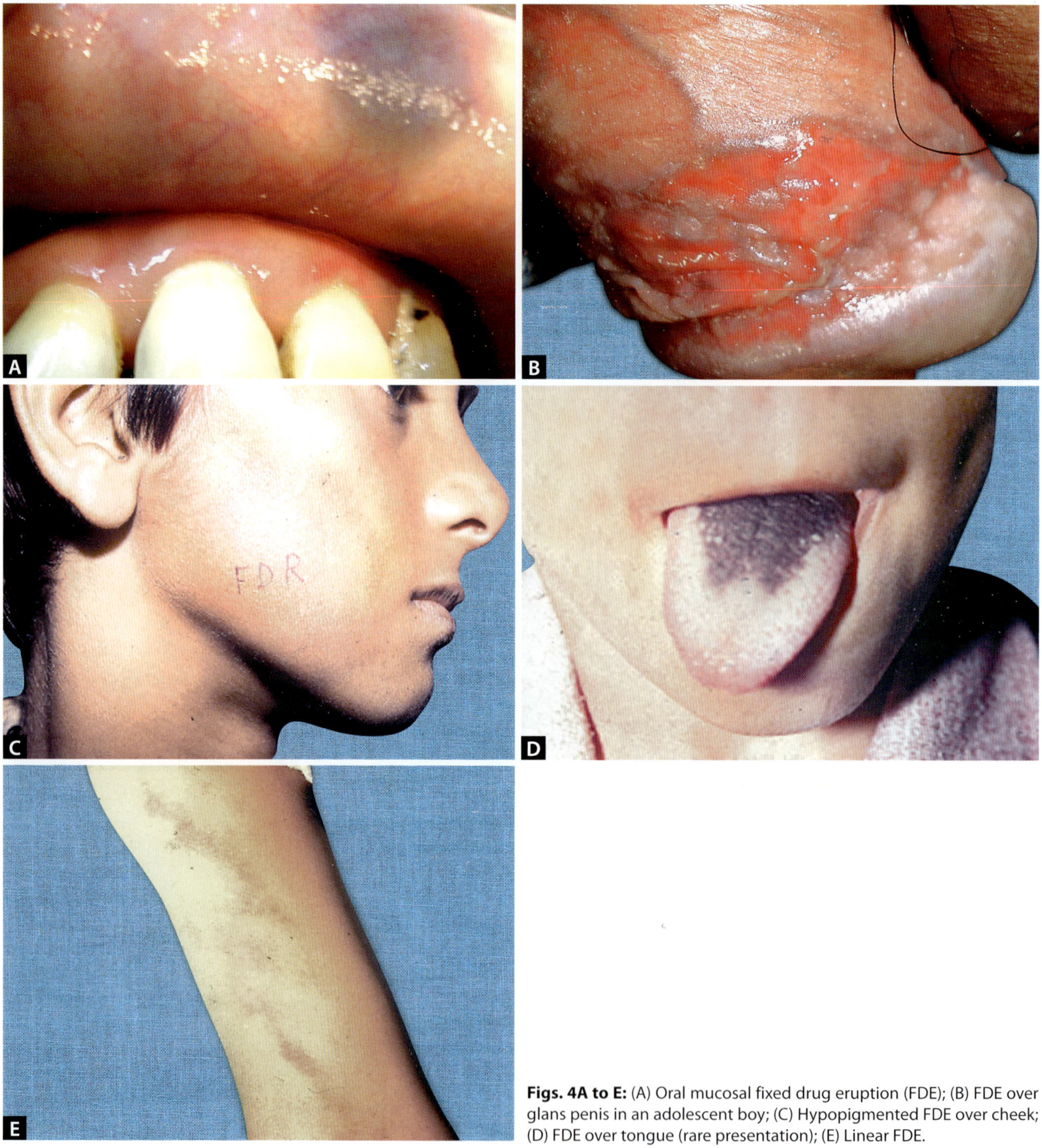

Figs. 4A to E: (A) Oral mucosal fixed drug eruption (FDE); (B) FDE over glans penis in an adolescent boy; (C) Hypopigmented FDE over cheek; (D) FDE over tongue (rare presentation); (E) Linear FDE.

Treatment

Advice regarding avoidance of the drug is very important. The post-inflammatory hyperpigmentation may take 6 months to 3 years or even more to subside. Topical 2% hydroquinone may be used over these pigmented patches for 6 months to 2 years. For initial inflammatory changes, topical steroids can be given. Oral steroids and cyclosporine have shown good improvement in generalized bullous FDE given over a period of 5–7 days.

"Out of difficulties grow miracles." —**Jean La Breyere**

ERYTHEMA MULTIFORME (FIGS. 5 TO 9)

As the nomenclature suggests, the rash manifests in various morphological forms, e.g., macular, papular, classical iris or target lesions, vesicular, and bullous. Atypical target lesions with flat macules may be present in EM. Drug-induced EM can downgrade to SJS or TEN. It can be part of type II, type III, or type IV reaction. As far as cases of only EM are concerned, there are other causes such as upper respiratory tract viral infection, bacterial infection, and collagen vascular diseases. Drug-induced EM develops within weeks after initiation of therapy. After re-exposure, the reaction may begin within hours. Drugs-causing EM are antibiotics (penicillin, amoxicillin, cephalosporins, and sulfonamides), anticonvulsants (carbamazepine, phenytoin), NSAIDs, fluconazole, terbinafine, and griseofulvin.

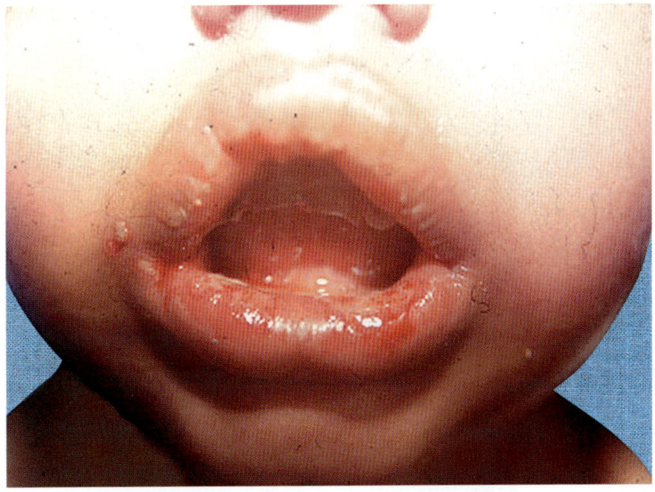

Fig. 6: Erosion of lips in erythema multiforme.

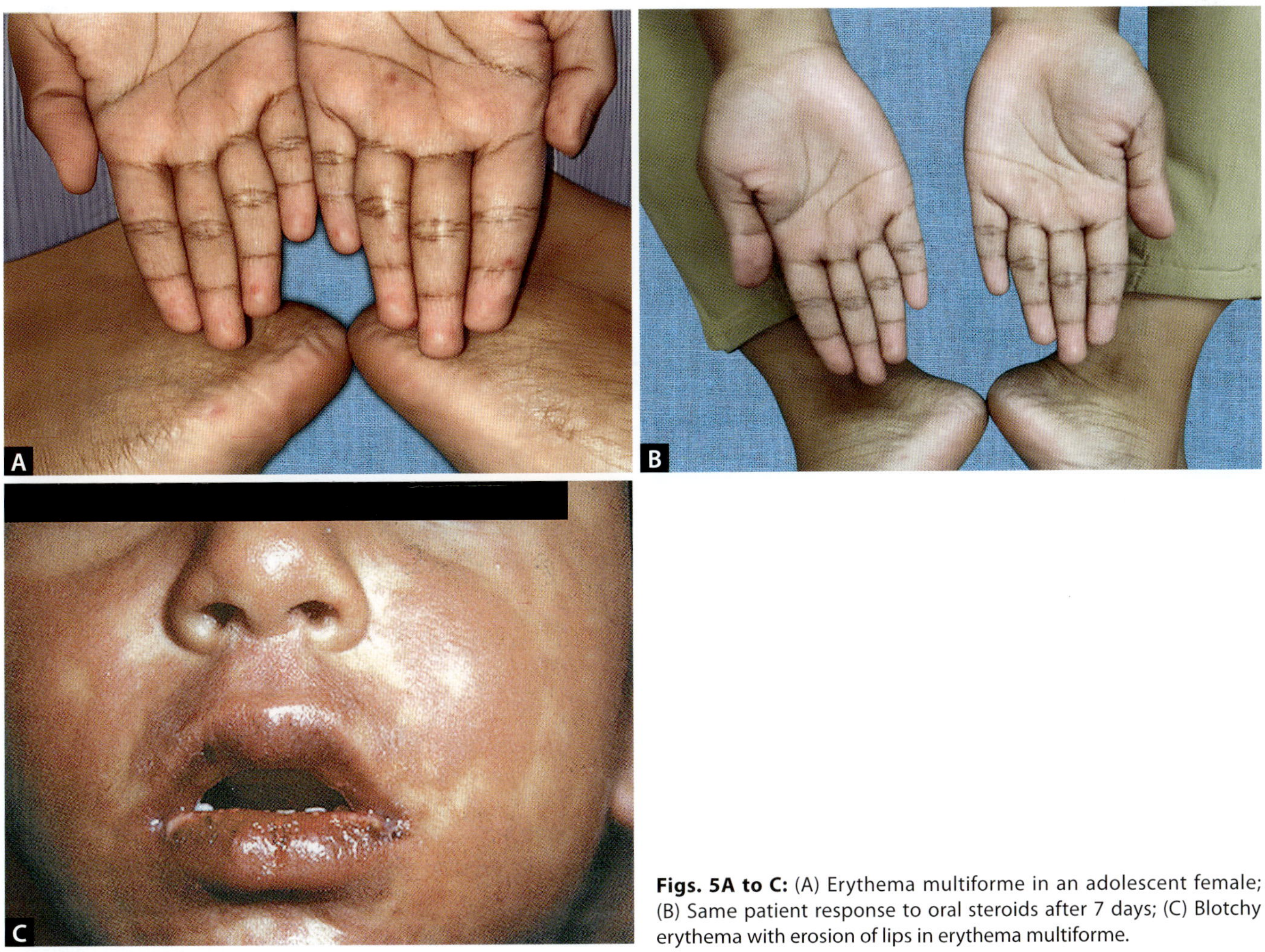

Figs. 5A to C: (A) Erythema multiforme in an adolescent female; (B) Same patient response to oral steroids after 7 days; (C) Blotchy erythema with erosion of lips in erythema multiforme.

"Hope is being able to see that there is light despite all of the darkness." —**Desmond Tutu**

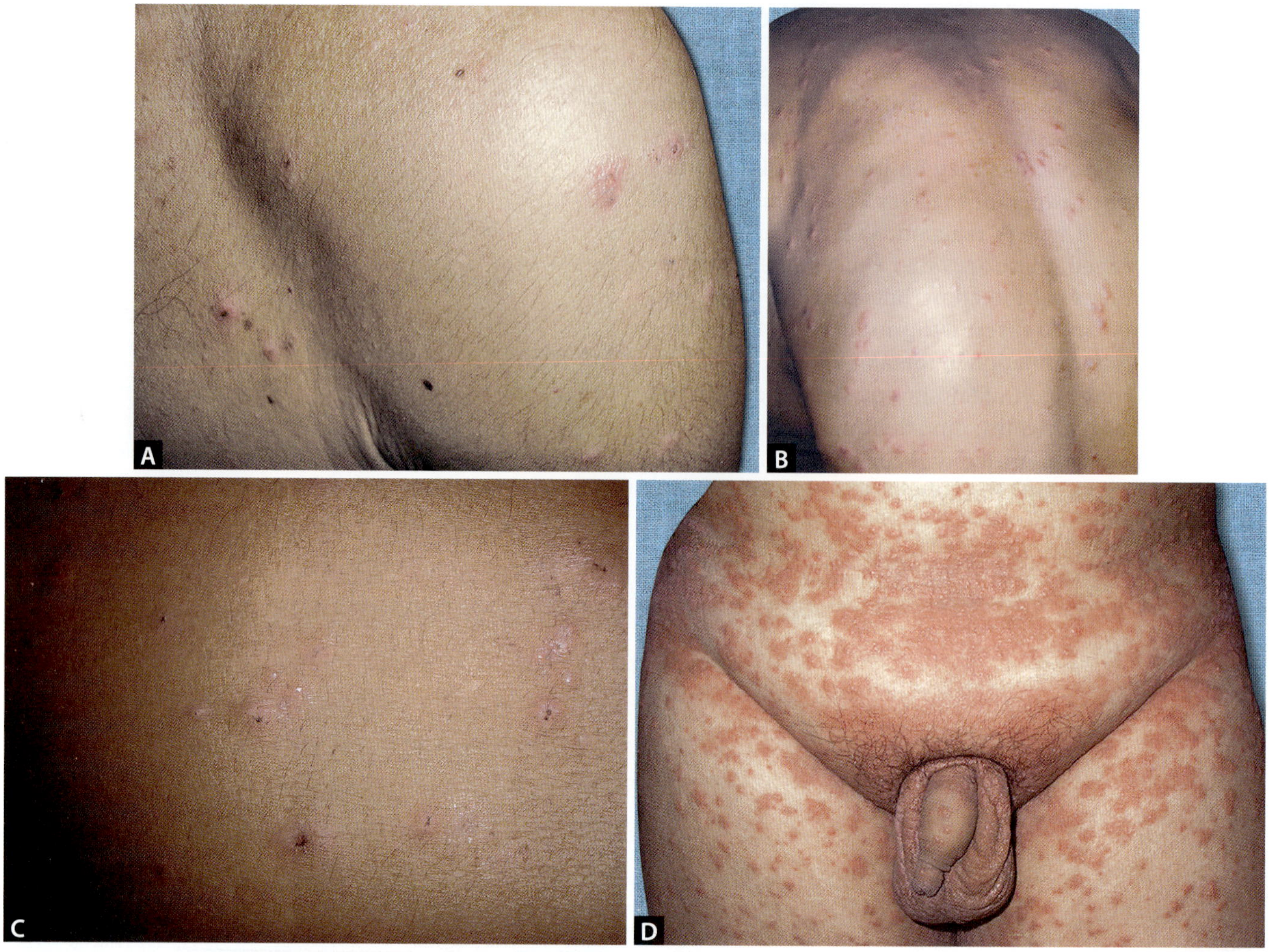

Figs. 7A to D: (A) Target lesions of erythema multiforme (EM); (B) EM lesions over back; (C) Close-up view; (D) Erythematous papules over lower trunk and thigh in a case of EM.

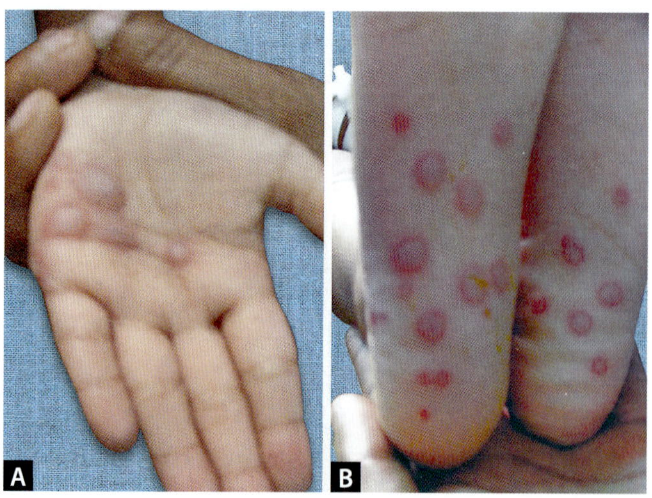

Figs. 8A and B: (A) Palmar lesions in erythema multiforme (EM); (B) EM lesions over soles.

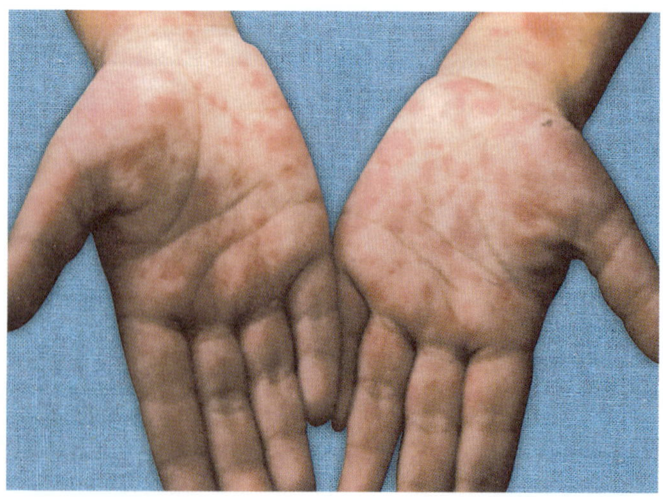

Fig. 9: Target lesions of erythema multiforme (EM) over palms.

STEVENS–JOHNSON SYNDROME (FIGS. 10 TO 12)

Stevens–Johnson syndrome is a severe and occasionally fatal drug eruption, sometimes develop downgrading from EM, while on other occasions develop as such. It is usually explosive in onset with associated fever, malaise, myalgia, headache, arthralgia, and injection of conjunctivae. Oral ulceration and erosion of lips are early features. Bullae, usually hemorrhagic, develop extensively all over the body, subsequently rupture to leave large areas of erosions. The patients usually run high-grade fever and look seriously ill. There is < 10% body surface area detachment.

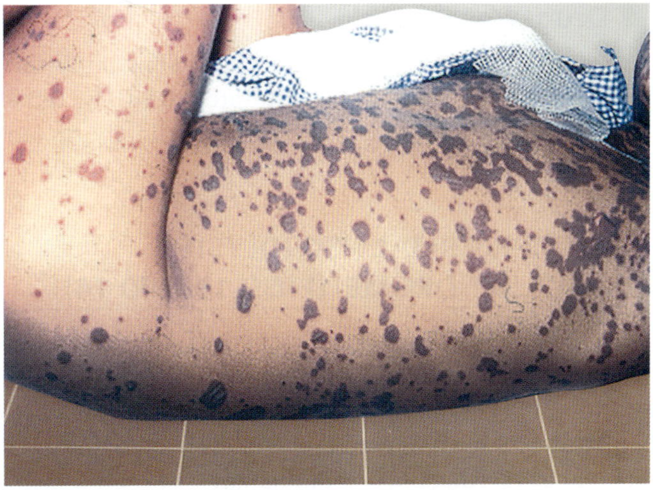

Fig. 10: Lesions of EM developing vesicles, downgrading to Stevens–Johnson syndrome.

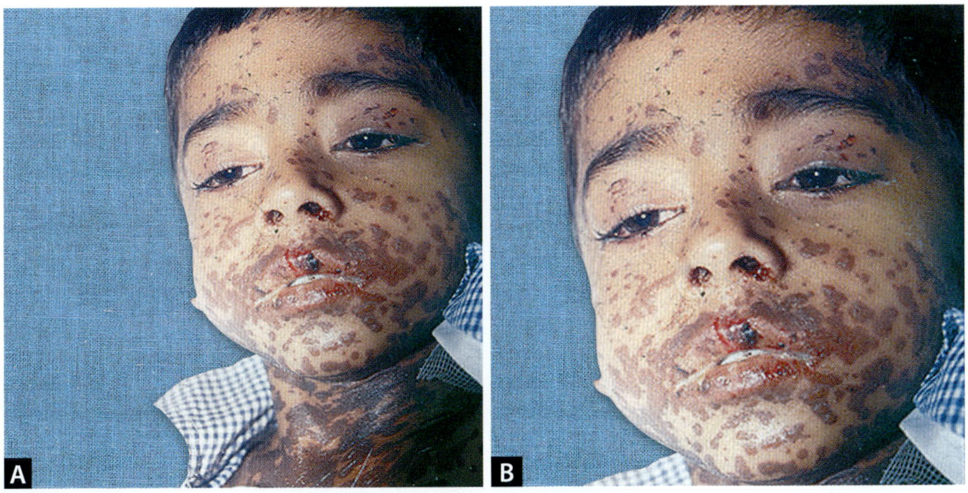

Figs. 11A and B: (A) Crusting in Stevens–Johnson syndrome (during recovery); (B) Same boy, close-up view.

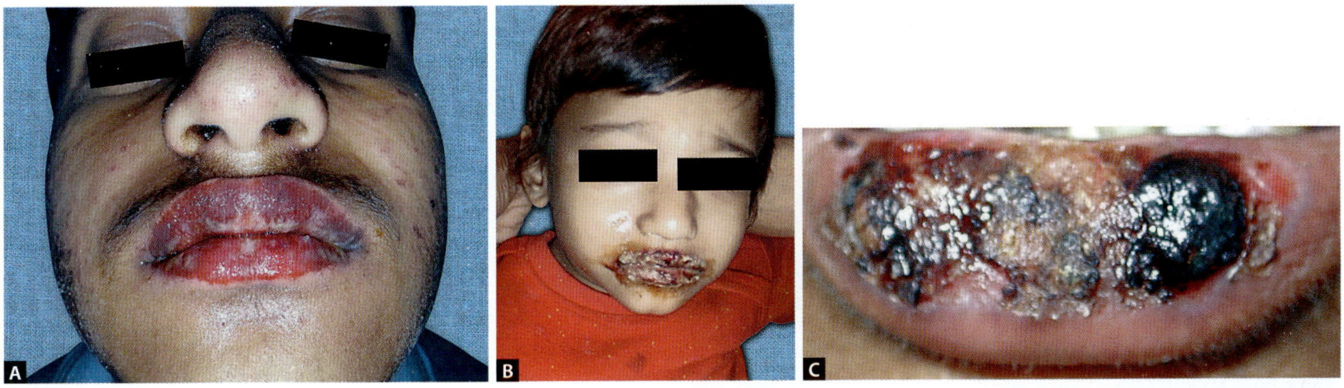

Figs. 12A to C: (A) Erosion of lips in Stevens–Johnson syndrome (SJS); (B) Hemorrhagic crusting over lips in SJS; (C) Close-up view of crusting of lips.

"Raise your words, not voice. It is rain that grows flowers, not thunder." —**Rumi**

Drugs Responsible

The drugs commonly implicated are penicillins, phenytoin sodium, carbamazepine, barbiturates, NSAIDs, tetracyclines, sulfonamides, isoniazid, rifampicin, ibuprofen, nimesulide, etc.

TOXIC EPIDERMAL NECROLYSIS (LYELL'S SYNDROME) (FIGS. 13 AND 14)

The condition is fairly uncommon in children as compared to adults. It is a serious and fatal rapidly progressive eruption of skin following intake of drug which leads to a picture like burn. It can rarely follow bacterial or viral infections, vaccination, or radiotherapy.

Drug-induced TEN usually develops within 48–72 hours after intake of a drug. However, in some cases, it may take 2–3 weeks and this is seen with anticonvulsants and

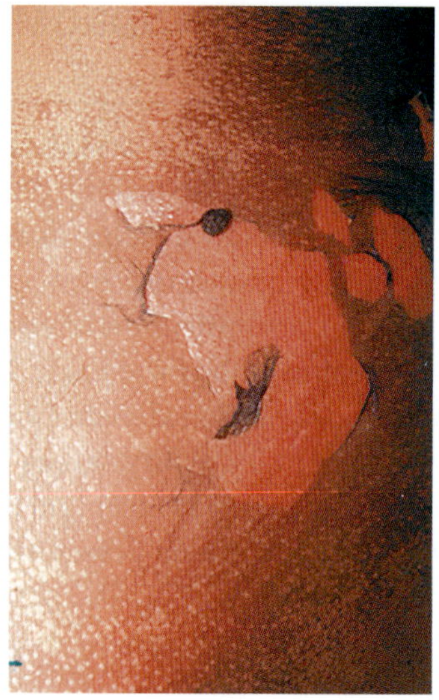

Fig. 13: Necrolysis showing easy peeling of skin in SJS/TEN (Nikolsky's sign).

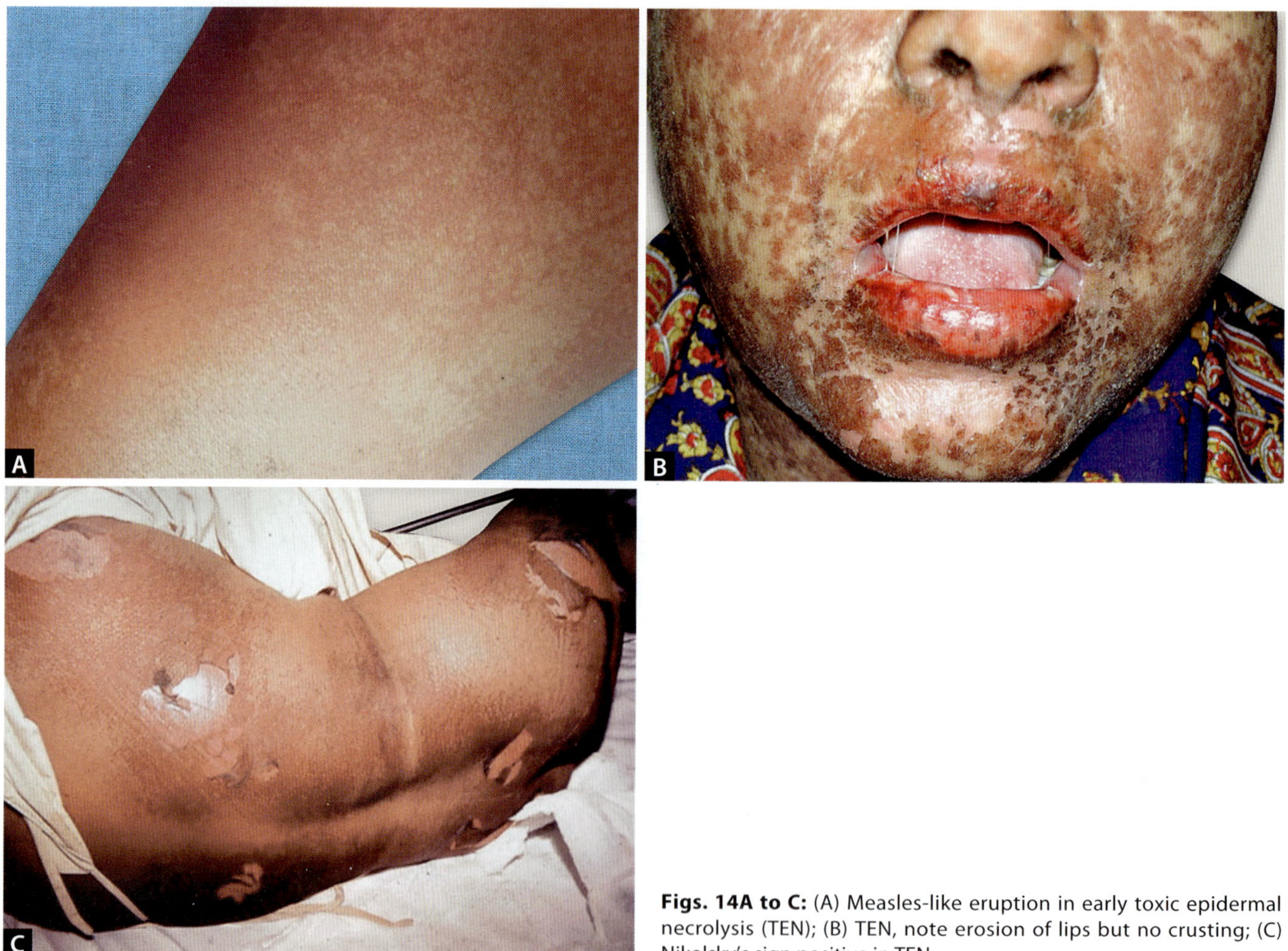

Figs. 14A to C: (A) Measles-like eruption in early toxic epidermal necrolysis (TEN); (B) TEN, note erosion of lips but no crusting; (C) Nikolsky's sign positive in TEN.

"Surround yourself only with people who are going to take you higher." —**Oprah Winfrey**

antitubercular drugs. The rash rapidly progresses to involve larger areas of the body (>30%) with extensive epidermal detachment. The skin becomes very tender because of necrolysis. High fever and associated symptoms are usual accompaniments. Mucosal involvement is not as common as SJS syndrome but there may be involvement of eyes, oral mucosa, and genitalia. The condition resembles second-degree burn and is associated with fever, vomiting, loose motion, and often chest pain. The condition may become life-threatening within hours of its onset. Complications include pneumonia, acute respiratory distress syndrome, anemia, esophageal erosions, septicemia, pigmentary changes, nail dystrophy, and contractures.

Drugs Responsible

Commonly implicated drugs are cotrimoxazole, sulfonamides, tetracyclines, isoniazid, hydantoin, carbamazepine barbiturates, phenothiazines, etc.

MANAGEMENT PROTOCOL FOR SJS/TEN

The fact that SJS and TEN are due to keratinocyte apoptosis, intravenous immunoglobulin (IVIg) is advocated to block apoptosis via the Fas pathway. Studies on the use of IVIg in TEN have reported good results. A study of ten consecutive patients with TEN of moderate severity were treated with different doses of IVIg (0.2–0.75 g/kg body weight per day for four consecutive days) and found that there was recovery in all cases. Blood transfusion in cases of SJS and TEN helps in many ways as toxic metabolites, cytotoxic T cells, and autoantibodies get diluted by hemotransfusion, and supplies immunoglobulins to fight infections. A benefit of plasmapheresis for treatment of TEN/SJS is also reported. Cyclophosphamide is also claimed to produce good results. A retrospective comparative study showed cyclosporine was safe and produced good re-epithelialization rate and a lower mortality. At present, it has become the first line of treatment in SJS/TEN. It is given at a dose of 3 mg/kg/day for 2–4 weeks. Tumor necrosis factor (TNF) is a mediator of cell death in TEN, and control of the progression of TEN with intravenous anti-TNF antibody infliximab yielded better outcomes. Systemic corticosteroids in TEN is controversial.

SERUM SICKNESS (FIG. 15)

Serum sickness, an allergic reaction, originally noted following administration of serum of horse or rabbit origin is now frequently observed with administration of drugs such as penicillins, other antibiotics, thiouracils, p-amino salicylic acid, and sulfonamides. It is mediated by circulating antigen-antibody complexes in which IgG is the predominant immunoglobulin. Following exposure to antigen, after 8–14 days in case of non-sensitized individuals and still earlier in presensitized persons, serum sickness is manifested by urticaria, maculopapular, or vasculitis eruptions, malaise, fever, lymphadenopathy, splenomegaly, and swollen and tender joints. Localized or generalized edema is common. Skin eruptions, the most common and characteristic features, are present in over 80% patients. The rash is urticarial in 90% cases. However, morbilliform and scarlatiniform eruptions, EM, erythema nodosum, and vasculitic purpura may be seen less commonly. Serum sickness may be a self-limiting disease that subsides within 2–3 weeks. Rarely death may occur due to coronary artery vasculitis or severe neuropathy.

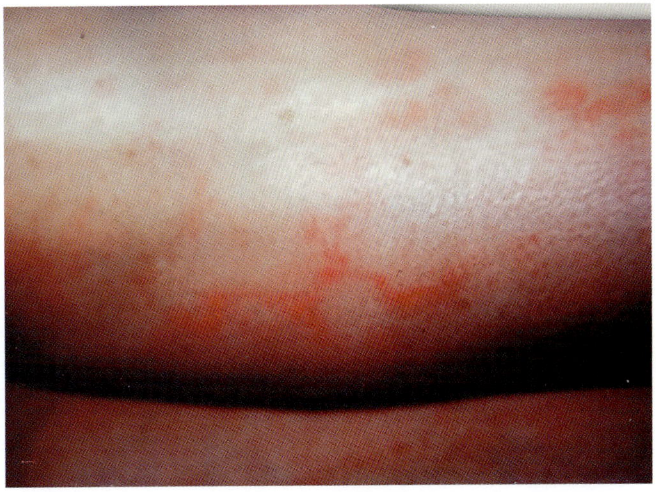

Fig. 15: Annular erythematous urticarial lesions of serum sickness.

Treatment

The condition is treated with adrenaline, antihistamines, and analgesics. Hydroxyzine is the most effective antihistamine in children for this condition. It is administered in a dose of 2 mg/kg/24 hours in three to four divided doses. Systemic corticosteroids are given in more severe cases. Tracheostomy may be life-saving in severe glottic edema.

DRESS SYNDROME (FIGS. 16A AND B)

DRESS, the acronym of Drug Reaction with Eosinophilia and Systemic Symptoms, is also referred to as DIDMOHS (drug-induced delayed multi-organ hypersensitivity

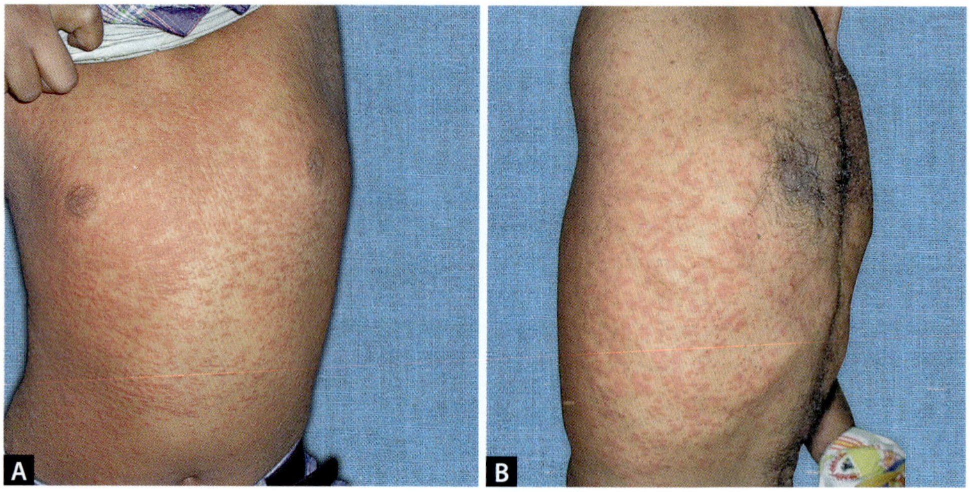

Figs. 16A and B: (A) Maculopapular rash of DRESS syndrome; (B) DRESS syndrome lateral view showing diffuse maculopapular rash.

syndrome) or drug hypersensitivity syndrome. This distinct type of ADR was initially described in association with aromatic anticonvulsants (phenytoin, carbamazepine, phenobarbital, lamotrigine and primidone). Other culprit drugs are sulfonamides, dapsone, minocycline, terbinafine, azathioprine, allopurinol, gold derivatives, cyclosporine, captopril, diltiazem, metronidazole, NSAIDs, and the antiretrovirals such as nevirapine and abacavir. The triad of fever, skin rash, and symptomatic or asymptomatic internal organ involvement characterizes this specific entity. The incidence is approximately 1 in 1,000 to 1 in 10,000 exposures. Reactions classically begin 1–8 weeks after initiation of therapy, but in previously sensitized individual, it appears within 1 day of rechallenge. It affects various organ and organ systems, with skin, liver, and hematological system being most commonly targeted. It presents with high, spiking fever followed in 1–2 days by other manifestations. Skin lesions are most commonly exanthematous and rarely generalized follicular pustules or more severe skin reactions, such as erythroderma, EM, SJS, or TEN may occur. Facial and periorbital edema is a characteristic sign of potentially serious reaction. Other manifestations are tender, local, or generalized lymphadenopathy, conjunctivitis, and various internal organ involvements in the form of hepatitis, nephritis, pneumonitis, neutrophilia, eosinophilia, atypical lymphocytosis, blood dyscrasias, hemolytic anemia, and changes in immunoglobulin levels, oral ulceration, exudative tonsillitis, oral ulcers, strawberry tongue, flu-like symptoms, myopathy, disseminated intravascular coagulopathy, pharyngitis, hypotension, pancreatitis, myocarditis, myositis, meningitis, parotitis, orchitis, arthralgia, and thyroiditis. Late-onset hypothyroidism has also been reported. Course is variable; with early diagnosis, outcome is favorable though not always. Fatality is mainly due to fulminant hepatitis.

Pathogenesis is multifactorial. Several factors act in concert in the causation and expression of this disease entity. Possible mechanisms explaining the pathogenesis are formation of drug metabolites and inherited defect in detoxification of such intermediates, intercurrent disease processes, and concurrent active viral infection (HIV, HHV-6/7, and EBV). Altered cytokine profile including raised level of IL-5 has also been suggested as a probable predisposing factor.

Diagnosis is mainly clinical, aided by histopathology, lymphocyte toxicity assay, and patch test. This entity should be distinguished from other mimicking conditions such as other cutaneous drug reactions, viral exanthem, lymphoma or pseudolymphoma, collagen vascular diseases, serum sickness-like reaction, Kawasaki disease, and hypereosinophilic syndrome. The main stay of therapy is discontinuation of the offending agent followed by systemic evaluation with necessary laboratory tests to ascertain degree of internal involvement. Antihistamines and topical steroids give symptomatic relief. Role of systemic steroids is controversial, although it gives encouraging result. Systemic steroids should be given for long term, probably for an year, due to frequent flares; hence, cyclosporine has become the treatment of choice in DRESS. It is given at a dose of 3–5 mg/kg body weight. Other therapeutic aids that can be tried are plasmapheresis and IVIg. Patients developing DRESS due to one aromatic anticonvulsant should be advised to avoid other arene oxide-producing anticonvulsants as cross-reactivity is seen in 80% cases. Long-term sequelae of DRESS has been reported to result in future development of autoimmune diseases (type III polyglandular autoimmune syndrome in pediatric age group).

TOXIC PALMAR ERYTHEMA AND FISSURING OF PALMS (FIGS. 17 TO 19)

Toxic palmar and plantar erythema is a common dermatological reaction associated with specific cytotoxic chemotherapy. It is also called as palmoplantar erythrodysesthesia (PPE) or hand foot syndrome. The incidence depends on the drug therapy, dosage, and route of administration.

Pathogenesis

The pathogenesis is still not clear. The common cytotoxic drugs known to cause this reaction are mercaptopurine, 5-fluorouracil, doxorubicin, docetaxel, capecitabine, vinorelbine, gemcitabine, and sorafenib. Various school of thoughts have been proposed such as deposition of drug in epidermis and dermal of palms and soles where there is rich vascular networks, rapid cell division rate in palms and soles, gravitational forces, increased drug concentration in the eccrine glands of palms and soles.

Clinical Features

Clinical manifestations vary from mild-to-severe forms. Initially there are prodromal symptoms of tingling, burning, and dysesthesia. Later, there is erythema of palms, fingers, and soles which later progress to dryness and desquamation. Papules, ulceration, edema, fissuring of the creases may occur. Rarely, sensory impairment, paresthesia, and pruritus have been reported. The National Center Institute has graded the severity of toxic rash **(Table 1)**.

Table 1: Severity of toxic rash according to the National Center Institute.

Grade	*Clinical symptoms*
1	Minimal skin changes (erythema, edema, and hyperkeratosis) without pain
2	Skin changes (peeling, blister, bleeding, edema, and hyperkeratosis) with pain not interfering with function
3	Severe skin changes with pain interfering with function

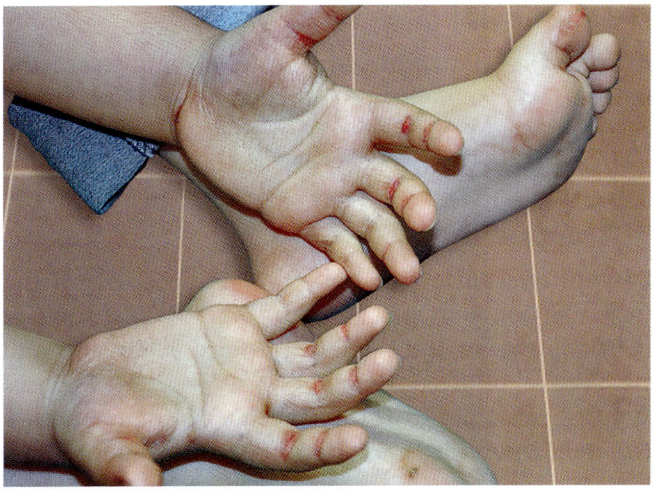

Fig. 17: Toxic palmoplantar erythema due to 6 mercaptopurine therapy in 5-year-old boy suffering from B-cell lymphoma.

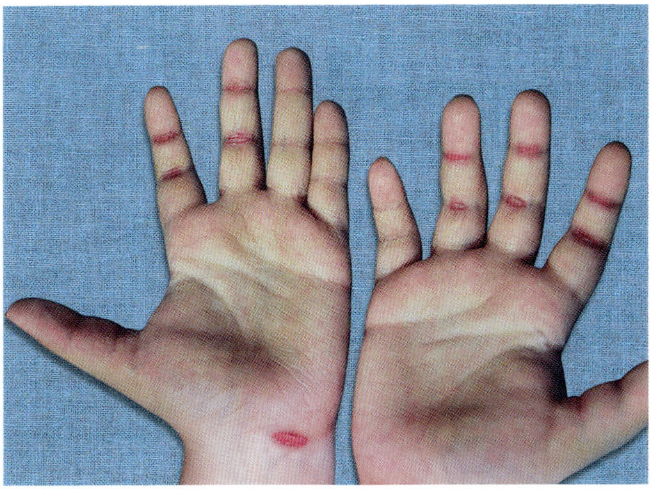

Fig. 18: Same boy, palms showing erythema and fissuring over inter-digital spaces of fingers

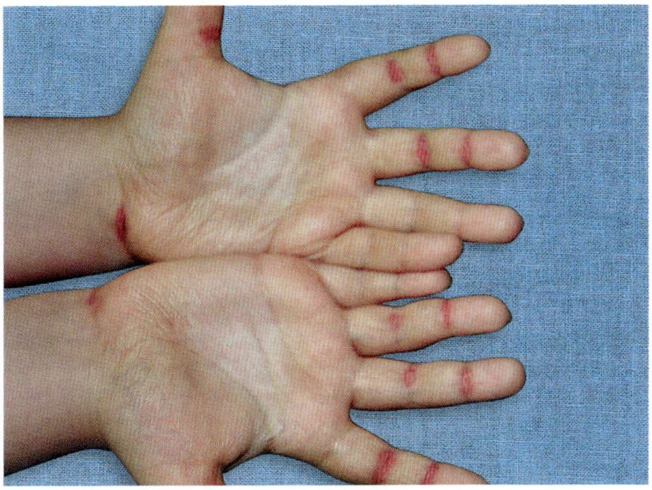

Fig. 19: Close-up view of palmar lesions.

"Having a soft heart in a cruel world is courage not weakness." —**Katherine Henson**

Diagnosis

It should be differentiated from neutrophilic eccrine hidradenitis, palmoplantar hidradenitis, and EM. Strong suspicion and awareness of this condition will help to diagnose the condition.

Treatment

Discontinuation of chemotherapy is necessary if the toxic reaction is in grade 2 or 3. Some advocate 50% of dose adjustment, if it is grade 2. Topical emollients and steroids can be given in grade 1. Oral pyridoxine at doses 800 mg daily has given good results in many studies. Other therapies tried are cyclooxygenase 2 inhibitors, oral vitamin E, and systemic steroids with variable response.

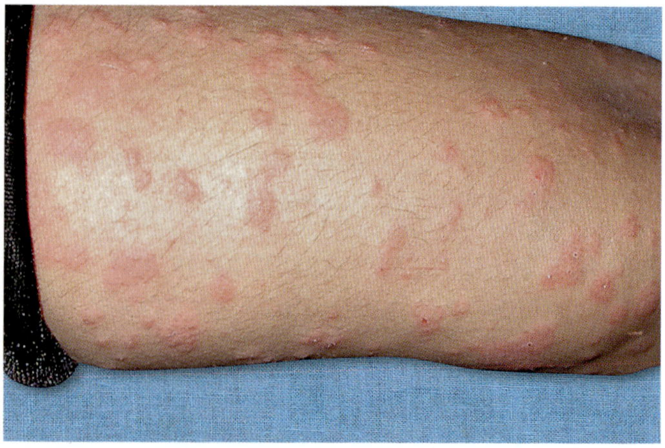

Fig. 21: Multiple erythematous, edematous papules and plaques over thigh in AGEP.

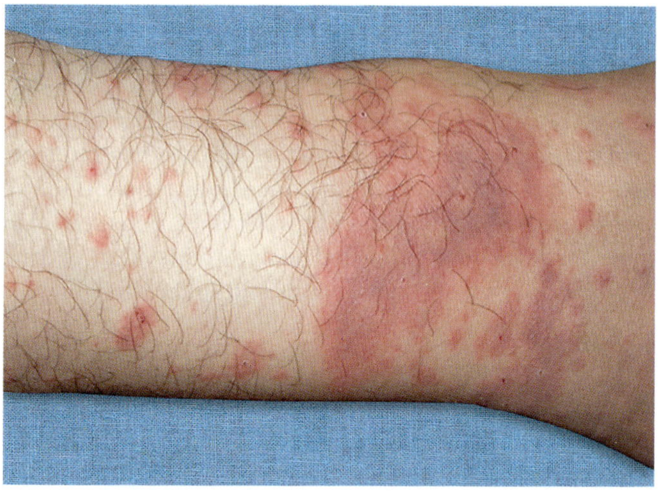

Fig. 22: Close-up view of AGEP lesions over leg.

ACUTE GENERALIZED EXANTHEMATOUS PUSTULOSIS (FIGS. 20 TO 22)

Acute generalized exanthematous pustulosis is a mostly severe drug reaction, characterized by an acute edematous erythema followed by numerous small nonfollicular pustules on an erythematous base and spontaneous resolution usually within 2 weeks. Various drugs incriminated are aminopenicillins, pristinamycin, sulfonamides, quinolones, hydroxychloroquine, terbinafine and diltiazem. However, a few cases due to bacterial, viral, parasitic, *chlamydial*, *Mycoplasma*, etc., infections are also on record. Systemic involvement occurs in about 20% of cases. The course is mostly benign, and only in rare cases, complications lead to life-threatening situations. Recent studies highlight the importance of genetic variations in interleukin-36 receptor antagonist (*IL-36RN*) gene in the pathogenesis of this disease. The pathophysiology of AGEP remains unclear, but an involvement of innate and acquired immune cells together with resident cells (keratinocytes), which recruit and activate neutrophils via production of cytokines/chemokines such as IL-17, IL-36, granulocyte-macrophage colony-stimulating factor (GM-CSF), TNF-α and chemokine (C-X-C motif) ligand 8 (CXCL8)/IL-8, has been postulated. Treatment is based on the removal of the causative drug, supportive care, infection prevention, and use of potent topical or systemic steroids.

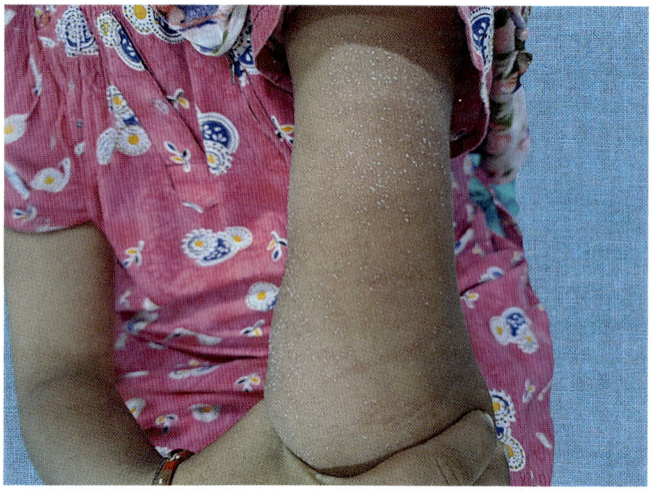

Fig. 20: Acute generalized exanthematous pustulosis in an adolescent girl.

FLAGELLATE PURPURA AND FLAGELLATE HYPERPIGMENTATION (FIGS. 23 TO 25)

Flagellate dermatoses or flagellate erythema, characterized by erythematous, linear, intermingled streaks of coalescent papules, purpuric macules, pustules,

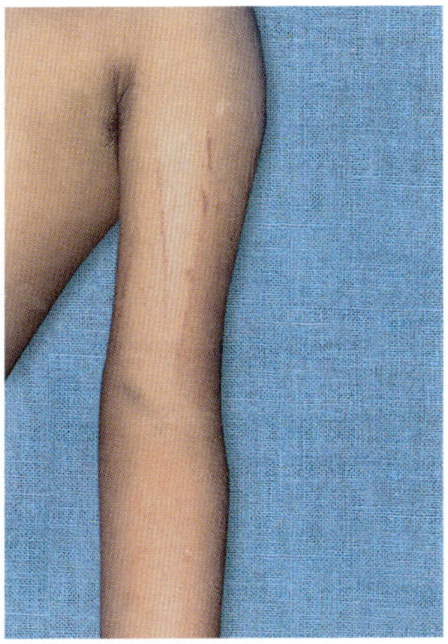

Fig. 23: Flagellate purpura in dengue.

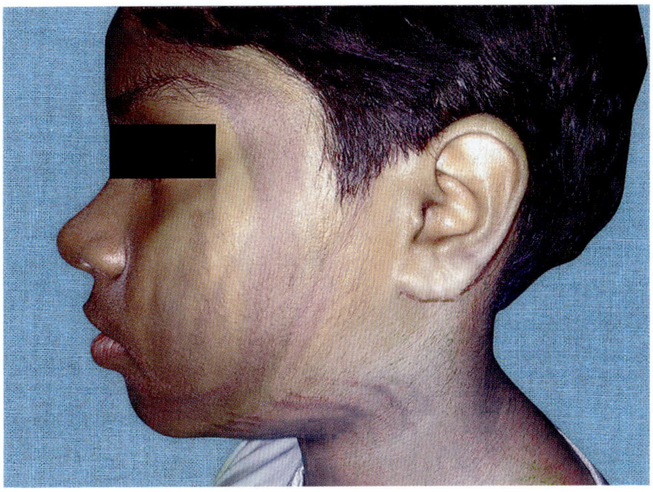

Fig. 25: Same girl, side view.

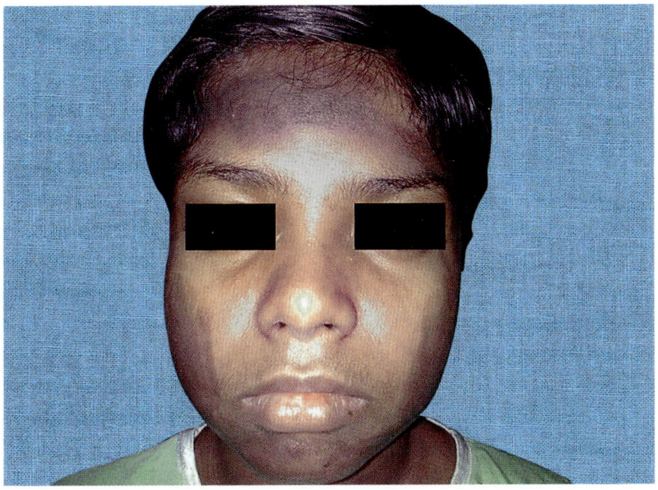

Fig. 24: Flagellate hyperpigmentation seen in dermatomyositis.

or bullae distributed in a whip-like pattern over the trunk, extremities, and face, simulating the marks of whiplash has classically been described in association with bleomycin and ingestion of Shiitake mushrooms. Subsequently, various other causes have been reported in association with flagellate dermatitis such as chikungunya fever (usually manifesting as flagellate hyperpigmentation), dengue fever (authors have recently reported in a child), other chemotherapeutic agents such as docetaxel, doxorubicin dermatomyositis and adult-onset Still disease.

Flagellate purpura has not been described in the literature apart from the flagellate edematous purpura caused by box-jellyfish stings. Recently, flagellate purpura has also been described in dengue infection (case reported by Authors). Histopathological features include spongiotic dermatitis, epidermal hyperpigmentation, necrotic keratinocytes with vacuolar degeneration of the dermoepidermal junction, superficial dermal inflammatory infiltrate (lymphocytic, neutrophilic, and eosinophilic) with edema, and melanophages in the papillary dermis. Lymphocyte-mediated vascular damage has also been reported.

WHAT'S NEW: SDRIFE

SDRIFE stands for symmetric drug related intertriginous and flexural exanthem. It was previously known as baboon syndrome. It is a type of systemic contact dermatitis, which manifests as exanthema on the buttocks and flexures after ingesting or absorbing a contact allergen. Commonly caused by antibiotics like amoxicillin, other culprits include antihypertensives and radiocontrast media. Diagnostic criteria involve exposure to the drug, erythema in gluteal or perianal areas, symmetrical involvement of other intertriginous sites, and absence of systemic toxicity. It affects all ages with a male bias, believed to be a delayed hypersensitivity reaction mediated by T-cells. Histological features range from inflammatory infiltrate to subcorneal pustules. Patch tests may not always confirm, but oral provocation tests are usually positive. Treatment is drug withdrawal along with short course of oral steroids.

"If you can change your mind, you can change your life." —**William James**

SUGGESTED READINGS

1. Alerhand S, Cassella C, Koyfman A. Stevens-Johnson syndrome and toxic epidermal necrolysis in the pediatric population: a review. Pediatr Emerg Care. 2016;32(7):472-6.
2. De A, Rajagopalan M, Sarda A, Das S, Biswas P. Drug reaction with eosinophilia and systemic symptoms: an update and review of recent literature. Indian J Dermatol. 2018;63:30-40.
3. Dhar S, Srinivas SM. Adverse drug reactions. In: Sharma N (Ed). Skin Clinical Dermatology. Jaypee Brothers Medical Publishers; 2019. pp. 595-601.
4. Dhar S, Srinivas SM. Cutaneous adverse drug reactions in children. In: Gupta LK (Ed). IADVL Textbook of Cutaneous Adverse Drug Reactions. Bhalani Publishing House; 2018. pp. 450-7.
5. Shokeen D. Cyclosporine in SJS/TEN management: a brief review. Cutis. 2016;97(3):E17-18.
6. Nguyen E, Gabel CK, Yu J. Pediatric drug eruptions. Clin Dermatol. 2020;38(6):629-40.
7. Perez CE, Dyer JA. Cutaneous Drug Eruptions in Pediatrics-A Primer. Pediatr Ann. 2020;49(3):e132-9.
8. Ramien M, Goldman JL. Pediatric SJS-TEN: Where are we now?. F1000Res. 2020;9:F1000 Faculty Rev-982.
9. Akbayrak A, Yazar C, Deresoy FA, Sencan M, Seckin HY, Kutlu O. Acute localized exanthematous pustulosis because of cefixime in a child: case report and review of pediatric cases. Int J Dermatol. 2022;61(6):707-9.

"Education costs money, but then so does ignorance." —**Claus Moser**

CHAPTER

19

Striae and Scars

IDIOPATHIC STRIAE DISTENSAE [FIGS. 1 TO 3A(iv)]

Striae are visible linear scars which form in areas of dermal damage produced by stretching of skin. In children, striae develop readily at puberty (growth spurts). Adolescent striae may first develop soon after the appearance of pubic hair. In boys, outer aspect of the thighs and lumbosacral region and in girls, breasts, buttocks and thighs are the most common affected sites. Early lesions may be raised and irritable but they soon become flat, smooth, and livid red or bluish in color. Their surface may be finely wrinkled. They are commonly irregularly linear, several centimeters long and 1–10 mm wide. After some years, they fade and become inconspicuous. The striae in Cushing's syndrome or those induced by steroid therapy may be larger and more widely distributed.

Natural History

Most striae which appear during late childhood or adolescence tend to become less prominent with time.

Treatment

Topical tretinoin (0.025% or 0.05%) once daily for 3–6 months may help in some patients. Weight reduction and avoidance of extreme stretching of skin are advised. Oral vitamin E may improve the condition but it has to be given for atleast 6–8 months.

HYPERTROPHIC SCAR (FIGS. 3B TO E)

Hypertrophic scars are overgrowth of fibrous tissue in the dermis and are considered to be an aberration of the wound-healing process. Clinically hypertrophic scar can be differentiated from keloid based on the following features: lack of claw-like projections, confinement to the site of original injury, spontaneous regression over time, lack of spontaneous occurence and improvement after appropriate surgery. Hypertrophic scars are usually asymptomatic, but sometimes similar to keloids, it can present with pain, pruritus, burning sensation and tenderness. Histopathological differentiating points from keloid are presence of thick, pale, glassy, and hyalinized collagen bundle arranged unidirectionally.

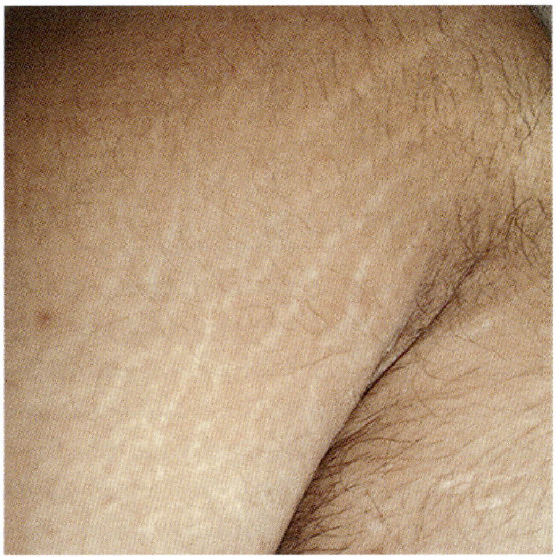

Fig. 1: Whitish atrophic lines of idiopathic striae distensae over axilla and shoulders.

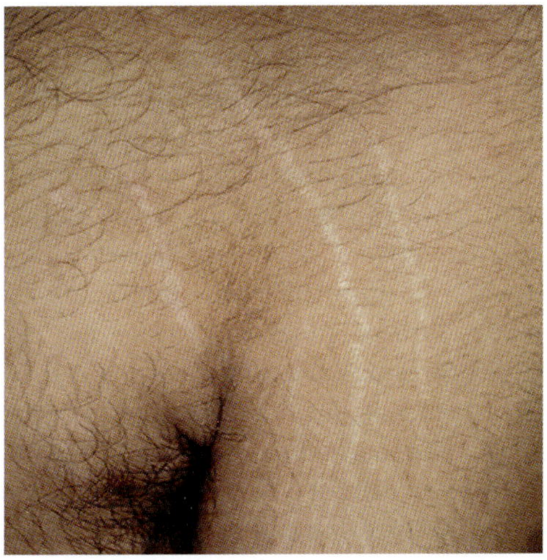

Fig. 2: Close-up view of idiopathic striae distensae.

"The only person you are destined to become is the person you decide to be." **—Ralph Waldo Emerson**

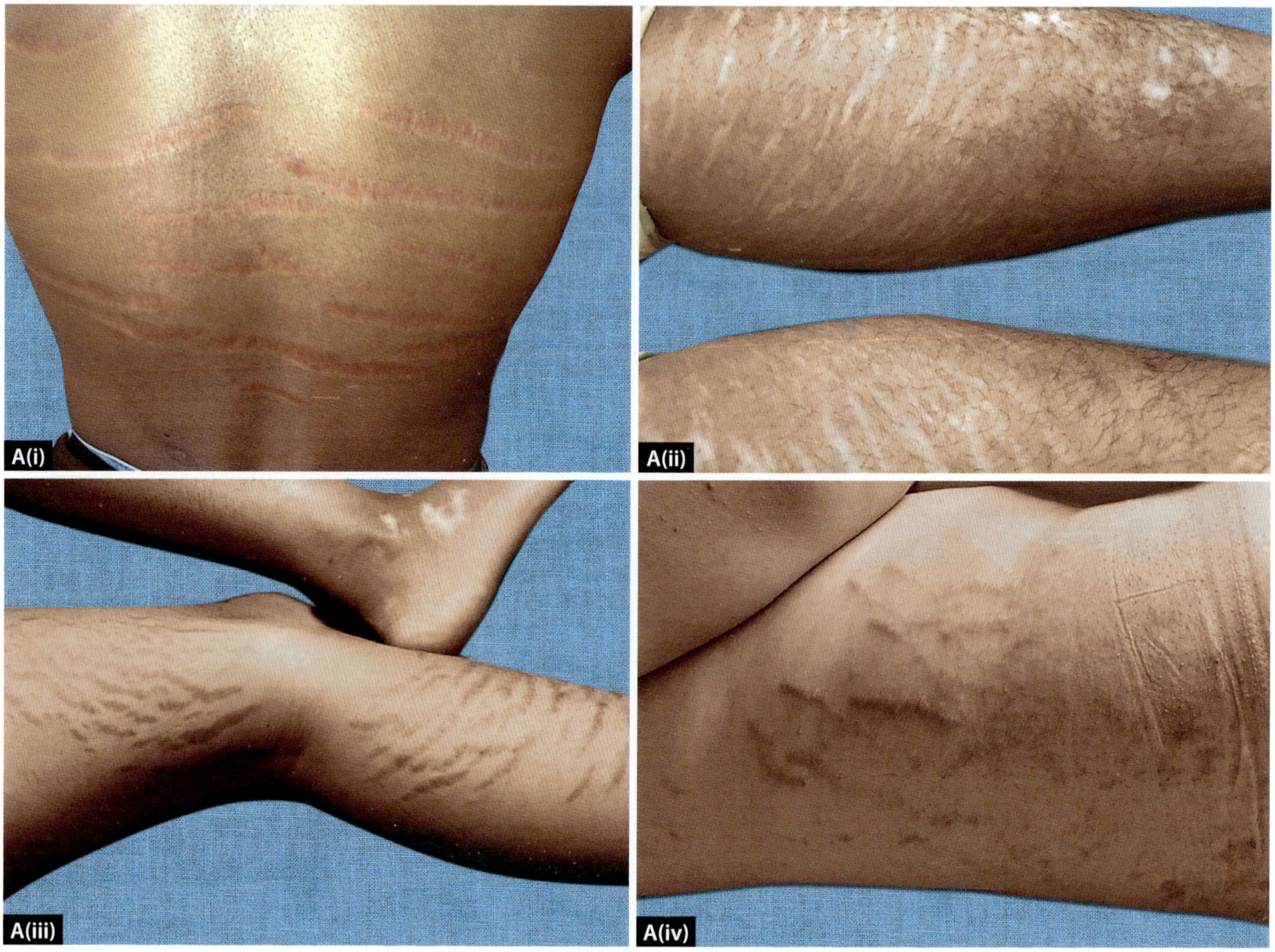

Figs. 3A(i) to (iv): A(i) Idiopathic striae distensae (ISD) over back in an adolescent boy; A(ii) ISD over legs; A(iii) ISD over thigh and legs in an adolescent girl; A(iv) ISD over side of upper thigh.

Pathophysiology is poorly understood. Any form of injury to the deep dermis such as surgery, ear piercing, burn, foreign body reaction, acne vulgaris, and herpes zoster can predispose to hypertrophy. Adverse wound healing factors such as improper wound closure, hematoma formation, excessive tension or infection of the wound also contribute to the same. The basic defect is imbalance between anabolic and catabolic process of wound healing leading to excessive production of collagen, fibronectin, and proteoglycan under the influence of mainly transforming growth factor-beta (TGF-β).

Preventive measures for keloid and hypertrophic scar include avoidance of nonessential cosmetic procedures, minimal tension during wound closure, and avoidance of incision across joint line and proper wound care.

Several treatment modalities have been tried including intralesional injection of steroid alone or in combination with 5-flurouracil, cryotherapy, compression therapy, silicone gel sheet, intralesional interferon gamma therapy, pulsed dye laser, verapamil, angiotensin-converting enzyme (ACE) inhibitors, imiquimod, and retinoic acid.

KELOID (FIGS. 4A TO E)

Keloid is a benign, well-demarcated area of fibrous tissue overgrowth that extends beyond the original defect. Keloids become raised and thickened within 3–4 weeks of the provocative stimulus. The lesions become a firm, pink or red plaque, which may grow for months or years. Lesions often assume a dumb-bell configuration, but sometimes become bizarre and irregular. The surface of a keloid becomes smoother and rounder extending beyond the area of the original lesion. It is often irritable,

"We can't help everyone, but everyone can help someone." —**Ronald Reagan**

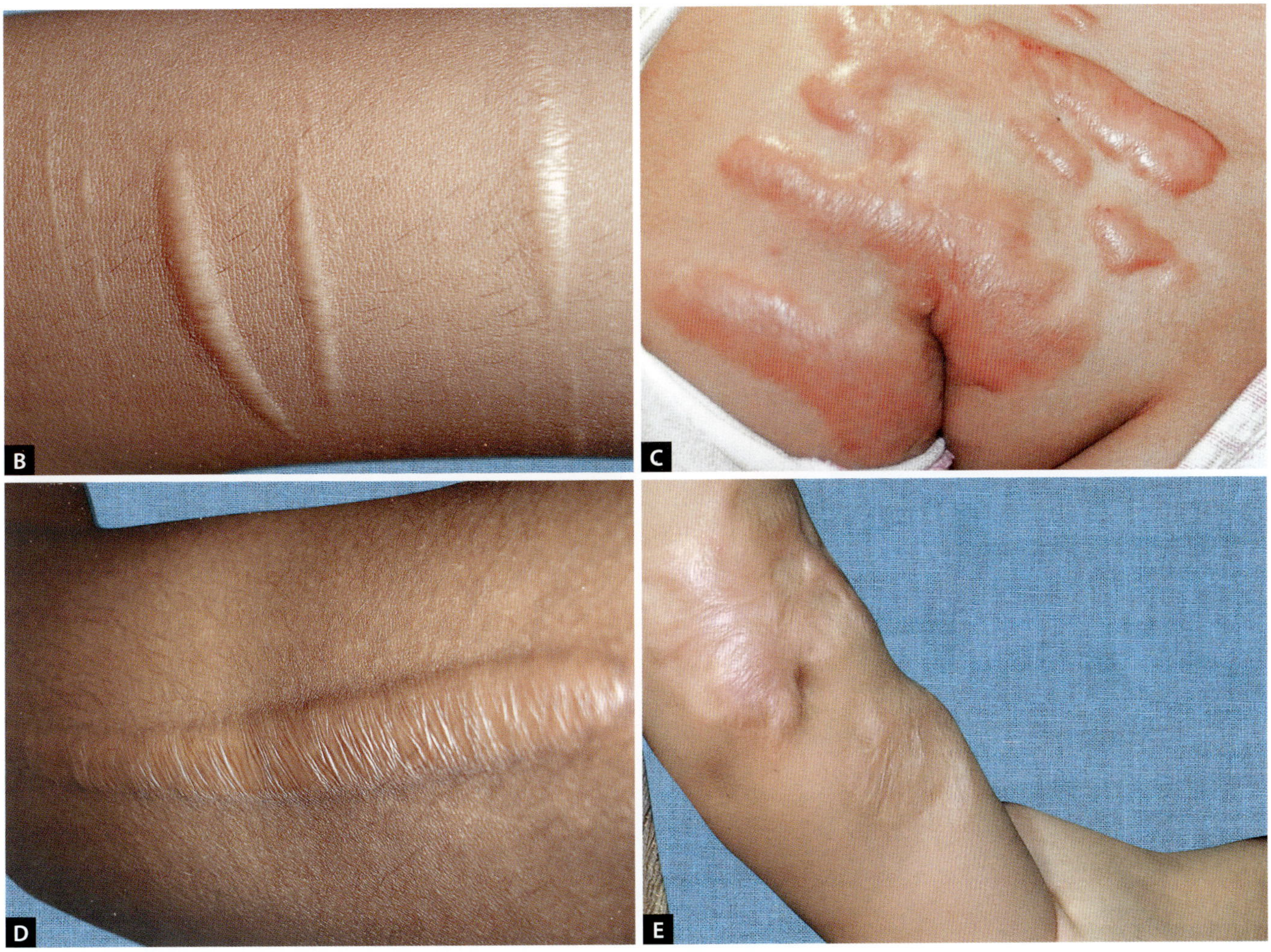

Figs. 3B to E: (B) Hypertrophic scars; (C) Multiple hypertrophic scars over sacral area; (D) Close-up view of hypertrophic scar; (E) Hypertrophic scars following scald injury.

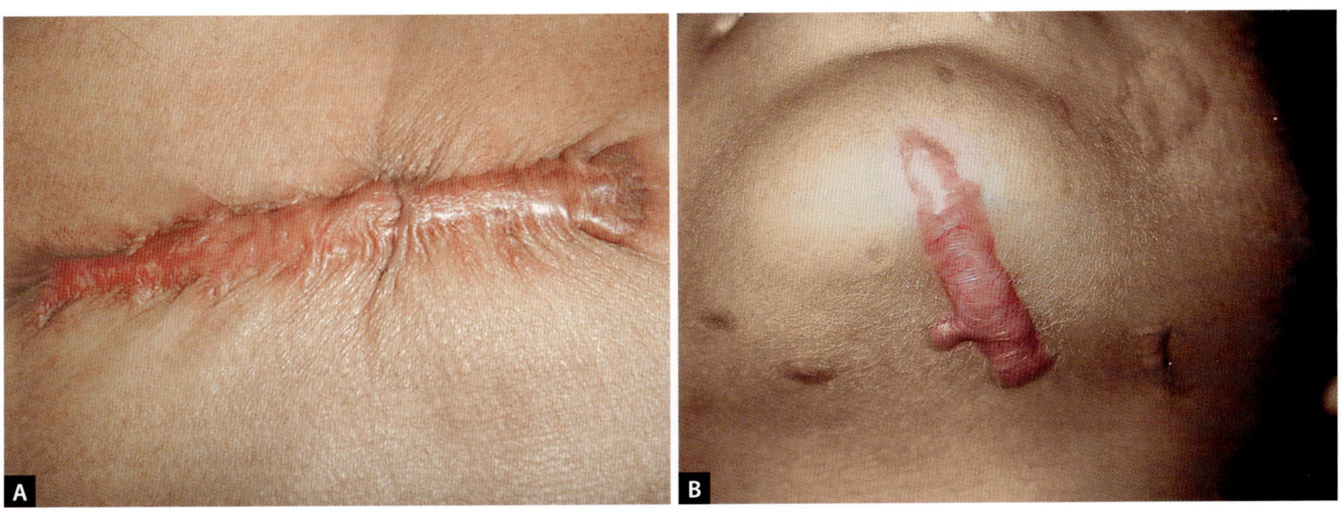

Figs. 4A and B: (A) Keloid over abdomen; (B) Keloid over chin.

"Everything you've ever wanted is on the other side of fear." —**George Addair**

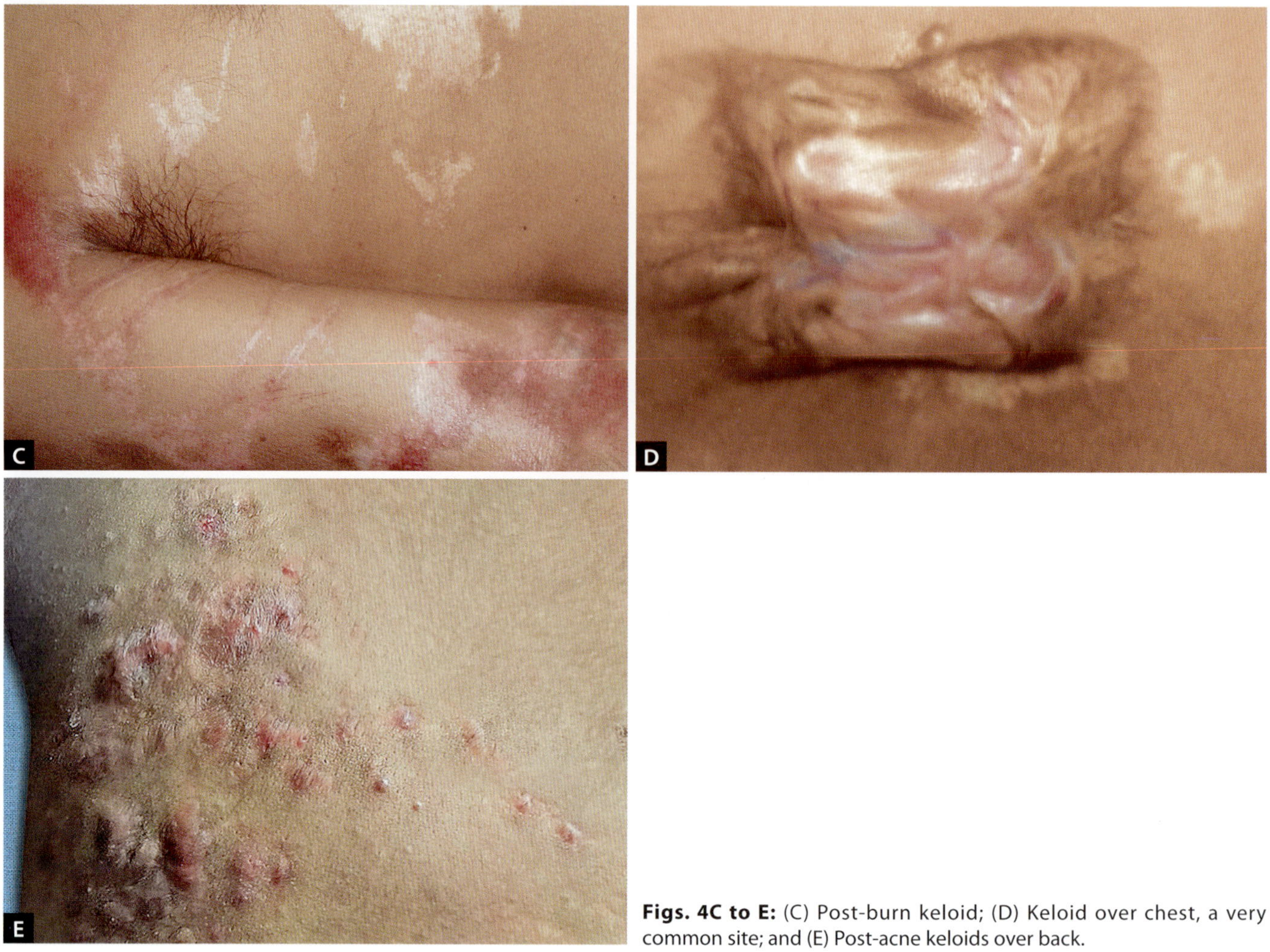

Figs. 4C to E: (C) Post-burn keloid; (D) Keloid over chest, a very common site; and (E) Post-acne keloids over back.

hypersensitive, and sometimes exquisitely tender. Keloids tend to regress after several years. Familial keloid has been reported to be associated with syndromes such as Rubinstein-Taybi syndrome, pachydermoperiostosis, Ehlers-Danlos syndrome, progeria, Turner syndrome, and Noonan syndrome.

Treatment

Intralesional triamcinolone acetonide injection every 3–4 weeks helps regression of keloid as well as alleviation of associated itching. Antihistamine ketotifen alleviates itching and it is said to be suppressing the growth of fibroblasts of keloids to some extent. However, since it is strongly sedative, it is to be given at night. Other treatment modalities are cryotherapy with liquid nitrogen, application of silicone gel sheet, topical application of heparin, allantoin, etc.

TOPICAL STEROID-INDUCED CUTANEOUS ATROPHY (FIGS. 5 AND 6)

Atrophy of the local site of application of a potent topical steroid is not uncommon. Atrophy is mostly seen over face and flexures when a potent topical steroid is applied for a considerable period of time. In most of the cases atrophy is associated with hypopigmentation/depigmentation and telangiectasia. The atrophy can be permanent and irreversible.

VERMICULATE ATROPHODERMA OF THE FACE (FIGS. 7 AND 8)

Atrophodermas are a group of disorders involving atrophy of skin. The different types are—follicular atrophoderma, vermiculate atrophoderma, atrophoderma of Pasini and Pierini, and linear atrophoderma. In vermiculate

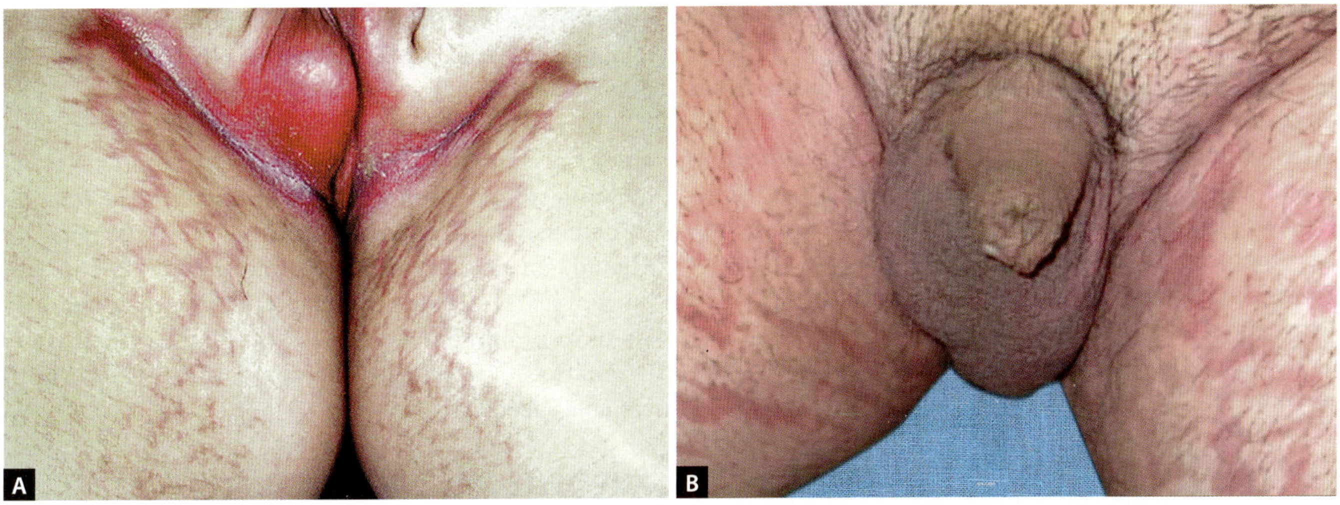

Figs. 5A and B: (A) Steroid-induced atrophy of skin over thighs; (B) Topical potent steroid-induced striae over groin.

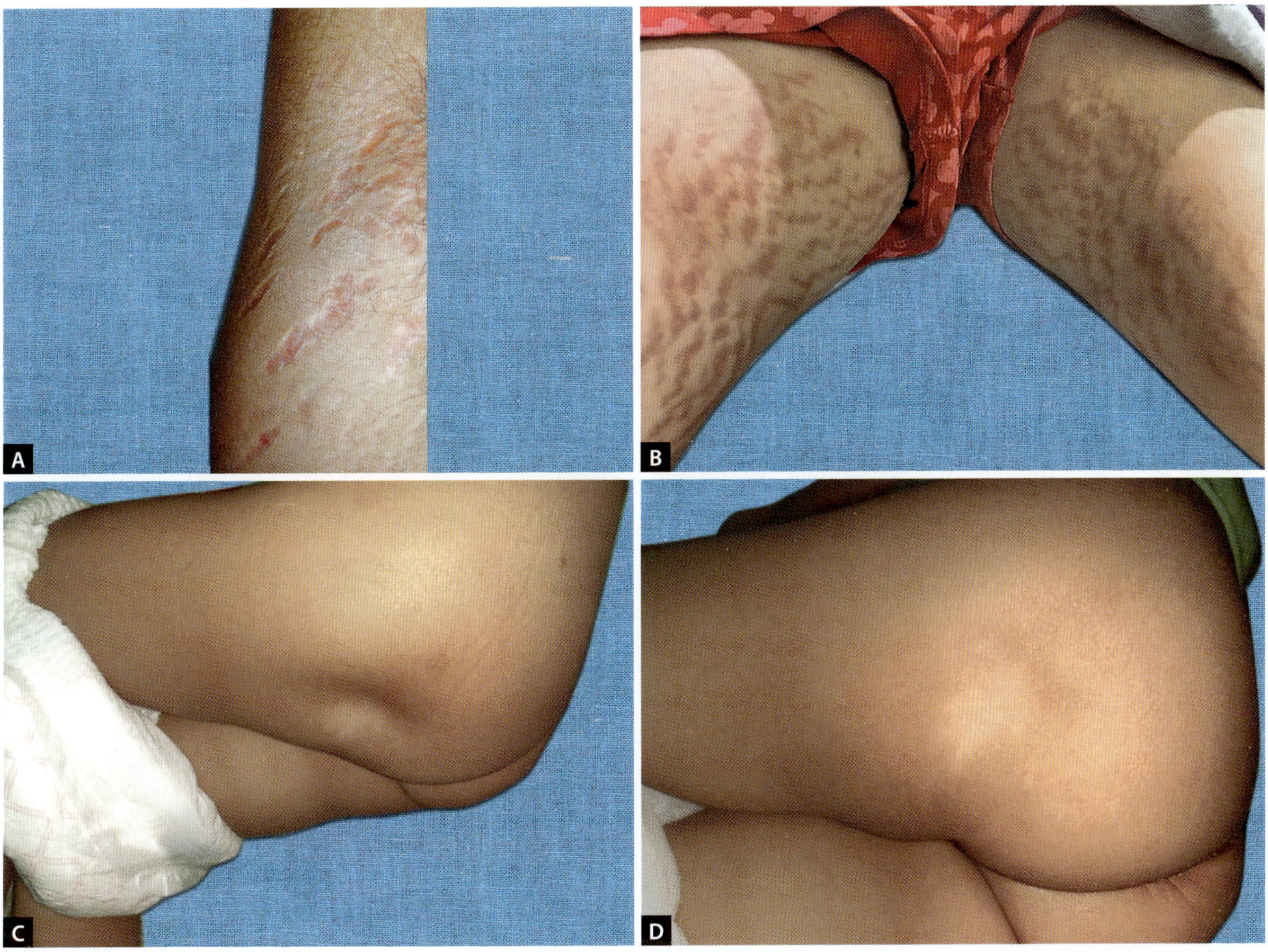

Figs. 6A to D: (A) Steroid-induced skin atrophy over axilla; (B) Topical potent steroid-induced striae over thighs and legs; (C) Steroid injection-induced atrophy over buttock; and (D) Same child, note steroid-induced hypopigmentation.

"Nothing will work unless you do." —**Maya Angelou**

atrophoderma (*syn.* Honeycomb atrophy/folliculitis ulerythematosa reticulata), there are bilateral atrophic pits in a reticular fashion on cheeks. The disease has an autosomal dominant mode of inheritance with an onset within 5–12 years of age. It is now recognized as a part of the keratosis pilaris atrophicans syndrome. It may be associated with other conditions such as neurofibromatosis, oligophrenia, congenital heart block, or Down syndrome. There have been reports of association with cataracts in unilateral lesions.

Clinically, there are symmetrically distributed multiple areas of atrophy, 1–3 mm in size, with intervening normal skin, giving a honeycomb or worm-like appearance. Common sites include the cheeks and preauricular areas but the forehead and ears may also be involved. The pathophysiology behind the lesions is possibly a late reaction to inflammation wherein reticulate or honeycomb atrophy develops around follicular plugging. When the follicular plugs are shed, atrophy results from the widely dilated hair follicles.

Histopathologic findings include atrophy of the epidermis, dilated capillaries, and mononuclear cell infiltrate around the vessels with basophilic degeneration of collagen with edema. Some hair follicles may be dilated, tortuous, and hyperkeratotic with occasional horn cysts. Treatment is unsatisfactory and sometimes lesions spontaneously regress or improve with time. Dermabrasion and laser therapy have been tried with variable success.

ANETODERMA (FIGS. 9 TO 12)

It is a term derived from a Greek word which means relaxed skin. It represents an idiopathic atrophic condition

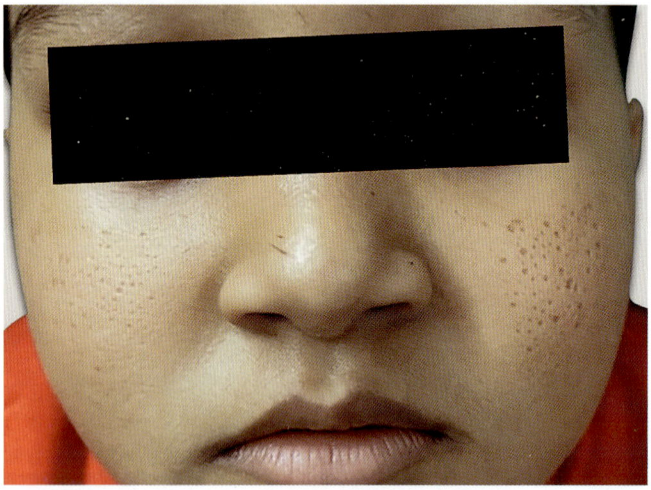

Fig. 7: Atrophoderma vermiculatum.

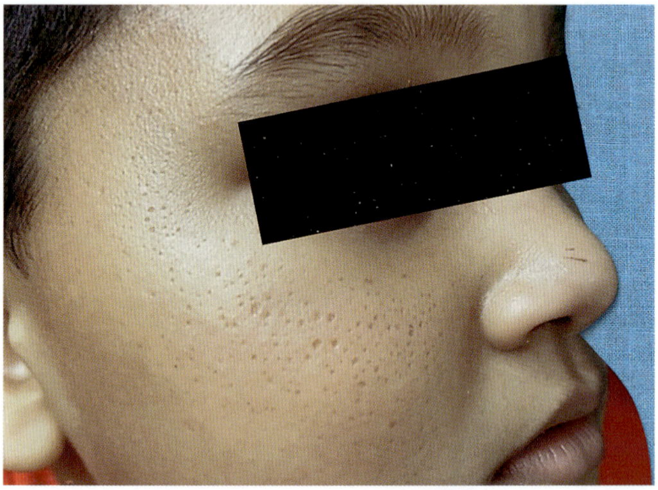

Fig. 8: Same patient, lateral view.

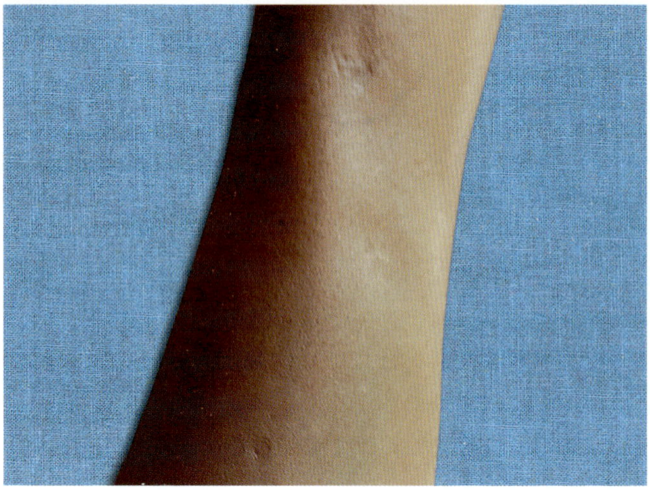

Fig. 9: Primary anetoderma over forearm.

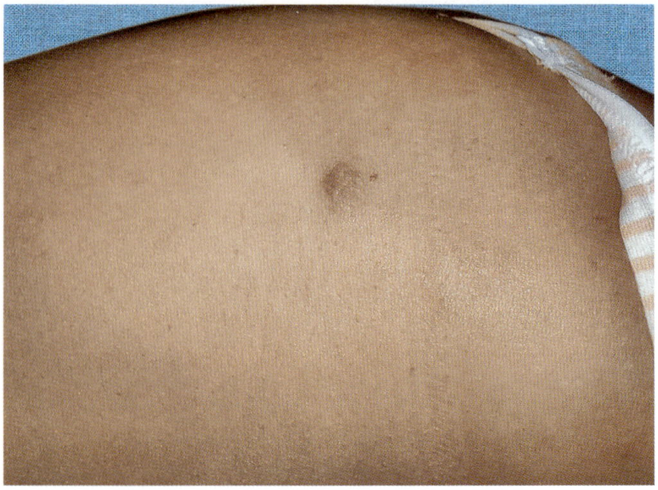

Fig. 10: Anetoderma.

"I alone cannot change the world, but I can cast a stone across the water to create many ripples." —**Mother Teresa**

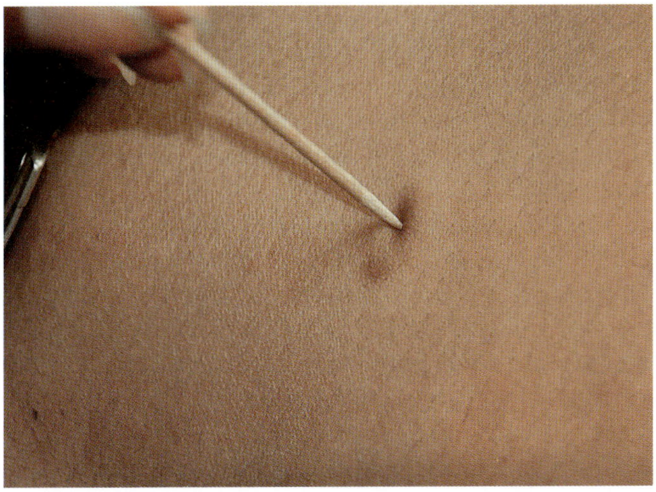

Fig. 11: Demonstration of depression in skin in anetoderma.

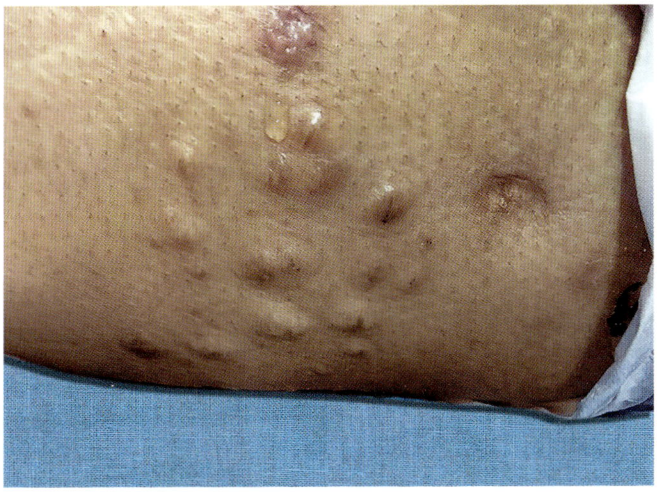

Fig. 12: Anetoderma secondary to panniculitis during phase of resolution.

leading to oval to rounded outpouchings of soft lax skin. The pathogenesis is unknown but immune mechanisms have been implicated.

Anetoderma can be divided into primary and secondary types. The causes for secondary anetoderma include lichen planus, antiphospholipid antibody syndrome, leprosy, sarcoidosis, tuberculosis, acne, varicella, and pilomatricoma to name a few.

Primary anetoderma can be further divided into two types:

1. *Jadassohn–Pellizzari anetoderma*: In this condition the lesions are preceded by inflammation. Females are more commonly affected than males. The onset is generally in the teens; however, patients up to the age of 30 years can be affected. The lesion starts as a red spot followed by depression with atrophy, wrinkling, and herniation.
2. *Schweninger–Buzzi anetoderma*: This type of primary anetoderma is not preceded by any inflammation. It presents with sudden appearance of large number of bluish white macular lesions which are protuberant. Females are more commonly affected than males. This condition is slowly progressive.

Anetoderma has been described in premature infants after gel electrocardiography and it has been postulated that the lesions occur due to local hypoxia and pressure from the electrodes.

Drugs such as penicillamine have also been implicated in the causation of anetoderma. Recurrent eye dermatitis leads to blepharochalasis. So far no therapy has been effective in this condition.

CUTANEOUS HORN (FIGS. 13 AND 14)

Cutaneous horns are elongated, keratinous projections from the skin, ranging in size from a few millimeters to many centimeters that resemble a miniature horn. The base of the horn may be flat, nodular, or crateriform. The horn is composed of compact keratin. The distribution of cutaneous horns is usually over sun-exposed areas, particularly the face, pinna, nose, forearms, and dorsal hands. Most cutaneous horns arise from actinic keratoses but they may also result from seborrheic keratoses, warts, molluscum contagiosum, keratoacanthoma, squamous cell carcinoma and basal cell carcinoma. Histologically, there is a greatly thickened stratum corneum with scattered areas of parakeratosis. The horn at the base will

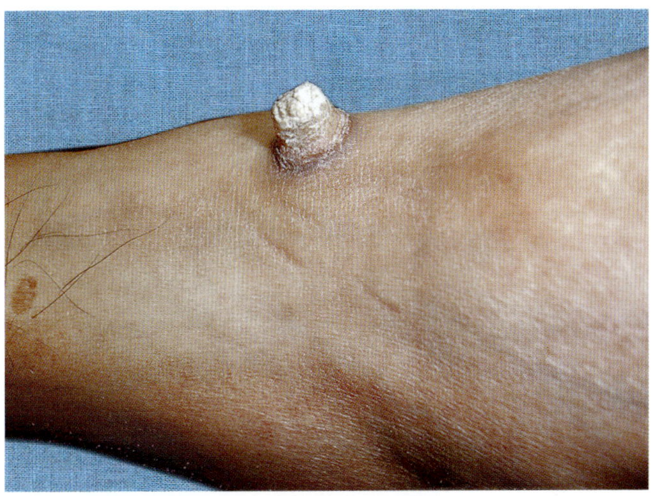

Fig. 13: Cutaneous horn.

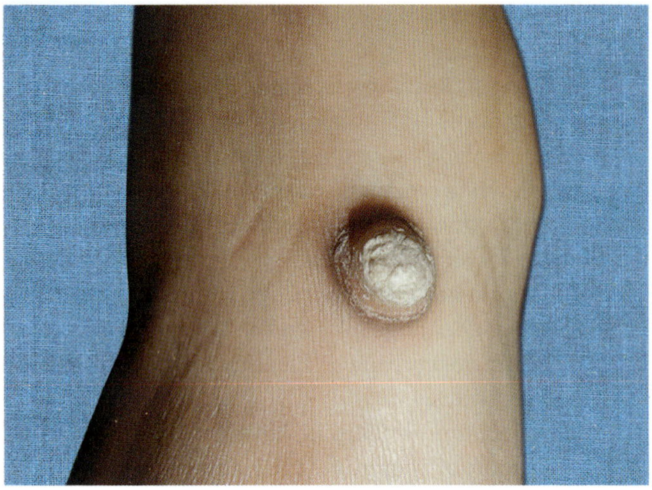

Fig. 14: Close-up view.

display features characteristic of the pathologic process responsible for the development of the horn. Malignancy may be present in up to 16–20% of cases, with squamous-cell carcinoma being the most common type. Tenderness at the base of the lesion and lesions of larger size favor malignancy.

Excision biopsy of the lesion and histopathological examination is recommended to rule out malignancy. Malignancies should be excised with appropriate margins and evaluated for metastasis. A careful physical examination of the lymph nodes draining the area of lesion may be adequate. Local destruction with cryosurgery is the first-line treatment for associated verruca vulgaris, actinic keratosis, and molluscum contagiosum. Other treatment options include wide surgical excision and CO_2, or neodymium-doped yttrium aluminum garnet (Nd:YAG) laser.

SUGGESTED READINGS

1. Coondoo A, Chattopadhyay C. Use and abuse of topical corticosteroids in children. Indian J Paediatr Dermatol. 2014; 15:1-4.
2. Dhar S, Srinivas SM, Parikh D. Use and misuse of topical corticosteroid in pediatric age group. In: Lahiri K (Ed). Treatise on topical corticosteroids in dermatology. Springer: 2018, DOI 10.1007/978-981-10-4609-4_10.
3. Lee YC, Son SJ, Han TY, Lee JH. A case of atrophoderma vermiculatum showing a good response to topical tretinoin. Ann Dermatol. 2018;30(1):116-8.

"It is a miracle that curiosity survives formal education." **—Albert Einstein**

CHAPTER 20

Sexual Abuse and Role of Patient Education and Counseling in Pediatric Dermatology Practice

SEXUAL ABUSE IN CHILDREN

Sexual abuse occurs when a child is engaged in sexual activities that he or she cannot comprehend, for which he or she is developmentally unprepared and cannot give consent or that violates the law or social taboos of society. Many studies have shown 12–25% of girls and 8–10% of boys are victims by the age of 18 years. Perpetrators may be males or females. It is underreported and underrecognized. In most cases, the perpetrator is well known or related to the victim. Children with sexual abuse present with behavioral changes such as sexual acting out (most specific indicator), insomnia, regression, depression, eating and sleep disturbances, or sexually transmitted diseases (STDs). Cutaneous findings seen are bruises, burns, bite marks, patterned injuries, hymenal changes, ecchymosis, hematomas, or oral injuries. Examination should include mouth, breasts, genitalia, perineum, medial thighs, buttocks, and anus. Strong suspicion is necessary to diagnose sexual abuse. Forensic evidence must be collected within 72 hours, if a recent abuse is suspected **(Figs. 1A and B)**. Cultures and serology must be done only if indicated. Differential diagnosis of skin lesions simulating child sexual abuse is described in **Table 1**.

Child sexual abuse differs from those of adult sexual abuse. In particular, children rarely disclose sexual abuse immediately after the event. The evaluation of children requires special skills and techniques in history taking, forensic interviewing, and examination. Definitive signs of genital trauma are seldom seen in cases of child sexual abuse, as physical force is rarely involved. Nonspecific vaginal findings include hymenal bumps, ridges and tags, and vulvovaginitis; nonspecific anal changes include erythema, fissures, venous congestion, minor anal dilatation, and lichen sclerosis. Findings suggestive of abuse also include acute abrasions, lacerations or bruising of the labia, perihymenal tissues, penis, scrotum, or perineum; condyloma in children over the age of 2 years; and significant anal dilatation or scarring. Definitive evidences of abuse or sexual contact are sperm or seminal fluid in, or on, the child's body;

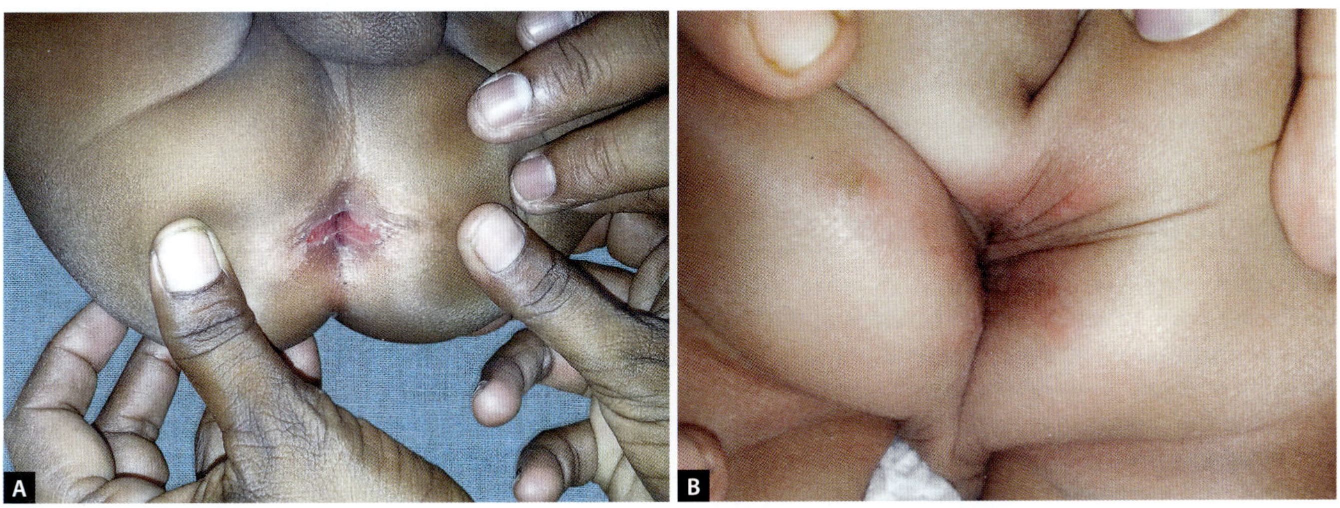

Figs. 1A and B: (A) Sexual abuse in a 1-year-old boy; note anal tear; (B) Sexual abuse in a 2-year-old boy, note funneling of perianal area.

"God grant me the serenity to accept the things I cannot change, courage to change things I can and wisdom to know the difference." **—Reinhold Niebuhr**

Table 1: Dermatological differential diagnosis of skin lesions of child sexual abuse.

Lesions of sexual abuse	*Differential diagnosis*
Genital trauma	• *Congenital abnormalities*: Perianal pyramidal protrusion, labial fusion, and failure of midline fusion • Lichen sclerosus • *Inflammatory dermatosis*: Seborrheic dermatitis, contact dermatitis, inverse psoriasis, and Kawasaki disease • *Ulcers*: Ulcerated vulval hemangioma, Behçet's disease • Crohn's disease • Anal fissuring and chronic constipation • Nonspecific vulvovaginitis
Sexually transmitted disease	• Innocently acquired infections which may have a sexual transmission: Human papillomavirus, herpes simplex, and molluscum contagiosum • Perianal streptococcal infections, staphylococcal infections, *Candida*, and pinworm infection

Source: Adapted from Srinivas SM, et al. (2018)[5]

positive culture for *Neisseria gonorrhoeae* or serologic confirmation of acquired syphilis; and intentional, blunt penetrating injury to the vaginal or anal orifice. Apart from physical and psychological problems, infections can be associated with sexual abuse in children. Sexually transmitted infection (STI) testing in children are not routinely done. Presumptive treatment of children for STIs is not generally recommended. Children and adolescents who test positive for a STI should be treated. A follow-up consultation is strongly recommended. It helps to assess any psychological problems and to ensure that the child and the caregiver are receiving adequate social support and counseling.

Any STI can be acquired by a child because of sexual abuse; the authors have commonly seen the following conditions.

CHANCRE OF PRIMARY SYPHILIS

Primary syphilis is characterized by hard sore or Hunterian chancre which usually develops at the site of entry of organism 10–90 days (average 21 days) following infection and young sexually active males are the usual victims. If the inoculum is large (10^7 organism), lesions can develop within 5–7 days. Initially, lesion starts as painless, dull red macule which transforms into papule and ulcerates. Asymptomatic nature of the lesion manages to skip attention of the unfortunate patient. Classically, the ulcer can be described as painless, nontender, rounded, well-defined, with button-like induration, raised or rolled out border and dull red granulation tissue-filled with clear floor. Any indurated lesion on coronal sulcus does not imply syphilis because other lesions on the same site are indurated too. Manipulation of the lesion exudes serous fluid. Regional lymph nodes which become palpable within a week can be described as painless, nontender, small, discrete, firm, rubbery in consistency, and nonsuppurative. In males, lesions are commonly present on coronal sulcus, glans penis, prepuce, frenulum, and shaft of the penis. Anorectal lesions are frequently observed in homosexual males. In females, common sites of involvement are labia, vulva, fourchette, clitoris, cervix, urethra, perineum, and vaginal wall. Among extragenital sites, lip, tongue, tonsils, fingers, and breast are frequently involved. Chancre spontaneously heals within 3–8 weeks with atrophic scar.

Clinical picture may be altered following drying of exudates, application of different topical medications, associated surrounding edema, secondary infection and mixed infection with *Haemophilus ducreyi* or *Chlamydia*. Other important atypical presentations are phimosis, balanoposthitis, and nongonococcal urethritis due to intrameatal chancre, proctitis, whitlow-like lesion, and multiple chancres.

Diagnosis is confirmed by demonstration of *Treponema pallidum* in exudate from ulcer base or lymph node aspirate by dark-field microscopy or by direct fluorescent antibody staining of *Treponema pallidum* (DFA-TP). Nontreponemal serological tests become positive 2–3 weeks after the appearance of chancre. If nonreactive, ideally should be repeated at 1 week, 1 month, and 3 months. Patients should be treated with benzathine penicillin (2.4 million units) in two divided intramuscular injection in two buttocks.

SKIN MANIFESTATIONS OF SECONDARY SYPHILIS

Manifestations of secondary syphilis usually develop 6–8 weeks after the appearance of the primary chancre. It is called the "great imitator" owing to its varied clinical manifestations. The most common clinical features include rash (75–100%), lymphadenopathy (50–86%), and mucosal lesions (6–30%). Classical skin lesion is a moist papule that often coalesce to form a plaque and is termed as condyloma lata. Syphilitic alopecia occurs

"If there is no struggle, there is no progress." —**Frederick Douglass**

infrequently. The patchy "moth-eaten" type alopecia is the most common. Macular syphilid or roseolar rash is the earliest generalized syphilid. It appears as symmetrical, coppery red, round, oval spots, and fades leaving a pattern of depigmented spots on a hyperpigmented background. Such a leukoderma syphiliticum is most commonly located on the back or sides of the neck and was earlier known as "necklace of Venus." Papular syphilid is the most common syphilid and the papules are dull red in color, rounded, discrete, symmetrically distributed, and usually polymorphic. These are commonly seen over palms and soles. Split papules found at the angles of the mouth, nasolabial folds, and behind the ears may become eroded and fissured. In warm moist areas, papules may become confluent, hypertrophic, pale-colored, broad, and flattened and are called condylomata lata which are highly infectious. Hyperpigmentation commonly occurs with healing of the skin lesions of secondary syphilis. Mucus patches have a dull red base and grayish slough. When the lesions become confluent with loss of slough, presenting as an erosion with serpiginous outline, it is called a 'snail-track' ulcer. To diagnose this stage of syphilis, a high index of clinical suspicion is essential.

CHANCROID

Chancroid is an infection of the genital skin or mucous membranes caused by *H. ducreyi*. It is transmitted in two ways.Sexual transmission through skin-to-skin contact with open sore and nonsexual transmission when pus-like fluid from the ulcer is transmitted to other parts of the body or to another person. After an incubation period of 3–7 days, small, painful papules appear and rapidly breakdown into shallow, soft, painful ulcers with ragged, undermined edges, and a red border. Ulcers vary in size and often coalesce. Inguinal lymph nodes become tender, enlarged, and matted together, forming a pus-filled abscess (bubo). The skin over the abscess may become red and shiny and may break down to form a sinus. The infection may spread to other areas of skin, resulting in new lesions. Diagnosis is usually based on clinical findings alone because culture of the bacteria is difficult. Serologic testing for syphilis and human immunodeficiency virus (HIV) and cultures for herpes should be done to exclude other causes of genital ulcers. Successful treatment for chancroid cures the infection, resolves the clinical symptoms, and prevents transmission to others. In advanced cases, scarring can result despite successful therapy. Antibiotics used to treat chancroid include azithromycin 1 g orally, ceftriaxone 250 mg intramuscularly, ciprofloxacin 500 mg orally, or erythromycin 500 mg orally.

CONDYLOMA ACUMINATA (FIGS. 2 AND 3)

Condyloma acuminata are anogenital warts caused by human papillomavirus. It is now increasingly seen in pediatric population. Girls are affected more than boys. Although the possibility of sexual abuse is considered in every case, other modes of acquiring the infection includes perinatal transmission, hetero-inoculation, and autoinoculation. The incubation period in children is not known. They are incidentally noted by the guardian. Perianal region is most commonly affected. It presents

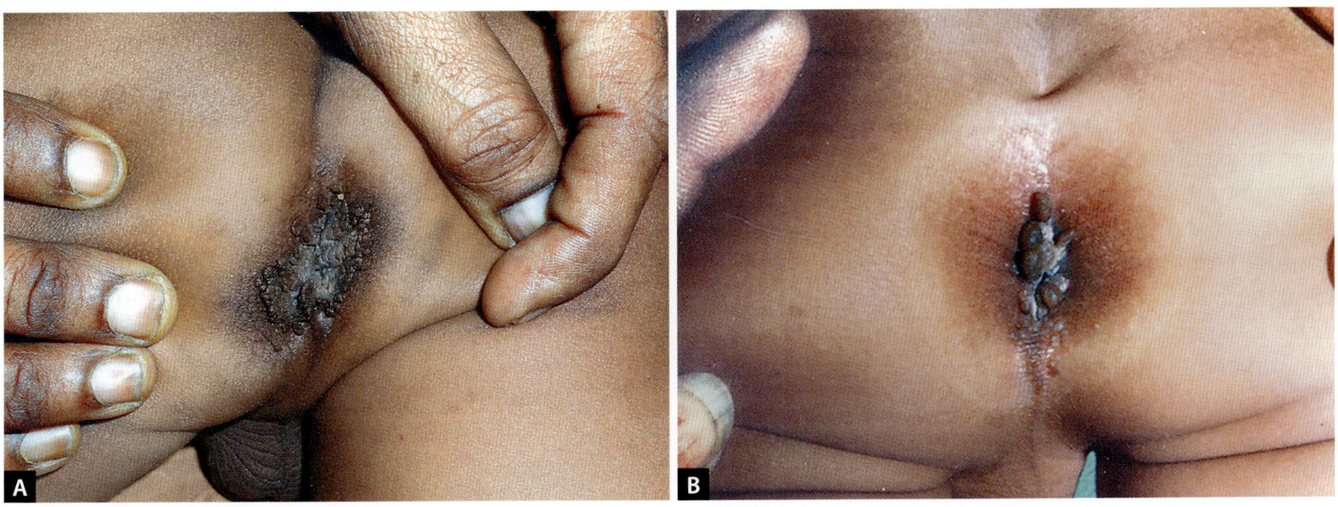

Figs. 2A and B: (A) Perianal condyloma acuminata in an 8-year-old boy; (B) Perianal condyloma acuminata in a 3-year-old boy.

"To improve is to change; to be perfect is to change often." **—Winston Churchill**

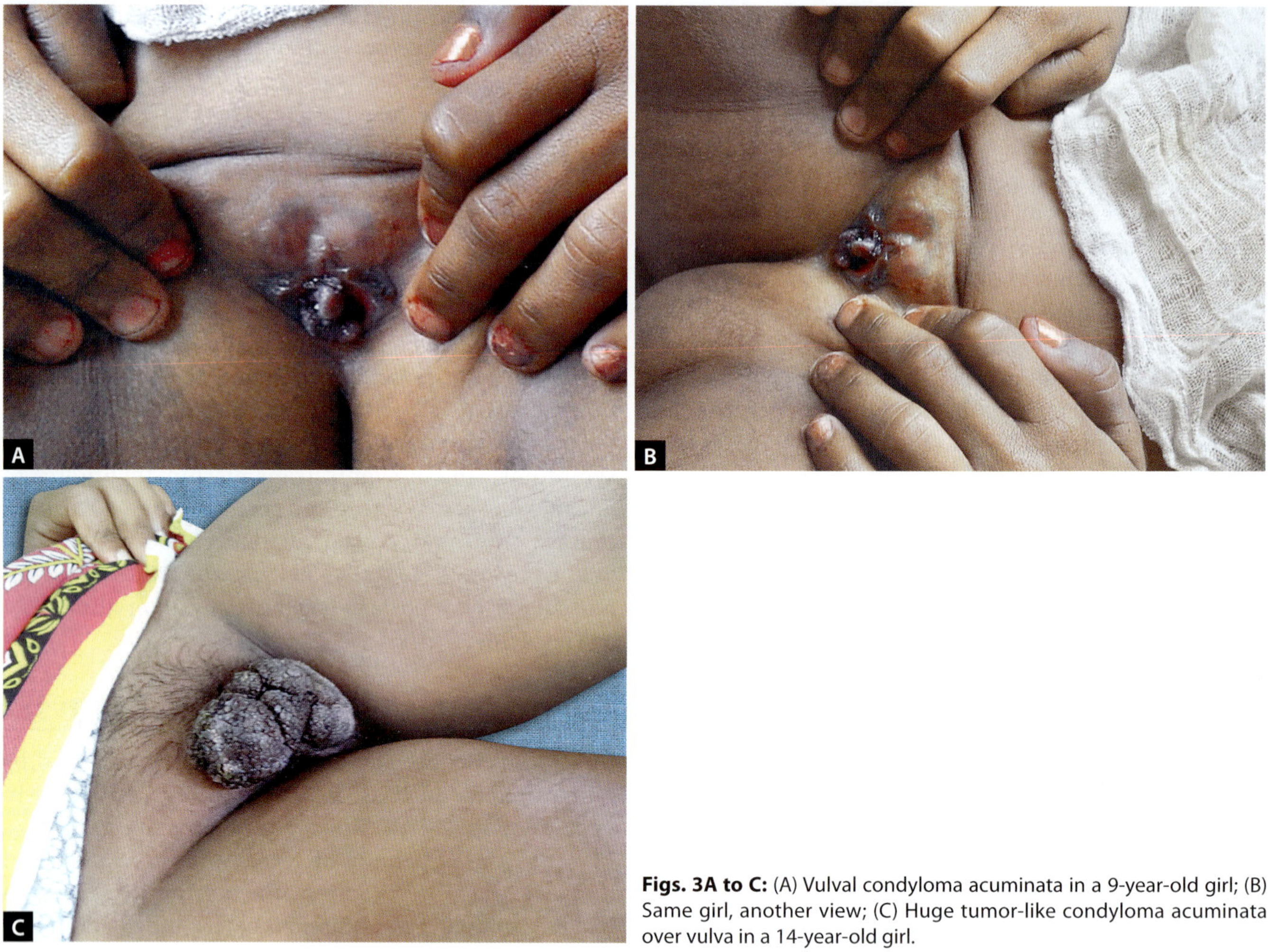

Figs. 3A to C: (A) Vulval condyloma acuminata in a 9-year-old girl; (B) Same girl, another view; (C) Huge tumor-like condyloma acuminata over vulva in a 14-year-old girl.

as asymptomatic flesh-colored, soft verrucous papules coalescing to form plaques. Lesions may rapidly enlarge to form an exophytic cauliflower-like mass. Sometimes they present with itching, pain, and bleeding. It can be seen in other areas such as glans penis, penile shaft, scrotum, and vulva.

The diagnosis is made on clinical grounds. Any child presenting with perianal warts should undergo a complete history and examination to rule out sexual abuse. Treating condyloma acuminata is challenging. Spontaneous resolution without treatment can occur in many cases. Lesions persisting for 2 years may not undergo spontaneous resolution. Destructive methods include cryotherapy, application of trichloroacetic acid or podophyllin. Immunomodulators include topical application of imiquimod. Laser therapy is rarely used in children.

HERPES GENITALIS INFECTION (FIGS. 4 AND 5)

Herpes simplex viruses (HSVs) are deoxyribonucleic acid (DNA) viruses that remain latent in the skin or mucosa after infection and undergo periodic reactivation. There are two types—HSV-1 which mainly causes orofacial disease and occasional genital disease and HSV-2 which primarily causes genital disease. Infection with HSV-1 occurs commonly in childhood but acquisition of HSV-2 correlates with sexual activity. In general, genital herpes is not common in childhood and thus it poses diagnostic dilemma as well as need for assessment of possible sexual abuse. A more common cause could be transmission during handling of the child by the parents or caregiver infected with HSV-1 or HSV-2 or the child having orofacial lesions of herpes.

"By changing nothing, nothing changes." **—Tony Robbins**

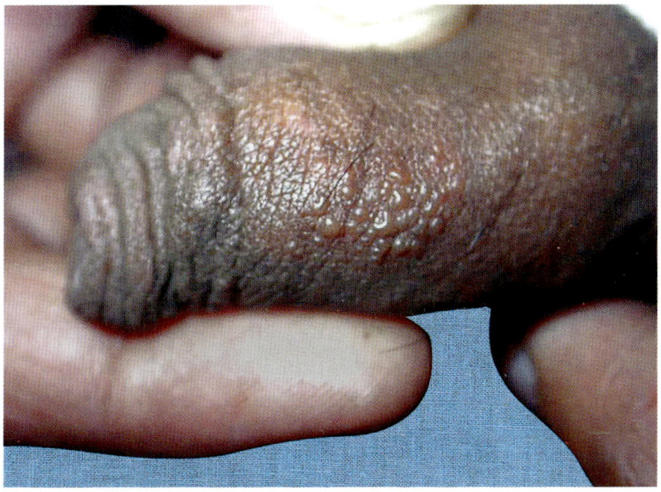

Fig. 4: Grouped vesicles over the shaft of penis.

Clinically, there is a prodrome which is most severe prior to the first episode with fever, malaise, headache, and myalgia. Subsequently, characteristic genital lesions appear in different stages of evolution, including vesicle, pustules, and erythematous ulcers that gradually heal. Lesions may be located over the glans penis or the shaft. In females, lesions may occur over the mons, perineum, vagina, or buttocks. There may be associated urinary retention and constipation.

Investigations include tzanck smear which is commonly done. The gold standard for diagnosis is viral cell culture. For the treatment of genital herpes, acyclovir may be given at a dose of 40–80 mg/kg/day for 7–10 days or until clinical resolution occurs. If the caregivers suffer from orofacial herpes, then they should be treated and asked

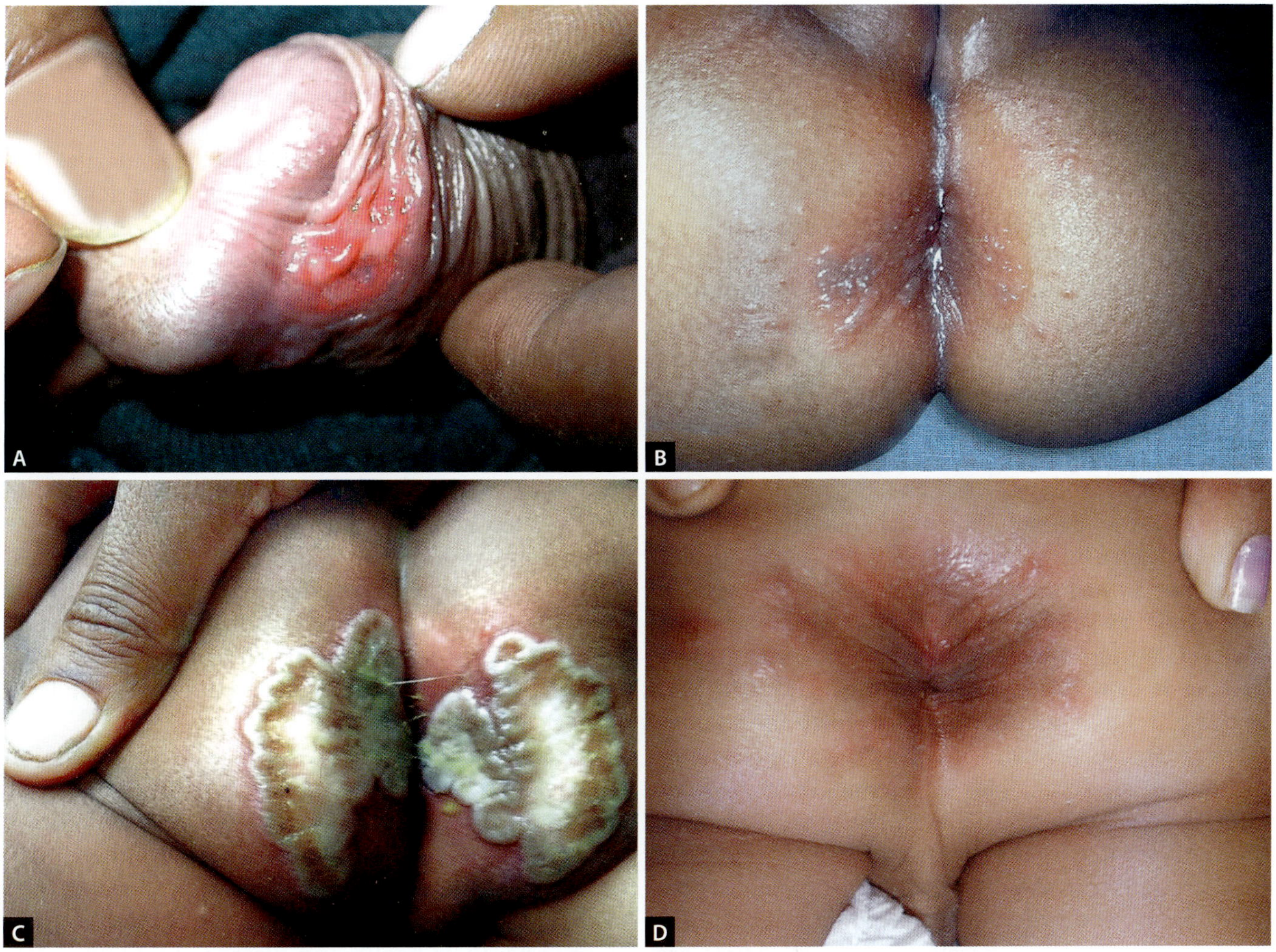

Figs. 5A to D: (A) Serpiginous ulcer of herpes genitalis; (B) Perianal herpes in a 5-month-old girl; (C) Macerated perianal herpes in a 3-month-old baby girl; (D) Perianal herpes in a 5-month-old boy.

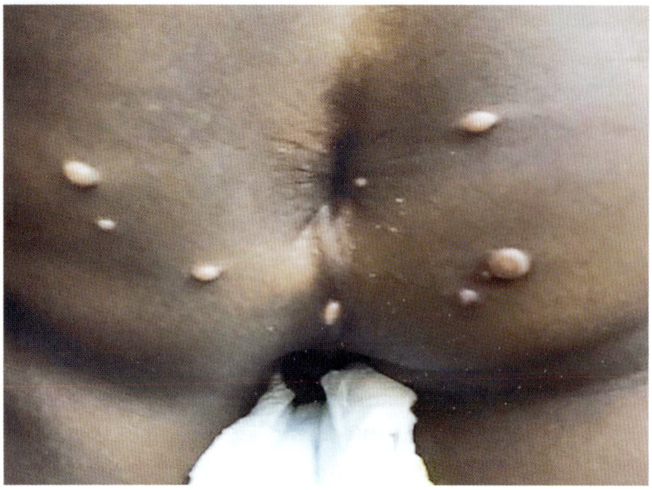

Fig. 6: Perianal molluscum contagiosum in an infant.

to avoid handling the child. If sexual abuse is suspected, then appropriate measures must be taken and counseling suggested.

PERIANAL MOLLUSCUM CONTAGIOSUM (FIG. 6)

Molluscum contagiosum (MC) is a self-limited infectious disease, frequent in the pediatric population. It is caused by molluscum contagiosum virus (MCV). In children, MCV-1 genotype infection is more frequent than in adults. MCV is transmitted by direct contact with infected skin, which can be sexual, nonsexual, or by autoinoculation. In children, perianal or genital lesions are mainly due to autoinoculation and are not pathognomonic of sexual abuse. It presents with firm rounded papules 2–5 mm, pink or skin-colored, with a shiny and umbilicated surface. The lesions may be single, multiple, or clustered. In most cases, they are self-limiting in a period of 6–9 months. It is described as a phenomenon called "beginning of the end" (BOTE) sign which refers to clinical erythema and swelling of an MC skin lesion when the regression phase begins. Children may develop eczematous plaques around one or more lesions of MC, a phenomenon known as "molluscum dermatitis" or "eczema molluscorum" which is more frequent in patients with atopic dermatitis. Diagnosis of MC is clinical but features with dermoscope are characteristic. It shows a central pore or umbilication, polylobular white-to-yellow amorphous structures, and peripheral crown vessels. General measures are recommended to prevent the spread such as not to scratch or rub the lesions. Cryotherapy and curettage can be effective treatment options. Potassium hydroxide which dissolves keratin, can be used in concentrations from 5 to 10%, two times a day or every other day for 4–6 weeks or until inflammation develops.

THE ROLE OF PATIENT EDUCATION AND COUNSELING IN PEDIATRIC DERMATOLOGY PRACTICE

Patient education and counseling are the cornerstones of effective management and patient care in different branches of modern medicine. Patient education is a technique through which doctors and health professionals provide easy to understand information and knowledge to their patients or their caregivers, which will ultimately help both the patient and their caregiver improve the health and also bring about a change in their healthcare-related behaviors. It can be effectively used as an instrument to prepare better care management plans, include both preventive measures and information regarding the disease, treatment, long-term follow-up, and complications.

It becomes even more relevant in the context of dermatologic practice because along with the various treatment modalities, the patient often needs to understand and follow do's and don'ts which help in quick recovery, prolonged remission as well as prevent exacerbations.

With respect to pediatric dermatologic practice, it is more of a challenge as the patient is sometimes too young to verbalize his or her symptoms and complaints and may not be able to take care of himself or herself. In such situation, the onus is on the parents and caregivers who must intuitively understand the needs of the child and respond accordingly. The situation is often further complicated in cases where the child has certain special needs or is either abandoned or orphaned and thus may always not have an attentive caregiver. Thus, counseling and patient (or rather parent) education becomes an important as well as challenging aspect of dermatologic practice and management.

There are a few elements of patient education counseling that are particularly important and can be suited to fit the patient and guardian in mind. These elements are skill building and responsibility. Skill building means making the patient and caregiver aware of the actions that they need to undertake in order to improve their health and disease condition, while understanding that ultimately it is they who are responsible for a favorable outcome of the treatment protocols and that they need to know about.

"Only when you can be extremely pliable and soft can you be extremely hard and strong." —**Zen Proverb**

DIFFICULTIES WITH PEDIATRIC PATIENT EDUCATION AND COUNSELING

The challenges that are faced in dermatology practice are often unique. For example, many skin disorders such as atopic dermatitis and psoriasis are chronic with extended periods of remissions and exacerbations. Patients and their caregivers thus become frustrated since they begin to understand that the disease can only be controlled to some extent and chances of a cure are minimal to say the least. Healthy and blemish-free skin is often associated with good health and patients approach the dermatologist with unrealistic expectations regarding the treatment of the disease. On top of that in a busy dermatology practice, the doctor often has little time to explain the treatment thus leaving little room for a healthy discussion regarding the psychosocial impact of that disease.

The most arduous obstacle in successful patient education and counseling is the use of technical medical jargon. Words and concepts which are often simple for dermatologists are incomprehensible to most parents and caregivers. Along with that instructions which are too elaborate or time-consuming are often either forgotten or skipped altogether by some. There also seems to exist wide variations in the perception of amount of topical medications required by many patients and caregivers alike. Hence, all attempts should be made to provide information in the simplest possible manner, with least number of steps and in a language that the caregiver understands best.

Parents (caregivers) are often burdened with their own lives and thus adherence to elaborate and intricate treatment protocols become difficult. This leads to a sense of guilt feeling among the parents and the child also suffers due to interruptions and disruptions to their treatment plan. The doctor too becomes confounded if the child does not respond to a treatment as he is often unaware that the parents (caregivers) may have been callous in following the instructions properly.

The second most important aspect is that children are a special subset of the patient population who are unique in certain aspects. They cannot verbalize their complaints or symptoms and in such cases, the dermatologist must have a keen eye and thorough clinical knowledge in pediatric dermatology so as to correctly identify the skin lesions and disease leading to the child's discomfort and treat accordingly. The only relevant clinical history that is available is from the parents, which can range from being highly accurate to completely erroneous depending on the educational status, economic condition, and family size among a few factors. In addition, the parents are often overconcerned and overcautious and all efforts must be taken to allay their fears and educate them about their child's illness.

In this aspect, the pediatric dermatologist can play a particularly important role by befriending the child. The doctor can try to communicate with the child at his or her own level and give them an opportunity to describe their symptoms and concerns. Children can often be afraid to speak up in front of the parents, especially if the parent has been negligent in adhering to the treatment. In such cases, the doctor must be diplomatic to gather truthful information from the child, while at the same time being sympathetic and tactful with the parents so that a mutual middle ground may be reached. The first author (SD) author of this book is extremely fond of interacting with his patients as his little friends. He spends as much time as possible with his young patients so as to gather maximum information in their own words and then discuss with parents to formulate a treatment plan individualized to suit the needs of that particular patient **(Figs. 7A and B)**.

Also, there are numerous social, religious, and cultural customs and rituals which are deep rooted in society and a cause for various dermatologic illnesses. For example, application of kohl to the eyes or face of the child can cause conjunctivitis, trachoma, and contact dermatitis; use of threads and talismans around the neck to protect from the evil eye can lead to candida intertrigo; use of cow dung or ash over the stump of the umbilical cord can lead to infection, omphalitis, and even death from neonatal tetanus. In all these cases, extreme care must be taken, explain and counsel in the most nonjudgmental manner as far as possible since these customs are often rooted in fear and not easy to overcome.

Lastly, since the child is often dependent on the parents or caregiver for physical, social, psychological, and economical support, they have little choice in decision-making regarding treatment. In such cases, it becomes doubly important to ensure that the child is well taken care of by the caregivers. In cases where the child is without a parent and is not being properly taken care of or being subjected to physical or mental abuse, it sometimes becomes the duty of the dermatologist to inform the social service authorities if the need so arises. Also, disease such as MC or herpes occurring over the genitalia may point toward sexual abuse and parents should be thoroughly counseled as children may often be unable to provide accurate history.

Children are not miniature adults and whenever possible, all attempts should be taken to customize treatment and counseling sessions according to their age. Play acting is a great way to bond with children and educate them at the same time. Presence of a parent may help gain the confidence of a young child too. Children are often sensitive to usage of certain words and whenever possible gentler and simpler sounding words must be used. A child may not be able to distinguish between itch and pain. Or clarify whether the oozing from lesion is hemorrhagic, serous, or serosanguinous. In all such situations, a thorough clinical examination becomes imperative. A soft and gentle tone of voice is quintessential to soothe a scared and apprehensive child. It has been seen that children above the age of 2 years can be taught to follow certain simple instructions and by age of 7 years can be trained to have a better understanding of their skin condition by explaining to them in simple and easy to understand words.

ADVANTAGES OF PATIENT EDUCATION AND COUNSELING

The advantages of successful patient education and counseling are numerous. On one hand, it makes the parent or caregiver equally responsible for the success or failure of any treatment modality and on the other hand, it builds their confidence and helps to improve adherence to therapeutic regimens.

There are certain key aspects of patient education which can be invaluable. Some of them are elaborated further. A little time spent educating the patient can lead to a better understanding of their disease or medical condition. In today's internet era, incorrect and often harmful information is freely available. A little explanation from a doctor can instill confidence in the patients' mind and protect them from gathering information from the wrong source.

It helps the patient and the caregiver about how they can manage the disease themselves since knowledge is empowering. Patient education is also helpful when the patient may need to be transferred to another specialist. Since the patient and their caregivers are adequately informed in advance, they are often at a better position to convey the relevant information and concerns to the next doctor. This is of immense help in continuing the treatment plan. A good level of communication also helps the patient and their caregivers to make better decisions along with their treating doctors. It also increases the compliance both with the treatment protocol and follow-up. An empowered patient is also more likely to comply with the doctor's instructions. There is also a legal aspect to adequate patient and caregiver education and counseling. An adequately informed patient is less likely to accuse a doctor of malpractice. There is also more effective utilization of health services as patients and their caregivers are going to make less phone calls or visits which may be unnecessary at times. Satisfied patients are also more likely to refer the doctor to other patients.

Dermatologic diseases often have a tendency for chronicity. Most diseases are marked with periods of remissions interspersed with episodes of exacerbations. With successful patient counseling and education, these periods can be prolonged, and the episodes are minimized. In totality, it improves patient compliance and decreases drop out and a tendency toward "doctor shopping."

It is true that in everyday dermatologic practice, there is immense constraints on proper time management and few precious minutes are available to diagnose and prescribe treatment to patients. But despite that, even a few moments spent in educating and counseling the patient and their caregivers can have a tremendous positive impact on the final treatment outcome. It also makes future follow-ups less time-consuming, since any queries regarding the disease or treatment would have been answered in the first visit itself. It thus becomes a win–win situation for both the patient (parent) and the doctor.

Several dermatologic diseases can be managed efficiently with proper education and counseling. For example, in atopic dermatitis, proper patient education and counseling are imperative to keep the disease process under control. Like use of adequate "barrier-repair" moisturizers, wet wraps, and wet dressings, use of hypoallergenic soaps and creams, avoidance of hot humid weather, woolen clothing, nuts, dairy products, etc. In infections and infestations, avoidance of sharing of items of personal use such as combs and towels. In disease such as acne vulgaris avoidance of comedogenic creams, cosmetics, and facial products by teenagers and young adults.

In cases of genodermatoses, education and counseling of parents assume significant importance. Many of these children are referred to a dermatologist for evaluation of the skin lesions since many genodermatoses have manifestations involving the skin, hair, nails, and mucosae most of the times. Parents are often also concerned about the probability of future offspring having the same disease. In all these cases, the different options must be discussed with the parents and their queries answered empathetically. They should be referred to other specialists for genetic and prenatal diagnosis whenever the need arises.

TYPES AND METHOD OF PATIENT EDUCATION AND COUNSELING

A wide variety of modalities are available for successful patient education and counseling. Each has its own advantage and disadvantage. In general, best results are achieved when there is bidirectional and interactive flow of information. Participation of the patients and their caregivers has shown to have greater adherence to instructions and improved treatment outcomes.

The most common type of education and counseling provided to patients and their caregivers is verbal. It is often casually offered within the time frame of the consultation. It is the simplest form of sharing information and time-saving. But it has the disadvantage of poor patient recall. Most patients and their caregivers have difficulty recollecting the verbal advice given to them. And since the dermatologist may not always be available for clarifications, it often leads to poor compliance to treatment and unsatisfactory outcomes.

The next most used medium is printed material. It is often made available to the patients in different local languages and describes the disease and treatment in a simple and easy to follow format. It has the advantage that it saves time spent in giving verbal advice and helps to overcome problems of recall, since the advice is available for easy reference. To be hugely successful, printed advice must be easy to read, with minimum text and maximum illustrations and preferably be colorful, have least possible number of steps, and must be self-explanatory. The disadvantage of printed material lies in the fact that the patient/parent/caregiver must be literate and have sufficient intelligence to comprehend the advice. Young children may not be able to read and if the caregiver is unable to understand and follow, then the whole purpose of the initiative fails.

Another important modality for counseling is group education. This is one of the most beneficial and productive methods. Here, the patient and the caregiver "learn by doing." This has the most successful and satisfying outcomes for both the patient and the dermatologist because there are no ambiguities or confusions. It boosts the morale and confidence of the patient and the caregivers. And since it is a group activity, there is interaction between different people, and they can form self-help and support groups. This has an immense positive effect on the psyche of the patients and their caregivers. This modality of patient and parent education and counseling is a preferred method of the author. As discussed previously, often the time available to a clinician is limited during a consultation. In that period, the child must be examined, relevant history elicited, treatment planned, and explained to the parents. And several patients during a single working day may present with the same disease. Thus, if each family is individually counseled, it takes up precious time which could have been used to examine and treat other patients. Thus, the author has a favorite approach, wherein biweekly or monthly seminars and workshops are arranged at auditoriums and halls, where families of children suffering from a specific dermatologic disease are invited and a detailed lecture is given. This is followed by an interactive session where anyone from the audience can ask any question to the author and all their queries are thoroughly and patiently answered **(Figs. 7C to E)**. These workshops are usually conducted on weekends to suit the schedule of both working parents and school-going children. Many interactive games are also arranged for the children so that they too may feel involved in the treatment plan. This approach has been extraordinarily successful and has also been covered by the media several times. Other clinicians too have started following this method after seeing the popularity and practicality of this approach.

This approach has been remarkably successful with various genodermatoses and other chronic conditions. Several international and national societies and groups have come up and the barriers of race, religion, language, and nationalities have been broken down and support is available throughout the world. The disadvantage of this modality lies in the fact that it might not be feasible to persons living in socially and economically backward areas. Also, sufficient commitment and interest is quintessential on the part of the caregivers to take part in group activities.

Lastly, the least informative and highly misleading source of information is the internet. Hordes of websites crop up each day that provide partial information and falsify facts. In the so-called "internet generation" parents

"Big changes come from hundreds of tiny steps and they all matter." —**Courtney Carver**

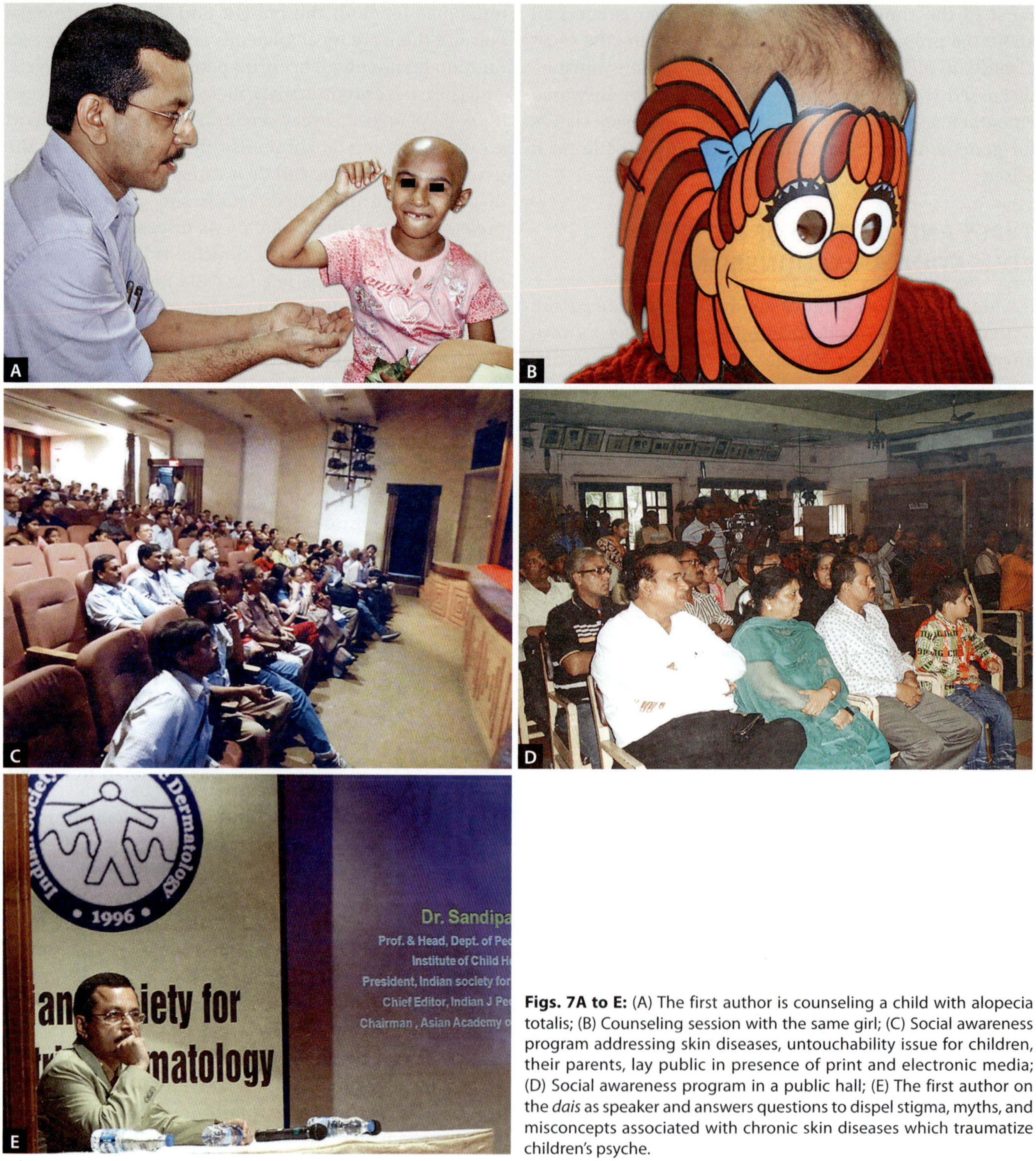

Figs. 7A to E: (A) The first author is counseling a child with alopecia totalis; (B) Counseling session with the same girl; (C) Social awareness program addressing skin diseases, untouchability issue for children, their parents, lay public in presence of print and electronic media; (D) Social awareness program in a public hall; (E) The first author on the *dais* as speaker and answers questions to dispel stigma, myths, and misconcepts associated with chronic skin diseases which traumatize children's psyche.

often come up with half-baked and misinterpreted facts and information acquired from different "medical websites" and attempt to guide the dermatologists regarding diagnoses and treatment options. Such situation should be dealt with humor as any confrontation is futile. An emphatic attitude must be maintained, and topmost priority to be given to dispelling myths and providing authentic and accurate information.

"Let us remember: One book, one pen, one child, and one teacher can change the world." **—Malala Yousufzai**

CONCLUSION

Successful treatment of any dermatological disorder requires equal participation from the dermatologist, affected children (barring neonates, infants, and young toddlers), and their parents or caregivers. Improvement or worsening of any dermatosis is often visual and the caregivers can be educated and trained to identify the various relieving and exacerbating factors. Also, positive behavioral outcomes can be reinforced as they get an understanding of the activities that help keep the disease within control and what action leads to worsening.

Different forms of educational and counseling modalities are available nowadays and should be customized depending on the needs of individual patients and their caregivers. Information should be shared, and counseling done in a nonjudgmental and nonconfrontational manner. Whenever possible, medical jargon should be avoided and instructions should be given in a simple and lucid fashion. Local customs and traditions must also be kept in mind. It is often said that "people learn best by doing." Thus, group demonstrations should be encouraged so that caregivers and parents may learn the techniques themselves as well as get to interact with others in similar situations.

Lastly, the greatest benefits of successful patient education and counseling is to the pediatric dermatologists themselves. Time is often a constraint in day-to-day clinical practice, but a few minutes spent in sharing educational information with the parents or the caregivers can have a multitude of positive outcomes. By involving the parents in the treatment of the child, it helps to gain their confidence and makes them aware of equal responsibility in therapeutic response. It also becomes easier to manage the child in subsequent follow-ups as the parent can often provide additional information to the clinical history. Lastly, the possibility of attrition is also reduced since the caregivers feel that they too can contribute to making the child get better faster and thus look forward to gaining more information from the dermatologist.

Worldwide, it has been observed that there is a blaring gap between the information that patient and their caregivers need and the information that they get. Doctors thus can play a key role in helping to disburse correct information. This has a multitude of benefits. On one hand, it ensures greater compliance and adherence along with better outcome to any treatment plan, while it also minimizes unnecessary and wasteful utilization of scarce health resources due to frequent hospitals visits and phone calls. Any form of education and counseling must be patient-centered and their health beliefs, local customs, and level of literacy must be kept in mind. The physician can choose any method of counseling which is best suited to his practice and personal choice. In fact, even other healthcare workers such as nurses and clinical assistants can be trained to provide basic information. Additionally, all information does not need to be given at one episode itself. This approach often burdens the caregivers with too much information, none of which is adequately retained. Thus, information sharing should be a gradual and step-by-step process so that the patient and their caregiver can utilize it to the best extent.

The relevance and essence of patient education and counseling in pediatric dermatologic practice can be beautifully summed up in the words of Confucius—"Tell me, and I will forget. Show me and I may remember. Involve me, and I will understand."

WHAT'S NEW?

The Protection of Children from Sexual Offences Act

The POCSO Act, 2012 was established to create a strong legal framework aimed at safeguarding children from acts of sexual assault, harassment, and pornography, while prioritizing the child's interests throughout the judicial process. The act was designed to be child-friendly, facilitating reporting, evidence recording, investigation, and swift trial of offenses through specialized Special Courts.

The POCSO defines various offenses punishable by law. It recognizes different forms of sexual penetration and prohibits indecent acts against children. These offenses encompass:

1. *Penetrative sexual assault*: Involving insertion of penis/object/another body part into a child's vagina/urethra/anus/mouth, or soliciting such acts from the child or another person.
2. *Sexual assault*: Involving any sexual contact initiated by a person toward a child or vice versa.
3. *Sexual harassment*: Including verbal or non-verbal sexually suggestive remarks, gestures, repeated stalking, indecent exposure, etc.
4. Child pornography
5. Aggravated penetrative sexual assault/aggravated sexual assault

"A mighty flame followeth a tiny spark." —**Dante Alighieri**

The act maintains gender neutrality for both children and the accused. It also criminalizes the viewing or possession of child pornography. Moreover, the act considers aiding child sexual abuse as an offense. In 2019, amendments were made to POCSO, increasing the minimum punishment for penetrative assault from 7 to 10 years and to 20 years if the victim was below 16 years old, with a maximum penalty of life imprisonment and provision for the death penalty for aggravated penetrative assault.

SUGGESTED READINGS

1. Langevin R, Kenny S, Kern A, Kingsland E, Pennestri MH. Sexual abuse and sleep in children and adolescents: A systematic review. Sleep Med Rev. 2022;64:101628.
2. Hailes HP, Yu R, Danese A, Fazel S. Long-term outcomes of childhood sexual abuse: an umbrella review. Lancet Psychiatry. 2019;6(10):830-9.
3. Adams JA. Sexual Abuse in Children: What the General Practice Ob/Gyn Needs to Know. Clin Obstet Gynecol. 2020;63(3):486-90.
4. Deb S, Dhar S, Parikh D. The role of patient (parent)education and counseling in pediatric dermatology practice. Ind J Ped Derm. 2015;16:117-21.
5. Srinivas SM, Moss S. Skin lesions simulating child abuse. Indian J Paediatr Dermatol. 2018;19:187-93.
6. Das S, De A, Sharma N, Sinha S, Dutta A, Nanda S. Sexual Abuse in Children and Relevance of POCSO Act-A Report of Four Cases. Indian J Dermatol. 2020;65(1):74-6.

"A room without books is a body without soul." —**Unknown**

CHAPTER 21

Skin and Systemic Diseases

INTRODUCTION

There are various skin diseases that remain restricted to skin such as superficial fungal and bacterial infections, but some of the skin diseases affect various organ systems of the body such as atopic dermatitis which often affects bronchial mucosa; psoriasis is now considered to be associated with "metabolic syndrome". In this chapter, we will discuss skin diseases which have a direct or indirect association with various systems of the body. We will also highlight some cutaneous malignancies and skin manifestations of some internal malignancies.

ACANTHOSIS NIGRICANS (FIGS. 1A TO E)

Acanthosis nigricans (AN) is characterized by hyperkeratosis and hyperpigmentation and the affected skin is covered by papillomatous elevations which give it a velvety texture. It is classified into six main types, each of which is now believed to be associated with insulin resistance. They are:

1. Hereditary benign AN
2. Benign AN
3. Pseudoacanthosis nigricans
4. Drug-induced AN
5. Malignant AN
6. Nevoid AN

It starts as pigmentation, dryness, and roughness of the skin which in the affected areas is gray-brown or black, palpably thickened and covered by small papillomatous elevations which give it a velvety texture. Gradually, the surface becomes mammillated or rugose and larger warty excrescences develop. The sites most commonly involved are the axillae, the back and sides of the neck, the anogenital region, and the groins.

Benign Forms

The skin lesions may be present at birth but usually develop during childhood or puberty. They may be unilateral and usually less severe than the malignant forms. Distal extremities are usually spared and the oral mucous membranes are rarely involved.

Malignant Forms

The lesions are more severe and more extensive. Pigmentation is more prominent and is not confined to hyperkeratotic areas. Thickening of the palms is frequent and the nails may be brittle or ridged. Hair loss may occur. Irritation is common. The mucous membranes and mucocutaneous junctions are involved in at least 50% of the cases, and warty papillomatous thickening around the lips and eyes may be a presenting symptom. The onset of the AN may precede other symptoms by as long as 5 years but the interval is usually considerably shorter. Many tumors have been reported including bladder, kidney, bile duct, thyroid, esophagus, bronchus, and rectum.

Natural History

Benign AN progresses very slowly, tends to become more severe at puberty, and then regresses in some patients and remains stationary in others.

Removal of the tumor in malignant AN may be associated with regression of the clinical signs but relapses are common.

Treatment

It is important to exclude associated endocrine disorder or internal malignancy by thorough clinical examination and necessary investigations. Associated obesity or endocrinopathy, if any, needs to be addressed. Topical retinoic acid (0.025–0.1%) either alone or in combination with salicylic acid or lactic acid in emollient base applied daily at night for 2–6 months usually helps to reduce the intensity of pigmentation as well as thickening of the skin. It is to be remembered that melanocyte or melanin has no role to play in the pigmentation of AN. Hence demelanizing

"Don't be trapped by Dogma-which is living with the results of other people's thinking." —**Steve Jobs**

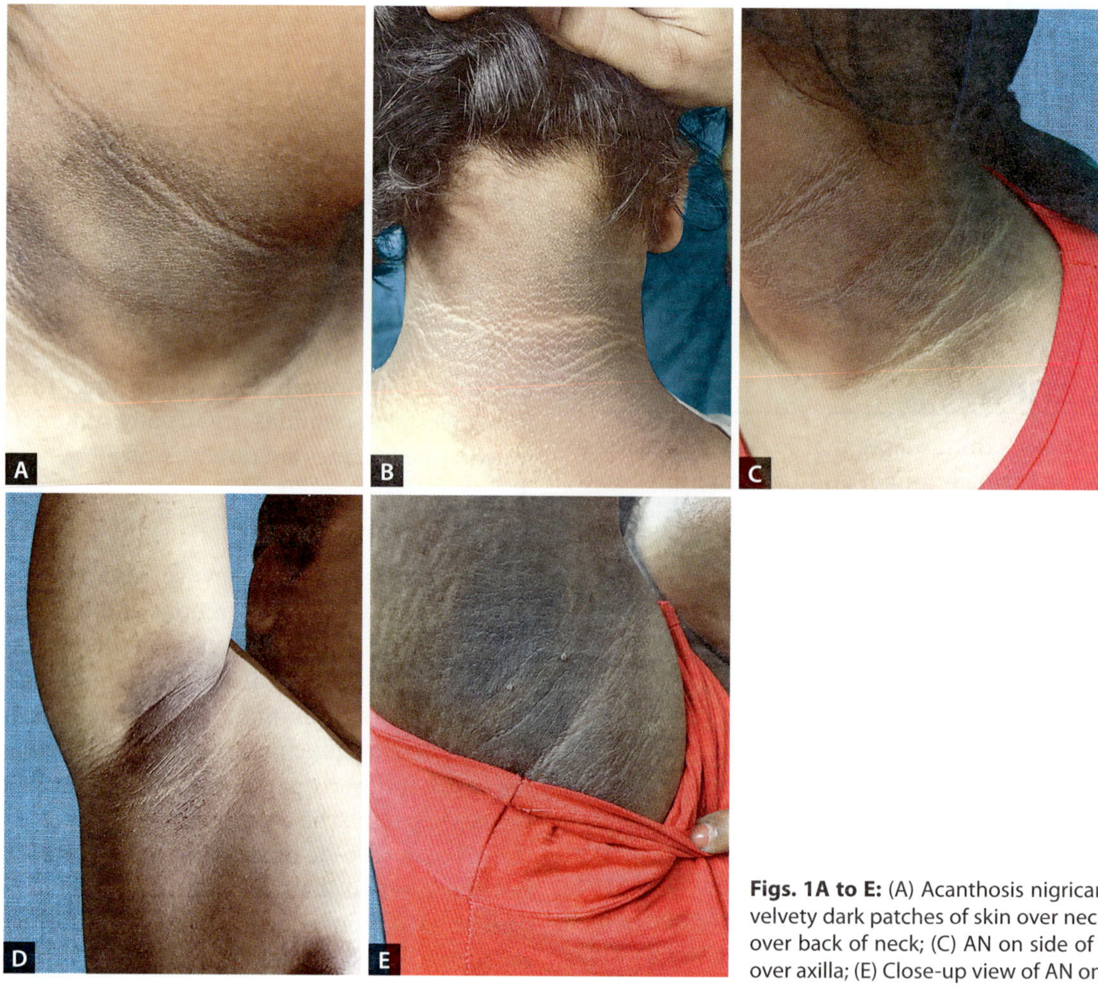

Figs. 1A to E: (A) Acanthosis nigricans (AN), note velvety dark patches of skin over neck fold; (B) AN over back of neck; (C) AN on side of neck; (D) AN over axilla; (E) Close-up view of AN on axilla.

creams containing 2% hydroquinone is of no use in such conditions. Topical steroids are better avoided as their application over body folds can lead to development of atrophic striae and telangiectasia. Oral metformin and topical tazarotene have been found useful in some cases.

DYSKERATOSIS CONGENITA (FIGS. 2A TO F)

Dyskeratosis congenita (DC) is a rare X-linked recessive disorder with some subtypes having autosomal dominant or recessive inheritance. It is characterized by atrophy and pigmentation of the skin, nail dystrophy, leukoplakia, bone marrow failure, and a predisposition to malignancy. The nails become dystrophic and are shed between the ages 5 and 13 years. Pigmentary changes appear simultaneously or 2–3 years after the nail changes and takes the form of fine, reticulate, gray-brown pigmentation on the neck, thighs, and trunk. The skin is atrophic with numerous telangiectasias. The lesions of mucous membranes take the form of blisters and erosions on the lingual and buccal mucous membranes succeeded by irregular patches of leukoplakia. Other features include palmoplantar keratoderma, absent dermatoglyphics, short stature, developmental delay, esophageal stenosis, urethral stenosis, pulmonary fibrosis, and pancytopenia.

Natural History

The incidence of carcinoma in the areas of leukoplakia is high. The prognosis is poor.

Treatment

Counseling of patients and early detection of malignancies are all that can be offered to these patients. In case malignancy is detected, a pediatric oncologist's consultation should be sought. Recommended disease surveillance includes biannual blood counts, hepatic ultrasound, annual bone marrow evaluation, pulmonary function tests, and skin cancer screening.

"When we learn how to become resilient, we learn how to embrace the beautifully broad spectrum of the human experience." —**Jaeda Dewalt**

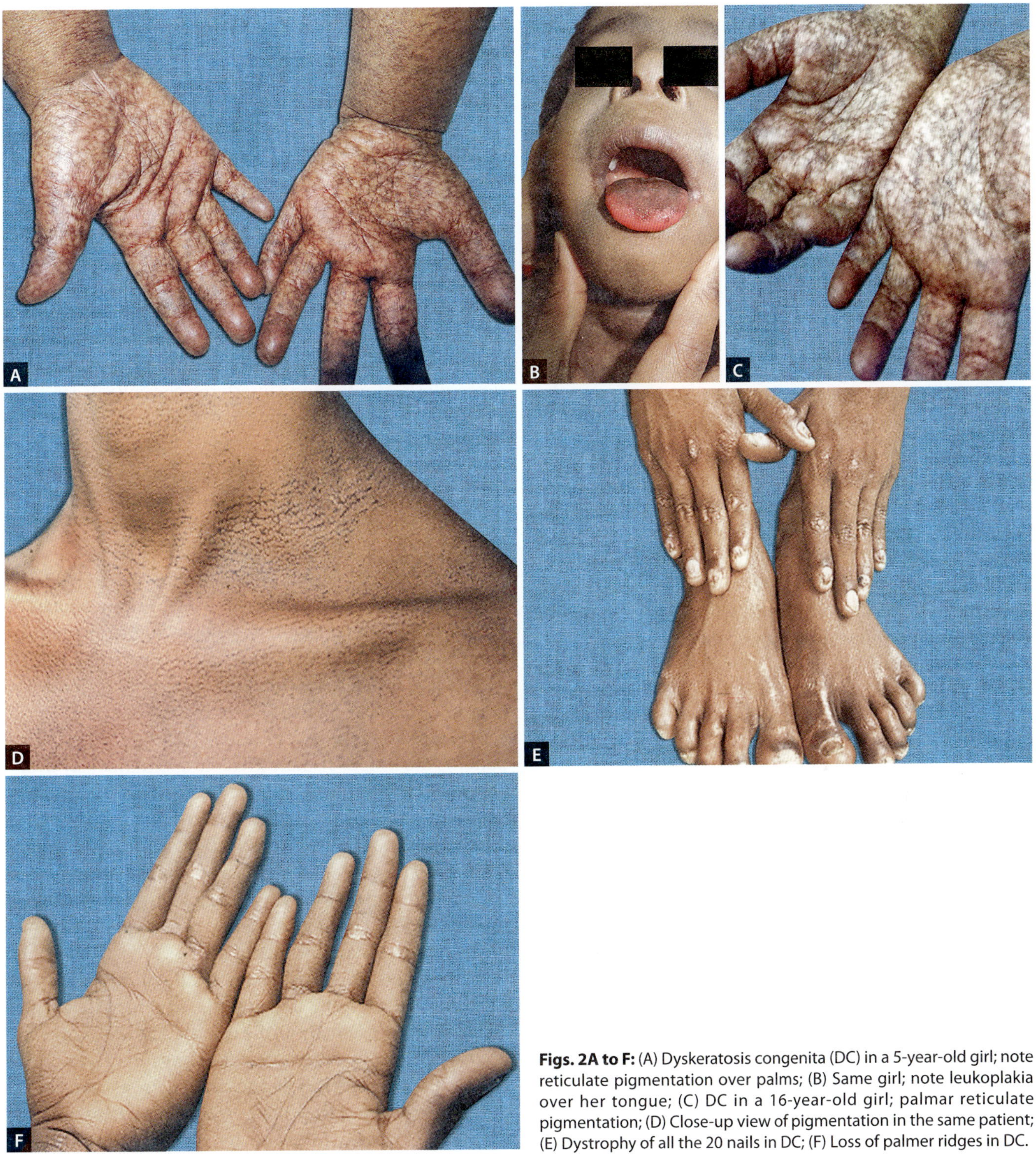

Figs. 2A to F: (A) Dyskeratosis congenita (DC) in a 5-year-old girl; note reticulate pigmentation over palms; (B) Same girl; note leukoplakia over her tongue; (C) DC in a 16-year-old girl; palmar reticulate pigmentation; (D) Close-up view of pigmentation in the same patient; (E) Dystrophy of all the 20 nails in DC; (F) Loss of palmer ridges in DC.

ERYTHEMA NODOSUM (FIGS. 3A TO C)

Erythema nodosum (EN) represents a delayed cell-mediated hypersensitivity reaction characterized by red, tender nodular lesions that usually occur on the pretibial surface of the legs and occasionally on the other areas of skin where subcutaneous fat is present.

Etiology

In children, streptococcal and other respiratory tract infections and tuberculosis (TB) are the most common causes of EN. Other disorders which can precipitate EN are leprosy, coccidioidomycosis, histoplasmosis, leishmaniasis, cat-scratch disease, *Mycobacterium marinum* infection, and fungal infections. Noninfectious causes of EN include sarcoidosis, Behçet's disease, ulcerative colitis, regional ileitis, and internal malignancies.

Erythema nodosum can occur as a reaction to various drugs such as sulfonamides, phenytoin, iodides, bromides (present in some cough syrups), and some hormonal preparations containing estrogen and progesterone.

Although a disease of adulthood, EN can occur in children but is seen rarely in children < 2 years of age. Girls are slightly more commonly affected than boys. Lesions, which are 1–1.5 cm in diameter, occur symmetrically, usually over the shins, occasionally on the knees, ankles, thighs, extensor aspects of the arms, the face and neck, and rarely on the palms. Initially red in color, these warm and tender nodules develop a purplish bruise-like appearance. The lesions last for 3–6 weeks. Recurrences may occur over a period of weeks to months and arthralgia may precede, coincide, or follow the development of eruptions.

Treatment

The management is directed at the identification and treatment of the underlying cause. Bed rest with leg elevation helps reduce pain and edema. Salicylates and other nonsteroidal anti-inflammatory drugs (NSAIDs) may reduce the pain and inflammation. Rarely intralesional corticosteroids can be helpful for refractory lesions. In persistent and recurrent eruptions, oral corticosteroids and immunosuppressants may be beneficial.

ERYTHEMA INDURATUM (FIGS. 3D TO F)

Erythema induratum (EI)/nodular vasculitis complex is a form of lobular panniculitis characterized by chronic, recurrent, tender erythematous to violaceous nodules and/or plaques, usually on the calves along with irregular and shallow ulcers which heal with scarring. Feet, thighs, buttocks, and arms may also be involved. It most commonly occurs in adult women, with peaks in incidence also reported during early adolescence. It has rarely been reported in children. It has been thought to be either an immune complex-mediated vasculitis or a type IV cell-mediated response to an antigenic stimulus.

It has been classified into three clinical subsets:

1. TB-associated EI
2. EI associated with other diseases and drugs
3. Idiopathic EI

The most commonly reported identifiable cause of EI is latent or active TB, called erythema induratum of Bazin (EIB), a tuberculid. Though it is uncommon in children, cases have been reported even in infants. Unlike in adults, surface ulceration is an uncommon finding in pediatric cases. Episcleritis has also been found to be associated with EIB in children. EIB is mostly a lobular or septolobular panniculitis with varying combinations of granulomatous inflammation, primary vasculitis, and subcutaneous necrosis with no histological evidence of *Mycobacterium tuberculosis*. Mantoux and interferon gamma release assay (IGRA) tests are positive but *M. tuberculosis* can seldom be cultured from the lesion. But *M. tuberculosis* can be identified by polymerase chain reaction (PCR) studies. EIB is differentiated from EN based on the location of the lesions on the anterior surface of the lower extremities which heals spontaneously in a few weeks and presence of septal panniculitis in the latter. Once a diagnosis of EIB is made, thorough evaluation for TB elsewhere should be done. The suspected TB focus is usually latent but there are many reports of active TB preceding or occurring with EIB. Very rarely, EIB has also occurred post-Bacillus Calmette-Guérin (BCG) vaccination. Treatment of underlying TB causes rapid clearance of the lesions, although in untreated patients the lesions usually involute spontaneously over a period of months or years.

Erythema induratum and EN are diverse entities in the group of panniculitis with distinct clinicopathological features. They have varying etiologies, of which TB is common to both. In majority of the patients, by meticulous history taking, cutaneous and systemic examination, a fairly accurate clinical diagnosis can be made, which is further confirmed by histopathology. EN is usually bilateral, with lesions developing on shins, knees, and ankles; and occasionally on the face, neck, trunk, arms, and thighs; while EI occurs more commonly on calves on the background of erythrocyanotic circulation. Lesions of EN never ulcerate, and they subside with hyperpigmentation within 3–6 weeks, followed by recurrences; while EI nodules usually ulcerate, resolve with atrophic scars, and have a more protracted course. The clinical diagnosis is further supplemented by a characteristic histopathology, which is distinctive for both entities. Various atypical forms of EI have been described that includes unilateral

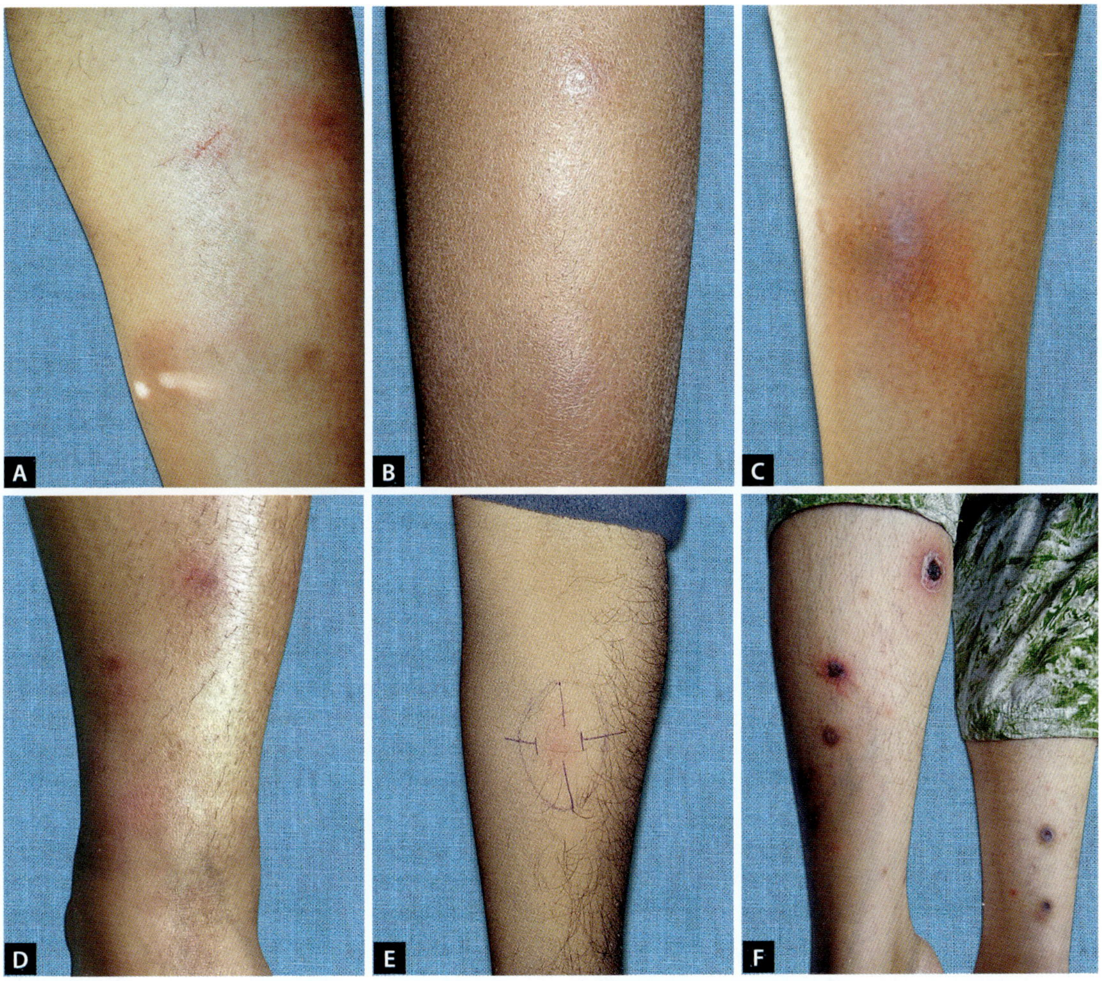

Figs. 3A to F: (A) Erythema nodosum (EN) over the shin, the most common site; (B) EN in another patient; (C) Close-up view of EN; (D) Erythema induratum in a 16-year-old girl; (E) Mantoux test positivity in the same girl with erythema induratum; (F) Erythema induratum.

lesions; lesions involving the shins, thighs, buttocks, arms, and other sites; and those resolving without ulceration.

SWEET'S SYNDROME (FIGS. 4A AND B)

Sweet's syndrome is an acute febrile neutrophilic dermatosis characterized by painful raised papules, plaques, nodules, and bullae on face, trunk, and extremities along with fever and leukocytosis. Pathergy is common. The criteria for Sweet's syndrome are summarized in **Table 1**. It is classified into classic/idiopathic (recurrent) form and secondary (58%) form. Secondary causes of Sweet's syndrome include parainflammatory and premalignant conditions which are described in **Table 2**. Skin lesions usually manifest along with malignancy, hence complete workup is necessary for malignancy at initial onset of skin lesions. Paraneoplastic Sweet's syndrome presents commonly on face and oral mucosa with well-defined erythematous, edematous papules, plaques, arcuate, and hemorrhagic or violaceous lesions. About 80–90% cases have leukocytosis. Systemic corticosteroids are the first-line of therapy (1–2 mg/kg/day) tapered over 2–3 months gradually. Other therapies include potassium iodide, colchicine, dapsone, methotrexate, and cyclosporine.

MELKERSSON–ROSENTHAL SYNDROME (FIGS. 5A TO E)

Melkersson–Rosenthal syndrome (MRS) is a triad of orofacial edema, recurrent facial nerve palsy, and scrotal tongue. It was described by Melkersson in 1928. It is rarely seen in children. Cheilitis granulomatosa is one of the components of this syndrome.

"I slept and dreamt that life was joy. I awoke and saw that life was service. I acted and behold, service was joy." —**Rabindranath Tagore**

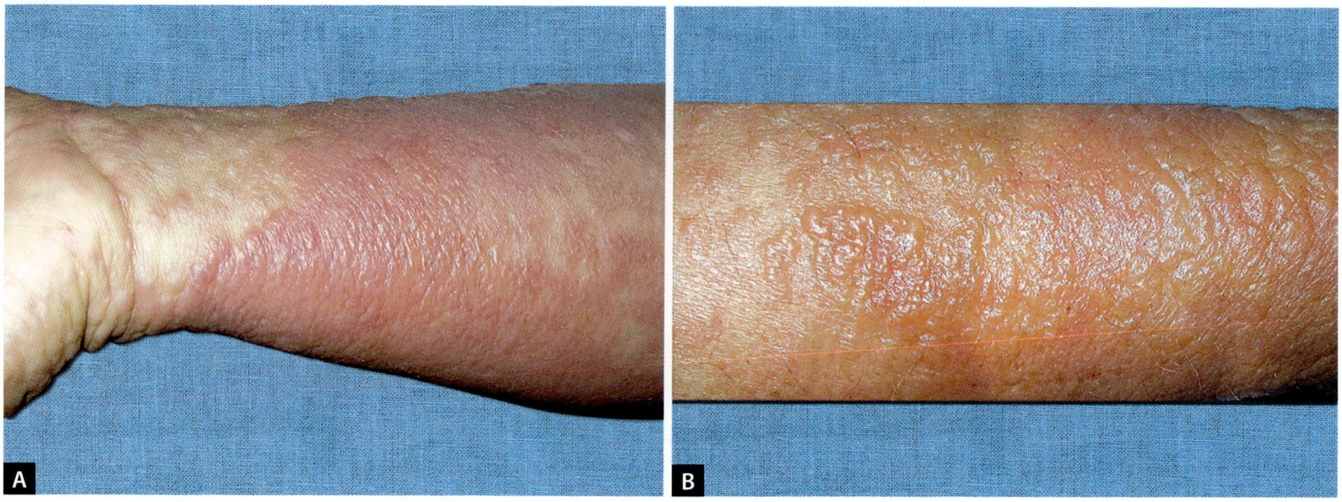

Figs. 4A and B: (A) Sweet's syndrome; (B) Close-up view of Sweet's syndrome.

Table 1: Criteria for Sweet's syndrome.

Major criteria	• Abrupt onset of tender or painful erythematous or violaceous plaques or nodules • Predominantly neutrophilic infiltration of the dermis without leukocytoclastic vasculitis
Minor criteria	• *Association with an underlying disorder*: (1) Respiratory tract infection, (2) gastrointestinal tract infection, (3) vaccination, (4) inflammatory disease, (5) hematoproliferative disorders, (6) solid malignant tumors, (7) pregnancy • Pyrexia (> 38°C) • *Abnormalities in at least three of the following four laboratory tests during onset*: (1) Elevated erythrocyte sedimentation rate (ESR) (> 20 mm), (2) positive C-reactive protein (CRP) result, (3) peripheral blood smear showing segmented nuclear neutrophils, bands > 70%, (4) leukocytosis (count > 8,000/μL) • Excellent response to treatment with systemic corticosteroids or potassium iodide

Table 2: Associated underlying disorders with Sweet's syndrome.

Disorder	Features
Parainflammatory	CNS vasculitis, arthritis, SLE, chronic multifocal osteomyelitis, dyserythropoietic anemia, and Takayasu arteritis
Immunodeficiency	T-cell deficiency, CVID, glycogen storage disorder with neutropenia, chronic granulomatous disease, humoral immune deficiency, and HIV
Premalignant	Juvenile chronic myelogenous leukemia, acute lymphoblastic anemia, fanconi anemia, myelodysplastic syndrome, osteosarcoma, and aplastic anemia

(CNS: central nervous system; CVID: common variable immunodeficiency; HIV: human immunodeficiency virus; SLE: systemic lupus erythematosus)

Etiology

The exact cause is not known. Various etiologies implicated are genetic factors and infective agents such as *Toxoplasma gondii, Treponema pallidum, M. tuberculosis, M. leprae,* herpes simplex, and *Borrelia burgdorferi*. It can be associated with Crohn's disease and sarcoidosis.

Clinical Features

Clinically, it presents as a nonpainful swelling of lips; gradually the swelling becomes hard in consistency like rubber. Erythema, erosions, ulceration, vesicles, and pustules may be present on oral cavity, vermillion border of lips, upper airways, gums, tongue, palate, pharynx, and larynx. Mucosal cobblestone appearance can occur. Facial paralysis may be unilateral, bilateral, partial, or complete. Fissured tongue is present only in 30% of pediatric cases.

Diagnosis

Diagnosis of this entity is mainly clinical. It should be differentiated from angioneurotic edema. Persistence of edema in between attacks and granulomatous pathology on skin biopsy confirms the diagnosis.

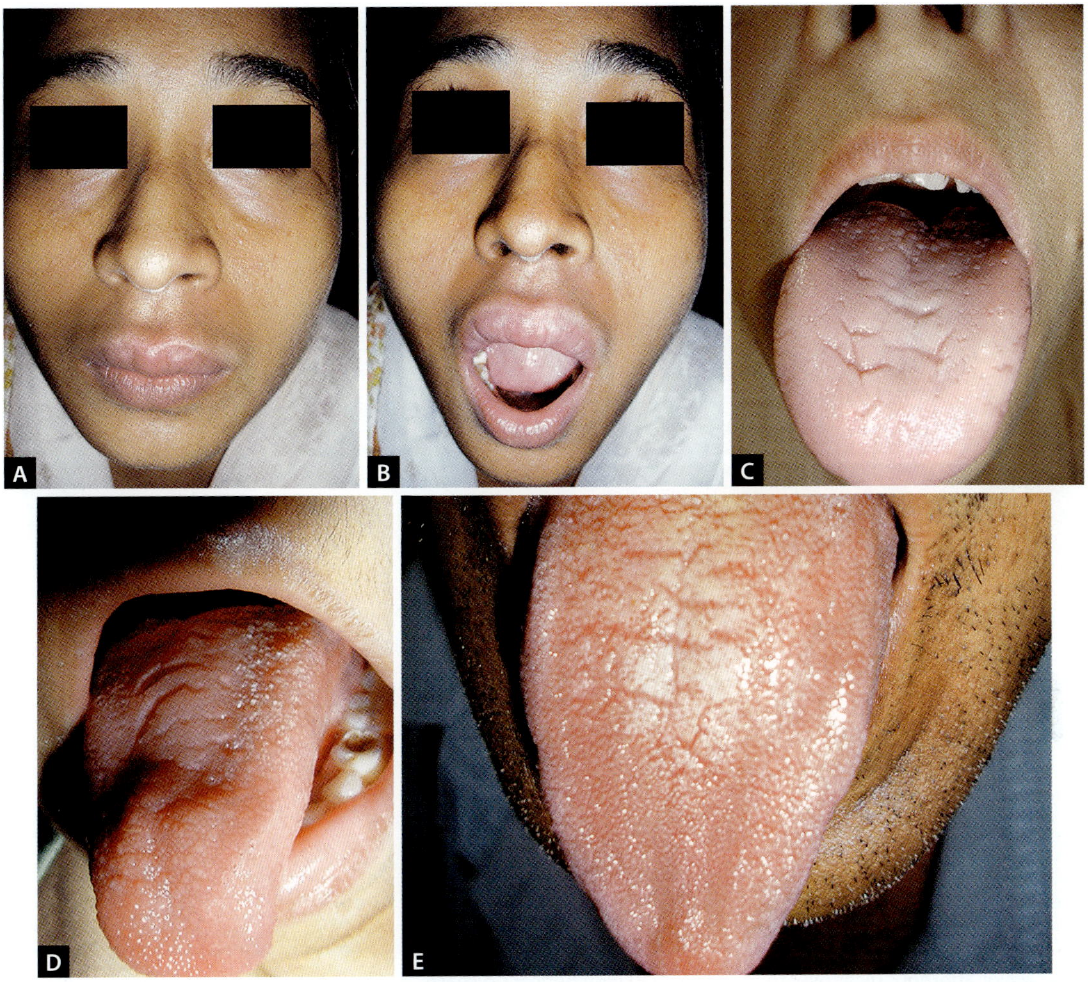

Figs. 5A to E: (A) Melkersson–Rosenthal syndrome (MRS), note swelling of lip (macrocheilia); (B) Same boy with MRS; (C) Scrotal tongue in MRS; (D) Brother of the boy having scrotal tongue; (E) Father of the boy having scrotal tongue.

Treatment

Treatment is mainly symptomatic. Oral steroids, intralesional steroids, immunosuppressants, clofazimine, metronidazole, and erythromycin have been tried with variable response. Cheiloplasty can be done.

BEHÇET'S DISEASE (FIGS. 6A TO D)

Behçet's syndrome is a rare, chronic multisystem, and vasculitis characterized by a triad of recurrent oral and genital ulcers along with inflammatory disease of the eye. The etiology is complex and is associated with HLA-B51. About 20% of pediatric cases have a family history of Behçet's disease. The onset of the disease is between 10 and 45 years. Neonatal Behçet's disease is seen in infants born to mother with the disease and characterized by skin lesions and aphthous stomatitis. Clinical features include recurrent painful oral ulcers (83%), genital ulcers (60%) along with systemic features such as fever, iritis, posterior uveitis, optic neuritis, retinal vessel thrombosis, and gastrointestinal (GI) and neurological symptoms. The criteria for pediatric Behçet's disease are described in **Box 1**. The treatment of choice is colchicine 0.5–1.5 mg daily. Other modalities of treatment include oral steroids, dapsone, methotrexate, cyclosporine, azathioprine, and pentoxifylline. For recalcitrant disease, tumor necrosis factor-alpha (TNF-α) inhibitors such as etanercept, infliximab, and adalimumab, interleukin-1 (IL-1) inhibitors (anakinra/canakinumab), antiCD20 monoclonal antibody (rituximab), and IL-6 inhibitors (tocilizumab) are helpful.

REITER'S DISEASE (FIGS. 7A TO I)

Reiter's disease presents as a classical triad of reactive arthritis, urethritis and conjunctivitis following a

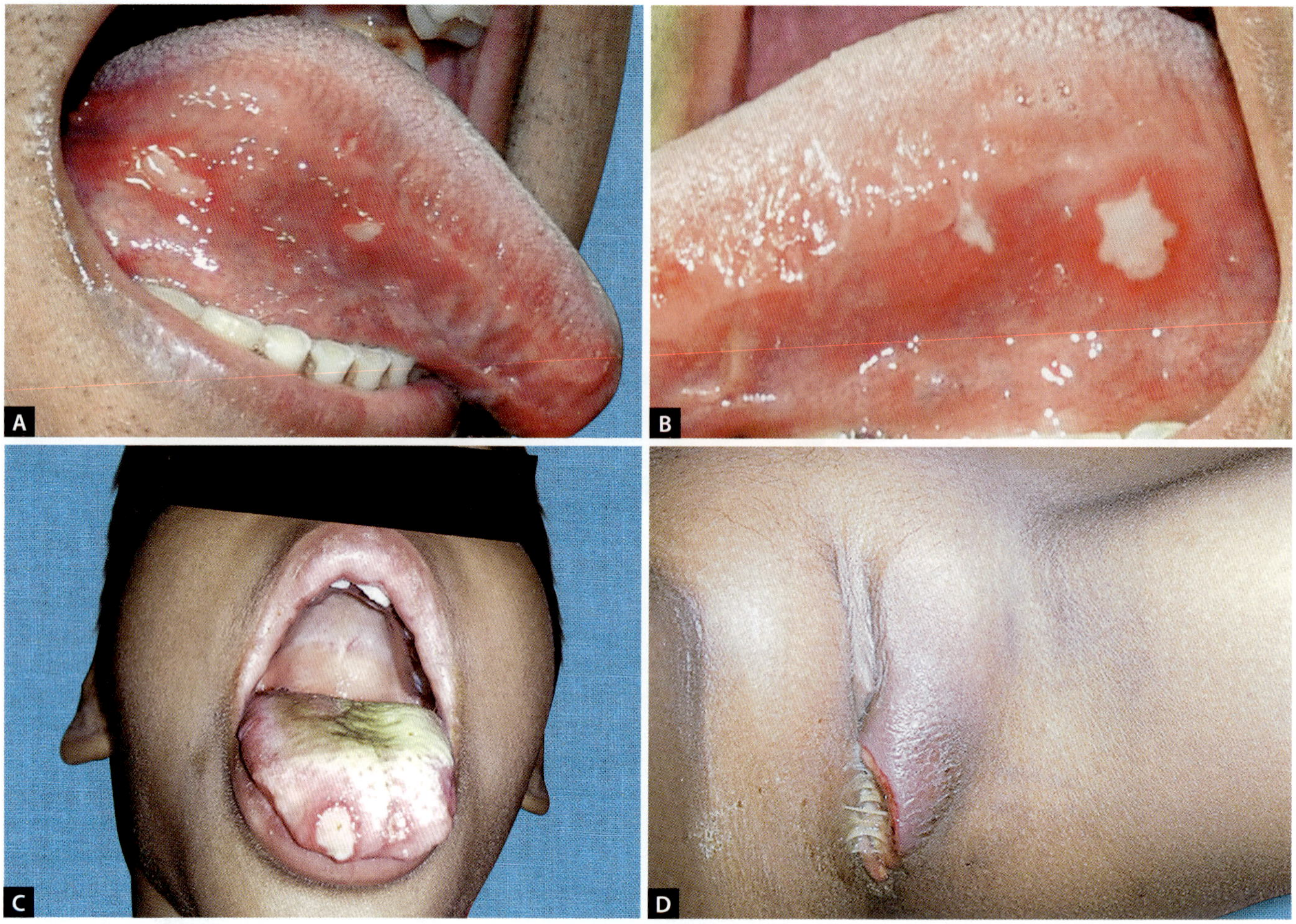

Figs. 6A to D: (A) Major aphthous ulcer over tongue in a child with Behçet's disease; (B) Close-up view of aphthous ulcer; (C) Multiple major aphthous ulcer in a 9-year-old girl; (D) Same girl with major aphthous ulcer over genitalia.

Box 1 | Proposed criteria for pediatric Behçet's disease.

Oral aphthous stomatitis, occurring at least three times yearly
Plus at least one of the following:
- Genital ulceration
- Erythema nodosum
- Pustular/Acneiform lesions
- Folliculitis
- Positive pathergy test
- Uveitis
- Venous/Arterial thrombosis
- Family history of Behçet's disease

genitourinary or GI infection. In children, they do not present as classical triad. It is thought to occur due to immune-mediated injury in a genetically predisposed patient associated with HLA-B27 positivity. Young children are more likely to acquire the postdysenteric form whereas, in adolescents, the posturethritic form is the most common. Conjunctivitis is the most common manifestation in children presenting as mild-to-severe inflammation. Conjunctivitis may be bilateral involving bulbar, tarsal, or angular.

Urethritis is usually nonspecific and is generally limited to a mild, painless, and nonpurulent urethral discharge. Balanitis and vulvitis are rarely seen in children. The characteristic cutaneous lesion in Reiter's disease is keratoderma blennorrhagica which manifests initially as macules and vesicles and later develop hyperkeratotic papules and plaques with a pustular center. Nails are usually thick, brittle with subungual hyperkeratosis. Mucosal erosions and ulceration can be seen. Sudden onset asymmetric arthritis affecting the weight bearing and peripheral joints is a prominent feature. There is no specific treatment for Reiter's disease.

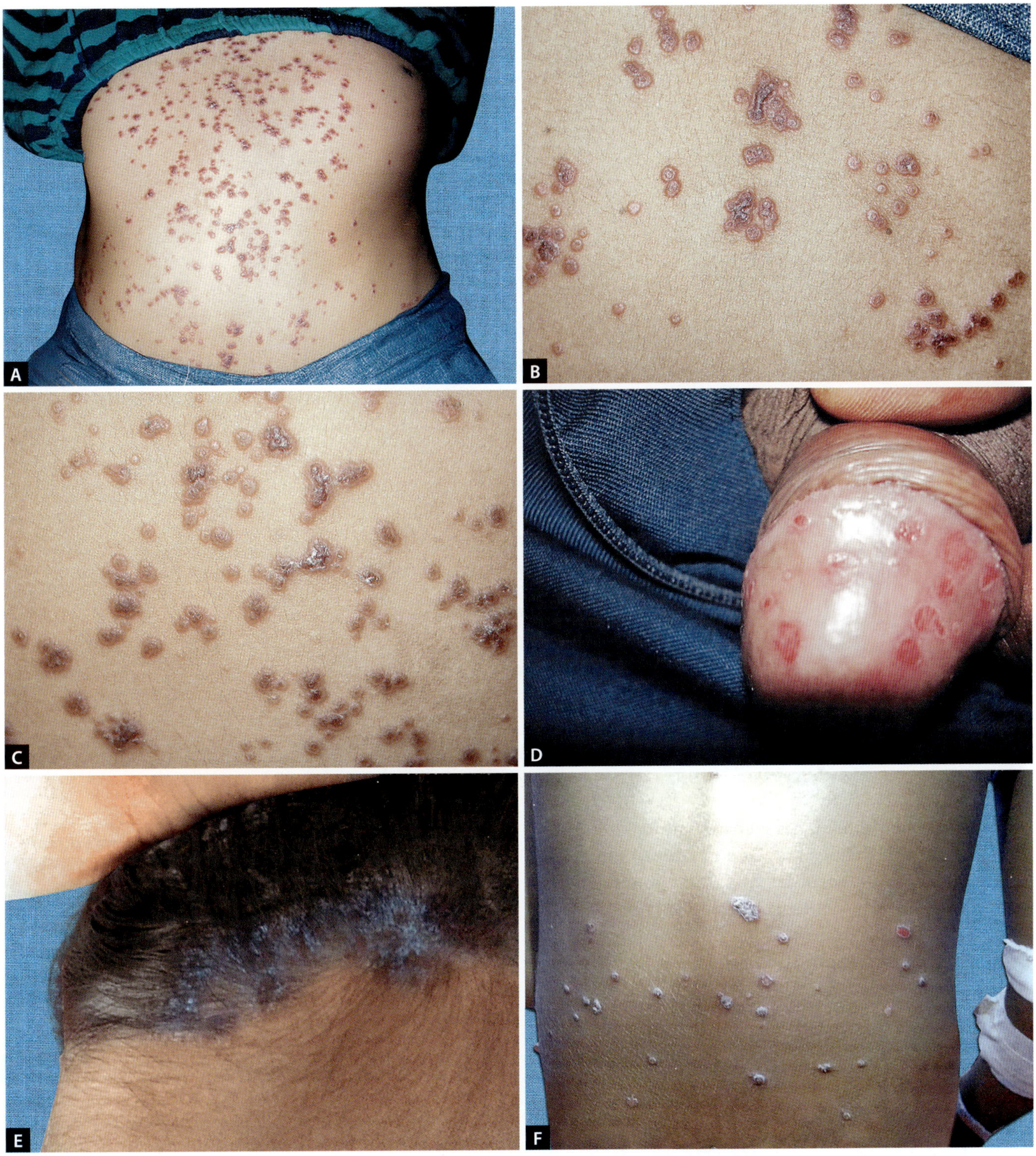

Figs. 7A to F: (A) Reiter's disease in a 18-year-old girl; (B) Close-up view of lesions; (C) Note moist but psoriasiform adherent limpet-like scales; (D) Circinate balanitis; (E) Scalp lesions having psoriasis-like appearance in Reiter's disease in a 8-year-old boy; (F) Limpet-like scales over back.

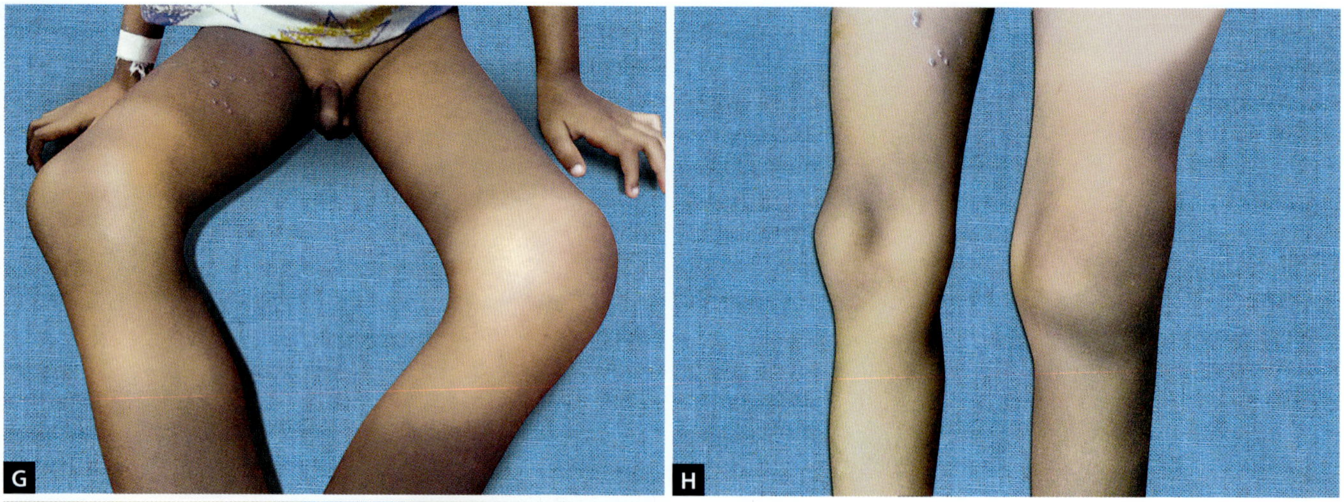

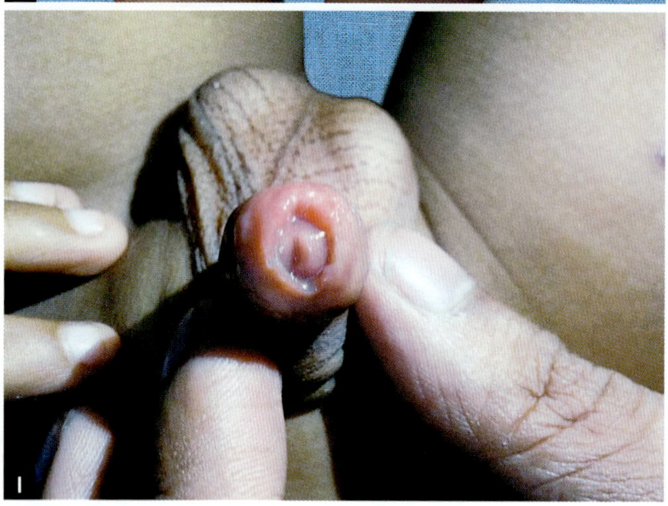

Figs. 7G to I: (G) Bilateral swelling of knees in Reiter's disease; (H) Bilateral knee arthritis in the same boy; (I) Inflammation of urethral meatus and prepuce in childhood Reiter's disease.

Spontaneous remission is seen in some children within 6 months. Tetracyclines are used to control underlying infections. NSAIDs, corticosteroids, and antimetabolites such as methotrexate and azathioprine have all been used depending on the severity of the disease and response. Refractory cases have been tried with infliximab, acitretin, and cyclosporine.

CUTANEOUS CROHN'S DISEASE

Crohn's disease is a chronic granulomatous disorder affecting any part of GI tract. It commonly affects adults, but is rarely seen in children. The etiology of Crohn's disease is multifactorial with immune-mediated inflammatory process. Varied cutaneous features are described in **Table 3**. In 25% cases, skin lesions precede the development of GI symptoms by months to years. Two-thirds of children suffering from Crohn's disease present with

Table 3: Mucocutaneous manifestations of Crohn's disease.

Specific	***Nonspecific***
• Perianal skin tags (75–80%) • Anal fissures • Fistulas • Abscesses • Cobblestoning of mucosa • Oral ulcerations • Cheilitis granulomatosis	• Erythema nodosum • Pyoderma gangrenosum • Aphthous stomatitis • Angular cheilitis • Erythema multiforme • Vasculitis • Polyarteritis nodosa
Metastatic	***Associated conditions***
• Swelling/ulceration/erythema/ edema of vulva, perineum • Isolated lymphedema of the genitalia • Sterile folliculitis • Nonspecific papules, pustules, plaques, ulcers, or abscesses on skin	• Vitiligo • Palmoplantar pustulosis • Clubbing • Palmar erythema

"That which does not kill us, makes us stronger." —**Friedrich Nietzsche**

genital involvement. Systemic features include diarrhea, weight loss, fatigue, fever, and growth failure. Skin biopsy is required to rule out other granulomatous disorders. Management includes topical steroids and tacrolimus for localized lesions and systemic immunosuppressants and biologics for multiple abscess and fistulae.

Orofacial Granulomatosis (Cheilitis Granulomatosa)

Cheilitis granulomatosa of Miescher is a rare, persistent, painless, recurrent swelling of both face and lip (macrocheilitis), and is the most common manifestation of MRS. It presents as a classical triad of relapsing facial paralysis, scrotal/fissured tongue (lingua plicata), and recurrent or persistent orofacial edema. Most of the cases of MRS present as incomplete triad. The exact etiology of cheilitis granulomatosa is not known and probably thought to be due to genetic predisposition, inflammatory, allergic, and microbial. Initially, children present with facial edema for several months or unilateral facial palsy. Lip swelling is firm; nonerythematous, painless, and may lead to drooling and speech difficulties. Crohn's disease can manifest as cheilitis granulomatosa. Histopathology shows noncaseating granulomas. Treatment includes topical and intralesional steroids, oral prednisone, antimalarials, minocycline, and metronidazole. Other therapies that have been tried include thalidomide, dapsone, azathioprine, clofazimine, and TNF-α inhibitors (infliximab).

SARCOIDOSIS (FIGS. 8A TO D)

Pediatric-onset sarcoidosis occurs in two groups—early onset (preschool children, <5 years) and late onset (older children, >5 years and adolescents). Early-onset

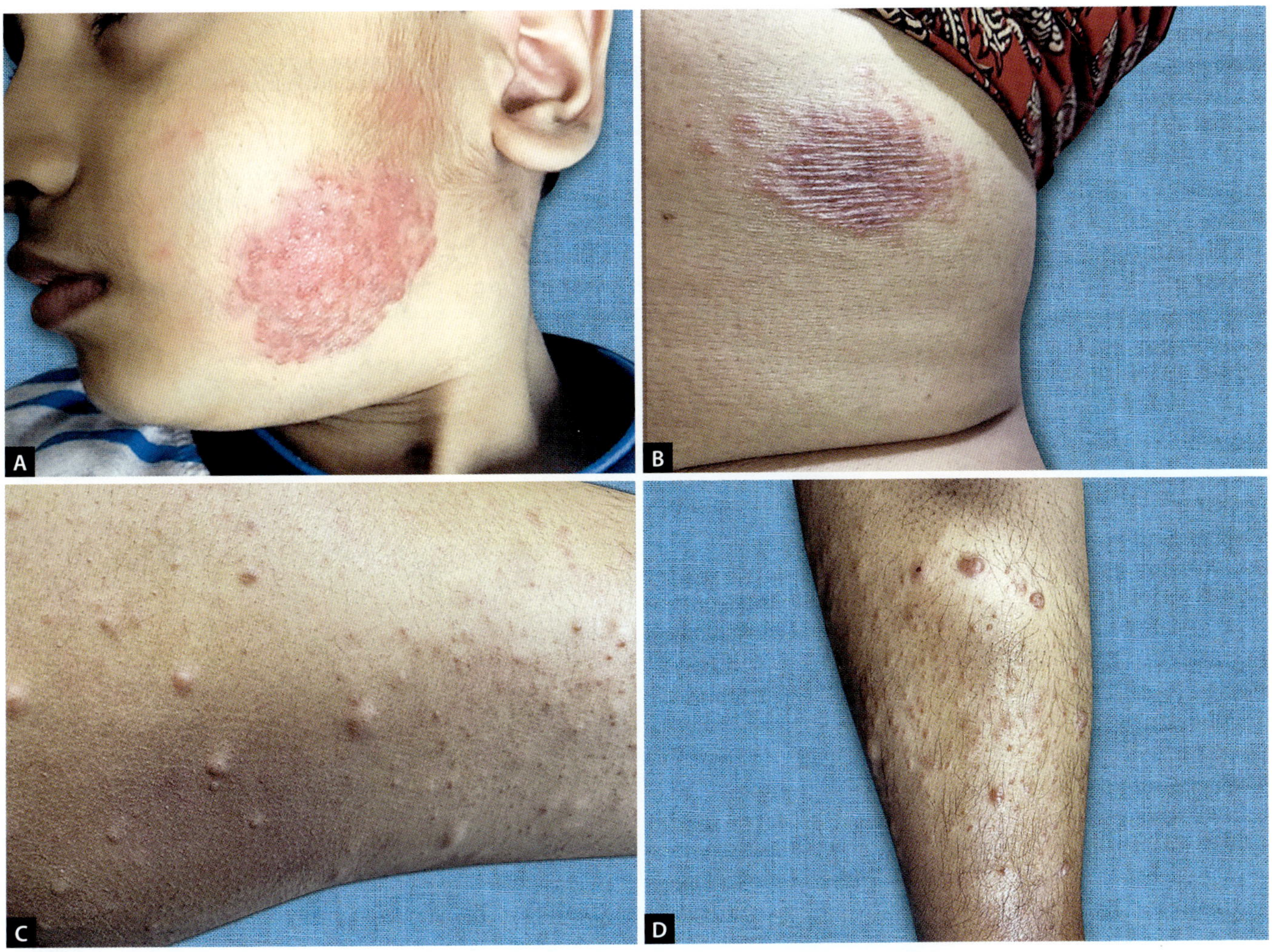

Figs. 8A to D: (A) Sarcoidosis over cheek in a 9-year-old boy; (B) Sarcoidosis over chest in a 18-year-old girl; (C) Lesions over thigh in the same girl; (D) Papular and nodular sarcoid in a 17-year-old boy.

"Life isn't as serious as the mind makes it out to be." —**Eckhart Tolle**

sarcoidosis also called as Blau syndrome (BS) is associated with heterozygous mutation in *NOD2* gene (*CARD15*). It is a triad of skin lesions, arthritis, and recurrent uveitis. Cutaneous features include multiple erythematous papules on trunk and extremities, eczematous, ichthyosiform lesions, EN, leukocytoclastic vasculitis, and pitted scarring. Systemic features include lymphadenopathy, iridocyclitis, anterior uveitis, parotid gland enlargement, splenomegaly, pneumonitis, and arthritis.

Clinically, late-onset sarcoidosis presents with constitutional symptoms such as fever, weight loss, cough, dyspnea, yellow-brown to red flat-topped papules, infiltrated plaques, nodules, annular plaques on face, ichthyosiform and erythroderma lesions, and hypopigmentation. Lung involvement is more common in older children. Other systemic features include anterior uveitis, hilar lymphadenopathy, hepatosplenomegaly, arrhythmias, congestive heart failure, hypercalciuria, facial paralysis, and arthritis. Multidisciplinary management is necessary.

AUTOINFLAMMATORY DISORDERS

Autoinflammatory disorders are group of monogenic inherited disorders, clinically characterized by repeated episodes of inflammation of the abdomen, skin, and joints manifesting as recurrent fever, serositis, osteoarticular symptoms, and mucocutaneous lesions. Cutaneous features include urticaria-like rash, recurrent cellulitis-like eruption, neutrophilic dermatoses-like lesions (nodules, ulcers, and pustules), leukocytoclastic vasculitis-like, purpura, and aphthous ulcer. The various types of autoinflammatory syndromes are described in **Table 4**.

Table 4: Autoinflammatory syndromes.

Disorders	*Clinical features*
Periodic fever syndrome	
Familial Mediterranean fever (FMF)	• Autosomal recessive • Childhood onset, recurrent fever, painful febrile attacks (short lasting), severe abdominal pain, serositis, orchitis, erysipelas-like skin eruption, pseudocellulitis, secondary amyloidosis • Treatment—colchicine
TNF receptor-associated periodic syndrome (TRAPS)	• Autosomal dominant • Recurrent prolonged fever (1–3 weeks), serositis, arthralgia, conjunctivitis, serpiginous, urticaria-like rash, periorbital edema, reticulate erythema, purpura, renal amyloidosis (10–25%) • Treatment—etanercept
Mevalonate kinase deficiency (MVK)/hyper-IgD syndrome	• Autosomal recessive • Early onset, recurrent fever, abdominal distress, diarrhea, headache, hepatosplenomegaly, aphthous stomatitis, urticarial eruption, petechiae, purpura • Treatment—steroids, NSAIDs, simvastatin, IL-1 blockade
Cryopyrinopathies	
Familial cold autoinflammatory syndrome (FCAS)	• Autosomal dominant • Early onset, cold triggered, urticarial eruption, arthritis, fever, and conjunctivitis • Treatment—IL-1 blockade
Muckle–Wells syndrome (MWS)	• Autosomal dominant • Recurrent urticaria, fever, progressive, and reactive amyloidosis • Treatment–IL-1 blockade
Chronic infantile neurological cutaneous and articular/neonatal-onset multisystem inflammatory disease (CINCA/NOMID)	• Autosomal dominant • Appears after birth, skin rash, urticaria, erythema, CNS abnormalities, arthralgia/arthritis, sensorineural hearing loss, and chronic aseptic meningitis • Treatment—IL-1 blockade
Pyogenic	
PAPA syndrome	• Autosomal dominant • Pyogenic sterile arthritis, pyoderma gangrenosum, acne, myositis
PFAPA syndrome	Periodic fever, aphthous stomatitis, pharyngitis, and cervical adenitis

Continued

Continued

Disorders	*Clinical features*
Deficiency of the IL-1 receptor antagonist (DIRA)	• Autosomal recessive • Fetal distress, joint swelling, severe osteopenia, lytic bone lesion, respiratory involvement, aphthae, pyoderma gangrenosum, and pustulosis • Treatment—IL-1 blockade
Deficiency of IL-36 receptor antagonist (DITRA)	Generalized pustulosis, fever, malaise, palmoplantar pustulosis nail dystrophy, arthritis, and cholangitis
CARD14–mediated pustular psoriasis	• Pityriasis rubra pilaris, plaque psoriasis, erythroderma • Treatment—TNF inhibitor
CANDLE (chronic atypical neutrophilic dermatosis with lipodystrophy and elevated temperature) syndrome	• Autosomal dominant • Fever, lymphadenopathy, purpura, and arthralgia • Treatment—JAK inhibitor
SAVI (STING-associated vasculopathy with onset in infancy) syndrome	• Autosomal dominant • Acral telangiectatic vasculopathy, pustules, fever, and adenopathy, interstitial lung fibrosis • Treatment—JAK inhibitor

(CNS: central nervous system; CARD14: caspase recruitment domain family member 14; IL: interleukin; JAK: Janus kinase; NSAIDs: nonsteroidal anti-inflammatory drugs; PAPA: pyogenic arthritis, pyoderma gangrenosum, and acne; PFAPA: periodic fever, aphthous stomatitis, pharyngitis, adenitis; TNF: tumor necrosis factor)

PYODERMA GANGRENOSUM (FIG. 9)

Pyoderma gangrenosum (PG) is a rare ulcerating, idiopathic, and inflammatory relapsing condition of the skin, resulting in severe scarring. Pediatric cases comprise 3–4% cases. About 50% cases are idiopathic. Secondary causes of PG include inflammatory bowel disease (ulcerative colitis and Crohn's disease), rheumatoid arthritis, lupus, leukemia, monoclonal gammopathy, multiple myeloma, Hodgkin's disease, myelodysplastic syndrome, immunodeficiency disorders, Takayasu's arteritis, necrotizing vasculitis, antineutrophil cytoplasmic antibody-associated vasculitides, human immunodeficiency virus (HIV), syphilis, malignancy, and diabetes.

Lesion starts as painful papulopustule or nodule, progresses quickly to form necrosis and ulceration healing with cribriform scarring. It can occur anywhere on the body but commonly affects lower extremity. In infants and younger children, it commonly affects scalp and anogenital areas. Treatment is not well-defined in children. Appropriate wound care along with treatment of underlying disease is the main stay of management in PG. Debridement is contraindicated. Systemic steroids are the drug of choice. Other immunosuppressants that have been used are tacrolimus, cyclosporine, etanercept, adalimumab, infliximab, dapsone, clofazimine, mycophenolate mofetil (MMF), and intravenous (IV) immunoglobulin.

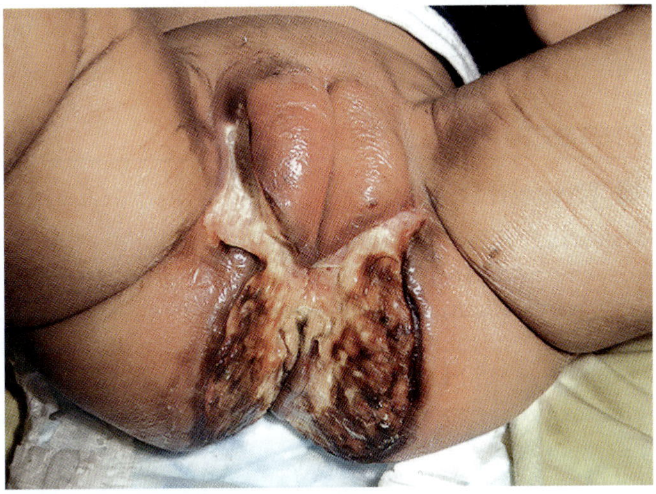

Fig. 9: Pyoderma gangrenosum in a 3-year-old girl.

RELAPSING POLYCHONDRITIS

Pediatric-onset relapsing polychondritis is very rare and represents <5% reported cases. It can be associated with a family history of autoimmunity. Clinical features include erythema, swelling, and pain in ear sparing the ear lobe, nasal cartilage inflammation, nonerosive arthritis, and eye changes such as conjunctivitis, episcleritis, uveitis, corneal ulceration, and optic nerve inflammation. In chronic disease, ear cartilage is destroyed resulting in scarred, "cauliflower"-like ear. Other features include aphthosis, EN, purpura, maculopapular rash, hoarseness, dyspnea, cough, and wheezing. Rarely relapsing polychondritis has been associated with renal and cardiac abnormalities. Management includes systemic corticosteroids (1 mg/kg/day), NSAIDs, TNF-α inhibitors, dapsone, and methotrexate.

ERYTHEMA MARGINATUM (FIG. 10A)

Erythema marginatum is a distinct form of annular erythema seen on trunk and extremities and is associated with active rheumatic fever. It is seen more commonly in children than adults. Erythema marginatum occurs after the onset of migratory arthritis or carditis by few days to months. Characterized by evanescent erythematous macules or papules that spreads centrifugally in concentric rings or in an annular pattern with elevated polycyclic or serpiginous borders resolving centrally in few hours to days to form pigmented center. Crops of lesions can occur in different areas. Recurrences occur for several months to years. Erythema marginatum should be differentiated from urticaria, tinea imbricata, erythema multiforme, and figurate erythema like erythema annulare centrifugum.

ENDOCRINE DISORDERS

Thyroid Disorders

Hyperthyroidism is caused by autoimmune thyroid disease and Graves' disease. Cutaneous features of hyperthyroidism include warm moist smooth skin, flushing, palmar erythema, hyperhidrosis, diffuse thinning of scalp hair, onycholysis, hyperpigmentation, chronic urticaria, periorbital edema, generalized pruritus,

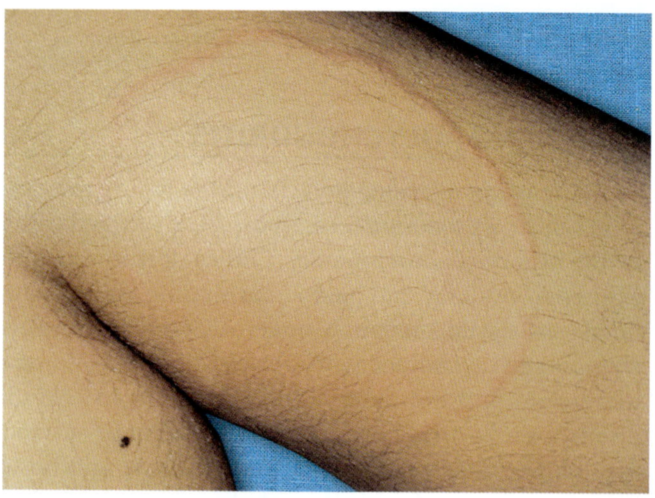

Fig. 10A: Erythema marginatum, note huge annular erythematous plaque over the thigh.

increased association with alopecia areata and vitiligo, and pretibial myxedema. Pretibial myxedema presents as nonpitting edema, nodules and plaques, shiny skin on the anterior tibial surface due to deposition of acid mucopolysaccharides. The varied cutaneous presentations of hypothyroidism are dry and coarse skin, carotenemia, myxedema, macroglossia, loss of lateral third of eyebrows, brittle hair, alopecia, telogen effluvium, urticaria, and pruritus.

Diabetes Mellitus

Type 1 diabetes mellitus (DM) [insulin-dependent DM (IDDM)] is more commonly seen in children, although type 2 DM has been increasing in younger population (adolescents). The type, severity, and frequency of skin changes in diabetes vary with age. The exact cause of many of the diabetic-associated skin changes is not known, but changes have been attributed to abnormal carbohydrate metabolism, metabolic alterations, atherosclerosis, microangiopathy, neuron degeneration, and impaired host mechanism. Xerosis is the most common skin change and was found in up to 15.8–22% of patients with type 1 DM. The most common infections seen in diabetes are fungal and bacterial infections, especially with *Candida*, dermatophytes, *Staphylococcus*, and *Streptococcus* species.

Skin changes associated with diabetes include hyperpigmentation, AN, diabetic dermopathy, necrobiosis lipoidica, bullae, skin tags, lipodystrophy, waxy skin syndrome, eruptive xanthoma, carotenemia, pruritus, yellow nails, infections, granuloma annulare, and scleredema diabeticorum. Diabetic dermopathy presents as well-defined, small, and light brown atrophic patches distributed bilaterally and asymmetrically on the pretibial area. Necrobiosis lipoidica presents as bilaterally symmetrical, asymptomatic, and irregular ovoid plaques with a yellow atrophic center and a red to purple periphery commonly on the pretibial skin. Lipoatrophy and lipohypertrophy are common complications of subcutaneous insulin injection and is attributed to the faulty technique of taking insulin injection.

Anorexia and Bulimia

Anorexia nervosa is seen in 3% of pubertal females and less common in prepubertal age group. Anorexia is associated with growth delay and developmental delay. Early recognition of cutaneous changes may detect hidden anorexia and bulimia. Mucocutaneous changes seen in anorexia and bulimia are xerosis, generalized pruritus,

"The future depends on how you do today." **—Mahatama Gandhi**

loss of subcutaneous fat, acne, purpura, callus on the dorsum of hand (Russell's sign), self-inflicted injuries, pellagra, scurvy, acrodermatitis enteropathica, seborrheic dermatitis, acrocyanosis, perniosis, livedo reticularis, cheilitis, aphthous stomatitis, telogen effluvium, and brittle hair.

H SYNDROME (FIGS. 10B TO D)

H syndrome, a rare autosomal recessive genodermatosis caused by the mutations in the *SLC29A3* gene which encodes the human equilibrative nucleoside transporter 3 (hENT3), is a novel inherited form of histiocytosis mainly characterized by hyperpigmentation, hypertrichosis, hepatosplenomegaly, heart anomalies, hearing loss, hypogonadism, low height, hallux valgus/flexion contractures and occasionally, hyperglycemia/DM. It was first described and named H syndrome by Molho-Pessach et al. in 2008, as most of the clinical features start with the letter "H". More than 20 different pathogenic mutations in *SLC29A3* have been documented. About 100 patients of H syndrome have been described worldwide, majority being of Arab descent and around 10 cases reported from India.

The pathognomonic skin findings, symmetrical cutaneous hyperpigmentation with sclerodermatous thickening, and hypertrichosis most often involve the lower limbs, especially the inner thighs, but can appear throughout the body. It usually begins in the first or second decade of life. The next most common feature seen is flexion contractures of fingers and toes followed by sensorineural hearing loss, short stature, hepatosplenomegaly, cardiac anomalies (pericardial involvement is most common), and hematological abnormalities (severe anemia with reticulocytopenia, pancytopenia, red cell aplasia, and myelofibrosis). Lymphadenopathy, insulin-dependent diabetes, and hypogonadism have also been described. Lymphadenopathy may be generalized or localized with inguinal, cervical, and axillary nodes being

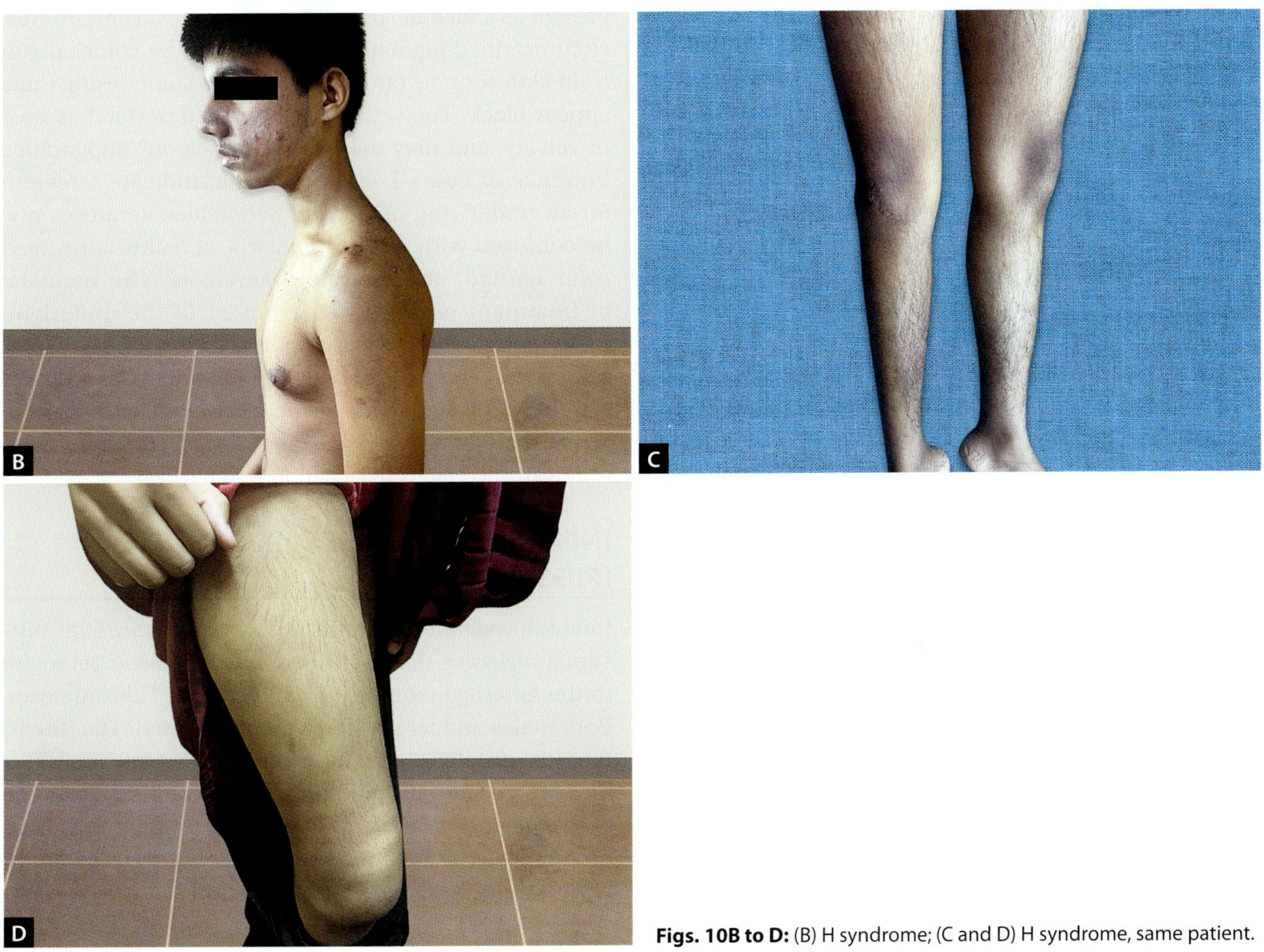

Figs. 10B to D: (B) H syndrome; (C and D) H syndrome, same patient.

"If you don't do anything, you risk even more." —**Erica Jong**

the most commonly involved. Other novel clinical features that have been described in various case reports are pancreatic exocrine deficiency, recurrent febrile episodes accompanied by joint inflammation, complete agenesis of the inferior vena cava with varicose veins, proptosis or exophthalmos, webbing of neck, sacroiliitis and uveitis, areas of hypopigmentation on the abdomen, and elevated serum amyloid level in blood.

Histopathological findings of cutaneous lesions include epidermal hyperplasia and increased basal pigmentation, and a dermal infiltrate including histiocytes, lymphocytes, and plasma cells, sometimes accompanied by hemosiderin deposition or calcification. H syndrome might have histopathological features similar to Rosai-Dorfman disease (RDD), including CD68+ S100+ CD1a- histiocytes with emperipolesis. Diagnosis is based on characteristic clinical findings and confirmed by genetic mutational analysis of *SLC29A3* gene. There is no definitive treatment. Multidisciplinary approach with proper genetic counseling is important. There is a poor response to agents directed against IL-1 or TNF-α (anakinra, canakinumab, and adalimumab) while colchicine or NSAIDs provide only partial relief. Systemic corticosteroids, methotrexate, cyclosporine, cyclophosphamide, tocilizumab, and radiotherapy have also been used primarily for the inflammatory features of the disorder. Treatment with tocilizumab (a humanized monoclonal antibody directed against the IL-6 receptor) has shown partial-to-complete response including reduction in hyperpigmentation and subcutaneous fibrosis, acceleration of growth velocity, and improvement in inflammatory indices.

H syndrome, pigmented hypertrichosis with insulin-dependent diabetes mellitus (PHID), Faisalabad histiocytosis, and familial RDD (also known as sinus histiocytosis with massive lymphadenopathy or SHML) are now considered to be part of the same disease spectrum.

LESER–TRÉLAT SIGN (FIGS. 11A AND B)

Leser–Trélat sign is a rare skin condition characterized by the sudden appearance of seborrheic keratoses that rapidly increase in number and size within weeks to months. The sign was first described in the 1800s by Edmund Leser and Ulysse Trélat; in 1900 Hollander was the first to describe seborrheic keratoses in association with malignancy. It is associated with particularly adenocarcinoma and lymphoma. The exact pathophysiology underlying the sign of Leser–Trélat remains elusive, but there is strong suspicion that the release of cytokines and growth factors from the neoplasm stimulates the eruptive growth of the seborrheic keratoses. The typical morphology of these lesions tends to vary extensively among patients and may present as a macule, papules, and plaques. They are well-circumscribed pigmented lesions with the color ranging from skin tone to tan or brown, and some lesions may appear black. The texture is typically described as waxy or velvety, and they may have a "stuck-on" appearance. Presence of Leser–Trélat sign would indicate screening for an underlying neoplasm. Seborrheic keratoses may be confused with verruca vulgaris, acrochordons, nevi, solar lentigo, and lichenoid keratosis. The mainstay of treatment involves management of the underlying malignancy which results in resolution of associated seborrheic keratoses in about 50% of patients. In addition, symptomatic lesions may be destroyed with various physical methods including cryotherapy, curettage, shave removal, and electrodesiccation.

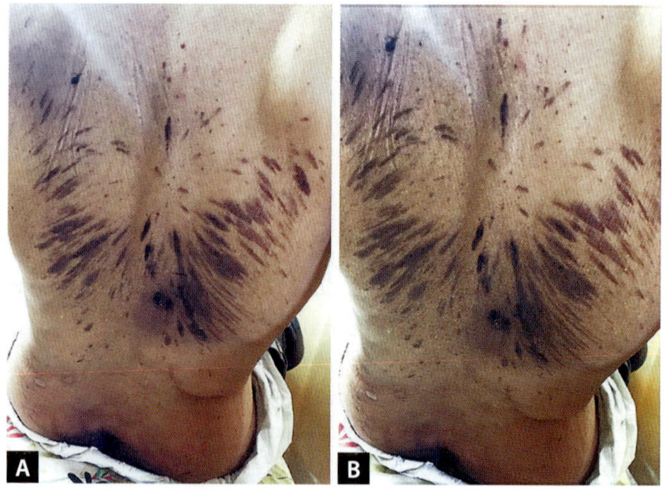

Figs. 11A and B: (A) Leser–Trélat sign; (B) Close-up view.

INFANTILE SYSTEMIC HYALINOSIS (FIGS. 12A TO K)

Infantile systemic hyalinosis (ISH) is a very rare fatal autosomal recessive disorder of connective tissue belonging to the heterogeneous group of disorders "fibromatoses". Both males and females are equally affected. The disease presents usually at birth or within the first few months of life with progressive painful joint contractures (presents as frog leg position), skin hyperpigmentation over bony prominences, and papules on the face (especially on the perioral and nasal area), scalp, and neck.

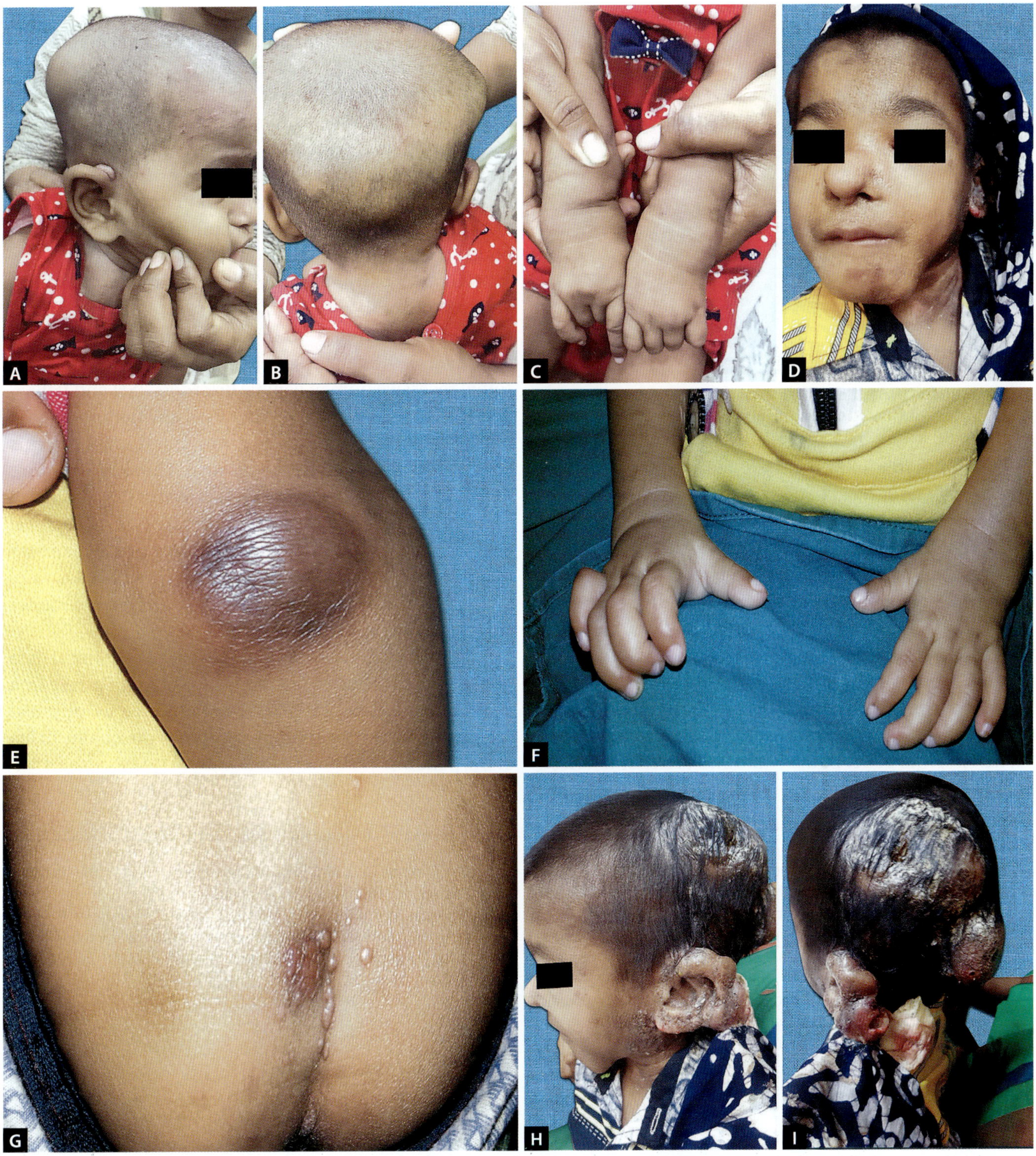

Figs. 12A to I: (A) Infantile systemic hyalinosis (ISH) in a 2-year-old girl; (B) Close-up view of scalp nodules; (C) Same child, note swollen and deformed wrists and hands; (D) A 5-year-old boy with ISH, note characteristic infiltrated nose and chin; (E) Nodule over the elbow; (F) Typical infiltrated hands in ISH; (G) Perianal fleshy nodules of ISH; (H) Gross noncancerous growths with secondary infection; (I) Close-up view of the same lesion.

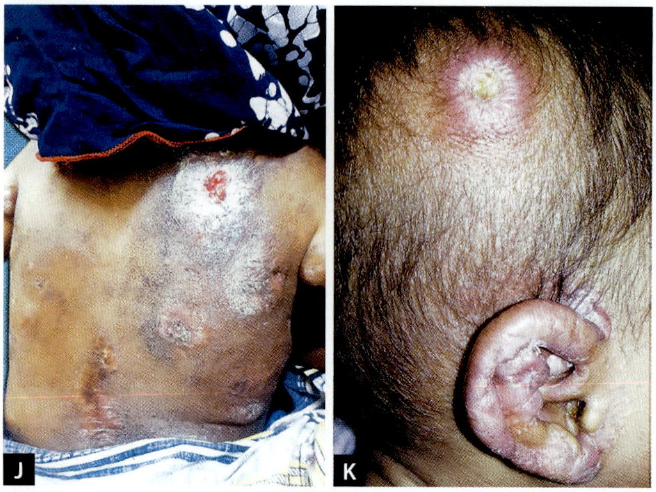

Figs. 12J and K: (J) Back lesion in the same boy; (K) Same boy, note infiltrated ear and plaque over scalp.

Other notable characteristic features are gingival hypertrophy and thickened skin. However, the children with ISH are found to be intellectually normal. Affected children suffer from osteopenia which results in increased susceptibility to bone fractures. Intractable diarrhea as a result of protein losing enteropathy and/or recurrent infections is commonly reported in children suffering from ISH. Because of multisystem failure resulting from complications, many patients die in infancy. ISH and juvenile hyaline fibromatosis (JHF) shares many clinical resemblances, both are caused by mutations in the *CMG2/ANTXR2* gene. Both syndromes are characterized by gingival hypertrophy, bilateral generalized joint contractures, and subcutaneous and perianal fleshy nodules. A progressive severe course, an earlier onset, and death in early childhood characterize ISH. They share characteristic histological similarities.

Histologically ISH and JHF are characterized by deposition of hyalinized fibrous material (glassy translucent substance and glycoprotein) in many tissues such as skin, skeletal muscle, cardiac muscle, GI tract, lymph nodes, spleen, thyroid, and adrenal glands.

Capillary morphogenesis gene 2—capillary morphogenesis protein 2 *(CMG2)*/anthrax toxin receptor 2 *(ANTXR2)*—mapped to chromosome 4q21.21, was identified as the gene responsible for these two rare autosomal recessive human genetic disorders, ISH and JHF.

Noncancerous tissue proliferation and nodules are the most outstanding external features found in all patients and are the hallmark of the disease. These nodules are not seen at birth but may develop in the first month of life. Since those nodules develop over areas of mechanical stress, upregulation of microtrauma repair mechanisms might be the suggested pathogenesis. The nodules were found to be rather cellular at the onset, while older ones contained mainly extracellular matrix.

Currently the diagnosis of ISH is based on clinical data but molecular genetic testing is available on a research basis only. Treatment of ISH is palliative as physical therapy and nutritional support improve the quality of life of the patients.

SUGGESTED READINGS

1. Lugović-Mihić L, Krišto M, Špoljar S, Novak-Bilić G, Bešlić I, Vučić M, et al. Can skin be a marker for internal malignancy? Evidence from clinical cases. Acta Clin Croat. 2021;60(4):711-21.
2. Gupta V, Ramam M. Monogenic autoinflammatory syndromes in children: through the dermatologist's lens. Indian J Paediatr Dermatol. 2018;19(3):194-201
3. Johnson KL, Jahnke MN. Cutaneous manifestations of systemic disease. In: Teng J, Marqueling A, Benjamin L (Eds). Therapy in Pediatric Dermatology. Switzerland: Springer; 2017.
4. McClanahan D, Funk T, Small A. Sweet Syndrome in the Pediatric Population. Dermatol Clin. 2022;40(2):179-90.
5. Navallas M, Inarejos Clemente EJ, Iglesias E, Rebollo-Polo M, Zaki FM, Navarro OM. Autoinflammatory diseases in childhood, part 1: monogenic syndromes. Pediatr Radiol. 2020;50(3):415-30.

CHAPTER

22

Psychodermatoses

INTRODUCTION

There is a complex interaction between the skin and the neuroendocrine and immune system. The exact prevalence of psychodermatoses in children is not known. The course of many cutaneous disorders is affected by stress and psychological events. Management often requires a multidisciplinary approach and includes a pediatrician, dermatologist, psychologist, and psychiatrist.

CLASSIFICATION

Psychodermatoses are broadly classified into psychophysiologic disorders, primary psychiatric disorders, and secondary psychiatric disorders. In psychophysiologic disorders, the skin diseases are affected by stress or anxiety such as atopic dermatitis, alopecia areata, vitiligo, acne, and psoriasis. In such cases, apart from treating primary skin disorder, it is important to manage with pharmacological and nonpharmacological therapy. In primary psychiatric disorders, there is an underlying psychological functional problem and the skin lesions are secondary and self-inflicted. Some of the factitious skin disorders described in this chapter such as dermatitis artefacta and delusions of parasitosis are examples of primary psychiatric disorders. In secondary psychiatric disorders, there are symptoms such as depression and social phobia that result from disfiguring skin conditions.

DERMATITIS ARTEFACTA (FIGS. 1A TO E)

Artefactual lesions in a child can be self-inflicted or caused by a perpetrator. Dermatitis artefacta is used to describe skin damage caused deliberately and secretly by the patient and presented as skin disease in order to satisfy a psychological need and in the pursuit of secondary gain. It is more commonly seen in adolescents and children but less commonly under 8 years of age. In children, it may be related to various situations such as school examination, relocation of school, bullying, discord in home, possible sexual abuse to draw attention to their plight, and other underlying psychiatric disorders. Hollow history (not able to give evolution) and unexplained symptoms such as headache, abdominal pain, and difficulty in walking disappearing mysteriously should raise the suspicion of dermatitis artefacta. Children avoid eye contact and put a "Mona Lisa" smile throughout the examination. Children use glue to produce desquamative lesions, natural colors and cosmetics for erythema, aerosols producing bullae, and tiny petechiae surrounding the mouth due to vacuum created by sucking beakers. Cutaneous lesions are often bizarre, linear, geometric arrangements, and have sharp demarcation with the surrounding skin. Lesions may be purpuric, excoriations, abrasions, crusting, necrosis, blisters, ulcers, erythema, nodules, and scarring on accessible parts of the body. Modes of injury include rubbing, picking, scratching, cutting, pinching, biting, and sucking. Bullous lesions can be seen in older children due to "salt and ice burn craze" or "aerosol challenge craze".

Dermatitis artefacta is a diagnosis of exclusion. It should be differentiated from other genuine skin disorders and factitious disease inflicted by others. Skin biopsy should be avoided as it shows nonspecific features. Strong suspicion of the disorder, early diagnosis, and multidisciplinary management are important. Confronting children is unhelpful in most of the cases. Disclosing to parents and counseling about the benign nature and addressing the underlying psychological issue are necessary.

DELUSIONS OF PARASITOSIS

Delusions of parasitosis, also called Ekbom's syndrome, is seen more commonly in adult females. Rarely, it can be seen in the adolescent age group. The patient has an adherence to possible yet implausible belief without any objective evidence. There is delusion that his or her own body is infested with parasites. The patients often

"What's meant to be will always find a way." —**Trisha Yearwood**

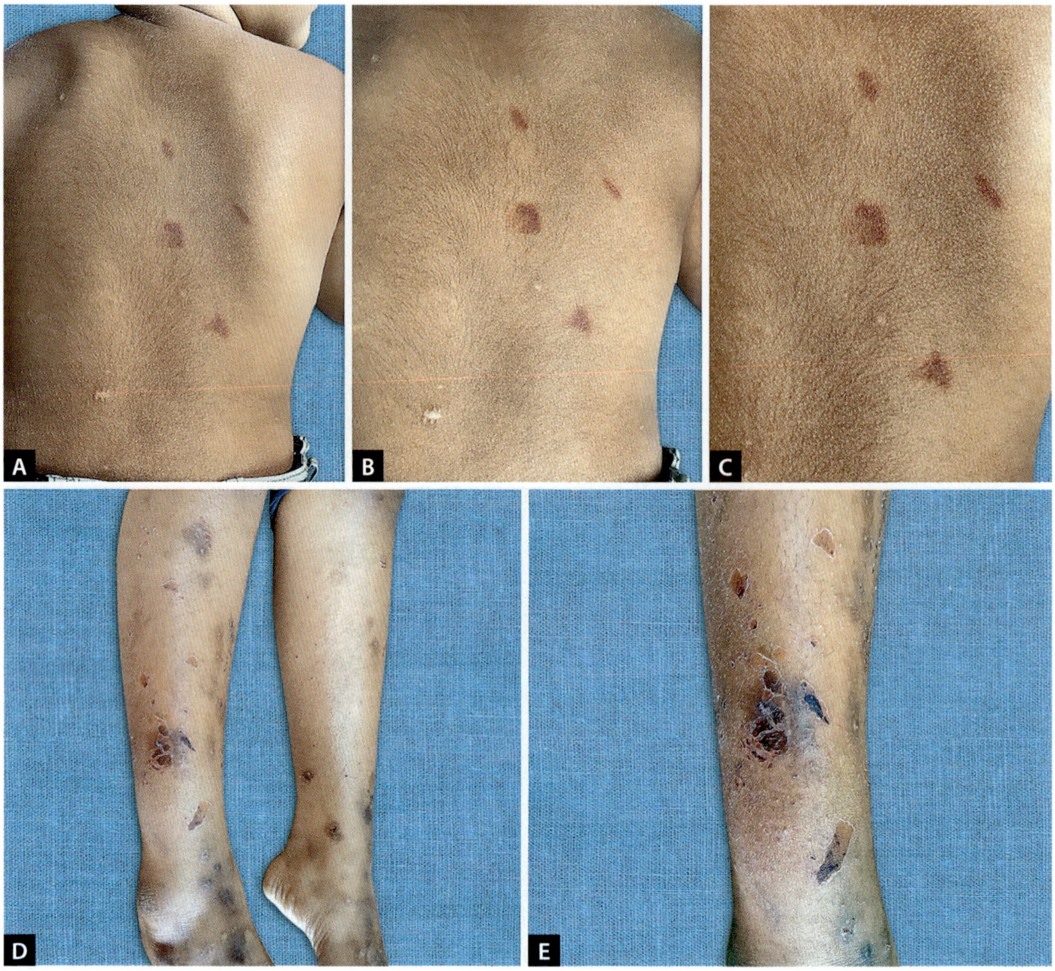

Figs. 1A to E: (A) Dermatitis artefacta in a 4-year-old boy, lesions over back; (B) Same boy, another view—note ecchymosis-like lesions; (C) Close-up view of lesions; (D) Dermatitis artefacta in a 9-year-old girl; (E) Close-up view, note cut/burn mark-like appearance of lesions.

complain of having a sensation of an insect crawling, burrowing, or biting on the skin. They are not satisfied with the dermatologist's opinion that they have underlying psychological issues. To prove themselves right, they often tend to collect samples of the parasite from the skin; however, when microscopically examined, it turns out to be dirt, lint, skin cells, scabs, and debris. Patients are not convinced even after counseling and investigations. Skin changes include excoriations, lichenification, prurigo nodules, pigmentation, and scarring. Sometimes, parents with delusion of parasitosis insist about the same symptoms on the child. Management by the dermatologist and psychiatrist is necessary. However, primary skin disorders and secondary psychiatric disorders such as depression, schizophrenia, formication without delusion, and organic causes should be ruled out before diagnosing delusions of parasitosis. Pimozide is the drug of choice in delusions of parasitosis.

OBSESSIVE-COMPULSIVE DISORDERS

Obsessive-compulsive disorder, though commonly seen in adults, can affect children. It is characterized by obsessions such as recurrent thoughts or images which could be disrupting and compulsions (repetitive and intentional behaviors) performed to decrease discomfort though it is senseless. The prevalence is 0.5–4% in children and 0.01% among 5–7 years of age. Symptoms can be seen as early as 2 years. It is more common in boys than girls in the prepubertal age group. Though children have repetitive behaviors as a part of normal development, they can become distressing, if they interfere in the daily activities. Symptoms have a waxing and waning course. Childhood obsessive-compulsive disorder may be associated with Tourette syndrome, tics, developmental delay, and hyperactivity. Some of the obsessive-compulsive disorders associated with dermatological disorders in children

"Sharing knowledge is not about giving people something, or getting something from them. That is only valid for information sharing. Sharing knowledge occurs when people are genuinely interested in helping one another develop new capacities for action; it is about creating learning processes." —**Peter Senge**

include trichotillomania, acne excoriée, irritant dermatitis due to repeated hand washing, lip-licker dermatitis, prurigo nodularis, neurotic excoriations, body dysmorphic disorder, onychophagia (nail biting), onychotillomania (picking cuticle/removal of nail), and nose picking.

Trichotillomania is a traumatic alopecia with an irresistible urge to pull the hair and sense of relief after the hair is pulled. Sometimes, the hair is swallowed, called trichophagia, resulting in trichobezoar (mass of undigested hair), causing gastric and intestinal obstruction. In acne excoriée, though the initial lesions are mild, they become excoriated and severe due to continuous squeezing resulting in permanent scarring. In neurotic excoriations, there is an irresistible urge to manipulate the skin leading to lichen simplex chronicus or prurigo nodularis. Sometimes, they may use a tool such as a pencil, stick, or point of knife to do the picking activity. Cognitive behavior therapy is the treatment of choice for obsessive-compulsive disorders in children. Selective serotonin reuptake inhibitors such as sertraline and fluoxetine have been successfully used in children. Counseling caregivers in handling and coping with the situation is important.

PSYCHOGENIC PURPURA/GARDNER–DIAMOND SYNDROME (FIG. 2)

Psychogenic purpura, also called autoerythrocyte sensitization syndrome or Gardner–Diamond syndrome, is characterized by recurrent episodes of painful ecchymoses. It is seen in young females with emotional disturbances, anxiety disorder, depression, or obsessive-compulsive disorder. There is autosensitization of patients to their own blood. Initially, there is a burning or stinging sensation followed by development of an erythematous to ecchymotic lesion resolving spontaneously by 7–10 days. Rarely, there could be associated hematuria and epistaxis. It should be considered in the differential diagnosis of recurrent painful purpura.

CAREGIVER-FABRICATED ILLNESS (MUNCHAUSEN SYNDROME BY PROXY) (FIGS. 3A AND B)

Caregiver-fabricated illness is also known as Munchausen syndrome by proxy or factitious disorder by proxy. It is a form of child abuse where parents or caregivers induce false illness in the child and substantiate by fabricating false physical signs. This is more often invented by the mother leading to unnecessary investigations and treatment in

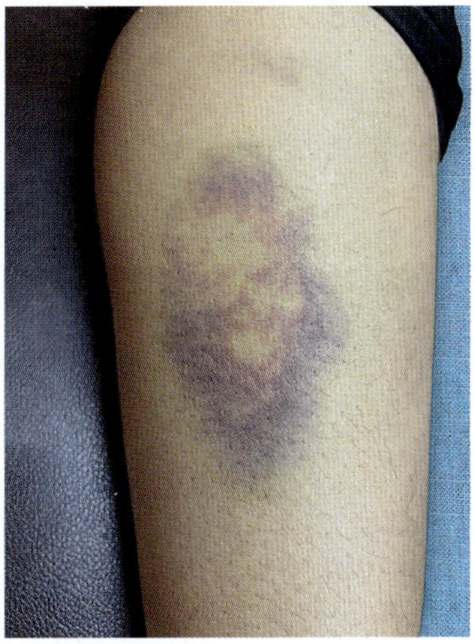

Fig. 2: Psychogenic purpura.

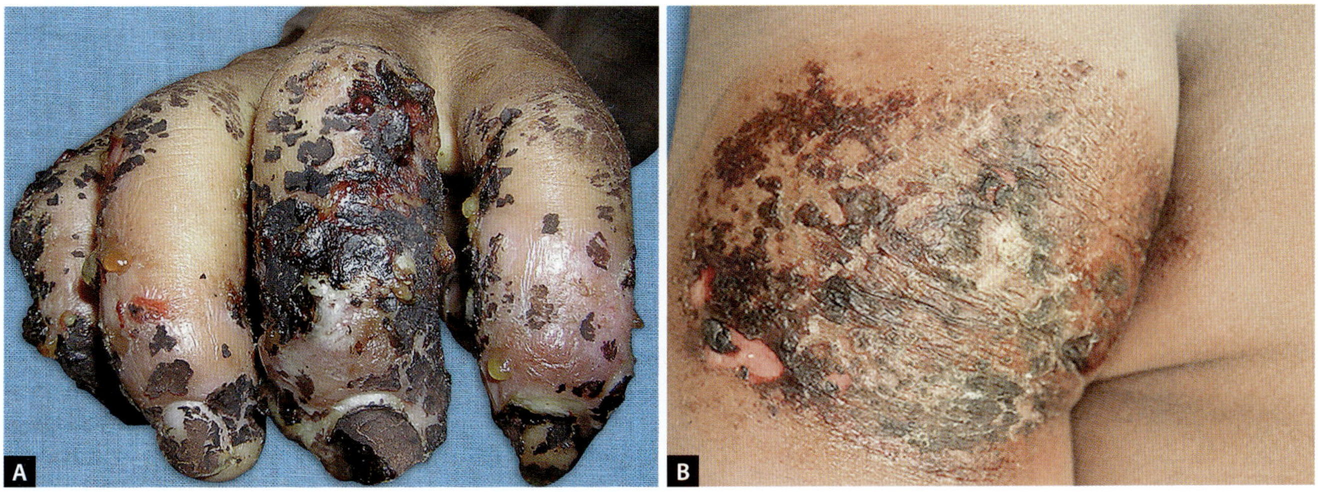

Figs. 3A and B: Caregiver-fabricated illness.

"Death is not extinguishing the light; it is only putting out the lamp because the dawn has come." —**Rabindranath Tagore**

the child. The perpetrator in this disorder mostly works in the healthcare field with familiar medical terminology and associated with underlying psychological issues. The physician in most of the times is unable to diagnose and the caregiver visits various hospitals for the same fabricated illness. The incidence is 0.4/100,000 children below 16 years of age and 2–2.8/100,000 below 1 year of age. The clinical clues to diagnosing fabricated illness include persistent symptoms unable to define medically, atypical symptoms, inconsistent history, unsatisfied caregiver even though the child improves, unnecessarily persist on investigations, signs and symptoms occurring in the presence of the same caregiver, lack of response to treatment, and history of somatic disorder in the caregiver. Varied clinical features seen in the child are failure to thrive, coagulopathy, hypoglycemia, sleep apnea, recurrent infections, and behavior problems. Skin findings have been reported in 3–9% cases and present with erythema, blisters, erosions, bruising, purpura, burns, lacerations, puncture wounds, and dermatitis. The child is almost symptom-free when separated from the caregiver. Careful approach, early diagnosis, and treatment of the perpetrator are important to prevent mortality and morbidity in the child.

MID-FACE TODDLER EXCORIATION SYNDROME (FIG. 4)

Mid-face toddler excoriation syndrome (MiTES) is a newly described entity in 2017 characterized by habitual scratching leading to excoriations, erosions, and chronic deep scarring wounds affecting mainly the mid-face region such as nose and eyes and the surrounding region such as medial cheeks and central forehead. It is an autosomal recessive disorder caused by homozygous biallelic mutations in a gene for hereditary sensory and autonomic neuropathy type VIII (HSAN8) and *PRDM12*. They are self-inflicted injuries that usually start in infancy, mostly within the first year of life. Some children may have associated neurological abnormalities without any evidence of insensitivity to pain. MiTES should be differentiated from child abuse or fabricated and induced illness. The lesions improve with age leaving only scarring.

EXFOLIATIVE CHEILITIS (FIG. 5)

Exfoliative cheilitis is a rare reactive condition presenting as continuous peeling of the lips. Factitial cheilitis can present as exfoliative cheilitis when it is due to attention-seeking or factitial behavior or an obsessive-compulsive tendency to pick or chap the lips. Exfoliative cheilitis is rarely reported but appears to affect both sexes equally and mainly affects young adults < 30 years of age. Occasionally, it affects children and adolescents. The condition may be painful, causing difficulty in eating and speaking. Other symptoms reported include sensations of tingling, itching, and dryness. In severe cases, fissuring and ulceration have been observed. Depression and personality disorders have been reported commonly in association with factitial exfoliative cheilitis. However, the cheilitis itself can be of such an unpleasant appearance that the patient avoids social situations, contributing to mood disturbance. The typical course of exfoliative cheilitis is chronic over several years. It may fluctuate, worsening with further stress. Spontaneous improvement has been reported, but it often recurs. Application of emollient once every 2 hours or even more frequently and counseling form the mainstay of treatment.

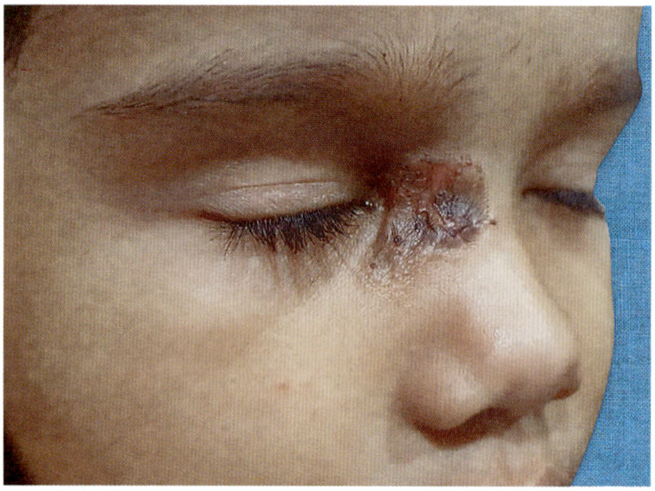

Fig. 4: Mid-face toddler excoriation syndrome (MiTES).

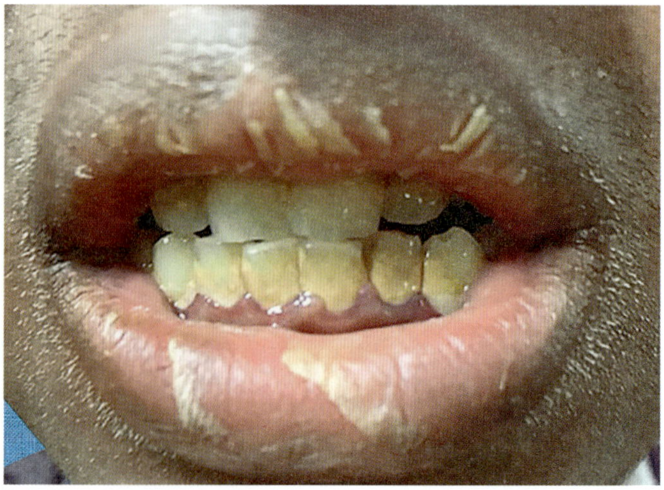

Fig. 5: Exfoliative cheilitis in a 17-year-old boy.

"One whose knowledge is confined to books and whose wealth is in the possession of others can use neither knowledge nor wealth when the need for them arises." —**Chanakya**

SUGGESTED READINGS

1. Hoffman JS, Koocher GP. Medical Child Abuse Hidden in Pediatric Settings: Detection and Intervention. J Clin Psychol Med Settings. 2020;27(4):753-65.
2. Glaser D. Fabricated or induced illness: From "Munchausen by proxy" to child and family-oriented action. Child Abuse Negl. 2020;108:104649.
3. Hassan I, Keen MA, Bhat YJ, Latif I. Psychodermatoses in children. Indian J Paediatr Dermatol. 2019;20:306-14.
4. Mosca M, Martin K, Hadeler E, Hong J, Brownstone N, Koo J. Review of the diagnosis and management of pediatric psychodermatologic conditions: Part I. Pediatr Dermatol. 2022; 39(1):17-21.
5. Mosca M, Martin K, Hong J, Hadeler E, Brownstone N, Koo J. A review of the diagnosis and management of pediatric psychodermatologic conditions: Part II. Pediatr Dermatol. 2022; 39(1):12-6.

"Setting goals is the first step in turning the invisible to the visible." —**Tony Robbins**

CHAPTER

23

Primary Immunodeficiency Disorders and Skin

INTRODUCTION

Primary immunodeficiency disorders (PIDs) are a group of disorders affecting the capability to fight against infection. These include defects in T cells and B cells affecting cell-mediated and humoral immunity, combined humoral and cell-mediated immunodeficiency, defects in phagocytosis, complement defects, and defects in cytokine or cytokine signaling pathways which are determinants for immune function. Depending upon the type and severity, age at onset of symptoms can vary from neonatal period to late childhood. Clinically, this group of disorders can involve any organ system of an individual such as respiratory system, gastrointestinal system, skin and mucous membrane, bone and joints, endocrine organs, and nervous system. The common skin manifestations of various PIDs include eczema [Wiskott–Aldrich syndrome (WAS) and autosomal dominant hyperimmunoglobulin E syndrome (HIES)]; erythroderma (Omenn syndrome); viral warts or molluscum contagiosum (autosomal recessive HIES); chronic mucocutaneous candidiasis (HIES, autoimmune polyendocrinopathy candidiasis ectodermal dysplasia syndrome, Th17 cell defects); recurrent non-healing ulcers (leukocyte adhesion defect); skin abscesses (antibody defects, HIES, and chronic granulomatous disease); petechial or purpuric spots (WAS).

Most PIDs cause symptoms in early life. However, the heterogeneous constellation of symptoms often results in delayed diagnosis. Adult presentations of PID tend to reflect polygenic diseases, such as common variable immunodeficiency disorder (CVID), or diseases in which environmental factors expose the underlying immunological phenotype [e.g., exposure to endemic mycobacteria can lead to the MonoMAC phenotype of GATA binding protein 2 (GATA-2) deficiency, characterized by monocytopenia and non tuberculous mycobacterial infection]. The advent of next-generation sequencing (NGS) has revolutionized clinical immunology by allowing detailed characterization of the genetic architecture of the immune system in healthy individuals and patients with significant immunological defects. Till date, more than 300 distinct, monogenic primary immunodeficiencies have been described.

The clinically heterogeneous presentations of PID can make them challenging to diagnose, and it is essential that all patients in whom PID is suspected are promptly referred to a clinical immunologist **(Box 1)**. Timely investigation and diagnosis are essential to allow early supportive interventions (prophylactic antimicrobials, avoidance of live vaccines, and immunoglobulin replacement), particularly in infants, in whom fitness for curative hematopoietic stem cell transplantation (HSCT) determines clinical outcome. A growing body of evidence supports the cost-effectiveness of newborn screening for severe combined immune deficiency (SCID).

Box 1 | Clinical features suggesting high risk for of primary immunodeficiency.

- A family history of primary immunodeficiency
- Unexplained infantile deaths
- Consanguinity
- Recurrent infections
- Four or more ear infections per year
- Two or more serious sinus infections per year
- Two or more pneumonia per year
- Two or more deep-seated infections (abscesses, osteomyelitis, and meningitis) or episodes of sepsis
- Infections with unusual/opportunistic organisms (e.g., nontuberculous mycobacteria, *Pneumocystis*, *Aspergillus*, mucocutaneous candidiasis)
- Requiring long courses of antimicrobials for resolution
- Requiring frequent courses of intravenous antibiotics
- Infections that have led to structural damage (e.g., bronchiectasis)
- Persistent viral infections (long-lasting warts, persistent molluscum)
- Early-onset eczematous skin rash
- Early-onset autoimmunity (e.g., cytopenias, polyendocrinopathies)
- Failure to thrive in infancy, especially chronic diarrhea or infection

"Whether you think you can or you think you can't, you're right." —**Henry Ford**

Various important entities of primary immunodeficiency diseases:

- Ataxia-telangiectasia (A–T)
- Cartilage—hair hypoplasia syndrome
- Chédiak-Higashi syndrome
- Griscelli syndrome
- Chronic granulomatous disease
- Chronic mucocutaneous candidiasis
- Complement deficiency disorders
- DiGeorge syndrome (DGS)
- Hyperimmunoglobulin E syndrome
- Immunoglobulin deficiencies
- IPEX syndrome (immune dysregulation, polyendocrinopathy, enteropathy, X-linked syndrome)
- Leukocyte adhesion deficiencies
- Severe combined immunodeficiency
- Wiskott-Aldrich syndrome

ATAXIA–TELANGIECTASIA (FIGS. 1A TO D)

(See also in Chapter 2)

About two-thirds of people with A–T have abnormalities of the immune system. The most common abnormalities are low levels of one or more classes of immunoglobulin (IgG, IgA, IgM, or IgG subclasses), failure to make antibodies in response to vaccines or infections, and lymphopenia, especially affecting T-lymphocytes. There are reduced numbers of new B cells leaving the bone marrow and new T cells leaving the thymus, reduced proportions of naive B and T cells, and reduced antigen receptor repertoire. A small percentage of people with A–T also may have elevated levels of IgM in combination with IgG and/or IgA deficiency. When this is the presenting symptom in infants or during childhood, the diagnosis of A–T can be

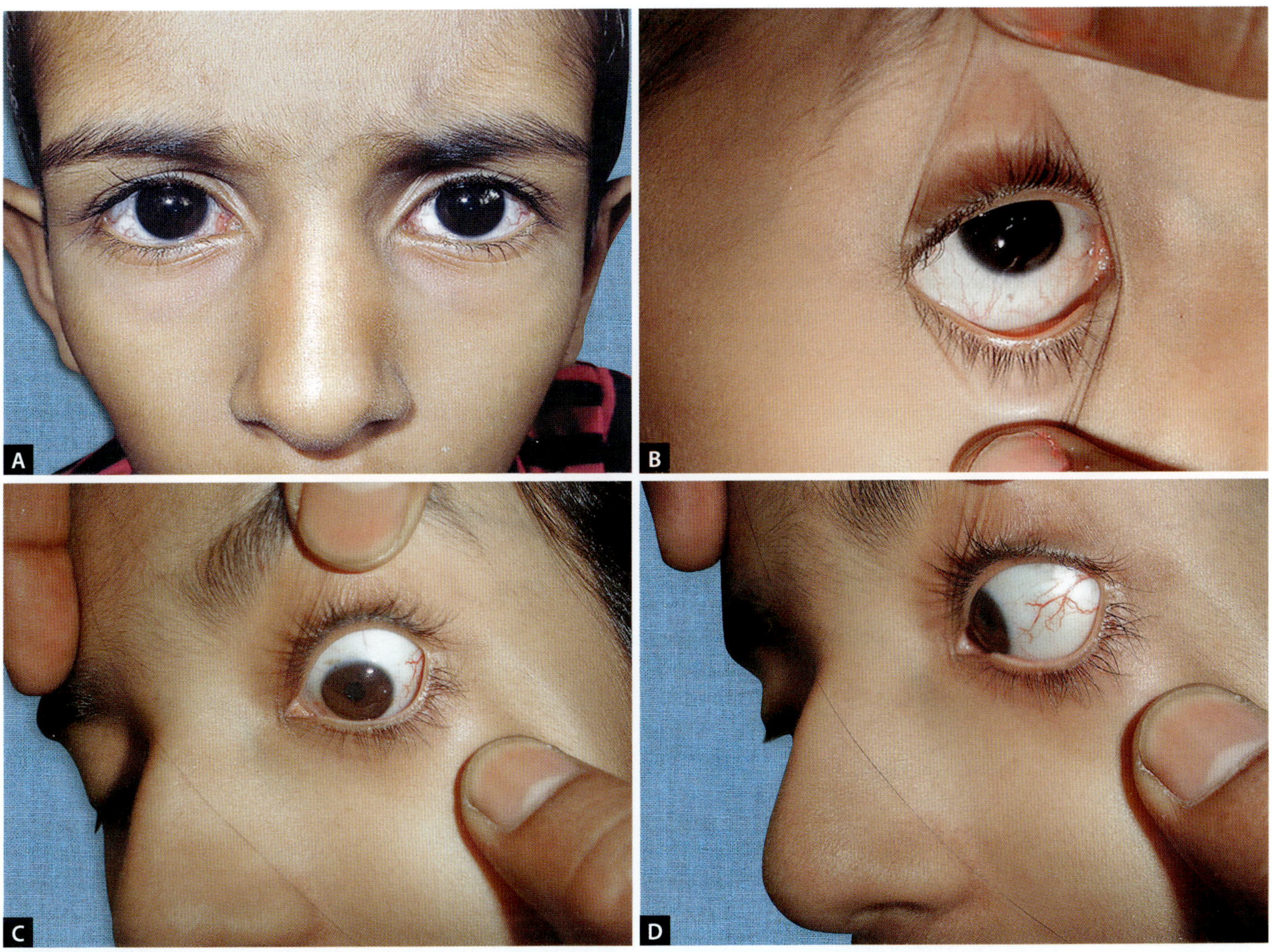

Figs. 1A to D: (A) Ataxia–telangiectasia, note conjunctival telangiectasia; (B) Ocular telangiectasia in a child with ataxia telangiectasia; (C) Ocular telangiectasia, close-up view; (D) Ocular telangiectasia, further close-up view.

"Perfection is not attainable, but if we chase perfection we can catch excellence." **—Vince Lombardi**

confused with that of hyper IgM syndrome. In the majority of individuals with A–T, the immunologic abnormalities do not deteriorate over time, but approximately 10% will develop more severe problems most often with humoral immunity. Sinopulmonary infections are common in people with A–T. All children with A–T should have their immune system evaluated to detect those with severe problems that require treatment to minimize the number or severity of infections. People with A–T have an increased risk of developing autoimmune or chronic inflammatory diseases. This risk is probably a secondary effect of their immunodeficiency and not a direct effect of the lack of ataxia telangiectasia mutated (ATM) protein. The most common examples of such disorders in A–T include immune thrombocytopenia (ITP), several forms of arthritis, and vitiligo. Fewer than 10% of people with A–T develop chronic cutaneous granulomas that are thought to be due to disordered inflammation.

CARTILAGE–HAIR HYPOPLASIA

Cartilage–hair hypoplasia is an autosomal recessive disorder, characterized by short stature, metaphyseal dysplasia, hypotrichosis, and immunodeficiency. More than 90 different biallelic mutations in *RMRP* gene have been identified to cause this condition. Three cases previously reported from India showed novel mutations in *RMRP* gene. It is a form of metaphyseal chondrodysplasia presenting with a variable degree of cellular immune impairment, bone marrow dysplasia, short-limbed dwarfism, Hirschsprung disease, and predisposition to malignancies and light-colored hypoplastic hair.

CHÉDIAK–HIGASHI SYNDROME

Refer Chapter 16

GRISCELLI SYNDROME

Refer Chapter 16

CHRONIC GRANULOMATOUS DISEASE (FIGS. 2 TO 4)

Chronic granulomatous disease (CGD) is a congenital immunodeficiency disorder of phagocyte bactericidal function with X-linked recessive inheritance, characterized clinically by granulomatous lesions in the skin, lymph nodes, lung, liver, gastrointestinal tract, and bones. The main pathology in this disease is a defect in the subunits of nicotinamide adenine dinucleotide phosphate oxidase, whose normal functioning is essential for killing phagocytosed bacteria by neutrophils using the myeloperoxide-halide system. They develop recurrent bacterial infections by *Staphylococcus aureus, Chromobacterium violaceum, Nocardia* species, *Serratia marcescens, Legionella,* and atypical mycobacteria. Fungal infection by *Aspergillus* is also common. The nitroblue tetrazolium test is used to confirm CGD.

The disease may become apparent in the first 2 years of life or may be delayed into the second decade of life. Neonatal pustulosis may be the initial manifestation. Impetiginized periorificial rash is highly characteristic and most commonly seen around the nostrils, ears, mouth, and eyes. Firm, translucent, and papular lesions may be

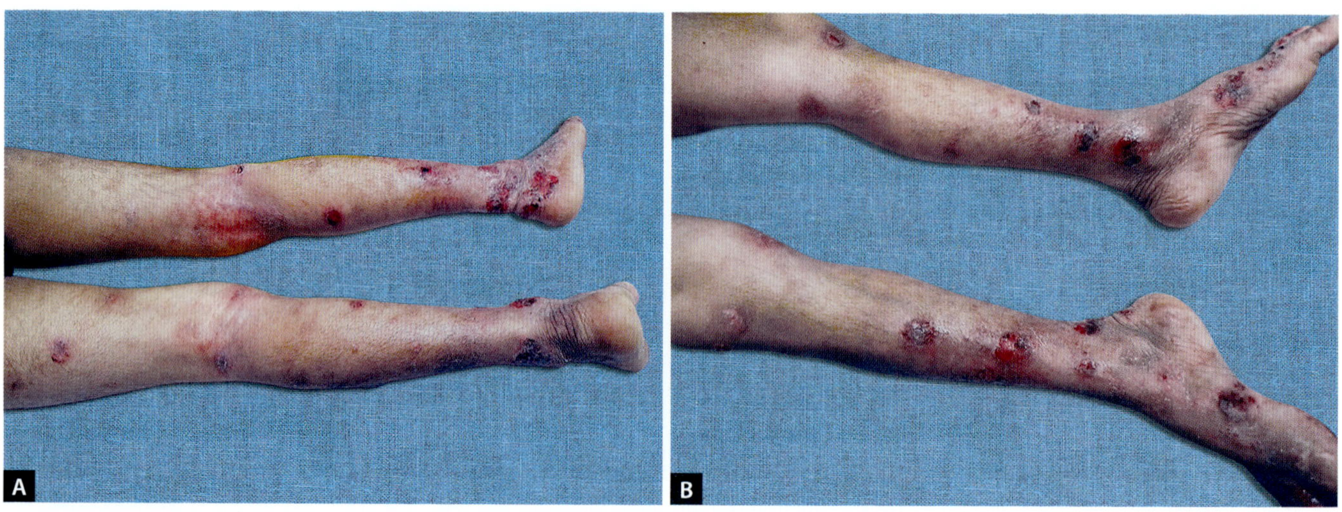

Figs. 2A and B: (A) Skin abscess in chronic granulomatous disease; (B) Same child, another view.

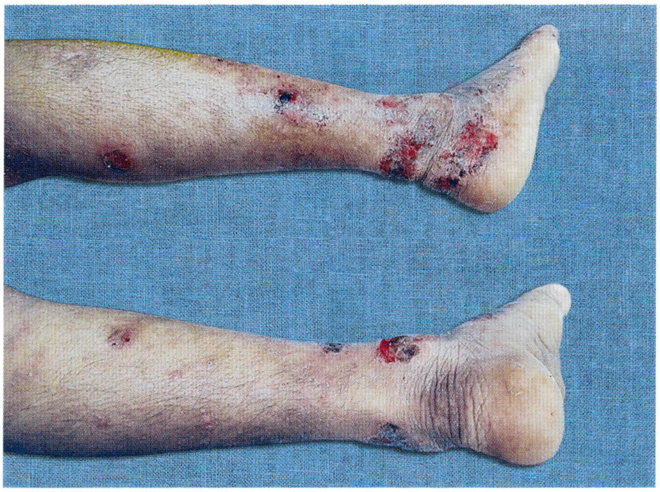

Fig. 3: Same child, close-up view of the lesions on legs.

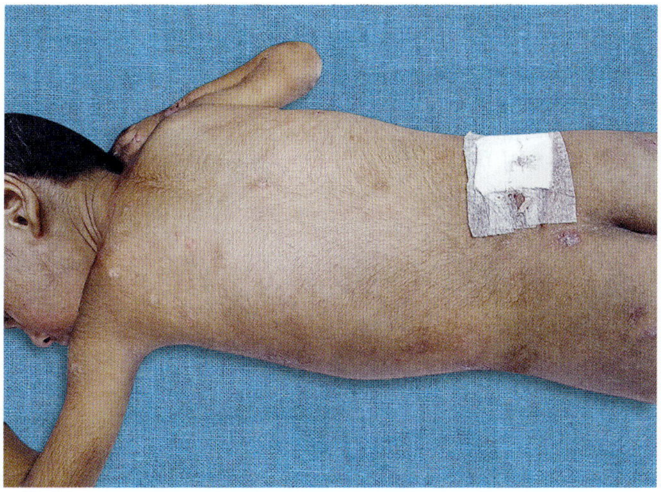

Fig. 4: Same child, back showing multiple healed pyogenic lesions.

found around the eyes, nose, lips, and on the cheeks. Other frequent pyogenic infections include liver abscesses, osteomyelitis, arthritis, pneumonia, skin sepsis, and perianal abscesses.

CHRONIC MUCOCUTANEOUS CANDIDIASIS

Refer Chapter 5

COMPLEMENT DEFICIENCY DISORDERS

The complement system represents far more than the originally thought function as a nonspecific defense mechanism against microorganisms. By virtue of extensive murine model studies and genome-wide association studies, our knowledge regarding the functions and hidden connections of complement has greatly expanded. Besides the protective role of complement, improper regulated activation of complement system can lead to extensive tissue damage. Local and systemic complement activation has been demonstrated in several skin diseases; however, whether complement activation has pathogenic significance in different skin diseases remains to be investigated. Although not all triggers of complement activation are fully elucidated in different skin diseases, antibody and immune complex deposition play an important role in (classical) complement activation. However, earlier and more recent experimental studies using mice deficient in complement components have shown involvement of complement in the pathogenesis of hypertension and psoriasis. Furthermore, preliminary results of a phase IIa clinical study in hidradenitis suppurativa (HS) shows promising results using a monoclonal anti-C5a antibody. These results indicate that complement mediates, at least in parts, in inflammatory skin diseases, in particular neutrophil-driven diseases. Therefore, inhibition of neutrophil recruitment through intervention in the C5a–C5aR axis might be the most interesting target of intervention in inflammatory skin diseases. There are various manifestations of complement deficiency disorders, e.g., skin, pulmonary, liver, reticuloendothelial system, kidney, and bone.

DiGEORGE SYNDROME

DiGeorge syndrome is a 22q11.2 microdeletion syndrome, associated with the classic triad of conotruncal cardiac anomalies, hypoplastic thymus (resulting in immunodeficiencies), and hypoplasia of the parathyroid glands (resulting in hypoparathyroidism and hypocalcemia). The other synonyms for DGS are 22q11.2 deletion syndrome (preferred terminology), velocardiofacial syndrome, conotruncal anomaly face syndrome, Sedlackova syndrome, and Cayler cardiofacial syndrome. In <1% of all patients with DGS, there is complete athymia, resulting in SCID. This is called "complete DGS." The remaining 99% are "partial" DGS, having some thymic function preserved. With a worldwide prevalence of between 1/2,000 and 1/4,000 live births, DGS is the most common microdeletion syndrome. The actual prevalence may be higher due to high clinical expressivity, accounting for underrecognition. DGS is caused due to the deletion of the genes in the DiGeorge chromosomal region (DGCR) on chromosome 22q11.2, secondary to a

"If you look at what you have in life, you'll always have more. If you look at what you don't have in life, "you'll never have enough." **—Oprah Winfrey**

nonallelic meiotic recombination during spermatogenesis or oogenesis. A great percentage (93%) of the probands has a *de novo* deletion of 22q11.2, while some (7%) inherit the 22q11.2 deletion from a parent in an autosomal dominant fashion. Rarely, <1% of the individuals with DGS have chromosomal rearrangements, such as a translocation between chromosome 22 and another autosome, involving 22q11.2. The clinical features of DGS are exceedingly variable, with over 190 features described in the literature, involving almost every organ system, thus underlining the need for sensitization among physicians and surgeons from all specialties. Of note, no phenotype occurs in 100% of the patients, as the penetrance of each clinical feature is diverse. Thus, one should be wary of excluding differential of DGS solely on the basis of absence of a particular feature. The presence of congenital heart disease (CHD; especially conotruncal anomalies), neonatal hypocalcemia (with hypoparathyroidism), and palatal defects can usually be picked up in the neonatal period, and should serve as red flags for early diagnosis. The authorities in this subject recommend that, given the high frequency of DGS among individuals with conotruncal anomalies, newborns with these heart anomalies should be routinely screened with fluorescence in situ hybridization (FISH) for 22q11.2 deletion, once other causes (Down syndrome, trisomy 13) have been ruled out. Other pointers for this condition, such as dysmorphisms, intellectual disability, and psychiatric disorders may appear only years later, often delaying the diagnosis. An emerging area of great interest is the high predilection of psychotic disorders (including schizophrenia and bipolar disorders) in adolescents and adults with DGS (25 times higher than the general population). Other than serving as a reminder to psychiatrists, this also underlines that pediatricians and geneticists dealing with DGS/suspected DGS should diligently excavate the psychiatric history of the pedigree in detail, along with the other relevant particulars.

HYPERIMMUNOGLOBULIN E SYNDROME (FIGS. 5 TO 11)

The HIES are rare primary immune deficiencies characterized by elevated serum IgE, dermatitis, and recurrent skin and lung infections. There are two forms of HIES: A dominant form caused by mutations in *STAT3* (signal transducer and activator of transcription-3), and a recessive form caused by mutations in *DOCK8* (dedicator of cytokinesis 8) or less commonly by mutations in *TYK2* (tyrosine kinase 2) gene. These two different syndromes

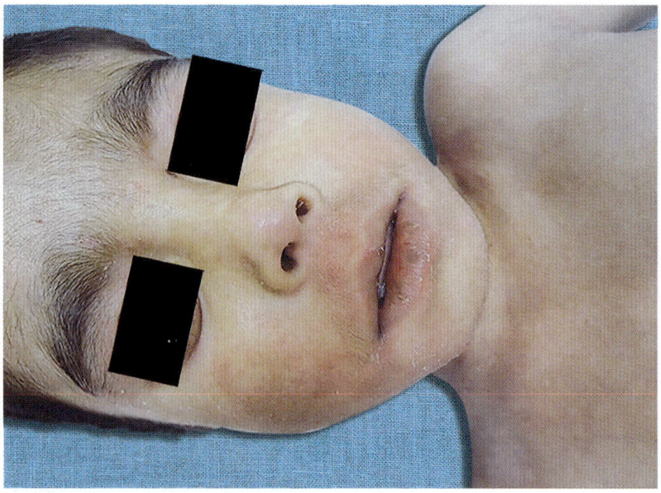

Fig. 5: Eczematous lesions over face in hyperimmunoglobulin E syndrome (HIES).

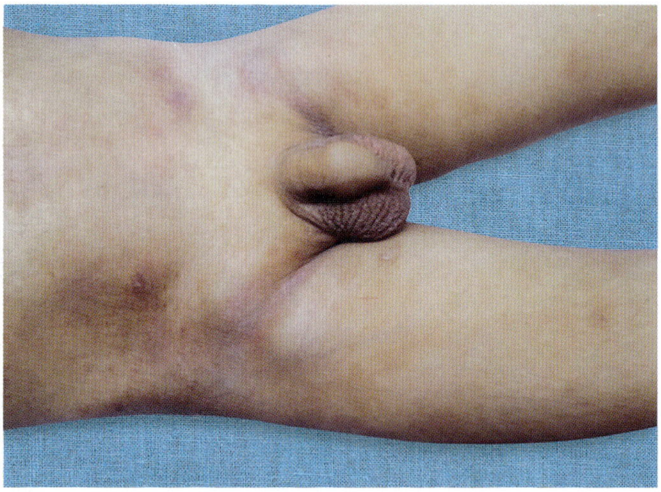

Fig. 6: Same child, eczematous lesions over lower abdomen and groin.

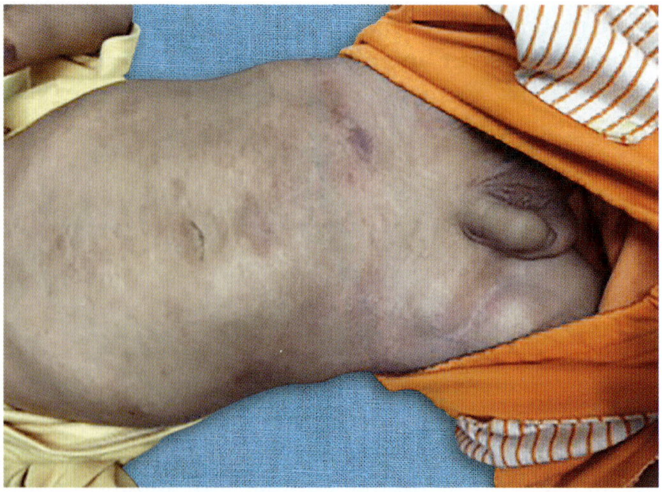

Fig. 7: Another child with hyperimmunoglobulin E syndrome (HIES) and gross inguinal lymphadenopathy.

"None of us is as smart as all of us." —**Ken Blanchard**

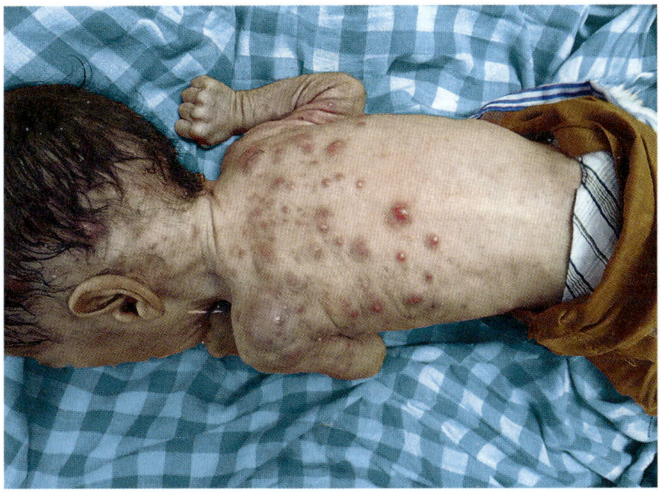

Fig. 8: Extensive abscesses in Job's syndrome.

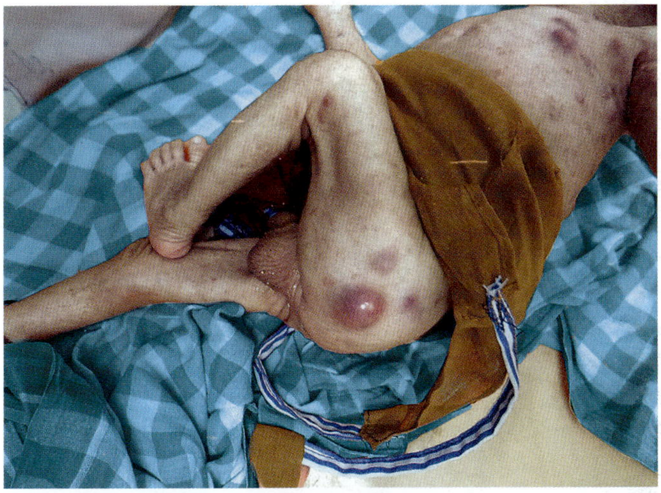

Fig. 9: Same baby, abscesses over buttocks.

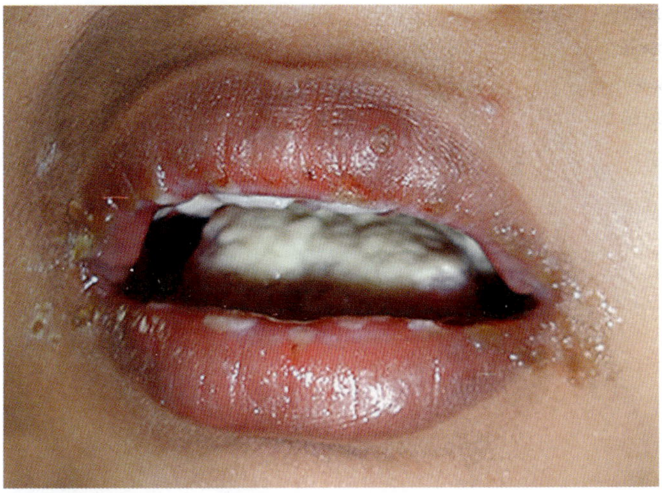

Fig. 10: Severe oral candidiasis in hyperimmunoglobulin E syndrome (HIES), note florid candidal growth over tongue and lips.

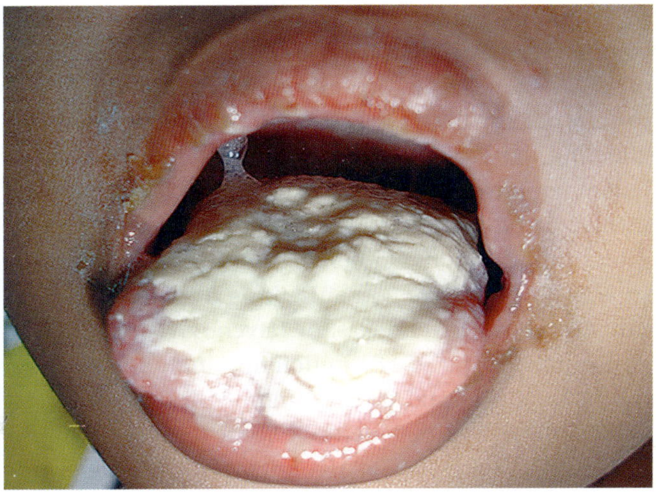

Fig. 11: Close-up view of same child.

have distinct presentation, course, and outcome, and share very little in terms of pathogenesis other than the IgE elevation. The dominant form has nonimmunologic features including skeletal, connective tissue, and pulmonary abnormalities in addition to recurrent infections and eczema. In contrast, the recessive form lacks the somatic features and has marked viral infections and neurologic complications.

AUTOSOMAL DOMINANT HIES (*STAT3* DEFICIENCY)

Hyper IgE syndrome was first described as Job's syndrome. Later on, it was found that there were extremely high serum IgE levels. Since that time, the classic triad of eczema, recurrent skin and lung infections, and high serum IgE has been expanded to include skeletal, connective tissues, cardiac and brain abnormalities. It has been found that *STAT3* mutations are responsible for most, if not all cases of autosomal dominant HIES, and these mutations have been able to explain the multisystem nature of the disease. To distinguish this dominant disease due to *STAT3* mutation from the recessive forms of HIES, and to distinguish this disease from other syndromes of IgE elevation, this disease is also referred to as *STAT3* deficiency. *STAT3* deficiency is a disease of multiorgan dysfunction. Although what brings patients to initial attention is usually eczema and recurrent infections, these individuals have abnormalities in vessels, connective tissue and skeleton. Prior to genetic testing, the diagnosis of HIES has typically been difficult to confirm unless both immunologic and somatic features exist.

"I can't change the direction of the wind, but I can adjust my sails to always reach my destination." —**Jimmy Dean**

In skin, eczema mimicking atopic dermatitis is common. A newborn rash is usually the first manifestation of *STAT3* deficiency. Pustular and eczematous rashes usually begin within the first month of life, typically first affecting the face and scalp. Boils without any sign of inflammation are characteristic of HIES type 1. Pulmonary involvement manifests in the form of recurrent pyogenic pneumonia. Mucocutaneous candidiasis is common in *STAT3* deficiency, manifesting typically as oral thrush, vaginal candidiasis, or onychomycosis. Skeletal abnormalities in *STAT3* deficiency include scoliosis, osteopenia, minimal trauma-induced fractures, hyperextensibility, and degenerative joint disease. Scoliosis occurs in about 75% of patients, typically emerging during adolescence in a pattern similar to that of idiopathic scoliosis. Hyperextensibility of both the large and small joints is frequent, and may be related to the early development of severe degenerative joint disease, particularly of the spine, that we have seen in several patients in their 20s to 40s.

IPEX SYNDROME (FIGS. 12 TO 14)

Immunodysregulation polyendocrinopathy enteropathy X-linked (IPEX) recessive disease/syndrome occurs due to defect in transcription factor FOXP3. The disorder is one of the autoimmune polyendocrinopathy syndromes. It manifests with autoimmune enteropathy, psoriasiform or eczematous dermatitis, autoimmune polyendocrine syndrome, etc. Presenting features may be lymphadenopathy, eczema, hypothyroidism, diarrhea, and a host of other conditions.

There is practically no treatment for IPEX syndrome. A successful bone marrow transplantation is the only hope.

LEUKOCYTE ADHESION DEFICIENCIES

Leukocyte adhesion deficiency 1 (LAD-1) is a rare autosomal recessive disorder of leukocyte function. LAD-1 affects about 1 per 10 million individuals and is characterized by recurrent bacterial and fungal infections and depressed inflammatory responses despite striking blood neutrophilia. Patients with the severe clinical form of LAD-1 express <0.3% of the normal amount of the β2-integrin molecules, whereas patients with the moderate phenotype may express 2–7%. Skin infection may progress to large chronic ulcers with polymicrobial infection, including anaerobic organisms. The ulcers heal slowly, require months of antibiotic treatment, and

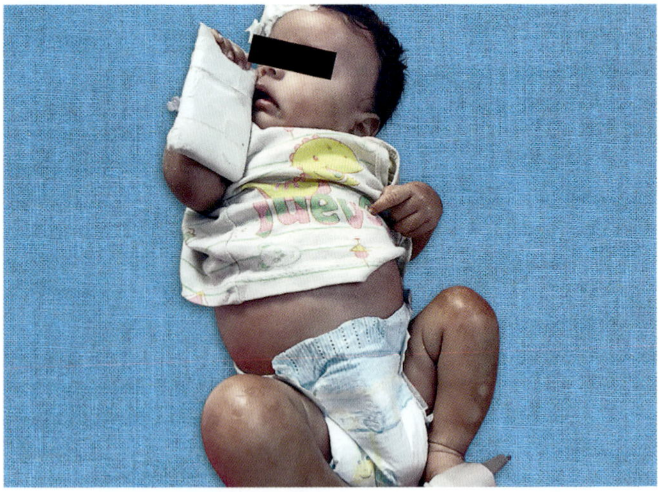

Fig. 12: IPEX syndrome in an 8-month-old baby. (IPEX: immune dysregulation, polyendocrinopathy, enteropathy, X-linked)

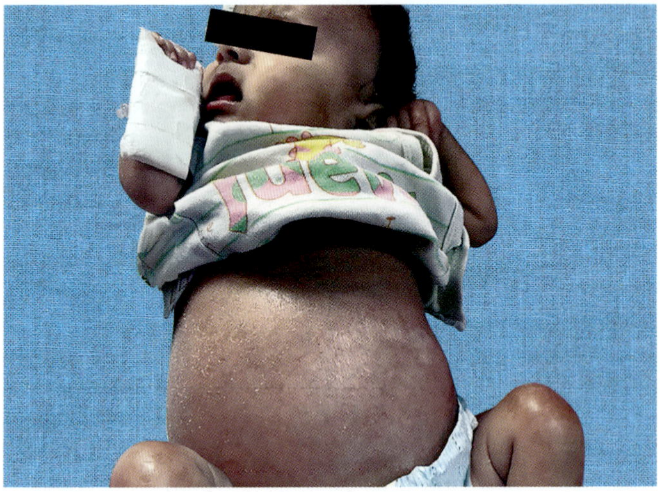

Fig. 13: Same baby, note psoriasiform lesions over abdomen.

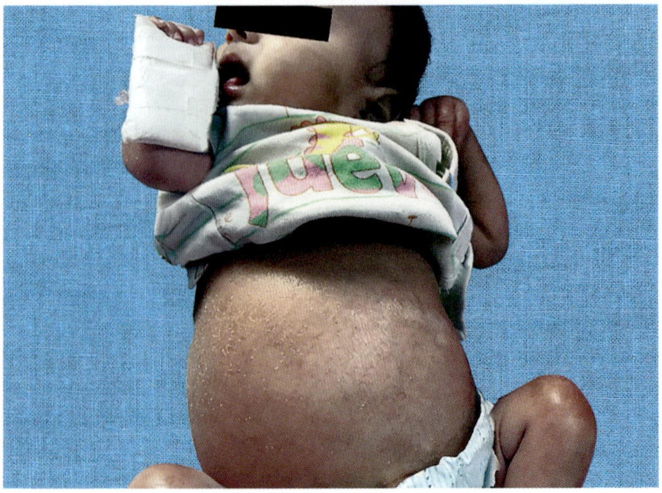

Fig. 14: Same baby, close-up view.

"Believe you can and you're halfway there." **—Theodore Roosevelt**

often require plastic surgical grafting. The diagnosis of LAD-1 is established most readily by flow cytometric measurements of surface CD11b in stimulated and unstimulated neutrophils using monoclonal antibodies directed against CD11b. Pyoderma gangrenosum (PG) is an uncommon condition characterized by recurrent sterile, inflammatory skin ulcers. Commonly, PG occurs in the context of inflammatory bowel disease or rheumatic, hematologic, or immunologic disorders.

SEVERE COMBINED IMMUNODEFICIENCY

Refer Chapter 7

WISKOTT–ALDRICH SYNDROME (FIGS. 15 TO 22)

Wiskott–Aldrich Syndrome is a genetically determined X-linked recessive disorder characterized by a triad of: (1) recurrent infections with a variety of organisms, (2) moderate-to-severe chronic microthrombocytopenia, and (3) eczema. The exact reason for the immunologic and platelet defect is unknown, but the absence of a 115,000-dalton glycoprotein from both platelet and lymphocyte membrane suggests that the basic problem lies in the pluripotent stem cell. Apart from the classical X-linked inheritance, sporadic cases have been described. The affected males invariably used to die in childhood at an average age of 4 years. But now there is hope for these children from allogenic bone marrow transplantation.

The most striking immunologic abnormality consistently found is an inability to form antibodies to carbohydrate antigens. As the disease progresses, poor

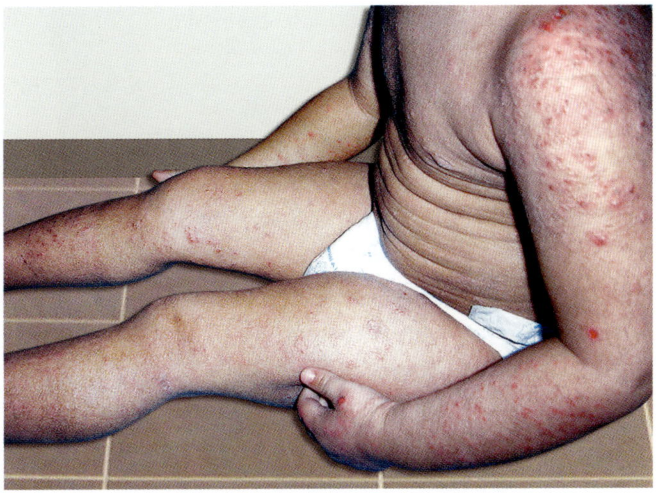

Fig. 16: Same girl, note eczema and hemorrhagic lesions.

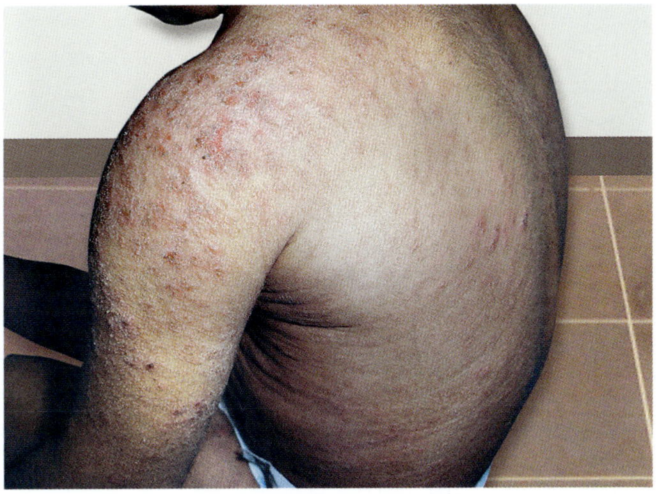

Fig. 17: Lesions over shoulder.

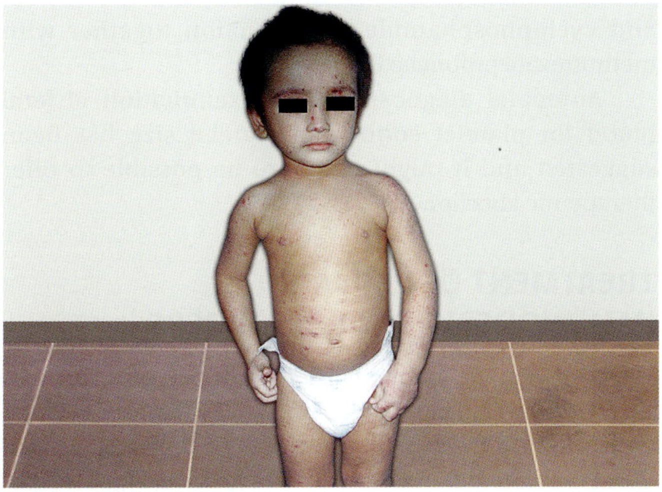

Fig. 15: Wiskott–Aldrich syndrome in a 3-year-old girl.

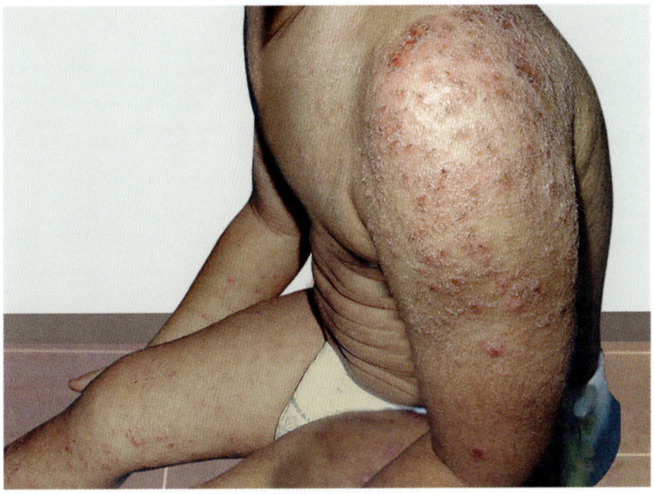

Fig. 18: Close-up view.

"To handle yourself, use your head; to handle others, use your heart." **—Eleanor Roosevelt**

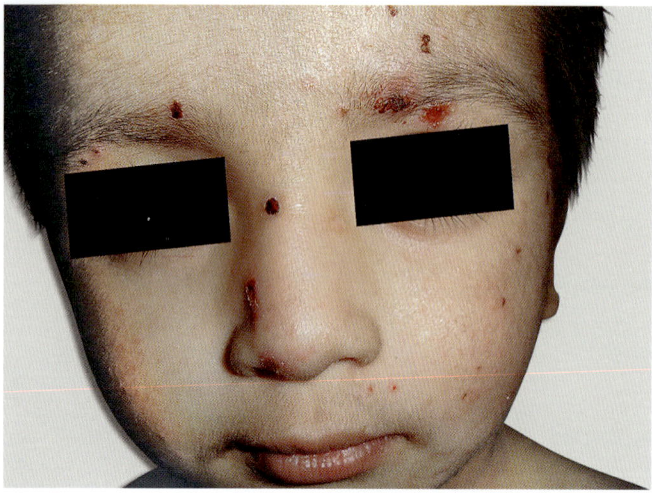

Fig. 19: Hemorrhagic lesions over face.

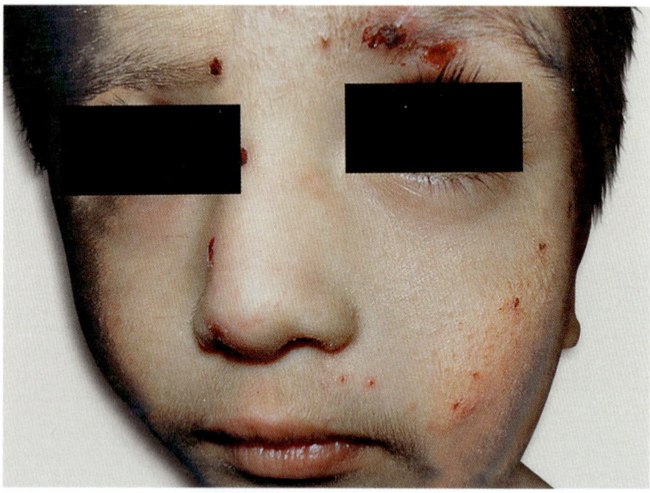

Fig. 20: Close-up view of face.

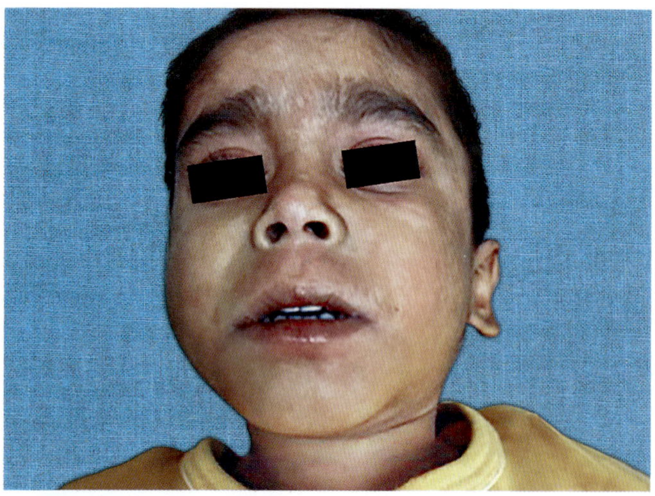

Fig. 21: Wiskott–Aldrich syndrome, note predominantly eczema over face.

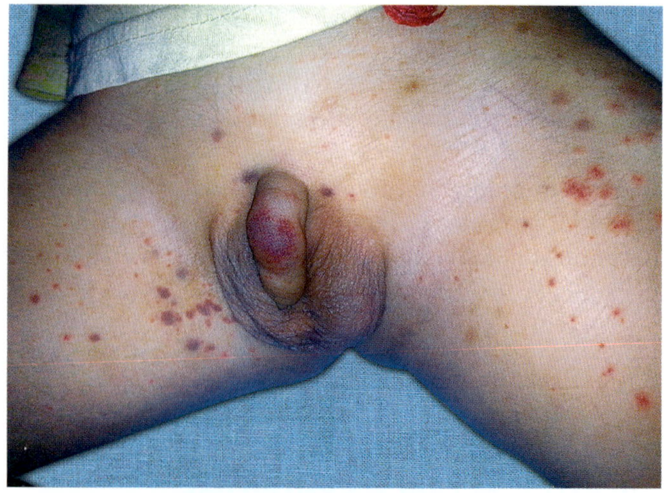

Fig. 22: Wiskott–Aldrich syndrome, note predominantly purpuric lesions over groin and thighs.

responses to other antigens are also found. In the first year of life, antibody levels are normal, sometimes with high IgA and IgE levels. Subsequently most patients have a low level of IgM with normal level of IgG and high levels of IgA and IgE.

The basic therapy includes antibiotics, pulmonary hygiene, and symptomatic treatment for the skin lesions. Platelet transfusions are helpful but all blood products should be irradiated with 3,000 rads before infusion to decrease the risk of graft-versus-host diseases.

Bone marrow transplantation is the treatment of choice when a normal histocompatible sibling donor is available. Complete hematologic and immunologic reconstitution has been achieved with allogenic bone marrow transplantation. Problems of graft-versus-host reaction have been overcome with the use of busulfan and cyclophosphamide, or diethyl-myelran and cyclophosphamide for induction together with methotrexate prophylaxis.

Antenatal diagnosis by the examination of fetal blood for platelet count and platelet size has been suggested and it might in future be possible to offer therapeutic abortion.

TREATMENT OF PRIMARY IMMUNODEFICIENCY DISORDERS

The treatment of immunodeficiencies depends on the type, severity, and clinical manifestations. The most common immunodeficiency, specific IgA deficiency, which affects one in 700 individuals, is usually asymptomatic, tends to be found incidentally, and requires no treatment. However, most immunodeficiencies do require treatment. With respect to infections, prophylactic antimicrobials (antibiotics, antifungals, and occasionally antivirals) are used to prevent infections, and the choice of agent should be guided by previous microbiological sensitivities. Aggressive treatment of breakthrough infection is necessary, often with prolonged courses of antimicrobials. When antimicrobials alone cannot prevent infections, immunoglobulin replacement therapy can be initiated in patients with antibody deficiency or dysfunction. Immunoglobulin can be delivered intravenously or subcutaneously, depending on comorbidities and patient preference. Adenosine deaminase (ADA) SCID can be partially treated with replacement ADA enzyme injections, restoring the function of the defective enzyme. HSCT remains the definitive treatment for all types of SCID and the preferred treatment option for many monogenic PIDs that present in childhood. The decision to undertake HSCT is influenced by multiple factors, not least the recipient's overall condition, their ability to tolerate myeloablative chemotherapeutic conditioning regimens and the availability of a haplotype-matched donor. Cell-based gene therapy remains in its infancy, but data from pediatric patients with SCID and chronic granulomatous disease show great promise. In the context of PID, the greatest advantage of gene therapy is that an autologous stem cell transplant can be performed with gene-modified hemopoietic stem cells, removing the requirement for a matched donor and the risk of graft rejection and graft-versus-host disease. An emerging field in PID is the management of complications of immune dysregulation. Immunosuppressive drugs are frequently required to treat complications of CVID such as lymphocytic infiltrative pneumonia, granulomatous disease, and autoimmune cytopenias. A delicate balance must be struck between the risks and benefits of immunosuppression in patients prone to infection who also have immune dysregulation. Special mention should be made of the role of genomics in PID. The rapid reduction in cost and the speed at which genomic investigations can now be performed has revolutionized PID diagnostics and approaches to treatment. Whole-exome and whole-genome sequencing have yielded molecular diagnoses in patients who previously had unclassified immune deficiencies, allowing informed genetic counseling for affected families and directing therapeutic management. Moreover, novel immune deficiencies defined by genomic techniques have improved our understanding of basic immunology, affording the opportunity to use rational therapeutics directly targeted at the underlying immunological defect (e.g., abatacept for *CTLA-4* and *LRBA* mutations).

CONCLUSION

Skin disorders are a prominent feature in PIDs. Earlier diagnosis of PIDs can be facilitated by recognition of specific skin conditions as signal function of PIDs in combination with the current warnings signs for PIDs or by recognizing PID-specific clusters of skin conditions. We provide a support tool to use in clinical practice that should raise awareness of PIDs based on the presenting skin manifestations. Limited data are available on *S. aureus*-associated skin disorders and atopy in PIDs. Since most of PIDs manifest for the first time in infancy or childhood, a thorough knowledge about them is mandatory for all practicing pediatricians, dermatologists, especially pediatric dermatologists.

SUGGESTED READINGS

1. Abdelhakim S, Cafone J, Basak RB. Cutaneous manifestations of primary immunodeficiency. Ind J Pediatr Dermatol. 2017;18:155-9.
2. de Wit J, Brada RJK, van Veldhuizen J, Dalm VASH, Pasmans SGMA. Skin disorders are prominent features in primary immunodeficiency diseases: A systematic overview of current data. Allergy. 2019;74:464-82.
3. Dhouib NG, Khaled MB, Ouederni M, Besbes H, Kouki R, Mellouli F, et al. Meditrr J Hematol Infect Dis. 2018; 10:e2018031.
4. Moin A, Farhoudi A, Moin M, Pourpak Z, Bazargan N. Cutaneous manifestations of primary immunodeficiency diseases in children. Iran J Allergy Asthma Immunol. 2006;5:121-6.
5. Shields AM, Patel S. The primary Immunodeficiency Disorders. Medicine. 2017;45:597-604.

"When you reach the end of your rope, tie a knot in it and hang on." —**Franklin D Roosevelt**

CHAPTER

24

Miscellaneous Dermatoses

ACROCHORDON (FIGS. 1 AND 2)

Acrochordons, also called as skin tags, are benign growths from the skin seen more commonly in adults, but recently the incidence has been increasing in children and adolescent age group. Acrochordons in children have been associated with childhood and teenage obesity, type 1 diabetes, abnormal lipid profile, and genetic disorders such as Birt–Hogg–Dube syndrome and tuberous sclerosis. They present as small-to-large, pedunculated hyperpigmented growths on the sides of neck, axillae, and groin region.

CHILBLAINS (FIGS. 3 TO 5)

Chilblains are mostly seen in extreme cold weather and environment and are very common among people living in hilly areas. They are more common in adolescents or adults rather than children. They mostly affect women/girls. Chilblains are the result of an abnormal reaction to cold and are usually localized to acral sites. The lesions are often itchy and usually tender, erythematous, and inflammatory, and in severe cases, they may blister or ulcerate. Many factors have been implicated in the etiology, varying from genetic, hormonal to increase in nerve bundles, persistent cold-induced constriction of the large cutaneous arterioles, and persistent dilatation of the smaller, more superficial vessels. Histopathologically, chilblains are characterized by edema of the papillary dermis, a perivascular lymphocytic infiltrate, and thickening of the blood vessel walls with intimal proliferation leading to obliteration of vascular lumen.

The treatment of chilblains remains unsatisfactory. Nifedipine and to a lesser extent, diltiazem, both calcium-channel blockers, are reported to be effective. Repeated intake of lukewarm water, milk, tea, coffee, etc., and wearing warm clothes and woolen gloves, particularly in the evening and at night time, are useful practice. Most importantly, the patients should be advised not to expose their hands and feet directly to heat (fire, room heater, hot water, etc.), as these are expected to aggravate the condition.

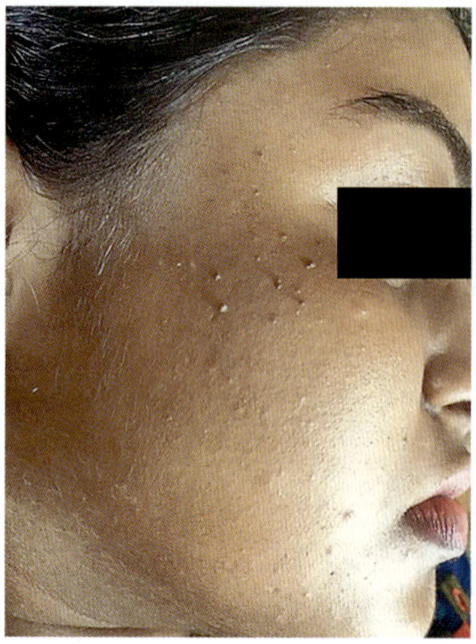

Fig. 1: Acrochordon over face.

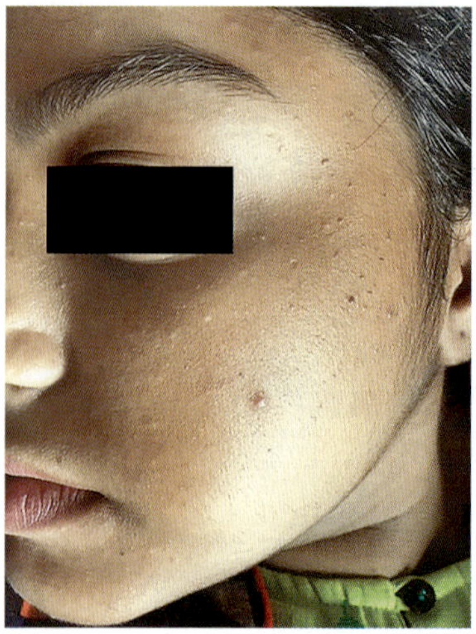

Fig. 2: Same girl—another view.

"If you don't like how things are, change it. You are not a tree." **—Jim Rohn**

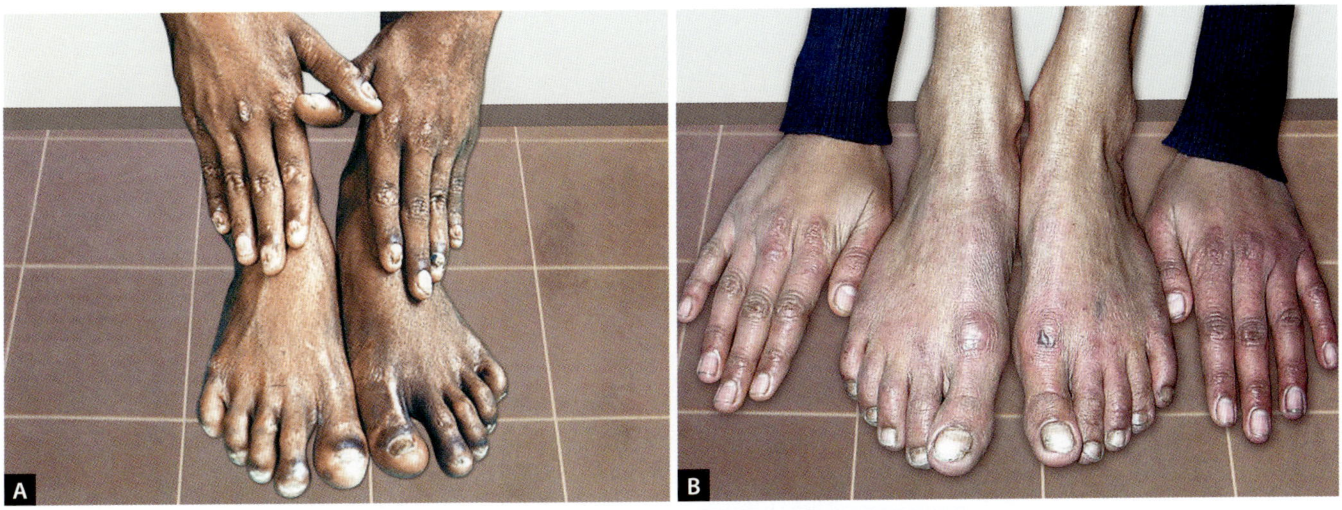

Figs. 3A and B: Chilblains—note both hands and feet involved.

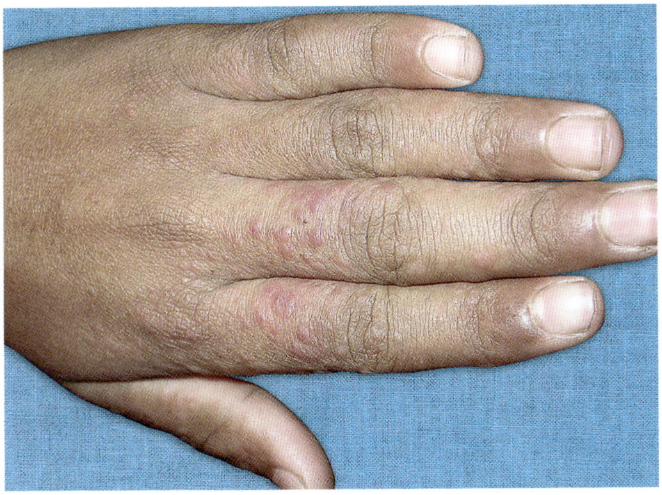

Fig. 4: Chilblains—erythematous papules over dorsum of hand.

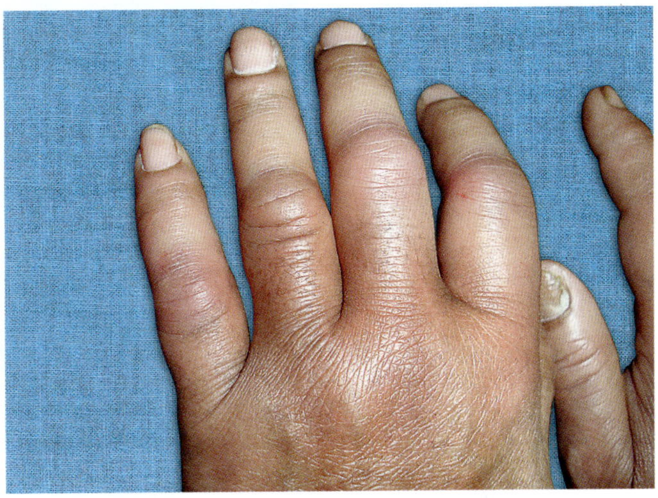

Fig. 5: Chilblains—erythematous swollen edematous fingers.

WISKOTT–ALDRICH SYNDROME (FIGS. 6 AND 7)

Wiskott–Aldrich syndrome is an X-linked recessive disorder characterized by microthrombocytopenic purpura, eczema, and recurrent infections. This triad becomes apparent during the first 6 months of life. Bloody diarrhea, epistaxis, and cutaneous petechiae are particularly common. Eczema usually appears during the first month; it most commonly affects the scalp, face, flexures, and napkin area and is essentially indistinguishable from atopic eczema apart from the frequent presence of purpura and excessive bleeding from excoriations.

Management

Genetic counseling and reassurance of the parents form the cornerstone of management. For eczematous eruptions, topical corticosteroids are used along with emollients. For excruciating pruritus, antihistamines such as cetirizine or hydroxyzine are prescribed. Rotational oral antibiotics are to be prescribed to prevent secondary infection from scratching. Periodic blood or fresh platelet transfusion or plasma transfusion often helps these children. Allogenic bone marrow transplantation following ablation of bone marrow with chemotherapeutic agents helps to prolong their life span.

INFANTILE DIGITAL FIBROMATOSIS (FIGS. 8 TO 11)

Infantile digital fibromatosis (IDF) is a benign tumor of myofibroblasts that presents clinically as firm, smooth, pink, or flesh-colored nodules on one or more fingers or toes at birth or may develop at any age up to the third year.

"What you do today can improve all your tomorrows." —**Ralph Marston**

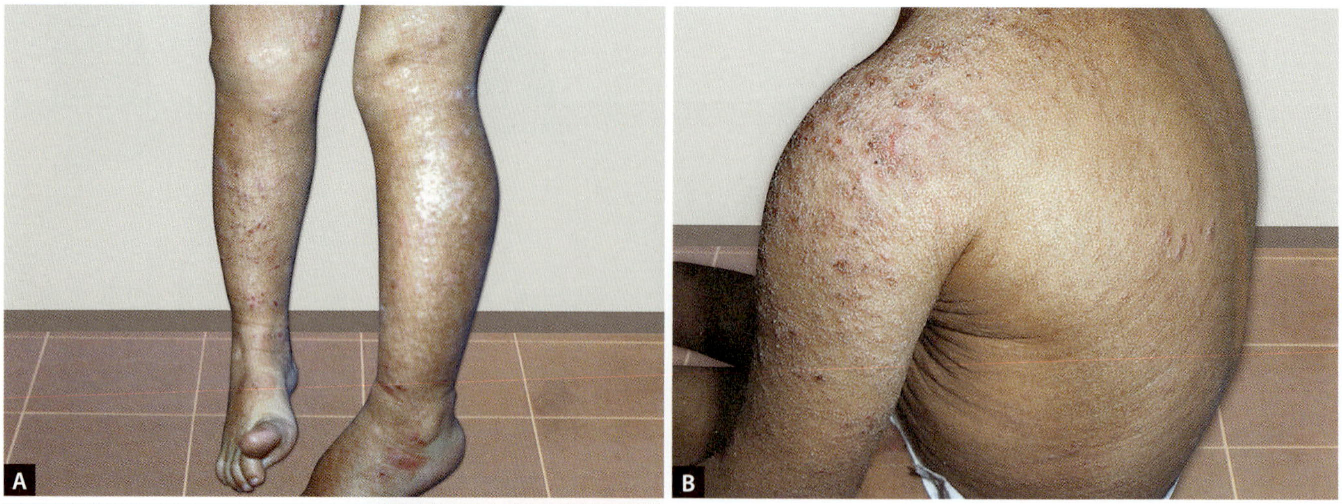

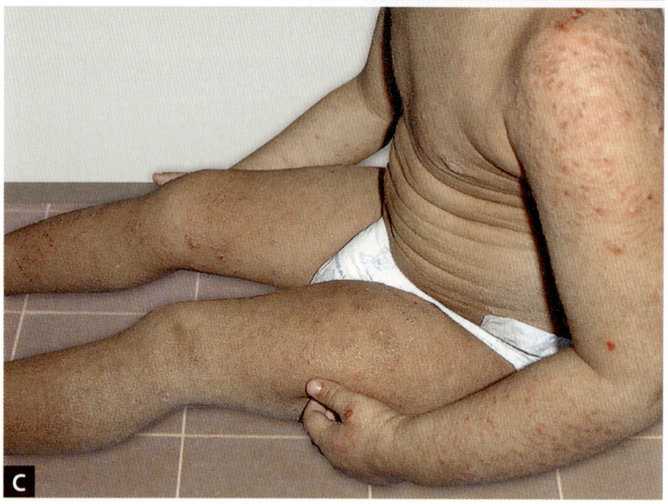

Figs. 6A to C: (A) Eczematous lesions with hemorrhagic crusts in a 3-year-old boy with Wiskott–Aldrich syndrome; (B) Upper arm and back in Wiskott–Aldrich syndrome; (C) Involvement of upper arms, thighs, and legs in Wiskott–Aldrich syndrome. Note excoriation and hemorrhagic lesions.

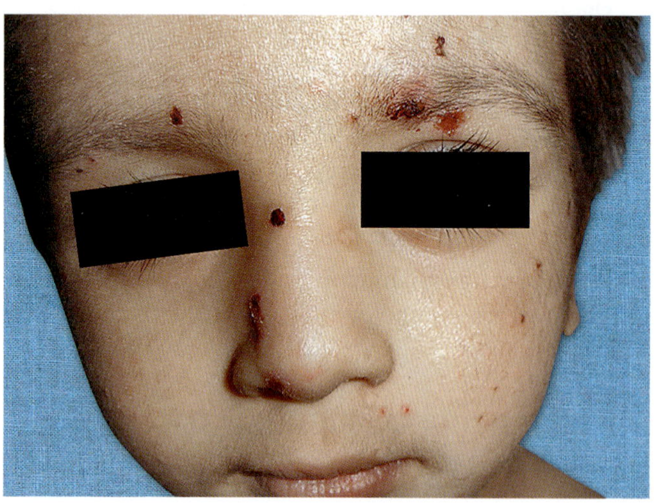

Fig. 7: Hemorrhagic papules over face in Wiskott–Aldrich syndrome.

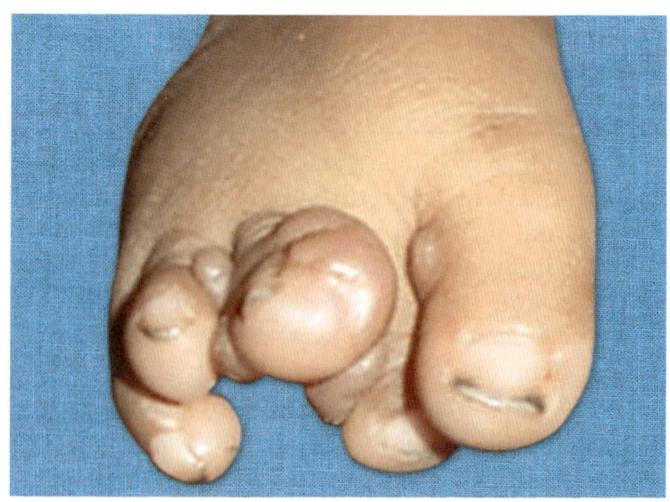

Fig. 8: Infantile digital fibromatosis; multiple skin-colored nodules on toes.

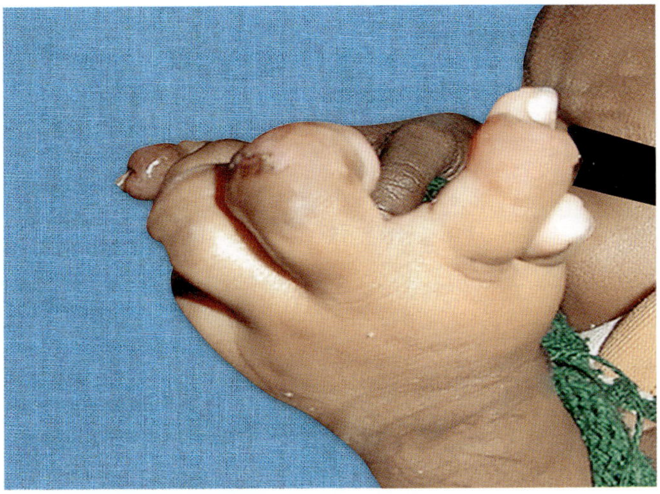

Fig. 9: Same baby with infantile digital fibromatosis. Note sparing of thumb.

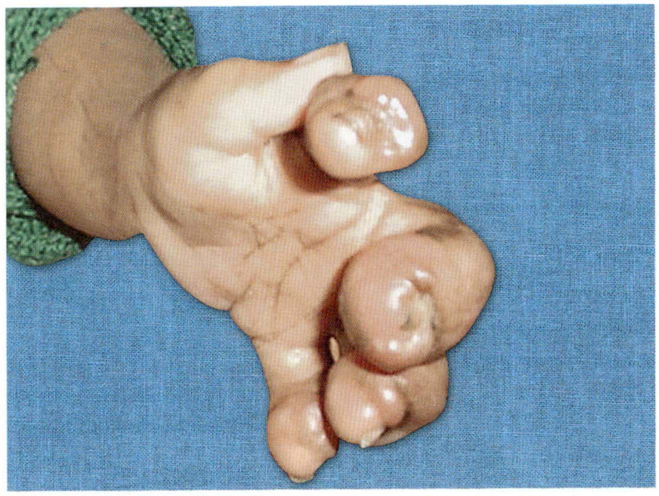

Fig. 10: Close-up view of infantile digital fibromatosis lesions.

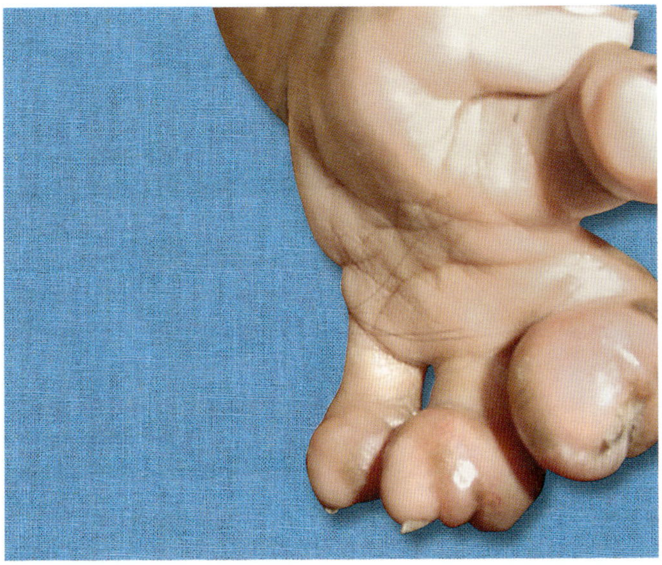

Fig. 11: Sparing of palm in infantile digital fibromatosis.

The thumbs and great toes are spared. The swellings are present on the extensor aspects or the side of the terminal phalanges and are firmly attached to the skin.

Natural History

Spontaneous regression may occur in 2–3 years.

Treatment

Explaining the condition to the parents and reassuring them are extremely important. They should be clearly told about the chances of spontaneous resolution of some of the lesions. This can avoid unnecessary and untimely surgery in them.

FRICTIONAL LICHENOID DERMATITIS (FIGS. 12 AND 13)

Frictional lichenoid dermatitis (FLD) presents in young children or adolescents as pin head-sized pale or white papules or warty lesions on the knees, elbows, and dorsal surface of the hands. The condition is mildly pruritic and has been more common in spring and summer. The probable etiology is friction from floor, walls, sand, or any other rough surfaces, and many of these children are atopic. The condition often recurs after treatment.

Treatment

The condition is treated with either a mildly potent topical steroid or tar ointment along with emollients.

HEMATOHIDROSIS (FIGS. 14 AND 15)

Hematohidrosis, also known as hemidrosis or hematidrosis, is an extremely rare episodic skin condition in which capillary blood vessels that feed the sweat glands rupture causing them to sweat blood. Historically, it has been reported by Da Vinci in a soldier under extreme stress and also in Jesus Christ at the time of crucifixion. It can occur at any part of the body with the face being the most common site. Other sites of involvement include trunk, limbs, and rarely palms, soles, and mucosa. There are also reports of bleeding from eyes and ears called as hemolacria and bloody otorrhea respectively. Bleeding can occur simultaneously at several points and the amount of bleeding is usually small. There might be weakness and mild-to-moderate dehydration from

"You will never win if you never begin." —**Helen Rowland**

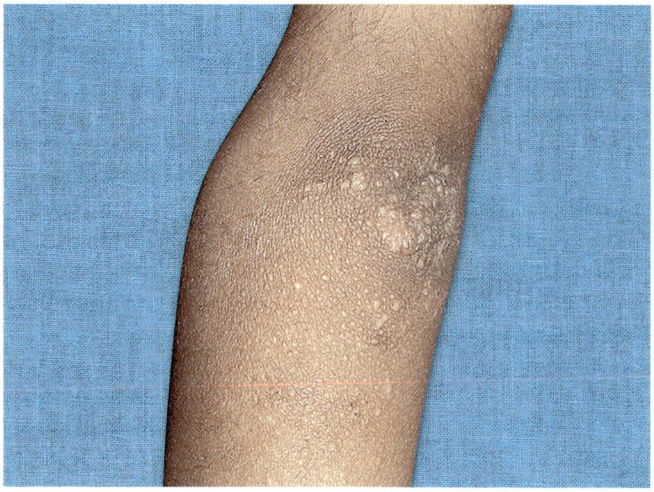

Fig. 12: Lichenoid skin-colored papules of frictional lichenoid dermatitis over elbow.

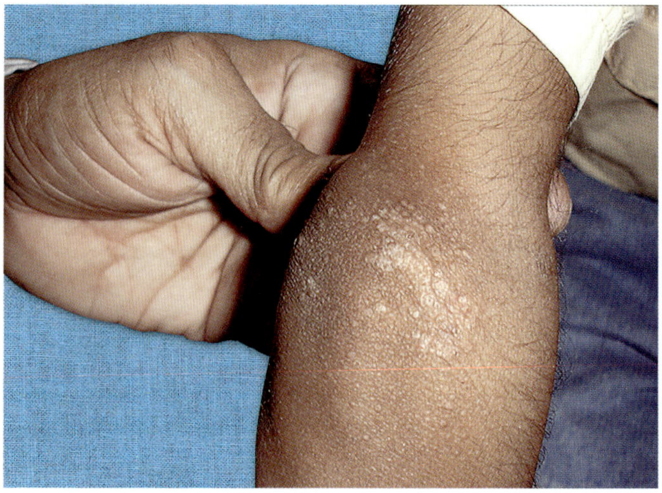

Fig. 13: Close-up view of frictional lichenoid dermatitis lesions over elbow.

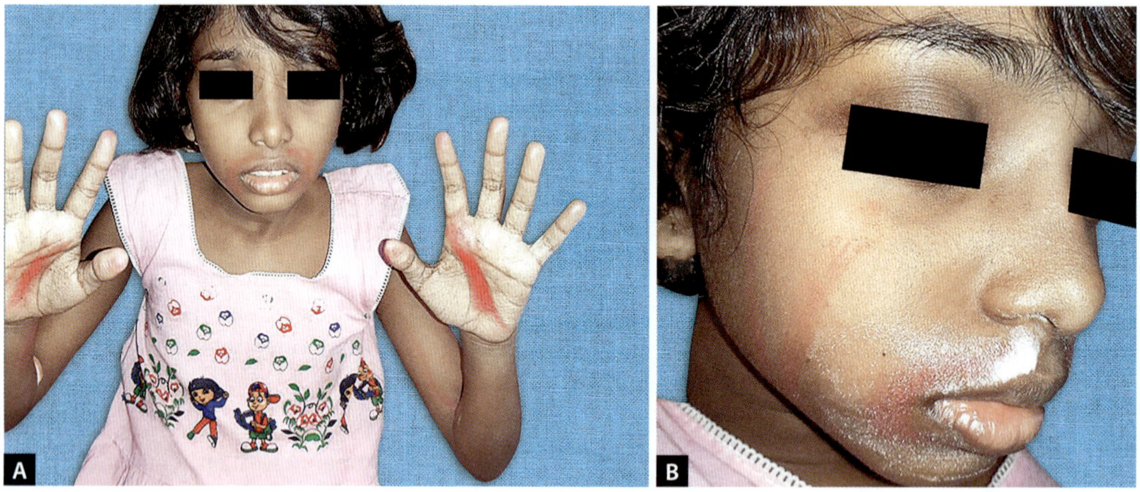

Figs. 14A and B: (A) Hematohidrosis—note blood-stained sweat over palms; (B) Same girl, look at face.

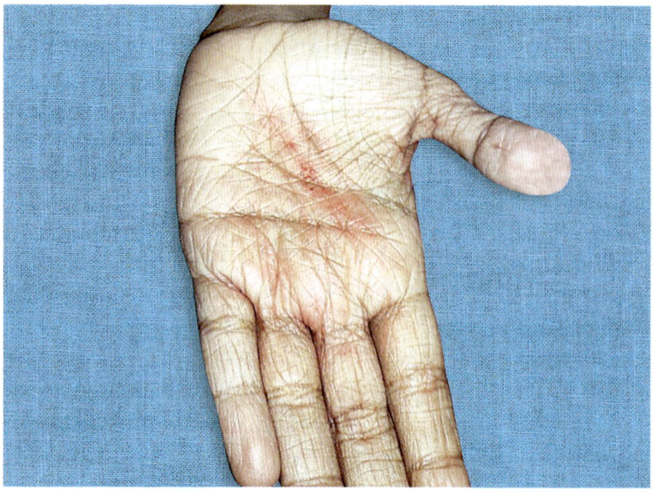

Fig. 15: Hematohidrosis, close-up view of palm.

the severe anxiety and from both blood and sweat loss in some cases. The term "hematofolliculohidrosis" has also been proposed because blood appeared along with sweat-like fluid and exuded via the follicular canals. Although the exact etiology is not known, various factors are attributed such as emotional or physical stress, systemic disorders such as vicarious menstruation and bleeding disorders such as primary thrombocytopenic purpura, psychogenic purpura, excessive exertion, trauma, psychogenic and idiopathic causes. However, even in cases with systemic etiology, psychological stressors act as a precipitating factor for bleeding. The presence of underlying bleeding disorders is called true hematohidrosis. The most common cause is acute physical or emotional stress. Few theories have been proposed explaining the

"Upon retiring, sleep as if you had entered your last sleep. Upon awakening, leave your bed behind you instantly as if you had cast away a pair of old shoes."

—Soyen Shaku

underlying mechanism of hematohidrosis. According to Dr Frederick Zugibe, multiple blood vessels arranged around the sweat glands in a net-like form constrict under pressure of stress due to activation of the sympathetic nervous system. As the anxiety passes the blood vessels dilate to the point of rupture leading the blood to go into the sweat glands which push the blood to the surface and present as droplets of blood mixed with sweat. Manonukul et al. proposed that some defects in the dermis may cause stromal weakness leading to communication of these defects with vascular spaces in the dermis which eventually dilate and enlarge as blood-filled spaces when the blood comes in. The blood then exudes out either via follicular canals or directly on to the skin surface whenever the positive pressure inside is enough. Thereafter, they collapse leaving no scar. This phenomenon waxes and wanes and thus explains why these bleedings are sometimes intermittent and self-limiting. A distinctive type of vasculitis as the underlying pathologic mechanism has also been proposed.

Diagnosis of hematohidrosis is made clinically by the presence of bloody discharge through intact skin without any obvious cause, and presence of blood components is confirmed by testing the discharge by Benzidine test. It is usually a self-limiting condition with a good prognosis. Currently, there is no specific treatment. Treatment of the underlying cause partly helps in the remission of symptoms. There are reports of good response to various drugs such as propranolol, antidepressants, atropine transdermal patch, and gauze wipes with adrenaline. Emotional support for the patient and family is important.

PALMOPLANTAR HYPERHIDROSIS (FIGS. 16A AND B)

Hyperhidrosis may be classified as primary or secondary. Primary hyperhidrosis is diagnosed after ruling out all other causes of secondary hyperhidrosis. Palmoplantar hyperhidrosis comes under the purview of localized hyperhidrosis. Emotional activity or stress increases sweating over palms and soles. Sometimes, it may be the manifestation of deep-seated mental disturbances. The sweating of palms and soles may be either phasic or continuous. The phasic hyperhidrosis is precipitated by emotional stress and strain and there is no difference in summer and winter. This type of hyperhidrosis is often complained by children and/or their parents during examinations as they face difficulty in holding pen in their hands. The continuous hyperhidrosis is more distressing in summer. Often, palmoplantar hyperhidrosis is associated with axillary hyperhidrosis. In some cases, there may be underlying thyrotoxicosis which needs to be ruled out.

Treatment

Explanation of the nature of the condition and reassurance are all that is necessary in many patients with hyperhidrosis. It is important to tell the children and their parents that it is going to improve slowly over many years. Various topical agents used are 1% formalin, 10% glutaraldehyde, and 20% aluminum chloride hexahydrate soaking for 15–20 minutes twice/day for 4–6 weeks. One of the more satisfactory methods of controlling continuous hyperhidrosis is by iontophoresis, using either tap water or anticholinergic drugs, e.g., glycopyrronium bromide.

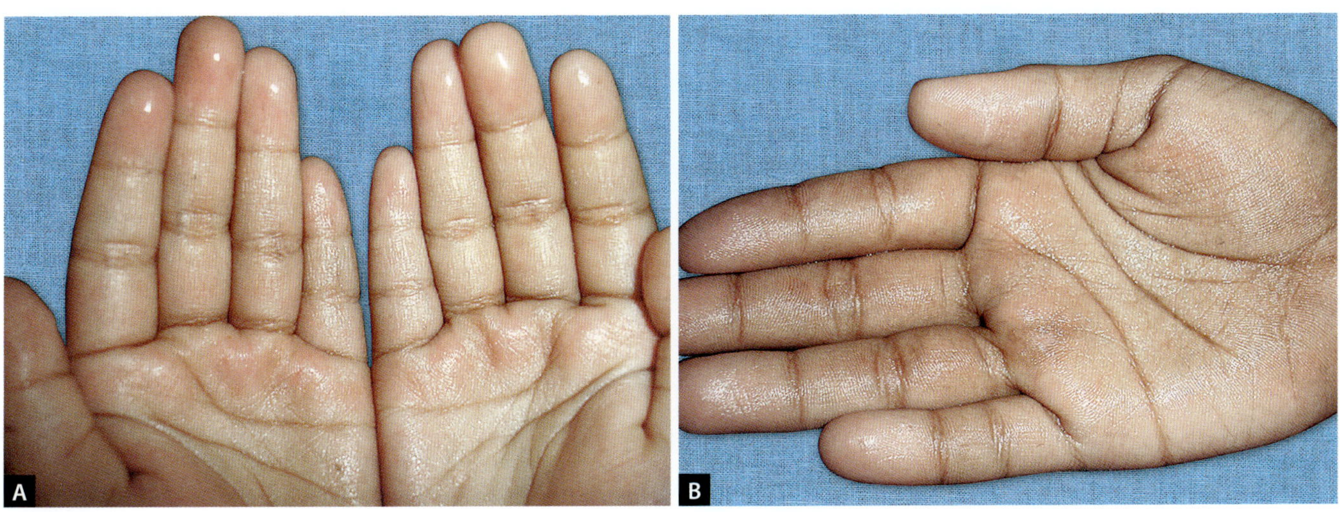

Figs. 16A and B: (A) Palmoplantar hyperhidrosis; (B) Palmoplantar hyperhidrosis, close-up view.

"One of the basic rules of the universe is that nothing is perfect. Perfection simply doesn't exist. Without imperfection, neither you nor I would exist."

—Stephen Hawking

Of late, botulinum toxin injection into the palms has been shown to reduce hyperhidrosis and the effect may last up to 6 months or even more. However, this is a painful and costly procedure. Various systemic anticholinergic atropine-like drugs are occasionally used to treat hyperhidrosis. However, their systemic adverse effects outweigh their efficacy. In very frustrating cases, even surgical methods such as sympathectomy may be undertaken.

GREEN ECCRINE HYPERHIDROSIS (FIGS. 17A AND B)

Chromhidrosis is a rare condition characterized by the secretion of colored sweat. It is caused by the deposition of lipofuscin in the sweat glands. Cases of red, blue, green, yellow, pink, and black sweat have been reported. Usually, chromhidrosis affects the apocrine glands, mainly on the face and axillae. A limited number of treatment options exist, including regular application of capsaicin cream, and prolonged relief may be provided by botulinum toxin treatment. Chromogenic pigments produced by bacteria (*Corynebacterium* in particular) are implicated in this condition, but their exact role still remains elusive. Chromhidrosis of the eccrine glands is rare; it occurs mainly after the ingestion of certain dyes and drugs.

MILIA (FIGS. 18 TO 20)

Milia are small epidermal inclusion cysts within the dermis. They are multiple, 1–2 mm, whitish, hard globoid

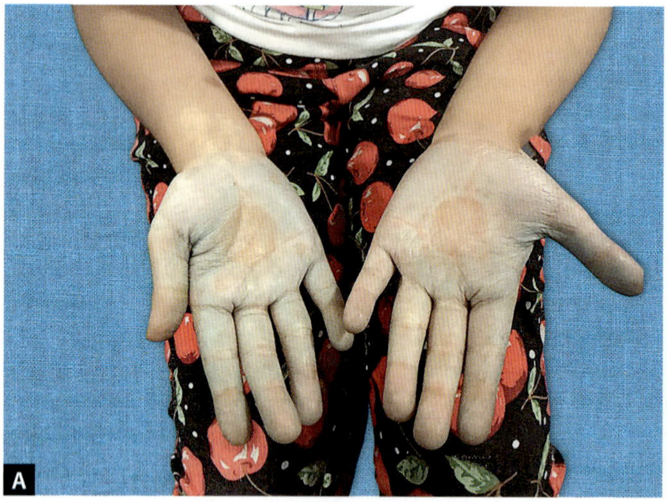
A

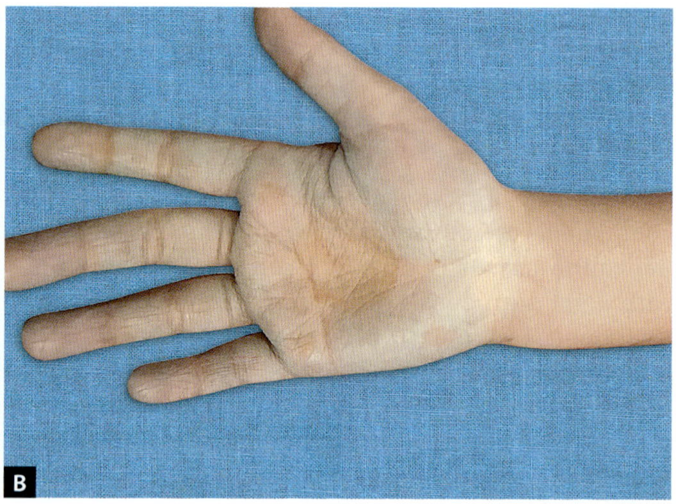
B

Figs. 17A and B: (A) Green eccrine chromhidrosis; (B) Close-up view of palm lesion.

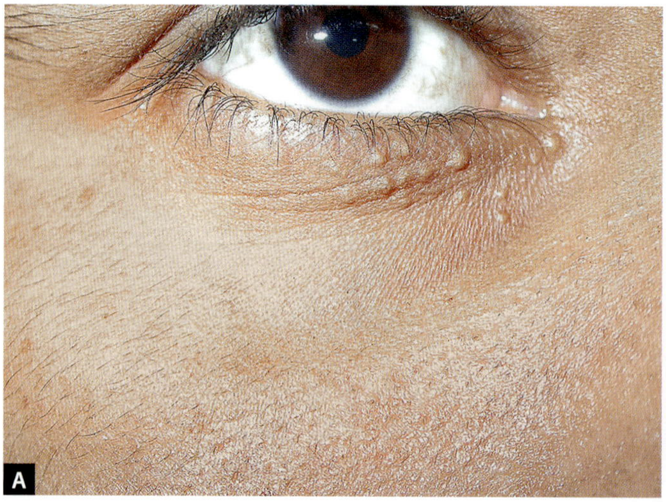
A

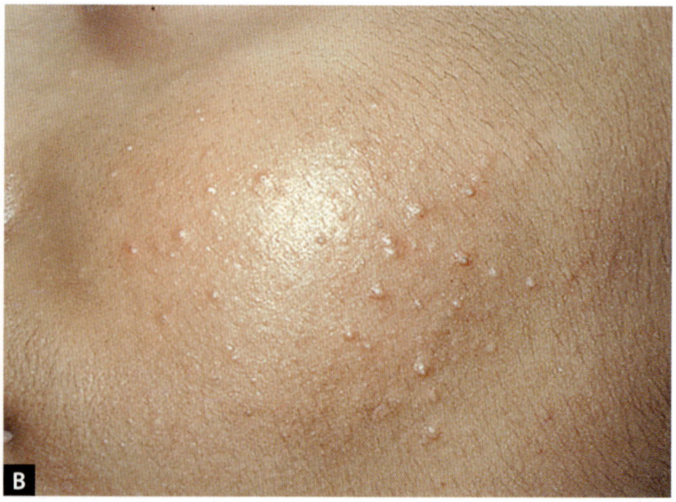
B

Figs. 18A and B: (A) Multiple milia over lower eyelid; (B) Primary milia over cheek in a young girl.

"Stop acting so small. You are the universe in ecstatic motion." —**Rumi**

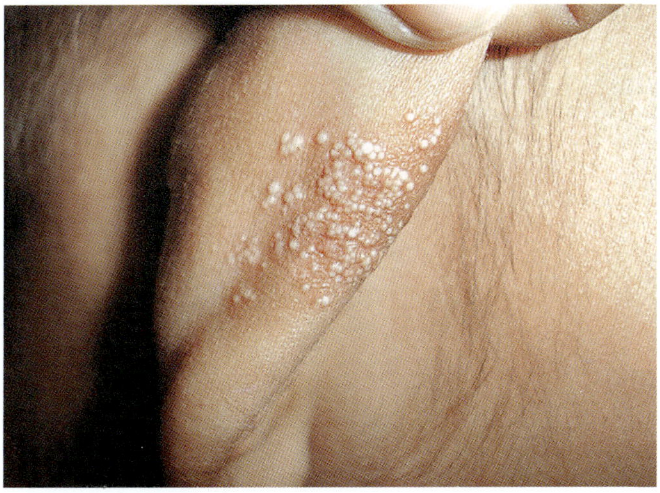

Fig. 19: Milia over pinna in a child with epidermolysis bullosa dystrophica.

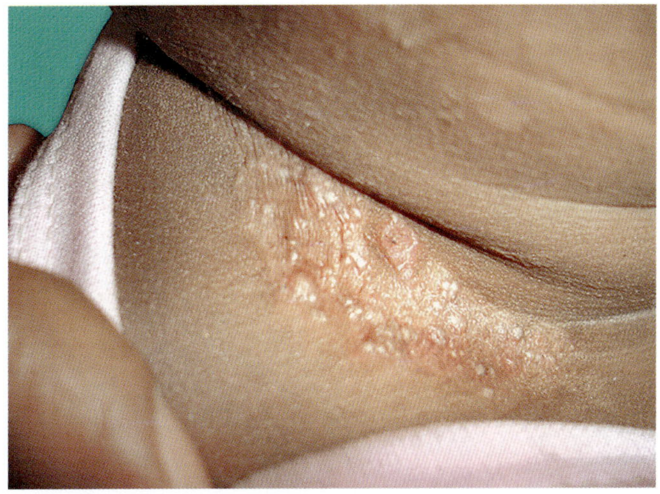

Fig. 20: Same child with milia at the border of a healed bullae in epidermolysis bullosa.

lesions arising spontaneously over face. In children and young adults, they arise following trauma or friction. Vigorous scrubbing and rubbing of face can lead to formation of milia. In some diseases where there is damage to the dermoepidermal junction, milia may form. These are often seen at the margins of the healed lesions of chronic bullous dermatosis of childhood, bullous pemphigoid, epidermolysis bullosa, etc.

Treatment

Milia can be self-resolving. It can be expressed out with a fine needle (24G or 26G) or can be destroyed by light electrodessication.

CHRONIC ARSENIC POISONING (FIGS. 21 TO 24)

Etiology and Epidemiology

Prolonged ingestion of inorganic arsenic may result in diffuse pigmentation, most intense on the trunk, where macular areas of depigmentation within areas of hyperpigmentation produce the distinctive raindrop appearance. Many cases also show arsenical keratosis. Severity of the two manifestations of arsenic poisoning is not necessarily proportionate and either may be present alone. Arsenic exposure in the first half of the 20th century was often caused by the ingestion of medical arsenic in the form of potassium arsenite (Fowler's solution) used to treat asthma and psoriasis. Today, arsenic exposure most frequently occurs because of high arsenic levels in well water either from natural sources or as a result of contamination from mining waste.

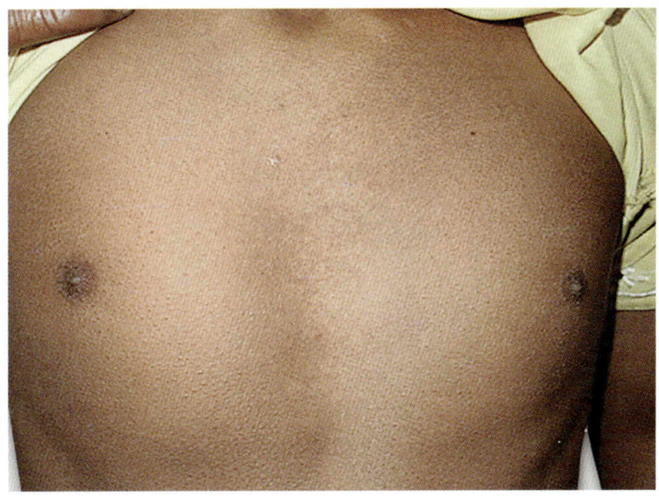

Fig. 21: Typical raindrop pigmentation in a young girl with chronic arsenic poisoning.

A considerable proportion of any population exposed to chronic arsenic intoxication develops keratosis. The frequency increases with the degree of intoxication and its tolerance. The condition is mostly reported from Bangladesh, West Bengal, and Taiwan resulting from well water contamination.

Clinical Features

The keratosis presents as corn-like punctate papules characteristically affecting the palms and soles. These gradually enlarge, thicken, and increase in number. The fingers, back of the hands, and proximal parts of the

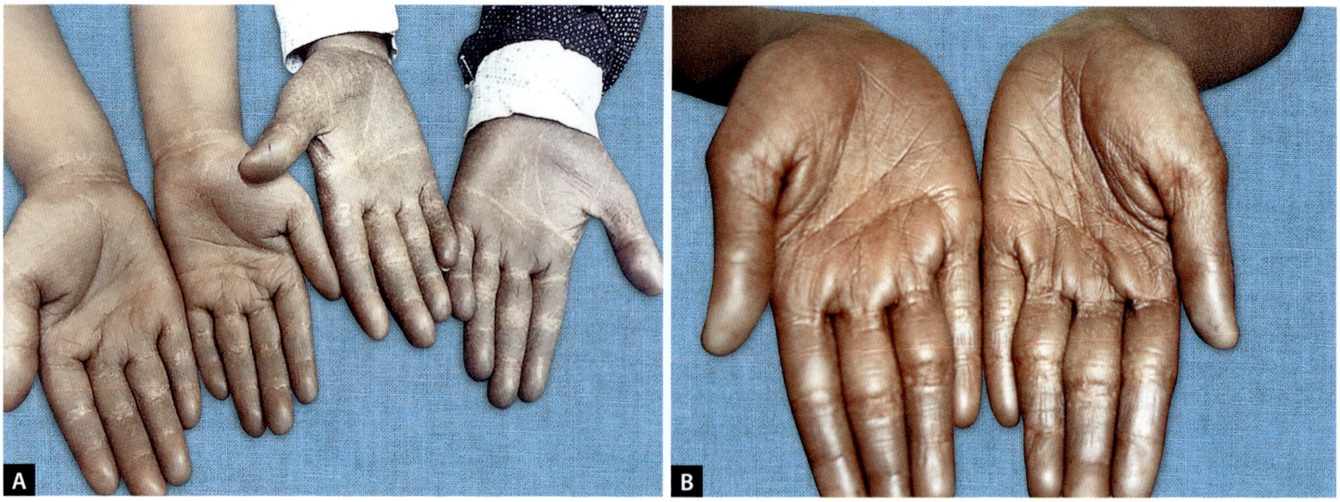

Figs. 22A and B: (A) Hands in chronic arsenic poisoning; (B) Palmar pigmentation in chronic arsenic poisoning.

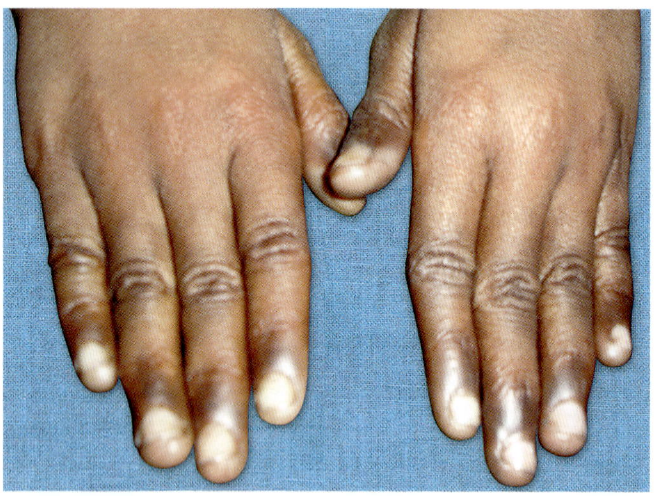

Fig. 23: Pigmentation over fingers in chronic arsenic poisoning.

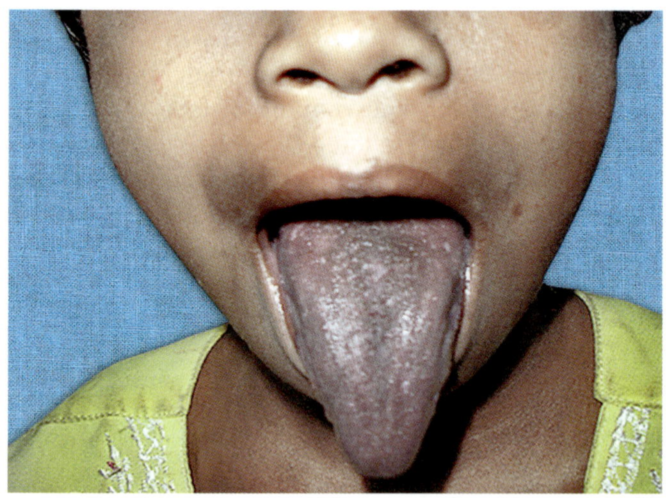

Fig. 24: Pigmentation of tongue in chronic arsenic poisoning.

extremities may be involved. Induration, inflammation, and ulceration occur when the lesions become malignant. They can be associated with Bowen's disease and multiple basal cell carcinomas on the trunk.

Differential Diagnoses

The palmar lesions have to be differentiated from the various types of punctate keratosis, e.g., disseminated punctate keratosis, Darier's disease, and lichen planus, which usually have characteristic lesions elsewhere. Plantar warts differ in being papillomatous.

Treatment

The multiplicity of the keratosis makes treatment difficult. Where it is necessary, the use of a keratolytic ointment and trimming down of the surface is helpful. Oral acitretin has shown to be beneficial in some cases. All affected patients should be examined periodically for evidence of malignant change and for signs of visceral malignancy. Stoppage of drinking contaminated water from the well is to be advocated in the patient and the community at large.

FORDYCE SPOTS (FIGS. 25 AND 26)

Fordyce spots (Fordyce disease) is a commonly observed benign condition characterized by minute yellowish macules and globoid papules that may form large plaques. They are often symmetrical and generally found on the vermilion border of the lips and oral mucosa and less commonly on glans penis or labia minora. The disorder is a manifestation of

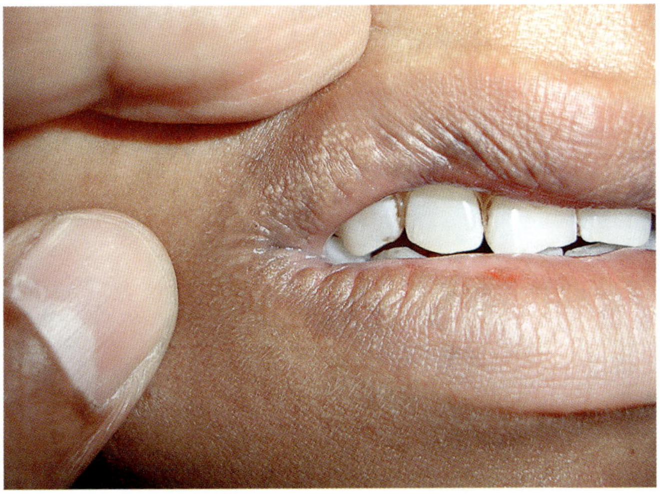

Fig. 25: Fordyce spots over lips.

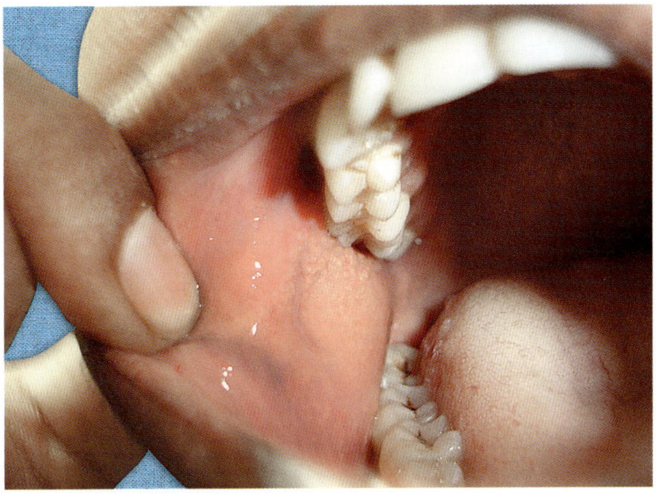

Fig. 26: Fordyce spots over buccal mucosa.

aberrant or ectopic sebaceous glands and is uncommon in young children. These become more apparent during adolescence. The disorder is asymptomatic. Explaining the condition and reassurance of the patients/parents are all that is necessary.

POLYMORPHOUS LIGHT ERUPTION (FIGS. 27 TO 31)

It is the most common of the idiopathic photosensitive disorders. It mostly occurs between 20 and 30 years of age and in lighter skin. However, these days the authors have been seeing quite a good number of children with polymorphous light eruption (PMLE). The exact etiology is not known but it is thought to be a delayed hypersensitivity reaction to UV rays in the wavelength of 290–480 nm.

The lesions usually present as polymorphic lesions usually after 24–72 hours' intense exposure to sunlight. Often a history of playing in the ground for 6–8 hours a day or going on vacation to seaside is available from the children or parents. The lesions in Indian patients mostly manifest as hypopigmented macules of various size and shape over face or extensor of the arms and forearms. The lesions are mildly itchy and a history of slight burning feeling on exposure to sun is often available. The lesions are to be differentiated with pityriasis alba and pityriasis versicolor.

The treatment is avoidance of direct sunlight exposure, application of mild-to-moderately potent corticosteroids for 2–4 weeks. For itching, antihistamines may be given. Use of a good chemical sunscreen is mandatory throughout the day (even when not going

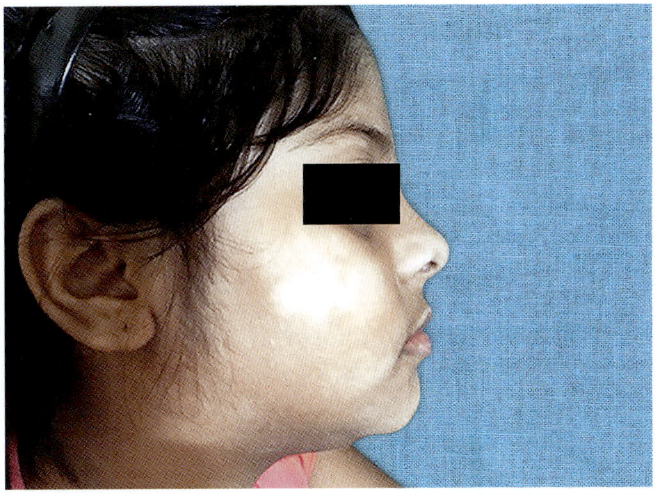

Fig. 27: Polymorphous light eruption over face, side view.

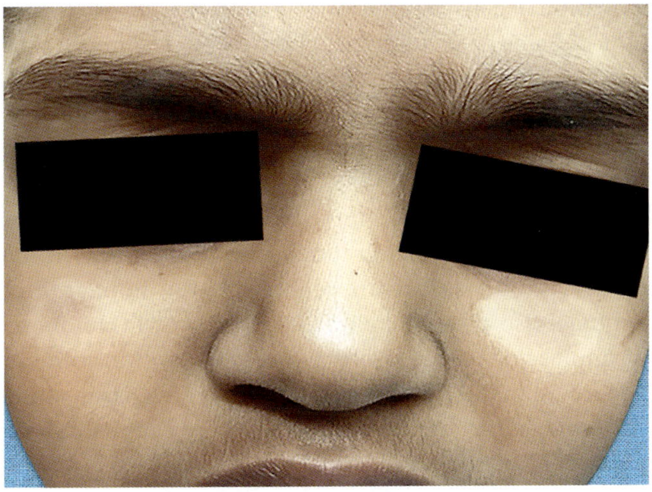

Fig. 28: Polymorphous light eruption over face, front view.

"Put your heart, mind and soul into even your smallest acts. This is the secret of success." —**Swami Sivananda**

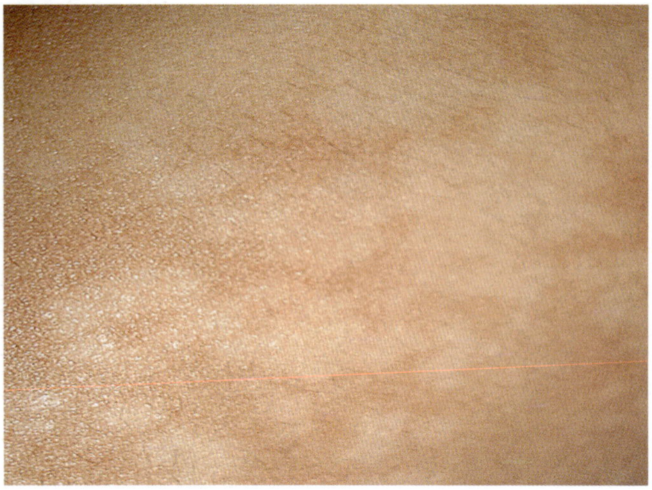

Fig. 29: Close-up view of polymorphous light eruption over face.

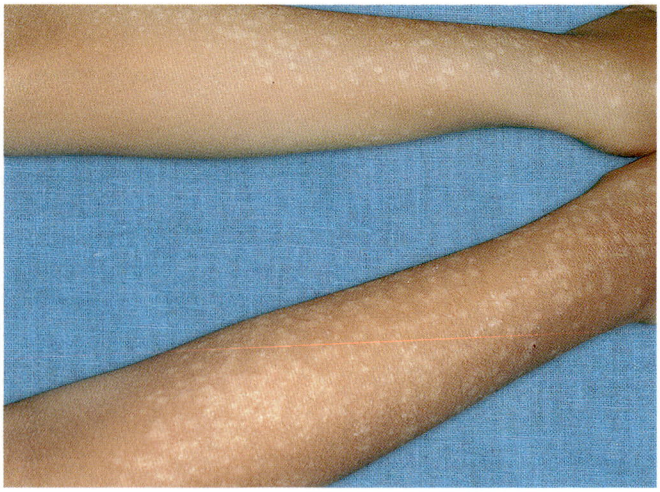

Fig. 30: Polymorphous light eruption over the outer aspect of forearms.

out). In severe cases, oral antioxidant containing betacarotene for months together is useful as an oral sunscreen. The condition often recurs and at times may be each year for few months. This may continue for a number of years. Counseling children/parents about the recurrent nature is important.

APHTHOUS ULCERS (FIGS. 32 TO 36)

Aphthous ulcers, also known as aphthae, aphthous stomatitis, or canker sores, is the most common cause of mouth ulcers characterized by recurrent episodes of ulceration from childhood to adolescence, each lasting from 1 to 4 weeks. A positive family history can be elicited in one-third of the cases. HLA-A2, HLA-A11, HLA-B12, and HLA-DR2 are the HLA associations documented. Nutritional causes such as low serum iron or ferritin and deficiency of folate or vitamin B_{12} are implicated in the causation. Ulcers similar to aphthae are seen in disorders such as Behçet's syndrome, Sweet's syndrome, human immunodeficiency virus (HIV) infection, or immunodeficiency.

A typical presentation is the presence of multiple, round-to-oval, well-circumscribed ulcers with an erythematous halo with yellow or grey floor. Minor aphthae, also called Mikulicz ulcers, are seen in childhood or adolescence measuring 2–4 mm up to 6 in number occurring mainly in the nonkeratinized mucosa of the vestibule, labial, buccal mucosa, and floor of the mouth. They heal within 10 days. Major aphthae, also called Sutton's ulcers **(Fig. 36)**, are larger than 10 mm and up to 3 cm in diameter, can involve any site, and usually heal

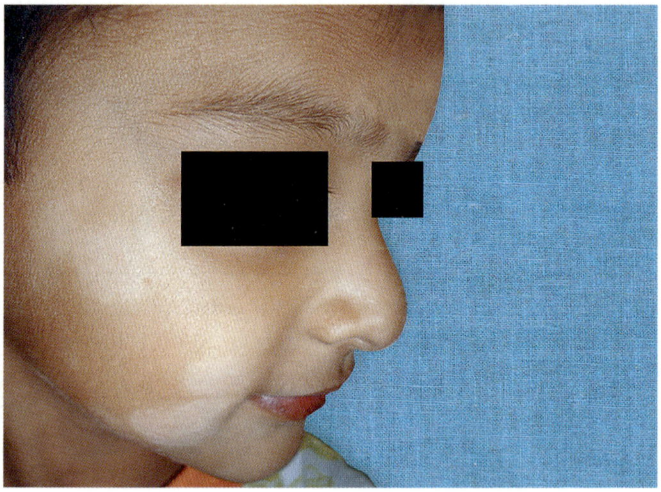

Fig. 31: Extensive polymorphous light eruption over face.

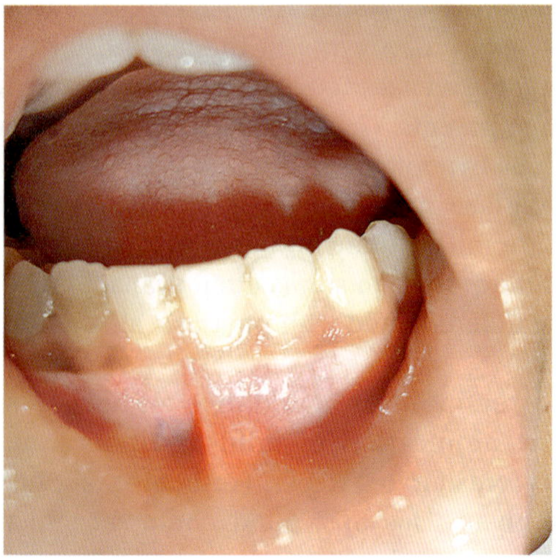

Fig. 32: Aphthous ulcer in a 4-year-old boy.

"Life is 10% what happens to you and 90% how you react to it." —**Charles R Swindoll**

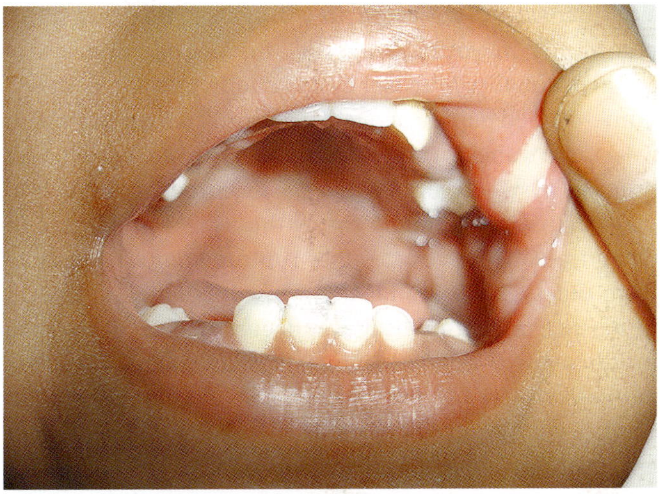

Fig. 33: Aphthous ulcer in a 3-year-old girl.

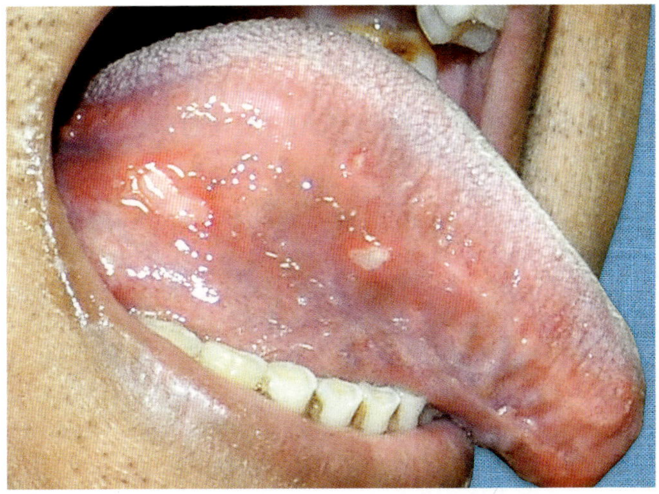

Fig. 34: Aphthous ulcer over tongue.

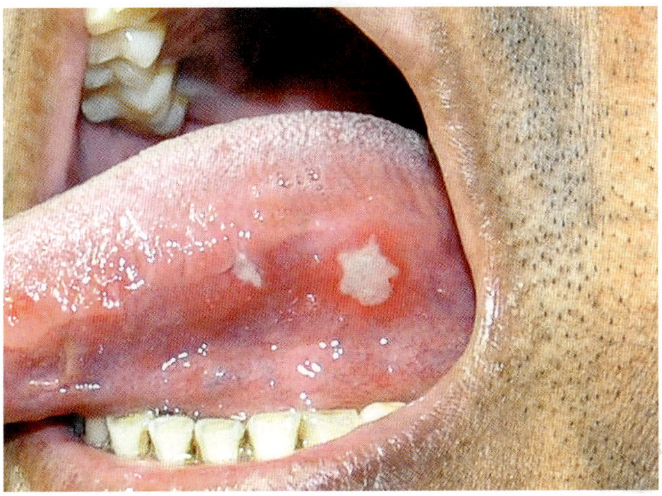

Fig. 35: Close-up view of a tongue lesion.

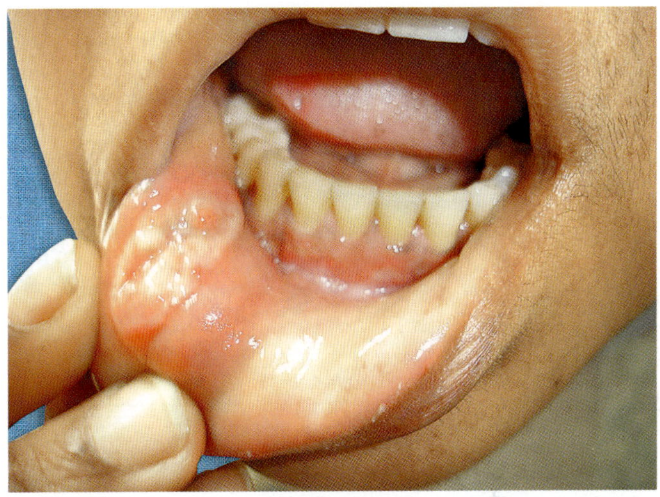

Fig. 36: Large necrotic aphthous ulcer (Sutton's aphthous ulcer).

over a month with scarring. Herpetiform aphthae begin as intensely painful tiny ulcers that coalesce together to form plaques with a herpetiform configuration. The number can vary from 10 to 100. Any site can be affected, but the most common site is the ventral aspect of the tongue. They usually heal within 10 days without scarring.

Treatment of aphthous ulcers is aimed at reducing pain and promoting rapid healing of the ulcers. Predisposing factors are corrected by improving oral hygiene, by decreasing the bacterial counts by use of chlorhexidine mouthwash and topical tetracycline or minocycline mouth rinse (to be carefully used in children because of swallowing which can lead to permanent staining of teeth). To decrease the pain associated with the ulcers and to accelerate healing, topical corticosteroids in an adherent vehicle such as carboxymethylcellulose (orabase) are recommended. In severe cases, systemic prednisolone can be tried. Other agents that are tried include sucralfate, colchicine, topical tacrolimus, dapsone, levamisole, pentoxifylline, and thalidomide in an attempt to induce remission.

STEATOCYSTOMA MULTIPLEX (FIG. 37)

Steatocystoma multiplex is an inherited benign skin disorder characterized by development of multiple cysts on different parts of the body. Steatocystoma simplex is the solitary counterpart to steatocystoma multiplex. It is associated with defects in keratin 17. The condition is inherited in an autosomal dominant manner. However, there are many reports of sporadic cases. The cysts can be removed via excision, though conventional cyst excision techniques have proven impractical, and a specialized

"No act of kindness, no matter how small, is ever wasted." —**Aesop**

regimen is required. Cryotherapy and electrodessication have also been tried with variable success.

MUCOSAL CYST OF ORAL MUCOSA (FIGS. 38A AND B)

Mucosal cysts are benign, mucus-containing cystic lesions of the oral mucosa. They are also called mucocele. Most of the mucocele are not true cysts as they do not have an epithelial lining. They arise following trauma to the minor salivary glands. Trauma is the main etiological factor for developing mucocele in children. Histological types include the mucus extravasation type, which is common in this age group and the rare retention type.

Mucosal cyst is seen in all age groups but more commonly in younger age. It affects both males and females equally. Mucosal cysts usually present as shiny, dome-shaped papule or a tense fluid-filled swelling which waxes and wanes for several months. There are two types of mucosal cyst—superficial and classic. Superficial mucosal cyst occurs immediately below the mucosa resulting in small translucent vesicles that rupture spontaneously to form ulcers. They are located on soft palate and buccal mucosa. Classic mucosal cyst occurs in the submucosa producing well-defined, dome-shaped papules. These are painless, situated on the lower lips, cheeks, floor of mouth, and palate. The upper lip is usually spared. Recurrences are common and may lead to fibrosis.

Management is usually reassurance to the parents. Cryotherapy and surgical removal of the cyst can be done.

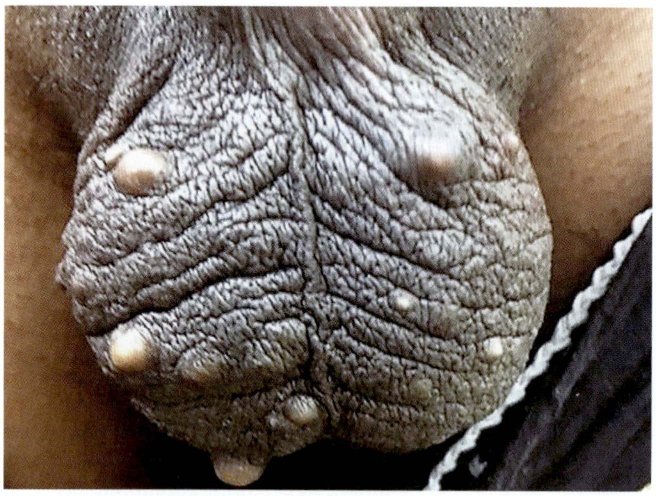

Fig. 37: Steatocystoma multiplex; note scrotal yellowish epidermal cysts.

GRANULOMA ANNULARE (FIGS. 39 TO 43)

Granuloma annulare is a common childhood dermatosis characterized by grouped dermal papules arranged in an annular or a ring fashion. The term was introduced by Radcliffe-Crocker in 1902. The exact cause is unknown and pathogenesis is poorly understood. The localized annular and subcutaneous form are common in children and young adults, but the disease is rare in infancy. Generalized forms are more common in adults. The various predisposing factors include nonspecific trauma such as insect bite reaction (since lesions are frequently located on extremities), infections and immunizations (infections with varicella-zoster virus, hepatitis B, hepatitis C, HIV virus, immunization for tetanus, diphtheria, etc.), sun exposure, drugs (gold,

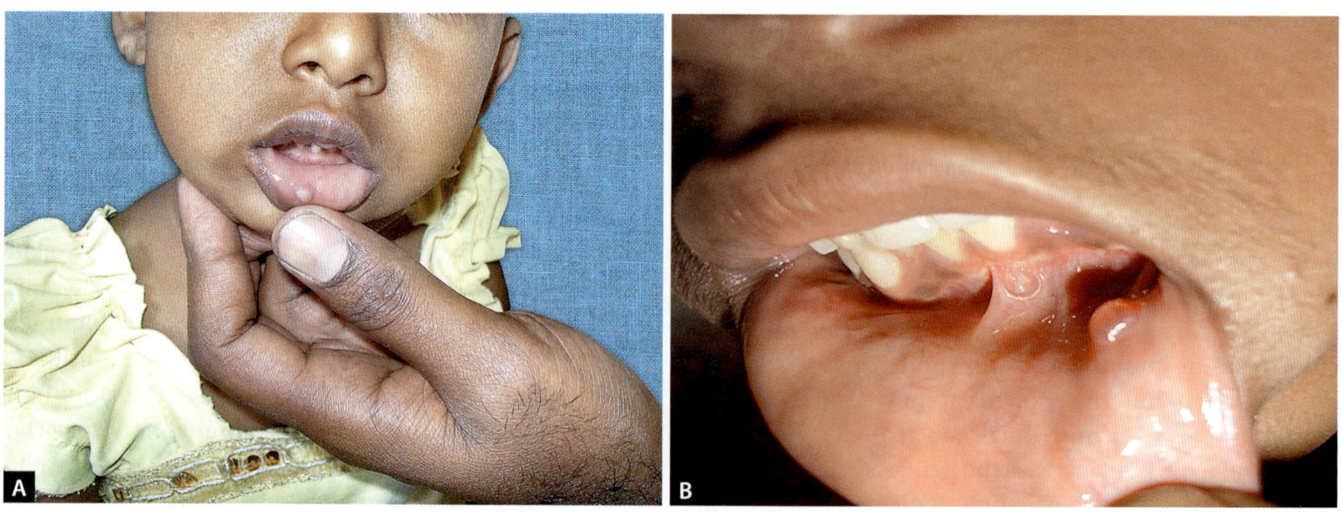

Figs. 38A and B: (A) Mucosal cyst lip; (B) Close-up view of a mucosal cyst.

"Don't judge each day by the harvest you reap but by the seeds that you plant." —**Robert Louis Stevenson**

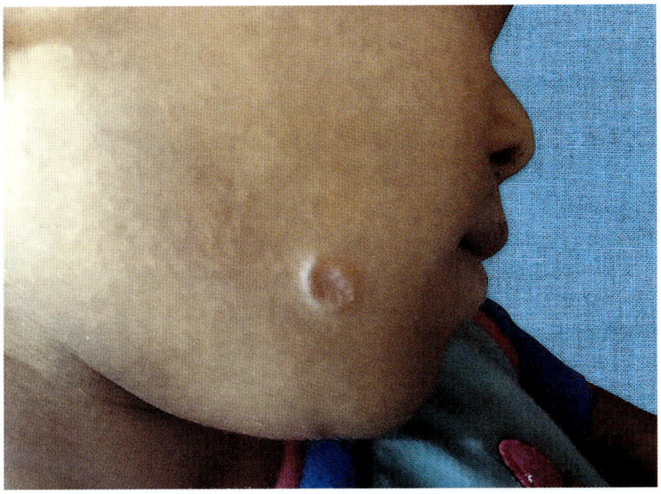

Fig. 39: Granuloma annulare, single lesion.

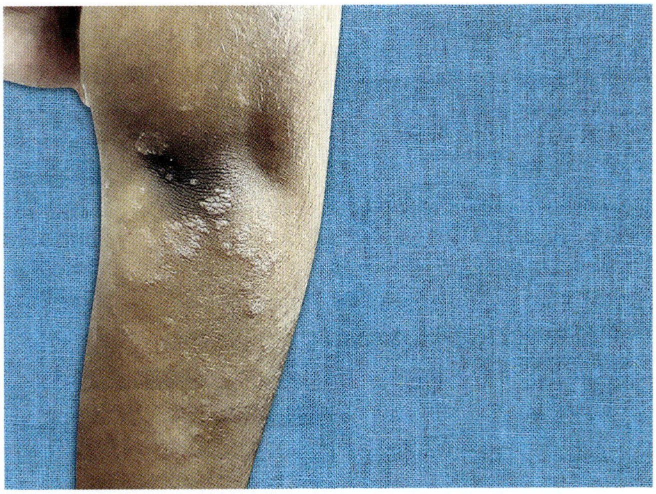

Fig. 40: Multiple lesions of granuloma annulare over elbow in a 15-year-old boy.

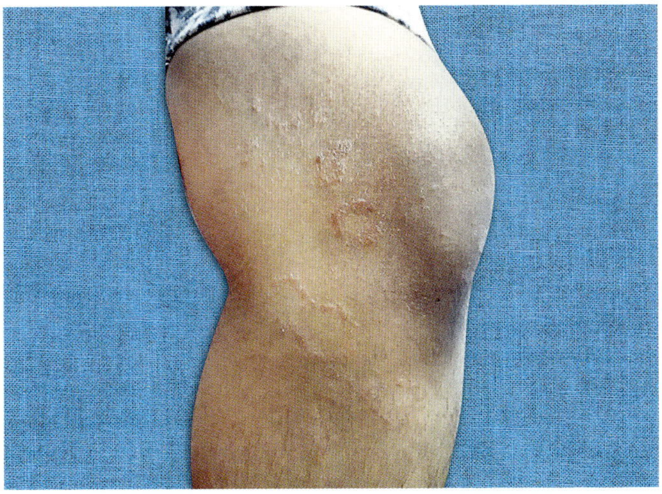

Fig. 41: Same boy, lesions over knee.

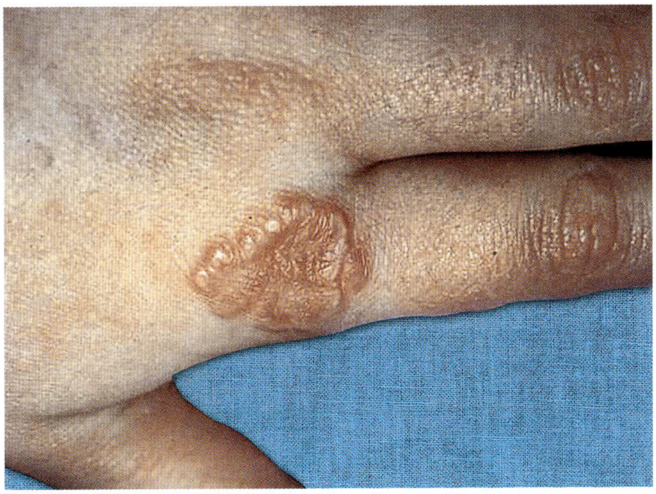

Fig. 42: Granuloma annulare over dorsum of hand.

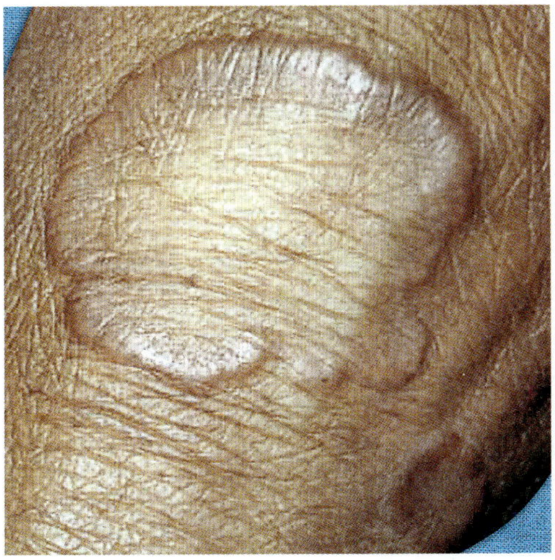

Fig. 43: Close-up view of granuloma annulare lesions.

diclofenac, amlodipine, etc.), endocrinal disorders (diabetes mellitus, thyroid), and malignancies.

Clinically, the child presents with asymptomatic papules arranged in an annular fashion commonly over the extremities such as dorsa of the hands and feet. The lesions enlarge centrifugally with central clearing. They are often treated for dermatophytic infection without success. In the localized form, skin-colored to slightly red papules appear over the extremities without scaling or epidermal change which enlarge peripherally to form annular or arcuate lesions. Multiple lesions may be present. An umbilicated form has also been described. The subcutaneous form is seen as a subcutaneous swelling in the lower legs in the pretibial region. Periocular granuloma annulare can be rarely seen in children.

"Knowledge speaks, but wisdom listens." **—Jimi Hendrix**

Histopathologic findings include focal degeneration of collagen in the dermis with reactive inflammation and fibrosis along with fragmented collagen bundles. Treatment is supportive as the lesions may undergo spontaneous resolution. Topical and intralesional steroids may be tried in some cases. In resistant and persistent lesions, cryotherapy or laser can be effective.

TRICHOEPITHELIOMA (FIG. 44)

Trichoepitheliomas are benign adnexal tumors of follicular differentiation. Familial cases have been reported. Multiple familial trichoepithelioma is an autosomal dominant disorder characterized by multiple skin-colored papules predominantly on the face. There are three types of trichoepitheliomas: solitary, multiple, and desmoplastic. Solitary and desmoplastic trichoepitheliomas are rarely seen in childhood. Multiple trichoepitheliomas present as small, firm, skin-colored papules and nodules measuring 2–5 mm on the nasolabial folds, nose, forehead, cheeks, upper lips, and eyelids. Occasionally scalp, neck, and trunk can be involved. Diagnosis is based on clinical and histological features. Since they are benign lesions, they can be left untreated. Treatment modalities include electrodessication, curettage, laser therapy, and surgical excision.

TERRA FIRMA-FORME DERMATOSIS (FIGS. 45 TO 47)

Terra firma-forme dermatosis is a benign condition of acquired dirt-like plaques. The name, "terra firma," is

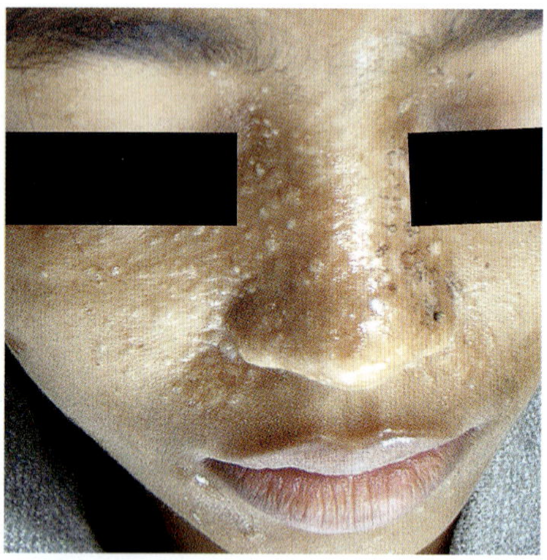

Fig. 44: Trichoepithelioma in a 15-year-old girl.

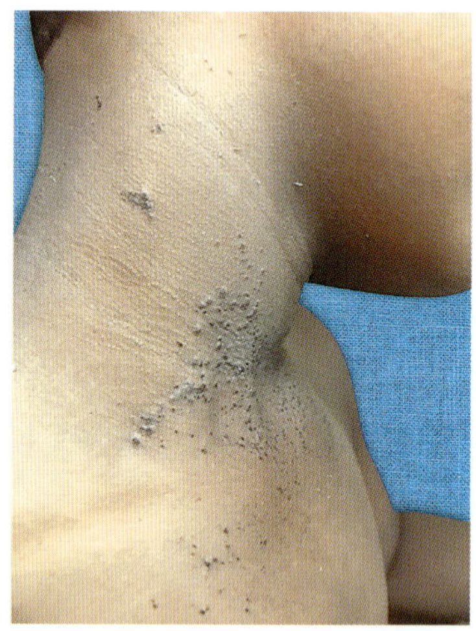

Fig. 45: Terra firma-forme dermatoses, neck lateral view.

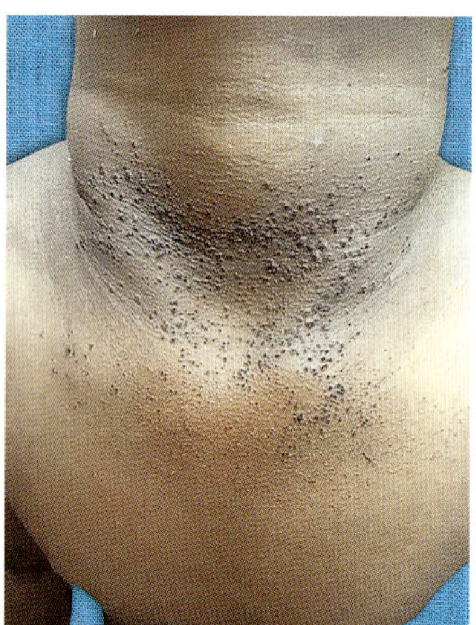

Fig. 46: Same boy, neck, front view.

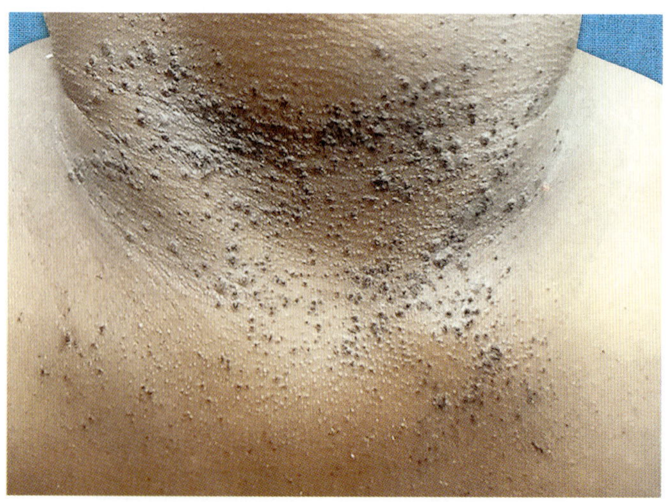

Fig. 47: Terra firma-forme dermatosis, close-up view.

"Patience is the companion of wisdom." —**Saint Augustine**

derived from the Latin word meaning "solid land." This condition affects people of all ages, with some reports of a higher incidence in children and young adults. Terra firma-forme dermatosis does not have a predilection for any particular gender. It is also unrelated to any known genetic condition or familial inheritance.

Terra firma-forme dermatosis usually presents as asymptomatic black or brown, dirt-like papules and plaques. It may also have a papillomatous, verrucous, or reticulate appearance. Lesions are usually located on the neck, face, trunk, and ankles, although they may involve any area of the body. The distribution of terra firma-forme dermatosis varies; it can be localized, generalized, bilateral, or unilateral. Lesions appear in patients with normal hygiene and are resistant to scrubbing with soap and water. They most often present during the warmer months of the year.

The treatment of terra firma-forme dermatosis consists of the application of 70% isopropyl alcohol; it is both diagnostic and therapeutic. Occasionally, lesions may recur after the initial complete removal of all hyperpigmentation. In this situation, additional wiping with isopropyl alcohol is recommended. Some patients may require weekly application of isopropyl alcohol to maintain resolution or for prophylaxis. Regular moisturization of the affected skin is important to prevent xerosis after regular treatments with isopropyl alcohol.

SACROCOCCYGEAL TERATOMA (FIG. 48)

Certain rare tumors arise at the base of the coccyx or sacrococcygeal region known as sacrococcygeal teratomas.

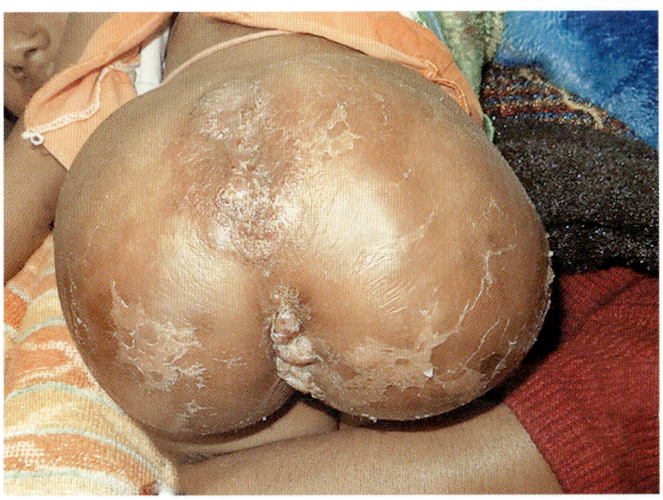

Fig. 48: Sacrococcygeal teratoma.

These are mostly benign in nature but can be quite large in size and require a surgical excision. They may be diagnosed prenatally with the help of ultrasound imaging. In very rare cases, they may be discovered only in adulthood with symptoms of low back pain, gastrointestinal, and genitourinary issues. The etiology of sacrococcygeal tumors is unknown. These are germ cell tumors and arise when germ cells, which are normally found in the ovary or testes, grow at other sites; the cause for this is unknown. They can contain cells that look like adult tissue or resemble embryonic tissue if undifferentiated. These are more common in females, but males have a higher incidence of malignancies.

The signs and symptoms of sacrococcygeal teratomas depend on their size and location. Very small teratomas are often asymptomatic.

If the teratoma grows too rapidly in utero, then there can be heart failure and hydrops due to increased blood supply demand, polyhydramnios, fetal hydronephrosis, bleeding into the tumor or amniotic space and dystocia.

Slowly growing tumors in adults may present with weakness of lower limbs, urinary tract infections, bowel movement dysfunctions, chronic low back pain, etc.

The diagnosis of sacrococcygeal teratoma can be made on routine ultrasound prenatally or at the time of birth. In doubtful cases, amniocentesis may be done to detect levels of alpha feto protein (AFP), a fetal plasma protein which may be elevated in sacrococcygeal teratoma. If detected, additional tests need to be done such as magnetic resonance imaging (MRI) and echocardiography to check the functioning of the heart. Many of these babies are born prematurely and need a cesarean section and specialized neonatal care.

In case of adults with symptoms and a suspicion of sacrococcygeal teratoma, per rectal examination can provide some clue. Fine needle aspiration cytology may be carried out to examine the tissue sample.

Sacrococcygeal teratomas can be classified according to the American Academy of Pediatrics Surgical Section:

Type I: The tumor is predominantly external with a very minimal internal component. Type I is rarely associated with malignancy.

Type II: The tumor is predominantly external but has some internal extension into the presacral space.

Type III: The tumor is visible externally but is predominantly located in the pelvic area with some extension into the abdomen.

"As knowledge increases, wonder deepens." —**Charles Morgan**

Type IV: The tumor is not visible externally and is located in the presacral space. Type IV has the highest rate of malignancy.

The management of sacrococcygeal teratomas involves early resection of the mass by specialist surgeons along with management of any comorbid conditions such as heart failure. Serial monitoring of AFP levels must be carried out for at least 3 years to rule out any recurrence.

Sacrococcygeal teratomas need to be differentiated from other tumors in this region such as tumors consisting of fat (lipomas), extrarenal Wilms' tumor, hamartomas, neuroblastomas, and pacinomas.

CAROTENEMIA (FIG. 49)

The yellowish discoloration of the palms and skin is reported under different terms: xanthoderma, hypercarotenemia, carotenemia, and carotenodermia. Yellow discoloration of the skin may be associated with carotenemia, hypothyroidism, diabetes mellitus, hyperlipoproteinemia, liver disease, and renal disease, meaning that carotenemia is not synonymous with yellow skin, but is rather one of the causes. In carotenemia, there is yellow discoloration of the palms and soles. The discoloration is uniformly distributed, symmetrically with no nail changes. There may be mild xerosis of palms.

INFANTILE PERIANAL PYRAMIDAL PROTRUSION (FIG. 50)

Infantile perianal pyramidal protrusion (IPPP), also called infantile perianal protrusion or infantile perineal protrusion, is a rare and benign condition, predominantly occurring in females and usually presenting at birth as a pyramidal-shaped protrusion covered with smooth red or rose-colored skin. It is most often located on the midline raphe of the perineum, usually anterior to the anus, though it may also be seen posterior to or concomitantly anterior and posterior to the anus. Papular, peanut-shaped, leak-like, tongue-like, and hen's crest-shaped lesions have also been described. Tenderness is absent. The exact pathogenesis of IPPP is unclear, but the recognition of three different types of IPPP may explain the underlying mechanism. These include the following:

1. *Constitutional IPPP (congenital and/or familial)*: It develops due to a pelvic floor and perineal weak points or may represent a remnant of the urogenital septum.
2. *Acquired IPPP*: It mainly occurs in association with constipation. Diarrhea, fistulas, and anal fissures have also been implicated in the formation of IPPP through mechanical stimulation of the perineum.
3. *IPPPs due to lichen sclerosus et atrophicus (LSA)*: IPPP might represent a peculiar form of LSA, probably an early manifestation, although in other cases it might coexist with LSA.

Histopathology may show epidermal acanthosis, upper dermal edema, dilated capillaries with fibrous tissue elements infiltrated by lymphocytes and eosinophils in the upper dermis, or an almost normal picture. In patients with LSA-associated IPPP, features suggestive of lichen sclerosus, such as patchy lichenoid infiltrates with vacuolar alteration and homogenization areas of the collagen in the papillary dermis, are present. Characteristic appearance and typical clinical course of recurrent swelling and eventual resolution differentiate it from other conditions

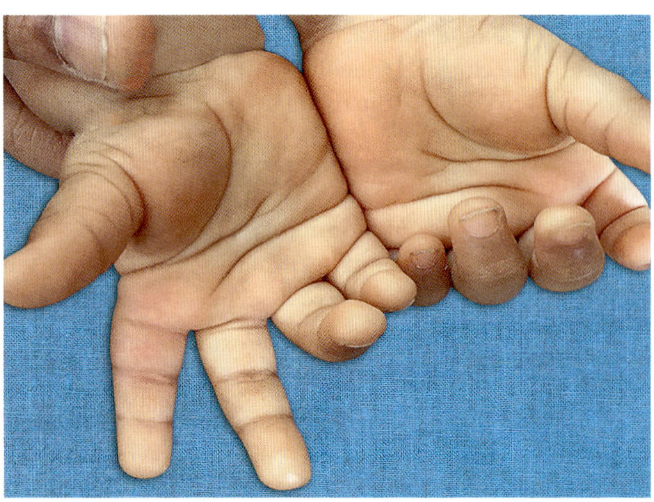

Fig. 49: Carotenemia, note yellowish discoloration of hands.

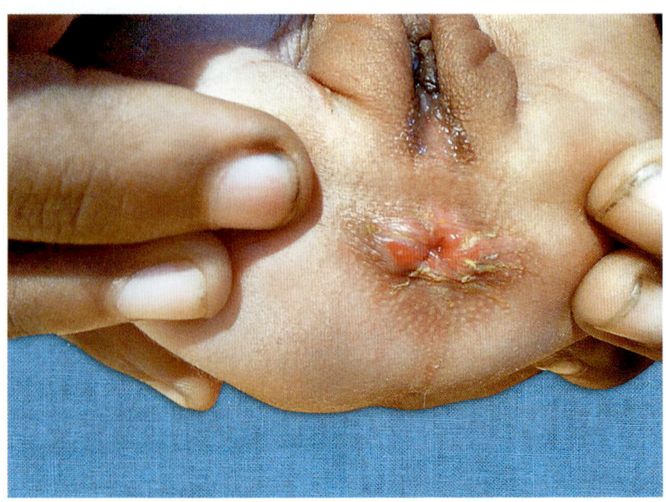

Fig. 50: Infantile pyramidal perineal protrusion.

"Things are as they are. Looking out into the universe at night, we make no comparisons between right and wrong stars, nor between well and badly arranged constellations." —**Alan Watts**

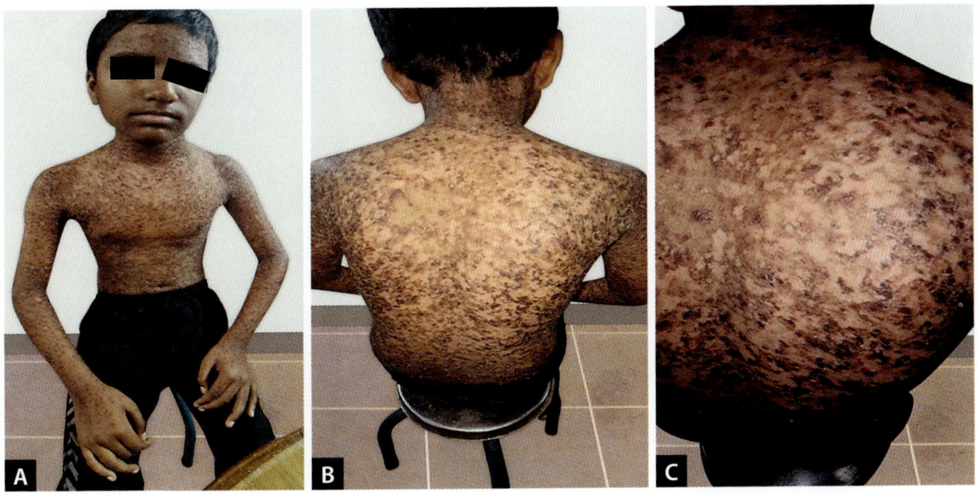

Figs. 51A to C: (A) Extensive pityriasis lichenoides et varioliformis acuta (PLEVA) in a young boy; (B) Same patient, back; (C) Close up view of back in same patient.

such as hemorrhoids, hemangiomas, rectal prolapse, granulomatous perineal lesions of Crohn's disease, sexual abuse, condyloma, molluscum contagiosum, and skin tags. Presence of LSA in other parts of the body might mean that IPPP is a manifestation of LSA. Ultrasonography and dermoscopy may be helpful in doubtful cases, thus avoiding the need for biopsy. Doppler imaging allows rapid identification of normal vessels and abnormal vascular structures. Dermoscopy shows presence of patchy structureless white areas consistent with fibrosis and a vascular pattern composed of red globular and dotted vessels correlating with the variably dilated capillaries.

Treatment is usually not necessary. Spontaneous resolution of the lesion occurs over time. In a few cases, it might remain unchanged over years. In an acquired form, management of the precipitating condition, instituting dietary changes and treating constipation or diarrhea when present usually, but not always, results in the regression of the lesion. IPPPs due to LSA can be treated with topical corticosteroids.

PLEVA

Pleva, or pityriasis lichenoides et varioliformis acuta, is a rare skin condition primarily affecting children and young adults. It exhibits a bimodal age distribution, with peaks in early childhood and early adulthood, though it predominantly affects children. The exact etiology remains elusive, with proposed triggers including infectious agents, immunological factors, and genetic predispositions. Clinically, it manifests as erythematous papules that evolve into vesicles and crusts, resembling a spectrum ranging from mild forms with few lesions to severe cases characterized by widespread involvement. Diagnosis relies on clinical assessment, often supplemented by histopathological examination, which typically reveals a dense infiltrate of lymphocytes in the dermis. Management of Pleva in children poses a challenge due to the self-limiting nature of the condition and the lack of standardized treatment guidelines. Symptomatic relief is often achieved through topical corticosteroids, phototherapy, or systemic immunomodulatory agents in severe or refractory cases. However, treatment decisions should be tailored to individual patients based on the extent and severity of lesions, as well as their overall health status. Prognosis of Pleva in children is generally favorable, with most cases resolving spontaneously within months to years. However, recurrence is not uncommon, necessitating long-term follow-up to monitor for disease progression or relapse. Furthermore, while Pleva typically does not result in significant morbidity or mortality, the impact on quality of life can be considerable, particularly in cases with extensive cutaneous involvement or associated systemic symptoms **(Figs. 51A to C)**.

Cydnidae Pigmentation (Burrowing Bug Pigmentation)

Cydnidae pigmentation in children, attributed secondarily to contact with Cydnidae bugs, presents a unique dermatological challenge. While Cydnidae pigmentation typically arises from sun exposure-induced melanin production, certain species of Cydnidae bugs contain

"The cure to boredom is curiosity." —**Dorothy Parker**

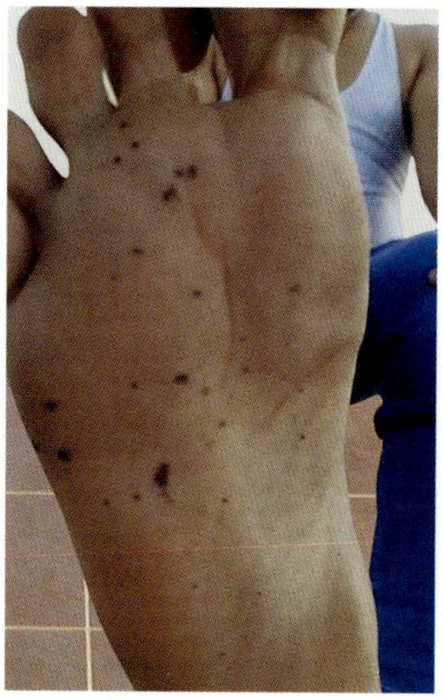

Fig. 52: Cydnidae pigmentation.

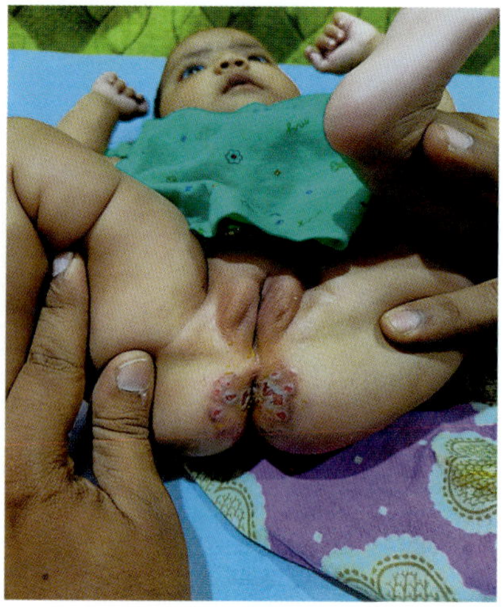

Fig. 53: Jacquet erosive dermatitis.

compounds capable of causing skin discoloration upon contact. These compounds may trigger localized hyperpigmentation, often manifesting as brownish spots or patches resembling freckles or lentigines. Diagnosis hinges on recognizing the association between bug exposure and subsequent pigmentation changes. Management involves meticulous hygiene practices, including prompt washing of affected areas to remove bug secretions and potential allergens. Topical treatments such as lightening agents or corticosteroids may aid in reducing pigmentation, though their efficacy varies. Preventive measures, such as avoiding contact with Cydnidae bugs and employing insect repellents, are crucial in minimizing the risk of further pigmentation episodes **(Fig. 52)**.

Jacquet Erosive Dermatitis

Jacquet erosive dermatitis, also known as diaper dermatitis is characterized by erythematous, erosive, and sometimes ulcerative lesions typically localized to the diaper area. While diaper dermatitis is multifactorial, with moisture, friction, and irritants playing significant roles, Jacquet erosive dermatitis represents a severe and potentially debilitating form. The condition is often exacerbated by prolonged contact with urine and feces, as well as by friction from diapers. In severe cases, secondary bacterial or fungal infections may develop, further complicating management. Diagnosis is primarily clinical, based on characteristic findings of erosive and ulcerative lesions in the diaper area, often accompanied by pain and discomfort in affected children. Management strategies focus on reducing moisture and friction through frequent diaper changes, gentle cleansing, and the use of protective barriers such as zinc oxide-based creams. Topical corticosteroids and antifungal agents may be indicated in cases of severe inflammation or superimposed infections. Prevention plays a crucial role, emphasizing proper diaper hygiene, regular diaper changes, and the use of hypoallergenic products **(Fig. 53)**.

CARD14 Mutation Psoriasis

CARD14 psoriasis, a subtype of psoriasis vulgaris, is a chronic inflammatory skin disorder characterized by well-demarcated, erythematous plaques with silvery scales. While psoriasis is typically associated with adults, its occurrence in children, particularly those with mutations in the *CARD14* gene, underscores its diverse clinical spectrum. The activation of CARD14 in keratinocytes leads to dysregulated immune responses, resulting in the proliferation of epidermal cells and the recruitment of inflammatory cells, ultimately culminating in the characteristic psoriatic lesions. Diagnosis of CARD14 psoriasis in children relies on clinical evaluation, including the presence of typical plaques, nail changes, and a family history of psoriasis. Management strategies encompass topical therapies, such as corticosteroids and vitamin D analogs, as first-line treatments for mild-to-moderate cases. In severe or refractory cases, systemic therapies, including biologic agents targeting specific inflammatory pathways, may be indicated. Comprehensive care involves a multidisciplinary approach, involving pediatric dermatologists, rheumatologists, and psychologists, to address the physical, emotional, and social aspects of the disease in affected

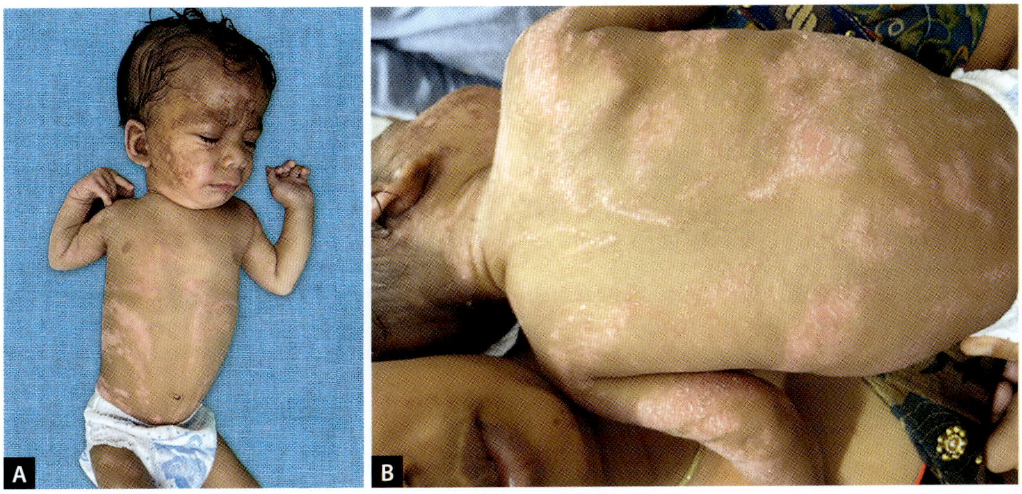

Figs. 54A and B: (A) CARD14 mutation in a 2-year-old boy; (B) Same boy back photograph.

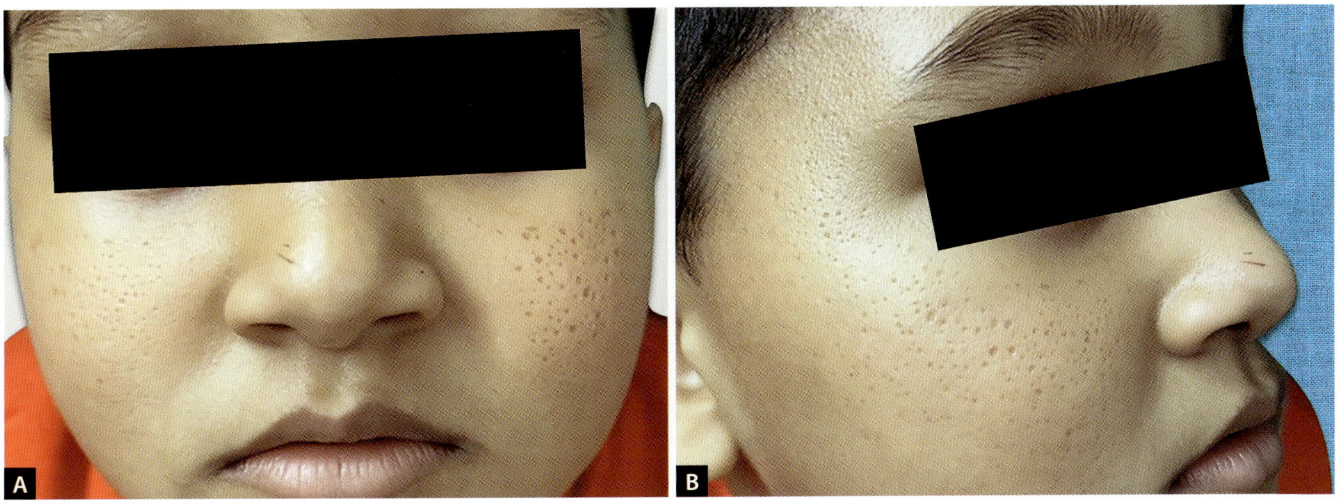

Figs. 55A and B: (A) Atrophoderma vermiculatum; (B) Same boy, right cheek, close up view.

children. Long-term follow-up is crucial to monitor disease progression, treatment response, and potential comorbidities, ensuring optimal outcomes and quality of life for pediatric patients with CARD14 psoriasis **(Figs. 54A and B)**.

ATROPHODERMA VERMICULATUM

Atrophoderma vermiculatum (AV) is a rare variant of keratosis pilaris (KP), characterized by distinctive clinical and histological features, primarily affecting children and adolescents. This dermatological condition presents with follicular papules, often accompanied by keratotic plugs, distributed symmetrically on the extensor surfaces of the extremities, particularly the arms and thighs. The pathogenesis of AV remains poorly understood, with proposed mechanisms involving abnormal keratinization, follicular plugging, and inflammatory responses. Histologically, AV exhibits follicular hyperkeratosis, perifollicular lymphocytic infiltrates, and atrophy of the dermis, distinguishing it from classical KP. Differential diagnoses include other follicular disorders such as lichen spinulosus and follicular mucinosis. Management of AV typically focuses on symptomatic relief and cosmetic improvement, utilizing emollients, keratolytics, topical corticosteroids, and retinoids. However, treatment outcomes vary, and there is limited evidence supporting the efficacy of specific interventions **(Figs. 55A and B)**.

"No one is perfect that is why pencils have erasers." —**Wolfgang Riebe**

SUGGESTED READINGS

1. Trai NN, Van Em D, Van BT, My LH, Tro CV, Hao NT, et al. Correlation of IL36RN and CARD14 mutations with clinical manifestations and laboratory findings in patients with generalised pustular psoriasis. Indian J Dermatol Venereol Leprol. 2023;89(3):378-84.
2. Reichel A, Grothaus J, Ott H. Pityriasis lichenoidesacuta (PLEVA) pemphigoides: A rare bullous variant of PLEVA. Pediatr Dermatol. 2020;37(4):710-12.
3. Coelho M, Tan JM, Ling N. Jacquet erosive dermatitis associated with commercial barrier cream. Australas J Dermatol. Published online December 22, 2023.
4. Amrani A, Sil A, Das A. "Transient pseudo-lentigines sign" in burrowing bug pigmentation. Pediatr Dermatol. 2021;38(5):1338-9.
5. Karimzadeh I, Namazi MR, Karimzadeh A. Trichoepithelioma: a comprehensive review. Acta Dermatovenerol Croat. 2018; 26(2):162-5.
6. Maguolo A, Maffeis C. Acanthosis nigricans in childhood: a cutaneous marker that should not be underestimated, especially in obese children. Acta Paediatr. 2020;109(3):481-7.
7. Webb K, Hlela C, Jordaan HF, Suliman S, Scriba T, Lipsker D, et al. A review and proposed approach to the neutrophilic dermatoses of childhood. Pediatr Dermatol. 2015;32(4):437-46.

CHAPTER

25

Principles of Vaccination in Immunosuppressed Children

INTRODUCTION

Vaccines represent one of the most successful public health advances of the 20th century. The vaccination of immunocompromised pediatric patients merits careful consideration because these children are at an increased risk for exposure to microbes from frequent visits to healthcare settings as compared to patients with normal immune function. The 2009 H1N1 influenza pandemic, the rise in the incidence of pertussis and antibiotic-resistant *Pneumococcus*, and recent outbreaks of measles and mumps in individuals with normal immune function further highlight the need for effective vaccination of immunocompromised patients. Other important considerations include safety concerns and the ability of immunocompromised individuals to generate a protective and sustained immune response. Some basic principles need to be followed while vaccinating immunocompromised children. In the practice of pediatric dermatology, where a host of chronic diseases, need to be treated with long-term oral steroid or various immunosuppressives such as cyclosporine, methotrexate, and biologics, it becomes very relevant to understand the intricate relationship between immunosuppression and vaccination. This also has tremendous medicolegal significance in current days' practice of medicine.

Box 1 highlights the basic principles of vaccination in immunocompromised children.

Vaccinating an immunocompromised child is a big challenge as one has to keep in mind so many diverse aspects. You can be caught on either side if you do not safeguard yourself with proper knowledge and practice **(Box 2)**.

In pediatric dermatology practice, there are various drugs which are known immunosuppressants but extremely useful to treat various chronic diseases (atopic dermatitis, vitiligo, psoriasis, lichen planus, disorders of keratinization, collagen vascular diseases, vasculitis, autoimmune bullous diseases, etc.), but can also have profound physical, psychological, emotional, moral, and social morbidity. These include systemic corticosteroids, cyclosporine, methotrexate, azathioprine, cyclophosphamide, mycophenolate mofetil and various biologics such as rituximab and omalizumab. Of all these, oral corticosteroid is most commonly used and is in use for the longest period of time. Hence, it is very important for all physicians in general and pediatric dermatologists in particular to learn finer nuances of its use, particularly when planned for long-term purpose.

Steroid therapy usually does not contraindicate administration of live-virus vaccines when such therapy is of short-term (<2 weeks); low-to-moderate dose; long-term, alternate-day treatment with short-acting preparations; maintenance physiologic doses (replacement therapy);

Box 1 Basic principles of vaccinating immunocompromised children.

- Determine immune status
- Carefully assess risks versus benefits. Understand that inactivated vaccines are generally safe and play an important role and that live vaccines are generally contraindicated, except in select circumstances for which safety and efficacy data are available
- Vaccinate contacts and healthcare workers
- Follow current vaccine recommendations. Administer vaccines before immunosuppression when possible (ideally 4–8 weeks before)
- Consider antibody testing to evaluate vaccine response

Box 2 Challenges in vaccinating immunocompromised children.

- Safety issues
- Immunogenicity
- Decreased vaccine efficacy
- Changing immune status
- Heterogeneous patient groups with variable immune deficits
- Increasing use of potent immunosuppressive regimens
- Preimmunosuppression immunization
- Vaccination of contacts to reduce exposure of the immunocompromised child
- Compliance

"Mastering others is strength, mastering yourself is true power." —**Lao Tzu**

or administered topically (skin or eyes), by aerosol or by intra-articular, bursal or tendon injection. The exact dose of systemic corticosteroids and the duration of their administration needed to suppress the immune system of an otherwise healthy child are not well defined. The immunosuppressive effects of steroid treatment vary, but many clinicians consider a dose equivalent to either 2 mg/kg body weight or a total of 20 mg/day of prednisolone as sufficiently immunosuppressive to raise concern about the safety of immunization with live-virus vaccines. Corticosteroids used in greater than physiologic doses also may reduce the immune response to vaccines. Physicians should wait for at least 3 months after discontinuation of therapy before administering a live-virus vaccine to patients who have received high-dose, systemic steroids for ≥2 weeks, 20 mg/day in children weighing ≥10 kg or >2 mg/kg/day in children weighing <10 kg. Treatment with high-dose steroids for >2 weeks duration will decrease immune function. The local administration of corticosteroids via the skin, the lungs, or the upper respiratory tract or by intra-articular injection will not be immunosuppressive **(Box 3)**.

- *Methotrexate (MTX)*: Good immunogenicity: Hepatitis B virus (HBV), Flu, Tetanus Toxoid (TT), MMR (measles, mumps, and rubella) with MTX <15 mg/m^2/week; lower response: Pneumococcal polysaccharide vaccine (PPV23) on MTX 15–25 mg/m^2/week; trend to lower response: Varicella zoster virus (VZV) on MTX 15–25 mg/m^2/week.
- *Azathioprine*: Like Methotrexate
- *Cyclosporine/Cyclophosphamide/Mycophenolate*: No live vaccines
- *Rituximab*: Good immunogenicity: TT—6 months after Rituximab; lower response: Flu, PPV23

If feasible, it is better to administer live vaccines before initiation of disease-modifying drugs.

Box 3 **Timing of live vaccines after steroid therapy and chemotherapy.**

- *United States*: At least 3 months
- *United Kingdom*: 6–12 months
- *Australia*: 12 months
- *Canada*: 12 months

Steroid dose

- *Topical (skin or respiratory tract)*: Can be given
- *Local injection*: Can be given
- *Physiologic*: Can be given
- *Systemic steroids (low or moderate dose)*: Can be given
- Systemic steroids (high dose, i.e., 2 mg/kg/day or 20 mg/day) for >2 weeks; after 3 months of stopping steroid (minimum 1 month)

Often, an important issue is raised, "when can live vaccination be started after stoppage of immunosuppressive therapy?" Although there is difference in guidelines practiced in India from abroad, and although all these are extrapolated from treatment of various malignancies or collagen vascular diseases in the pediatric age group and use of immunosuppressives, no data or guidelines exist about the use of immunosuppressives in various difficult-to-treat and chronic dermatoses. Here, we have to remember that the dose of various immunosuppressives used in the treatment of malignancies or collagen vascular diseases is much higher than the dose of the same drug used in dermatologic conditions, e.g., psoriasis, atopic dermatitis, and lichen planus.

Monitoring of the vaccination, i.e., whether the vaccine is working or not, is done on the basis of the antibody level. The degree of immunosuppression is estimated by the following parameters: Conserved/no immunosuppression: CD4+ T-lymphocytes > 25%; moderate immunosuppression: CD4+ T-lymphocytes 15–24%; severe immunosuppression (impaired, absent): CD4+ T-lymphocytes < 15%.

LIVE VACCINES

Both bacterial and viral live vaccines are generally contraindicated for severely immunocompromised individuals because of the risk of disease caused by vaccine strains.

Oral poliovirus vaccine: Use of live oral poliovirus vaccine (OPV) is contraindicated in patients with acquired immunodeficiency and their household contacts because of the risk of vaccine-associated polio in immunocompromised children. Viral shedding may occur in OPV recipients for 8–12 weeks after vaccine administration. Inactivated poliovirus vaccine is recommended when immunization is appropriate in both immunocompromised patients and their contacts. If OPV is introduced into the household of an immunosuppressed child, to minimize exposure to OPV, household members should practice proper hand hygiene before and after contact with the child and the person who received the OPV should avoid changing diapers for the immunosuppressed child **(Box 4)**.

KILLED AND COMPONENT VACCINES

Killed and component vaccines do not pose a risk to immunocompromised patients, and these vaccines

Box 4 Vaccines which are safe and which are to be avoided in immunocompromised children.

Safe	*Avoid*
• Influenza (inactive)	• Measles
• Pneumococcal	• Mumps
• Diphtheria	• Rubella
• Tetanus	• Oral poliomyelitis (OPV)
• Pertussis	• Bacillus Calmette–Guérin (BCG)
• *Haemophilus Influenzae* type b (Hib)	• Yellow fever
• Hepatitis A	• Nasal influenza vaccine
• Hepatitis B	• Chickenpox vaccine
• Japanese encephalitis	
• Meningococcal	
• Inactivated poliomyelitis (IPV)	
• Rabies	
• Conjugate typhoid	
• Typhoid Vi polysaccharide	
• Human papillomavirus (HPV)	

are not generally contraindicated. However, the immunocompromised patient's ability to develop an adequate immune response is a significant clinical consideration that the physician should weigh against the risk of contracting a vaccine-preventable disease when making clinical decisions about when to immunize.

Influenza vaccine: Patients and close contacts of immunosuppressed patients who are 6 months old should receive an annual dose of the inactivated influenza vaccine. Immunosuppressed patients are at a higher risk of complications from influenza, including prolonged hospitalization and intensive care stays than the general population. The live influenza vaccine is contraindicated in patients with immune suppression because of the risk of disease from the vaccine strain.

FAMILY MEMBERS, HOUSEHOLD CONTACTS, AND HEALTHCARE WORKERS

All close contacts who live in the same household as the immunocompromised child should be immunized with all routinely recommended vaccines, including the live-attenuated MMR, varicella, and rotavirus vaccines because the transmission of the live vaccine virus is rare. The transmission of the live varicella vaccine virus from vaccine recipients to close contacts who are not immunosuppressed has occurred, but only from vaccine recipients who developed a rash. Household contacts who develop a vesicular rash after varicella vaccination should avoid contact with immunosuppressed individuals until the rash resolves. Immunocompromised patients should be instructed to avoid exposure to stools from rotavirus-immunized contacts, and all members of the family should practice good hand hygiene for at least 1 week after vaccination. In addition, the trivalent inactivated influenza vaccine should be administered annually to all close contacts of immunocompromised individuals. Vaccinating siblings, family members, and other close contacts is an important strategy to protect immunocompromised patients against vaccine-preventable diseases, especially those transmitted in households, such as pertussis and influenza.

Live-attenuated vaccines such as the oral polio vaccine are contraindicated in household contacts.

VACCINATING THE PRIMARY IMMUNODEFICIENT CHILD

Immunization is an important active protection instrument against infections in children with congenital immunodeficiencies, but B-cell and T-cell deficiencies may alter the effectiveness of vaccines and increase the risk of adverse postvaccine events. Among the congenital immunodeficiencies, severe combined immunodeficiencies are the most feared, as Bacillus Calmette–Guérin (BCG) vaccine complications are frequently the first event to indicate this condition. BCG vaccine in these children may lead to systemic dissemination. With the purpose of preventing this BCG vaccine complication, which may be fatal, children with a family history suggestive of immunodeficiency (siblings who died prematurely from undefined causes or who had an extremely exuberant vaccine lesion) must have BCG vaccination postponed until their immunocompetence has been defined.

Oral poliomyelitis vaccine (live-attenuated virus) must not be given to children with congenital immunodeficiencies, because of the increased risk of developing paralytic poliomyelitis associated with vaccination, in addition to continuing to excrete the virus for long periods. In severely immunosuppressed patients, household contacts must also not receive this vaccine, because of the risk of vaccine virus dissemination through feces, which may last for up to 4 weeks. Other live-virus vaccines, such as measles/rubella/mumps vaccine, and yellow fever vaccine are also contraindicated for children with T-cell immunodeficiency. Live-attenuated vaccines against measles, mumps, and rubella may be considered for children with minor antibody immunodeficiency.

"He who has a why to live can bear almost any how." —**Friedrich Nietzsche**

The varicella vaccine may be given to children with humoral immunodeficiency but is contraindicated in those with cellular immunodeficiency.

Yearly influenza (inactivated) immunization is safe and is indicated in congenitally immunodeficient patients who have greater influenza morbidity and mortality. The vaccine must also be offered to the patient's household contacts. Children with complement deficiency may receive all the vaccines in the routine calendar; there is specific indication for immunization against meningococci, *Haemophilus influenzae* type b (Hib), and pneumococci. Children with phagocytosis defects must not receive BCG vaccine, but they may receive the other vaccines in the routine calendar. The protective response obtained with immunization of those congenital immune deficiency children may be inadequate: the antibody titers obtained may be insufficient and they may drop more quickly than usual. Thus, even though vaccinated, these patients may remain susceptible to infectious diseases, which make it advisable to perform serologic tests to assess the antibody levels obtained after vaccination; additional or higher doses of vaccines may be necessary and even so, the response obtained may not be optimal. Taking all these into consideration, in the event of exposure to infectious diseases, these patients must be considered susceptible and passive immunization, if available, must be indicated.

The bottom line is that vaccination can be considered on a case-to-case basis weighing the risk of infection versus hypothetical risks of vaccination. Live-attenuated vaccines should be withheld in patients on high-dose glucocorticoids and on biologics.

SUGGESTED READINGS

1. Jansen MH, Rondaan C, Legger GE, Minden K, Uziel Y, Toplak N, et al. EULAR/PRES recommendations forvaccination of paediatric patients with autoimmune inflammatory rheumatic diseases: update 2021. Annals of the rheumatic diseases. 2023;82(1):35-47.
2. Munshi MA, Noe MH, Chiu YE, Streicher JL. Vaccines: considerations for pediatric dermatology patients on immunosuppressive agents. Pediatric dermatology. 2021;38(5):1040-6.
3. Martinez-Cabriales SA, Kirchhof MG, Constantinescu CM, Murguia-Favela L, RamienML. Recommendations for Vaccination in Children with Atopic Dermatitis Treated with Dupilumab: A Consensus Meeting, 2020. Am J Clin Dermatol. 2021;22(4):443-55.
4. Immunisation Recommendations for Children and Adult Patients Treated with Immune-suppressive Medicines.Br Asso Dermatol May;2018.[online]Availablefromwww.bad.org.uk/leaflets.
5. Moulik NR, Mondal P, Chandra J, Bansal S, Jog P, Sanjay S, et al. Immunization of Children with Cancer in India Treatedwith Chemotherapy: Consensus Guideline from the Pediatric Hematology-Oncology Chapter and the Advisory Committee on Vaccination and Immunization Practices of the Indian Academy of Pediatrics. Indian Pediatr. 2019;56:1041-8.

"Graduation is not the end, it is the beginning." —**Unknown**

CHAPTER

26

Cutaneous Manifestations in Pediatric COVID

INTRODUCTION

The coronavirus disease-2019 (COVID-19) pandemic has had a profound impact on global health, affecting people of all ages, including children. While children are often less severely affected by the virus itself, they present with some unique symptoms, which include a range of cutaneous manifestations. The prevalence of these cutaneous manifestations in children with COVID-19 varies widely, with some studies reporting rates as high as 20%. The most common among these is chilblains which are also known as "COVID toes" but other manifestations such as urticaria, maculopapular rash, erythema multiforme (EM)-like rash, and symptoms associated with multisystem inflammatory syndrome have also been reported. This chapter aims to provide a comprehensive overview of the prevalence and various cutaneous manifestations of COVID-19 in the pediatric population, contributing to the broader understanding of this novel virus's impacts on children.

CHILBLAIN

Chilblains are the most common cutaneous manifestation of pediatric COVID-19 which appear as red or purple lesions on the toes and can be accompanied by mild itching or burning. These lesions, often referred to as COVID toes or chilblains-like lesions, have been widely reported in children and adolescents since the onset of the pandemic. It occurs most notably in people exposed to the cold and damp, as well as those who participate in cold weather sports such as hockey, figure skating, and speed skating.

Most patients test negative for infection using both serology and reverse transcription-polymerase chain reaction (RT-PCR), despite a temporal correlation between the start of chilblain-like lesions and the pandemic. This raises questions about whether the lesions are associated with severe acute respiratory syndrome coronavirus 2 (SARS-CoV-2).

It is characterized by the presence of multiple erythematous, violaceous and/or purpuric macules predominantly over the finger and toes. Majority of cases affect the toes without crossing the metatarsophalangeal joint. The reported mean age of patients is above 10 years. Children are commonly asymptomatic unlike adults where these lesions are predominantly painful.

Pathogenesis

- *Role of interferon type 1 (INF-1)*: INF-1 is a part of the innate immunity which is responsible for the first line of defense against viral infections. The levels of INF-1 are higher in infants and children. A study by Hubiche et al. found that there was a significantly higher IFN-1 response in chilblains patients with mild COVID in comparison to patients with moderate or severe COVID-19 explaining the rarity of chilblain-like lesions.
- *Thrombotic or embolic hypothesis*: The presence of fibrin microemboli blocks the smaller vessels leading to acral ischemia and subsequently chilblain-like lesions. In a study by Hachem et al., microthrombi were observed on histopathological analysis in three patients with chilblains. This supports the possibility of a thrombotic or embolic event precipitating chilblain-like lesions.

Dermoscopy

- Red to purple globules over an erythematous background
- Gray-brown reticular network in the periphery (30%)

Histopathology

Lymphocytic vasculitis ranging from endothelial swelling to fibrinoid necrosis is the hallmark of lesions resembling chilblains. In addition, perieccrine and superficial perivascular lymphocytic infiltrates are observed, which is comparable to idiopathic perniosis.

"Nothing will work unless you do." —**Maya Angelou**

URTICARIA (FIGS. 1 AND 2)

Urticaria is commonly known as hives presents as red, itchy welts on the skin and can appear anywhere on the body.

Pediatric patients frequently develop urticaria, which has a variety of etiologies that typically vary by age group. Cases of urticaria have been observed in patients of all ages during the COVID-19 pandemic, including infants as young as 2 months. Majority of patients came to the dermatologist or pediatrician with urticaria as their only symptom.

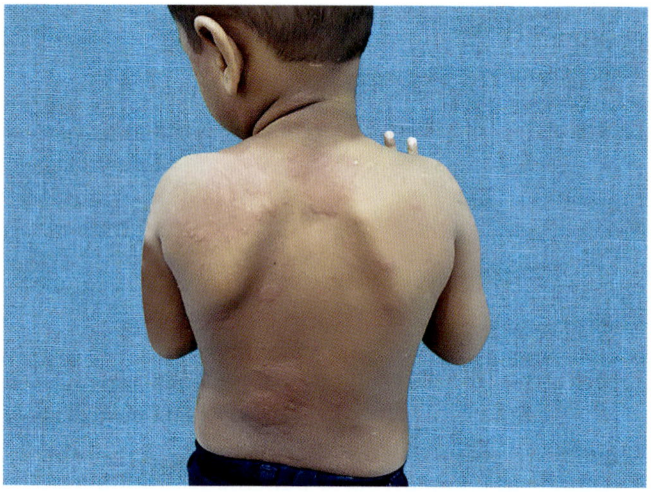

Fig. 1: A 7-year-old boy positive for coronavirus disease 2019 (COVID-19) presenting with urticaria.

The exact cause of urticaria in COVID-19 patients is unknown. However, it is believed to be a result of the body's immune response to the virus.

- Interaction between viral immunoglobulin M (IgM) and immunoglobulin G (IgG) with mast cell immunoglobulin E (IgE) causes mast cell degranulation.
- Immune complexes stimulate basophils into producing vasoactive amines, which activates complement, leading to increased vascular permeability.
- Interleukin-6 (IL-6), a cytokine that is elevated in COVID-19 patients directly causes mast cell degranulation, leading to urticaria in conjunction with angiotensin-converting enzyme 2 (ACE2) receptor stimulation.

Antihistamines and corticosteroids are the mainstay treatment options of urticaria in COVID-19 patients. The urticaria usually disappears on the subsidence of COVID-19 infection.

ERYTHEMA MULTIFORME-LIKE RASH (FIG. 3)

Erythema multiforme is an acute onset hypersensitivity disorder characterized by the presence of target lesions. Three distinct kinds of EM or EM-like rash have been described during the COVID-19 pandemic—drug-induced EM, elder classical EM rash (age > 55 years), and juvenile virus-associated EM-like rash (age < 30 years) **(Table 1)**.

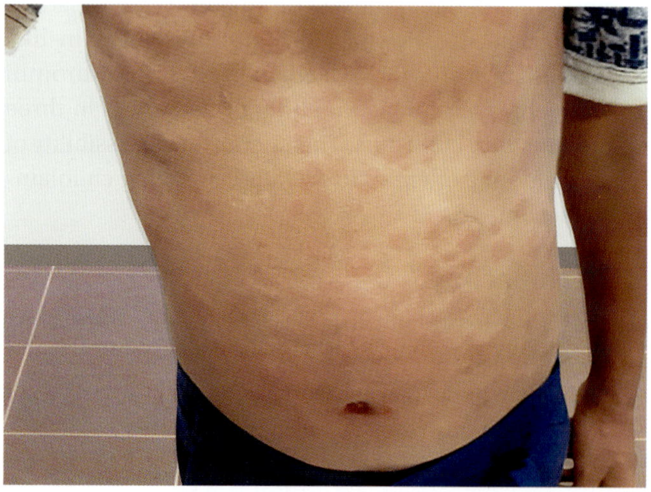

Fig. 2: Another patient presenting with urticaria later diagnosed to be coronavirus disease 2019 (COVID-19) positive.

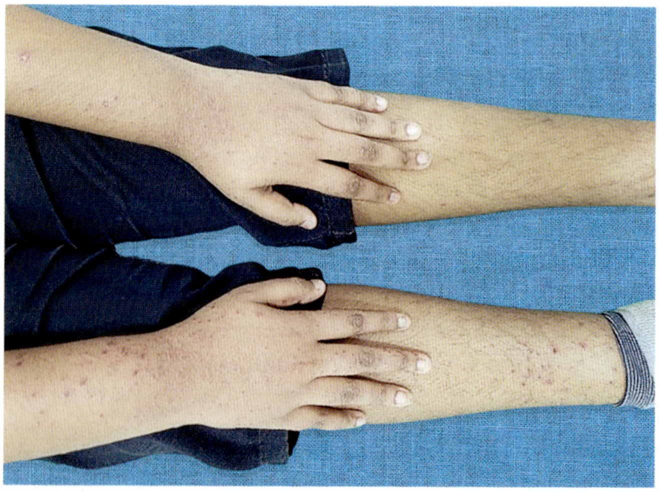

Fig. 3: Erythema multiforme-like rash over all four extremities in a 8-year-old boy who later tested positive for coronavirus disease 2019 (COVID-19).

Table 1: Clinical features of coronavirus disease 2019 (COVID-19)-associated erythema multiforme.

	Virus-related juvenile type	*Drug-induced type*	*Virus-related older type*
Age	<30 years of age	>30 years of age	>55 years of age
Presentation	No systemic involvement, the lesions are acrally distributed	Associated with patients taking hydroxychloroquine	Starts on the trunk and then spreads to the entire body
Histopathology	Mild superficial perivascular dermatitis, without necrosis	Subepidermal blistering occurring due to infiltration of CD8+ lymphocytes into the epidermis also causing necrosis of the keratinocytes	• *Epidermis*: Mild spongiosis • *Dermis*: Extravasation of red blood cells, and lymphocytic perivascular and interstitial infiltrate in the dermis

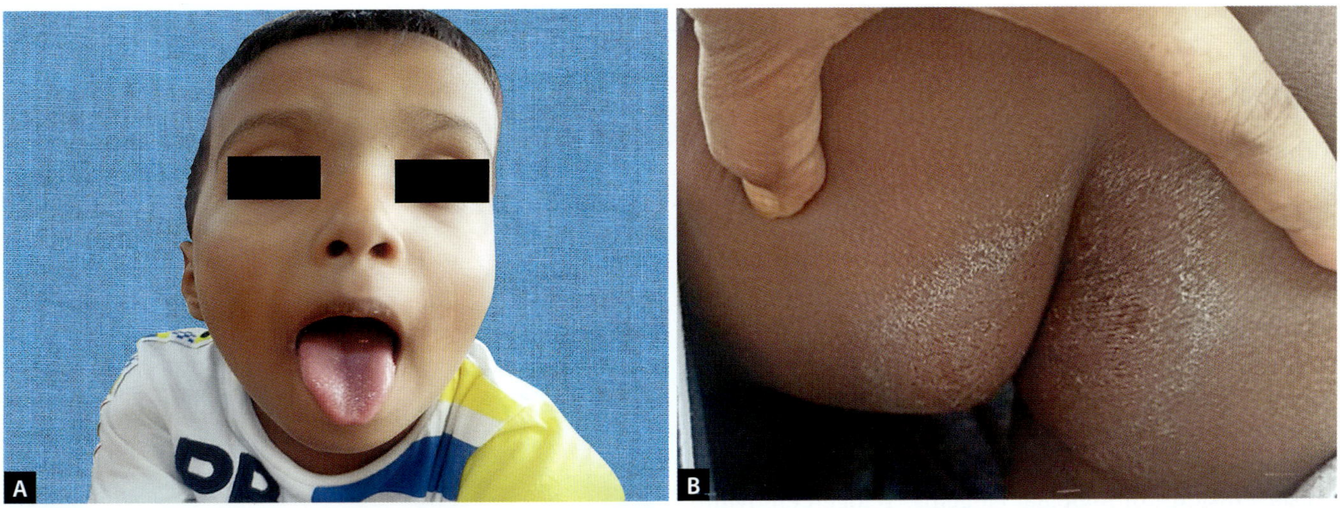

Figs. 4A and B: (A) A 5-year-old presenting with cheilitis and strawberry tongue 4 weeks after being positive for coronavirus disease 2019 (COVID-19). His antibody titers were positive for COVID-19. He was diagnosed as a case of multisystem inflammatory syndrome in children (MIS-C); (B) Same boy, perianal desquamation can be appreciated.

In most cases, the rash is an unusual target lesion that is limited to the palms and soles. The frequency of the acral involvement may indicate type III and/or IV hypersensitivity, which targets the small arteries that are involved in dermal and perivascular lymphoid infiltration, and endothelial activation. The lesions are smaller, less widespread, and may be itchy or painful and are associated with a latency of few days to 3 weeks between COVID-19 infection and EM-like rash.

Overall, EM or EM-like rash is not associated with a severe course of SARS-CoV-2 infection among children and the lesions subside with topical or oral corticosteroids in most of the cases.

MULTISYSTEM INFLAMMATORY SYNDROME IN CHILDREN (FIGS. 4A AND B)

A common COVID-19 consequence that mimics Kawasaki disease and toxic shock syndrome clinically is multisystem inflammatory syndrome in children (MIS-C). The majority of children test positive for COVID-19 and negative for PCR indicating that immunological dysregulation following acute infection is likely the cause of this illness. It is commonly known that in children and adolescents, age <1 year, obesity, and preexisting comorbidities such as chronic respiratory and heart disorders are linked to more severe clinical outcomes. Some studies also identified the presence of diarrhea and significantly elevated C-reactive protein (CRP) as predictors of severe disease in children with COVID-19. According to reports, MIS-C can present with a very broad range of signs and symptoms ranging from a persistent fever to some traits common to Kawasaki disease. Due to similarities in clinical characteristics, MIS-C was mistaken for toxic shock syndrome, secondary hemophagocytic lymphohistiocytosis, and Kawasaki disease. SARS-CoV-2 antibodies are seropositive in the majority of MIS-C patients, which are related to severe shock and multiorgan failures. The two mainstays of MIS-C treatment are high-dose corticosteroids as an adjuvant and intravenous immunoglobulin (IVIG). The cutaneous symptoms are temporary subside once MIS-C is treated.

"A little progress each day adds to big success." —**Satya Nani**

Table 2: Nail changes in pediatric COVID patients.

Author	Condition	Description
Neri et al.	Red half-moon sign	Observation of a red convex lesion at the distal margin of the lunula on the fingernail beds, noted 2 weeks after symptoms with a confirmed diagnosis of COVID
Tammaro et al.	Transverse orange nails	Orange discolorations at the distal tips of the fingernail beds, observed 16 weeks after symptoms, coinciding with a positive IgG test for SARS-CoV-2
Fernandez-Nieto et al.	Transverse leukonychia (Mees' lines)	White, transverse lines across the fingernail beds, appearing concurrently with symptoms and a confirmed diagnosis of COVID
Alobaida et al.	Beau's lines	Transverse grooves along the proximal finger and toenail beds, occurring 3.5 months after symptoms with a confirmed diagnosis of COVID

(COVID: coronavirus disease; IgG: immunoglobulin G; SARS-CoV-2: severe acute respiratory syndrome coronavirus 2)

HAIR AND NAIL CHANGES

Although hair changes are not frequently reported in pediatric COVID-19 patients, there have been a few cases documented in the literature. Hayran et al. reported two post-MIS-C children with distinct patterns of hair loss. A 10-year-old kid who suffered from telogen effluvium (TE) was the first patient. The second patient had alopecia areata and was a 13-year-old boy. The hair loss started 4 weeks ago, and dermatological examination revealed no discernible alopecic spots but a decrease in hair volume. Dermoscopic examination revealed no erythema, scaling, crusts, erosions, or follicular clogging. Telogen effluvium was identified as the patient's cause of diffuse hair loss, and a thorough laboratory workup was carried out to rule out alternative possibilities. The nail changes found in pediatric COVID patients have been given in **Table 2**.

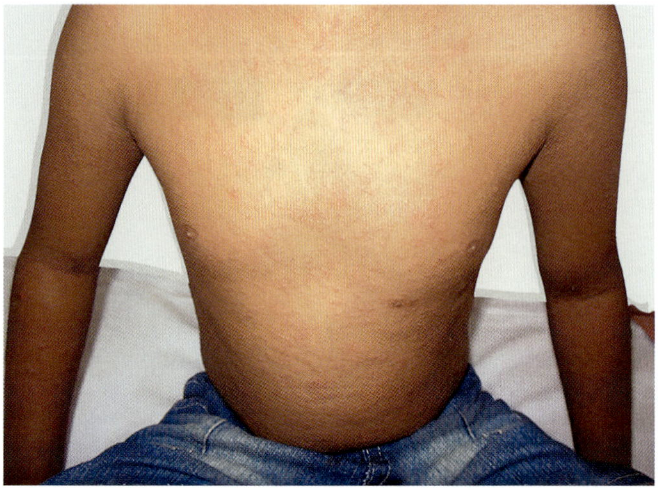

Fig. 5: Maculopapular rash in a patient with coronavirus disease 2019 (COVID-19) positivity.

NONSPECIFIC CHANGES (FIG. 5)

A wide spectrum of signs and symptoms were reported in association with novel COVID-19. Carreras-Presas et al. reported three cases of vesiculobullous lesions associated with COVID-19. All cases presented ulcers or blisters in the oral cavity, appearing and advancing during the isolation period. In two of these cases, lesions affected keratinized tissue, as seen in herpes simplex lesions; in the third case, oral lesions affected both keratinized and non-keratinized tissue and were more compatible with EM. In our pediatric cohort, we found the following oral lesions: Hyperemic pharynx, oral pseudomembranous candidiasis, geographic tongue, and coated tongue. Cutaneous manifestations in patients with COVID-19 infection are being more and more frequently reported. Several patterns have been described since the initial report by Recalcati, including erythematous maculopapular, urticarial, chickenpox-like, purpuric periflexural, transient livedo reticularis, and acro-ischemic or chilblain-like lesions. Considering these findings, it is possible that COVID-19 provokes common viral exanthematous lesions, such as those caused by adenoviruses, enteroviruses, influenza A, or parainfluenza type 3.

CONCLUSION

In conclusion, the cutaneous manifestations of pediatric COVID-19 represent a multifaceted aspect of the disease, providing clinicians with valuable diagnostic clues and insights into the virus's impact on the pediatric population. The incidence of these dermatologic symptoms emphasizes the importance of considering COVID-19 in the differential diagnosis of pediatric patients with unexplained skin changes. Early recognition of these cutaneous manifestations not only aids in the timely diagnosis of SARS-CoV-2 infection but also plays a crucial role in the treatment of the affected children.

"Teachers open the door, but you must enter yourselves." **—Chinese quote**

SUGGESTED READINGS

1. Panda M, Agarwal A, Hassanandani T. Dermatological Manifestations of COVID-19 in Children. Indian Pediatr. 2022;59(5):393-9.
2. Shah S, Akhade K, Ganguly S, Nanda R, Mohapatra E, Goel AK. Cutaneous manifestations associated with COVID-19 in children: A systematic review. J Family Med Prim Care. 2021;10(1):93-101.
3. Larenas-Linnemann D, Luna-Pech J, Navarrete-Rodríguez EM, Rodríguez-Pérez N, Arias-Cruz A, Blandón-Vijil MV, et al. Cutaneous manifestations related to COVID-19 immune dysregulation in the pediatric age group. Curr Allergy Asthma Rep. 2021;21(2):13.
4. Chang TH, Wu JL, Chang LY. Clinical characteristics and diagnostic challenges of pediatric COVID-19: A systematic review and meta-analysis. J Formos Med Assoc. 2020;119(5):982-9.
5. Sati H, Alzraikat N, Milan M, Saliba M, Fawaz AA, Boueri M, et al. Skin manifestations in children with MIS-C and COVID-19: a narrative review. Int J Dermatol. 2024;63(1):32-40.
6. Preda-Naumescu A, Penney K, Pearlman RL, Brodell RT, Daniel CR, Nahar VK. Nail manifestations in COVID-19: insight into a systemic viral disease. Skin Appendage Disord. 2021;7(6):433-8.

"You can cross the sea merely by by standing and looking at the waves." —**Rabindranath Tagore**

CHAPTER

27

Pediatric Dermatology–Oncology Interface

INTRODUCTION

Cutaneous manifestations in pediatric oncology patients may occur either due to primary cutaneous malignancy or the adverse effects of the treatment. In this chapter, we have discussed about various primary cutaneous malignancies in pediatric patients, chemotherapy-induced cutaneous adverse effects, and transplant-associated cutaneous adverse effects.

PEDIATRIC CUTANEOUS MALIGNANCIES

Primary cutaneous malignancies such as squamous cell carcinoma (SCC), basal cell carcinoma (BCC), and melanoma occurring de novo in pediatric age group is usually less common which accounts for 3–4% of the skin cancers. However, these occur in the presence of various other predisposing conditions such as genetic disorders and connective tissue disorders.

Squamous Cell Carcinoma (Figs. 1 and 2)

Squamous cell carcinoma is a relatively uncommon malignant tumor observed in children, particularly those with skin of color. Various factors can predispose individuals to SCC, including chronic injury, exposure to sunlight, thermal burns, chronic inflammation, human papillomavirus (HPV) infection (especially in immunocompromised children), organ transplantation, immunosuppression, and chemotherapy. Additionally, several genetic skin disorders, such as xeroderma pigmentosum, genodermatoses associated with photosensitivity, dystrophic epidermolysis bullosa, dyskeratosis congenita, and pansclerotic morphea, can increase the risk of SCC development. Malignant transformation, such as SCC, is a rare complication occasionally observed in long-standing discoid lupus erythematosus (DLE).

Squamous cell carcinoma most commonly occurs on the scalp and lips, often attributed to prolonged exposure to sunlight. Other common sites of presentation include the face, dorsal hands, forearms, and occasionally the oral mucosa. Lesions may present as red, scaly papules, indurated plaques, ulcerations, telangiectasias, and necrosis. Prolonged and persistent lesions carry a higher risk of metastasis.

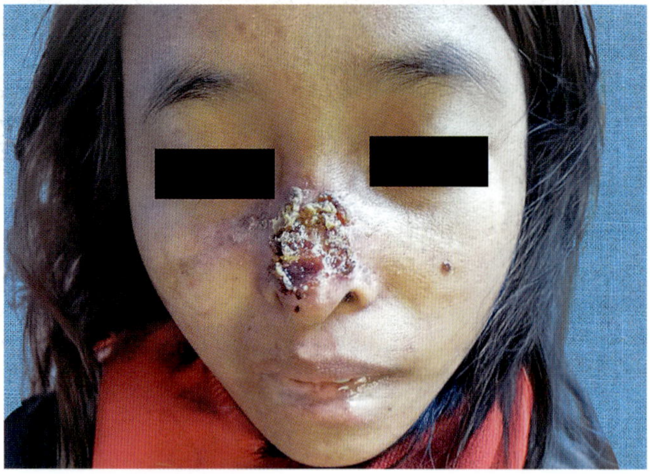

Fig. 1: Squamous cell carcinoma over a plaque of discoid lupus erythematosus (DLE) over nose.

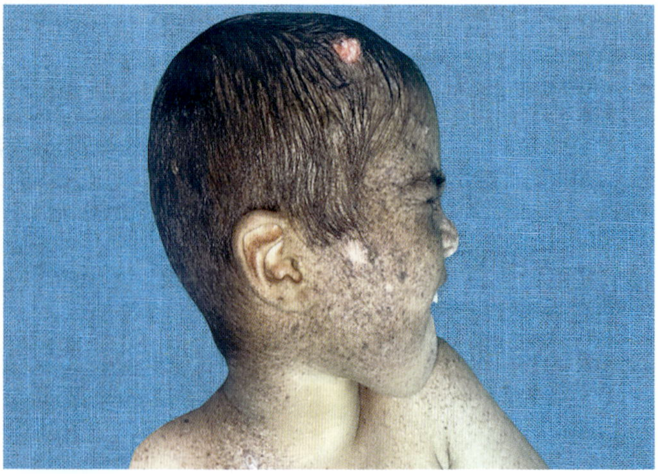

Fig. 2: Squamous cell carcinoma (SCC) in a patient of xeroderma pigmentosum.

"Life isn't about finding yourself. Life is about creating yourself." —**George Bernard Shaw**

Management typically involves complete excision, electrodessication, cryotherapy, and curettage for smaller lesions. In children with genodermatoses, predisposing them to SCC and sun protection measures, including the use of broad-spectrum sunscreens, are crucial for prevention. Counseling parents about the importance of regular skin examinations is essential for early diagnosis and management to reduce mortality associated with SCC. Early detection and intervention play a significant role in improving the prognosis of SCC cases.

Certain other dermatological condition like DLE can predispose the patient to SCC in long-standing lesions.

Syndromes associated with development of BCC are basal cell nevus syndrome, Bazex-Dupré-Christol syndrome, and Schöpf-Schulz-Passarge syndrome.

Malignant Melanoma (Figs. 3A and B)

Childhood malignant melanoma, though rare, is increasing in incidence in West than in India. It is a potentially aggressive tumor of melanocytic origin derived from the neural crest stem cells. It comprises 3% of all skin cancers diagnosed each year, but accounts for approximately 75% of all skin cancer-related deaths. It is seen more in adolescent age group than in prepubertal age. Congenital melanoma represents a small subset of melanoma and is extremely rare. Though majority of the cases occur sporadically, risk factors include fair skin, genetic susceptibility, ultraviolet (UV) radiation, pigmentation, age, nevi pattern, family history, and xeroderma pigmentosum. Around 65% cases of melanoma arise from preexisting nevus. Mutations in *CDKN2A* and *CDK4* have been associated with atypical nevi and early-onset melanoma. Familial cases account for 1% cases of melanoma. The classic signs of melanoma follow the ABCDE rule—asymmetry, irregular borders (notched/scalloped), color change (blue/red/black/white), diameter > 6 mm, and enlargement. The most common forms are superficial and spreading type. Malignant melanoma starts initially as papule or nodule, brown to brown-black in color and rapidly enlarges. Rarely a halo of depigmentation can be present surrounding the primary lesion. Boys show head and neck distribution whereas girls show arm and leg distribution. Lymph node enlargement indicates poor prognosis.

A high index of suspicion is important in recognizing pediatric melanoma as they go unrecognized. Dermoscopy helps to differentiate melanoma from nevi. Full-thickness excision biopsy with histopathological examination is necessary. Staged surgical excision is the treatment of choice. For advanced lesions, combination of chemotherapy, radiotherapy, and immunotherapy have been tried with nonsatisfactory results. Consensus on the overall prognosis still does not exist in pediatric melanoma. The prognosis of melanoma depends on the initial stage. The 5-year overall survival for all stages is 87–95%. Studies have shown children <10 years present with higher stage of the disease. Sun protection methods (using sunscreen, staying in the shade, wearing wide brim hats, and wearing protective clothing) can be helpful in preventing early acquisition and UV-related deoxyribonucleic acid (DNA) damage.

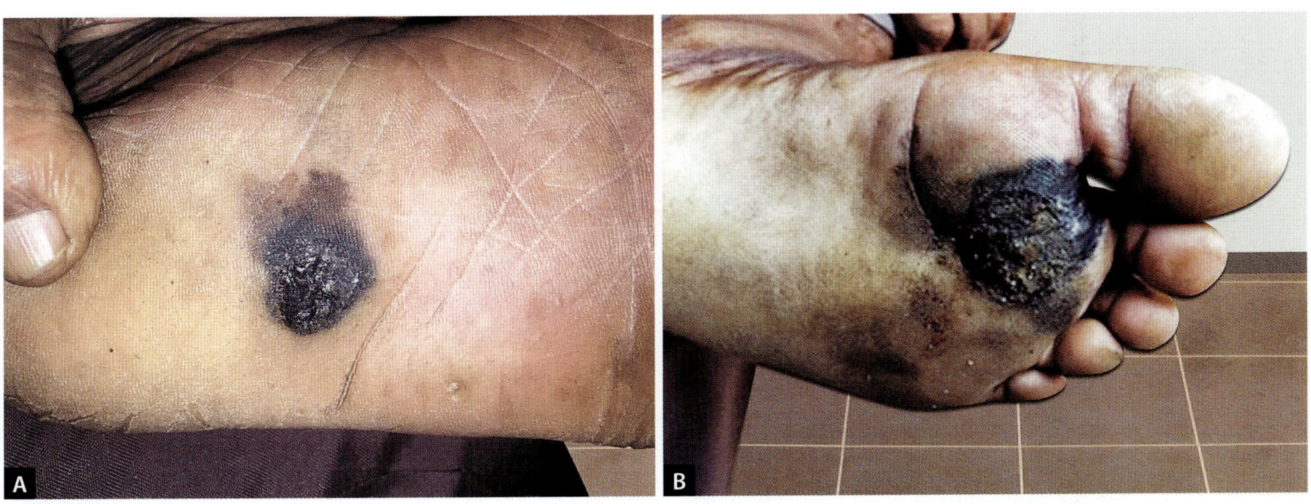

Figs. 3A and B: (A) Malignant melanoma over sole in a 18-year-old boy; (B) Another young boy with malignant melanoma of the sole.

"We can have all the knowledge in the world, but it means nothing without the wisdom to know what to do with it." **—Marie Osmond**

Angiosarcoma in Children (Fig. 4)

Angiosarcoma is a soft tissue tumor and is extremely rare in children. The age of presentation ranges from 3 months to 16 years. The characteristic features of pediatric angiosarcoma are aggressive clinical behavior, local recurrences, and metastasis. They present as firm and painful enlarging multinodular mass with ill-defined margins distributed on the head, neck, trunk, and mediastinum. Visceral organs such as liver and heart may be involved. Other features include acute hemorrhage, anemia, and coagulopathy. Mortality is high as they are high-grade tumors capable of invading peripheral tissue and metastasis. Differential diagnoses include Kaposi sarcoma, hemangiopericytoma, and epithelioid and spindle cell hemangioendothelioma. Surgical resection, radiotherapy, chemotherapy, and paclitaxel have been tried in the management of angiosarcoma in children. The prognosis is poor and mortality is high.

Cutaneous T-cell Lymphomas

They are a group of heterogeneous disorders characterized by neoplastic lymphocytic infiltration of skin which is commonly seen in adults and elderly, and is rare in children. Mycosis fungoides (MF) is the most prevalent form of cutaneous lymphoma in children. Juvenile MF classically presents as erythematous patches and plaques with epidermotropism of lymphocytes. It may also be associated with lymphomatoid papulosis or pityriasis lichenoides-like lesions. Hypopigmented variant is the most common in adolescent/childhood age group where diagnosis is usually delayed. Other atypical variants are hyperpigmented, solitary, follicular, poikilodermic, ichthyosiform, and intraoral. Majority of the cases show partial clearance within 1 year of staring the therapy. Next common variant in children is lymphomatoid papulosis which is characterized by chronic recurrent papules and nodules similar to the presentation in adults. Three unusual presentations in children are localized presentation for years before becoming generalized, presenting with hundreds of lesions, and dwindling outbreaks after initial presentation. Pruritus is present in almost 40% of the cases.

Subcutaneous Panniculitis-like T-cell Lymphoma (Fig. 5)

Subcutaneous panniculitis-like T-cell lymphoma (SPTCL) is a rare form of peripheral T-cell lymphoma in which neoplastic cytotoxic alpha/beta CD9+ T cells infiltrate subcutaneous adipose tissue. It may affect both children and adults with approximately 20% of patients presenting under the age of 20 years. Pediatric SPTCL is rare, with extremely few cases reported in infants. Hemophagocytic lymphohistiocytosis (HLH) observed in 20% of cases is associated with poor prognosis and may be the leading cause of death. SPTCL in patients without HLH follows an indolent course. The etiology of SPTCL was mostly unknown. However, germline mutations causing loss of function of T-cell immunoglobulin mucin-3 (TIM-3) has been identified recently in 60–85% of SPTCL patients.

Clinically, it presents as slowly progressive subcutaneous nodules and plaques, usually involving multiple areas at the same time. Ulcerating skin lesions are rare. Systemic manifestations such as fever, asthenia, and weight

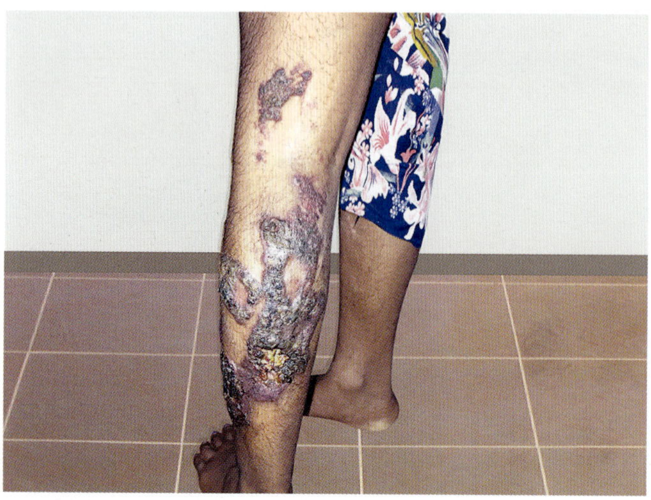

Fig. 4: Angiosarcoma over left thigh and leg in a 18-year-old girl.

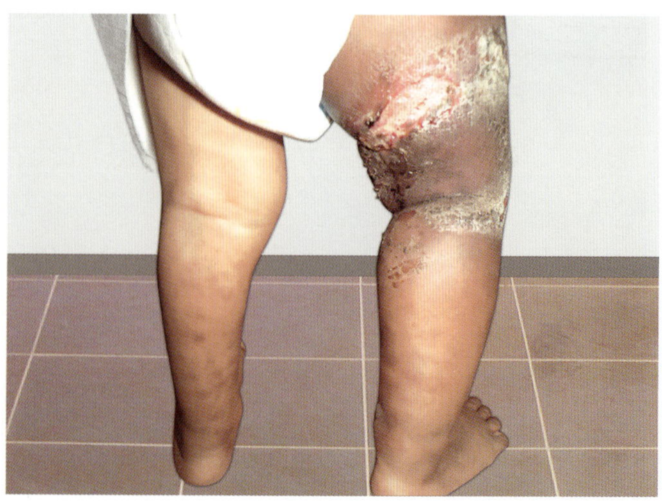

Fig. 5: Subcutaneous panniculitis-like T-cell lymphoma in a 2-year-old boy.

loss, associated with cytopenias and liver dysfunction are common. In infantile SPTCL, there is a low rate of systemic symptoms and HLH complications, compared with other age groups. Diagnosis of SPTCL is based on histopathological and immunophenotyping findings. There is lobular panniculitis without dermal invasion. Atypical lymphocytes rim the adipocyte with infiltrates expressing cytotoxic markers (CD3+, CD8+, CD4–, and CD56–). T-cell gene rearrangement regularly shows a clonal infiltrate, though a polyclonal result does not exclude this diagnosis. Pediatric patients have been observed to display a higher incidence of plasmacytosis in histopathology, which may potentially be confused with lupus panniculitis. Many patients with SPTCL may also have underlying connective tissue disease. So, clinical and serological data along with histopathology may be necessary to arrive at a definitive diagnosis. There is no standardized therapy for SPTCL alone or in association with HLH. Various therapies include corticosteroids, immunosuppressive therapy, chemotherapy, and radiotherapy showing variable response. Intensity-reduced therapy may be used as the initial treatment for pediatric SPTCL, especially in infants, without HLH in order to avoid treatment-related complications. Limited cutaneous involvement with no other symptoms can be treated with radiotherapy and low-dose steroids. In cases of SPTCL-associated HLH, prompt treatment is required. High-dose chemotherapeutic regimens, stem cell transplantation, and ruxolitinib may be used in these cases.

Hematological Malignancy (Figs. 6A to G)

Cutaneous manifestations of hematological disorders in children are different from adults. Cutaneous features can present due to disorders of red blood cells, white blood

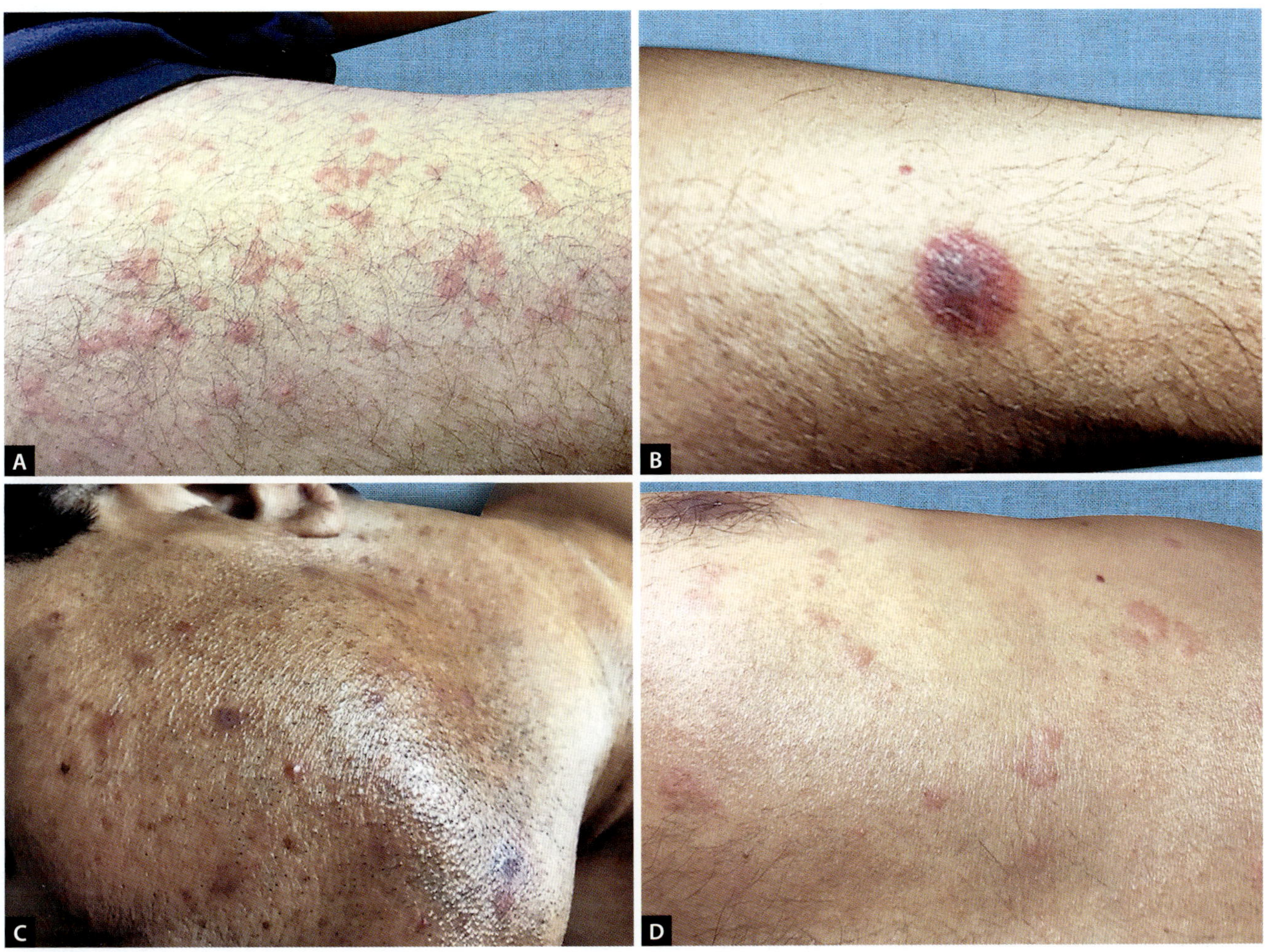

Figs. 6A to D: (A) Acute lymphoblastic leukemia (ALL) with leukemic infiltrate; (B) Close-up view of infiltrate; (C) ALL with leukemic filtrate over the face; (D) Same patient, infiltrate over the trunk.

"You can't stop a teacher once they want to do something, they just do it." — **JD Salinger**

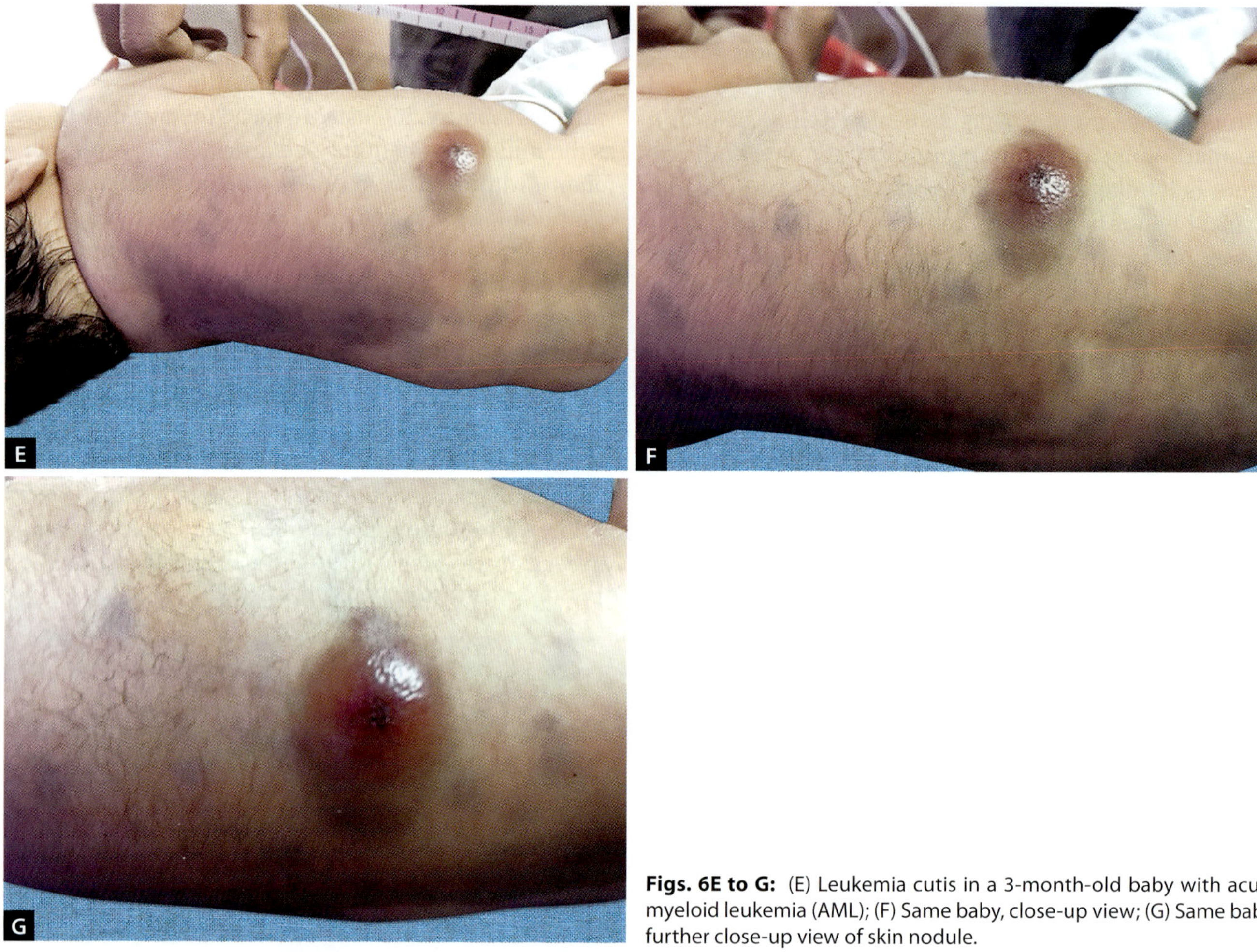

Figs. 6E to G: (E) Leukemia cutis in a 3-month-old baby with acute myeloid leukemia (AML); (F) Same baby, close-up view; (G) Same baby, further close-up view of skin nodule.

cells, platelet and clotting mechanism, hematological malignancy, and immunodeficiencies. Nonspecific changes include anemia secondary to deficiency of iron, folate, and vitamin B_{12}, pruritus, purpura, pigmentation of hands, feet and face, nail pigmentation, ulceration, vasculitis, vesiculobullous lesions, and recurrent cutaneous infections. The most common hematological malignancies in children are leukemia and lymphoma. Cutaneous findings in leukemia may be primary (leukemia cutis) and secondary skin lesions (Sweet's syndrome, pyoderma gangrenosum, and opportunistic infections). Leukemia cutis is the most common malignancy of childhood. There is infiltration of neoplastic leukocytes (myeloid or lymphoid) in the epidermis, dermis, or subcutaneous tissue. Leukemia cutis is seen both in acute myeloid leukemia (3–30%) and acute lymphoblastic leukemia (1–3%). In one-third of patients, it can manifest along with systemic leukemia where skin manifestation can precede the bone marrow or peripheral blood involvement. Leukemia cutis has varied presentation such as macules, papules, plaques, nodules, ecchymoses, erythroderma, ulcers, purpura, vesiculobullous, and urticarial lesions. Rarely, seborrheic dermatitis-like presentation and mastocytosis-like lesion have been reported. Leukemia cutis mimics various disorders and hence skin biopsy along with immunophenotyping and examination of peripheral smears and bone marrow aspirates are necessary.

There has been association of juvenile chronic myelogenous leukemia with juvenile xanthogranuloma. It is estimated that children with neurofibromatosis with juvenile xanthogranuloma have 20- to 32-fold risk of association with chronic myelogenous leukemia. Congenital leukemia cutis presents as blueberry muffin lesions and indicates extramedullary hematopoiesis. Leukemia cutis has poor prognosis and 88% patients die

"Just one positive thought in the morning can change your whole day." **—Dalai Lama**

within 1 year of diagnosis. Systemic chemotherapy is indicated in leukemia cutis.

The most common form of cutaneous lymphoma is cutaneous T-cell lymphoma (CTCL) (mycosis fungoides). Around 0.5–5% of mycosis fungoides cases occur in children. It has been reported in infants also. As compared to adults, children may have indolent course with slow progression. The average time for diagnosis of lymphoma reported in children is around 5 years. It presents as erythematous scaly patches, plaques, papules, atrophic patches, and eczematous lesions on the buttocks and non-photo-exposed areas. Rare presentations include erythroderma or poikiloderma changes. Hypopigmented variant of CTCL is a common variant seen in children and adolescents. Clinical features include asymptomatic, round to arcuate hypopigmented macules with mild scaling. It often resembles pityriasis alba, vitiligo, and postinflammatory hypopigmentation. MF should be differentiated from atopic dermatitis, psoriasis, or systemic lupus erythematosus. Although follicular mucinosis is a feature of CTCL, it is considered as a benign condition in children. Diagnosis is mainly by histopathological examination and immunophenotyping. Immunohistochemical studies show an infiltrate of CD4+ T-cells with loss of CD7+ cells. For localized lesions, topical steroids are given. Other modalities of treatment include topical bexarotene, topical carmustine, imiquimod, tazarotene, and phototherapy [psoralen ultraviolet-A (PUVA)/narrowband UVB (NBUVB)]. Systemic treatments include chemotherapy, interferon, and photopheresis. Prognosis depends on the stage, extent, and extracutaneous involvement.

Lymphomatoid papulosis is a chronic, recurrent, self-healing papulonecrotic and papulonodular skin lesions with histopathological features of lymphoma. It manifests as numerous reddish-brown papules, vesiculopustules, and nodules and necrotic lesions on trunk, scalp, and extremities. They may resolve with varioliform scarring. Differential diagnoses include arthropod bites, pseudolymphoma, pityriasis lichenoides et varioliformis acuta (PLEVA), and lymphoma. They are at increased risk of developing nonlymphoid malignancies. Many of the cases resolve spontaneously. Therapies include topical steroids, low-dose methotrexate (5–20 mg/week), systemic steroids, phototherapy, and topical immunotherapy.

Eosinophilic Leukemia (Fig. 7)

The hypereosinophilic syndrome (HES) including eosinophilic leukemia is a group of disorders with persistent and elevated eosinophil levels with systemic involvement. These diseases have high morbidity. Although the spleen, bone marrow, and liver are the organs initially affected, mucocutaneous manifestations are also important in the diagnosis of this rare group of illnesses.

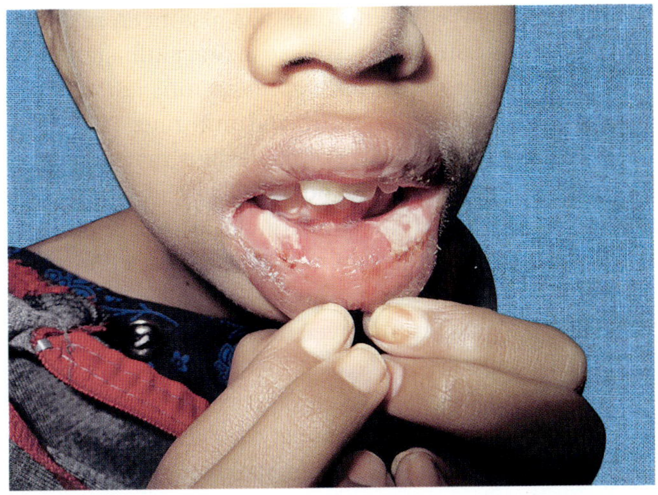

Fig. 7: Mucocutaneous manifestation of chronic eosinophilic leukemia.

The lymphocytic HES (L-HES) variant is most commonly associated with cutaneous features. Whenever skin lesions are present, it becomes easier to take a biopsy and the presence of numerous eosinophils can help make a diagnosis of this rare condition. There are many types of skin lesions which may be found in patients with eosinophilic leukemia. Up to 60% of cases can present with skin manifestations. These include itching or pruritus, urticaria which can be recurrent, angioedema, erythema with scaling, papular eruptions, pruritic nodules, and bullous lesions.

More severe manifestation can include petechiae and vasculitis, and leukemic infiltrations.

Erythema annulare centrifugum, necrotizing vasculitis, livedo reticularis, purpura, erythroderma, and even Well's syndrome has been reported.

Biopsies from these lesions show a lymphocytic pattern with increased eosinophils in the affected tissues. The infiltrate may be deep or superficial, perivascular, or interstitial. Biopsies from uninvolved tissue or after starting therapy may not show these changes and needs to be kept in mind.

Some specific patterns are as follows:

- *Angioedema*: This has angioedema along with urticaria and suggests a benign course of the disease with favorable response to steroids. Both the eyelids may show periorbital swelling with darkening. Urticarial cellulitis or Well's syndrome has also been reported and has a diminished response to oral antihistamines.

- *Pruriginous papules and papulonecrotic lesions*: This has a nonvasculitic and mixed infiltrate. It is more prevalent in L-HES. Size of the lesions may vary from small papules to large nodules. The chief complaint is of severe pruritus. The large lesions may become plaque type and the skin may become pachydermic—known as pachydermatous eosinophilic dermatitis. These patients respond well to treatment with steroids and dapsone.
- *Eczematous lesions*: These appear as thin, red, and scaly plaques which look like atopic dermatitis or precursor lesions of MF. These may coalesce together leading to erythroderma. Associated lymphadenopathy can occur and pruritus is severe. There is usually no family or personal history of atopy. Topical steroids along with photochemotherapy are effective in these patients.
- *Mucosal ulcers*: These are uncommonly reported manifestation of HES. There are recalcitrant and debilitating ulcers of the mucocutaneous surfaces and interfere with hygiene and nutrition. These patients will often have a poorer prognosis. Imatinib mesylate is often indicated in these cases.
- *Splinter hemorrhages*: These are seen on the nail fold and may indicate thromboembolic complications and endomyocardial involvement.

Although it remains unexplained, if there is a correlation between eosinophilic malignancies and subsequent mucocutaneous involvement, it has been observed that mucocutaneous involvement may indicate a poorer prognosis compared to those who do not have skin involvement.

CHEMOTHERAPY-INDUCED CUTANEOUS ADVERSE EFFECTS

Pediatric oncology patients usually present with varied cutaneous features, out of which majority are chemotherapy-induced adverse effects. These cutaneous changes can impose both social and psychological effect on patients. Hence, every dermatologist should be aware of the common as well as the specific adverse effects caused by various chemotherapeutic agents. Anagen effluvium is the most common adverse effect seen due to chemotherapy. All the cutaneous adverse effects are categorized as following:

- *Cutaneous changes*: Commonly seen cutaneous changes include xerosis, inflammatory dermatosis, exanthematous rash, hyperpigmentation, toxic erythema of chemotherapy, urticaria, and leukocytoclastic vasculitis in the order of occurrence. Among inflammatory dermatosis, diaper dermatitis is the most common followed by seborrheic dermatitis, contact dermatitis, and perioral dermatitis. Toxic erythema of chemotherapy is characterized by erythematous and edematous patches or plaques confined to intertriginous areas associated with pain, tenderness, paresthesias, burning sensations, and sometimes petechiae and erosions can also be seen. This occurs due to excretion of the chemotherapeutic drug into the eccrine glands causing local toxic effects which appears 2 days to 3 weeks after starting the therapy and subsides spontaneously. Recurrence is seen is the same drug is reintroduced.
- *Mucosal changes*: Mucositis and oral aphthous ulcers are the commonly seen mucosal changes. Mucosal hyperpigmentation is also seen in many cases.
- *Hair changes*: Alopecia is the most common chemotherapy-induced adverse effect, among which anagen effluvium is the most common. Trichomegaly or hypertrichosis is also seen in few cases **(Fig. 8)**.
- *Nail changes*: Beaus lines, nail hyperpigmentation, transverse ridging of nails, nail fragility, and paronychia are the frequently seen nail changes. Nail pigmentation is the most common adverse effect observed **(Fig. 9)**.
- *Cutaneous infections*: Bacterial infections such as acute paronychia and bacterial folliculitis were noted in few patients. Viral infections included herpes simplex (mostly orolabialis) and verruca vulgaris. Most common were the fungal infections, including extensive pityriasis versicolor, mucocutaneous candidiasis, and some patients also had systemic candidiasis. Skin eruptions in systemic candidiasis were maculopapular rash or nodular where hyphae were found in biopsy from these lesions **(Figs. 10 and 11)**.
- *Specific changes*: Trametinib, a MAPK extracellular signal-regulated kinase inhibitor (MEKI), seen to cause a centrofacial acneiform eruptions which is the early cutaneous adverse effect and truncal furunculosis. Other specific changes seen due to trametinib are new-onset androgenetic alopecia, drug reaction with eosinophilia and systemic symptoms (DRESS) and psoriasiform reaction. BRAF inhibitors (dabrafenib and vemurafenib) are known to cause keratosis pilaris-like reactions most commonly followed by

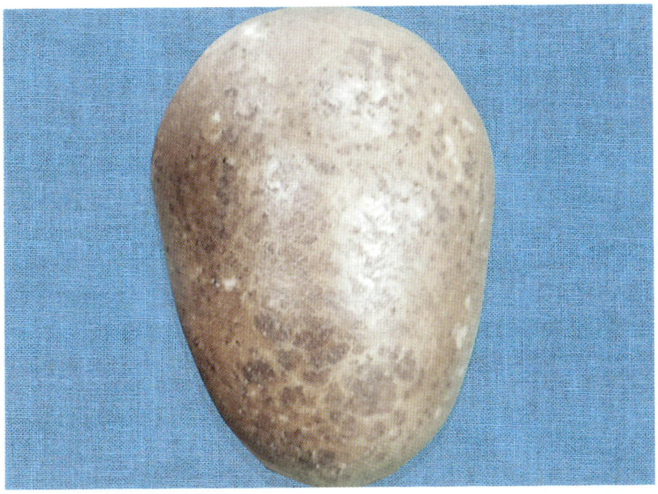

Fig. 8: Seborrheic dermatitis with anagen effluvium in a B-cell acute lymphoblastic leukemia (B-ALL) child on induction chemotherapy with vincristine, daunorubicin, L-asparaginase, and dexamethasone.

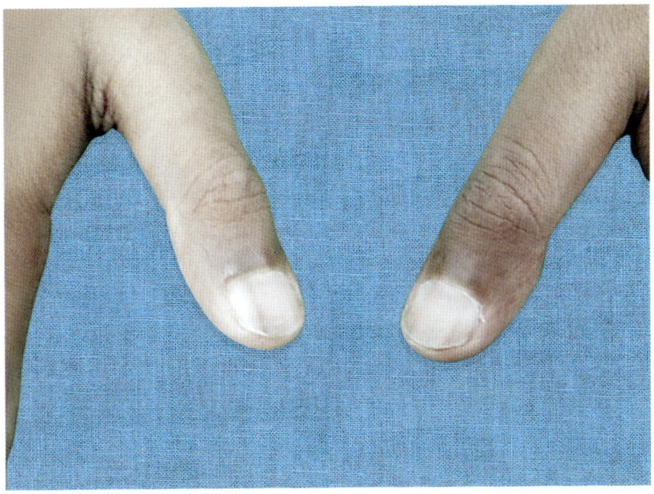

Fig. 9: Melanonychia following cyclophosphamide-based chemotherapy.

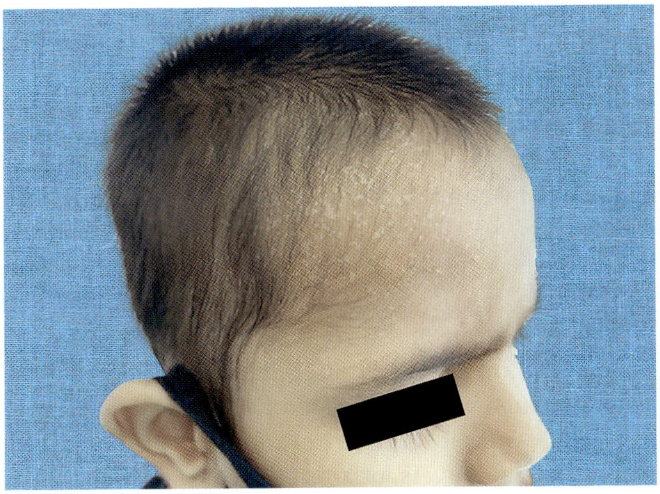

Fig. 10: Verruca plana in a B-cell acute lymphoblastic leukemia (B-ALL) patient on antimetabolites.

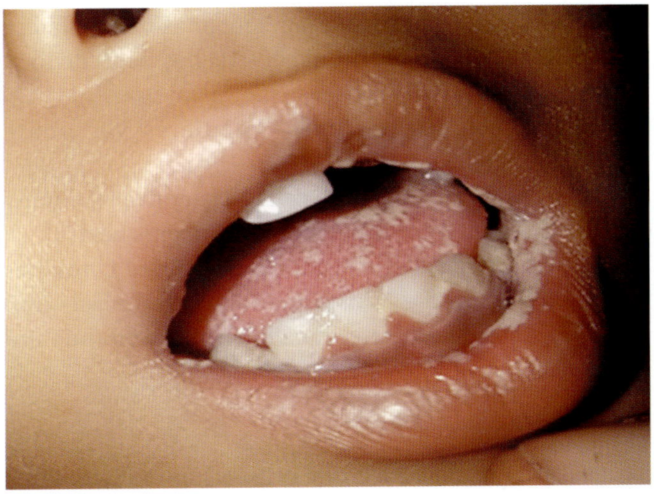

Fig. 11: Oral candidiasis in a Hodgkin lymphoma patient on adriamycin, bleomycin, vinblastine, and dacarbazine (ABVD) induction chemotherapy.

photosensitivity and palmoplantar hyperkeratosis. Panniculitis is another cutaneous adverse effect seen mostly with BRAF inhibitors with or without MEK inhibitors, but few cases have been reported due to only MEK inhibitors. Dabrafenib-specific reactions include hand-foot syndrome (manifests as acquired keratoderma), erythema multiforme-like reaction, and eruptive nevi.

TRANSPLANT-ASSOCIATED ADVERSE EFFECTS

Cutaneous adverse effects associated with transplantation are mostly related to hematological stem cell transplant (HSCT) and less due to solid organ transplantation. Major adverse effects are graft-versus-host disease (GVHD), increased risk of cutaneous malignancies, and cutaneous infections.

Graft-versus-host Disease

It is the most common complication in posttransplant patients. Target organs are skin, gut, liver, and lungs among which skin is the most common and earliest organ affected. It is broadly classified into acute and chronic forms based on the duration of manifestation. Acute GVHD occurs within 100 days of transplant whereas chronic GVHD occurs after 100 days usually but sometimes can occur

"The whole purpose of education is to turn mirrors into windows." —**Sydney Harris**

beyond the time frames. Risk factors include disparities in minor human leukocyte antigen (HLA), older age of recipient and donor, genetic polymorphisms, gender mismatch, donor multiparity, myeloablative conditioning (MAC), recipient seropositivity for cytomegalovirus (CMV), and nonconventional GVHD prophylaxis. The National Institute of Health (NIH) has proposed a consensus criteria classifying GVHD into four forms:

1. Classic acute GVHD
2. Persistent or late-onset acute GVHD
3. Classic chronic GVHD
4. Overlap syndrome (mixed acute and chronic features)

Pathogenesis

Both acute and chronic forms are immune mediated, where acute GVHD is mostly the inflammatory state whereas chronic GVHD is both inflammatory and fibrotic states. Acute GVHD pathogenesis is further divided into three stages, i.e., conditioning, afferent phase, and efferent phase. Pathogenesis of chronic GVHD has been divided into three steps by NIH consensus:

1. Firstly, innate immunity mediates an acute inflammation
2. Dysregulation of B- and T-cells in adaptive immunity which causes chronic inflammation occurs next
3. The activated T-cells produce profibrotic cytokines which help in the transformation of fibroblasts into myofibroblasts in the extracellular matrix in the third stage.

Clinical Features

Acute GVHD characteristically presents as erythematous to violaceous morbilliform rash initially over palms and soles, face, trunk, and gradually becomes generalized. Acral erythema and erythroderma with or without bullous lesions resembling toxic epidermal necrolysis are other variants. Atypical variants such as psoriasiform plaques, acquired ichthyosis, and diffuse erythematous perifollicular rash are most commonly seen in pediatric cases. Mucosal involvement can be present, especially conjunctival mucosa.

Chronic GVHD has wide variety of manifestations from nonspecific lesions such as xerosis, keratosis pilaris, and ichthyosis to diagnostic features such as poikiloderma, lichenoid lesions, and sclerotic changes. Lichenoid variant, which is rare in children, usually presents as violaceous, flat-topped papules, and plaques resembling lichen planus. Sclerotic variant, which is the major source of morbidity, generally occurs in the late stages. Sometimes bullous lesions or ulcerations can also be seen. Rare variants of chronic GVHD include atopic dermatitis-like, psoriasiform, verrucous wart-like, and erythema multiforme-like. Mucosal involvement is common in chronic GVHD than in acute forms where oral and genital mucosae are most commonly involved. Lichen planus-like lesions in both oral and genital mucosa are diagnostic along with phimosis, urethral meatal stenosis in males and vaginal scarring and labial/clitoral agglutination in females. Ocular mucosa can be involved in some cases showing punctate keratopathy and keratoconjunctivitis sicca. Nail changes include onycholysis, splitting, brittle nails, pterygium, dystrophy, and anonychia. Vitiligo-like depigmentation and alopecia areata were also found to occur in chronic GVHD patients **(Figs. 12A and B)**.

Based on histopathology, GVHD is further graded into four grades:

1. Grade 1—focal/diffuse basal cell vacuolization
2. Grade 2—dyskeratotic squamous cells in epidermis and/or hair follicle with basal cell vacuolization
3. Grade 3—subepidermal clefting with dyskeratosis and spongiosis
4. Grade 4—complete separation of epidermis from dermis

Treatment

Treatment of acute and chronic forms of GVHD depends on the grading and location. Mild cases (Grade 1) are usually treated with topical steroids. Grade 2 and above requires systemic corticosteroids like prednisolone 1–2 mg/kg per day. As long-term steroids possess severe side effects, second-line treatments under investigating are low dose methotrexate, mycophenolate mofetil, infliximab [tumor necrosis factor-α (TNF-α) inhibitor], alemtuzumab (anti-CD52 monoclonal antibody), and pentostatin [adenosine deaminase (ADA) inhibitor]. Extracorporeal photopheresis (ECP) is a well-established alternative for systemic steroids both in acute and chronic cases, reducing the use of steroids with >80% complete response rates. In lichenoid and sclerotic variants, phototherapy especially UVA1 phototherapy was found to be very effective in refractory cases. Newer therapies such as Treg therapy, maraviroc, bortezomib, and mesenchymal stem cell therapy are under trials. Imatinib mesylate, a tyrosine kinase inhibitor, has been tried and found to be effective in steroid refractory sclerosant type of chronic GVHD.

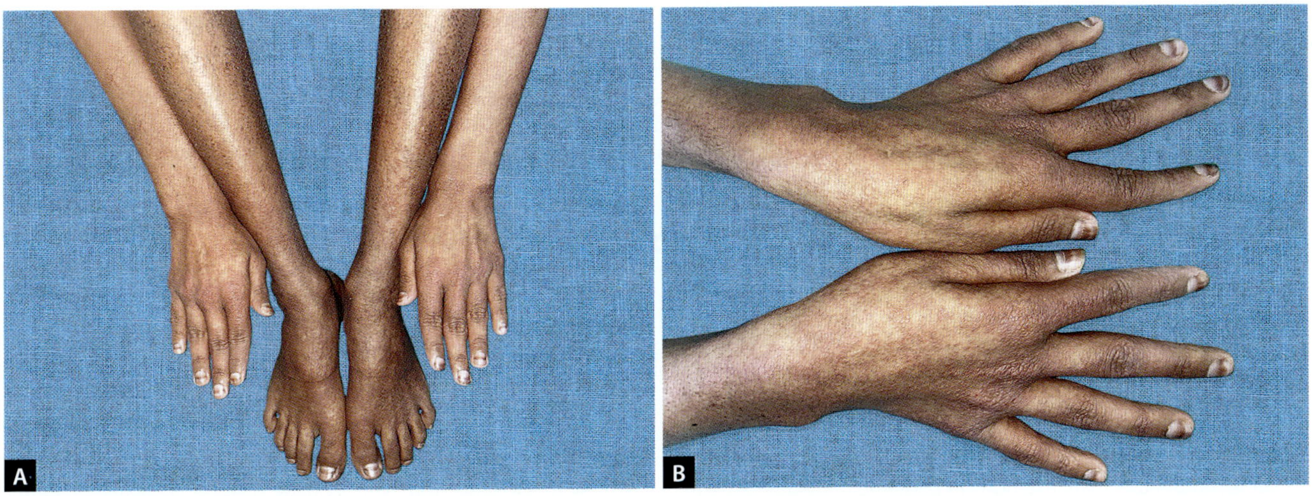

Figs. 12A and B: (A) Chronic graft-versus-host disease (GVHD): Lichenoid variant in a post-hematopoietic stem cell transplant child occurring 120 days after transplant; (B) Same patient close-up view.

Infections

Severe immunosuppression in the posttransplant patients predisposes them to various cutaneous and systemic infections. Risk factors associated are age >10 years, acute GVHD, patients who have received allogenic HSCT and total body irradiation as the conditioning regimen. Among all the infections, reactivation of varicella zoster virus (VZV) is the most common and a major cause of morbidity. Reactivation is not limited to a particular dermatome and usually presents as a disseminated variant and sometimes as visceral VZV can occur. Visceral VZV usually presents with severe abdominal pain mostly in the right upper quadrant (due to the stretching of hepatic capsule) and sometimes severe hyponatremia. Chronic GVHD can be a possible risk factor in the viral reactivation due to several alterations in the humoral and cell mediated immunity. Other viral reactivations associated with GVHD are CMV and human herpesvirus (HHV)-6 and 7. A rare occurrence of cutaneous toxoplasmosis postallogenic HSCT is reported which presents as 3–4 mm erythematous, round, nonscaling macules, and papules over trunk without lymphadenopathy and mucosal involvement.

Cutaneous Malignancy

The incidence of secondary solid tumors after HSCT is twice the expected rate in the general population. Cutaneous malignant neoplasms accounts for 0–58.5% of secondary neoplasms. BCC and cutaneous SCC have a 20-year cumulative incidence of 6.5% and 3.4%, respectively. Melanomas usually appear 1–4 years post-HSCT. The multifactorial pathogenesis involves patient-related, primary disease-related, transplantation-related, and immunosuppression-related factors. Risk factors include age at transplantation, male sex, genetically determined skin pigmentation, skin cancer incidence differences in Asian populations, and certain medical conditions such as Fanconi anemia, alkylating agents, immunosuppressive treatments (usually azathioprine), and radiation.

Posttransplant lymphoproliferative disorders (PTLDs) are a wide spectrum of B and T lymphocyte proliferations in the background of iatrogenic immunosuppression. The basic pathogenesis lies in the chronic immunosuppression which leads to modification of antitumor surveillance system causing lymphoproliferation. Epstein–Barr virus (EBV) infection is the most common trigger of PTLDs in pediatric patients, mostly associated with B-cell lineage. CTCLs are extremely rare in posttransplant patients with MF being the most common among them. Secondary cutaneous changes in peripheral T-cell lymphoma include morbilliform lesions, folliculitis-like lesions, and generalized eczematous lesions. Biopsy reveals atypical lymphocytes infiltrate with immunohistochemistry positive for CD2, CD3, and CD5, negative for CD7. The World Health Organization (WHO) has classified PTLDs as nondestructive, monomorphic, polymorphic, and classical Hodgkin lymphoma. In B-cell PTLDs, prednisolone was found to be highly efficacious in moderate-to-severe cases. Novel targeted therapies such as cytokine inhibitor therapy, anti-B-cell antibodies, and anti-EBV cytotoxic T lymphocytes seem to be promising in B-cell PTLDs. Localized T-cell PTLDs were effectively treated with surgery and radiotherapeutic therapies, while disseminated T-cell PTLDs needed intensive chemotherapy with an increased risk for infections and end-organ damage.

Post-HSCT should avoid carcinogenic agents such as alcohol and tobacco while adhering to the use of sun protection measures. Consensus-based guidelines suggest regular dermatologist assessments every 12 months for whole skin and mucous membranes. For patients with history of cutaneous malignancies or GVHD, screening intervals should be at least every 6 months.

SUGGESTED READINGS

1. Fogel AL, Sarin KY, Teng JMC. Genetic diseases associated with an increased risk of skin cancer development in childhood. Curr Opin Pediatr. 2017;29(4):426-33.
2. Wu JH, Cohen BA, Sweren RJ. Mycosis fungoides in pediatric patients: Clinical features, diagnostic challenges, and advances in therapeutic management. Pediatr Dermatol. 2020;37(1):18-28.
3. Özkur E, Sert C, Kıvanç Altunay İ, Yıldırırmak ZY, Genç DB, Vural S, et al. Cutaneous manifestations in pediatric oncology patients. Pediatr Dermatol. 2021;38(1):58-65.
4. Boull CL, Gardeen S, Abdali T, Li E, Potts J, Rubin N, et al. Cutaneous reactions in children treated with MEK inhibitors, BRAF inhibitors, or combination therapy: A Multicenter Study. J Am Acad Dermatol. 2021;84(6):1554-61.
5. Shi CR, Huang JT, Nambudiri VE. Pediatric Cutaneous Graft Versus Host Disease: A Review. Curr Pediatr Rev. 2017;13(2):100-10.
6. Koc Y, Miller KB, Schenkein DP, Griffith J, Akhtar M, DesJardin J, et al. Varicella zoster virus infections following allogeneic bone marrow transplantation: frequency, risk factors, and clinical outcome. Biol Blood Marrow Transplant. 2000;6:44-9.
7. Peritz DC, Duncan C, Kurek K, Perez-Atayde AR, Lehmann LE. Visceral varicella zoster virus (VZV) after allogeneic hematopoietic stem cell transplant (HSCT) in pediatric patients with chronic graft-versus-host disease (cGVHD). J Pediatr Hematol Oncol. 2008;30(12):931-4.
8. Szlauer-Stefańska A, Kamińska-Winciorek G, Giebel S, Bagłaj M. Secondary skin neoplasms in patients after autologous and allogeneic hematopoietic stem cell transplantation procedures. Adv Clinw Exp Med. 2020;29(10):1221-30.

"Educations's purpose is to replace an empty mind with an open one." —**Malcom Forbes**

Index

Page numbers followed by *b* refer to box, *f* refer to figure, and *t* refer to table.

B

C

F

G

H

I

J

K

L

M

N

Q

R

S

T

U

V